American Academy of Orthopaedic Surgeons

Atlas of Amputations and Limb Deficiencies
Surgical, Prosthetic, and Rehabilitation Principles

Edited by

Douglas G. Smith, MD
John W. Michael, MEd, CPO
John H. Bowker, MD

Published 2004 by the
American Academy of Orthopaedic Surgeons
6300 North River Road
Rosemont, IL 60018

Third Edition (Previous editions published under the title *Atlas of Limb Prosthetics.*)

ISBN 0-89203-313-4
Printed in the USA

Library of Congress Cataloging-in-Publication Data

Atlas of amputations and limb deficiencies: surgical, prosthetic and rehabilitation principles/ American Academy of Orthopaedic Surgeons; edited by Douglas G. Smith, John W. Michael, John H. Bowker.

p. cm.

Includes bibliographical references and index.
ISBN 0-89203-313-4

1. Amputation. 2. Amputees--Rehabilitation. 3. Artificial limbs. I. Smith, Douglas G. II. Michael, John W. III. Bowker, John H. IV. American Academy of Orthopaedic Surgeons.

RD553.A87 2004
617.58--dc22
2004046436

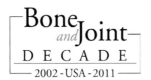

Editorial Board

Dedicated to our wives,
Kathryn Ponto Smith, Linda Michael, and Alice Bowker,
and to our children,
Tina, Ali, and Kevin Smith,
David and Kate Michael,
and Thomas Bowker.
With heartfelt gratitude for their support and forbearance
during the long development of this volume.

Contributors

Christopher H. Allan, MD
Assistant Professor
Department of Orthopaedics and Sports Medicine
Section of Hand and Microsurgery
Harborview Medical Center
University of Washington School of Medicine
Seattle, Washington

Randall D. Alley, CP*
Director of Clinical Development
Innovative Neurotronics, Inc
Hanger Orthopedic Group, Inc
Thousand Oaks, California

Michael T. Archdeacon, MD, MSE
Director, Orthopaedic Trauma
Assistant Professor
Department of Orthopaedic Surgery
University of Cincinnati Medical Center
Cincinnati, Ohio

Diane J. Atkins, OTR
Clinical Assistant Professor
Department of Physical Medicine and Rehabilitation
Baylor College of Medicine
Houston, Texas

Gary M. Berke, MS, CP
Private Practitioner and Adjunct Clinical Instructor
Department of Orthopaedic Surgery
Stanford University
Redwood City, California

Allen T. Bishop, MD
Professor of Orthopedic Surgery, Mayo Medical School
Consultant in Orthopedic, Hand, and Microvascular Surgery
Mayo Clinic
Department of Orthopedic Surgery
Mayo Foundation
Rochester, Minnesota

David Alan Boone, CP, MPH
Associate Professor
Rehabilitation Engineering Centre
The Hong Kong Polytechnic University
Kowloon, Hong Kong

Roy Bowers, SR ProsOrth
Lecturer
National Centre for Training and Education in Prosthetics
  and Orthotics
University of Strathclyde
Glasgow, Scotland

John H. Bowker, MD
Professor Emeritus
Department of Orthopaedics and Rehabilitation
University of Miami School of Medicine
Miami, Florida

Rickard Brånemark, MD, MSc, PhD
Centre of Orthopaedic Osseointegration
Department of Orthopaedics
Sahlgren University Hospital
Gothenburg, Sweden

Carl D. Brenner, CPO
Director of Prosthetic Research
Michigan Institute for Electronic Limb Development
Livonia, Michigan

Kevin M. Carroll, MS, CP
Vice President, Prosthetics
Department of Prosthetics
Hanger Prosthetics and Orthotics, Inc.
Oklahoma City, Oklahoma

Howard A. Chansky, MD
Associate Professor
Department of Orthopaedics and Sports Medicine
University of Washington School of Medicine
Chief, Section of Orthopaedics
Veterans Affairs Puget Sound Health Care System,
  Seattle Division
Seattle, Washington

Dudley S. Childress, PhD
Professor and Senior Research Health Care Scientist
Department of Physical Medicine, Rehabilitation,
  and Biomedical Engineering
Prosthetics Research Laboratory and Rehabilitation Engineering
  Research Program
Northwestern University and VA Chicago Health Care System
Chicago, Illinois

Curtis R. Clark, PT
University of Miami
Supervisor of Amputee Service
Jackson Memorial Hospital
Miami, Florida

Mary Williams Clark, MD
Clinical Professor of Orthopedics and Pediatrics
Sparrow Regional Children's Center
Michigan State University
Lansing, Michigan

David N. Condie, CEng
Consultant Clinical Engineer
Honorary Senior Lecturer
Department of Orthopaedic and Trauma Surgery
University of Dundee
Dundee, Scotland

Colleen Coulter-O'Berry, PT, MS, PCS
Senior Physical Therapist
Team Leader, Limb Deficiency Program
Department of Orthotics and Prosthetics
Children's Healthcare of Atlanta
Atlanta, Georgia

Donald R. Cummings, CP, LP
Director, Prosthetics
Department of Prosthetics
Texas Scottish Rite Hospital for Children
Dallas, Texas

Wayne K. Daly, CPO, LPO
Center for Prosthetics Orthotics
Seattle, Washington

Hans Dietl, PhD
Managing Director
Otto Bock HealthCare Products GmbH
Vienna, Austria

Kim Doolan
Patient Advocate Clinical Coordinator
Allen Orthotics and Prosthetics
Midland, Texas

John P. Dormans, MD
Chief of Orthopaedic Surgery
Children's Hospital of Philadelphia
Professor of Orthopaedic Surgery
University of Pennsylvania School of Medicine
Philadelphia, Pennsylvania

Paul J. Dougherty, MD
Chief
Department of Surgery
Program Director
Orthopaedic Surgery Residency
William Beaumont Army Medical Center
El Paso, Texas

Joan E. Edelstein, MA, PT
Special Lecturer
Department of Physical Therapy
Columbia University
New York, New York

Dawn M. Ehde, PhD
Assistant Professor
Department of Rehabilitation Medicine
University of Washington School of Medicine
Seattle, Washington

James Engels, MD
Pediatric Orthopaedic Consultant
Center for Limb Differences
Mary Free Bed Hospital
Grand Rapids, Michigan

Bülent Erol, MD
Research Fellow
Division of Orthopaedics
The Children's Hospital of Philadelphia
Philadelphia, Pennsylvania

John R. Fergason, CPO
Director, Division of Prosthetics and Orthotics
Department of Rehabilitation Medicine
University of Washington
Seattle, Washington

John R. Fisk, MD
Professor
Department of Surgery
Southern Illinois University School of Medicine
Springfield, Illinois

Charles M. Fryer, MS
(deceased)

Robert S. Gailey, PhD, PT
Assistant Professor
University of Miami School of Medicine
Department of Orthopaedics and Rehabilitation
Division of Physical Therapy
Miami, Florida

Brian J. Giavedoni, MBA, CP
Senior Prosthetist
Orthotics and Prosthetics Department
Children's Healthcare of Atlanta
Atlanta, Georgia

Gerard L. Glancy, MD
Associate Professor
Department of Orthopaedic Surgery
The Children's Hospital
Denver, Colorado

Frank Gottschalk, MD, FRCSEd, FCS(SA)
Professor
Department of Orthopaedic Surgery
University of Texas Southwestern Medical Center at Dallas
Dallas, Texas

Gregory S. Gruman, CP
President
The Winkley Company
Minneapolis, Minnesota

Kenneth J. Guidera, MD
Assistant Chief of Staff
Department of Medical Staff
Shriners Hospital for Children
Tampa, Florida

James T. Guille, MD
Co-Director, Spine and Scoliosis Service
Department of Orthopaedic Surgery
Alfred I. DuPont Hospital for Children
Wilmington, Delaware

Brian J. Hartigan, MD
Clinical Instructor
Department of Orthopaedic Surgery
Northwestern University, Feinberg School of Medicine
Chicago, Illinois

Craig W. Heckathorne, MSc
Research Engineer
Upper-Limb Prosthetic Specialist
Rehabilitation Engineering Research Program
Northwestern University
Chicago, Illinois

Alice L. Kahle, PhD
Psychologist
Department of Psychology
The Children's Hospital of Philadelphia
Philadelphia, Pennsylvania

Susan L. Kapp, CPO
Associate Professor and Director
Prosthetics-Orthotics Program
University of Texas Southwestern Medical Center at Dallas
Dallas, Texas

S. Jay Kumar, MD
Clinical Professor of Orthopaedic Surgery
Department of Orthopaedic Surgery
Thomas Jefferson University
Philadelphia, Pennsylvania

Julian E. Kuz, MD
Upper Extremity Consultant
Center for Limb Differences
Mary Free Bed Hospital
Grand Rapids, Michigan

Chris Lake, CPO
Southwest Clinical Director
Advanced Arm Dynamics, Inc.
Dallas, Texas

S. William Levy, MD
Clinical Professor of Dermatology
Department of Dermatology
University of California School of Medicine
San Francisco Medical Center
San Francisco, California

Terry R. Light, MD
Dr. William M. Scholl Professor and Chairman
Department of Orthopaedic Surgery and Rehabilitation
Loyola University Chicago Stritch School of Medicine
Maywood, Illinois

Janet G. Marshall, CPO
Orthotics and Prosthetics
Shriners Hospital for Children
Tampa, Florida

Peter T. McCollum, MCh, FRCSI, FRCSEd
Professor of Vascular Surgery
Vascular Unit
Hull Royal Infirmary
Hull, England

John W. Michael, MEd, CPO*
President
CPO Services, Inc.
Portage, Indiana

John M. Miguelez, CP
President and Senior Clinical Director
Advanced Arm Dynamics, Inc.
Rolling Hills Estates, California

Michelle D. Miguelez, JD
Redondo Beach, California

Walid Mnaymneh, MD
Professor of Orthopaedics and Oncology
Department of Orthopaedics and Rehabilitation
University of Miami School of Medicine
Miami, Florida

Sara J. Mulroy, PhD, PT
Director
Pathokinesiology Laboratory
Rancho Los Amigos National Rehabilitation Center
Downey, California

John J. Murnaghan, MD, MSc, MA, FRCSC
Assistant Professor Surgery
University of Toronto
Division of Orthopaedic Surgery
Orthopaedic and Arthritic Institute
Toronto, Ontario, Canada

Christopher B. Nelson, CPO
Prosthetist Orthotist
Department of Orthotics and Prosthetics
The Children's Hospital
Philadelphia, Pennsylvania

Cara D. Novick, MD
Orthopaedic Surgeon
Shriners Hospital for Children
Tampa, Florida

Mary P. Novotny, RN, MS
Nurse, Advocate, and Consultant
Knoxville, Tennessee

E. Anne Ouellette, MD, MBA
Professor, Chief
Division of Hand Surgery
Department of Orthopaedics and Rehabilitation
University of Miami School of Medicine
Miami, Florida

Patrick Owens, MD
Assistant Professor of Clinical Orthopaedics
University of Miami School of Medicine
Miami, Florida

Thomas Passero, CP
President and Clinical Director
LIVINGSKIN® Aesthetic Concerns Prosthetics, Inc
Middletown, New York

Joanna G. Patton, OTR/L
Clinical Occupational Therapist and Instructor
Child Amputee Prosthetics Project
Shriners Hospital for Children
Los Angeles, California

Jacquelin Perry, MD
Chief Emeritus, Pathokinesiology Service
Professor Emeritus of Orthopaedics, USC
Department of Pathokinesiology
Rancho Los Amigos National Rehabilitation Center
Downey, California

Michael S. Pinzur, MD
Professor
Department of Orthopaedic Surgery and Rehabilitation
Loyola University Medical Center
Maywood, Illinois

Pradip D. Poonekar, MD
Prosthetic Surgeon
Artificial Limb Centre
Pune, India

Charles H. Pritham, CPO
Practice Manager
Carolina Orthotic and Prosthetic Lab, Inc.
Hanger Prosthetics and Orthotics, Inc.
Wilmington, North Carolina

John C. Racy, MD
Professor of Psychiatry
Department of Psychiatry
University of Arizona College of Medicine
Tucson, Arizona

Robert Radocy, MS*
President, CEO
TRS, Inc.
Boulder, Colorado

Zahid Raza, MD, FRCSEd, FRCS
Specialist Registrar in Vascular Surgery
Department of Vascular Surgery
Royal Infirmary of Edinburgh
Edinburgh, Scotland

Kingsley Peter Robinson, MS, FRCS
Consultant Advisor in Osseointegration
Queen Mary's Hospital
Roehampton, London, England
Visiting Professor in Biomedical Engineering
University of Surrey
Guildford, Surrey, England

Rebekah Russ, CPO, LPO
Department of Prosthetics and Orthotics
Texas Scottish Rite Hospital for Children
Dallas, Texas

Roy Sanders, MD
Chief, Department of Orthopaedics
Tampa General Hospital
Tampa, Florida

Shahan K. Sarrafian, MD
Clinical Associate Professor, Emeritus
Department of Orthopaedic Surgery
Northwestern University, Feinberg School of Medicine
Chicago, Illinois

Michael L. Schmitz, MD
Pediatric Orthopaedic Surgeon
Children's Orthopaedics of Atlanta
Children's Healthcare of Atlanta at Scottish Rite
Atlanta, Georgia

C. Michael Schuch, CPO
Vice President of Clinical Services
Assistant Clinical Professor
Center for Orthotic and Prosthetic Care
Duke University Medical Center
Durham, North Carolina

Alexander Y. Shin, MD
Consultant, Hand Surgery
Assistant Professor, Orthopedic Surgery
Department of Orthopedic Surgery
Mayo Clinic
Rochester, Minnesota

Douglas G. Smith, MD*
Associate Professor
Department of Orthopaedic Surgery and Sports Medicine
University of Washington & Harborview Medical Center
Director, Prosthetics Research Study
Medical Director, Amputee Coalition of America
Seattle, Washington

Gerald E. Stark Jr, CP*
Director of Education and Technical Support
The Fillauer Companies, Inc.
Chattanooga, Tennessee

H. Thomas Temple, MD*
Professor of Orthopaedics and Pathology
Division of Orthopaedic Oncology
Department of Orthopaedics and Rehabilitation
University of Miami School of Medicine
Miami, Florida

Jose J. Terz, MD
Clinical Professor of Surgery
Department of Oncologic Surgery
University of Southern California
Los Angeles, California

Jack E. Uellendahl, CPO
Hanger Prosthetics and Orthotics, Inc.
Phoenix, Arizona

Lawrence D. Wagman, MD
Chair, Division of Surgery
City of Hope Cancer Center
Duarte, California

David A. Ward, FRCS Orth
Consultant Orthopaedic Surgeon
Kingston Hospital NHS Trust
Kingston-Upon-Thames
Surrey, England

Robert L. Waters, MD
Clinical Professor Orthopedic Surgery
University of Southern California
Department of Surgery
Rancho Los Amigos National Rehabilitation Center
Downey, California

Hugh Watts, MD
Clinical Professor of Orthopedics
University of California at Los Angeles
Shriners Hospital for Children, Los Angeles
Los Angeles, California

Richard F. *ff.* Weir, PhD
Research Healthcare Scientist
Department of Veterans Affairs
Northwestern University Prosthetics Research Laboratory
VA Chicago Healthcare System
Chicago, Illinois

Saeed Zahedi, OBE, FIMechE
Head of Technology
PDD Group, Ltd.
London, England

---

* Has received something of value from a commercial or other party related directly or indirectly to the subject of his/her chapter.

Foreword

Limb amputations and congenital limb deficiencies are as old as humanity. Amputation represents an irreversible loss of physical integrity that is very often considered a form of punishment both for the patient and indirectly for the patient's family and society. In some cultures, an amputee is even believed to be denied Paradise. In medieval law, amputation was a common penalty, a sort of partial execution, and is still practiced in certain countries. As recently as the year 2000, terrorist rebels in Sierra Leone, West Africa, cut off the hands of an estimated 10,000 civilians. The need for limb replacement is, therefore, as old as civilization itself. The earliest known prosthesis, a beautifully designed hallux made some 4,000 years ago in Egypt, was probably not the first one ever made.

Today, despite great progress in medicine and technology, the basic considerations with regard to amputation and prosthetics remain constant. The disability increases with each more proximal level of amputation, particularly with the loss of major joints. For example, the bilateral transfemoral amputee suffering from peripheral arterial occlusive disease will never be able to walk effectively again, even with the most sophisticated prostheses. And despite advances in electronically controlled prostheses, bilateral short transhumeral amputees will always require help for daily activities, such as personal hygiene, eating, and writing. For these amputees, technical aids for daily living and professional activities—such as the devices developed by Ernst Marquardt and Eberhard Franz in Heidelberg, Germany, in 1976 that allow an armless person to drive a car—become more important for rehabilitation than does any prosthetic replacement. With regard to congenital deficiencies, surgeons should be particularly aware that, in most cases, it is better not to remove more than is already missing because even rudimentary limbs can become highly functional in the hands of a knowledgeable, creative prosthetist.

Unfortunately, most surgeons who perform amputations are not aware of their responsibility in selecting the most distal possible amputation level and creating a residual limb that is free of pain and is functional with or without a prosthesis. Some surgeons may consider amputation rather a nuisance—as an operation with little social and economic reward or, even worse, an unsupervised surgical opportunity for the beginner. This widespread attitude results in the selection of amputation levels that are much too proximal, increasing the disability unnecessarily, and in the creation of residual limbs of poor quality. For these reasons, I wish I had been confronted more often with the opportunity for primary amputations rather than surgical revisions. Limb amputation is not to be considered a self-learning experience for unsupervised beginners, but rather a challenge even for the experienced surgeon, whether a general, orthopaedic, pediatric, vascular, or plastic and reconstructive surgeon. It is also true that the best results will usually be achieved by surgeons who have some basic knowledge of prosthetics and amputee rehabilitation.

As in any medical specialty, there are limits to surgery and to prosthetics that should be recognized. This is because amputation is far more than simply a surgical and prosthetic affair. In surgery, the limits are set by physiology, bacteriology, immunology, and, last but not least, by ethical considerations. All these factors come to the fore, to varying degrees, in any discussion of "future developments" such as osseointegration and hand transplantation. The question of whether there is a future for these controversial procedures remains open. It seems logical that bacteria would be grateful for the open door offered by osseointegration, although it works wonderfully in maxillofacial surgery. The constraints imposed by Wolff's Law in regard to the mechanical strains to bone at the implant-bone interface are also considerable. Because of the multiplicity of tissue types involved in hand transplantation, the future of this field remains firmly tied to future developments in the field of immunology. The questionable safety of long-term use of current forms of immunosuppression as well as the psychological stress associated with this entirely elective procedure require careful consideration. Nonetheless, the cautious and factual presentation of the latest information on these techniques in this text, including the current barriers to their success, serves a very useful purpose in avoiding unrealistic expectations of their current applicability on the part of both the medical and lay communities. Whether the barriers remain insurmountable remains to be seen.

American Academy of Orthopaedic Surgeons

In regard to the virtually total prosthetic replacement of an upper limb, results of long-term follow-up of upper limb amputees fitted with the most sophisticated electronically controlled, electrically powered arm prostheses are needed. In these cases, technical aids, although much less spectacular, are usually far more important for a useful rehabilitation result.

Above all, amputation is a challenge not only to the surgeon and the prosthetist, but to many other professionals as well. For the best results in rehabilitation, the team approach is of utmost importance, although coordination of effort is sometimes frustratingly difficult to achieve. As in an orchestra, the various specialists must each play their part at the appropriate time, with one person prepared to play the role of the conductor. In this third edition of the *Atlas*, the orchestra, consisting of specialists recognized in their respective fields who have made contributions in 79 chapters, has been conducted by three internationally known experts. Most of the contributors also play an active role in the highly respected International Society for Prosthetics and Orthotics (ISPO).

I would like to congratulate the editors and the contributors for the immense work they have accomplished. This *Atlas* represents the state of the art, particularly in North America. Being an orthopaedic surgeon who has been fascinated by amputation surgery, prosthetics, and rehabilitation throughout a professional lifetime in Switzerland and in Germany, I am most interested to learn what is going on elsewhere. I am particularly grateful to the editors for having given me the chance to contribute a foreword to this *Atlas*. Like its predecessors, this edition will be the manual to be consulted the world over.

July 15, 2003
René F. Baumgartner, MD
Emeritus Professor of Orthopaedic Surgery
University of Muenster, Germany
Department of Prosthetics, Orthotics, Rehabilitation
and Related Surgery
Address:
Langwisstrasse 14
CH-8126 Zumikon, Switzerland
rabaumgart@bluewin.ch

Preface

With the third edition of this *Atlas*, the American Academy of Orthopaedic Surgeons (AAOS) continues a commitment that began in 1960 with the publication of Volume 2 of *The Orthopaedic Appliances Atlas: Artificial Limbs*. Now, as then, the goal of the Academy is to provide its members and all amputee rehabilitation team members with the latest knowledge relating to amputation surgery, congenital deficiencies, prosthetics, and rehabilitation. In that first text, the emphasis was on prosthetics, perhaps in deference to Donald Slocum's highly regarded and encyclopedic *Atlas of Amputations*, which had appeared in 1949. The *Orthopaedic Appliances Atlas* did, however, include brief sections on amputation surgery and rehabilitation, setting the precedent for the increasingly holistic approach of later editions. A much greater emphasis on surgery was apparent in the first edition of the current series, *The Atlas of Limb Prosthetics: Surgical and Prosthetic Principles*, which appeared in 1981. The second edition of 1992 featured, in addition to advances in surgical technique and prosthetics, an in-depth review of the latest physical and occupational therapy methods used in the prosthetic and nonprosthetic rehabilitation of amputees, an emphasis reflected in the book's subtitle, *Surgical, Prosthetic, and Rehabilitation Principles*.

In this latest edition, we have sought to present the major advances of the past decade. A number of new authors have been recruited to provide additional chapters on amputee care in wartime, the role of the Krukenberg procedure in developing countries, the rise of the amputee consumer movement, and the rapidly expanding role of sports and recreation for amputees, as well as the more controversial topics of osseointegration and transplantation. Contemporary European contributions to partial foot amputation surgery have been included for the first time. The major influence of orthopaedic surgeons on the development of both amputation surgery and prosthetics is noted in the greatly expanded chapter on the history of these fields. Several new pediatric issues are covered, including the psychological impact, not only on the child but also on the family, of a congenital or acquired limb deficiency. A chapter on absence of the lumbar spine and sacrum has been added, as well as a chapter on surgical revision.

We hope that both the new and the expanded chapters will enhance the book's usefulness to all members of the amputee rehabilitation team, including surgeons (whether general, vascular, pediatric, plastic, or orthopaedic), physiatrists, prosthetists, physical and occupational therapists, recreational therapists, bioengineers, rehabilitation nurses, social workers, and amputees and their families.

The support of the Academy's Board of Directors has made this volume possible and is gratefully acknowledged. The work of the authors and editors has been greatly enhanced by the deft touch of the Academy's publication staff, resulting in what we trust is a cohesive and readable text.

Douglas G. Smith, MD
John W. Michael, MEd, CPO
John H. Bowker, MD

Table of Contents

Section I: Introduction

1 *The History of Amputation Surgery and Prosthetics* .3
John H. Bowker, MD
Charles H. Pritham, CPO

2 *General Principles of Amputation Surgery* 21
Douglas G. Smith, MD

3 *Vascular Disease: Limb Salvage Versus Amputation* 31
Peter T. McCollum, MCh, FRCSI, FRCSEd
Zahid Raza, MD, FRCSEd, FRCS

4 *Infection: Limb Salvage Versus Amputation* 47
John H. Bowker, MD

5 *Tumor: Limb Salvage Versus Amputation* 55
Walid Mnaymneh, MD
H. Thomas Temple, MD

6 *Trauma: Limb Salvage Versus Amputation* 69
Michael T. Archdeacon, MD
Roy Sanders, MD

7 *Wartime Amputee Care* 77
Paul J. Dougherty, MD

Section II: The Upper Limb

8 *Kinesiology and Functional Characteristics of the Upper Limb* 101
Brian J. Hartigan, MD
Shahan K. Sarrafian, MD

9 *Body-Powered Components* 117
Charles M. Fryer, MS
Gerald E. Stark Jr, CP
John W. Michael, MEd, CPO

10 *Harnessing and Controls for Body-Powered Devices* 131
Charles M. Fryer, MS
John W. Michael, MEd, CPO

11 *Components for Electric-Powered Systems* 145
Craig W. Heckathorne, MSc

12 *Control of Limb Prostheses* 173
Dudley S. Childress, PhD
Richard F. ff. Weir, PhD

13 *Partial Hand Amputation: Surgical Management* 197
E. Anne Ouellette, MD, MBA

14 *Partial Hand Amputation: Prosthetic Management* 209
Chris Lake, CPO

15 *Wrist Disarticulation and Transradial Amputation: Surgical Management* 219
Patrick Owens, MD
E. Anne Ouellette, MD, MBA

16 *Wrist Disarticulation and Transradial Amputation: Prosthetic Management* 223
Carl D. Brenner, CPO

17 *The Krukenberg Procedure* 231
Pradip D. Poonekar, MD

18 *Elbow Disarticulation and Transhumeral Amputation: Surgical Management* 239
Patrick Owens, MD
E. Anne Ouellette, MD, MBA

19 *Elbow Disarticulation and Transhumeral Amputation: Prosthetic Management* 243
Wayne K. Daly, CPO, LPO

20 *Amputations About the Shoulder: Surgical Management* 251
Douglas G. Smith, MD

21 *Amputations About the Shoulder: Prosthetic Management* 263
John M. Miguelez, CP
Michelle D. Miguelez, JD
Randall D. Alley, CP

22 *Prosthetic Training.* 275
Diane J. Atkins, OTR

23 *Brachial Plexus Injuries: Surgical and Prosthetic Management* 285
Alexander Y. Shin, MD
Allen T. Bishop, MD
John W. Michael, MEd, CPO

24 *Aesthetic Prostheses* 303
Thomas Passero, CP
Kim Doolan

25 *Bilateral Upper Limb Prostheses* 311
Jack E. Uellendahl, CPO

26 *Prosthetic Adaptations in Competitive Sports and Recreation.* 327
Robert Radocy, MS

27 *Future Developments: Hand Transplantation.* 339
Christopher H. Allan, MD

28 *New Developments in Upper Limb Prosthetics* 343
Hans Dietl, PhD

Section III: The Lower Limb

29 *Normal Gait* 353
Jacquelin Perry, MD

30 *Amputee Gait.* .367
Jacquelin Perry, MD

31 *Visual Analysis of Prosthetic Gait* 385
Susan L. Kapp, CPO

32 *Energy Expenditure of Walking in Individuals With Lower Limb Amputations* 395
Robert L. Waters, MD
Sara J. Mulroy, PhD, PT

33 *Prosthetic Suspensions and Components* 409
John W. Michael, MEd, CPO

34 *Amputations and Disarticulations Within the Foot: Surgical Management* 429
John H. Bowker, MD

35 *Amputations and Disarticulations Within the Foot: Prosthetic Management* 449
David N. Condie, CEng
Roy Bowers, SRProsOrth

36 *Ankle Disarticulation and Variants: Surgical Management* 459
John H. Bowker, MD

37 *Ankle Disarticulation and Variants: Prosthetic Management* 473
Gary M. Berke, MS, CP

38 *Surgical Management* 481
John H. Bowker, MD

39 *Transtibial Amputation: Prosthetic Management* 503
Susan L. Kapp, CPO
John R. Fergason, CPO

40 *Knee Disarticulation: Surgical Management* 517
Michael S. Pinzur, MD

41 *Knee Disarticulation: Prosthetic Management* 525
Donald R. Cummings, CP, LP
Rebekah Russ, CPO, LPO

42 *Transfemoral Amputation: Surgical Management* 533
Frank Gottschalk, MD, FRCSEd, FCS(SA)

43 *Transfemoral Amputation: Prosthetic Management* 541
C. Michael Schuch, CPO
Charles H. Pritham, CPO

44 *Hip Disarticulation and Transpelvic Amputation: Surgical Management* 557
Howard A. Chansky, MD

45 *Hip Disarticulation and Transpelvic Amputation: Prosthetic Management* 565
Kevin M. Carroll, MS, CP

46 *Translumbar Amputation: Surgical Management* 575
Lawrence D. Wagman, MD
Jose J. Terz, MD

47 *Translumbar Amputation: Prosthetic Management* 583
Greg Gruman, CP
John W. Michael, MEd, CPO

48 *Physical Therapy* 589
Robert S. Gailey, PhD, PT
Curtis R. Clark, PT

49 *Bilateral Lower Limb Prostheses* 621
Jack E. Uellendahl, CPO

50 *Prostheses for Sports and Recreation* 633
John R. Fergason, CPO
David Alan Boone, CP, MPH

51 *Physical Therapy for Sports and Recreation* 641
Robert S. Gailey, PhD, PT

52 *Research in Lower Limb Prosthetics* 661
Saeed Zahedi, OBE, FIMechE

Section IV: Management Issues

53 *Future Developments: Osseointegration in Transfemoral Amputees* 673
Kingsley Peter Robinson, MS, FRCS
Rickard Brånemark, MD, MSc, PhD
David A. Ward, FRCS Orth

54 *Musculoskeletal Complications* 683
John J. Murnaghan, MD, MSc, MA, FRCSC
John H. Bowker, MD

55 *Skin Problems in the Amputee* 701
S. William Levy, MD

56 *Chronic Pain Management* 711
Dawn M. Ehde, PhD
Douglas G. Smith, MD

57 *Psychological Adaptation to Amputation* 727
John C. Racy, MD

58 *The Art of Prosthesis Prescription* 739
John H. Bowker, MD

59 *Rehabilitation Without Prostheses* 745
Joan E. Edelstein, MA, PT

60 *Special Considerations: Consumer Movement* 757
Mary P. Novotny, RN, MS

Section V: Pediatrics

61 *The Limb-Deficient Child* 773
John R. Fisk, MD
Douglas G. Smith, MD

62 *Terminology in Pediatric Limb Deficiency* 779
John R. Fisk, MD

63 *Developmental Kinesiology* 783
Joan E. Edelstein, MA, PT

64 *General Prosthetic Considerations* 789
Donald R. Cummings, CP, LP

65 *Psychological Issues in Pediatric Limb Deficiency* 801
Alice L. Kahle, PhD

66 *Occupational Therapy* 813
Joanna G. Patton, OTR/L

67 *Physical Therapy* 831
Colleen Coulter-O'Berry, PT, MS, PCS

68 *Acquired Amputations in Children* 841
John P. Dormans, MD
Bülent Erol, MD
Christopher B. Nelson, CPO

69 *Hand Deficiencies* 853
Terry R. Light, MD

70 *Radial Deficiencies* 863
Terry R. Light, MD

71 *Longitudinal Ulnar Deficiency* 869
Julian E. Kuz, MD
James Engels, MD

72 *Humeral Deficiencies* 875
Mary Williams Clark, MD
Chris Lake, CPO

73 *Foot Deficiencies* 885
Mary Williams Clark, MD

74 *Fibular Deficiencies* 889
Gerard L. Glancy, MD

75 *Tibial Deficiencies* 897
Michael L. Schmitz, MD
Brian J. Giavedoni, MBA, CP
Colleen Coulter-O'Berry, PT, MS, PCS

76 *Femoral Deficiencies* 905
Kenneth J. Guidera, MD
Cara D. Novick, MD
Janet G. Marshall, CPO

77 *Absence of the Lumbar Spine and Sacrum* 917
James T. Guille, MD
S. Jay Kumar, MD

78 *Multiple Limb Deficiencies* 923
Hugh Watts, MD

79 *Surgical Modification of Residual Limbs* 931
Hugh Watts, MD

Appendix: Terminology in Acquired Limb Loss 945
John H. Bowker, MD

Index 947

Index of Manufacturers 965

Section I

Introduction

Chapter 1

The History of Amputation Surgery and Prosthetics

John H. Bowker, MD
Charles H. Pritham, CPO

Introduction

The distinct but interdependent fields of amputation surgery and prosthetics have historical roots extending back to about 1800 BCE when, according to the Rig-Veda, the Indian warrior-Queen Vishpla had her leg amputated following a battle, was fitted with a prosthesis made of iron, and subsequently returned to lead her troops. The oldest archeologic evidence of amputation dates to 45,000 years ago. Study of a male Neanderthal skeleton, found in present day Iraq, indicated that he had survived to age 40 years with an atrophic right upper limb that had been amputated just above the elbow. The oldest surviving prosthesis (roughly 1000 BCE) is an artistically carved wooden hallux found on a female mummy in the west Theban Necropolis. It is held in place by a laced leather band around the forefoot and shows signs of wear from use.

To present the many changes that have occurred in these two fields over time, we will separately examine the evolution of those individual aspects of prime interest to the amputation surgeon, prosthetist, therapist, and other members of the rehabilitation team. The political, social, and economic forces that influenced both advances and regression are mentioned where appropriate. We begin with the development of amputation surgery.

History of Amputation Surgery
Expansion of Indications for Amputation

Early surgeons were strongly influenced by the writing of Hippocrates (460 to 377 BCE), the greatest medical authority of antiquity. He considered gangrene the only indication for amputation and recommended cutting through insensate necrotic tissue, preferably the knee joint, analogous to a débridement rather than a definitive procedure. Any attendant bleeding was controlled by cauterization. Battle wounds were, of course, another matter. Hippocrates wisely observed that "war is the only proper school for the surgeon." This was true because of the battle surgeon's intense exposure to wide varieties of injuries inflicted by the assorted cutting, piercing, and crushing weapons then in use. Although surgeons of that time could do little for soldiers with severe wounds of the trunk or head, they frequently encountered combatants with limb injuries whose lives could, at times, be saved by amputation. Judicial amputation of criminals' hands was also widely practiced, sanctioned by both the Babylonian Code of Hammurabi and the Mosaic law.

The next reference to surgical indication was by the Roman physician Celsus (25 BCE to 50 CE). While still restricting amputation to cases of gangrene, he recommended transosseous division at the junction of viable and gangrenous tissue. He also advocated vessel ligation, invented earlier by Alexandrian surgeons, as well as wound compression for hemostasis. Both techniques made surgery considerably safer. Celsus considered cauterization of vessels by hot irons as the last resort. Over the next half century, indications were expanded much further by Archigenes and Heliodorus to include chronic leg ulcers, tumors, trauma, and congenital malformations. This extension of indications to include even semielective problems was made possible by the use of a tight bandage proximal to the site of the amputation. Larger vessels were controlled with ligatures and smaller ones with compression and torsion. Additional indications mentioned in the Talmud were leprosy and other incurable infections. Thereafter, through the influence of the plentiful writings of the Roman physician Galen (131 to 201 CE), there was a return to the teachings of Hippocrates, including amputating only through necrotic tissue or the knee joint, although Galen did use ligatures for hemostasis.

Following the decline of Roman influence during the third and fourth centuries CE, Roman advances in medicine made before those of Galen

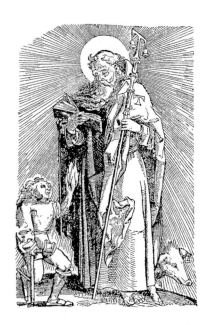

Figure 1 St. Anthony, patron saint of ergotism, is shown with a victim of the disease. The flames emanating from the victim's left hand symbolize the burning pain of severe vasoconstriction caused by ergotism, or "St. Anthony's fire." He uses a kneewalker peg-leg because of the loss of his right foot. *(Reproduced from Hans von Gersdorff:* Field-Book of Wound Surgery. *Strassberg, 1540.)*

did not pass into the succeeding Byzantine and Arabic medical traditions. Instead, with the rise of Islam, the numerous works of Hippocrates and Galen were translated from Greek into Arabic by Persian scholars in the seventh and eighth centuries. This perpetuated their influence for the next thousand years, aided by belief in their infallibility on the part of both Muslims and Christians. Other influences maintaining the status quo were the conservatism of the Christian church regarding anatomic studies, a prohibition against surgery, and the feuding of rival medical groups. These factors led to widespread discrimination against surgery and its practitioners, who were held in low esteem.

Nonetheless, in Europe during the Middle Ages (circa 476 to 1453 CE), indications for amputation continued to expand and now included limbs damaged by leprosy and ergotism. Leprosy, a mycobacterial infection introduced to Europe by returning Crusaders (11th to 13th centuries), is characterized by loss of limb sensation. Repetitive trauma frequently results in painless injury to the hands and feet, leading to ulceration and deep infection. Ergot poisoning follows ingestion of bread made from rye flour contaminated with an alkaloid produced by the fungus *Claviceps purpurea*. In 857, the first of many European pandemics occurred among the poor, for whom rye bread was a staple food. Ergotism is manifested by the painful burning sensation of prolonged arterial vasoconstriction, hence the names ignis sacer (sacred fire) or St. Anthony's fire (Figure 1). Autoamputation or surgical ablation of gangrenous hands and feet was usually followed by recovery, while vasoconstriction of mesenteric arteries was rapidly fatal. Although far from a new indication, amputations from battle wounds greatly increased in number following the introduction of the cannon at the Battle of Crecy in 1346 and of muskets at Perugia in 1364. The wounds incurred were so severe, compared to those from cutting or piercing weapons, that surgeons became newly interested in amputations as a worthy endeavor.

During the Renaissance (14th to 16th centuries), the original works of Hippocrates, Galen, and, most significantly, Celsus were rediscovered in cloister libraries and widely circulated with the aid of the printing press. Prior to this, European physicians had only Latin translations of Arabic translations made from the original Greek, with many attendant inaccuracies. With the rise of Humanism and a relative decline in ecclesiastical authority, DaVinci (1452 to 1519) was able to undertake detailed anatomic studies that refuted some of Galen's revered notions. Unfortunately, DaVinci's work was suppressed for another century.

Ambroise Paré (1509 to 1590) contributed greatly to the development of modern amputation surgery during this period by reintroducing Celsus' principles, namely, amputation through viable tissue and using ligatures for hemostasis, rather than cauterization with hot irons—two ideas lost for a millennium. He also abandoned the use of boiling oil for cauterization of wounds contaminated by gunpowder, which was thought to be poisonous, after he fortuitously ran out of oil during a battle. The immediate improvement in his results reinforced his resolve to abandon this excruciatingly painful measure. Paré's other great contribution was making Vesalius' monumental anatomic treatise *De Fabrica Humani Corporis Libri Septem* (1543) readily accessible to his contemporaries by publishing an epitome in vernacular French.

The Napoleonic Era (1792 to 1815) produced two great military surgeons: George Guthrie on the British side and Dominique-Jean Larrey on the French. Larrey concurred with Guthrie that prompt primary amputation on the battlefield resulted in fewer fatalities than waiting the commonly recommended 3 weeks before secondary amputation. To permit rapid access to injured solders, Larrey introduced "flying ambulances" to pick up the wounded during battle and transport them to an aid station (Figure 2). Using this method, Larrey was able to provide truly expeditious care for the men of Napoleon's Imperial Guard. During one battle, only 43 of 12,000 casualties brought to his aid station died, a record far better than that of other French army units.

During the American Civil War (1861 to 1865), the severity of limb wounds increased markedly with the introduction of the French minié ball, a conical bullet with a hollow base that expanded as it left the rifle barrel, splintering bone on impact. The extensive damage to both soft and bony tissue led to a refinement of indications for primary amputation. These included, in both the Union and the Confederate Armies, comminuted open fractures, open joints with fracture, major nerve or blood vessel injury, extensive soft-tissue injury, and crush. The modern introduction of blood replacement, aseptic surgery, antibiotics, primary vascular repair, and external skeletal fixation, augmented by helicopter evacuation to well-equipped forward hospitals, has since narrowed this list of absolute indications for amputation while expanding the indications for attempts at limb salvage. Nonetheless, the list remains basically valid in many less than ideal circumstances.

Advances in Level Selection

As mentioned above, Hippocrates recommended amputation through gangrenous tissue, thereby averting much of the pain of surgery as well as reducing the likelihood of exsanguination. Celsus' use of ligatures for hemostasis allowed him to amputate through viable tissue, but this technique was lost for a millennium after the fall of Rome. Hieronymus Brunschwig (1425 to 1520) recommended amputation below the knee whenever possible and considered knee disarticulation the most proximal level consistent with survival. Within a half century, however, Paré's reintroduction of the ligature allowed him to report the first successful transfemoral amputation. The English surgeon James Kerr, in 1774, was the first to report survival of a patient following hip disarticulation for 18 days, at which point she succumbed to tuberculosis. During the Napoleonic wars, Larrey, and later Guthrie, performed successful hip disarticulations on the battlefield. A consummate anatomist, Larrey was able to complete the open disarticulation within 15 seconds of ligating the femoral vessels. It should be noted that, prior to the discovery of effective anesthetic agents, the most sought-after surgeons combined a profound knowledge of anatomy with dexterity and speed to shorten the patient's period of extreme pain. Fortunately, this is no longer necessary, and more attention now can be focused on reconstruction of a residual limb that will interface comfortably with a modern prosthesis. As to the preferred length for a transtibial amputation, both Larrey and Guthrie opted for a short transtibial limb of 8 to 10 cm to more conveniently fit

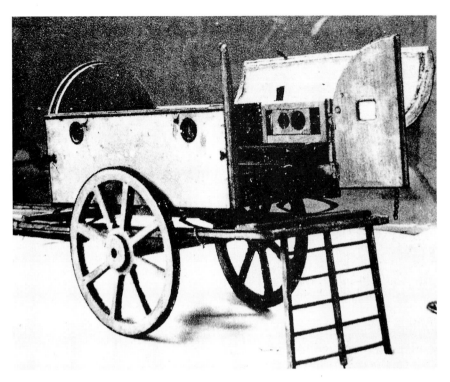

Figure 2 Ambulance volante (flying ambulance) invented by Larrey to rapidly collect wounded men during a battle for transfer to an aid station. *(Reproduced from van der Meij WKN:* No Leg to Stand On. *Groningen, AE Brinkman, 1995, p 84.)*

the kneewalker peg-leg then in use. If only a very short level could be salvaged, Larrey advocated removing the fibula entirely.

A number of end–weight-bearing ablations were developed about this time that either eliminated the need for a prosthesis entirely or permitted fitting of a simplified, less expensive one. These were important developments because the transtibial amputee who could not afford a prosthesis that permitted knee motion was relegated to a kneewalker peg-leg. The first of these procedures was the midtarsal disarticulation described by Francois Chopart in 1792, followed closely by Jacques Lisfranc's tarsometatarsal disarticulation in 1815 and James Syme's ankle disarticulation in 1843. Nikolai Pirogoff, a Russian surgeon who admired Syme's innovation, found that he was unable to provide Russian peasant-soldiers with a prosthesis that would control an unstable heel pad following that procedure. Therefore, in 1854, he stabilized the heel pad by fusion of an attached

calcaneal fragment to the distal tibia, allowing the use of standard work boots. In 1939, the American orthopaedist Harold Boyd reported a similar procedure. Despite the development of these new distal techniques, the transfemoral level remained dominant throughout World War I. In 1914, Blake reported that 70% of amputations were at that level, while J.S. Speed's series was 58.6% transfemoral. Overall, of the total 42,400 lower limb amputations sustained by the Allied Forces, 39.6% were transfemoral. The first successful transpelvic amputation was carried out by the French surgeon Mathieu Jaboulay in 1894. Immediately following World War II, basic research into normal human gait, under United States Federal government sponsorship, was begun by Verne Inman and Howard Eberhart at the University of California at Berkeley. Their studies demonstrated that amputees' gait would benefit by retention of as much healthy bone and soft tissue as possible. This conclusion was in sharp contrast to the

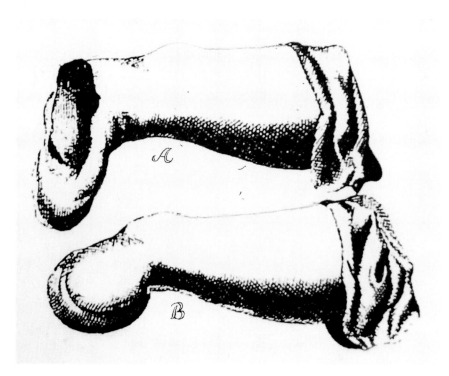

Figure 3 The transtibial amputation of Verduyn (1696) showing his posterior myofasciocutaneous flap. **A,** The flap. **B,** The completed residual limb. He also designed a prosthesis with a movable knee specifically to permit the full benefit of this advanced surgical technique. *(Reproduced from Heister L:* Chirurgie. *Nuremberg, 1718.)*

time-honored practice of amputating at fixed sites in each limb segment as agreed on by surgeons and prosthetists.

Turning to the upper limb, Paré performed the first elbow disarticulation in 1536; Henri-Francois LeDran, the first successful shoulder disarticulation in 1731; and John Cuming, a British naval surgeon, is credited with the first successful forequarter amputation. The concept of cineplasty as a means to capture the power of arm and forearm muscles to control a prosthetic hand was developed in chickens by the Italian Giuliano Vanghetti in 1896. His associate A. Ceci first applied it to Italian soldiers whose hands had been amputated while war prisoners of the Ethiopians. The following briefly describes the steps in cineplasty. First, a transverse tunnel is made in a muscle, then its insertion is severed. After healing has occurred while keeping the tunnel patent, a rod is passed through the tunnel and harnessed to a cable attached to the prosthetic hand. When the muscle contracts, it pulls on the cable activating the hand. In 1916, Sauerbruch and ten Horn refined the procedure by lining the tunnel with a medially based skin flap. Thereafter, it was used during both world wars, but with the widespread availability of myoelectric prostheses, it is now rarely used even though some researchers believe that this surgery may prove useful in the future to control prosthetic hands with multifunctional fingers.

Evolving Techniques for Bone Coverage

From the time of Hippocrates until the first century, the recommended technique for limb amputation was division of all tissues at the same level. As these open wounds healed by secondary intention, the soft tissues contracted, resulting in a conical residual limb with the bone prominent distally. Early in the first century, however, Celsus advocated cutting the bone at a higher level than the soft tissues. This double circular incision allowed the skin to be drawn distally to cover the end of the bone. With the decline of Rome, this advancement was lost, only to be rediscovered during the Renaissance. A number of new techniques based on Celsus' principle appeared in the 18th century. During 1717 and 1718, the contemporaries Jean Louis Petit, Lorenz Heister, and William Cheselden favored making a circular incision through skin and fat, pulling these tissues proximally, then dividing the muscle and bone. Edward Alanson (1779) created a less bulky residuum by following the skin and fat incision with an oblique cut through muscle from distal to proximal, followed by division of the bone at the apex of the muscle cone.

The triple circular incision was introduced by Henri-Francois LeDran (1731) and Benjamin Bell (1787). Following succeeding circular divisions of the skin and subcutaneous tissue and a muscle layer, both were pulled proximally to the level of bone division. This was the method used by both Dominique-Jean Larrey and George Guthrie during the Napoleonic Wars. Although double and triple circular incisions remained the most common methods used to ensure that bone remained well covered, other surgeons were developing flaps for wound closure, beginning in 1679 with James Yonge, a British naval surgeon. Shortly thereafter, in 1696, Pieter Verduyn described the first long posterior myofasciocutaneous flap for transtibial amputation (Figure 3). H. Ravaton (1739) and Vermale (1756) reported the first use of sagittal flaps consisting of skin and muscle. In addition, the French surgeon Raphael Bienvenu Sabatier in 1796 described a myofasciocutaneous flap raised from the anterior leg to close a knee disarticulation. In 1915, during World War I, Fitzmaurice-Kelly performed emergent flapless open amputations at the most distal level of viable tissue to save limb length. He considered this the first stage of a two-stage procedure, using skin traction in the interim. The American surgeon Kellogg Speed modified this technique by incising the skin longitudinally on each side in preparation for the secondary closure. Using this method, he found that the wounded could be moved safely to a rear hospital 1 week after amputation.

Although these incremental improvements in technique tended to produce marginally better residual limbs, the bone would often become prominent over time as soft-tissue atrophy occurred, leading to distal discomfort and ulceration with use of a prosthesis. This was noted to be especially common following transfemoral amputation if the muscles were not attached stably over the end of the femur. After World War II, the myoplasty methods of the German surgeons F. Mondry and R. Dederich, in which the distal femur is covered by suturing opposing muscles over its end, were widely adopted. In 1960, the Polish surgeon Marian Weiss introduced myodesis, in which the muscles are reattached to bone or periosteum to restore some of their motor function. This concept was carried further by Frank Gottschalk, who in 1990 demonstrated the value of preserving the adductor power of a transfemoral residuum by myodesing the adductor magnus tendon to the lateral femoral cortex. Ample padding is then provided by suturing the quadriceps muscle over the distal femur. Distal coverage of a transtibial residual limb with a posterior myofasciocutaneous flap, introduced by Verduyn in 1696, was first used in the United States by William Bickel in 1943 and later was widely promoted by Ernest Burgess.

Mortality Related to Amputation

From the earliest records, it is clear that amputation commonly resulted in death from blood loss during surgery or some days later from septicemia, which was often associated with secondary hemorrhage. These known risks led to the conservatism of Hippocrates and his adherents who accepted gangrene as the only proper

indication with the transection to be done through necrotic tissue to decrease the chance of fatal hemorrhage. In addition, because hemorrhage was more easily controlled by cauterization or bandaging at distal levels, only transtibial amputation or, at most, knee disarticulation was recommended.

It remained largely for military surgeons to gradually improve the outlook for survival by controlling blood loss during amputation. The evolution of intraoperative hemostasis evolved over many centuries, beginning with the introduction of ligatures by Celsus, and their reintroduction by Paré during the Renaissance. A precursor of tourniquets was a circular bandage placed proximal to the site of amputation, used by Archigenes and Heliodorus in the first century. The French army surgeon Etienne Morel, however, introduced the first true tourniquet, tightened by a stick, in 1674. Because the stick often obstructed the surgical site, it was quickly displaced by Petit's screw tourniquet (roughly 1700) (Figure 4). Nonetheless, mortality rates following battle wounds remained so high that Louis XIV (1638 to 1715) complained that "For my soldiers, the amputation knife of my surgeons is far more dangerous [than] the enemie's [sic] fire."

It was eventually accepted that mortality following amputations for battle wounds was closely linked to the interval between wounding and surgery. Initially, opinion was sharply divided between those who advocated primary amputation on the battlefield and those who would wait 2 to 3 weeks until it was clear that the patient was able to survive this initial period without surgical intervention. By delaying treatment, these latter surgeons were able to claim a lower rate of surgical mortality because most of the wounded had died of sepsis or hemorrhage while waiting the prescribed interval. Larrey's use of "flying ambulances" during the Napoleonic Wars to bring the wounded directly to a surgical station during the battle for primary amputation mark-

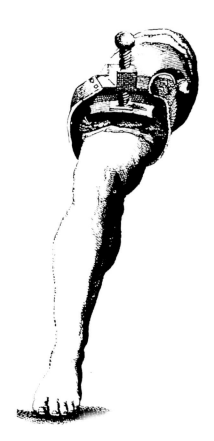

Figure 4 The screw tourniquet, invented by Petit in the early 18th century, was a great improvement on Morel's windlass tourniquet because of its security. *(Reproduced from Heister L:* Chirurgie. *Nuremberg, 1718.)*

edly decreased intraoperative death rates as well as death from wound infection and secondary hemorrhage. Guthrie's experience with British casualties was similar. During the Crimean War (1853 to 1856), primary amputation resulted in a 37% mortality rate, compared to 60% for secondary ablation. The Union Army had a similar experience with 20,500 amputations during the American Civil War, with a mortality rate of 35.7%. This was a marked improvement from the battle of Fountenoy in 1745, when the mortality rate from amputation was 90%.

The other major cause of death following amputation was septicemia. Although Hippocrates had recommended that surgeons clean their hands and nails and use boiled water for wound cleansing, this advice was

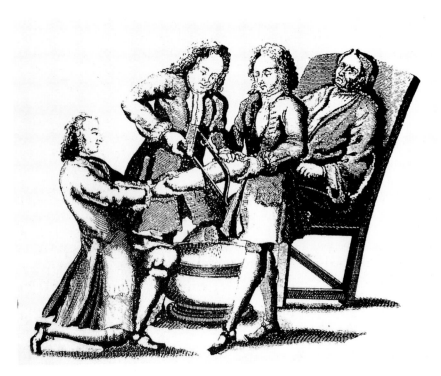

Figure 5 Typical 18th century transtibial amputation, performed swiftly without anesthesia. The assistant on the right compressed the thigh to control hemorrhage. All tissues were divided at the same level, commonly resulting in a residual limb of poor quality. *(Reproduced from Heister L:* Chirurgie. *Nuremberg, 1718.)*

rarely heeded, either on the battlefield or even in hospitals. Early attempts at wound lavage with purported antiseptics included the use of wine by Avicenna in the Middle Ages and turpentine by Paré during the Renaissance. The concept of asepsis progressed with Ignaz Semmelweis' 1848 report of the reduction in puerperal sepsis mortality from nearly 10% to 1.3% by enforced hand washing in a solution of calcium chloride for all personnel before any patient contact.

In 1865, Joseph Lister, appalled by the high mortality rate from septicemia associated with open fractures and thoroughly familiar with the work of Louis Pasteur, began treating fracture wounds with carbolic acid dressings in an attempt to sterilize them, rather than doing primary amputations as commonly recommended. Following successful salvage of several limbs by this method, he applied the principle of antisepsis to his surgical cases. This included preoperative washing of hands and instruments, as well as intraoperative

spraying of wounds with a carbolic acid solution. By using antisepsis, Lister was able to reduce his 48% surgical mortality rate for amputations performed from 1864 to 1866 to 15% for amputations performed from 1867 to 1870. Antisepsis opened a new era of safety for elective surgery as well. By 1877, it was widely accepted by most, including American military surgeons. Antisepsis still retains applicability for lavage of contaminated wounds as exemplified by the continued use of Carrel-Dakin solution (dilute sodium hypochlorite) and its various successors.

The progression from antisepsis to asepsis was also based on the work of Pasteur. Ernst Von Bergmann, a prominent surgeon of the Franco-Prussian war (1870 to 1871), introduced steam sterilization of surgical instruments in 1886. Then, in 1891, he began the gradual introduction of asepsis as we know it today, including sterile gowns and gloves and the use of masks. During World War I, British, French, and American surgeons

achieved an overall amputation survival rate of 85%, using a combination of extensive wound débridement, early open amputation, and wound irrigation with Carrel-Dakin solution. The availability of sulfonamides from the beginning of World War II and the introduction of penicillin in 1943 marked the beginning of the antibiotic era.

Surgical Analgesia and Anesthesia

In the fourth century, Dioskorides, a military surgeon under Nero, compiled the first *Materia Medica*, describing the medical uses of more than 600 plants, including the anesthetic effects of mandragora and opium for surgical procedures. The Talmud later mentions the specific use of anesthesia for amputation as well. During the Middle Ages, the Spongia Soporifica, invented by Ugo di Borgognoni of the University of Bologna, was widely used for surgical anesthesia. A sponge was soaked in a mixture containing, among other ingredients, opium, mandragora, hyoscyamus, and hemlock, providing both narcotic and atrophine-like effects when inhaled or swallowed. When dried after preparation, the sponge became easily portable, being reconstituted with water when needed. For the next four centuries, however, from the end of the Middle Ages (roughly 1450) until the mid 19th century, amputations were done without benefit of analgesia, placing a premium on the speed of the surgeon to lessen the duration of suffering. Because of these circumstances, little thought was given to the quality of the resulting residual limb (Figure 5).

The evolution of modern anesthesia began with two notable events: Humphrey Davey's description of the pain-killing property of nitrous oxide in 1792, and Michael Faraday's demonstration of a similar effect from nitrous ether inhalation in 1818. The first amputation using ether anesthesia was transfemoral, done for tuberculosis of the knee by John Collins

Warren at the Massachusetts General Hospital in Boston in 1846. Six weeks later, having heard of Warren's success, Robert Liston performed the first amputation using ether anesthesia in Britain at the University College of London Hospital. Although he accomplished this transfemoral ablation with his usual dispatch, the necessity for extreme speed was over, to be succeeded by a new luxury, the availability of sufficient time to carefully execute a deliberate surgical plan and deal with unexpected findings without the sometimes violent struggles of a patient in extreme pain. The use of ether anesthesia was quickly adopted in 1847 by both Syme in Edinburgh and Pirogoff in Russia. Chloroform was widely used by military surgeons during the American Civil War as a safer alternative to ether under battlefield conditions.

Education and Training in Amputation Surgery

From ancient times, the place of surgery and surgeons in society has been dictated by forces that directly or indirectly affected its advances and declines. In Rome, the role of physicians seems to have included surgery, especially by those with military experience. During the Middle Ages, Ali Ibn Sina, or Avicenna (980 to 1037 CE), the leading Islamic medical scholar of his era, put forth two doctrines that, through the influence of Latin translations of his voluminous writings, became institutionalized by both the Christian church and the universities. The first tenet was that methodical and logical reasoning (ratiocination) was superior, in medical treatment, to first-hand experience and investigation. The second was that surgery, as a hands-on profession, was an inherently inferior and separate branch of medicine. Thus, university medical education in the Middle Ages became purely theoretical, leaving practical treatment of illness and injury to nonacademically trained "popular physicians," barbers, surgeons, bath-stove attendants, and assorted quacks.

France gradually led the way out of this morass during the 13th to 18th centuries. The first attempts to legitimize surgery and to raise the status of surgeons occurred circa 1250 through the political influence of Jean Pitard, the personal barber-surgeon to the King. With royal support, Pitard founded a surgeon's guild called the College of St. Cosmas. To ensure that new applicants to the college had reached an acceptable level of knowledge and experience, Pitard organized a 4-year apprenticeship that encompassed not only practical surgery but theoretical lessons, given for the first time in the French language. After passing an examination, the apprentices were called "master surgeons" and entitled to enter the college, open an office, and train their own apprentices. Despite these advances, however, real progress was stymied throughout much of the Middle Ages because of the rivalries among the university medicine faculties, the master-surgeons' guild, and the barber surgeons, characterized by constant bickering and ever-shifting alliances as each group sought to control the others. The result of this divisive turmoil was a delay in the application of new knowledge such as Servetus' discovery (circa 1550) of the pulmonary (lesser) circulation and William Harvey's discovery (1628) of the systemic (greater) circulation, advances characteristic of the rise of scientific medicine.

A few foresighted physicians, however, who found their theoretical education useless for rendering aid on the battlefield, went to the best-regarded barber-surgeons for further training. On becoming physician-surgeons, they returned to the universities to teach surgery. Three physician-surgeons of the period, Henri de Mondeville, Guy de Chauliac, and Lanfranc, wrote surgical texts. Lanfranc, the founder of surgery in France, sought to bring the opposing camps together, teaching that "no one can be a good physician who has no idea of surgical operations, and that a surgeon is nothing if ignorant of

medicine." Richelieu, the Prime Minister of Louis XIII, helped raise the standards and social status of army surgeons by making them members of the College of St. Cosmas. Surgical education, at least in France, was finally brought to the same academic level as university medicine in the mid 1700s with the founding of the Royal Academy of Surgery by Mareschal, the personal surgeon of Louis XIV. In England, the development of surgery lagged behind that of France, but surgeons and barbers finally became differentiated, culminating in the 1800 founding of the Royal College of Surgeons of London and later the Royal College of Surgeons of England.

From the earliest times, military surgeons learned the art of amputation surgery while treating wounded combatants. In fact, the first two illustrated books that discussed amputation were written by experienced military surgeons from Strassberg. The first was *The Book of Wound Surgery* by Brunschwig in 1497, followed by Hans von Gersdorff's *Field-Book of Wound Surgery* in 1517, which contained the first illustration of an amputation (Figure 6). Both of these books dealt with wounds caused by firearms. Many other books dealing with amputations followed. One by Paré was the first to provide designs for a "wooden leg for the poor." In 1815, Guthrie published an epoch-making treatise, *Gunshot Wounds of the Extremities Requiring Amputation*, which enjoyed six editions. Formal education in amputation surgery on a sustained basis did not materialize until after World War II, but interest in this topic has been waning in recent years among surgeons in general.

History of Prosthetics

Whether a result of conflict, accident, disease, or judicial decree, amputations have always been a part of human experience, as has been the desire to replace the lost part for

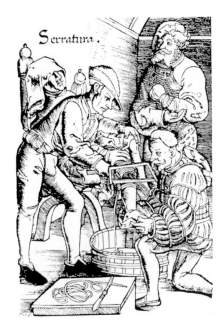

Figure 6 "Serratura" (sawing off)—the first known illustration of amputation surgery. Note the hemorrhage despite the tight bandages above and below the incision. The scalpel lies in the foreground. The person behind wears the Tau cross of St. Anthony, indicating that he may have lost the fingers of his left hand from ergotism. *(Reproduced from Hans von Gersdorff: Field-Book of Wound Surgery. Strassberg, 1517.)*

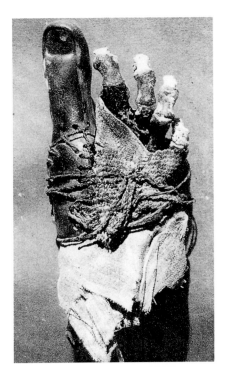

Figure 7 Cosmetic wooden hallux prosthesis found on female mummy circa 1000 BCE. Note laced leather band around forefoot. *(Reproduced with permission from Nerlich A, Zink A: Eine Zehenprothese an einer altaegyptischen Mumie. Med Orth Tech 2002;122:32-33.)*

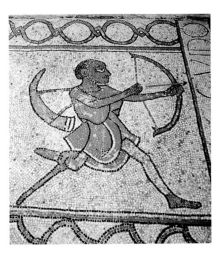

Figure 8 A Gallo-Roman mosaic depicting a hunter with a transtibial peg-leg. *(Courtesy of Professor R. Baumgartner, MD, Zumikon/Zürich, Switzerland.)*

functional, cosmetic, or protective reasons or some combination of these. The word prosthesis (plural prostheses), the proper name for an artificial limb, derives from the Greek roots meaning "to place an addition," whereas prosthetics is the professional field that deals with the construction and custom-fitting of prostheses.

Evolution of Prosthetic Design

The earliest example of a prosthesis for which we have visual evidence is the cosmetic hallux fitted in Egypt about 1000 BCE (Figure 7). A Roman transtibial prosthesis circa 300 BCE had a wooden socket reinforced with bronze sheets. A mosaic found in France, of the Gallo-Roman era, depicts a hunter pursuing game on a transtibial peg-leg (Figure 8). Prostheses made by armorers for officer-amputees had the additional benefit of concealing the warriors' deficit

from enemies. These included the iron hands of the Roman Marcus Sergius and that of the Teutonic knight Goetz von Berlichingen, which were designed to firmly lock onto a sword or shield in battle (Figure 9).

Despite the awakening of intellectual curiosity in the Renaissance (14th to 16th centuries), the development of prosthetics during its first 200 years did not keep pace with that of amputation surgery. The poor continued to use crude crutches, peg-legs, or rolling platforms as they had for centuries before (Figure 10). The increasing use of cannons and muskets, meanwhile, made battle wounds an ever-increasing cause of amputation as survival rates improved. Prosthetic innovation finally began in the 16th century, closely linked to the constant warfare of that period. The first major advance made during the Renaissance (circa 1560) was by the French surgeon Paré who devised both an inexpensive wooden kneewalker peg-leg

for the poor private soldier and a sophisticated transfemoral prosthesis resembling armor for wealthy officers, as well as cleverly crafted prosthetic hands with locking fingers. Although peg-legs had been known since ancient times, Paré's design featured elevated sides with straps to securely attach the prosthesis to the thigh (Figure 11). His endoskeletal transfemoral prosthesis featured a leather socket, a foot with a spring-loaded midfoot hinge, and a knee that could be unlocked for sitting. The whole device was covered with thin iron plates shaped to match the contours of the opposite limb and was suspended from an undervest (Figure 12). The most significant prosthetic design of the Renaissance, however, was the transtibial prosthesis introduced by the Dutch surgeon Verduyn in 1696. With this prosthesis, the amputee was able to fully use the benefits of Verduyn's revolutionary posterior myofasciocutaneous flap. It consisted of a copper socket lined with leather, a solid ankle wooden foot, and a leather thigh corset attached to the socket with jointed metal bars. The tightly laced thigh corset aided in both suspension and weight bearing, while the joints allowed free knee motion (Figure 13). This became the prototype for functional transtibial prostheses

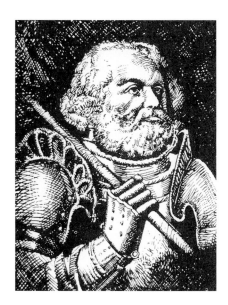

Figure 9 The Teutonic knight Goetz von Berlichingen holding a staff with his prosthetic right hand, which featured jointed, locking fingers to hold a weapon. *(Reproduced from American Academy of Orthopaedic Surgeons: Atlas of Orthopaedic Appliances. Ann Arbor, MI, JW Edwards, 1960, vol 2, p 3.)*

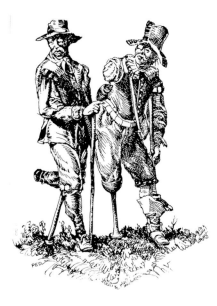

Figure 10 Typical prostheses made for their own use by army veteran amputees of the Renaissance period. The ankle disarticulate uses a kneewalker peg-leg and cane. The knee disarticulate has a weight-bearing peg-leg and a crutch. *(Reproduced from American Academy of Orthopaedic Surgeons: Atlas of Orthopaedic Appliances. Ann Arbor, MI, JW Edwards, 1960, vol 2.)*

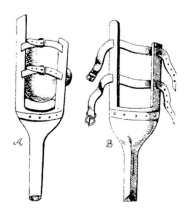

Figure 11 Paré's kneewalker peg-leg for poor private soldier-amputees. **A,** Front view shows the flexed limb between medial and lateral uprights resting on a cushion. **B,** Posterior view. *(Adapted from Paré A: Ten Books of Surgery. 1563. Reproduced from the University of Georgia Press, Athens, GA, 1969.)*

until the introduction of the patellar tendon–bearing (PTB) prosthesis in 1961 by Charles Radcliffe and James Foort at the University of California at Berkeley. Nonetheless, the kneewalker peg-leg was still in common use during the first half of the 19th century. It was so ubiquitous, in fact, that the ideal length of a transtibial amputation was held to be no more than 8 to 10 cm below the knee joint to more conveniently fit this design.

Conceptual progress in upper limb prosthetic design continued with Gavin Wilson's artificial hand (circa 1790), capable of holding a knife, fork, or pen. Peter Baliff, a Berlin dentist, (circa 1816) developed the first body-powered prosthetic hand activated by elbow and shoulder motion (Figure 14). The concept of harnessing the remaining muscles of a limb to operate a terminal device remained central to all development in upper limb prosthetics until the practical introduction of myoelectrically controlled external power, beginning in 1958.

With the increase in higher-level gunshot injuries and the prevalence of transfemoral amputees, there was a growth of interest in the design of prostheses for this level with many ingenious devices as a result. The concept of an ischial weight-bearing socket had already been introduced by Gavin Wilson in 1790. In 1810, J.G. von Heine, considered the founder of German orthopaedics, introduced ball-and-socket knee and ankle joints. The knee joint was locked except when sitting. In 1816, Peter Baliff also introduced a prosthesis with an ingenious knee joint that unlocked on toe-off to allow knee flexion during swing phase and relocked on heel contact to give stability during stance.

In 1816, James Pott of London made a hollow-shanked wooden transfemoral prosthesis with partially restrained ball-and-socket knee and ankle joints and a toe hinge. The joints were connected by cords so that knee flexion would dorsiflex the ankle. This leg became known as the

Anglesey leg after one was fitted to H.W. Bayly, Marquess of Anglesey, who lost his leg in the closing moments of the battle of Waterloo in 1815 (Figure 15). Various modifications of this leg remained the standard British design until after World War I. In 1839, the design was brought to the United States by William Selpho, a limb-maker in Pott's factory, as the "American" leg and was thereafter modified by competitors. Martin and Charrière, in 1842, introduced another concept fundamental to contemporary prosthetic and orthotic design by offsetting the knee joint center posterior to the line of weight bearing, greatly improving stance phase stability. In 1860, capitalizing on the 1839 invention of vulcanized rubber by Charles Goodyear, A.A. Marks of New York produced a foot made of this material. This became the precursor of several designs of flexible feet popularized since World War II. Vulcanized rubber was also quickly formed into rubber bumpers to limit and cushion the motion of prosthetic joints by American, British, and Continental prosthetists. It is of interest that Marks was also the first to shrink-wrap wooden sockets and hollow shanks in rawhide for added strength and durability.

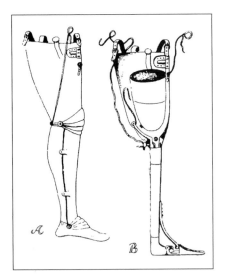

Figure 12 Paré's transfemoral prosthesis designed for wealthy officer-amputees. **A,** External view. **B,** Note the leather socket and metal shank and foot before coverage with iron plates to resemble armor. *(Adapted from Paré A: Ten Books of Surgery.1563. Reproduced from the University of Georgia Press, Athens, GA, 1969.)*

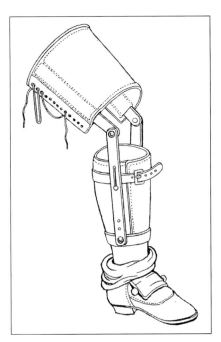

Figure 13 Transtibial prosthesis designed by Verduyn especially for amputees with a posterior myofasciocutaneous flap. This remained the prototype for transtibial prostheses until the introduction of the patellar-tendon-bearing PTB prosthesis by Radcliffe and Foort in 1961. *(Reproduced from American Academy of Orthopaedic Surgeons: Atlas of Orthopaedic Appliances. Ann Arbor, MI, JW Edwards, 1960, vol 2.)*

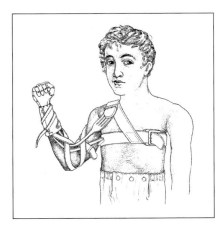

Figure 14 Transradial prosthesis designed by Baliff circa 1816. Fingers are activated by elbow and shoulder motion. *(Reproduced from American Academy of Orthopaedic Surgeons:* Atlas of Orthopaedic Appliances. *Ann Arbor, MI, JW Edwards, 1960, vol 2.)*

The American Civil War resulted in large numbers of amputees, augmented by the accident toll from the expansion of industry and the railroad system. After the war, the United States experienced much more growth in the development of prosthetic design and manufacture than did Europe. One entrepreneur was James E. Hanger, a Confederate officer who lost his leg early in the war, made a prosthesis for himself, and returned to battle. In 1861, he introduced a single-axis ankle joint controlled by vulcanized rubber bumpers rather than cords. He went on to found the prosthetics company that bears his name to this day. Also, during the war, in 1863, Dubois Parmelee of New York was issued a patent for the first transfemoral prosthesis using a suction suspension socket, eliminating the need for elaborate body harnesses or corsets. His prosthesis also featured a polycentric roller knee joint, a multiarticulated foot, and endoskeletal construction at a time when most contemporary prostheses were of exoskeletal design (Figure 16).

Neither suction suspension nor endoskeletal construction became widely accepted in the prosthetics field until the latter part of the 20th century.

Despite the many profound conceptual changes in prosthetic design of 19th-century innovators, the resulting limbs were affordable only by the rich and by government-subsidized war amputees. Civilian amputees, who greatly outnumbered military ones, could not afford these advanced limbs. With this age-old problem in mind, the Comte de Beaufort designed two inexpensive transtibial prostheses, made entirely of wood and leather, for working men in 1867. One was a kneewalker peg-leg, and the other had wooden side joints and a leather thigh lacer; each featured a rocker foot that made walking much easier. The latter prosthesis, improved with steel side joints, continued in use until about 1929 as the "French" leg (Figure 17).

Progress in prosthetics made during the 19th and early 20th centuries as a result of the Napoleonic, Crimean, American Civil, and First World Wars was influenced by a number of critical factors that would continue to play a role thereafter. Because prosthetics has always been a small field that serves relatively few people, it has not always been possible, especially for prosthetists themselves, to devote the necessary time and financial resources to fully develop their concepts on any scale. In addition, there was initially a limited number of materials available from which to construct limbs, namely, wood, leather, and iron. Nonetheless, both prosthetists and amputees have always placed a premium on reliability, strength, comfort, and low weight as worthwhile goals, with cost of secondary importance. By necessity, prosthetists have had to borrow new techniques, devices, and materials, as they became affordable, from other fields that value these attributes and then adapt them to their own use. Innovations of the Industrial Revolution provided many opportunities for exploitation of new materials, meth-

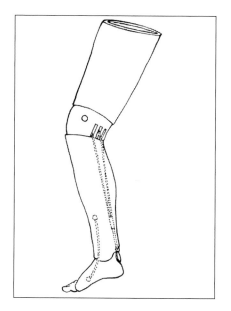

Figure 15 Pott's Anglesey Leg of 1816, in various modifications, was one of the most popular transfemoral prostheses for the next century. Internal elastic straps are used to control movement of the knee and ankle. *(Reproduced from American Academy of Orthopaedic Surgeons: Atlas of Orthopaedic Appliances. Ann Arbor, MI, JW Edwards, 1960, vol 2.)*

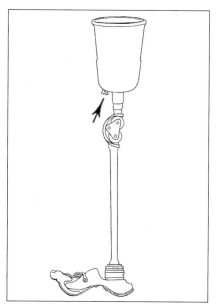

Figure 16 Parmelee's endoskeletal transfemoral prosthesis of 1863, featuring a suction suspension socket, eliminating the need for body harnessing. The lateral view shows the valve *(arrow)* placed in the distal-anterior socket, a polycentric roller knee joint, and a multiarticulated foot. *(Reproduced from American Academy of Orthopaedic Surgeons: Atlas of Orthopaedic Appliances. Ann Arbor, MI, JW Edwards, 1960, vol 2.)*

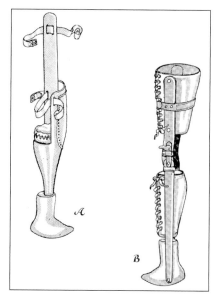

Figure 17 The inexpensive Beaufort transtibial prostheses of 1867 are made entirely of wood and leather. **A,** Knee-walker peg-leg. **B,** Prosthesis featuring leather thigh lacer, locking knee joints, and adjustable leather socket. Both designs have a rocker foot. *(Reproduced from American Academy of Orthopaedic Surgeons: Atlas of Orthopaedic Appliances. Ann Arbor, MI, JW Edwards, 1960, vol 2.)*

ods, and devices such as steel, vulcanized rubber, and machine tools.

Another material that was adapted to prosthetic use was aluminum, which combines reasonable strength with light weight. Although Hermann of Prague had substituted aluminum for steel components as early as 1865, it remained for a fortuitous mishap to lead to its fullest use in prosthetics. In about 1912, British test pilot Marcel Desoutter lost his leg in a flying accident. Unhappy with heavy contemporary prostheses, he enlisted the help of his brother Charles, an aeronautical engineer and his partner in the aircraft manufacturing firm Desoutter Brothers. Charles designed an exoskeletal prosthesis weighing only 3.5 pounds using the newly available aluminum alloy named duralumin. Word spread and soon Desoutter Brothers became a prosthetic design and manufacturing firm. Demand increased rapidly, despite the initial reluctance of the British government to purchase these prostheses for war amputees because of their high cost. Alu-

minum exoskeletal prostheses remained the British standard until well after World War II.

Building on Parmelee's concept of suction suspension for transfemoral limbs, Ernest Underwood, a British war amputee, designed a wooden socket with annular spiral grooves that closely fit the bare skin of the residual limb. Fashioned of duralumin and with a valve added, this became a successful design of the Blatchford firm. German designers were also active between the two world wars. The prosthetist Oesterlee of Ulm designed his own suction-suspension socket, followed in 1932 by one with an improved valve from the surgeon Felix of Dusseldorf. The use of suction suspension was sufficiently widespread in Germany by the end of World War II to capture the attention of an American commission charged with improving prosthetic care for US veterans. Another German development

was the design of three- and four-bar linkage knee joints by Alfred Habermann. Probably the most important American advance during this period was the split hook for body-powered upper limb prostheses, invented and promoted by D.W. Dorrance, a transradial amputee. Terminal devices based on his original design remain among the most commonly prescribed options.

During World War II, returning military amputees quickly became dissatisfied with the design and function of available prostheses, especially those for the upper limb, which combined excessive weight with little function. In response to these persistent complaints, Army Col. John Loutenheiser enlisted the help of Northrop Aviation engineers in 1943 to develop lighter weight and more functional upper limb prostheses. Using a plastic laminate, socket weight and bulk were significantly reduced. The Bowden cable, used to activate aircraft control surfaces, was adapted to operating upper limb prostheses, replacing stretchable, fragile leather thongs. Northrop engineers also invented a shoulder-operated locking elbow for transhumeral amputees. That same year, the first prosthetic research laboratory was organized by the Navy at Mare Island, California.

Before the war ended, a concerted national campaign was launched to address these same concerns, led by the amputee veterans themselves, strongly supported by Representative Edith Nourse Rogers, Chairman of the House Veterans Committee, and Secretary of War Stimson. The goal was to marshal the efforts of academia and private industry to improve prosthetic design. The redevelopment of this partnership, which had been so productive in the war effort, would lead to a new intellectual and clinical foundation for contemporary prosthetics. The program eventually came under the auspices of the National Academy of Sciences (NAS) with its Committee on Prosthetics Research and Development (CPRD) and Committee on Prosthetics and Orthotics Education.

In January 1945, the NAS organized a meeting in Chicago of leading surgeons, engineers, and prosthetists, among them orthopaedists Paul Magnuson of Northwestern University and P.D. Wilson of the Hospital for Special Surgery, to establish standards for upper and lower limb prostheses. It was soon determined that there was insufficient scientific basis on which to formulate any meaningful standards. They recommended the organization of a government-funded program to undertake fundamental studies related to prosthetic design, fitting, and usage. Under the aegis of this program, basic studies of normal human gait were conducted at the University of California (UC) under the direction of Verne Inman, Professor of Orthopaedic Surgery at UC Medical School in San Francisco, and Howard Eberhart, Professor of Civil Engineering at UC Berkeley (UCB), himself an amputee. They attached

metal pins with reflective targets to bony prominences of the lower limbs and pelvis of volunteers. Using interrupted-light photography, these markers allowed the accurate measurement of the relative motions of limb segments in three dimensions during walking. These and other innovations formed the basis for the field of biomechanics as we know it today. Additional studies by J. Perry, M.P. Murray, and others over the next decades further enhanced our understanding of normal and amputee gait.

Within a short time, a network of biomechanics laboratories was established, each with a particular mission. UCB would continue to study the lower limb, while UC Los Angeles (UCLA) would initiate a parallel biomechanical research program for the upper limb. Two major advances occurred at UCLA. One was the development of a rationale for socket and harness design for every level of upper limb amputation. The second was the design and testing of commercially available components that could be assembled to meet the individual needs of amputees. The Veterans Administration Prosthetics Research Laboratory in New York City, under the direction of E. Murphy, would seek to apply the results of the UC research directly to war veterans with amputations. The Army Prosthetics Research Laboratory at Walter Reed Hospital and the navy counterpart at Oakland, California, would serve their respective populations, the army concentrating their efforts on upper limb prosthetic development and the navy on lower limb. This aggregate body of work provided a solid rationale not only to guide the future design and use of prostheses but to encourage surgeons to save all possible limb length and thus preserve more function than considered feasible before.

Following reports of the widespread, successful fitting of transfemoral prostheses with suction suspension by prosthetists in postwar West Germany, the US Surgeon General dispatched a group of surgeons and engineers to study this application.

Actually, the Germans had been using this method since the early 1930s, based on Parmelee's American patent of 1863. This technology was promptly reintroduced to American amputees. With the reintroduction of the intimately fitting suction suspension socket, the fixed-position hip joint and pelvic belt were no longer required, and coronal plane alignment of the prosthesis became more critical. To meet this requirement, C. Radcliffe of UCB developed both an adjustable knee alignment unit and an alignment-duplication jig to ensure accurate transfer of the three-dimensional configuration achieved during standing and walking to the finished prosthetic limb.

Significant improvements in prosthetic knee joints soon followed. J. Stewart, an engineer who was a transfemoral amputee, developed a superior seal for a hydraulic shank unit of his design, which integrated ankle dorsiflexion with knee flexion to clear the foot during swing phase. The seal also proved to be a great advance for aircraft hydraulic systems. This latter application, as well as the prosthetic one, was supported by Vickers Corporation of Detroit. Immediately after the war, Hans Mauch, an engineer in charge of developing the German V-1 military rocket, came to the United States and resumed work on another hydraulic knee unit with his orthopaedic colleague, Ulrich Henschke. The final result was a knee with hydraulic control of both swing and stance, which is still in production. The excessive weight of early hydraulic units led the UCB laboratory to develop a lighter pneumatic swing control knee unit, variations of which remain in use.

By 1950, the UCB laboratory, based on its anatomic studies, had developed the ischial weight-bearing quadrilateral socket to replace the historic plug-fit. The original concept had been brought to England by the New Zealand prosthetist Nugent 5 years earlier. Another major advance of that decade for both upper and lower limb prosthetics was the in-

ety of myoelectric hands, grippers, and elbows to fit both adults and children. This expansion became possible with the availability, from industrial applications, of solid-state circuits, efficient small motors, energy-dense batteries, and more recently, microprocessors. Since 1976, technologic growth and development have continued unabated, and indeed, accelerated, due in large part to the incorporation of spin-off technology from the rapidly advancing cell phone, pager, and handheld video game industries.

Socioeconomic Forces Affecting the Provision of Prostheses

From ancient times until the mid-1800s, a prosthesis was a luxury available only to the wealthy. The relatively few poor who survived a major amputation managed with homemade crutches, peg-legs, kneewalkers, or rolling platforms, such as those seen in the paintings of Pieter Brueghel the Elder (1528-1569). Recognizing the huge socioeconomic disparity between wounded officers and common peasant soldiers, Paré devised an inexpensive wooden kneewalker peg-leg for the poor. The organization of special funds for the medical care of disabled workers started in the early 1600s, with the European guilds. With the decline of the guilds a century later, a variety of health funds were established by manufacturers and trade unions, but none paid for prostheses.

The situation began to change, at least for military amputees, during the American Civil War, when both the Federal and Confederate governments began to provide prostheses at public expense. The original Federal legislation of 1862 was amended in 1870 to allow a new prosthesis every 5 years, and later to every 3 years. The Prussians and British quickly followed suit, providing both an articulated prosthesis and a peg-leg to wear during repairs on the primary prosthesis. These measures substantially increased the number of prostheses

fitted, thus encouraging further development of the field. During World War I, British philanthropists established Queen Mary's Hospital for the Limbless at Roehampton. Beset with wartime shortages and short-staffed facilities, British firms alone were unable to cope with the surge in demand for prostheses created by the two most common mechanisms; scything machine gun fire and shrapnel. To supply the necessary expertise and prostheses in sufficient quantity, the British, as the French had before them, turned to American prosthetic firms to fill the void. They, along with their British counterparts, were invited to locate facilities on the hospital grounds. For the first time, prosthetists and surgeons met at the patients' bedside to discuss their prosthetic restoration. The cumulative experience gained and knowledge shared made Roehampton renowned worldwide for excellence. At the same time, the field of prosthetics began its transformation from a cottage industry to a multinational business. The Americans introduced designs, materials, and production techniques that were new to the British and French. The characteristic feature of the "American" leg included shoulder suspenders for control of the knee in swing phase, construction of the shank from a single piece of wood, a single-axis foot controlled by rubber bumpers, and external reinforcement of wooden shank and thigh segments with shrink-wrapped rawhide.

The huge numbers of battle amputations forced the Central Powers (Germany and Austria-Hungary) to drastically change their methods of prosthesis manufacture and provision. For the first time, anthropomorphic measurements of the lower limbs, developed by the Berlin orthopaedist Professor Gocht, were used to help design simple prosthetic components that could be produced quickly. In this way, wounded soldiers could be rapidly deployed to supportive agricultural or war factory work. The Hungarian military surgeon Dollinger produced the "Arbeitsprothese" (work

prosthesis) while the Germans made the "Behelfsprothese" (temporary prosthesis). Both were simple designs resembling von Hessings' 19th-century knee-ankle-foot orthosis with jointed metal uprights, connected by bands encompassing a leather socket. To provide a proper fit, the socket of the Arbeitsprothese was molded about a plaster model of the amputee's residual limb.

Prior to World War I, limb-fitting firms were vertically integrated, including the fabrication of components for their own use on a custom or semicustom basis on demand. With the experience gained by government-sponsored prosthetic facilities attached to amputee hospitals, it became clear that greater production capacity and cost-containment could be achieved by a horizontal reorganization, allowing mass production of uniform components to be purchased and used by many firms. The new efficiency would also allow component manufacturers to devote the necessary capital to exploit new materials and techniques beyond the reach of individual prosthetic fitters. With the 1919 founding of Orthopaedische Industrie GmbH in Berlin, Otto Bock introduced mass production of prosthetic components together with the techniques for their alignment. The three major lower limb modules were a socket block, a knee joint with shank, and an ankle-foot assembly.

In anticipation of the need for a greatly increased number of prostheses for American war amputees, the chief medical officer of the Council of National Defense convened a meeting of the 10 leading American prosthetic firms in 1917. This meeting resulted in the formation of the Association of Limb Manufacturers of America that eventually became the American Orthotic and Prosthetic Association, which remains the preeminent trade organization for these fields in the United States. Because of the late entry of the American Expeditionary Force into the war, however, the number of US amputations totaled 4,403, of which 2,635 were considered major, as compared to 42,000 for the British, allowing the redeployment of American prosthetists to the United Kingdom as described previously.

During World War II, United States forces sustained 17,130 amputations. With thousands of American amputees returning home throughout World War II, the Army and Navy responded by establishing specialized centers for their overall care, including all aspects of prosthetic rehabilitation; ten for the Army and two for the Navy. These centers incorporated the work of surgeons, prosthetists, and therapists working as a team. By 1945, the Army Center in Walter Reed Hospital was receiving up to 1,500 amputees each month. In 1965, the Medicare program began to provide prostheses for US citizens older than age 65 years and younger persons permanently disabled by amputation. This trend reversed in the 1990s, when managed care organizations either began excluding prostheses from coverage or limited benefits to "one per lifetime" or an annual maximum reimbursement of as little as $1,000.

With advances in prosthetic design, manufacture, and provision well underway for the war amputee population, attention turned to another group whose care badly needed reorganization: children with limb deficiencies. In 1952, the United States Children's Bureau assisted the Michigan Crippled Children's Commission in organizing the first Child Amputee Program in the United States. It was located in Grand Rapids, Michigan, under the direction of orthopaedists C.H. Frantz and G.T. Aitken. A similar program was established in 1955 at UCLA and both continue to serve this population today. In 1956, the Committee on Prosthetic Research and Development (CPRD) of the National Academy of Sciences established the Subcommittee on Child Prosthetic Problems (SCPP), chaired successively by Drs. Frantz and Aitken. To further evaluate devices and techniques resulting from these projects, a Child Prosthetics Studies program was funded the same year at

New York University under the direction of Sidney Fishman. To assist in the widest possible dissemination of this new knowledge in a timely manner, the Child Amputee Clinic Chiefs inaugurated an annual meeting and SCPP began publication of the Inter-Clinic Information Bulletin (ICIB). With the dissolution of CPRD in 1976 and with it SCPP, the Association of Child Prosthetic and Orthotic Clinics (ACPOC) was formed to fill the void and continue publication of the ICIB, later known as the *Journal of the Association of Child Prosthetic and Orthotic Clinics*. Unfortunately, the journal ceased publication in 1994.

Education and Training in Prosthetics

Prior to World War II, training in prosthetics was largely based on informal apprenticeships. The widespread and vocal dissatisfaction of war amputees with the available prosthetic designs led to a massive government-sponsored research and development program. In 1949, UCB gave a pilot course in the prescription, fabrication, and alignment of the suction-suspension transfemoral socket recently readopted from Germany. This was followed by local courses in key areas of the country, sponsored jointly by the Veterans Administration (VA) and the limb manufacturers' association that is now known as the American Orthotic and Prosthetic Association (AOPA). Thereafter, the VA organized 30 amputee clinic teams for their hospitals, each consisting of a surgeon, prosthetist, physical and occupational therapist, and a VA prosthetic representative. As a result of these actions, a strong desire arose on the part of prosthetists to elevate their educational and professional status to match that of other team members. In 1949, the American Board for Certification in Prosthetics and Orthotics (ABC) was formed to establish standards for examination and certification of individual practitioners and the accreditation of prosthetic and orthotic facilities.

Further VA-sponsored courses for clinic teams followed. UCLA presented 12 six-week courses on upper limb prosthetics during 1953 and 1954. The response was so great that prosthetics education programs were established at New York University's Postgraduate Medical School in 1956 and in 1959 at Northwestern University. The national program reached its peak in the late 1980s when 12 universities offered preparatory programs in prosthetics and orthotics. Five were at the baccalaureate level, while seven offered postgraduate certificates in prosthetics, orthotics, or both disciplines. By 2000, fledgling master's level programs had begun and doctoral programs existed in Scotland, Hong Kong, and Australia. Unfortunately, chronic reductions in federal funding for prosthetic and orthotic education led to the demise of three entry-level baccalaureate programs by the new millennium.

The first English-language periodical for prosthetists appeared in 1946 as the *Orthopaedic and Prosthetic Appliance Journal*, published by the forerunner of AOPA. In 1976, the American Academy of Orthotists and Prosthetists (AAOP) began their own journal. The two journals merged in 1988 to become the quarterly *Journal of Prosthetics and Orthotics*. The Prosthetic and Sensory Aids Service of the Department of Veterans Affairs in 1964 began publishing what has become the *Journal of Rehabilitation Research and Development*, which appears bimonthly with additional supplements. In the late 1950s, having realized the need for an international exchange of information on prosthetics, orthotics, and amputation surgery, The International Committee on Prosthetics and Orthotics (ICPO) began publication of a technical journal. ICPO evolved into the present-day International Society for Prosthetics and Orthotics (ISPO), and its publication became *Prosthetics and Orthotics International*, published three times a year. In cooperation with the World Health Organization (WHO) and the International Committee of the Red Cross (ICRC), ISPO has developed standards for prosthetic and orthotic education programs and clinical care delivery systems for developing nations. ISPO also sponsors a triennial World Congress and periodic international consensus conferences and update courses throughout the world, cosponsored by local prosthetic and orthotic organizations. The charitable German Society for Technical Cooperation (Deutsche Gesellschaft fuer technische Zusammenarbeit [GTZ]) has been one of the most effective prosthetic and orthotic outreach groups. GTZ has organized prosthetic and orthotic training programs in several countries in Africa, Asia, and Latin America, successfully turning them over after a time to local instructors whom they have trained.

In 1970, the AAOP was formed with a primary focus on education, modeled after the American Academy of Orthopaedic Surgeons. Shortly thereafter, in 1972, ABC commissioned the development of standards for educational programs in prosthetics and orthotics. These standards are carried out by a new independent body, now called the National Commission on Orthotic and Prosthetic Education, which approves education and residency programs in these fields, in cooperation with the Commission on Accreditation of Allied Health Education Programs. The AAOP has been a major force in advancing the level of practitioner education and clinical practice in prosthetics and orthotics, sponsoring an ever-growing array of continuing education conferences and review courses each year. In 2003, the AAOP inaugurated an ongoing series of consensus conferences to develop clinical standards of practice, patterned after the successful multidisciplinary consensus conferences hosted by ISPO.

Emergence of Amputee Rehabilitation

Until the 19th century, the governments that recruited men to fight their wars typically turned away from those too disabled to serve again, leaving them to beg for subsistence. Even for the few who obtained prosthetic limbs, there was no organized care with a goal of societal reintegration. In 1867, the Prussian government was the first to legislate not only prosthetic restoration but hospitalization for accommodation to walking with the prosthesis. The British also began providing prostheses for the war wounded during this period, but it was not until 1915 that Queen Mary's Hospital for the Limbless (Roehampton) was established where physicians and prosthetists were brought together with the patient. During this time, the Central Powers also began fitting early temporary prostheses to speed the return of war amputees to useful work in factories and farms. The US government also established seven widely dispersed stateside amputee centers at Walter Reed General Hospital in Washington, DC; Letterman General Hospital in San Francisco, California; Fort Des Moines in Iowa; Fort Snelling in Minnesota; Fort McPherson in Georgia; General Hospital 3 in New Jersey; and General Hospital 10 in Boston, Massachusetts. Another concept that would later be resurrected after World War II was the fitting of an immediate postoperative prosthesis (IPOP), begun by the Frenchman Depage in 1917. Berlemont and Weber resumed this method in 1957, followed by Marian Weiss of Poland who reported on his extensive experience in 1963, stimulating research by E.M. Burgess in Seattle, A. Sarmiento in Miami, and the Navy Prosthetic Research Laboratory in Oakland.

During their World War II occupation, the Dutch set up a rehabilitation center for their wounded soldiers. The program included physical therapy, sports therapy, and job placement. During this time, a similar program was in operation at Roehampton in England. The Dutch program of amputee rehabilitation was expanded in the 1950s to include injured workers. In the United States, the Army Surgeon General established specialized centers for the rehabilitation of amputees prior to their separation from military service. By 1945, the army had 10 amputee centers and the navy had two.

Success in these military programs was replicated for civilians by the establishment of interdisciplinary amputee clinics. Many of the advances in amputee rehabilitation in the latter half of the 20th century resulted from this close collaboration between physician, surgeon, prosthetist, therapist, and other professionals who shared a commitment to amputee care. In recent years, changes in the economics of health care have reversed this trend, as postoperative hospitalizations become increasingly brief and outpatient treatment becomes the norm for new amputees. It has proven difficult to replicate the fertile interchange of ideas among team members that was inherent in the formal amputee clinic, now that they often function in geographic isolation from one another.

Summary

Historically, advances in amputation surgery have been closely linked to armed conflict, in turn spurring improvements in prosthetic technology and care. These trends have accelerated during postwar periods whenever attention and resources have been focused on amputee veterans. Advances in military rehabilitation have, in turn, been incorporated into civilian practice and developed further whenever adequate funding has been established. Better surgery and sockets after World War II led to demands for more sophisticated components, which were first developed based on government research funding and later from commercial investment. The level of prosthetic education has gradually risen since World War II, along with the technical sophistication of the materials, methods, and components used, while education in amputation surgery has declined. Only time will tell whether the recent fragmentation of the clinic team and reduction in funding for prosthetic rehabilitation and training in amputation surgery is a temporary setback or the harbinger of a new era in which the pace of advancement in amputee care will diminish.

Acknowledgment

The authors wish to express their thanks to Mrs. Eugenie Henry for her expert preparation of this manuscript.

Selected Readings

Ellis H: *Famous Operations*. Media, PA, Harwal Publishing, 1984.

Furman B: *Progress in Prosthetics*. Washington, DC, US Government Printing Office, 1962.

Garrison FH: *An Introduction to the History of Medicine*, ed 4. Philadelphia, PA, WB Saunders, 1929.

Guyatt M: Better legs: Artificial limbs for British veterans of the first World War. *J Design Hist* 2001;14:307-325.

Historical development of artificial limbs, in *Orthopaedic Appliances Atlas*. Ann Arbor, MI, JW Edwards, 1960, vol 2, pp 1-22.

Nerlich A, Zink A: Eine Zehenprothese an einer altaegyptischen Mumie. *Med Orth Tech* 2002;122:32-33.

Paré A: *On Gangrenes and Mortifications*, book VII in *Ten Books of Surgery With the Magazine of the Instruments Necessary for It, 1563*. Translated from the French by RW Linker and N Womack. Athens, GA, University of Georgia Press, 1969.

Phillips G: *Best Foot Forward: Chas. A. Blatchford & Sons Ltd (Artificial Limb Specialists) 1890-1990*. Cambridge, England, Granta Editions, 1990.

Sanders GT: *Lower Limb Amputations: A Guide to Rehabilitation*. Philadelphia, PA, FA Davis, 1986.

Weir RFff, Heckathorne CW, Childress DS: Cineplasty as a control input for externally powered prosthetic components. *J Rehabil Res Dev* 2001;38:357-363.

van der Meij WKN: *No Leg to Stand On. Historical Relation Between Amputation Surgery and Prostheseology*. Gronigen, the Netherlands, AE Brinkman, 1995.

Wilson AB Jr: History of amputation surgery and prosthetics, in Bowker JH, Michael JW (eds): *Atlas of Limb Prosthetics: Surgical, Prosthetic, and Rehabilitation Principles*, ed 2. American Academy of Orthopaedic Surgeons, Rosemont, IL, 2002, pp 3-15. (Originally published by Mosby-Year Book, 1992.)

Chapter 2

General Principles of Amputation Surgery

Douglas G. Smith, MD

Introduction

Arms and legs, hands and feet: These unique and wonderful extensions of the body allow humans to touch, to feel, and to manipulate the environment. They provide the invaluable capability of propulsion and allow free movement. The word limb hardly captures the essence of these magnificent structures.

Loss of part or all of a limb forever changes how a person moves, touches, works, and plays. The individual who loses a limb faces enormous emotional, psychological, and physical challenges and may perceive himself or herself as no longer whole. To regain lost function, the most common option is to supplement the newly altered physical body with a prosthesis. This is how many amputees find peace and wholeness.

One young transfemoral amputee recently advanced her vision for those with limb loss.[1] Her hope is that in the future, amputees will be offered not "artificial" limbs but "replacement" limbs. Replacement limbs would be so comfortable, natural, and functional that limb loss would become a much less significant event, similar to the loss of an appendix or a gallbladder. This goal, of minimizing the impact of an amputation on the patient, is one toward which surgeons, prosthetists, and rehabilitation specialists all strive.

Amputation surgery severs all the varied tissues of the limb. Each tissue must heal in its own particular manner, and the knowledgeable surgeon considers the unique role of each tissue when planning the course of reconstruction. This careful calculation is essential to create the most functional residual limb possible. Limb loss is not only a major physical and functional loss, it also presents the patient with an enormous psychological and emotional challenge. Limbs not only are a major part of the physical being but also contribute to the individual's body image and self-image. Losing a limb alters all these aspects of the amputee's life. When a limb or portion of a limb is removed, the brain continues to perceive sensations, movement, and even pain in the tissues no longer physically present. As Burgess[2] has pointed out, no amount of psychological testing and evaluation can completely measure the effects of limb loss on a given individual. Only the amputee knows what it is like to lose a limb and how that loss impacts his or her life.[3]

The surgeon has a unique responsibility to achieve two goals, both of which are critical to the success of an amputation. The first goal is the removal of the diseased, damaged, or dysfunctional portion of the limb. The second goal is the reconstruction of the residual limb. Reconstruction must promote primary or secondary wound healing as well as create the most functional residual limb possible. The reconstructive nature of amputation surgery and the positive impact proper technique can have on an individual's postamputation function cannot be overemphasized. The success of every amputation surgery depends on the balance between removal and reconstruction. To provide the best care for each patient, the surgeon must thoroughly understand not only surgical principles but also all the aspects of healing, rehabilitation, and residual limb physiology and the nature of prosthetic devices.

The team approach to amputee rehabilitation leads to more successful healing and a better informed patient. Communication among team members is essential. The surgeon is but one member of the amputation rehabilitation team and can benefit from the wisdom and perspectives of the other team members throughout all phases of the process—the preoperative evaluation, during surgery, during the early postoperative healing phase, and through management of late complications long after the definitive surgery is complete. Surgeons would be wise to encourage opinions from their teammates and take these opinions into consideration.

Surgical Considerations
General Considerations

Amputation is a broad term that has been used to cover the entire range of body-part loss, from the loss of part of a finger to scapulothoracic amputation and from the loss of a toe to a pelvic or even a translumbar amputation. However, it is more precise to reserve the term amputation for the process of removing a limb by dividing through one or more of the bones and to use the term disarticulation for the process of removing a limb by dividing between joint surfaces. Each particular site throughout the upper or lower limbs has unique anatomy involving bone shape, nerves, musculature, and blood vessels, as well as available muscles and skin and soft-tissue envelope available for padding, protection, and reconstruction. When deciding where and how to amputate, the surgeon should have an intimate understanding of the anatomy of the different sites and the various attributes and characteristics that affect healing and prosthetic rehabilitation.

Limb Salvage Versus Amputation

The decision between limb salvage and amputation depends on different considerations for the upper and lower limbs.[4] For example, the upper limbs are not weight bearing and can function with minimal sensation. A salvaged upper limb, even with only minimal assistive function, is often better than the upper limb prostheses available today. In contrast, weight bearing is an essential function of the lower limb, so a salvaged lower limb must provide durability and protective sensation sufficient to hold up to the demanding forces of walking and weight bearing if it is to function as well as or better than a prosthesis. When salvage is not possible and amputation is the best course of action, the patient and the rehabilitation team should be aware of these differences between upper and lower limbs.

Levels of Amputation

Amputation levels developed through tradition, as surgeons passed down knowledge and lessons learned about specific techniques. The best techniques provided the fastest healing, as well as a residual limb that was well padded and could best retain its physiology. Specific amputation levels were determined by how well they accommodated prosthetic fitting.

Controversies still exist concerning the most appropriate level of amputation. As would be expected, not all surgeons agree on the best course of action in specific cases. In instances of lower limb injury, an ankle disarticulation and a knee disarticulation both have advantages and disadvantages. This makes selecting between these levels controversial, not because the techniques are questionable—most surgeons agree that the techniques are practicable—but because success rates and ease of prosthetic fitting remain disputed. In the past decades, improvements in design and engineering of prosthetic devices have made these amputation levels much more successful. Today, even conservative surgeons are apt to consider ankle and knee disarticulations to be viable surgical procedures.

In each case, the surgeon faces a vast number of decisions and has considerable latitude to exercise personal judgment. All options must be weighed thoughtfully and thoroughly. The initial and most basic decision is the choice between amputation and salvage. Once amputation has been decided upon, the surgeon must determine the most distal level of amputation still compatible with wound healing and subsequent satisfactory prosthetic fitting. Level selection requires detailed clinical evaluation combined with appropriate laboratory and radiographic studies. Except in special circumstances, as discussed in chapters on each particular level, surgeons should select the most distal amputation level that successfully removes diseased or damaged tissue. Preserving functional residual limb length is a basic principle of modern amputation surgery. Nevertheless, the surgeon must balance skeletal length and soft-tissue reconstruction to provide a well-healed, nontender, physiologic residual limb.

In determining amputation level, the goal is to create the best environment for the rapid return of mobility and function, and this ideal environment will be different for each patient. For example, the patient's nutritional status will play a role in wound healing. For patients with diabetes mellitus, controlling blood glucose levels is essential. In all cases, minimizing edema, optimizing vascular inflow, and eliminating bacteremia through appropriate use of antibiotics are essential to determining amputation level. All surgical procedures must be coordinated with rehabilitation plans to minimize deconditioning. Amputee management requires a multidisciplinary approach to address these issues. Medical, surgical, social, rehabilitative, prosthetic, and economic factors all play an important role in each case. Planning for optimum function in amputation surgery requires continual evaluation and reevaluation of preoperative, surgical, and short- and long-term postoperative goals.

Skin

In amputation, the general principles of plastic and reconstructive surgery apply to incision location and scar placement. A painless, pliable, and nonadherent scar is a primary goal in most surgeries, but in amputation, the prosthetic interface and socket design may make the location of the scar even more important. When uncomplicated primary healing occurs and the resulting scars are nontender, pliable, mobile, and durable, then scar location does not really matter. When healing is less than ideal, however, and the scars become adherent, tender, thin, nondurable, thick, or prominent, then location matters a great deal. The wise surgeon plans scar placement to minimize potential future complications in the event of less-than-perfect healing.

With lower limb amputations, the amputation site functions as the patient's foot and, therefore, requires reconstructive design to provide a durable interface with the socket for walking and the transfer of body weight. With upper limb amputations, the amputation site becomes, in essence, the patient's hand. The skin should therefore be managed as carefully as it would be in hand surgery to ensure the most successful outcome.

Fasciocutaneous Flaps

Fasciocutaneous flaps should be made as broad based as possible to maximize perfusion and avoid compromising blood supply.[15] The skin closure must be without tension but also without redundancy. Particularly in the dysvascular limb, care must be taken to avoid separating the skin from the underlying subcutaneous tissue and fascia. Care should be taken not to place scars over a bony prominence or the subcutaneous bone. The more skin surface that is available for contact with the prosthetic socket, the less pressure will be applied to each unit area of skin surface. A cylindrically shaped residual limb with muscular padding presents fewer skin problems than a bony, atrophic, tapered residual limb.

Skin Grafts

Along with fasciocutaneous flaps and free-flap techniques, skin grafts can be a viable option. Split-thickness skin grafts can withstand forces applied by a prosthesis, but grafts will be most successful when they do not adhere to bone. Application of the graft over a cushioned, mobile muscle bed is ideal. Without the fine layer of subcutaneous fat to absorb shear, however, grafts are not as durable as normal skin. Fortunately, socket liners made of elastomeric materials have improved prosthetic success for individuals with scar and skin grafts. This is especially helpful for burn survivors because amputations on burned limbs often require skin grafts. The

grafted skin and burn tissue will tolerate more pressure over time if the shear and skin stretch are minimized by careful prosthetic fitting. A gradual introduction to wearing the prosthesis will also help establish tolerance. The amount of time wearing the prosthesis, the amount of force applied, and the activity levels must be carefully controlled and slowly increased. Even a badly burned residual limb with free graft coverage may become accustomed to a prosthetic device over a period of many months, allowing it to provide optimum function and thereby avoiding reamputation at a higher anatomic level.

Long-Term Concerns

Skin problems remain a major concern for amputees throughout their lives. The surgeon needs to be familiar with the many different types of potential short- and long-term skin and wound-healing problems. Postoperative infections, wound dehiscence, and partial skin flap failure occur with unfortunate frequency in the early postoperative phase. Contact dermatitis, skin irritation, reactive hyperemia, callus formation, verrucous hyperplasia, folliculitis, epidermoid cysts, hidradenitis, fungal infections, and chronic breakdown are potential long-term skin ailments. Complicated skin problems often require multidisciplinary approaches involving prosthetists, wound care specialists, dermatologists, and the original surgical team.

Muscle

Muscle makes up the bulk of the soft tissues of the residual limb. A muscular, well-padded, and balanced residual limb is less prone to chronic pain. Maximum retention of functioning muscles is essential to provide the residual limb with effective strength, size, shape, circulation, metabolic exchange, and proprioception. Proper muscle function depends on the anatomic origin and insertion of the muscle. Without fixed resistance against which a muscle can forcefully

contract, progressive weakness and atrophy develop. Distal muscle stabilization is therefore a primary goal of amputation surgery. Whenever possible, the sectioned muscle should be attached and stabilized in order to retain muscle function and improve coverage and distal padding of the bone.

Four types of muscle stabilization can be accomplished surgically, including simple myofascial closure, myoplasty, myodesis, and tenodesis. These have varying degrees of efficacy and efficiency in terms of muscle stabilization and preservation of function.

Myofascial Closure

The first of these techniques, myofascial closure, encases the bone and transected muscle by simply closing the outer fascial envelope over the top of the muscles. Myofascial closure itself does not effectively stabilize muscle because it provides only minimal stabilization for the most superficial muscles and it does not provide adequate distal attachment of the muscle tissue to the bone. Myofascial closure is used primarily when severe ischemia prevents more effective distal muscle fixation.[6-8] Even in most dysvascular and diabetic amputations, however, more effective muscle stabilization is almost always technically possible and should be attempted.

Myoplasty

In most diaphyseal amputations, which includes most transfemoral and transtibial amputations, the muscle bellies themselves are transected, making it more difficult to attach the muscle to the bone than when the thicker distal fascia, aponeuroses, or tendons are still present. In these instances, myoplasty has been employed. In myoplasty, the surgeon brings the muscles over the end of the bone and sews them to opposing muscle groups. Unfortunately, unless these muscles become firmly stabilized by scar tissue, the attachment can work antagonistically as a muscular sling, sliding back and forth over the distal end of the bone. This sliding of muscle over bone creates bursal tissue and can cause severe pain. Such a scenario is easy to detect on physical examination because both the motion and the accompanying crepitance will be palpable over the end of the bone. Because of the frequency of these complications, simple myoplasty by itself is not usually recommended. The surgeon should instead attempt to secure the tissue directly to the distal end of the bone. This is called myodesis and, used with myoplasty, can be a very effective means of muscle stabilization.

Myodesis

In myodesis, the muscle groups themselves are attached directly and securely to the periosteum or the bone. Typically, the deepest layers of muscle are secured directly to the bone and the more superficial layers of muscle are sewn to each other as a myoplasty. The myofascial envelope is then closed over the top of this muscular reconstruction.[4]

Tenodesis

A final muscle stabilization technique is tenodesis. Tenodesis involves the firm distal attachment of the severed tendon to the bone and is the most physiologic and effective way to stabilize muscle. However, it is often not possible anatomically. It is possible only when the muscle belly itself is not transected and the tendon is intact. Tenodesis is most commonly used in disarticulations. It is the primary method used in knee disarticulations, in which the patellar tendon is secured to the origin of the cruciate ligaments on the distal femur. Whenever anatomic circumstances permit, distal attachment of the muscles, tendons, fascia, or aponeuroses directly to the bone should be performed.

Stabilization

To optimize effective muscle activity in the residual limb, the muscle should be stabilized under near-physiologic tension. Correct muscle tension varies in different situations,

and determining the appropriate tension level does not follow a set of hard-and-fast rules. Studied clinical judgment and adherence to the principles of muscle tension provide the best results. Determining correct muscle tension in an amputation is similar to determining the tension of tendon transfers in the hand or foot. In general, most surgeons err on the side of too lax rather than too tight. Excessive or unbalanced tension can cause severe pain. For example, excessive tension can occur in transfemoral amputation if a surgeon advances the quadriceps too far distally, leading to hip flexion contracture.

Nerves

The management of sectioned nerves remains a controversial aspect of amputation surgery. The free end of a divided nerve heals by forming a neuroma. This intertwined mass of scar and nerve tissue can become painful to pressure, stretching, and other types of physical manipulation. Even when the neuroma is completely undisturbed, electrical potentials may arise within the mass, causing negative local and distant sensory and motor phenomena that can be bothersome and painful to the amputee. Numerous techniques have been devised to minimize neuroma formation, but none has proven uniformly successful. Methods include cauterizing the nerve ends using chemicals or heat, burying the nerve in bone, encasing the nerve in impervious material, ligating the nerve, or injecting the nerve with a variety of chemicals. Other methods include sewing the sectioned nerves to other nerves or sewing them back onto themselves, thereby creating a nerve loop, or simply dividing the nerve and allowing it to retract.

Because none of the new methods has demonstrated a lower rate of symptomatic neuromas or phantom pain, the generally accepted procedure is to draw the nerve distally, section it, and allow it to retract away from areas of pressure, scarring, and

pulsating vessels. Nerve ligation is indicated if the nerve is likely to bleed, as is the case with the sciatic nerve. When a nerve is severed in the amputation, the surgeon's goal is to position the nerve ending in a well-cushioned area of soft tissue away from the incision and any scar tissue, where the nerve will not be irritated by traction, pressure from the prosthetic socket, or any other potential sources of contact.

Neuromas that form in very scarred and adherent areas are the most symptomatic. When working in these areas, the surgeon should apply moderate tension to the nerve and section it cleanly, allowing it to retract away from the site of amputation and into the proximal soft tissues. This prevents scarring of the distal end of the nerve to the surgical site, where traction and pressure are more likely. Traction on the nerve at the time of sectioning should not be excessive because too much tension can lead to proximal pain and neuropathy. As with the conservation of muscle tissue in the residual limb, the surgeon's goal is to retain and employ as much useful nerve function in the residual limb as possible. Care should be taken to avoid disturbing the nerve fibers innervating limb structures that are still intact, particularly those innervating the muscles and skin.

The theory that the proximity of nerves and blood vessels can cause symptoms is attracting renewed interest. When a nerve is unintentionally ligated with a pulsing artery, the nerve endings may sense the vessel's cadence and become a source of painful throbbing. In the transtibial amputation, the two nerves most commonly ligated with a vessel are the deep peroneal nerve and the tibial nerve. This happens if the deep peroneal nerve is not separated from the anterior tibial vessels or if the tibial nerve is not separated from the posterior tibial vessels. A revision surgery in which the nerve is separated and divided away from the vessels can relieve the throbbing. Extra caution concerning the nerves should always be exercised in high-level upper limb amputations. Unfortunately, particularly in surgeries involving the brachial plexus, nerves are often inadvertently included in the ligatures with the axillary vessels.

Blood Vessels

Adequate hemostasis and the management of blood vessels and bleeding sites are of utmost importance in amputation surgery. Major arteries and veins should be isolated and ligated securely. Double ligation of large arteries should be standard, especially when the blood supply is normal. Cauterization should be reserved for smaller bleeding points only. The central artery of a large nerve, such as the sciatic nerve, can be a source of troublesome bleeding. In this instance, excessive bleeding can be avoided by ligation with absorbable suture. Bleeding from the sectioned bone end is best controlled by pressure. Occasionally, critical intraosseous vessels will require cauterization or a small amount of bone wax. Bone wax should be used as infrequently as possible because it remains as foreign material within the surgical site and can lead to complications. Fortunately, bone wax is only rarely required.

Adequate blood supply to the distal tissues and to the wound margins facilitates proper healing. For appropriate blood supply, the surgeon should avoid dissecting the subcutaneous tissue, keeping the muscle and the muscle-investing fascia with the skin whenever possible. The surgeon should take care to avoid damaging proximal blood vessels. The skin, or preferably fasciocutaneous flaps, even when broad based, should be developed with careful attention to blood supply. Preservation of blood supply is especially important in patients with vascular disease and diabetes mellitus. Careful attention to hemostasis and managing the vascular supply to the flaps can make the difference between healing and failure,

particularly when blood supply is marginal.

Amputation sites are usually closed over suction drainage because sectioned muscle and bone can often result in a surgical site that is not perfectly dry. The surgeon should make every effort to avoid a postoperative hematoma; however, in the event one does form, it must be identified early and treated quickly. A postoperative hematoma can predispose the patient to infection, delayed wound healing, or complete failure. Revision surgery and higher level amputation have been required because of hematomas. If a large postoperative hematoma is identified, therefore, the patient should be returned to the operating room for evacuation, irrigation, débridement, and hemostasis. Complete hemostasis should be achieved before the patient leaves the operating room.

Bone Tissue

The forces passing between prosthesis, residual limb, and the rest of the body are in large part transmitted through the retained bone in the residual limb. Therefore, the surgeon must keep this in mind when choosing the amputation level and shaping the bone. Diaphyseal bone should be sectioned at the length consistent with optimal reconstructive soft-tissue closure. Careful management of the severed bone, including careful contouring and rounding of the sharp cortical bone edges and irregularities, is essential to pain-free healing. Bone transection and shaping should take into account the prosthetic devices available for that particular level of amputation. Familiarity with the most frequent bone-related problems at the planned amputation level will help the surgeon avoid future problems. For example, in transtibial amputations, anterior cortical beveling to remove the distal corner of the tibia is one method of proactive management. Removing the distal plantar corner of the calcaneus in a hindfoot

amputation can also help prevent future complications.

Proper attention to bone preparation eliminates potential areas of high pressure at the bone-socket interface. In the normal anatomy, there are no sharp, angular surfaces in the palm of the hand or the sole of the foot, and retained distal bone in the residual limb, which will function as a hand or foot, should come as close to this natural state as possible. Occasionally in disarticulations, it is wise to narrow the distal metaphyseal flare of the bone to prevent an overly bulbous and enlarged distal end. For example, in the Syme ankle disarticulation, surgical contouring of the distal tibia and fibula are mandatory because a bulbous and noncontoured distal end will cause difficulties in prosthetic fitting. In general, however, bone resection is kept to a minimum in most disarticulations.

Protocol for the successful management of the periosteum is less concretely defined. In instances of diaphyseal amputation in children, new bone tends to form with periosteal and endosteal bone overgrowth at the end of the amputation. Capping the end of a diaphyseal amputation with osteochondral bone surface (often obtained from the amputation specimen) has been shown to minimize bony overgrowth. These techniques are addressed in the pediatric chapters.

In its natural state, diaphyseal bone has an outer covering, or cortex. Thus, it would seem logical to seal the end of the bone after amputation, and techniques have been refined for forming an osteoperiosteal bone cap over the end of diaphyseal bone. Even without a surgical osteoperiosteal flap, however, the end of the bone naturally heals by formation of callus and fibrous tissue. When a periosteal cuff is available, it may be sutured over the end of the bone, but excessive use of periosteal strips can cause problems. As occasionally seen in traumatic amputations or when the periosteum is circumferentially peeled off the bone before sectioning, the residual periosteal strips can slowly form irregular bone spurs, which can cause painful pressure points. The surgeon should be aware of this potential problem and attempt to minimize its occurrence.

Wound Closure

The standard protocols for skin closure in any other surgery also apply to closing the wound after an amputation. Dead space should be eliminated and drain systems used when necessary. To close the wound, opposing tissue layers are sewn under physiologic tension, and care must be taken to ensure the final closure is neither too tight nor too loose. As with all surgery, careful judgment is necessary in the selection of suture material and closure technique, and the surgeon must be aware of the options and differences between various techniques. Many patients have only marginal blood supply, and the utmost surgical care and technique is required in such cases to maximize the wound healing potential.

Staged Amputations

If primary closure of the wound is not advisable, amputation should be carried out in two or more stages. An initial amputation may be done to provide adequate drainage of infection. This is the recommended course for a preliminary open ankle disarticulation involving sepsis with a severely infected, nonsalvageable diabetic foot. Patients presenting with such a scenario are frequently febrile and bacteremic. The initial open amputation helps to control the infection, eliminate the bacteremia, and provide a safer wound environment for a definitive amputation at a later date. Leaving the bone long and avoiding transecting the muscle bellies will minimize the postoperative swelling and edema that often complicate middiaphyseal open amputations. When left long, the bone can act as an internal splint, protecting the remaining soft tissue. This will fa-

cilitate the later definitive amputation.

Often a contaminated, open amputation is the result of the original traumatic injury. Contaminated amputations can be treated in a similar fashion to other open amputations. As always, the first consideration in performing the amputation is how it will eventually be shaped and closed. Often in trauma cases, there is an intermediate zone of injured tissue that usually needs time to either recover or demarcate, and multiple secondary surgeries may be required before it becomes evident whether the involved tissue is viable or must be removed.

Open amputations are not guillotine amputations. They should follow the same surgical principles as other amputations, with the same care taken to allow for a healthy, functional residual limb. In past times of war, guillotine amputation was used to avoid infection. In a guillotine amputation, all the different tissues are transected at the same level, much as a guillotine blade would sever a limb. No flaps are fashioned, no muscle for myodesis is retained, and no fasciocutaneous closure is planned. The postoperative plan following guillotine amputation is not to perform a secondary closure, but instead to apply skin traction, change the dressing daily, and administer prolonged wound care. Distal healing with skin traction results in fragile, thin distal coverage with poor durability. Revision is usually required many months later. The guillotine technique is no longer recommended. In its War Surgery Extremity Course, the US Army now teaches the concepts and techniques of open, length-preserving amputation. Even in instances of grave trauma, open amputation with a thoughtful plan for closure is the best option.

Revision Amputation

The general principles of primary amputation also apply to revision amputation. Revision is necessary if the primary amputation fails to heal or if

the residual limb is unsatisfactory for prosthetic fitting. Revision may also be necessary if the residual limb does not serve the patient's functional requirements. Thanks to advances in prosthetic devices and interfaces, limbs that would have been difficult to fit with prostheses in the past can now be accommodated reasonably well. Unfortunately, many amputations are still poorly done, leading to complications during the healing process or requiring revision surgery later. Better education of surgeons, more research, and additional refinement of surgical technique are the keys to avoiding unnecessary revision amputations.

Revision amputation for pain is a viable option only when the cause of the pain can be clearly identified. Pain problems amenable to surgical treatment include redundant tissue, infolded skin, painful scars, bone prominence, bone spurs, heterotopic ossification, failure of myodesis, distinct and identifiable symptomatic neuromas, and some chronic skin conditions, such as epidermoid cysts and chronic skin breakdown or ulceration. Surgery specifically to treat phantom pain or pain without clear pathologic cause has not been successful.

When revising an amputation, the surgeon manages each tissue type with the same goals as primary amputation but must manage new challenges. In revision cases, the muscles may be scarred and atrophic and muscle stabilization, while technically possible, tends to be less effective with each successive operation. Nonetheless, muscle stabilization should always be considered an essential goal of secondary reconstruction. Whatever muscle stabilization can be achieved is better than none at all.

Postoperative Management

Most surgical procedures are considered complete when the wound is healed. This is not the case in amputation surgeries. Every amputee should be considered for functional restoration with an appropriate limb substitute or prosthesis, and until rehabilitation has been completed, the process remains unfinished. Although some amputees may choose not to use a prosthesis, in most cases, an empty sleeve or trouser leg is an arresting testimony to incomplete postoperative management. Because the residual limb must interface with and control the prosthetic device, surgical responsibility ends only when maximum functional restoration has been achieved. The surgeon must always remember the ultimate goal: to replace the limb and restore independence.

The primary goals of postoperative amputation management include prompt, uncomplicated wound healing, control of edema, control of postoperative pain, prevention of joint contractures, and rapid rehabilitation to optimum levels of activity. During the first year of prosthetic fitting, the residual limb changes shape and volume, muscles readapt, and the limb "matures." Time and maturation are necessary to avoid a mismatch between the shape of the residual limb and the prosthetic socket.

Postoperative protocols can be designed to actively rehabilitate individuals and manage the dramatic changes in volume and shape that inevitably occur. Without patience and careful planning, a definitive prosthesis may be fabricated too early, only to become incompatible with the residual limb when it changes shape. The patient is left with a fancy, expensive prosthesis that is useless, and often must wait to obtain funding for a new prosthesis. This is followed by another lengthy process of socket fabrication, assembly, and alignment. It is far wiser to use progressive protocols that allow frequent modification, adjustment, and replacement of check sockets or other temporary devices. These protocols allow for the inevitable volume changes without interrupting rehabilitation until the definitive fitting can be made. Fitting is a

gradual process that cannot be rushed while the shape and volume of the limb are still changing.

Soft Dressings

Compressive wound dressings have long been recognized as essential for controlling swelling, minimizing postoperative pain, and promoting stable limb volume. Even when nurses, therapists, and other health care providers are carefully trained in the protocol and techniques of residual limb wrapping and bandaging, these techniques are not always problem free. Soft dressings are sterile and compressible and cover the wound beneath a layer of elastic bandages. The bandages support the amputation site under compressive pressure, but care must be taken to ensure they are not so tight as to cause proximal constriction, or a tourniquet effect. Careful judgment, technical skill, and vigilance are required. Although unquestionably beneficial to the healing process, elastic bandages need frequent changing and require close monitoring to maintain the correct amount of pressure.

The advantages of soft dressing management include the apparent ease of application and, because they provide easier access to the wound, the surgeon can inspect the wound site frequently as it heals. Complications can arise, however, from poor wrapping of the residual limb, and it is not uncommon for the patient to develop joint contractures. When used exclusively, soft dressings can make muscle conditioning and pain control more difficult. Even though some surgeons consider simple soft dressings outdated in comparison with the semirigid and rigid postoperative prosthetic techniques available, soft dressings are still preferred by many surgeons.

Rigid Dressings

For many years, both open and closed amputations have been treated with early application of rigid dressings. This technique was first described immediately after World War I, and these

first experiences were documented in comprehensive writings charting both clean and infected lower limb amputation procedures. Wilson[9] first described his experiences with early weight bearing and the treatment of amputations of the lower limbs in 1922. He applied the first simple functional prosthetic units to the rigid dressings and allowed his patients to ambulate with some degree of weight bearing on the healing amputated limb. Wilson's methods received little attention until surgeons in France and Poland resurrected his work after World War II, when thousands of soldiers were left with unhealed or poorly healed amputations. In response to this increase in patient population, Berlemont in France, Weiss in Poland, and later Burgess in the United States revived medical interest in the use of rigid dressings and the refining of early postoperative prosthetic techniques.[10-12]

Injured tissues heal best and are less painful when they are supported and placed at rest. When the injured limb or amputation site is immobilized and the appropriate local pressure and elevation protocols are applied, the inflammatory response and edema associated with early healing are minimized. Immobilization, application of gentle distal pressure, and infrequent dressing changes are three tenets of good postoperative care. It is essential that each new generation of surgeons be schooled on the importance of these tenets. The surgeon's curiosity can prompt overly frequent dressing changes and unnecessary wound inspection, generally doing more harm than good.

Rigid dressings can be fabricated from a variety of materials, including conventional plaster of Paris, elastic plaster of Paris, fiberglass cast material, thermoplastic materials, or other splinting materials. The dressing is applied at the end of surgery and is typically changed at intervals of 5 to 14 days. Proper rigid cast protocol requires that a therapeutic degree of terminal pressure and a sterile, dry wound surface be maintained with no restrictions to hinder circulation. No proximal constriction should be applied to the dressing, and the dressing must be adequately suspended to maintain distal pressure. Placing a compressible material, such as closed-cell foam or distal end pads, at the site of surgery helps maintain distal pressure. Suspension is managed initially by molding the cast as it sets and is later reinforced by devices such as waist belts or shoulder harnesses. Careful attention to suspension will minimize the likelihood of the cast "falling away," or slipping down and away from the end of the residual limb. When a cast falls away, terminal edema can develop, often with dire results. At this point in the healing process, patients should try straight-leg raises and towel-pull exercises to provide intermittent pressure and control edema.

The primary objection to rigid dressings as a postoperative form of management is that the dressing prohibits frequent inspection of the surgical site. In most cases this is advantageous, however, because a surgical site heals best when it is properly supported and is undisturbed and uncontaminated, which a rigid dressing accomplishes. Unusual pain, temperature elevation, leukocytosis, or other evidence of complications, however, does require cast removal and wound inspection, which are indeed somewhat more difficult with a rigid dressing.

Some surgeons are daunted by the rigid dressing application process, but although application does require some skill, it requires no more skill than the proper application of soft dressings and supportive wraps. Compared with soft dressings, rigid dressings have the advantages of improved patient comfort and easier mobility as well as an improved wound healing environment. Regardless of dressing choice, surgeons must have a firm grasp of modern postoperative amputation management and the proper application of postoperative dressings.

The Immediate Postoperative Prosthesis

The immediate postoperative prosthetic device can serve as a socket and temporary prosthetic limb in both upper and lower limb amputations. There are tremendous physical and psychological rehabilitative advantages to applying a prosthesis immediately. It minimizes the potentially psychologically traumatic period when the limb is absent because some degree of functional restoration can begin immediately. The patient's general physical and mental state benefit from early physical activities. Comparative studies show that, in cases in which postoperative prostheses are employed immediately, patients have less pain and mobilize faster. The overall amputee rehabilitation period, including hospitalization and the time allotted for limb maturation, is shorter with immediate-fit systems. The positive effects of the encouragement and enthusiasm of the amputation team during this period are very important, as is the support of family and friends. Positive voices and encouragement are essential in speeding the patient's return to regular activity levels.

Although some of the benefits of the immediate-fit systems have not been statistically documented, positive experiences reported worldwide support many of the assertions made by its advocates.[12,13] Areas of disagreement center on the possibly injurious effects of early function, particularly weight bearing and its effect on wound healing. Some surgeons feel that early application of a prosthesis limits access to the surgical site, thereby preventing inspection and the ability to identify infections early. The major concern associated with immediate fitting is potential tissue damage and wound breakdown when excessive stresses are applied to the amputation site early in the healing process. In general, the application of some distal intermediate pressure reduces edema and, in many circumstances, facilitates early healing. Tissue dam-

age can occur, but experience has shown that if early weight bearing is individualized according to the patient's skill, understanding, and ability to comply, trouble can be avoided. As always, the surgeon must take into account the particular patient, the wound, and the circumstances of the healing environment.

Finally, in addition to immediate postoperative prosthetic devices fit by traditional casting techniques, prefabricated and custom-fabricated devices for immediate fittings are also available. The manufacturers of these devices emphasize that rehabilitation and the return of function is the primary goal of treatment.

The First Year of Amputee Care

It is essential that the surgeon be familiar with the course of amputee care and the elaborate nature of the prosthetic fitting process.[14,15] The surgeon must understand that the first postoperative year is very different from the later years. The amputee's needs regarding components and prosthetic technology can change radically after the limb is mature and the activity level has increased. For example, traumatic amputees are typically younger patients with more muscle mass than commonly seen in the dysvascular and diabetic amputee group. They often experience more swelling and more dramatic volume changes in the residual limb. Because the volume of the residual limb is changing dramatically, this can make the first year of socket fitting particularly difficult.

It is the surgeon's job to help supervise prosthetic care. When a leg is swollen and not fully mature, even if the patient and the prosthetist are eager to move ahead, the surgeon must resist the urge to prescribe a definitive prosthesis. This intermediate period is essential to the healing process, and acting impatiently will only cause later disappointment. One patient had five definitive sockets made during the first year after amputation.

Because of these successive failures, the insurance provider refused to fund further prosthetic care just when the patient needed it most, and the patient was ultimately left with a prosthesis that did not fit and could not be used. This is far from the appropriate standard of prosthetic care, and scenarios like this should be avoided. Similarly, it is a grave disappointment when a patient has limited insurance coverage for prosthetic care and the funds are exhausted too early. Some patients are left with a prosthetic device that looks great and has technologically advanced components but no longer fits. Patience and financial caution will avoid this predicament.

Some centers have successfully used reinforced, multiple check-socket prostheses. The patient walks on each temporary socket for 2 to 8 weeks. Ambulatory activity over several months in a check socket or temporary socket can help relieve edema. Expanded polyethylene foam liners are also an excellent option for the first socket fitting. Instead of fabricating a brand new socket, the liner can be padded in appropriate locations. These pads compensate for changes in volume in the appropriate location, thereby saving both time and money.

Typically, when the residual limb in a recent traumatic transtibial amputee loses volume, redness and pain develop at the end. The first step to remedy pain is to increase the ply and number of socks to modify fit. The second step is to pad the anteromedial and the anterolateral tibial flare regions of the socket or the liner. These regions support the tibia and push the distal tibia up and away from the front of the socket, thus protecting the distal end of the tibia. Skillful padding can maintain a successful fit during periods of volume change with fewer new socket fabrications. When volume decreases more substantially, the posterior region of the socket can be padded or the tibial regions can be padded a second time. It is not uncommon to pad the liner up to four times before fabricating a new

socket. Padding techniques can save time, keep the course of rehabilitation smooth and continuous, and delay the hassle of reauthorizing a new prosthetic limb until absolutely necessary.

The elastomeric liners recently introduced on the prosthetic market have gained in popularity. Soft and pliable, these liners have immediate tactile appeal to the amputee, but they can cause skin reactions in some patients and are not universally tolerated. Complications reported include skin irritation, discomfort from constriction, and distal traction edema. One randomized study revealed that patients might actually ambulate less in the elastomeric locking liner systems than they do in traditional systems.[16] Although many protocols have been advanced for the use of elastomeric liners and total-contact socket shapes early in the postoperative period, these techniques can sometimes be more difficult to adjust and modify than other systems. No scientific studies to date have fully assessed the benefits and limitations of these protocols. I do not typically use elastomeric liners during the first year of care because the changes in residual limb volume may be too dramatic to make fittings routinely successful. Elastomeric liners can be appropriate for select cases in which very fragile soft tissue or scarring is involved or if traditional systems have failed. In these instances, an expandable polyethylene foam liner can be fabricated to fit over the locking liner to provide padding and adjust to volume changes.

Transition between prosthetic systems can be difficult, and the anticipated benefits are not always realized. Many surgeons or rehabilitation teams unfortunately transition their patients into new socket shapes or new suspension systems after 12 to 18 months without testing the proposed changes. Again, ambulatory check-socket protocols can allow the patient 2 to 8 weeks to decide if the change is indeed beneficial. This trial period keeps the patient from getting "stuck"

with a new system that sounds appealing at first but is not successful for him or her in practice.

Choice of Prosthetic Components

Many young traumatic amputees are adamant about obtaining state-of-the-art prosthetic components. The prosthesis becomes a part of their body, and their desire for the "finest" is indeed understandable. However, many components may not be optimal for the first year of amputee care. Some of the highest-end foot and ankle components may be too stiff for the first 6 to 12 months of ambulation. Less technologically advanced components may make adapting to the prosthetic device easier.

Ideally, a new prosthetic prescription should be generated only after the amputee has established a steady symmetric gait, can engage in impact activities, and is ready to advance to a higher level of activity. The amputee should be able to maneuver barriers, manage stairs, and negotiate inclines and ramps. Typically, this does not happen until 9 to 18 months after surgery. Only at this point is a new, more technologically advanced prosthesis useful. The old prosthesis can often be refurbished to become a spare prosthesis or to be used with water activities.

Conclusions

It is essential that the thoughtful surgeon understand the entire course of the amputation process, from the preoperative stage to the final selection of the perfect prosthesis. As devastating as it is for the patient, amputation will always be a difficult and a complex process for the surgeon as well. It asks the surgeon to successfully balance existing surgical technique and knowledge, intimate familiarity with the entire course of the amputee care, and human understanding of each unique patient. The surgeon capable of making an amputation successful can indeed help make the patient whole.

Acknowledgment

I owe much to the wisdom, writings, and personal mentorship of Dr. Ernest M. Burgess (1911-2000). Much of this material was updated from Burgess EM: General principles or amputation surgery, in *Atlas of Limb Prosthetics: Surgical and Prosthetic Principles*, St. Louis, MO, CV Mosby, 1981, pp 14-18.

References

1. Willingham L: *A New Vision for Limb Loss.* Seattle, WA, Prosthetics Research Study, 2002.

2. Burgess EM: General principles of amputation surgery, in *Atlas of Limb Prosthetics: Surgical and Prosthetic Principles.* St. Louis, MO, CV Mosby, 1981, pp 14-18.

3. Legro MW, Reiber GE, del Aguila M, et al: Issues of importance reported by persons with lower extremity amputations and prostheses. *J Rehabil Res Dev* 1999;36:155-163.

4. Smith DG, Fergason JR: Transtibial amputations. *Clin Orthop* 1999;361: 108-115.

5. Humzah MD, Gilbert PM: Fasciocutaneous blood supply in below-knee amputations. *J Bone Joint Surg Br* 1997; 79:441-443.

6. Burgess EM, Romano RL, Zettl JH, Schrock RD Jr: Amputations of the leg for peripheral vascular insufficiency. *J Bone Joint Surg Am* 1971;53:874-890.

7. Pedersen HE: Treatment of ischemic gangrene and infection in the foot. *Clin Orthop* 1960;16:199-202.

8. Pedersen HE: The problem of the geriatric amputee. *Artif Limbs* 1968; 12(suppl 2):1-3.

9. Wilson PD: Early weight-bearing in the treatment of amputations of the lower limbs. *J Bone Joint Surg* 1922;4: 224-247.

10. Berlemont M: Ten years of experience with immediate application of prosthetic devices to amputations of the lower extremity on the operating table. *Prosthet Orthot Int* 1969;3.

11. Burgess EM, Romano RL, Zettl JH (eds): *The Management of Lower-Extremity Amputations: Surgery, Immediate Postsurgical Prosthetic Fitting, Patient Care.* Washington, DC, Prosthetic and Sensory Aids Service, 1969.

12. Burgess EM, Romano RL: The management of lower extremity amputees using immediate postsurgical prostheses. *Clin Orthop* 1968;57:137-146.

13. Mooney V, Harvey JP, McBride E, Snelson R: Comparison of postoperative stump management: Plaster vs soft dressings. *J Bone Joint Surg Am* 1971;53:241-249.

14. Fergason JR, Smith DG: Socket considerations for the patient with a transtibial amputation. *Clin Orthop* 1999; 361:76-84.

15. Smith DG: Amputations, in Skinner H (ed): *Current Diagnosis and Treatment in Orthopedics*, ed 2. New York, NY, Lange Medical Books/McGraw Hill, 1999, pp 577-601.

16. Coleman K, Boone D, Smith DG, Laing L, Mathews D, Czerneicki J: Crossover trial comparing alpha liner with pelite liner for trans-tibial prostheses using ambulatory activity and questionnaire responses, in *Transactions of the Tenth World Congress of the International Society for Prosthetics and Orthotics, July 4, 2001*, Glasgow, Scotland, International Society for Prosthetics and Orthotics, 2001, p W05.

Chapter 3

Vascular Disease: Limb Salvage Versus Amputation

Peter T. McCollum, MCh, FRCSI, FRCSEd
Zahid Raza, MD, FRCSEd, FRCS

Introduction

The most common cause of major lower limb amputation in developed countries is peripheral vascular disease (PVD), which is often associated with diabetes mellitus. Indeed, more than 90% of limb amputations are associated with PVD. Other causes of lower limb amputations include trauma, tumor, or severe infection. The predominant cause of PVD is atherosclerosis, and its most common manifestation is intermittent claudication (IC) caused by inadequate arterial blood supply to the legs. This chapter explores the issues relating to the choice between amputation and reconstructive surgery for the threatened limb in patients with end-stage PVD.

The estimated prevalence of PVD is 3% to 6% of the Western population; this increases to 8% in persons older than 55 years.[1,2] IC usually runs a benign course, with less than 6% of patients requiring intervention 1 year after diagnosis.[3] Persons with IC have the same life expectancy as a healthy person 10 years older.[4] However, approximately 30% of patients will have died 5 years after onset of IC, and the mortality rate increases to 70% by 10 years after onset. Despite this benign course, many patients require hospitalization and surgery, which has a substantial impact on health care resources.[3] Symptoms worsen with disease progression, and IC can severely limit physical and social activity.

In the United Kingdom, 5,000 amputees are referred for prosthetic assessment each year. There are no data regarding the number of patients who undergo amputation in the United Kingdom without being referred for a prosthesis. However, based on the estimated incidence of critical limb ischemia (CLI) in the general population of 500 patients per million, more than 25,000 cases of CLI occur annually in the United Kingdom, and up to 25% of patients (6,250) with CLI will require a major amputation. This implies that each year, more than 1,000 patients who undergo amputation are not referred for prosthetic assessment.[5]

Patients with IC commonly experience pain in the thigh and calf muscles when walking or exercising. Leg pain is usually relieved by rest, but pain that persists while the patient is at rest is generally indicative of severe vascular disease. Severe PVD could result in gangrene and the need for limb amputation. Patients with both PVD and diabetes mellitus have the greatest risk for limb loss. The prognosis is less favorable if the leg is critically ischemic.[6] The number of patients with limb-threatening ischemia is steadily increasing as a result of the increasing mean age of the general population and the growing number of patients with diabetes mellitus. Pa-

TABLE 1 The Fontaine Classification of PVD

Stage	Characteristics
I	Atherosclerosis without clinical symptoms
II	Claudication
	• Claudication at > 200 m No rest pain
	• Claudication at < 200 m No rest pain
III	Rest pain
	• Ankle pressure > 50 mm Hg (patients without diabetes mellitus)
	Toe pressure < 30 mm Hg (patients with diabetes mellitus)
	• Ankle pressure < 50 mm Hg (patients without diabetes mellitus)
	Toe pressure < 30 mm Hg (patients with diabetes mellitus)
IV	Tissue loss
	• Ulceration/gangrene with local inflammation
	• Ulceration/gangrene with widespread inflammation

TABLE 2 Indications for Major Limb Amputation in PVD

Incapacitating rest pain
Ulceration or gangrene that is extending and results in disability
Life-threatening sepsis
Failed limb salvage operation (nonfunctioning graft/angioplasty)
Nonhealing minor amputation

tients with limb-threatening ischemia are often the elderly, who lack social support and are prone to neglect their health care needs.

Classification of PVD

The first widely used classification of PVD was developed by Fontaine[7] and provides a good, albeit simplistic, classification based on the severity of symptoms. This classification was revised to provide subcategories for patients with and without diabetes mellitus (Table 1). The classification of Fontaine is not without problems. Its simplicity suggests that each patient fits neatly into a specific category. The fact that a change in Fontaine classification does not necessarily occur only during medical intervention compounds this problem. Most studies of medical treatment of patients with PVD equate improvement in symptoms, such as healed ischemic ulcer or increased claudication distance, with success of the treatment; therefore, the use of the Fontaine classification can affect the interpretation of clinical trials.

Fontaine stage III or stage IV PVD is considered end-stage PVD. Symptoms include leg pain at rest as a result of CLI. A small but significant proportion of patients with advanced CLI has stable symptoms or will even improve without intervention.[8] The classification of end-stage PVD, however, is complicated by the inclusion of diabetic patients who have a different disease process and prognosis.[9] For this reason, the European consensus document uses a separate category for diabetic patients with CLI.[10] Another category known as subcritical limb ischemia includes patients who have rest pain but a more favorable prognosis with regard to limb loss.[11] Another group includes patients suffering from traumatic injury that causes acute limb ischemia. If blood flow is insufficient to keep the limb perfused, these patients are at risk of limb loss without immediate intervention. Limb reperfusion injury and the systemic effects of toxic metabolites are more pronounced in the absence of a background of PVD. Patients with otherwise normal vasculature have the greatest risks associated with limb reperfusion injury because they will have little if any collateral circulation, unlike patients with previous underlying PVD, who effectively undergo a process of ischemic preconditioning.

General Considerations

All patients who are candidates for amputation should be assessed by a vascular surgeon.[12,13] New techniques and a more aggressive approach to limb salvage provide the potential for limb salvage in many patients who are potential candidates for amputation. For patients who require amputation, advances in prosthetics, the establishment of centers that specialize in treatment of amputees, and improved methods of rehabilitation offer a better chance for the functional use of a prosthesis, rather than only using a wheelchair.[14-16] Factors such as younger age at amputation, absence of significant vascular disease in the contralateral limb, and prompt rehabilitation following amputation are associated with a better prognosis for successful ambulation and overall rehabilitation.[17]

Limb salvage is neither feasible nor desirable for a minority of patients who are usually elderly, have pain while at rest, and are ill with sepsis (Table 2). Patients in such circumstances often have very advanced PVD and can be described as having total body failure. Thus their immediate and short-term prognosis is extremely guarded.[18,19] If a patient obviously requires a major lower limb amputation, time-consuming and often invasive investigations such as angiography are not required. A prompt decision to amputate based on clinical assessment and simple pressure measurements will quickly relieve severe ischemic pain and improve sepsis.

In some patients, it may be appropriate to avoid all surgical intervention if the inevitable conclusion is early death. This situation is generally obvious to the attending physician; however, both the patient and the patient's relatives should be involved in making the decision to limit surgical intervention. The pain team and palliative care physicians provide guidance for the optimal management of these patients. Good analgesic support, nursing care, and help with planning a dignified death are essential. In such circumstances, the patient's relatives can be reassured that the care of their loved one involved a planned approach to relieve pain and make the patient comfortable. In addition, the patient is not subjected to mutilating surgery that would not have altered the eventual outcome. Clearly, subjecting patients to a prolonged hospital stay, inappropriate surgery, continuing pain, sepsis, and a miserable death is unacceptable.

Psychological Aspects of Amputation

Health care workers can be so engrossed in the physical well-being of patients that the psychological aspects of amputation are overlooked, but they must remember that the prospect of undergoing an amputation often comes as a deep shock to the patient and the patient's family. The patient should be reassured that the procedure is necessary and that it is a positive step toward rehabilitation back into the community. A patient's reaction to the loss of a limb depends on personality factors and may include a period of grief similar to that following the death of a loved one.

After lower limb amputation, patients often have poor social support and multiple medical problems. These patients are likely to experience social isolation, lethargy, pain, and sleep disturbances.[20] Poor mobility is a feature that exacerbates most of these symptoms.[21] Indeed, patients who eventually face bilateral amputation are unlikely to be ambulatory after the second amputation unless they are mobilized immediately after the first amputation.[22,23] Any amputation for lower limb arterial disease should be performed at the most distal level possible. The rehabilitation process and psychological support should begin before or immediately after amputation.

Setting Realistic Goals

For successful rehabilitation, the health care team must ensure that the patient's overall needs are met so that the patient can enjoy life with maximal independence. The goals set for and by the amputee should be realistic, as unrealistically high expectations will lead to disappointment, negatively affecting the patient's quality of life. The health care staff should have a balanced and realistic approach to patient rehabilitation and be able to determine that the expectations of both the patient and family are not exaggerated.

The long-term prognosis for patients with end-stage PVD is generally poor compared with that of the healthy age-matched population.[4,24] Adequate patient follow-up is essential. In addition, patients and their families should have easy access to re-

habilitation facilities and prosthetic management.

Financial Considerations

Unfortunately, the financial implications of treating patients with end-stage PVD must be addressed. The most cost-effective option for the vascular patient is revascularization rather than primary amputation.[25] However, this situation is complicated by the costs of multiple failed revascularizations and subsequent amputation compared with the costs of primary amputation.

Comparisons of costs of limb salvage and primary amputation are fraught with difficulties. Nonetheless, the median cost of successful revascularization in a patient with criteria favorable for distal bypass is more than $10,000 in Great Britain. The inpatient cost of a primary amputation is $16,000. Repeated failed revascularizations with a subsequent amputation, however, nearly doubles the overall costs of treatment.[26] Patients with preoperative morbidity require prolonged hospital care, which is more expensive than the costs associated with uncomplicated limb revascularization of previously healthy patients with CLI.

Patients should be selected carefully to exclude those unlikely to have a successful reconstruction. Important determinants of a successful distal bypass include the use of an autologous vein, characteristics of inflow vessels, and the number of patent blood vessels in the calf.[27] Selection of patients is likely to subject unfit patients to amputation rather than limb revascularization.

Patients selected for amputation are usually older, in poor medical condition, and regarded as inoperable compared with those selected to undergo reconstructive surgery. Primary amputation may be the treatment of choice in patients who have extensive tissue loss, are elderly with decreased life expectancy, or in whom rehabili-

tation is very unlikely.[28] The costs of a major amputation are significantly greater than those of a successful arterial reconstruction. The costs of an inpatient hospital stay, physiotherapy, and nursing care contribute to the added expenditures. Admission to a nursing home during the rehabilitation phase can also contribute to the overall cost. Provision of a prosthesis, a wheelchair, or other technical equipment and modification of the amputee's home can add to the cost.[25] Overall costs might be reduced if an efficient outpatient rehabilitation program is developed.

Ethical Considerations and Informed Consent

The ethical debate of whether to subject a patient to treatment of end-stage PVD is paramount. The clinician must address the practical aspects of intervention. Should limb salvage be attempted when it is likely to prolong the hospital stay and increase suffering? What is the true benefit of repeated revascularizations when there is some doubt regarding limb salvage? In most patients, such decisions will be straightforward. In certain patients, however, the clinician must ultimately select the treatment option based on the goal of reducing patient morbidity by limiting the mental and surgical trauma to the patient. Thus, the decision to limit procedures might be appropriate when there is likely to be a diminishing return with successive limb salvage procedures. Subjecting such patients to the repeated trauma of surgery will have devastating consequences on the patient's psyche and long-term prognosis. Also, the strain on the patient's family and caregivers must not be overlooked. Such considerations are of real importance and must be applied to decisions regarding each patient.

Both the patient and his or her family should be fully aware of any anticipated surgical intervention. The decision should always be in the patient's best interest. All options of intervention and nonintervention must be explained clearly in terms of the potential complications and prognosis. If amputation is ultimately required, the patient should be fully informed that all limb salvage options were explored. Patients should understand that if surgery is not possible or has failed, amputation and fitting of a prosthesis is a logical and natural progression. Discussing the procedures with a positive attitude helps the patient to deal with the amputation.

Management

The decision to perform either a major amputation or major reconstructive surgery should not be based solely on clinical parameters or unduly influenced by past experience. Vascular surgery has developed as a full-fledged specialty in many countries, and enormous strides have been made in specific areas, such as managing the patient with CLI. In such patients, distal arterial bypass surgery performed at specialized vascular centers and using prosthetic material or autologous vein results in satisfactory graft patency and rates of limb salvage.[29] Patency rates vary considerably according to the type of conduit, length of conduit, state of the inflow vessel, and resistance to any outflow vessel. Factors related to both surgical technique and the patient determine the long-term success of a bypass procedure. In general, the patency rate for an infrainguinal vein graft can be up to 80% at 5 years. In contrast, a synthetic graft will function with a patency rate of less than 50% at 5 years.[30] In planning surgical outcome, it must be recognized that patients with gangrene and rest pain often require a prolonged hospital stay as well as subsequent rehabilitation after initial distal revascularization and/or primary or delayed toe amputation.

Nonsurgical Management of Critical Limb Ischemia

The use of drugs to treat intermittent claudication and CLI has generated much interest. The goals of pharmacotherapy for patients with CLI include stabilizing symptoms in the hope of postponing amputation and relieving rest pain by improving local blood flow and/or the development of collateral circulation. A number of drugs have been studied, including anticoagulants,[31] thrombolytics,[32] antiplatelet agents,[33] and other vasoactive agents.[34] The prostacycline analogues are the most promising drugs for the treatment of ischemic rest pain.[35,36] Prolonged intravenous infusions of prostacycline analogues can potentially salvage a small proportion of limbs from amputation,[35] with a resultant increase in walking distance and diminished rest pain.[36] Most studies of prostacycline analogues did not select patients using the strict criterion of CLI giving rise to rest pain.[10] Although lack of consistent criteria may have complicated the interpretation of study results, treatment is clearly beneficial in some patients. Prostacycline analogue treatment regimens are labor intensive and involve infusions that must be administered over a 6-hour period each day for several days. Gradual increases of dosage are titrated against side effects, which include hypotension, facial flushing, abdominal pain, and headaches. The effects of prostacycline analogues have been evaluated in several worldwide multicenter randomized controlled trials and summarized in a meta-analysis that showed some benefit for patients with CLI with an overall reduction in amputation rate.[37] This benefit is most likely to be seen in patients with subcritical ischemia.

Percutaneous Transluminal Angioplasty

A small number of patients may be suitable for percutaneous transluminal angioplasty (PTA). In PTA, with the use of a guidewire, a balloon catheter is placed across an arterial steno-sis or occlusion and is inflated to fracture the atheromatous plaque and recreate a lumen. Often performed under local anesthesia, PTA has a lower morbidity and mortality than surgical reconstruction. The best results of PTA are obtained in larger blood vessels, such as the iliac and femoral arteries. In general, the long-term patency is lowest for the most distal lesions that require PTA. Combining PTA with stenting of stenotic or previously occluded arteries can also be considered. Like PTA, stents work better in more proximal lesions. Indications to combine stenting with PTA include recurrent stenosis following an angioplasty, prevention of recoil of an artery, high risk of embolization after PTA, and flow limitation caused by dissection of the artery during PTA. PTA with or without stenting generally has an inferior patency rate compared to that of open surgery.[38] Thus, the use of PTA can be reserved for patients with uncomplicated and discrete lesions or those unfit for surgery.

Subintimal Angioplasty

Subintimal angioplasty is being investigated for the recanalization of longer occlusions. Inadvertently entering the subintimal space is not an indication to abandon an angioplasty procedure, despite previously being a common cause of primary recanalization failure. A successful outcome could be salvaged if the subintimal passage dissection was continued until reentry into the true lumen beyond the distal extent of the occlusion[39] (Figure 1). Subintimal angioplasty may offer an alternative to femorodistal grafting in elderly patients with CLI. However, before the role of subintimal angioplasty in clinical practice can be established, acceptable patency and limb salvage rates need to be documented by long-term follow-up studies performed at multiple centers.

Lumbar Sympathectomy

Lumbar sympathectomy has been used in an attempt to increase the blood flow of the lower limb. A

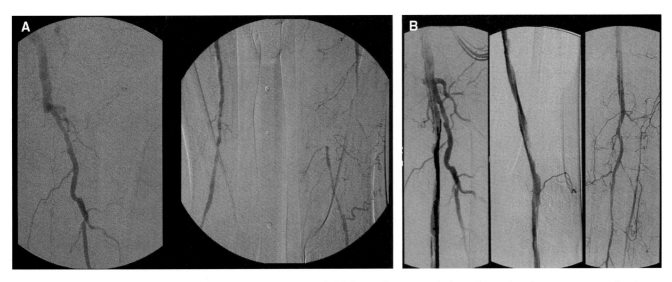

Figure 1 **A,** Angiography of a patient with CLI showing a superficial femoral artery occlusion. The patient has a patent popliteal segment with a two-vessel runoff. **B,** Recanalization of the occluded segment and reentry into the true lumen were successful following subintimal angioplasty. There was a complete resolution of rest pain.

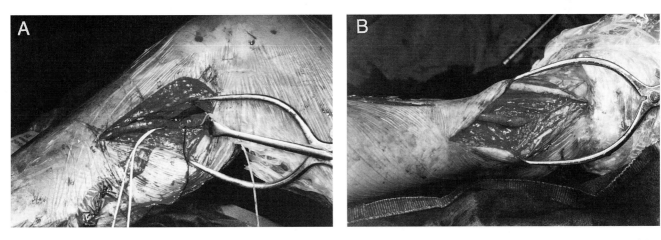

Figure 2 A popliteal-to-distal anterior tibial/dorsalis pedis bypass. This 71-year-old patient with diabetes mellitus had gangrene of the toes and also rest pain. The greater saphenous vein has been harvested from the opposite leg and used to bypass from the below-knee popliteal artery, which was widely patent. The dead toes were subsequently amputated and healed well with complete resolution of the rest pain. **A,** The medial aspect of the upper exposure, with the foot to the left. **B,** The lateral aspect of the lower exposure, with the foot to the right.

warmer foot following sympathectomy is mainly a result of the opening of nonnutritional arteriovenous shunts. In some patients, a chemical or surgical sympathectomy[40] may help relieve ischemic rest pain by a direct effect on pain perception pathways. This effect has also been achieved with the use of epidural spinal cord stimulation involving transmission of low-voltage impulses to the epidural space from a pulse generator. Most of the trials of lumbar

sympathectomy are uncontrolled, but some have shown an improvement in microcirculatory effect. Rates of limb salvage in these studies are similar to those described for the natural history of CLI.[41]

At present, the role of sympathectomy is limited to patients who have end-stage vascular disease with no options for reconstruction. These patients fall into two categories: those without tissue loss, and those who have ulceration, necrosis, and/or ex-

tensive tissue loss. Long-term studies show that patients who have diabetes mellitus with no tissue loss and have an ankle pressure greater than 35 mm Hg gain the most benefit from this technique.[42,43] Overall, only 50% of patients have an initial favorable response to sympathectomy.

Vascular Reconstruction

The optimal reconstructive vascular procedure varies according to the disease process. In selected patients, PTA

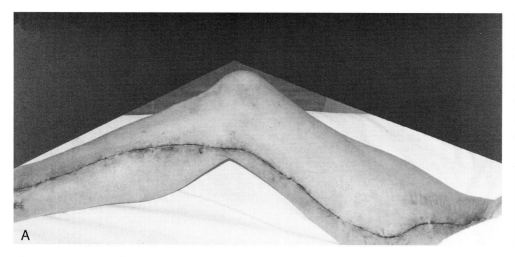
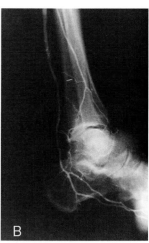

Figure 3 A 78-year-old patient underwent in situ saphenous vein femoroposterior tibial bypass grafting. Rest pain was completely relieved. **A,** The long length of the wounds can be seen in this medial view of the right leg. **B,** The completion angiogram shows the vein graft anastomosed to the posterior tibial artery just above the ankle.

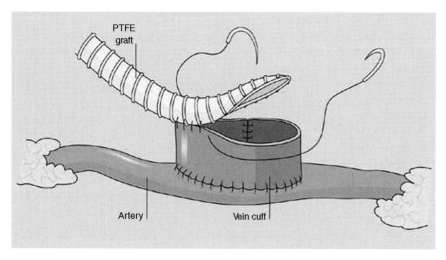

Figure 4 The Miller vein cuff technique for creating an autologous vein cuff at an infrageniculate distal anastomosis of a PTFE bypass. *(Reproduced with permission from Corson JD, Williamson RCN (eds): Surgery. London, England, Mosby International, 2000.)*

is suitable for short (< 6 cm) occlusions. Correction of short lesions by PTA will be sufficient to relieve rest pain in some patients. Vascular reconstructive surgery should be considered for the treatment of longer occlusions that are not likely to be treated effectively with PTA. This type of surgery might involve the aorta (aortofemoral, aortoiliac) or the iliac vessels. Vascular reconstruction can also be an infrainguinal procedure, such as a femoropopliteal or femorodistal bypass. An extra-anatomic bypass, such as a femorofemoral crossover graft or an axillofemoral bypass,

can be considered if there is doubt that the patient is fit for a prolonged major procedure (Figure 2).

The choice of material for a bypass conduit is of paramount importance. In most patients, a long saphenous vein can be harvested and either reversed or used in situ (Figure 3). Vein grafts have superior patency rates compared to any other form of bypass material. In patients who have no usable leg or arm vein, the use of either a prosthetic conduit or human umbilical vein might be considered. The use of human umbilical veins has become problematic because of the possibility

of slow virus infection, biodegradation of grafts, their cumbersome handling characteristics, and expense. For these reasons, human umbilical veins are generally unacceptable to most surgeons. Most surgeons use either Dacron or expanded polytetrafluoroethylene (PTFE) graft material.

The use of vein cuffs at a distal transtibial anastomosis improves primary patency rates[44] (Figure 4) to approximately 52% at 2 years compared with approximately 29% without the use of the cuff. For distal bypass surgery, a vein cuff results in better patency rates compared with prosthetic graft to the crural vessels alone.[45,46] Good salvage rates can be expected from vascular surgeons who regularly perform distal bypass surgery. Unfortunately, because this is a specialized area, consistently good results tend to occur only in dedicated vascular units.

Treatment of Patients With Infection

In patients with PVD, dry gangrene is a result of reduced arterial inflow or stasis in the circulation of the limb or toe. After revascularization, demarcation usually is readily observed without evidence of infection in the area of mummification (Figure 5). Autoamputation of the toe may readily occur without systemic effects, particularly where the limb has been revascularized. Alternatively, simple toe amputation can be performed where the limb has adequate blood supply. In contrast, "wet" gangrene may be a consequence of arterial or venous obstruction and often occurs in diabetic patients. Infection and putrefaction are invariably present during this process. Early revascularization may help to reduce the volume of tissue lost in wet gangrene, although graft infection is a concern in patients with bypass surgery, especially with prosthetic grafts. This risk is even more serious in situations where the patient is positive for methicillin-resistant *Staphylococcus aureus* (MRSA) infection.[47] The decision to amputate or to attempt limb salvage can be extremely difficult, but in the case of life-threatening sepsis, primary amputation is usually indicated.

Treatment of Trauma and Acute Vascular Insufficiency

In managing serious limb insult in which vascular compromise is evident, urgent treatment is critical. Rapid but careful assessment by the primary care team and prioritizing the medical issues are paramount. The patient as a whole should be assessed first, followed by evaluation of the injured limb. The level of priority with respect to the traumatized limb is generally vessels, nerves, bones, and then soft tissues. In reality, surgery is often required to repair the bones before vascular reconstruction can be attempted in an effort to protect the vessel repair from stress.

Any patient with a limb with signs of acute CLI should, if possible, be referred to a specialist in this field. Prompt referral of such patients is vital. Full and careful evaluation by an experienced vascular surgeon followed by appropriate investigation and subsequent treatment will provide the greatest chance of limb salvage. These patients should be treated by a specialist, rather than by the occasional vascular surgeon, although this may be necessary in the absence of immediate specialist resources.

Of patients admitted with CLI, those with an otherwise normal vascular tree are most at risk because there is little if any collateral circulation, unlike patients with previous underlying PVD. Of all those admitted with evidence of acute CLI of the legs, approximately 60% to 70% of patients will leave the hospital with an intact limb.[48] Up to 15% of surviving patients require amputation.[49] Surgical treatment depends on the specific circumstances, but general principles include the use of autologous vein as a bypass material if at all possible and generous decompression fasciotomies to reduce the risk of reperfusion injury. Selection of the level of amputation, when necessary, is defined by the available viable tissue and depends entirely on clinical assessment with the emphasis on preserving limb length.

Intravenous drug abuse is a problem in the medical management of patients with vascular conditions. An increasing number of drug abusers are admitted to the vascular unit following inadvertent intra-arterial injection and microembolization of various substances. These injuries do not seem serious initially, but within a few hours the injected limb can show signs of severe ischemic injury that is sometimes irreversible. In such a situation, opening of the diseased artery will show only intraluminal reaction with massive edema causing significant hemodynamic stenosis in the artery. In general, treatment consists of decompression fasciotomies, intravenous anticoagulant therapy, and prostacycline infusions, followed by observation. Vascular exploration has a very limited role. Major amputation is often the final outcome. This group of patients also has a high rate of infection with hepatitis and HIV.

Prediction of Healing

Predicting whether an amputation is likely to heal is challenging. Accurate prediction of amputation healing

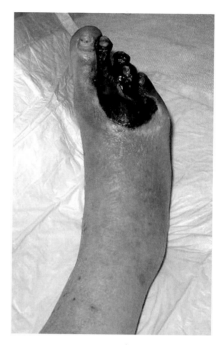

Figure 5 Dry gangrene showing demarcation of part of the toes and forefoot.

would be beneficial as patients could be spared additional revision surgery. Patients who have a single amputation and are predicted to have adequate healing could be ambulatory immediately following surgery, which is likely to improve both their physical and psychological state.[21]

Selection of Level of Amputation

Three levels of amputation are commonly used for patients with PVD: (1) transfemoral, (2) transtibial, and (3) transmetatarsal. Unless prior revascularization has been performed or if the patient has diabetes mellitus, amputation should generally be performed at the transtibial level or higher. If a more distal level is selected, such as a transmetatarsal amputation, and healing occurs, at least one distal vessel must have been suitably patent and therefore amenable to a distal revascularization procedure rather than an amputation.

Obviously, the level of the amputation is important to the patient. Compared with transfemoral or transmetatarsal amputation, a transtibial amputation is likely to allow the patient to be more independent, provide a better cosmetic result, allow lower energy expenditure during ambulation, and be associated with lower mortality and morbidity.[18,19]

McCollum and associates[50] proposed that if clinical decisions are complemented with tests to help determine the optimal level of amputation, a wound healing rate of greater than 90% can be achieved with a ratio of transtibial to transfemoral amputations of 3:1. Malone and associates[51] and Moore and associates[52] achieved the proposed healing rates with a transtibial to transfemoral amputation ratio of 3.3:1.

An ideal method would be noninvasive, quick, have a high degree of accuracy, and be patient friendly, but this has not been achieved. For this reason, many centers advocate the use of more than one method to increase the chances of predicting whether a certain level of amputation has healing potential. No one test has achieved widespread popularity, and clinical judgment may play the biggest role in amputation decision-making.[53]

The ability of a surgeon to determine an amputation level that is likely to heal based only on clinical parameters is poor. The absence of pulses and capillary bleeding are unsatisfactory indicators for healing and tissue viability.[54] Various techniques have been used to assess skin blood flow. Care must be taken to ensure that the measured flow reflects nutritional blood flow rather than secondary flow attributed to the opening of nonnutritional arteriovenous shunts, as may occur after lumbar sympathectomy.

Tests

Tests commonly used in clinical practice are reviewed here. No single method has 100% sensitivity and specificity. The methods described are often used in combination with other tests to increase the potential predictive value.

Angiography

Virtually all patients being considered for amputation should have angiography or some form of imaging, such as arterial duplex or magnetic resonance angiography. Any type of angiography alone has been reported to be a poor predictor of wound healing in major lower limb amputation.[55] In contrast, a correlation between level of amputation and angiographic scoring has also been observed.[56] A patent profunda femoris appears to be of major importance in the presence of a superficial femoral artery occlusion and should be ensured before attempting a transtibial amputation.[57] An occlusion of both the profunda femoris and the superficial femoral artery indicates a poor prognosis for the healing of a transtibial amputation.

Doppler Ultrasound

The Doppler ultrasound principle is used to detect the movement of red blood cells in vessels in order to assess systolic pressure, with the transcutaneous Doppler flow velocity detector, the instrument most commonly used for this purpose. Moving red cells cause a backscatter of a transmitted sound undergoing a Doppler shift in frequency that is directly related to the velocity of the red blood corpuscles. As ultrasound waves contact the skin, they are backscattered as either from stationary structures or from moving red blood cells. The signals from these components mix to produce interference. The frequency at which this interference occurs is the Doppler shift frequency. This shift is directly related to the velocity of red blood cells and the cosine of the angle between the direction of blood flow and the ultrasound beam. When the Doppler angle approaches 90° (cosine 90° = 0), the detection of the Doppler shift is jeopardized. The ideal Doppler angle is 0° (cosine 0° = 1), but this angle is rarely achieved. In practice, Doppler angles between 45° and 60° produce satisfactory results. Two types of continuous-wave Doppler machines are available. These are the nondirectional and the

directional velocity meters; the latter is able to differentiate forward from reverse movement of blood and to calculate blood flow.

Ankle Brachial Pressure Index and Segmental Pressures

The waveform of the arterial pulse can be detected in the lower limb using a Doppler ultrasonic probe. A cuff is placed around the limb and inflated to determine the systolic pressure by listening to the sound transmitted by the Doppler probe. When comparing measurements at the thigh, calf, and ankle, a gradient is observed, with the greatest amount of pressure at the thigh and the least amount at the most distal end of the limb, usually the ankle. The patient's brachial pressure is also taken so that a standardized ratio can be calculated to allow direct comparisons. This value is expressed as the Ankle Brachial Pressure Index (ABPI).

Ankle pressures are slightly higher than arm pressures. When comparing lower limb pressures with brachial pressures, a resting ABPI greater than 1.0 is considered normal. An ABPI less than 1.0 suggests stenotic disease. Patients with IC generally have an ABPI in the range of 0.5 to 0.7, and patients with rest pain or other severe ischemic symptoms generally have an ABPI ≤ 0.3. A pressure less than 50 mm Hg at the ankle is associated with limb-threatening ischemia. A decrease of 30 mm Hg or more in pressure from the lower thigh to the ankle suggests a severe stenotic or an occlusive process. Because measuring segmental pressures is discontinuous, the ability to measure rapid changes in blood flow with this method is limited. The ABPI seldom correlates with the severity of symptoms. Although it provides good baseline values of arterial pressure and serves as a guide to the extent of ischemia, the ABPI is useless for selecting amputation level.

Carter[58] evaluated distal systolic pressures in patients with and without diabetes mellitus. In patients with foot ulceration, the risk of amputation was greater if the ankle pressure was less than 55 mm Hg. In patients with diabetes, amputation was still a strong possibility with higher pressures because spuriously high pressures can be present in these patients as a result of calcification of the arterial media. Toe pressure measurements are a more reliable test in patients in whom calcification of the smaller blood vessels of a toe is not usually a problem.[59] More recently, pulsed-wave assessment of the toes has provided information relative to risk of amputation.[60]

Several investigators have demonstrated that a transtibial amputation will go on to heal if the popliteal pressure is greater than 70 mm Hg.[61,62] This finding is of limited use in the patient with a popliteal pressure less than 70 mm Hg, however, as healing is still possible in these patients.[62] Identifying which patients are likely to heal is of utmost importance. One problem is that the pressure measured before amputation is not necessarily reflective of that after amputation. Although skin blood flow is more important than muscle blood flow after major lower limb amputation, it is difficult to separate skin and muscle components because the blood flow of the whole limb is measured. Physiologic changes after amputation play a determining role in whether healing occurs.

Treadmill stress testing can also be performed in patients in whom the resting ankle/brachial pressure is near normal to determine if exercise causes a redistribution of blood that results in a decrease in the ABPI. At best, however, this index provides only a very crude estimate of the vascular status of a patient.

Transcutaneous Oxygen Partial Pressure Measurement

Transcutaneous oxygen partial pressure measurement ($TcPo_2$) was initially developed to determine the arterial partial pressure in neonates,[63,64] but it is also used to measure the transcutaneous oxygen partial pressure of adults with PVD. With this technique, an electrode is placed on the patient's skin on the area of interest. The electrode should be warmed to 44°C to achieve maximal local hyperemia by vasodilation and improve the conditions for oxygen to diffuse to the surface. This warming relaxes the resistance vessels and abolishes local autoregulatory mechanisms.[65] A partial pressure greater than 35 mm Hg always predicts wound healing; however, values less than 35 mm Hg do not always predict failure of tissue healing.[66] In a patient with severe ischemic rest pain, it is not uncommon to observe a $TcPo_2$ value of 0 mm Hg despite a toe pressure greater than 50 mm Hg. An explanation for this situation is that a very low blood supply gives rise to constant, but total, oxygen extraction at the capillary bed, resulting in a $TcPo_2$ measurement of 0 mm Hg at the skin.[67] Patients with ischemic limbs often have $TcPo_2$ values at the thigh similar to those of healthy age-matched individuals, but the values decrease significantly as measurements are taken closer to the ankle,[68] which correlates well with ankle segmental pressures. Healing can potentially occur in areas of skin with extremely low or 0 mm Hg $TcPo_2$ and, therefore, in situations of severe ischemia, the $TcPo_2$ is an insensitive indicator of the nutritional supply of the skin. Difficulties in calibration of the instrument are often encountered and result in large variations in $TcPo_2$ values.

The initial enthusiasm for transcutaneous oximetry as a major tool for assessment of limb viability has not been vindicated by clinical studies. Many problems arise with interpretation of the results of this technique, mainly related to the nature of the electrode.[69] In addition, several characteristics of ischemic skin contribute to these difficulties. The skin in these patients is likely to be maximally vasodilated already, and thus local heating provides little or no augmentation of skin blood flow. Also, oxygen availability at the electrode may be compromised in ischemic skin because of the increased oxygen extraction that occurs in such tissues. These factors, combined with a small but potentially significant oxygen consumption by the electrode itself, may produce erroneously low or even zero transcutaneous oxygen readings in severely ischemic skin, which may actually be viable in terms of healing potential.[70] Inhalation of 100% oxygen during the measurement of $TcPo_2$ can significantly improve the predictive value and sensitivity in defining tissue viability.[71] Thus, the inhalation of oxygen helps delineate an interface between viable and nonviable tissues.

Radioisotope Clearance Technique

Freely diffusible radioactive isotopes that have a short half-life can be injected into the skin. The washout rate, often denoted by its half-life, is proportional to the skin blood flow. This method was initially developed by Kety in 1949.[72] After intramuscular injection of radioactive sodium, the rate of clearance can be measured, which also correlates with skin blood flow.

The most widely used radioisotope is xenon Xe 133, which has been shown to be especially well suited to measurement of blood flow in the brain.[52] One of the drawbacks of using xenon Xe 133 is that it has a high affinity for fat, which leads to an underestimation of skin blood flow. The clearance of this isotope in skin is biphasic. Despite these disadvantages, this radioisotope has been used to select the amputation level for transtibial amputation (TTA) and transfemoral amputation (TFA), as well as amputations at more distal and proximal sites.[51,52]

The injection of radioisotopes is invasive and produces some tissue damage. Several measurements often have to be made when isolated areas of abnormally high or low skin blood flow are encountered.[73] Patients also are required to lie completely still during measurements, which can be difficult for a patient with ischemic rest pain. Finally, repeated injections of radioisotopes are not possible because of the potential accumulation of relatively large amounts of radiation, which may cause local and systemic cell damage.

Other compounds commonly used include antipyrine labeled with iodine I 125 (4-iodoantipyrine)[74] and thallium Tl 201.[75] These isotopes have different solubilities, redistributions, and blood and tissue partition coefficients. The radiopharmaceutical 4-iodoantipyrine I 125 deserves special mention because of its favorable pharmacokinetic properties, which include a monoexponential clearance and lower fat solubility than other compounds.

The invasive nature and the risks of anaphylaxis, however, remain a problem with the radioisotope washout technique. The intradermal injection is also painful for the patient. In addition, recent legislation has greatly increased the cost of production for many of these isotopes, making them unaffordable in many hospitals.

Laser Doppler Velocimetry

A laser source providing a monochromatic light can be used instead of sound waves to measure the Doppler effect. The potential for its use in PVD is established.[76,77] There appears to be a reasonable correlation between laser Doppler measurements and radioisotope skin blood flows,[78] but results are inconsistent because each method measures different entities. With the laser Doppler, the movement of red blood corpuscles is recorded at a depth of approximately 1.5 mm. With a radioisotope, blood flow is measured at a depth determined by the depth of the injection. A major disadvantage of the laser Doppler is that it only evaluates blood flow with measurements at individual points and thus does not necessarily represent the same flux value in the rest of the limb. Laser Doppler velocimetry is most valuable in assessing changing conditions in the skin. Examples of relevant situations include monitoring skin flaps and local or systemic pharmacologic interventions that cause changes in skin blood flow.

A more recently introduced method of assessing laser Doppler flux is the scanning laser Doppler (Moor Instruments, Devon, England). This device allows readings to be taken without actual skin contact. Furthermore, it allows a larger area of the body to be scanned. The scanning laser Doppler produces a high-quality anatomic image from which smaller areas can be examined in more detail.

Thermography

Thermography is not only valuable for determining level of amputation[50,79,80] but also is useful in the assessment of wound healing,[81] deep venous thrombosis, and the evaluation of vasoactive drugs.[82] The infrared thermogram obtains images by detecting heat that is radiated from the tissues. Skin temperature depends not only on blood flow but also is a function of arterial and venous blood temperature as well as tissue metabolism. Any inflammation and variations in environmental temperature are likely to affect the thermographic image. Heat transported to the skin by arterial perfusion and exchanged at the deep dermal plexus as a result of opening the pre- and postcapillary sphincters may indicate high blood flow through arteriovenous anastomosis in the skin, rather than a high nutrient blood flow; this result provides a false impression of healing potential.

Thermography is useful to complement findings from other tests such as radioisotope tracers,[83] as opposed to use as the only test. Thermography is useful for the assessment of the viability of skin flaps. A medial-to-lateral thermal gradient is often present in a lower limb requiring a transtibial amputation. This result suggests that a medially skewed flap is more likely to undergo healing, as the vascular pedicle is more likely to be viable.[83,84]

The advantages of thermography are the lack of physical contact with the patient and the resulting images over a large surface area. Disadvantages include the need for a specialized room kept at a standard condition and specialized skills to interpret the thermograms. In addition, the initial costs of the equipment for thermography are high. Maintenance costs also contribute to the overall expense of this technique.

Fluorometry

Initially described by Lange and Boyd,[85] this method uses a fiber-optic fluorometer to measure tissue fluorescence after the intravenous administration of fluorescein. The movement of fluorescein in the bloodstream equates to blood flow. Both the uptake and the elimination of fluorescein can be measured.[86] This method relied heavily on subjective findings until a quantitative approach to measuring fluorescence was developed in 1980.[87] This method of measurement also eliminated problems with light transmission caused by pigmented skin. A dual-channel fiber-optic light guide is used; one transmits a blue light to excite the fluorescein in the skin, and the other channel receives the emitted fluorescence, which is measured by a photomultiplier tube.

Impressive results have been reported by Silverman and associates[88,89] in predicting amputation wound healing and selection of level of amputation. Fluorometry has not gained widespread acceptance, however, because of its failure to reproduce meaningful results from other studies, its invasive methodology, false positive results with cellulitic or edematous tissue, and a real, albeit small, risk of anaphylaxis.

Light Guide Spectrophotometry

Light guide spectrophotometry is a new method that is noninvasive and easy to perform. A halogen or xenon light source is shone on the surface of the skin and absorbed by the hemoglobin in the blood. Computer analysis of the reflected light enables measurement of the oxygen saturation of the hemoglobin. Spectrophotometers with different sensitivities and light guides can be used so that light can be detected at either superficial or deep levels of the skin. These are referred to as micro- and macro-light guide spectrophotometers, respectively (Diehl GmbH and Co, Nürnberg, Germany). These spectrophotometers are designed for in vivo measurements.[90] No heating of the epidermis occurs, and continuous recordings can be made at one site. The relatively expensive equipment and difficulties in the interpretation of measurements limit this technique to experimental use until the system is fully validated.

Macro- and micro-light guide spectrophotometers produce different results for oxygen saturation because of differing penetration of the light guides and methods of analysis of the reflected light beam. Spectrophotometry compares favorably with the radio-isotope technique of measuring skin blood flow for the selection of level of amputation.[91] Encouraging results have been observed for the use of spectrophotometry for predicting wound healing following amputation for critical limb ischemia.[92] A clear advantage of spectrophotometry is the speed at which measurements can be taken, eliminating the need for a patient with a painful limb to keep absolutely still when recordings are taken. In addition, the technique is pain free, noninvasive, and provides immediate results.

Summary and Conclusions

The optimal level of amputation should be based on assessment of limb viability by specialized techniques and clinical judgment.[93] An aggressive approach to knee joint preservation in major lower limb amputation should be pursued in all patients. More than 70% of all major lower limb amputations should be at the transtibial level, and these procedures should be accompanied by a primary healing rate

greater than 90%. All too often, an equal number of transtibial and transfemoral amputations are performed with good primary healing rates, indicating that a disproportionate number of patients are being subjected to proximal amputations. There are no grounds for performing an initial transfemoral amputation to spare the patient an additional operation; however, the ratio of transtibial to transfemoral amputations performed varies tremendously by institution, region, and country. This variation is likely attributable to surgeons electing to perform a transfemoral amputation in borderline patients in an attempt to limit residual limb failure. The possibility that ill-planned distal amputations have been performed by inexperienced surgeons on tissue that is of dubious viability may have contributed to the impression that a transfemoral amputation is necessary and that distal procedures inevitably require revision to a more proximal level. Furthermore, the level of amputation selected is often incorrect, resulting in the conservative option of amputating proximally rather than attempting a TTA after careful assessment of the patient. This is especially true in centers that do not have a comprehensive amputation service and when the level of amputation is based mainly on clinical judgment.

All too often, the need for amputation is considered a failure by the surgical team and any additional care of these patients is left to the most junior of surgeons. As with all surgical procedures, amputation surgery involves a learning curve for any trainee. As one surgeon leaves the training program, another inexperienced surgeon replaces him or her. Unless amputations are directly supervised by an experienced surgeon, the ratio of transtibial to transfemoral amputations and the primary healing rates of all amputations will remain poor. Junior trainees should not perform amputation procedures as their initial training in orthopaedic or vascular surgery. Senior trainees or con-

sultants should perform these procedures.[94]

Not all studies, however, agree that rehabilitation rates and mobility will improve if an appropriate TTA:TFA ratio is achieved.[95] Partial foot amputations performed in an attempt to preserve maximum limb function are now more common, especially in diabetic patients who are more likely to heal after a forefoot amputation in the absence of concomitant revascularization. Diabetic vascular disease affects the very distal vessels, a factor that influences healing. Therefore, a forefoot amputation in a patient who does not have diabetes mellitus is unlikely to heal in the absence of prior revascularization.

At present, no established test can completely predict healing after amputation. The predictions made by the tests described are purely quantitative and are mainly used to help determine the level of amputation. An ideal test would not only accurately predict the viability of the residual limb but also would be quick, easy to perform, painless, reproducible, and cost effective. Regardless of predictions based on laboratory tests, the skill of the surgeon is an important determinant of residual limb failure or success. These limbs are already deprived of oxygen, and poor surgical technique can certainly contribute to failure of the amputation wound to heal.

Ideally, the patient should be transferred to a special unit devoted exclusively to the care of amputees as soon as possible after amputation. Successful ambulation after amputation is best achieved in specialized rehabilitation centers that are experienced in caring for amputees. Typically, up to 80% of patients will be able to ambulate successfully after transtibial amputation, but only 30% of transfemoral amputees will achieve independent mobility.[16] A patient who undergoes any type of amputation should start rehabilitation immediately postoperatively. Amputations are predominantly performed in the elderly, and the overall quality of life for these patients is poor unless rehabilitation is aggressive. Sadly, many surgeons fail to appreciate the importance of level selection and appear to be unaware of the considerable advantages in retaining the knee joint, which conserves energy expenditure during ambulation. The more proximal the level of amputation, the more energy that is required during ambulation.[96] The amount of energy needed to walk is a crucial factor for elderly patients who already have a low energy reserve. Another aspect of level selection is that an amputee is far more likely to make use of a prosthesis if amputation is at the transtibial level.[97] These patients are also subjected to a higher level of morbidity and mortality because of the nature of their systemic vascular disease.[18] Preservation of the knee joint is generally more acceptable to the patient, is associated with better cosmesis, and often allows increased mobility.

Most lower limb amputations in the developed world are performed for severe PVD or complications of diabetes mellitus. A significant number of patients may be denied a full and formal assessment by the rehabilitation team based on the decision of physicians who think that the patient cannot be rehabilitated. All patients subjected to amputation surgery, however, should be referred for formal assessment. Assessment for rehabilitation will determine the patient's capabilities, which can range from bed to wheelchair transfer only to full mobility with a prosthesis without a walking aid.

In summary, amputation should be regarded as a reconstructive procedure that is designed to restore function and attempt to allow the patient to return to an independent lifestyle. Despite the initial shock at the prospect of a lower limb amputation, most patients have a successful rehabilitation. Ambulation after amputation, with or without the use of aids, represents a major achievement. Preservation of as much of the knee joint as possible greatly facilitates successful rehabilitation. Patients should have early access to a multidisci-

plinary team experienced in the care of amputees. Early involvement of such a team allows the amputee the best chance to live as pain free and as independently as possible. Rehabilitation, however, is an ongoing process for all amputees.

References

1. Criqui MH, Fronek A, Barrett-Conner E, Klauber MR, Gabriel S, Goodman D: The prevalence of peripheral arterial disease in a defined population. *Circulation* 1985;71:510-515.

2. Fowkes FG, Housley E, Cawood EH, Macintyre CC, Ruckley CV, Prescott RJ: Edinburgh Artery Study: Prevalence of asymptomatic and symptomatic peripheral arterial disease in the general population. *Int J Epidemiol* 1991;20:384-392.

3. Dormandy JA, Murray GD: The fate of the claudicant: A prospective study of 1969 claudicants. *Eur J Vasc Surg* 1991; 5:131-133.

4. Bevan EG, Waller PC, Ramsay LE: Pharmacological approaches to the treatment of intermittent claudication. *Drugs Aging* 1992;2:125-136.

5. Dormandy JA, Ray S: The fate of the amputees. *Vasc Med Rev* 1995;5:331-346.

6. Norgren L: Life expectancy for critical limb ischaemia, in Greenhalgh RM (ed): *The Durability of Vascular and Endovascular Surgery*. London, England, WB Saunders, 1999, pp 163-173.

7. Fontaine R, Dubost C (eds): *Les Greffes Vasculaires*. Paris, France, Brodard et Taupin, 1954.

8. Sillesen H: Conservative treatment, amputation or revascularisation for critical limb ischaemia. *Ann Chir Gynaecol* 1998;87:159-161.

9. Tseng CH, Tai TY, Chen CJ, Lin BJ: Ten-year clinical analysis of diabetic leg amputees. *J Formos Med Assoc* 1994;93:388-392.

10. Second European Consensus Document on chronic critical limb ischaemia. *Eur J Vasc Surg* 1992;6(suppl A):1-32.

11. Wolfe JH, Wyatt MG: Critical and subcritical ischaemia. *Eur J Vasc Endovasc Surg* 1997;13:578-582.

12. Lepantalo M, Biancari F, Tukiainen E: Never amputate without consultation of a vascular surgeon. *Diabetes Metab Res Rev* 2000;16(suppl 1):S27-S32.

13. Lindholt JS, Bovling S, Fasting H, Henneberg EW: Vascular surgery reduces the frequency of lower limb major amputations. *Eur J Vasc Surg* 1994; 8:31-35.

14. Campbell WB, Ridler BM: Predicting the use of prostheses by vascular amputees. *Eur J Vasc Endovasc Surg* 1996; 12:342-345.

15. Moore TJ, Barron J, Hutchinson F III, Golden C, Ellis C, Humphries D: Prosthetic usage following major lower extremity amputation. *Clin Orthop* 1989;238:219-224.

16. Stewart CP, Jain AS: Dundee revisited: 25 years of a total amputee service. *Prosthet Orthot Int* 1993;17:14-20.

17. Traballesi M, Brunelli S, Pratesi L, Pulcini M, Angioni C, Paolucci S: Prognostic factors in rehabilitation of above knee amputees for vascular diseases. *Disabil Rehabil* 1998;20:380-384.

18. Stewart CP, Jain AS: Cause of death of lower limb amputees. *Prosthet Orthot Int* 1992;16:129-132.

19. Stewart CP, Jain AS, Ogston SA: Lower limb amputee survival. *Prosthet Orthot Int* 1992;16:11-18.

20. Matsen SL, Malchow D, Matsen FA III: Correlations with patients' perspectives of the result of lower-extremity amputation. *J Bone Joint Surg Am* 2000;82:1089-1095.

21. Pell JP, Donnan PT, Fowkes FG, Ruckley CV: Quality of life following lower limb amputation for peripheral arterial disease. *Eur J Vasc Surg* 1993;7:448-451.

22. De Fretes A, Boonstra AM, Vos LD: Functional outcome of rehabilitated bilateral lower limb amputees. *Prosthet Orthot Int* 1994;18:18-24.

23. Fusetti C, Senechaud C, Merlini M: Quality of life of vascular disease patients following amputation. *Ann Chir* 2001;126:434-439.

24. Criqui MH, Langer RD, Fronek A, et al: Mortality over a period of 10 years in patients with peripheral arterial disease. *N Engl J Med* 1992;326:381-386.

25. Myhre HO: Socioeconomic costs of limb-threatening critical ischaemia. *Crit Isch* 1998;8:49-55.

26. Panayiotopoulos YP, Tyrrell MR, Owen SE, Reidy JF, Taylor PR: Outcome and cost analysis after femoro-crural and femoropedal grafting for critical limb ischaemia. *Br J Surg* 1997; 84:207-212.

27. Panayiotopoulos YP, Reidy JF, Taylor PR: The concept of knee salvage: Why does a failed femorocrural/pedal arterial bypass not affect the amputation level? *Eur J Vasc Endovasc Surg* 1997;13: 477-485.

28. Johnson BF, Evans L, Drury R, Datta D, Morris-Jones W, Beard JD: Surgery for limb threatening ischaemia: A re-appraisal of the costs and benefits. *Eur J Vasc Endovasc Surg* 1995;9:181-188.

29. Jamsen T, Tulla H, Manninen H, et al: Results of infrainguinal bypass surgery: An analysis of 263 consecutive operations. *Ann Chir Gynae* 2001;90: 92-99.

30. Klinkert P, Schepers A, Burger DH, van Bockel JH, Breslau PJ: Vein versus polytetrafluoroethylene in above-knee femoropopliteal bypass grafting: Five-year results of a randomized controlled trial. *J Vasc Surg* 2003;37:149-155.

31. Bounameaux H, Verhaeghe R, Verstraete M: Thromboembolism and anti-thrombotic therapy in peripheral arterial disease. *J Am Coll Cardiol* 1986;8 (suppl B):98B-103B.

32. Verstraete M, Vermylen J, Donati MB: The effect of streptokinase infusion on chronic arterial occlusions and stenoses. *Ann Intern Med* 1971;74:377-382.

33. Hess H, Mietaschk A, Deischel G: Drug-induced inhibition of platelet function delays progression of peripheral occlusive arterial disease: A prospective double-blind arteriographically controlled trial. *Lancet* 1985;1: 415-419.

34. Smith FB, Bradbury AW, Fowkes FG: Intravenous naftidrofuryl for critical limb ischaemia. *Cochrane Database Syst Rev* 2000;2:CD002070.

35. Treatment of limb threatening ischaemia with intravenous iloprost: A randomised double-blind placebo controlled study: U.K. Severe Limb Ischaemia Study Group. *Eur J Vasc Surg* 1991;5:511-516.

36. Arosio E, Sardina M, Prior M, De Marchi S, Zannoni M, Bianchini C: Clinical and circulatory effects of Ilo-prost either administered for 1 week or 4 weeks in patients with peripheral obstructive arterial disease at Leriche-Fontaine stage III. *Eur Rev Med Pharmacol Sci* 1998;2:53-59.

37. Loosemore TM, Chalmers TC, Dormandy JA: A meta-analysis of randomized placebo control trials in Fontaine stages III and IV peripheral occlusive arterial disease. *Int Angiol* 1994;13:133-142.

38. Whatling PJ, Gibson M, Torrie EP, Magee TR, Galland RB: Iliac occlusions: Stenting or crossover grafting? An examination of patency and cost. *Eur J Vasc Endovasc Surg* 2000;20:36-40.

39. Bolia A, Miles KA, Brennan J, Bell PR: Percutaneous transluminal angioplasty of occlusions of the femoral and popliteal arteries by subintimal dissection. *Cardiovasc Intervent Radiol* 1990; 13:357-363.

40. Holiday FA, Barendregt WB, Slappendel R, Crul BJ, Buskens FG, van der Vliet JA: Lumbar sympathectomy in critical limb ischaemia: Surgical, chemical or not at all? *Cardiovasc Surg* 1999;7:200-202.

41. Ubbink DT, Jacobs MJHM: Spinal cord stimulation in critical limb ischaemia, in Branchereau A, Jacobs M (eds): *Critical Limb Ischemia*. Armonk, NY, Futura, 1999, pp 75-84.

42. Mashiah A, Soroker D, Pasik S, Mashiah T: Phenol lumbar sympathetic block in diabetic lower limb ischemia. *J Cardiovasc Risk* 1995;2:467-469.

43. Walker PM, Key JA, MacKay IM, Johnston KW: Phenol sympathectomy for vascular occlusive disease. *Surg Gyn Obs* 1978;146:741-744.

44. Stonebridge PA, Prescott RJ, Ruckley CV: Randomised trial comparing infrainguinal polytetrafluoroethylene bypass grafting with and without vein interposition cuff at the distal anastomosis: The Joint Vascular Research Group. *J Vasc Surg* 1997;26:543-550.

45. Veith FJ, Gupta SK, Ascer E, et al: Six-year prospective multicenter randomized comparison of autologous saphenous vein and expanded polytetrafluoroethylene grafts in infrainguinal arterial reconstructions. *J Vasc Surg* 1986;3:104-114.

46. Wijesinghe LD, Beardsmore DM, Scott DJ: Polytetrafluoroethylene (PTFE) femorodistal grafts with a distal vein cuff for critical ischaemia. *Eur J Vasc Endovasc Surg* 1998;15:449-453.

47. Grimble SA, Magee TR, Galland RB: Methicillin resistant Staphylococcus aureus in patients undergoing major amputation. *Eur J Vasc Endovasc Surg* 2001;22:215-218.

48. Gaines PA, Beard JD: Radiological management of acute lower limb ischaemia. *Br J Hosp Med* 1991;45:343-344, 346-353.

49. Lusby RJ, Wylie EJ: Acute lower limb ischemia: Pathogenesis and management. *World J Surg* 1983;7:340-386.

50. McCollum PT, Spence VA, Walker WF, Swanson AJ, Turner MS, Murdoch G: Experience in the healing rate of lower limb amputations. *J R Coll Surg Edinb* 1984;29:358-362.

51. Malone JM, Leal JM, Moore WS, et al: The 'gold standard' for amputation level selection: Xenon-133 clearance. *J Surg Res* 1981;30:449-455.

52. Moore WS, Henry RE, Malone JM, Daly MJ, Patton D, Childers SJ: Prospective use of xenon Xe-133 clearance for amputation level selection. *Arch Surg* 1981;116:86-88.

53. Wagner WH, Keagy BA, Kotb MM, Burnham SJ, Johnson G Jr: Noninvasive determination of healing of major lower extremity amputation: The continued role of clinical judgment. *J Vasc Surg* 1988;8:703-710.

54. Burgess EM, Matsen FA III: Determining amputation levels in peripheral vascular disease. *J Bone Joint Surg Am* 1981;63:1493-1497.

55. Robbs JV, Ray R: Clinical predictors of below-knee stump healing following amputation for ischaemia. *S Afr J Surg* 1982;20:305-310.

56. van den Broek TA, Dwars BJ, Rauwerda JA, Bakker FC: A multivariate analysis of determinants of wound healing in patients after amputation for peripheral vascular disease. *Eur J Vasc Surg* 1990;4:291-295.

57. Roon AJ, Moore WS, Goldstone J: Below-knee amputation: A modern approach. *Am J Surg* 1977;134:153-158.

58. Carter SA: The relationship of distal systolic pressures to healing of skin lesions in limbs with arterial occlusive disease: With special reference to diabetes mellitus. *Scand J Clin Lab Invest* 1973;31(suppl 128):239-243.

59. Carter SA: Ankle and toe systolic pressures: Comparison of value and limitations in arterial occlusive disease. *Int Angiol* 1992;11:289-297.

60. Carter SA, Tate RB: The value of toe pulse waves in determination of risks for limb amputation and death in patients with peripheral arterial disease and skin ulcers or gangrene. *J Vasc Surg* 2001;33:708-714.

61. Schwartz JA, Schuler JJ, O'Connor RJ, Flanigan DP: Predictive value of distal perfusion pressure in the healing of amputation of the digits and the forefoot. *Surg Gynecol Obstet* 1982;154:865-869.

62. Spence VA, McCollum PT, Walker WF, Murdoch G: Assessment of tissue viability in relation to the selection of amputation level. *Prosthet Orthot Int* 1984;8:67-75.

63. Huch A, Huch R, Lübbers DW: Quantitative polarographic measurement of the oxygen pressure on the scalp of the newborn. *Arch Gynakol* 1969;207:443-448.

64. Huch R, Lübbers DW, Huch A: The transcutaneous measurement of oxygen and carbon dioxide tensions for the determination of arterial blood-gas values with control of local perfusion and peripheral perfusion pressure: Theoretical analysis and practical application, in Payne JP, Hill DW (eds): *Oxygen Measurements in Biology and Medicine.* London, England, Butterworths, 1975, pp 121-138.

65. Rooth G, Hedstrand U, Tyden H, Ogren C: The validity of the transcutaneous oxygen tension method in adults. *Crit Care Med* 1976;4:162-165.

66. Ratliff DA, Clyne CA, Chant AD, Webster JH: Prediction of amputation wound healing: The role of transcutaneous pO2 assessment. *Br J Surg* 1984;71:219-222.

67. Tonnesen KH: Transcutaneous oxygen tension in imminent foot gangrene. *Acta Anaesthesoal Scand Suppl* 1978;68:107-110.

68. Clyne CA, Ryan J, Webster JH, Chant AD: Oxygen tension of the skin of ischemic legs. *Am J Surg* 1982;143:315-318.

69. Spence VA, McCollum PT, McGregor IW, Sherwin SJ, Walker WF: The effect of the transcutaneous electrode on the variability of dermal oxygen tension changes. *Clin Phys Physiol Meas* 1985;6:139-145.

70. Melillo E, Catapano G, Dell' Omo G, et al: Transcutaneous oxygen and carbon dioxide measurement in peripheral vascular disease. *Vasc Surg* 1995;29:273-280.

71. McCollum PT, Spence VA, Walker WF: Oxygen inhalation induced changes in the skin as measured by transcutaneous oxymetry. *Br J Surg* 1986;73:882-885.

72. Kety SS: Measurement of regional circulation by the local clearance of radioactive sodium. *Am Heart J* 1949;38:321-328.

73. McCollum PT, Spence VA, Walker WF: Circumferential skin blood flow measurements in the ischaemic limb. *Br J Surg* 1985;72:310-312.

74. McCollum PT: Antipyrine clearance from the skin of the foot and lower leg in critical ischaemia: Clinical implications, in *Practical Aspects of Skin Blood Flow Measurement.* London, England, Biological Engineering Society, 1985.

75. Siegel ME, Stewart CA, Kwong P, SakimuraI: 201 Tl perfusion study of 'ischemic' ulcers of the leg: Prognostic ability compared with Doppler ultrasound. *Radiology* 1982;143:233-235.

76. Holloway GA Jr, Burgess EM: Preliminary experiences with laser Doppler velocimetry for the determination of amputation levels. *Prosthet Orthot Int* 1983;7:63-66.

77. Stern MD, Lappe DL, Bowen PD, et al: Continuous measurement of tissue blood flow by laser-Doppler spectroscopy. *Am J Physiol* 1977;232:441-448.

78. Holloway GA Jr, Watkins DW: Laser Doppler measurement of cutaneous blood flow. *J Invest Dermatol* 1977;69:306-309.

79. Lee BY, Trainor FS, Kavner D, McCannWJ, Madden JL: Noninvasive hemodynamic evaluation in selection of amputation level. *Surg Gynecol Obstet* 1979;149:241-244.

80. Spence VA, Walker WF, TroupI M, Murdoch G: Amputation of the ischemic limb: Selection of the optimum site by thermography. *Angiology* 1981;32:155-169.

81. Kliot DA, Birnbaum SJ: Thermographic studies of wound healing. *Am J Obstet Gynecol* 1965;93:515-521.

82. Henderson HP, Hackett ME: The value of thermography in peripheral vascular disease. *Angiology* 1978;29:65-75.

83. McCollum PT, Spence VA, Walker WF, Murdoch G: A rationale for skew flaps in below-knee amputation surgery. *Prosthet Orthot Int* 1985;9:95-99.

84. Jain AS, Stewart CP, Turner MS: Transtibial amputation using a medially based flap. *J R Coll Surg Edinb* 1995;40:263-265.

85. Lange K, Boyd LJ: Use of fluorescein method in establishment of diagnosis and prognosis of peripheral vascular diseases. *Arch Intern Med* 1944;74:175-184.

86. Weisman RA, Silverman DG: Fiberoptic fluorometer for skin flap assessment. *Otolaryngol Head Neck Surg* 1983;91:377-379.

87. Silverman DG, LaRossa DD, Barlow CH, Bering TG, Popky LM, Smith TC: Quantification of tissue fluorescein delivery and prediction of flap viability with the fiberoptic dermofluorometer. *Plast Reconstr Surg* 1980;66:545-553.

88. Silverman DG, Roberts A, Reilly CA, et al: Fluorometric quantification of low-dose fluorescein delivery to predict amputation site healing. *Surgery* 1987;101:335-341.

89. Silverman DG, Rubin SM, Reilly CA, Brousseau DA, NortonKJ, Wolf GL: Fluorometric prediction of successful amputation level in the ischemic limb.*J Rehab Res Dev* 1985;22:23-28.

90. Newton DJ, Harrison DK, Delaney CJ, Beck JS, McCollum PT: Comparison of macro- and micro-lightguide spectrophotometric measurements of microvascular haemoglobin oxygenation in the tuberculin reaction in normal human skin. *Physiol Meas* 1994;15:115-128.

91. Harrison DK: Clinical application of light-guide diffuse reflectance spectrophotometry in vascular disease. *Proc Biomed Optoelectronic Devices Syst* 1993;2084:195-203.

92. Harrison DK, McCollum PT, Newton DJ, Hickman P, Jain AS: Amputation level assessment using lightguide spectrophotometry. *Prosthet Orthot Int* 1995;19:139-147.

93. Coffman JD: Editorial: Intermittent claudication: Be conservative. *New Engl J Med* 1991;325:577-578.

94. White SA, Thompson MM, Zickerman AM, et al: Lower limb amputation and

grade of surgeon. *Br J Surg* 1997;84: 509-511.

95. McWhinnie DL, Gordon AC, Collin J, Gray DW, Morrison JD: Rehabilitation outcome 5 years after 100 lower-limb amputations. *Br J Surg* 1994;81:1596-1599.

96. Waters RL, Perry J, Antonelli D, Hislop H: Energy cost of walking of amputees: The influence of level of amputation. *J Bone Joint Surg Am* 1976;58:42-46.

97. Pohjolainen T, Alaranta H, Karkkainen M: Prosthetic use and functional and social outcome following major lower limb amputation. *Prosthet Orthot Int* 1990;14:75-79.

Chapter 4

Infection: Limb Salvage Versus Amputation

John H. Bowker, MD

Introduction

Most limb-threatening infections occur in the foot, mostly in patients with long-standing diabetes mellitus. Among the risk factors for infection found in this population, sensory neuropathy appears to be the most important.[1,2] Sensory neuropathy is also seen in Hansen's disease (leprosy), alcoholic neuropathy, myelomeningocele, syphilis, congenital indifference to pain and spinal cord or peripheral nerve trauma, among others. Because they are unable to perceive a correct fit, patients with neuropathy tend to wear shoes that are too tight, thus inducing ulcer formation by direct pressure and shear forces. These patients may also see no harm in walking without shoes, at least in their homes, and thereby expose themselves to penetrating wounds from various objects left on the floor and other minor environmental trauma. The latter may include hard objects striking the foot such as containers of food, either in cans or frozen, and "stubbing" of bare toes. Swelling and venous congestion of the toes can result in loss of tissue. Motor neuropathy may affect the foot and toe dorsiflexors and allow a rapid uncontrolled descent of the forefoot following heel contact. This slapping gait can result in damage to the skin under the metatarsal head area. This effect will be aggravated by shifting of the metatarsal fat pad distally as the toes assume a clawed position, thus leaving the skin under the metatarsal heads with little protective fat padding. In addition, autonomic neuropathy results in extremely dry skin in which fissures may develop, providing sites of entry for bacteria.

In the absence of normal pain sensation, patients commonly exhibit marked denial even in regard to open sores, resulting in failure to seek medical care during the early stages of an infection. Yancey and Brand[3] ascribed this behavior to a change in body image/ownership that sometimes accompanies the loss of pain sensation. In addition, these patients may exhibit a displaced locus of control manifested by an inability to take responsibility for care of their feet and/or medical condition in general. They often become quite depressed, especially if they have experienced chronic problems with their feet, becoming quite fearful of amputation as an outcome. All of these basically psychological difficulties are likely to result in poor compliance with a preventive foot care regimen. In diabetic patients, especially those in a state of chronic hyperglycemia, infection is further complicated by decreased phagocytosis and chemotaxis of leukocytes.[4]

The approach to management of foot lesions in the diabetic patient is greatly simplified by use of the Brodsky depth-ischemia foot grading system[5] (Figure 1). This method classifies the depth of the wound by a number from 0 to 3 and the level of perfusion of the foot by a letter from A to D. The combination of number and letter provides a concise description of the foot that is useful in planning treatment. For example, a lesion in a grade 1-A foot may be expected to heal with suitable off-loading by a total contact cast or a specially designed shoe. A grade 3-A foot, in contrast, will require inpatient wound débridement and intravenous antibiotics. The depth of an ulcer is easily determined by probing the wound. In the clinic, this can be done with a sterile applicator, probe, or hemostat. If bone is contacted with the instrument or is visually exposed in the depths of the wound, osteomyelitis with or without septic arthritis is usually present.[6] Radiographs are useful in determining the extent of bony involvement. Bone scans are not necessary in the usual assessment of most penetrating lesions.

Any wound with clinical signs of infection should be cultured and the patient initially given intravenous antibiotics that cover a wide range of organisms, including gram-positive, gram-negative, and anaerobic bacteria.[7,8] The choice of definitive antibiotics will be determined by culture sensitivities. Gentle probing will also give a good idea of the extent of any abscess that has developed in the forefoot. Neuroarthropathic (Charcot) changes in the foot are com-

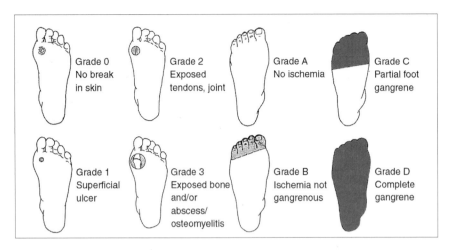

Figure 1 The depth-ischemia classification. Each foot is graded with both a number from 0 to 3 indicating wound depth and a letter from A to D indicating foot vascularity. *(Reproduced from Bowker JH, Pfeifer MA (eds):* Levin & O'Neil's The Diabetic Foot, *ed 6. St. Louis, MO, Mosby, 2001, p 277. Reproduced with permission of James W. Brodsky, MD. Copyright © James W. Brodsky, MD.)*

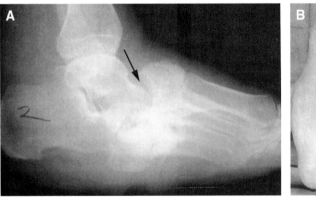

Figure 2 A, Radiograph of the left foot of a severely neuropathic diabetic patient with Charcot neuroarthropathy. Fracture-dislocation at the midtarsal joint (arrow) has resulted in a prominent bony mass. B, Note the large plantar ulcer, which probed to a bony mass. MRI or leukocyte scanning may help avoid an erroneous diagnosis of osteomyelitis.

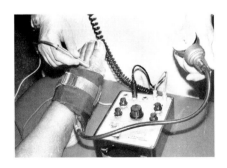

Figure 3 Doppler determination of systolic blood pressure at the level of the metatarsal necks. Note the placement of a child-sized blood pressure cuff.

(^{111}In) may be useful in diagnosis.[9-13] In general, however, the presence of bone infection becomes quite clear over a short period of time with the aid of serial radiographs and close clinical observation.

Surgical Management of Diabetic Foot Infections
Patient Evaluation

Prior to embarking on a definitive surgical solution, the surgeon should determine the patient's potential for wound healing. This includes evaluation of blood flow to the foot, nutritional status, and immunocompetence. Several methods are available that will give an indication of blood flow to the distal part of the foot, but the simplest remains the bedside Doppler ultrasound test. This can be done very easily by first applying an adult-width blood pressure cuff just above the malleoli and determining systolic pressure over the dorsalis pedis and posterior tibial arteries. A child-sized cuff is then placed around the midfoot and pressures are determined at the level of the metatarsal necks (Figure 3). If the ischemic index (foot systolic pressure divided by the brachial systolic pressure) is greater than or equal to 0.5, foot salvage may be feasible, with the caveat that calcification of the muscular wall of small arteries may result in falsely elevated values, especially in patients with diabetes. If the ischemic index is less than 0.5 and the problem is one of low-grade infection or distal dry gangrene, the patient should be referred to a vascular surgeon regarding the possibility of vascular reconstruction before limited distal amputations. When Doppler data are unreliable because of severe vessel calcification, transcutaneous oxygen measurements will give reliable information regarding local tissue perfusion, especially when tested during inhalation of 100% oxygen. Nutritional status is considered adequate with a serum

monly mistaken for acute osteomyelitis. Infection usually can be excluded on clinical examination alone: patients with neuropathic arthropathy will not be systemically ill and will exhibit only moderate local skin warmth and discomfort relative to the bony destruction seen on radiographs. On occasion, however, Charcot deformity may have an overlying ulcer that penetrates to the bony mass, leading to an erroneous diagnosis of osteomyelitis (Figure 2). In such cases, a bone biopsy, MRI, or leukocyte scanning with Indium-111

albumin level greater than or equal to 3 g/dL, while a total lymphocyte count of at least 1,500/mm^3 is considered evidence of immunocompetence.[14,15]

Surgical Approach

The goal of any surgical procedure in the infected insensate foot is the prompt removal of all necrotic and infected tissue while preserving as much of the forefoot lever as possible. If an operating room is not immediately available, an abscess should be opened widely in the emergency department to reduce its internal pressure. This may be accomplished by using ankle block anesthesia or, in many cases, no anesthesia at all if the patient's sensory neuropathy is profound. Whether the procedure is done in the emergency department or in the operating room, the surgeon should use longitudinal incisions to preserve as many neural and vascular structures as possible. Normal weight-bearing surfaces such as the heel pad, lateral portion of the sole, and metatarsal head areas should be respected. The surgeon should not compromise a later ablation, such as a Syme ankle disarticulation, by unnecessarily extending a midsole incision into the heel pad or a dorsal incision proximal to the ankle joint. It is helpful, even for an experienced surgeon, to first draw one or more possible surgical approaches on the skin before incision to avoid such unintended consequences. The surgeon should also begin an open amputation with a tentative plan for its ultimate closure, whether secondarily or by wound contraction with or without split-thickness skin grafting. Multiple dorsal and plantar incisions may be required to gain full, open drainage of all abscess pockets. For deep infections, the central plantar spaces, described by Grodinsky,[16] can be opened by a single extensile plantar incision as demonstrated by Loeffler and Ballard.[17] Although the complete exposure begins posterior to the medial malleolus and ends between the first and second metatarsal heads,

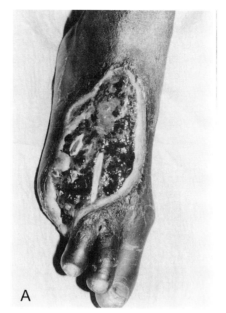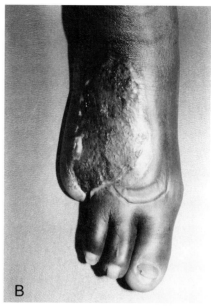

Figure 4 A, Right foot of a 52-year-old woman with diabetes mellitus following disarticulation of the fourth and fifth toes and excision of necrotic dorsal skin resulting from wet gangrene. The wound is well covered with granulation tissue and ready for split-thickness skin grafting. **B,** Same foot 3 months after grafting. At the time of publication, the graft had tolerated shoe wear for many years. (*Reproduced with permission from Bowker JH: Partial foot amputations and disarticulations.* Foot Ankle Clin N Am *1997;2: 153.*)

only part of it may be used, depending on the extent of the infection. Tissues to be removed include grossly infected bone and soft tissue, as well as poorly vascularized tissues exposed in the area of infection such as cartilage, tendon, joint capsule, and volar plates of the metatarsophalangeal joints. The wound is then lightly packed with gauze to allow free wicking of infective fluids to the surface.

Dressing changes two to three times daily will remove residual wound detritus and encourage granulation tissue growth. Healthy wounds can often be secondarily closed 10 to 14 days postoperatively, thus greatly reducing patient morbidity. If doubt exists as to the condition of the wound, dressing changes should be continued twice daily as the wound slowly granulates and contracts over a period of 3 to 6 months. When a healthy granulating wound shows no further volume contraction for 2 to 3 weeks, coverage with a split-thickness skin graft is appropriate, particularly in non–weight-bearing areas (Figure

4). To ensure prompt incorporation of split-thickness skin grafts, dependent edema as well as direct and shear forces are to be avoided. If a graft has been placed across a mobile joint, its immobilization in a well-padded cast may be necessary to prevent displacement of the graft.

Wound Closure in Chronic Osteomyelitis

In selected chronic, nonpurulent cases of chronic osteomyelitis, following removal of infected and necrotic tissue, primary loose closure of the wound should be considered. The surgeon should individually assess the feasibility of closed versus open management for each case. The criteria for this method include a wound with minimal or no pus, remaining tissues that are not inflamed, and a grossly clean wound. The methodology originally described by Kritter[18] is quite simple. A small polyethylene irrigation tube is placed in the depths of the wound and tacked to the skin. No deep sutures are used, and skin su-

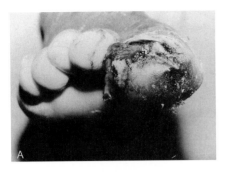

Figure 5 A, Wet gangrene of the right great toe in a man with diabetes mellitus. Both phalanges were infected, but some lateral toe skin was salvageable. Forefoot systolic pressure was adequate. B, Closure using a lateral toe flap after disarticulation of the great toe. Note the use of the Kritter irrigation system, including widely spaced sutures to allow egress of irrigation fluid and fixation of irrigation catheter to skin.

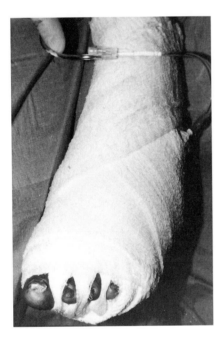

Figure 6 Bulky bandage used to absorb fluid from the Kritter irrigation system. The outer of two rolls of bandages is replaced every few hours.

tures are placed at wide intervals. One liter of irrigation fluid is run through the wound every 24 hours for a period of 3 days. The fluid passes from the wound between the skin sutures and is absorbed by the dressing. The outermost wrap is changed every 4 to 5 hours (Figures 5 and 6). If pus formation is noted on gentle wound compression after discontinuation of the irrigation, the wound is reopened and packed at the bedside. The advantage of this method is that primary healing of the wound will usu-

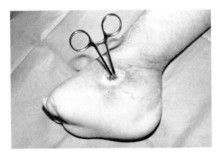

Figure 7 Foot of a 53-year-old patient with Hansen's disease. Note the absorption of bony and soft-tissue structures of the forefoot. The hemostat is placed in a deep sinus leading to a large area of chronic osteomyelitis in the midfoot and hindfoot.

ally occur in a 3- to 5-week period. The alternative is the prolonged morbidity associated with several months of healing by secondary intention while the wound is packed open. Better cosmesis is also generally achieved by eliminating the need for skin grafting of residual defects. The patient should avoid direct weightbearing for a minimum of 5 to 6 weeks. If a significant portion of the forefoot remains, changes in footwear may be limited to simple fillers attached to an insole, combined when necessary with a sole stiffener and rocker sole on an in-depth shoe. Well-designed shoe wear should provide the partial-foot amputee with a stable platform, proper padding of bony prominences, and protection of the foot from external trauma.

Types of Infections

Several other infections may result in lower limb amputation. In Hansen's disease, infection of peripheral nerves with *Mycobacterium leprae* will cause loss of foot sensation. As in diabetes mellitus, loss of sensation commonly leads to ulceration from repetitive minor trauma. Progressive absorption of bone and soft tissue aggravated by intractable deep infection following a skin ulceration may require transtibial amputation for control (Figure 7). Mycetoma (Madura foot) is a localized, chronic infection caused by Nocardia and other actinomycetes in more than 50% of cases, with the remainder culturing many different fungal species. Mycetoma occurs chiefly in agricultural workers who go barefoot in the tropics and subtropics, including the southern United States. Characteristic "grains" of clumped organisms exude from multiple subcutaneous sinuses. If the chronic infection is not treated, eventual systemic bacterial superinfection can be fatal. Progressive destruction of the pedal skeleton may necessitate a transtibial amputation (Figure 8). Other major infections that sometimes necessitate lower limb amputation include chronic osteomyelitis and life-threatening forms of infectious gangrene such as necrotizing fasciitis and clostridial myonecrosis (gas gangrene).

Chronic Osteomyelitis

Patients with chronic osteomyelitis usually present with a long-standing draining sinus. The sinus can be probed; radiographs, including a sinogram, will determine its full extent. To obtain a useful preoperative or intraoperative sample for biopsy, the surgeon must take tissue from the hypertrophic edge of the lesion, not from the central area of tumor necrosis. When a careful physical examination reveals palpable popliteal or inguinal lymph nodes, a preoperative tumor-staging evaluation should be done, including CT of the pelvis, abdomen, and chest. Material from an excisional

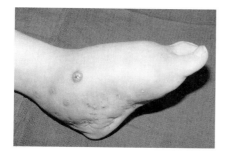

Figure 8 Right foot of a 54-year-old man with mycetoma. As a political prisoner, he was forced to work barefoot in soil. Over a 22-year period, progressive destruction of the pedal bones occurred.

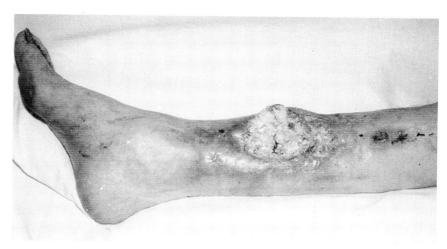

Figure 9 Right leg of a man with a 46-year history of a draining sinus from chronic osteomyelitis of the tibia. Biopsy of the mass revealed squamous cell carcinoma that had developed in the sinus. No enlarged inguinal nodes and no local or remote recurrence was found after short transtibial amputation.

biopsy of the sinus and infected bone must be carefully examined microscopically for evidence of squamous cell carcinoma (Figure 9). If the biopsy is positive, amputation above the level of tumor and excision of any suspicious lymph nodes will be necessary.

Necrotizing Fasciitis

Necrotizing fasciitis is a life-threatening, rapidly invasive bacterial infection of the subcutaneous tissue and fascia. It appears most commonly as a mixed aerobic and anaerobic infection or may be caused by group A streptococcus alone.[19] It is seen most commonly following a traumatic, surgical, or infectious break in the skin of an immunocompromised older person in association with diabetes mellitus, obesity, end-stage renal disease, cancer chemotherapy, critical limb ischemia, or use of immunosuppressive drugs for allografted organs.[20] High mortality rates (20% to 70%) from necrotizing fasciitis are related to delay in diagnosis as well as delay in definitive treatment (Figure 10). In its early stages, it is commonly confused with cellulitis, but necrotizing fasciitis does not respond to antibiotics within the first 48 hours as cellulitis should. Palpable crepitus due to gas formation is present and can be confirmed by radiographs showing gas in the soft tissues. As infection spreads, subcutaneous vessels are occluded and dermal gangrene ensues. The patient becomes progressively toxic, and diabetic patients may be-

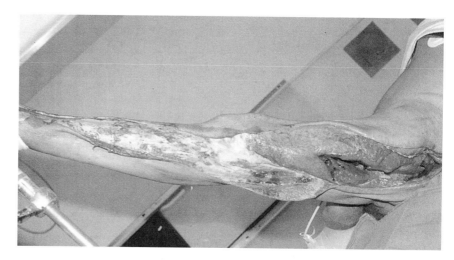

Figure 10 Left lower limb of a 68-year-old man with diabetes mellitus following extensile débridement of necrotizing fasciitis that followed internal fixation of a hip fracture 2 weeks earlier. The patient became comatose and died 48 hours after transfemoral amputation.

come ketotic as well. Elevated muscle compartment pressures, leading to a compartment syndrome, may be associated. Compartment pressure measurements, therefore, should be strongly considered.

Once the diagnosis is suspected, bedside biopsy and frozen section will provide a positive diagnosis. This is followed promptly by aggressive débridement, broad-spectrum antibiotic coverage, and adjunctive hyperbaric oxygen treatments.[21] The affected area should be excised widely in an extensile manner, as the infection often spreads from the limb to the trunk. The incision is extended to the point where a finger can no longer readily separate the skin and subcutaneous tissue from the investing fascia. The subcutaneous tissue will often have a gelatinous appearance. When the investing fascia is incised, a similar-appearing material may overlie the muscle. All of this material as well as the isolated fascia and any gangrenous involved skin must be excised. A repeat débridement should be done 1 to 2 days later to ensure that all infected tissue has been excised. Riseman and associates[22] reported on a nonrandomized series of patients with necrotizing fasciitis. Of 29 patients, 12 received débridement and antibiotics alone, and the remaining 17 received hyperbaric oxygen treatments in addition. Despite being much more ill on admission, those who received adjunctive hyperbaric oxygen therapy had only a 23% mortality rate compared with 66% of those treated with surgery and antibiotics alone. Also of interest, the hyperbaric group required an average of only 1.2 débridements versus 3.3 for the other cohort.[22] Based on this and other studies, the Undersea and Hyperbaric Medical Society strongly recommends the routine use of hyperbaric oxygen treatments as an adjunct to thorough débridement, repeated as needed, and specific antibiotic therapy.[23] Because few communities possess or are located near a hyperbaric center, the temptation exists to transfer the patient immediately. Nonetheless, supportive care provided by a skilled internist remains the third most important element of good treatment in this condition, after surgery and antibiotics. If these capabilities are present locally, it would be unwise, given the rapid course of this infection, to delay the prompt application of these basic measures by transfer of a critically ill patient long distances to a hyperbaric center. Even within centers with hyperbaric capabilities, physically coordinating these treatments in a safe manner for such unstable patients may not be possible. Although the limbs of surviving patients are usually salvaged, their function may be compromised by limited joint motion and loss of cutaneous sensation from skin grafts and scar, joint contractures from associated compartment syndrome, and paralysis from loss of muscle tissue. A customized orthosis may be beneficial in restoring walking function.[24]

Gas Gangrene

Progressive gas gangrene (clostridial myonecrosis) may sometimes be confused with necrotizing fasciitis in a se-

verely toxic patient. A major diagnostic difference, however, is that gas gangrene usually develops in a limb with devitalized tissue hours or days after a severe penetrating or crushing trauma. Infection spreads rapidly, producing gas and a brown exudate with progressive toxicity as the myonecrosis extends.[25] In most advanced cases, crepitus due to gas formation can be readily felt. Early exploration to confirm suspicion of gas gangrene is essential. Radiographs may demonstrate gas in muscle tissue, and the full extent of involvement can be defined by MRI and CT imaging. Thorough débridement of all necrotic tissue remains the keystone of treatment. Massive doses of penicillin are specific for clostridial infection, but a mixed flora may be present and require additional agents. Tetanus prophylaxis is given, and polyvalent gangrene antitoxin may be necessary. Hyperbaric oxygen therapy should be started immediately following débridement to prevent further myonecrosis. Holland and associates[26] reported on 49 patients with clostridial myonecrosis. In 33 (67%), this followed closure of wounds: elective surgery in 11, and early closure of trauma wounds in 22. This latter statistic emphasizes the importance of delayed closure of wounds resulting from trauma. The overall survival rate was 73.5%. Of 28 patients receiving at least five hyperbaric oxygen treatments, 24 (86%) survived. The amputation rate was 59.4%.[26]

Summary

The prevention of major lower limb amputation by salvage of all or most of the foot in patients with foot infections associated with diabetes mellitus has become a reality in recent years. Success in this endeavor depends on timely presentation of the patient and control of infection and hyperglycemia by a combination of early and complete débridement and appropriate antibiotics and insulin. When gangrene or poor healing is related to limb ischemia, a vascular surgeon should be consulted regarding the fea-

sibility of vessel recanalization or reconstruction. Once healing is achieved, the patient should be actively engaged in a program devoted to prevention of further lesions by the use of proper footwear, tight control of diabetes, and education in foot care with emphasis on assumption of responsibility for self-care. A similar approach to treatment applies to foot infections occurring in other conditions associated with loss of protective sensation. Necrotizing fasciitis and clostridial myositis/myonecrosis are two major life- and limb-threatening infections, the control of which depends heavily on thorough, repeated débridement of infected and necrotic soft tissue. Combined with appropriate antibiosis and hyperbaric oxygen therapy, débridement can avert amputation if diagnosis is early and treatment prompt.

Acknowledgment

The author wishes to express thanks to Ms. Patsy Bain for her expert preparation of this manuscript.

References

1. Reiber GE, Vileikyte L, Boyko EJ, et al: Causal pathways for incident lower extremity ulcers in patients from two settings. *Diabetes Care* 1999;22: 157-162.

2. Boulton AJM, Malik RA: Diabetic neuropathy. *Med Clin North Am* 1998; 82:909-929.

3. Yancey P, Brand P: *The Gift of Pain: Why We Hurt and What We Can Do About It*. Grand Rapids, MI, Zondervain Publishing House, 1997.

4. Calvet HM, Yoshikawa TT: Infection in diabetes. *Infect Dis Clin North Am* 2001;15:407-421.

5. Brodsky JW: An improved method for staging and classification of foot lesions in diabetic patients, in Bowker JH, Pfeifer MA (eds): *The Diabetic Foot*, ed 6. St Louis, MO, Mosby-Year Book, 2001, pp 273-282.

6. Grayson JL, Gibbons GW, Balogh K, et al: Probing to bone in infected pedal ulcers: A clinical sign of underlying

osteomyelitis in diabetic patients. *JAMA* 1995;273:721-723.

7. Lipsky BA: Evidence-based antibiotic therapy of diabetic foot infections. *FEMS Immunol Med Microbiol* 1999;26: 267-276.

8. Lipsky BA, Berendt AR: Principles and practice of antibiotic therapy of diabetic foot infections. *Diabetes Metab Res Rev* 2000;16(suppl 1):S42-S46.

9. Wang A, Weinstein D, Greenfield L, et al: MRI and diabetic foot infections. *Magn Reson Imaging* 1990;8:805-809.

10. Maurer AH, Millmond SH, Knight LC, et al: Infection in diabetic neuroarthropathy: Use of indium-111 labeled leukocytes for diagnosis. *Radiology* 1986;161:221-225.

11. Schon LC, Easley ME, Weinfeld SB: Charcot neuroarthropathy of the foot and ankle. *Clin Orthop* 1998;349: 116-131.

12. Beltran J, Campanini DS, Knight C, et al: The diabetic foot: Magnetic resonance imaging evaluation. *Skeletal Radiol* 1990;19:37-41.

13. Devendra D, Farmer K, Bruce G, et al: Diagnosing osteomyelitis in patients with diabetic neuropathic arthropathy. *Diabetes Care* 2001;24:2154-2155.

14. Dickhaut SC, DeLee JC, Page CP: Nutritional status: Importance in predicting wound healing after amputation. *J Bone Joint Surg Am* 1984;66:71-75.

15. Pinzur MS, Smith D, Osterman H: Syme ankle disarticulation in peripheral vascular disease and diabetic infection: The one-stage versus two-stage procedure. *Foot Ankle Int* 1995; 16:124-127.

16. Grodinsky M: A study of fascial spaces of the feet. *Surg Gynecol Obstet* 1929; 49:739-751.

17. Loeffler RD Jr, Ballard A: Plantar fascial spaces and a proposed surgical approach. *Foot Ankle* 1980;1:11-14.

18. Kritter AE: A technique for salvage of the infected diabetic foot. *Orthop Clin North Am* 1973;4:21-30.

19. Brook I, Frazier EH: Clinical and microbiological features of necrotizing fasciitis. *J Clin Microbiol* 1995;33:2382-2387.

20. Brandt M-M, Corpron CA, Wahl WL: Necrotizing soft tissue infections: A surgical disease. *Am Surg* 2000;66: 967-971.

21. Majeski J, Majeski E: Necrotizing fasciitis: Improved survival with early recognition by tissue biopsy and aggressive surgical treatment. *South Med J* 1997;90:1065-1069.

22. Riseman JA, Zamboni WA, Curtis A, et al: Hyperbaric oxygen therapy for necrotizing fasciitis reduces mortality and the need for debridements. *Surgery* 1990;108:847-850.

23. Hampson NB (ed): *Necrotizing Soft Tissue Infections. Hyperbaric Oxygen Therapy.* Committee Report, Undersea and Hyperbaric Medical Society, Kensington, MD,1999, pp 42-43.

24. Speers D, Shurr D: Necrotizing fasciitis: An overview. *J Prosthet Orthop* 2001;13:83-86.

25. Hart GB, Lamb RC, Strauss MB: Gas gangrene. *J Trauma* 1983;23:991-1000.

26. Holland JA, Hill GB, Wolfe WG, et al: Experimental and clinical experience with hyperbaric oxygen in the treatment of clostridial myonecrosis. *Surgery* 1975;77:75-85.

Chapter 5

Tumor: Limb Salvage Versus Amputation

Walid Mnaymneh, MD
H. Thomas Temple, MD

Introduction

Limb salvage for patients with bone and soft-tissue tumors is not a new concept; however, its widespread application was made possible by effective multiagent chemotherapy[1-8] and adjuvant radiation therapy[2,9-11] as well as improved diagnostic imaging and surgical advances in skeletal reconstruction. Studies have found local tumor control and overall patient survival rates are equivalent whether limb-sparing surgery or amputation is performed.[12-21] Requirements for successful limb-sparing surgery include adequate tumor resection, reconstruction of bone and soft-tissue defects, and restoration of function. If all of these goals of limb salvage cannot be achieved, amputation is necessary.

Tumor staging is a process that identifies the tumor type and its extent. It involves a thorough history and physical examination, careful interpretation of radiographic studies, and finally a biopsy. A multidisciplinary approach is critical in diagnosing and treating sarcomas and, ideally, should be implemented in an oncology center by a group of individuals dedicated to these rare cancers.[22] Treatment is dictated by tumor stage, which, in turn, is based on tumor type, size, location, and distant spread.[23-25] Prognosis is linked to tumor stage, and it is likely that future staging systems will also account for quantifiable measurements of tumor response to adjuvant treatment as well as the presence or absence of molecular markers expressed by tumor cells.

Biopsy errors are common, and possible adverse effects on the subsequent surgical treatment may preclude successful limb-saving surgery.[22] The incision for the biopsy should be longitudinal, not transverse, and should be placed in line with the planned incision for the definitive resection so that the entire field of the biopsy can be excised with the resected tumor. Deeper dissection should avoid intermuscular planes, joints, and major neurovascular structures. Direct bone biopsy should be avoided if possible to reduce risk of pathologic fracture, but if such a biopsy is necessary, it should be done through an oval or round cortical window. The intraosseous biopsy site may be plugged with methylmethacrylate cement to prevent spread of tumor cells to soft tissues from the resulting hematoma. Frozen section analysis of tissue removed in the biopsy is necessary to ensure that adequate material is available for diagnosis. In a multicenter study, Mankin and associates[22] reported significant problems in patient management caused by inappropriate biopsy technique in nearly 20% of patients. It was found that 8% of the biopsy procedures altered the prognosis adversely and that 4.5% of the patients who might have had a limb-saving procedure required an amputation as a result of an ill-planned biopsy. Moreover, errors in diagnosis occurred twice as often when the biopsy was done in a community hospital rather than an oncologic center. Hence, it is recommended that patients be transferred to a specialty center before the biopsy, not after.

The surgical staging system that has been adopted by the Musculoskeletal Tumor Society[23-25] applies to

TABLE 1 Staging of Malignant Tumors

Stage	Grade	Compartment	Metastases*
IA	low	intracompartmental	none
IB	low	extracompartmental	none
IIA	high	intracompartmental	none
IIB	high	extracompartmental	none
III	any	any	present

*Metastases to other organs and lymph nodes; skip metastases in bone

bone as well as soft-tissue tumors. It separates benign tumors into three stages: stage 1 (latent), stage 2 (active), and stage 3 (aggressive). Malignant tumors are stratified into three stages based on grade, compartment location, and the presence or absence of metastases (Table 1).

Treatment depends on tumor characteristics such as type and grade. For example, patients with high-grade, chemotherapy-sensitive bone tumors, such as osteosarcoma and Ewing's sarcoma, are treated with adjuvant chemotherapy,[2,3,5-7] whereas patients with chondrosarcomas and low-grade sarcomas of bone require only surgery. A similar strategy is followed in soft-tissue tumors: high-grade soft-tissue sarcomas are treated preoperatively with either chemotherapy,[13,14] radiation therapy,[9-11] or both[2]; however, patients with low-grade soft-tissue sarcomas generally are not given chemotherapy, and any requirement for radiation therapy is based on the adequacy of tumor margins. Definitive surgical treatment is then performed, consisting of resection with limb preservation if feasible, or amputation. A notable exception is fibromatosis, a benign but aggressive disease that can be treated with chemotherapy or radiation therapy alone or in conjunction with surgery.[26,27]

The beneficial effect of preoperative chemotherapy is reflected by the degree of tumor necrosis seen in histologic specimens from the resected tumor.[5,6] The degree of necrosis is significant to the prognosis and is helpful in selecting the postoperative chemotherapeutic regimen. An additional advantage of preoperative chemotherapy is the possible reduction of tumor size, decrease in perilesional edema, and containment of the tumor in a well-defined pseudocapsule. Sometimes the effects of chemotherapy on the tumor are dramatic and improve the prospect of successful limb salvage and survival. Postoperative chemotherapy, radiation therapy, or both are usually administered, depending on the type of tumor and the surgical procedure performed.

Surgical Treatment

The ultimate goal of treatment of patients with limb sarcomas should be to maximize the patient's survival by minimizing the risks of metastasis and local recurrence. Thus, the importance of complete tumor resection cannot be overemphasized. The advantages of limb salvage versus amputation in the lower limb are the preservation of a sensate plantigrade foot and more energy-efficient ambulation, a factor that becomes increasingly important with advanced age and more proximal levels of skeletal resection. Other important factors include the psychological impact of the surgical treatment in terms of the resultant body image, quality of life, and the anticipated function of the limb. In the upper limb, the main advantage of limb-sparing surgery is superior function with a sensate hand and opposable thumb; other advantages are improved cosmesis and self-image.

Amputation is associated with fewer surgical complications, shorter hospital stays, and better functional restoration for patients with tumors below the knee. Although the initial cost of limb salvage is high, the cost of amputation is considerable over the lifetime of an amputee because multiple prosthetic devices will be required as a result of wear and tear and inevitable changes in the size and contour of the residual limb.

Recently, some researchers have examined the true advantages of limb-saving procedures over amputations with regard to psychological and quality-of-life parameters. Sugarbaker and associates[28] and Weddington and associates[29] found no significant difference between patients who underwent amputations and those who had limb-saving procedures. Otis and associates[30] showed that patients whose limbs were salvaged by knee arthroplasty walked at a higher velocity and a lower net energy expenditure than patients who had transfemoral amputations. In contrast, Harris and associates[31] compared groups of patients with distal femoral resections who underwent three different procedures: amputation, arthrodesis, and arthroplasty. A fourth group of healthy control subjects was compared with the study group patients. The authors found that, for this level of resection, all three groups walked at comparable energy efficiency at three different velocities and that energy consumption was not significantly different than that of the normal control subjects. Patients who underwent amputation were very active but had difficulty walking on uneven surfaces. Patients with arthrodeses had more stable limbs and performed the most demanding physical activity but had trouble sitting. Patients with arthroplasty led sedentary lives and were the most protective of the limb but were the least self-conscious.[31] Moreover, there was no significant difference in psychological functioning among the studied groups.

Obviously, further comparative studies that consider the level of amputation, age, premorbid functional status, and response to adjuvant therapy and that use more sensitive measurements of gait and function are needed to resolve whether amputation or limb salvage is more appropriate.

We believe that limb-sparing procedures are superior to more proximal amputations around the hip and shoulder where body image and function are severely affected, energy costs of ambulation are higher, and prosthetic fitting is more difficult. Conversely, patients with large and high-grade tumors below the knee may be better served by amputation and early prosthetic fitting because in these patients energy costs are low, prosthetic fitting is relatively easy, and function is superior to that after most limb-saving procedures.

Indications for Limb-Saving Procedures

Conceptually, limb-saving procedures are indicated if all of the following criteria are deemed attainable: (1) an

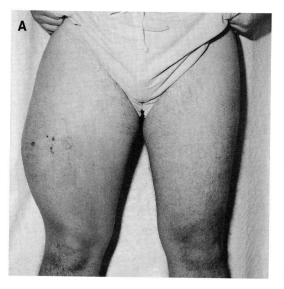
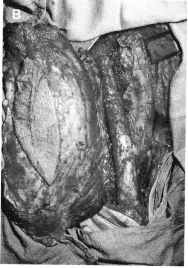
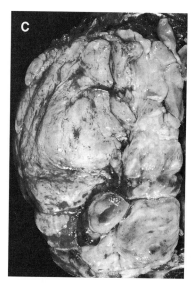

Figure 1   A 50-year-old man presented with a large liposarcoma involving the quadriceps muscle compartment of the right thigh. **A,** Preoperative photograph. **B,** Intraoperative photograph shows wide resection of the entire quadriceps compartment. Note the biopsy site that was removed with the specimen and the bare anterior surface of the femur. **C,** Cut section of the resected specimen.

oncologically adequate resection of the tumor can be achieved; (2) limb reconstruction is technically feasible; and (3) the cosmetic and functional results are anticipated to be superior to those of an amputation, with consideration given to the patient's lifestyle and occupational and recreational demands. The ultimate goal is not merely salvaging the limb but reconstructing a functional and cosmetically acceptable limb. If any of these goals is not attainable, amputation is the preferred option.

Tumors that lend themselves to limb-saving procedures include malignant tumors and some recurrent aggressive benign tumors (stage 3). Obviously, early diagnosis is important for successful limb salvage because delays in diagnosis lead to increased tumor size, making limb salvage more difficult.

Limb-saving procedures are technically more complex than amputations and result in more surgical complications and subsequent procedures. For patients with bone tumors, two major surgical procedures are necessary: one to resect the tumor and another to reconstruct the defect and to provide durable soft-tissue coverage. Patients with soft-tissue tumors often require muscle transfers to fill large dead spaces and occasionally require bone, joint, and vascular reconstruction for extensive tumors that efface or invade these structures.

Tumor Resection

Malignant and aggressive benign musculoskeletal tumors should be resected according to strict oncologic surgical principles. The recommended procedure for malignant tumors is either radical or, more frequently, wide resection of the tumor.[24] Radical resection involves removal of an entire compartment; the entire bone, including the joint above and below; or the entire muscle compartment, including muscle origins and insertions. Wide excisions involve resections outside of the reactive zone or tumor pseudocapsule. It is unclear how much healthy tissue around the tumor must be removed to constitute an adequate resection. The type of tissue is also important in assessing the adequacy of the margin of resection. For example, fascia is an effective barrier to tumor extension, but fat and muscle fibers are relatively poor barriers (Figure 1). Most orthopaedic oncologists now accept the idea that wide margins are adequate to achieve local disease control and

advocate wide resection with adjuvant chemotherapy and radiation therapy for most high-grade tumors. The need for an adequate resection cannot be overemphasized because close and positive margins of resection are believed to be associated with local recurrence, which in patients with high-grade malignant bone tumors often is associated with distant metastases and death from disease.[32]

Tumor resectability is determined by the intraosseous and extraosseous extent of the tumor as based on radiologic staging studies. Previous biopsy scars are excised along with the underlying tumor. The resected bone should include a margin of healthy bone ranging from 3 to 5 cm beyond the intraosseous tumor extent. For epiphyseal or metaphyseal tumors, an intra-articular resection including the articular surface is necessary. If the tumor extends into the joint, an extra-articular resection including the whole joint is necessary. In all cases, a cuff of soft tissues around the bone is also resected.

Displacement or frank invasion of adjacent neurovascular structures is not an absolute contraindication to resection, ie, an indication for amputation. If a major vessel is compressed but not directly involved by the tu-

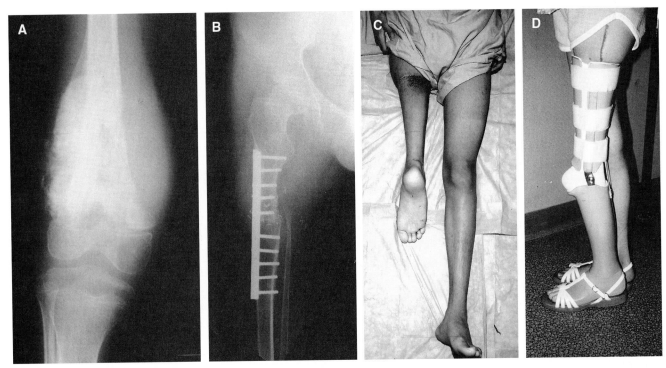

Figure 2 A 15-year-old boy presented with an osteosarcoma of the right distal femur. **A,** Preoperative radiograph. **B,** Radiograph taken 4 months after wide resection of the distal femur and the knee joint followed by tibial rotationplasty shows fixation of the ti-biofemoral junction with a plate and screws. **C,** Appearance of the lower limbs after the rotationplasty. The patient is lying supine with his right foot pointing backward. **D,** Another patient wearing a prosthesis designed for rotationplasty, which provides a special socket for the foot. The patient is fully functional and ambulates without support.

mor, a careful subadventitial dissection is performed to preserve the vessel. Under certain circumstances, a vessel directly invaded or circumferentially surrounded by tumor can be resected with the tumor specimen and replaced by a reverse vein or synthetic graft. If necessary, major nerves invaded by tumor may be resected. In the upper limb, protective sensation can be restored with nerve grafts, and motor function can be restored with appropriate tendon transfers. Sciatic nerve deficits in the lower limb are debilitating but can be partly compensated for by well-fitting orthoses and assistive ambulatory devices.

The surgeon and pathologist should inspect the resected tumor together to identify areas in which tumor appears to be surrounded by scant healthy soft tissue. These areas should be inked and examined microscopically to confirm the absence of tumor at the margin. If tumor is seen, more tissue from the involved area should be excised and reexamined

microscopically to ensure the absence of tumor.

Skeletal Reconstruction

Skeletal reconstruction following tumor resection constitutes the second stage of the surgical procedure. The type of reconstruction is determined preoperatively. However, in most cases where expendable or nonessential bones are resected, no reconstruction is needed to preserve function. The scapula (except the glenoid portion), clavicle, rib, proximal part of the radius, distal end of the ulna, metacarpal, phalanx, ischium, pubis, patella, fibula, and metatarsal bone can be resected with minimal disturbance of function. However, for nondispensable or essential bones, skeletal reconstruction is necessary to preserve the limb and its function.

Rotationplasty is an alternative to high transfemoral amputation in skel-

etally immature patients with large tumors around the knee. It involves an extra-articular resection of the knee joint in addition to the lower part of the femur and upper part of the tibia. The lower limb is then rotated 180°, and the vessels and nerves are coiled medially. If the vessels have to be removed with the tumor, anastomosis should be performed. Osteosynthesis of the distal femoral shaft to the residual tibial shaft in proximal tibial tumors is performed using a plate and screws. The ankle joint should be placed at or just below the level of the contralateral knee joint, depending on how much growth remains in the normal limb, so that the knee joints are at the same level after skeletal maturity. A special prosthesis is constructed to take advantage of the mobile ankle to restore knee function (Figure 2). The patient and parents must be counseled preoperatively because the appearance of the lower limb following surgery may be disturbing and cause significant psychological problems. This is, however, a durable, oncologically sound, and highly functional reconstruction.

The choice of a particular reconstructive procedure depends on the tumor location, the size of the postresection defect, anticipated patient survival, perioperative use of cytotoxic drugs, patient lifestyle and occupation, social and financial considerations, and the surgeon's preference and expertise. There are three major methods of skeletal reconstruction: (1) intercalary (segmental) reconstruction, (2) arthrodesis, and (3) arthroplasty. By and large, the commonly used constructs for these reconstructive methods include autografts, allografts, and metal prostheses.

Intercalary reconstruction, which is needed after diaphyseal resection, uses allografts, autografts (vascularized and nonvascularized), and, rarely, metallic prostheses. Arthrodesis, used to reconstruct the limb after extra-articular resection of a joint such as the knee, shoulder, or wrist, also uses allografts, autografts, or, rarely, metal prostheses. Arthroplasty, used to replace a resected hemijoint or whole joint with an articulating joint surface such as the knee, hip, shoulder, elbow, or wrist, uses allografts, metallic prostheses, or allograft-prosthesis composites.

Autografts are desirable bone substitutes because they incorporate more readily than allografts and, once incorporated, do not loosen over time like metal implants. However, their use is limited because autografts cannot replace large bone segments, are associated with donor site morbidity, and offer only limited articular joint surfaces (eg, proximal fibula articular cartilage for distal radius reconstruction). Vascularized and nonvascularized autografts can be used for radiocarpal (Figure 3) and tibiotalar arthrodeses following tumor resection. Two other surgical techniques that use large autografts can be applied in selected patients. One is resection-arthrodesis of the knee.[33,34] Following wide resection of the prox-

imal third of the tibia or distal part of the femur, arthrodesis of the knee is achieved by inserting a long intramedullary nail and bridging the resection defect with a combined construct made up of the ipsilateral fibula and half of the proximal end of the tibia (to replace a resected distal femur) or half of the distal part of the femur (to replace a resected proximal tibia). When successful, this technique results in a stable, pain-free, and functional reconstruction. However, most patients prefer to have a movable rather than a fused knee. The other surgical technique is the use of a vascularized free fibular autograft as an intercalary graft to reconstruct a diaphyseal defect.[35] The healing potential is greatly improved over that of an avascular fibular allograft because it is similar to fracture healing. The graft is more readily incorporated, heals more rapidly following fracture, and can remodel and hypertrophy with time.

In contrast to autografts, both allografts and prostheses can replace large segments of bones and provide movable joints. Conceptually, allografts have certain advantages over metal prostheses.[36-39] These advantages are related to the biologic nature of the allograft, which allows healing at the graft-host junction by a process of creeping substitution, and the presence of soft-tissue attachments that serve as anchors to which host tendons and ligaments can be reattached,

thus restoring critical motor function and joint kinematics. Moreover, an osteoarticular allograft replaces only the involved half (or quarter) of the joint, thus sparing the uninvolved normal portions of the joint, whereas a joint prosthesis requires removal of the normal uninvolved half of the joint to accommodate the prosthesis. Joint preservation in whole or part may result in improved proprioception that may translate into improved long-term function. Finally, bone substrate on which future reconstructions can be based is retained.

Widespread allograft use is mitigated in part by limited availability, potential risk of virally transmitted disease,[40] inconsistent healing, fracture,[41] and a relatively high risk of infection.[42,43] Limb-saving reconstructive procedures using massive allografts are often complex and lengthy procedures with relatively high rates of complications. Hornicek and associates[44] reported 72% satisfactory overall results in 840 patients treated at the Massachusetts General Hospital. Major complications included fractures in 19%, nonunion in 18%, infection in 12%, and joint instability in 5% of the patients. Some of the patients had more than one complication. Forty-seven percent of the patients required additional surgery, and most complications occurred within the first 2 years postoperatively. These data are similar to our

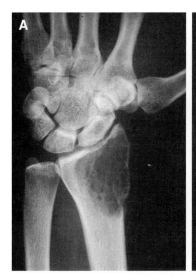
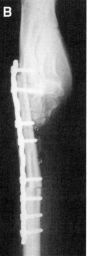

Figure 3 A 44-year-old woman presented with a stage 3 giant cell tumor of the distal radius. The tumor extended into the radiocarpal joint. **A,** Preoperative radiograph. **B,** Radiograph taken 4 months after wide resection of the distal radius and reconstruction using a vascularized ipsilateral fibular autograft. The graft healed completely and the patient resumed her work as a secretary.

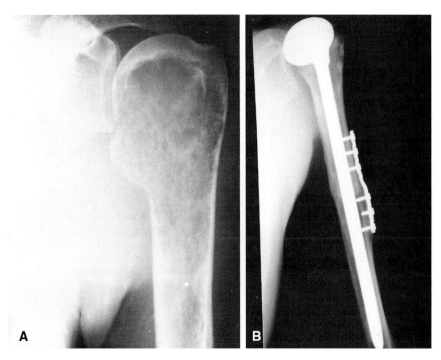

Figure 4 A 25-year-old man presented with a large giant cell tumor of the proximal humerus. **A,** Preoperative radiograph. **B,** Radiograph taken 5 years after wide resection of the proximal humerus and reconstruction using a humeral allograft-prosthesis composite shows that the host-graft junction is completely healed. The patient was doing well 14 years postoperatively, working as a carpenter. *(Reproduced with permission from Mnaymneh W, Malinin T: Massive allografts in surgery of bone tumors.* Orthop Clin North Am *1989;20:455-467.)*

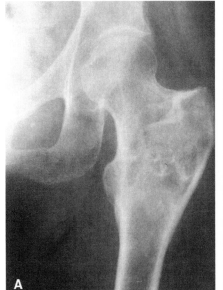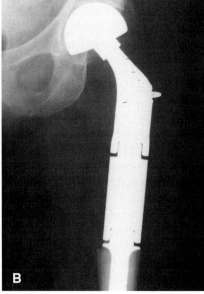

Figure 5 A 73-year-old woman presented with a chondrosarcoma of the proximal femur. **A,** Preoperative radiograph. **B,** Radiograph taken 3 years after wide resection of the proximal femur and reconstruction with a modular oncologic proximal femoral prosthesis.

own. Moreover, several of the complications of allograft use could be salvaged by subsequent surgery, such as adding an autograft to a fractured or nonunified allograft, replacing a fractured allograft with a new allograft, or using a metal prosthesis. We believe that the incidence of complications can be significantly reduced with meticulous surgical techniques, proper preoperative planning, and good postoperative management.

The advantages of reconstruction using metal prostheses include an easier surgical procedure with fewer complications, especially fracture; more rapid recovery; and easier rehabilitation in contrast to the long rehabilitation following reconstruction with an allograft. Improved metallurgy, rotating-hinge designs, improved cement technique, and modularity are factors that have improved outcomes in patients undergoing reconstruction with metal prostheses. In the largest series of patients receiving metal implants following tumor resection, Unwin and associates[45] reported survival of 32.6% of prostheses in patients with distal femoral replacement and 6.2% in patients with proximal femoral reconstruction at a mean follow-up of 120 months. Longer resections resulted in worse outcomes in patients undergoing distal femoral replacement. In addition, younger patients had a higher rate of aseptic loosening, the most common problem in patients undergoing reconstruction with metal prostheses. Malawer and Chou[46] reported survival of prostheses in 83% of all patients undergoing segmental reconstruction at 5 years of follow-up and 67% at 10 years. No differences in 5- and 10-year survival rates were seen on comparison of sex, age, or diagnosis. However, prosthetic reconstruction of the proximal part of the tibia had the worst survival rates. Wirganowicz and associates[47] reported that reconstructions in which custom endoprostheses were used to replace tumors failed in 64 of 278 patients (23%) with 2-year minimum followup. For patients with endoprosthetic failures, aseptic loosening and fatigue fracture were the most common causes of failure, occurring in 44% and 16% of patients, respectively.

Although we generally favor allografts, we prefer to use metal prostheses in conjunction with intercalary allografts (allograft-prosthesis composite) in lieu of osteoarticular allografts to replace the proximal femur and the proximal humerus (Figure 4) because, in our experience, there has been an unacceptably high incidence of fragmentation and collapse of the allograft femoral and humeral heads.[36,38] We use prostheses in older patients with high-grade tumors and relatively short life expectancies (Figure 5) as well as in patients with metastatic tumors that cause significant bone and periarticular destruction. We also prefer reconstruction with metal prostheses in patients requiring resection of the entire bone including the joints above and below.

To help solve some of the problems encountered with customized prostheses,[48-50] such as fracture, loosening, need of customized implants, improper size, and high cost, new modular segmental defect replacement prostheses have been developed for the proximal and distal ends of the femur (Figure 6) and proximal parts of the tibia and humerus. This system depends on dual fixation, with initial fixation of the solid intramedullary stem by methylmethacrylate bone cement and long-term fixation by extracortical bone bridging and ingrowth over the porous shoulder region of the segmental prosthesis.[48,50] The bone bridging around the prosthesis is accomplished by applying autogenous iliac grafts over the porous segment. Bone grafting at the prosthesis-bone junction is believed to transmit forces from the body of the prosthesis through cortical bone instead of the stem. The grafting also creates a biologic envelope that theoretically impedes the ingress into the bone-cement interface of wear debris that may be partly responsible for aseptic loosening. Initial clinical results seem to be promising.

Expandable metal prostheses have been successfully used in children with malignant limb tumors.[51,52] Previously, when epiphyseal growth plates of long bones had to be removed with the resected tumor in young children, limb salvage was not

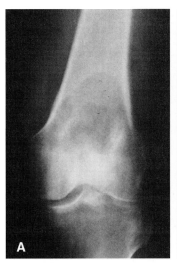 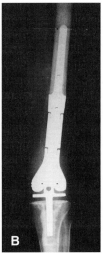 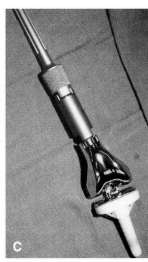

Figure 6 A 61-year-old man presented with a leiomyosarcoma of the distal femur. **A,** Preoperative radiograph. **B,** Radiograph taken after wide resection of the distal femur shows that the defect was reconstructed using a modular oncologic rotating-hinge distal femoral prosthesis. The patient was doing well 5 years postoperatively. **C,** A photograph of the prosthesis used (Manufactured by Howmedica, East Rutherford, NJ).

recommended because of the expected significant shortening of the limb. These expandable prostheses can be lengthened periodically to gradually keep up with the growth of the contralateral limb.

Allograft Procedures

We have used four types of allografts in procedures to reconstruct large skeletal defects in bone tumors. These are massive osteoarticular allografts, allograft-prosthesis composites, intercalary allografts, and intercalary allograft-arthrodesis. The indication for each of these allografts is dictated by the skeletal location and extent of tumor resection. Sterilely harvested osteoarticular allografts that are glycerol-treated and frozen are used most commonly. They are usually used as hemijoints to reconstruct the knee, wrist, shoulder, and elbow joints. Whole-joint allografts have proved unsatisfactory because of articular cartilage degeneration and bone fragmentation reminiscent of Charcot (neuropathic) joints.[53,54] Intercalary allografts are either frozen or freeze-dried and are used to reconstruct diaphyseal defects, to achieve arthrodesis following knee or shoulder joint resection, or as allograft-

prosthesis composites to reconstruct the hip or shoulder joints.

Allograft reconstructions are often complex and lengthy. Technical factors that improve surgical outcomes include size matching of the graft to the resected segment; rigid fixation of the graft-host junction; congruent joint fit; reconstruction of ligaments, tendons, and joint capsule; and adequate skin and soft-tissue coverage by using, if necessary, local muscle transfers, skin grafts, or free flaps. The following are examples of allograft reconstruction of the limbs.

Scapula

The whole scapula or the functionally important glenoid and neck portion can be replaced by a scapular allograft with satisfactory cosmetic and functional results.[55]

Humerus

The proximal two thirds of the humerus can be successfully replaced by an osteoarticular allograft. However, we have observed a relatively high incidence of late fracture or fragmentation of the humeral head.[38,39] This has not been a problem with distal humeral allografts. Accordingly, we now recommend using an allograft-prosthesis composite consisting of a

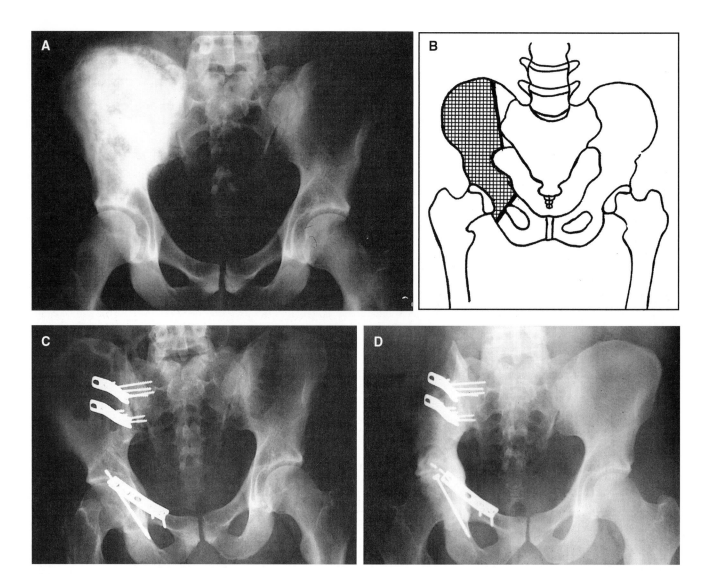

Figure 7 A 23-year-old man presented with a large chondrosarcoma of the ilium. **A,** Preoperative radiograph. **B,** Drawing showing the internal hemipelvectomy resection (shaded area). **C,** Postoperative radiograph showing the pelvic reconstruction using a pelvic allograft that included the ilium and acetabulum. Internal fixation of the allograft, using plates and screws for the ilium and pubis as well as a long lag screw for the ischial host-graft junction. **D,** Radiograph taken 12 years postoperatively shows complete healing of the host-graft junction. Note the partial resorption of the graft iliac crest and the narrowing of the hip joint space. The patient ambulates with no support. *(Reproduced with permission from Mnaymneh W, Malinin T, Mnaymneh LG, Robinson D: Pelvic allograft: A case report with a follow up evaluation of 5.5 years.* Clin Orthop *1990;255:128-132.)*

long-stem endoprosthesis combined with an intercalary humeral allograft to replace the proximal end of the humerus (Figure 4). When evaluation necessitates resection of the whole glenohumeral joint or resection of the deltoid muscle and rotator cuff, we recommend an allograft-arthrodesis using a proximal humeral allograft with fusion to the scapula.

Radius

The distal end of the radius can be replaced by a size-matched osteoarticu-lar allograft that is fixed to the host radius by a dorsally placed compression plate. We have observed a late complication of volar subluxation of the carpus on the allograft radius with progressive degenerative changes in the radiocarpal articulation. To prevent this complication, we use a contralateral distal radius allograft (right graft in left arm or vice versa) and then rotate it 180° on the longitudinal axis. By rotating the allograft, the normally long dorsal lip of the articular surface of the radius becomes volar, thus acting as a buttress against volar subluxation of the carpus.

Pelvis

In selected patients with tumors of the bony pelvis, a partial or complete internal hemipelvectomy can be as effective as a conventional transpelvic amputation. However, this procedure produces significant disability in terms of loss of hip function and stability. We favor the use of a massive pelvic osteoarticular allograft to replace the resected hemipelvis. When

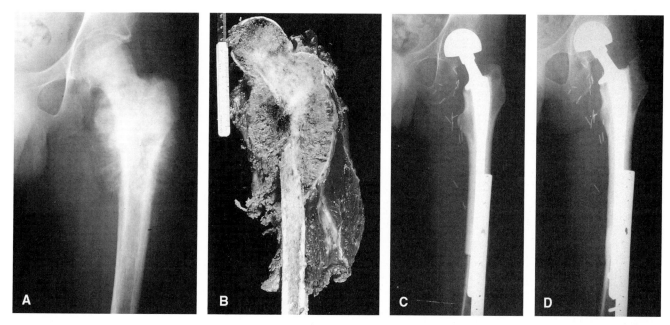

Figure 8   A 16-year-old boy presented with an osteosarcoma of the proximal femur. **A,** Preoperative radiograph. **B,** A coronal section of the resected proximal femur shows the bone destruction by the tumor and the large extraosseous tumor mass. **C,** Postoperative radiograph after wide resection of the proximal femur and reconstruction with allograft-prosthesis composite. The long-stem prosthesis was cemented to the allograft but not to the patient's femur. The host-graft junction was fixed with a plate and screws. **D,** Radiograph taken 2 years postoperatively shows complete healing of the host-graft junction.

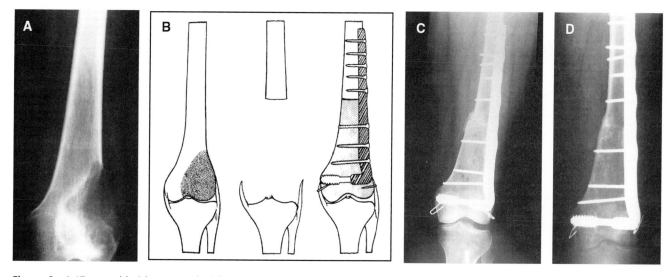

Figure 9   A 17-year-old girl presented with a twice-recurrent giant cell tumor of the distal femur. **A,** Radiograph shows tumor at second recurrence. **B,** Drawing illustrating the wide resection of the distal femur and reconstruction using a distal femoral osteoarticular allograft. **C,** Radiograph taken 6 months postoperatively shows the healing callus over the host-graft junction. **D,** Radiograph taken 12 years postoperatively shows complete healing of the host-graft junction and preservation of the knee joint space. The patient was still doing well 22 years postoperatively. *(Reproduced with permission from Mnaymneh W, Malinin T, Lackman RD, Hornicek FL, Ghandur-Mnaymneh L: Massive distal femoral osteoarticular allografts after resection of bone tumors. Clin Orthop 1994;303:103-115.)*

successful, the pelvic allograft restores anatomy, stability, function, and limb length[56] (Figure 7). This procedure is associated with many complications including neurovascular injury, hemorrhage, infection, hip dislocation, and fracture.[57,58] If the femoral head and neck have to be included in the resection, a bipolar femoral prosthesis is used rather than a proximal femoral allograft.

Femur

In the proximal end of the femur, we favor the use of a proximal femoral allograft combined with a long-stem femoral prosthesis instead of an osteoarticular allograft (Figure 8). This allograft-prosthesis composite is stable and provides a good osseous bed for reattaching tendons.

In the distal third of the femur, osteoarticular allografts have often re-

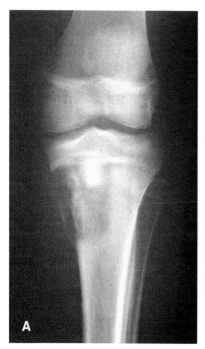
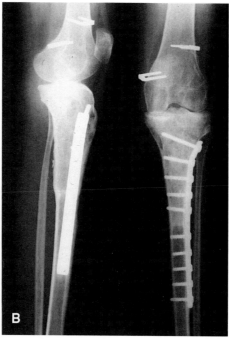

Figure 10 An 18-year-old man presented with an osteosarcoma of the proximal tibia. **A,** Preoperative radiograph. **B,** Radiograph taken 3 years after wide resection of the proximal tibia and reconstruction using a proximal tibial osteoarticular allograft. The host-graft junction has healed completely.

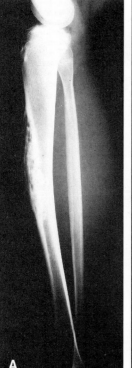
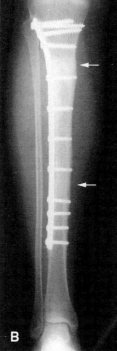

Figure 11 A 14-year-old girl presented with an adamantinoma of the tibial diaphysis. **A,** Preoperative radiograph. **B,** Radiograph taken 4 years after wide resection of the tumorous segment of the tibial diaphysis and reconstruction using an intercalary tibial allograft that was fixed with a long plate and screws. Arrows indicate the completely healed proximal and distal host-graft junctions.

repair are critical. The remnants of the allograft collateral and cruciate ligaments are sutured to the corresponding remnants of the patient's ligaments. In the absence of these attachments, we have reconstructed the ligaments by using a hemi-Achilles tendon allograft.[37,38] Repair of the posterior cruciate ligament along with reconstruction of the anterior cruciate ligament using a tibial bone tunnel and over-the-top technique has resulted in superior stability and function in our patients.

When the whole knee joint has to be resected, we have successfully used distal femoral and proximal tibial allograft-prosthesis composites with a rotating hinged-knee prosthesis. For extra-articular resections in which the extensor mechanism can be saved, however, metal prosthetic reconstruction is an easier alternative.

Tibia

Proximal tibial osteoarticular allografts have been used successfully (Figure 10). Ligament reconstruction of the joint is similar to that used with the distal femoral allograft. The detached patellar tendon is sutured to the stub of the patellar tendon of the allograft. To avoid the risk of wound dehiscence and infection resulting from scarcity of skin and soft tissues on the anterior surface of the tibial allograft, it is highly recommended to transpose the medial or lateral head of the gastrocnemius muscle anteriorly to cover the anterior surface of the graft. The transposed muscle is then covered with a skin graft. Although patients with proximal tibial allograft reconstruction have a relatively high risk of fracture compared with patients with metal reconstruction, they have better extensor function and improved gait mechanics. Diaphyseal tumors can be resected preserving the knee and ankle joints, and the defect is reconstructed with an intercalary tibial allograft (Figure 11).

sulted in acceptable and durable function. The entire distal femur (Figure 9) or one femoral condyle can be re-

placed. To restore joint stability and function, size matching of the allograft, joint fit, and ligamentous

Postoperative Management

Because of the increased risk of infection, antibiotic treatment is continued postoperatively for about 3 months; parenteral antibiotics are given perioperatively and oral antibiotics on discharge. There is no scientific evidence, however, that prolonged antibiotic coverage in these patients decreases the risk of infection. Decreased surgery time and blood loss, perioperative antibiotics, and adequate soft-tissue coverage are probably more important in preventing infection than long-term oral antibiotic therapy. The operating surgeon should pay close attention to the source of the grafts and the methods by which they are harvested and processed.

In proximal femoral allograft-prosthesis composites, the patient walks by using an abduction hip brace and crutches for 2 to 3 months, followed by a crutch or a cane.

For patients with allograft reconstructions about the knee, we immobilize the limb in a long leg plaster cast for 8 weeks to allow soft-tissue and ligament healing. This is followed by protection of the limb in a knee-ankle-foot orthosis and gradual mobilization of the knee joint. The orthosis is used until evidence of union at the allograft-host junction is seen on radiographs. The patient uses crutches to avoid weight bearing on the affected leg until early signs of union are evident.

In patients with proximal humeral allograft reconstruction, a shoulder abduction splint is used for 6 weeks, followed by protection in a sling and gradual mobilization of the shoulder joint. Patients with distal radial allograft reconstruction have the forearm immobilized in a short arm plaster cast for 6 to 8 weeks, followed by protection in a volar splint and gradual mobilization of the wrist joint.

Conclusion

Despite potential complications, the biologic advantages of allografts, including the presence of soft-tissue attachments and their versatility (either alone or in combination with metal prostheses), make them useful for limb-salvage procedures following wide resections of bone tumors. Recent improvements in metallurgy and prosthetic design have led to increased use of oncologic megaprostheses. No single reconstructive procedure is optimal for all situations. The orthopaedic oncologist must be familiar with all aspects of limb salvage because the biology and location of the tumor, as well as patient desires, age, and comorbid conditions must be taken into consideration to ensure optimal outcomes.

References

1. Gherlinzoni F, Bacci G, Picci P, et al: A randomized trial for the treatment of high-grade soft-tissue sarcomas of the extremities: Preliminary observations. *J Clin Oncol* 1986;4:552-558.

2. Goodnight JE Jr, Bargar WL, Voegeli T, Blaisdell FW: Limb-sparing surgery for extremity sarcomas after preoperative intraarterial doxorubicin and radiation therapy. *Am J Surg* 1985;150:109-113.

3. Jaffe N: Chemotherapy for malignant bone tumors. *Orthop Clin North Am* 1989;20:487-503.

4. Link MP, Goorin AM, Miser AW, et al: The effect of adjuvant chemotherapy on relapse-free survival in patients with osteosarcoma of the extremity. *N Engl J Med* 1986;314:1600-1606.

5. Rosen G: Preoperative (neoadjuvant) chemotherapy for osteogenic sarcoma: A ten year experience. *Orthopedics* 1985;8:659-664.

6. Rosen G, Caparros B, Huvos AG: Preoperative chemotherapy for osteogenic sarcoma: Selection of postoperative adjuvant chemotherapy based on the response of the primary tumor to preoperative chemotherapy. *Cancer* 1982;49:1221-1230.

7. Rosen G, Marcove RC, Huvos AG, et al: Primary osteogenic sarcoma: Eight-year experience with adjuvant chemo-

therapy. *J Cancer Res Clin Oncol* 1983;106(suppl):55-67.

8. Weiner MA, Harris MB, Lewis M, et al: Neoadjuvant high-dose methotrexate, cisplatin, and doxorubicin for the management of patients with nonmetastatic osteosarcoma. *Cancer Treat Rep* 1986;70:1431-1432.

9. Lindberg RD, Martin RG, Romsdahl MM, Barkley HT Jr: Conservative surgery and postoperative radiotherapy in 300 adults with soft-tissue sarcomas. *Cancer* 1981;47:2391-2397.

10. Rosenberg SA, Tepper J, Glatstein E, et al: The treatment of soft-tissue sarcomas of the extremities: Prospective randomized evaluations of (1) limb-sparing surgery plus radiation therapy compared with amputation and (2) the role of adjuvant chemotherapy. *Ann Surg* 1982;196:305-315.

11. Suit HD, Proppe KH, Mankin HJ, Wood WC: Preoperative radiation therapy for sarcoma of soft tissue. *Cancer* 1981;47:2269-2274.

12. Eckardt JJ, Eilber FR, Dorey FJ, Mirra JM: The UCLA experience in limb salvage surgery for malignant tumors. *Orthopedics* 1985;8:612-621.

13. Eilber FR, Mirra JJ, Grant TT, Weisenburger T, Morton DL: Is amputation necessary for sarcomas? A seven-year experience with limb salvage. *Ann Surg* 1980;192:431-438.

14. Eilber FR, Morton DL, Eckardt J, Grant T, Weisenburger T: Limb salvage for skeletal and soft tissue sarcomas: Multidisciplinary preoperative therapy. *Cancer* 1984;53:2579-2584.

15. Malawer M: Surgical technique and results of limb sparing surgery for high grade bone sarcomas of the knee and shoulder. *Orthopedics* 1985;8:597-607.

16. Rao BN, Champion JE, Pratt CB, et al: Limb salvage procedures for children with osteosarcoma: An alternative to amputation. *J Pediatr Surg* 1983;18:901-908.

17. Potter DA, Kinsella T, Glatstein E, et al: High-grade soft tissue sarcomas of the extremities. *Cancer* 1986;58:190-205.

18. Shiu MH, Turnbull AD, Nori D, Hajdu S, Hilaris B: Control of locally advanced extremity soft tissue sarcomas by function-saving resection and brachytherapy. *Cancer* 1984;53:1385-1392.

19. Sim FH, Beauchamp CP, Chao EY: Reconstruction of musculoskeletal defects about the knee for tumor. *Clin Orthop* 1987;221:188-201.

20. Sim FH, Bowman WE Jr, Wilkins RM, Chao EY: Limb salvage in primary malignant bone tumors. *Orthopedics* 1985;8:574-581.

21. Simon MA, Aschliman MA, Thomas N, Mankin HJ: Limb-salvage treatment versus amputation for osteosarcoma of the distal end of the femur. *J Bone Joint Surg Am* 1986;68:1331-1337.

22. Mankin HJ, Lange TA, Spanier SS: The hazards of biopsy in patients with malignant primary bone and soft-tissue tumors. *J Bone Joint Surg Am* 1982;64:1121-1127.

23. Enneking WF: A system of staging musculoskeletal neoplasms. *Clin Orthop* 1986;204:9-24.

24. Enneking WF: Surgical procedures, in Enneking WF (ed): *Musculoskeletal Tumor Surgery*. New York, NY, Churchill Livingstone, 1983, pp 89-122.

25. Enneking WF, Spanier SS, Goodman MA: The surgical staging of musculoskeletal sarcoma. *J Bone Joint Surg Am* 1980;62:1027-1030.

26. Weiss AJ, Lackman RD: Therapy of desmoid tumors and related neoplasms. *Compr Ther* 1991;17:32-34.

27. Weiss AJ, Lackman RD: Low-dose chemotherapy of desmoid tumors. *Cancer* 1989;64:1192-1194.

28. Sugarbaker PH, Barofsky I, Rosenberg SA, Gianola FJ: Quality of life assessment of patients in extremity sarcoma clinical trials. *Surgery* 1982;91:17-23.

29. Weddington WW Jr, Segraves KB, Simon MA: Psychological outcome of extremity sarcoma survivors undergoing amputation or limb salvage. *J Clin Oncol* 1985;3:1393-1399.

30. Otis JC, Lane JM, Kroll MA: Energy cost during gait in osteosarcoma patients after resection and knee replacement and after above-the-knee amputation. *J Bone Joint Surg Am* 1985;67:606-611.

31. Harris IE, Leff AR, Gitelis S, Simon MA: Function after amputation, arthrodesis, or arthroplasty for tumors about the knee. *J Bone Joint Surg Am* 1990;72:1477-1485.

32. Bacci G, Ferrari S, Mercuri M, et al: Predictive factors for local recurrence in osteosarcoma: 540 patients with extremity tumors followed for minimum 2.5 years after neoadjuvant chemotherapy. *Acta Orthop Scand* 1998;69:230-236.

33. Enneking WF, Shirley PD: Resection-arthrodesis for malignant and potentially malignant lesions about the knee using an intramedullary rod and local bone grafts. *J Bone Joint Surg Am* 1977;59:223-236.

34. Campanacci M, Cervellati C, Guerra A, Biagini R, Ruggieri P: Knee resection: Arthrodesis, in Enneking WF (ed): *Limb Salvage in Musculoskeletal Oncology*. New York, NY, Churchill Livingstone, 1987, pp 364-378.

35. Weiland AJ: Vascularized free bone transplants. *J Bone Joint Surg Am* 1981;63:166-169.

36. Mankin HJ, Doppelt S, Tomford W: Clinical experience with allograft implantation: The first 10 years. *Clin Orthop* 1983;174:69-86.

37. Mnaymneh W, Malinin TI, Lackman RD, Hornicek FJ, Ghandur-Mnaymneh L: Massive distal femoral osteoarticular allografts after resection of bone tumors. *Clin Orthop* 1994;303:103-115.

38. Mnaymneh W, Malinin T: Massive allografts in surgery of bone tumors. *Orthop Clin North Am* 1989;20:455-467.

39. Mnaymneh W, Malinin TI, Makley JT, Dick HM: Massive osteoarticular allografts in the reconstruction of extremities following resection of tumors not requiring chemotherapy and radiation. *Clin Orthop* 1985;197:76-87.

40. Buck BE, Malinin TI, Brown MD: Bone transplantation and human immunodeficiency virus: An estimate of risk of acquired immunodeficiency syndrome (AIDS). *Clin Orthop* 1989;240:129-136.

41. Berrey BH Jr, Lord CF, Gebhardt MC, Mankin HJ: Fractures of allografts: Frequency, treatment, and end-results. *J Bone Joint Surg Am* 1990;72:825-833.

42. Lord CF, Gebhardt MC, Tomford WW, Mankin HJ: Infection in bone allografts: Incidence, nature, and treatment. *J Bone Joint Surg Am* 1988;70:369-376.

43. Dick HM, Strauch RJ: Infection of massive bone allografts. *Clin Orthop* 1994;306:46-53.

44. Hornicek FJ, Gebhardt MC, Sorger JI, Mankin HJ: Tumor reconstruction. *Orthop Clin North Am* 1999;30:673-684.

45. Unwin PS, Cannon SR, Grimer RJ, Kemp HB, Sneath RS, Walker PS: Aseptic loosening in cemented custom-made prosthetic replacements for bone tumors of the lower limb. *J Bone Joint Surg Br* 1996;78:5-13.

46. Malawer MM, Chou LB: Prosthetic survival and clinical results with use of large-segment replacements in the treatment of high-grade bone sarcomas. *J Bone Joint Surg Am* 1995;77:1154-1165.

47. Wirganowicz PZ, Eckardt JJ, Dorey FJ, Eilber FR, Kabo JM: Etiology and results of tumor endoprosthesis revision surgery in 64 patients. *Clin Orthop* 1999;358:64-74.

48. Chao EY: A composite fixation principle for modular segmental defect replacement (SDR) prostheses. *Orthop Clin North Am* 1989;20:439-453.

49. Bradish CF, Kemp HB, Scales JT, Wilson JN: Distal femoral replacement by custom-made prostheses: Clinical follow-up and survivorship analysis. *J Bone Joint Surg Br* 1987;69:276-284.

50. Ward WG, Johnston KS, Dorey FJ, Eckardt JJ: Loosening of massive proximal femoral cemented endoprostheses: Radiographic evidence of loosening mechanism. *J Arthroplasty* 1997;12:741-750.

51. Lewis MM: The use of an expandable and adjustable prosthesis in the treatment of childhood malignant bone tumors of the extremity. *Cancer* 1986;57:499-502.

52. Eckardt JJ, Kabo JM, Kelley CM, et al: Expandable endoprosthesis reconstruction in skeletally immature patients with tumors. *Clin Orthop* 2000;373:51-61.

53. Thompson RC Jr, Manivel C: Neuropathic arthropathy as a possible cause of failure of a whole joint allograft: A case report. *Clin Orthop* 1988;234:124-128.

54. Mnaymneh W, Malinin T, Head W, et al: Massive osseous and osteoarticular allografts in non-tumerous disorders. *Contemp Orthop* 1986;13:13-24.

55. Mnaymneh W, Temple HT, Malinin T: Allograft reconstruction after resection of malignant tumors of the scapula. *Clin Orthop* 2002;405:223-229.

56. Mnaymneh W, Malinin T, Mnaymneh LG, Robinson D: Pelvic allograft: A case report with a follow-up evaluation of 5.5 years. *Clin Orthop* 1990; 255:128-132.

57. Bell RS, Davis AM, Wunder JS, Buconjic T, McGoveran B, Gross AE: Allograft reconstruction of the acetabulum after resection of stage-IIB sarcoma: Intermediate-term results. *J Bone Joint Surg Am* 1997;79: 1663-1674.

58. Harrington KD: The use of hemipelvic allografts or autoclaved grafts for reconstruction after wide resections of malignant tumors of the pelvis. *J Bone Joint Surg Am* 1992;74:331-341.

Chapter 6

Trauma: Limb Salvage Versus Amputation

Michael T. Archdeacon, MD
Roy Sanders, MD

Introduction

Salvage of the severely traumatized lower limb is a modern concept, possible only since sterile techniques and vascular reconstruction were developed. Before amputation became common, an open fracture was a virtual death sentence. Until the late 19th century, most patients died even if amputation was performed. In 1832, Malgaigne reported that the mortality rate for amputations performed in the hospital was 52% for major amputations and 62% for thigh amputations.[1] This is not surprising considering the methods used.

Surgery was conducted on unwashed patients in their beds with the rest of the ward looking on. Before 1846, all surgery was performed without anesthesia.[2] Speed was of the essence, and amputations were usually completed within 3 minutes while strong men held the patient down and casual onlookers put their hands in the wound. Instruments were simply wiped clean, often on the surgeon's shirt. Surgeons also performed autopsies and would not wash their hands between prosection and amputation. Wounds were packed with dressings made of old bed sheets and rags. The same pus bucket was used postoperatively to wash wounds of every patient on the ward.[1]

War was even worse. The mortality rate for open fractures in the Franco-Prussian War (1870 to 1871) was 50% for transtibial and 66% for transfem-

oral amputations.[1] In the American Civil War, the mortality rate was 33% for transtibial amputations and 54% for transfemoral amputations. In 1874, von Nussbaum recorded a 100% mortality rate for 34 consecutive knee disarticulations.

The development of the germ theory, bringing with it hand washing, proper sanitation, and nursing virtually eliminated mortality from open fractures. In World War I, Orr's protocol for treating open wounds used wound extension, cleaning, stable reduction of the fracture, and application of plaster with the wound left open.[2] As a result, his mortality and amputation rates were extremely low. Using this technique, Trueta achieved a 0.6% septic mortality rate in 1,069 open fractures in the Spanish Civil War. It is interesting to note that these two men simply used the principles of Paré, who in 1540 advocated irrigation, débridement, stabilization, and packing of open fractures.[1,2]

As death from wound sepsis virtually disappeared and salvage of the mangled limb became possible, the next important hurdle was vascular reconstruction. In World War II, De-Bakey and Simeone[3] reported an amputation rate of 75% for popliteal artery injuries associated with fractures. The Korean War paved the way for successful arterial repair. By the Vietnam war, the overall amputation rate

for open fractures with vascular injury was negligible.[4]

Advances in all fields of medicine have made salvage of the massively injured lower limb a reality. Since the 1970s, orthopaedic traumatology has developed into a subspecialty. Highly skilled in salvage and reconstruction, these surgeons began to view amputation of a mangled lower limb as an admission of defeat.[5] With even the most complex injury, salvage became possible. Guidelines for deciding between amputation and salvage did not exist, however, nor had the social and economic consequences of limb salvage been addressed.

Quality-of-Life and Economic Considerations

The patient's potential function and the quality of life need to be considered in the decision to amputate or salvage the mangled limb. Factors such as donor site morbidity, joint stiffness, neurologic impairment, and prolonged rehabilitation times should be taken into account. Studies comparing the long-term functional outcomes of amputation and salvage are ongoing and not yet definitive.

In addition, the cost and socioeconomic impact of limb salvage are increasing concerns. Between 1992 and 1994, the estimated annual expenditure for the care of musculoskeletal conditions in the United States was $149.4 billion, and the annual cost for fracture care was estimated at approximately $24 billion.[6] Because medical costs are rising, the predictability and financial burden of a treatment modality need to be thoroughly investigated before it can be universally recommended. Several studies have attempted to address these particular issues.

In 1988, Bondurant and associates[7] reported on the cost of limb salvage in open grade IIIB and IIIC tibial fractures. Of 263 patients, 43 ultimately underwent amputation. Fourteen patients had a primary amputation and averaged 22.3 days in the hospital, 1.6 surgical procedures, and $28,964 in hospital costs. Patients who underwent attempts at limb salvage averaged 53.4 days in the hospital, 6.9 surgical procedures, and $53,462 in hospital costs. The authors suggested that early amputation based on appropriate criteria would improve function, shorten hospitalization, and lessen the financial burden placed on both the patient and the institution.

Similarly, in 1990, Sanders and associates[8] evaluated the results of a salvage protocol in 11 grade IIIB ankle and talus injuries. All patients required anterior plating, multiple-level fusions, free flaps, and bone grafts. All patients had at least three separate hospitalizations, with an average of 8.2 surgical procedures per patient (range, 5 to 12). The total inpatient hospital stay averaged 61.6 days (range, 20 to 107 days), and inpatient costs averaged $62,174 per patient (range, $33,535 to $143,847). Overall hospital cost averaged $1,009 per day. All injuries healed; the fusion rate and muscle flap success was 100%; no osteomyelitis or nonunion occurred; and no patient required subsequent amputation. Nevertheless, when asked about their functional outcome in detail, all patients stated that the injury had significantly altered their lifestyle. Five patients returned to a modified job, and the other six became permanently disabled. All stated that their relationships with spouses or immediate family members had become strained. Patients with children or grandchildren stated that they could no longer play with them even occasionally because this required too much activity. Shopping at the mall or going out at night was equally difficult, with most patients participating in these activities only if absolutely necessary. All stated that they were unhappy with the appearance of their limb, their gait, and their shoes. At the time of final interview, all patients were offered an amputation as a definitive procedure, yet all refused.

Georgiadis and associates[9] performed a comparable investigation in 1994. They compared results of limb salvage with those of early amputation in 45 patients with open tibial fractures and concomitant soft-tissue loss, 27 of whom underwent salvage and 18, early amputation. Amputation was ultimately required for 5 of the 27 limb salvage patients. Limb salvage patients also had more complications and underwent more surgical procedures, resulting in longer hospitalization, than did patients who underwent early amputation. At 35 months follow-up, the 16 limb salvage patients available for follow-up were less able to work and had significantly higher hospital charges than early amputation patients. In addition, limb salvage patients had more problems with occupational activities, and more of them considered themselves to be disabled.

Butcher and associates[10] evaluated disability in 319 patients who had sustained high-energy lower limb trauma and compared outcomes at 12 and 30 months. At 30 months follow-up, 20% of the patients had not returned to work; 64% of the patients had no disability (as assessed with the Sickness Impact Profile), 17% had mild disability, 12% had moderate disability, and 7% had severe disability. The actual physical impairments at 12 months follow-up did not change significantly, and this measure was not a predictor of return to work or disability. These results demonstrate that good outcomes can be achieved after significant lower limb trauma, but it is difficult to predict which patients will not have a good outcome.

Pezzin and associates[11] assessed long-term outcomes in 146 patients with trauma-related amputations. Approximately 25% of the patients reported ongoing problems with the residual limb, including phantom pain and wounds on the limb. The number of days in rehabilitation directly correlated with increased vitality, reduced bodily pain, and positive vocational outcomes.

In a recent publication, MacKenzie and associates[12] compared the demographics and socioeconomic characteristics of patients with high-energy lower limb trauma with those of the general population. More than 70% of the trauma patients were white men between the ages of 25 and 40 years, of whom only 70% had graduated from high school, compared with 86% nationally. Twenty-five percent lived below the federal poverty line, and 38% had no health insurance. In comparison, 16% of the general population lived below the federal poverty line, and 20% were uninsured. In addition, the rate of heavy alcohol consumption in the patient population was more than twice the national average.

In another study, MacKenzie and associates[13] assessed rates of return to work in 312 patients with severe lower limb trauma. The results were 26% at 3 months, 49% at 6 months, 60% at 9 months, and 72% at 12 months. The characteristics that were most closely associated with return to work were younger age, higher education, higher income, a strong support system, and employment in a job that was not physically demanding. In addition, receiving disability income had a strong negative effect on returning to work. These characteristics further demonstrate that limb salvage and amputation patients suffer significant economic and quality-of-life losses.

In this era of managed care, it is imperative that medical decision-making be based on medical evidence rather than on financial considerations alone. Nevertheless, limb salvage surgeons need to take into account the economic burden on the patient and the institution in addition to quality-of-life issues. Hansen[14,15] and others have noted that when posttraumatic limb salvage patients were candid, they frequently stated that, although their limbs were saved, their lives were ruined by the prolonged and costly attempts at reconstruction. Hansen has termed this approach the "triumph of technique over reason." Several authors[1,7,14-20] now suggest that early amputation and prosthetic fitting are preferable to salvage of a questionably functional lower limb. The goal of this chapter is to offer information to orthopaedic surgeons that will help them make rational decisions when faced with these difficult injuries.

Evolution of Limb Salvage Scoring Indices

To determine when amputation is not only justified but also beneficial, an objective tool to predict outcome is required. In 1976, Gustilo and Anderson[21] based their prognostic classification scheme for open fractures on wound size. They found the type III open fracture to have the worst prognosis, with a high rate of infection, nonunion, and secondary amputation. In 1984, Gustilo and associates[22] subclassified the type III open fracture into type IIIA, adequate soft-tissue coverage of a fractured bone despite extensive soft-tissue laceration or flaps; type IIIB, extensive soft-tissue injury with periosteal stripping and bony exposure usually associated with massive contamination; and type IIIC, an open fracture with an arterial injury requiring repair.

Caudle and Stern[23] found this classification to be prognostic (Table 1). In their review of 62 type III open tibial fractures, type IIIA injuries had a low complication rate and type IIIB open fractures had significant complications; however, type IIIB open fractures with soft-tissue coverage within 1 week (group 1 in Table 1) had fewer complications than those covered after 1 week (group 2 in Table 1). Type IIIC open tibial fractures had disastrous rates: 100% of patients had major complications, and 78% required secondary amputation. These authors began to question the wisdom of salvage in type IIIB and IIIC injuries.

Lange and associates[20] analyzed 23 cases of open tibial fractures with limb-threatening vascular compromise. Fourteen patients (61%) underwent amputation; none had complications or functional disability at 1-year follow-up. In contrast, those patients who underwent limb salvage required several operations and had persistent wound or tibia healing problems at 1-year follow-up. The authors suggested that a realistic appraisal of functional outcome needs to be made when considering salvage for limbs with type IIIC injuries because the overall amputation rate for these injuries approached 60%.[19,20] Other investigators[18,19,23-26] have cited amputation rates from 8% to as high as 87% in high-energy lower limb trauma (Table 2). Lange and associates[20] also consider more than 6 hours of warm ischemia time and a complete disruption of the tibial nerve to be an absolute indication for

TABLE 1 Treatment Outcomes in Grade III Tibial Fractures

Type of Open Fracture	Number of Fractures / Patients	Number of Nonunions / Fractures (%)*	Number of Infections / Fractures (%)†	Number of Secondary Amputations / Fractures (%)
IIIA	11/10	3/11 (27)	0/11 (0)	0/11 (0)
IIIB	42/42	15/35 (43)	12/41 (29)	7/42 (17)
Group 1‡	24/24	5/22 (23)	2/24 (8)	2/24 (8)
Group 2‡	17/17	10/13 (77)	10/17 (59)	4/17 (24)
IIIC	9/9	5/5 (100)	4/7 (57)	7/9 (78)
Total	62/61	23/51 (45)	16/59 (27)	14/62 (23)

*Fractures that were treated with amputation before 6 months after injury were excluded in calculating the percentages for nonunion.

†Fractures that were treated with amputation within 72 hours after injury were excluded in calculating the percentages for infection.

‡Group 1 defined as early wound coverage within 1 week of injury. Group 2 defined as delayed wound coverage after 1 week from injury.

(Reproduced with permission from Caudle RJ, Stern PJ: Severe open fractures of the tibia. J Bone Joint Surg Am 1987;69:801-807.)

TABLE 2 Amputation Rates for High-Energy Lower Limb Trauma

Study	Number of Limbs	Number of Immediate Amputations	Number of Delayed Amputations	Total Amputations (%)
Caudle and Stern[23]	9	0	7	7 (78)
Lancaster et al[24]	15	11	2	13 (87)
Lange[19]	23	5	9	14 (61)
Edwards et al[25]	12	0	1	1 (8)
Helfet et al[18]	54	15	6	21 (39)
Bosse et al[26]	556	63	86	149 (27)
Total	669	95	110	205 (32)

TABLE 3 Mangled Extremity Syndrome Index (MESI)		Points
Injury Severity Score		
	0-25	1
	25-50	2
	>50	3
Integument		
	Guillotine	1
	Crush / Burn	2
	Avulsion / Degloving	3
Nerve		
	Contusion	1
	Transection	2
	Avulsion	3
Vascular		
	Artery	
	Transected	1
	Thrombosed	2
	Avulsed	3
	Vein	1
Bone		
	Simple fracture	1
	Segmental fracture	2
	Segmental–Comminuted fracture	3
	Segmental–Comminuted fracture with bone loss < 6 cm	4
	Segmental fracture, intra-/extra-articular	5
	Segmental fracture intra-/extra-articular with bone loss > 6 cm	6
	Bone loss > 6 cm	Add 1
Lag time	Every hour after 6 hours	Add 1
Age		
	40-50 years	1
	50-60 years	2
	60-70 years	3
Preexisting disease		1
Shock		2
MESI Score		Sum of points

amputation in patients with a severe crush injury. MacKenzie and associates[27] also confirmed that severe soft-tissue injury and the absence of plantar sensation have the greatest impact on the decision to salvage or amputate the severely injured lower limb.

Not all patients present with these findings, however, so complex scoring systems have been developed to help the surgical team decide whether to perform limb salvage or a primary amputation. Daines and associates (unpublished data) evaluated 26 lower limb fractures with vascular injuries based on four variables, including extent of soft-tissue damage, duration and severity of ischemia, presence of shock, and age of the patient. They developed a score that predicted amputation and had no overlap in the variables. They also thought that soft-tissue grading was the most important variable.

Gregory and associates[16] proposed a Mangled Extremity Syndrome Index (MES or MESI) based on a point system for the severity of injury to four major organ systems of the limb (integument, nerve, vessel, and bone).

This injury severity scale considered time from injury, age, preexisting disease, and shock. In this system, a score of 20 was the dividing line: below 20, limb salvage could be reliably achieved, and above 20, amputation rate was 100%. This initial series, however, was limited to only 12 patients, fracture type was not identified, and an unspecified number of primary amputations were included (Table 3).

Based on most of the abovementioned studies, Johansen and associates[17] developed a modified version of the MESI they termed the Mangled Extremity Severity Score (MESS) to predict amputation (Table 4). This scoring system was used only in documented type IIIC open tibial fractures; first retrospectively in 26 cases and then prospectively in 26 more. The score was assigned after the salvage versus amputation decision had been made. In both groups there was a significant difference in the mean MESS scores between those limbs that were amputated and those that were salvaged successfully and thus did not require an amputation. A score of 7 or greater was 100% predictive of amputation.

Evaluating Limb Salvage Indices

The limb salvage indices in current use have been undergoing critical evaluation. These include the MES or MESI;[16] the Predictive Salvage Index (PSI);[28] MESS;[17,18] the Limb Salvage Index (LSI);[29] the Nerve Injury, Ischemia, Soft-Tissue Injury, Skeletal Injury, Shock and Age of Patient Score (NISSSA);[30] and the Hannover Fracture Scale-97 (HFS-97).[31] Durham and associates[32] attempted to evaluate four of these indices (MESI, MESS, PSI, and LSI) by applying them in a retrospective review of all severe upper and lower limb injuries at their institution over a 10-year period. The indices predicted amputation in most patients, but none of the indices could predict functional

TABLE 4 The Mangled Extremity Severity Score (MESS)

Skeletal / Soft-Tissue Injury		Points
Low-energy	Stab wounds, simple closed fractures, small-caliber gunshot wounds	1
Medium-energy	Open/segmental fractures, dislocations, moderate crush injuries	2
High-energy	Shotgun blast (close range), high-velocity gunshot wounds	3
Massive crush	Logging, railroad, oil rig accidents	4
Shock		
Normotensive hemodynamics	Blood pressure stable in the field and the operating room	0
Transiently hypotensive	Blood pressure unstable in the field but responsive to intravenous fluids	1
Prolonged hypotension	Systolic pressure < 90 mm Hg in the field; responsive to intravenous fluids only in the operating room	2
Ischemia		
None	A pulsatile limb, no signs of ischemia	0
Mild	Diminished pulse, no signs of ischemia	1
Moderate	No Doppler pulse, sluggish refill, paresthesias, diminished motor activity	2
Advanced	Pulseless, cool, paralyzed, no refill	3
Age		
< 30 years		1
30–50 years		2
> 50 years		3
MESS Score		Sum of points

outcome. This emphasizes the difficulty of developing reliable limb salvage scoring indices. Because no index has been validated, a multicenter study,[26] the Lower Extremity Assessment Project (LEAP), was begun to attempt to develop reliable criteria for salvage and amputation.

LEAP, funded by the National Institutes of Health (NIH), was begun in 1994 to evaluate severe lower limb injuries at eight level 1 trauma centers. Clarification of the open fracture classification systems is critical to assess the clinical utility of limb salvage scoring systems. The LEAP authors modified the classification system of Gustilo[21,22,33] so that final grading of open fractures was determined at the time of definitive closure or amputation. Type III open fractures definitively closed with delayed primary closure and/or split-thickness skin grafting were classified as type IIIA

injuries. Injuries requiring local flap coverage or free tissue transport were classified as type IIIB injuries. Only injuries requiring a vascular procedure for limb viability were categorized as type IIIC injuries.

Analysis of the prospectively collected data for 556 high-energy lower limb injuries revealed that none of the previously developed scoring systems (MESS, PSI, LSI, NISSSA, and HFS-97) was clinically valid. In addition, although low scores were highly specific for performing limb salvage, their sensitivity was low. Currently, no limb salvage index has been statistically confirmed to be reliable in the evaluation and treatment of patients with severely mangled lower limbs. Therefore, current recommendations center on early assessment of the extent of injury, along with frank discussions with the patient to explain

the potential risks and benefits of salvage and amputation in each case.

Managing the Salvaged Limb

When the decision to salvage a mangled lower limb is made, the first step is to evaluate the wound and then sterilely cover it in the emergency department. Tetanus prophylaxis should be performed, prophylactic systemic antibiotics should be administered immediately, and the wound should not be exposed again until the patient is in the operating room. For type III open fractures in the mangled lower limb, a first generation cephalosporin is used. We advocate cephazolin 1 to 2 g every 8 hours. An aminoglycoside such as gentamycin 2 to 6 mg/kg in divided daily doses should be given as well. For massively contaminated wounds or wounds at risk of clostridial infection, aqueous penicillin 4 to 6 million U every 4 to 6 hours should also be given. Vascular surgery consultation should be obtained when appropriate and the patient taken to the operating room as quickly as possible. Depending on the recommendation of the consulting vascular surgeon, angiography is done preoperatively or intraoperatively.

The next step in the management of these injuries is proper surgical débridement and lavage. In no other injury is complete and meticulous débridement so important. All necrotic and contaminated tissue must be excised. Elliptical excision of the necrotic wound edges is performed. This is followed by wound extension, both proximally and distally, to expose and identify all deep devitalized tissues. With a mangled limb, extensive injury to the surrounding muscle envelope is inevitable, so the surgeon should resist the urge to preserve some of the muscle to allow for better function. Retained necrotic muscle increases the risk of infection and provides a nidus for heterotopic ossification.

When addressing the bone, the soft-tissue débridement should be used as a guide for the bony débridement. All bony tissues that have marginal soft-tissue attachments or fail to demonstrate adequate bleeding are necrotic and should be excised. This reduces the risk of infection or the development of osteomyelitis.

The difficulty is trying to determine when a bony fragment has lost its blood supply. Free-floating cortical fragments completely stripped of periosteum or muscle attachments are devitalized and should be discarded. Diaphyseal bone that is stripped but remains in continuity with the remaining shaft or metaphyseal region may be more difficult to evaluate. In addition, metaphyseal fragments and periarticular fragments with attached cancellous bone may retain their ability to revascularize through the abundant vascular bed of the cancellous bone. We would recommend retaining any periarticular fragments, provided they can be stabilized adequately with internal fixation. Thereafter, copious pulsatile lavage with saline irrigation is necessary to remove all particulate matter.

Once a clean surgical wound bed has been created, stabilizing bone is the next step. Early stabilization with external fixation, intramedullary rods, or open reduction and internal fixation is used. The choice of external or internal fixation depends on the wound and bony injury. The fixation method should not further disrupt the wound or limit future débridements. Osseous defects are filled with antibiotic-impregnated polymethylmethacrylate beads made by mixing 1.2 g of tobramycin with one 40-g package of polymethylmethacrylate. The beads are then strung over a braided 26-gauge wire or a No. 5 braided suture. In addition to providing a high concentration of local antibiotics, these beads provide a space for a later bone graft.[34] Surgical extensions of all wounds should be primarily closed, whereas traumatic wounds can be loosely approximated or temporarily covered with a synthetic biologic dressing, dressing sponges, or a vacuum-assisted closure device (V.A.C. Sponge, Kinetic Concepts, Inc, San Antonio, TX).

Once stable, the limb will require additional débridements to further assess tissue viability. All necrotic or contaminated tissue must be excised. If significant contamination or myonecrosis exists, formal surgical débridements may need to be performed every 24 hours. If the wound is not grossly contaminated, débridements performed every 48 to 72 hours should be sufficient. The initial antibiotic regimen of aminoglycoside and penicillin is continued for 48 to 72 hours after the first débridement and discontinued if a clean wound bed is obtained at the second surgical débridement. Typically, antibiotic coverage is provided for 48 hours after each subsequent surgical débridement. Although the patient receives intravenous antibiotics during this period, débridement is the most important treatment to prevent infection.

Once a stable, adequately vascularized, clean wound bed is obtained, the soft-tissue wound should be aggressively covered and closed, ideally within 5 to 7 days after the injury. Closure can be accomplished either with a delayed primary closure, split-thickness skin graft, local flaps, or a vascularized free-tissue transfer. If this treatment regimen is successful, the surgeon has transformed a massively contaminated open fracture into a clean closed fracture that may require only treatment of a bony defect. Usually, this can be accomplished with bone grafting, vascularized bone transplantation, or distraction osteogenesis.

Conclusions

When massive trauma to the lower limb occurs, the orthopaedic surgeon must make difficult decisions. Although treatment has changed significantly over the past 200 years, many of the dilemmas remain the same. It is the obligation of the physician to treat the entire patient and not the limb in isolation. What is technically feasible may not be in the best interest of the patient. Amputation should not be considered a failure but rather another therapeutic modality. To return an individual to preinjury function while limiting pain and suffering is the goal of treatment. If this cannot be accomplished by limb salvage, then amputation must be considered seriously. We hope that ongoing multicenter prospective studies will produce clinically validated guidelines for amputation and salvage.

References

1. Border J, Allgower M, Hansen ST, et al: *Blunt Multiple Trauma: Comprehensive Pathophysiology and Care.* New York, NY, Marcel Dekker, 1990.

2. Wangensteen O, Wangensteen S: *The Rise of Surgery From Empiric Craft to Scientific Discipline.* Minneapolis, MN, University of Minnesota Press, 1978.

3. DeBakey ME, Simeone FA: Battle injuries of the arteries in World War II: An analysis of 2471 cases. *Ann Surg* 1946; 123:534-579.

4. Rich NB, Baugh JH, Hughes CW: Popliteal artery injuries in Vietnam. *Am J Surg* 1969;118:531-534.

5. Hicks JH: Amputation in fractures of the tibia. *J Bone Joint Surg Br* 1964;46: 388-392.

6. Yelin EH, Trupin LS, Sebesta DS: Transitions in employment, morbidity, and disability among persons ages 51-61 with musculoskeletal and non-musculoskeletal conditions in the US, 1992-1994. *Arthritis Rheum* 1999;42: 769-779.

7. Bondurant FJ, Cotler HB, Buckle R, Miller-Crotchett P, Browner BD: The medical and economic impact of severely injured lower extremities. *J Trauma* 1988;28:1270-1272.

8. Sanders R, Helfet DL, Pappas J, Mast J, et al: The salvage of grade IIIB open ankle and talus fractures. *J Orthop Trauma* 1990;14:585.

9. Georgiadis GM, Behrens FF, Joyce MJ, Earle AS, Simmons AL: Open tibial fractures with severe soft-tissue loss: Limb salvage compared with below-the-knee amputation. *J Bone Joint Surg Am* 1994;76:1594-1595.

10. Butcher JL, MacKenzie EJ, Cushing B, et al: Long-term outcomes after lower extremity trauma. *J Trauma* 1996;41: 4-9.

11. Pezzin LE, Dillingham TR, MacKenzie EJ: Rehabilitation and the long-term outcomes of persons with trauma-related amputations. *Arch Phys Med Rehabil* 2000;81:292-300.

12. MacKenzie EJ, Bosse MJ, Kellam JF, et al: Characterization of patients with high-energy lower extremity trauma. *J Orthop Trauma* 2000;14:455-466.

13. MacKenzie EJ, Morris JA Jr, Jurkovich GJ, et al: Return to work following injury: The role of economic, social, and job-related factors. *Am J Public Health* 1998;88:1630-1637.

14. Hansen ST: Overview of the severely traumatized lower limb. *Clin Orthop* 1989;143:17-19.

15. Hansen ST: The type IIIC tibial fracture. *J Bone Joint Surg Am* 1987;69:799-800.

16. Gregory RT, Gould RJ, Peclet M, et al: The mangled extremity syndrome (M.E.S.): A severity grading system for multi-system injury of the extremity. *J Trauma* 1985;25:1147-1150.

17. Johansen K, Daines M, Howey T, Helfet D, Hansen ST: Objective criteria accurately predict amputation following lower extremity trauma. *J Trauma* 1990;30:568-572.

18. Helfet DL, Howey T, Sanders R, Johansen K: Limb salvage versus amputation: Preliminary results of the Mangled Extremity Severity Score. *Clin Orthop* 1990;256:80-86.

19. Lange RH: Limb reconstruction versus amputation decision making in massive lower extremity trauma. *Clin Orthop* 1989;243:92-99.

20. Lange RH, Bach AW, Hansen ST Jr, Johansen KH: Open tibial fractures with associated vascular injuries: Prognosis for limb salvage. *J Trauma* 1985;25:203-208.

21. Gustilo RB, Anderson JT: Prevention of infection in the treatment of one thousand and twenty-five open fractures of long bones: A retrospective and prospective analysis. *J Bone Joint Surg Am* 1976;58:453-458.

22. Gustilo RB, Mendoza RM, Williams DN: Problems in the management of type III (severe) open fractures. *J Trauma* 1984;24:742-746.

23. Caudle RJ, Stern PJ: Severe open fractures of the tibia. *J Bone Joint Surg Am* 1987;69:801-807.

24. Lancaster SJ, Horowitz M, Alonso J: Open tibial fractures: Management and results. *South Med J* 1986;79:39.

25. Edwards CC, Simmons SC, Browner BD, Weigel MC: Severe open tibial fractures: Results treating 202 injuries with external fixation. *Clin Orthop* 1988;230:98-115.

26. Bosse MJ, MacKenzie EJ, Kellam JF, et al: A prospective evaluation of the clinical utility of the lower-extremity injury-severity scores. *J Bone Joint Surg Am* 2001;83 :3-14.

27. MacKenzie EJ, Bosse MJ, Kellam JF, et al: Factors influencing the decision to amputate or reconstruct after high-energy lower extremity trauma. *J Trauma* 2002;52:641-649.

28. Howe HR Jr, Poole GV, Hansen KJ, et al: Salvage of lower extremities following combined orthopaedic and vascular trauma: A predictive salvage index. *Am Surg* 1987;53:205-208.

29. Russell WL, Sailors DM, Whittle TB, et al: Limb salvage versus traumatic amputation: A decision based on a seven-part predictive index. *Ann Surg* 1991; 213:473-481.

30. McNamara MG, Heckman JD, Corley FG: Severe open fractures of the lower extremity: A retrospective evaluation of the Mangled Extremity Severity Score (MESS). *J Orthop Trauma* 1994; 8:81-87.

31. Tscherne H, Oestern HJ: A new classification of soft-tissue damage in open and closed fractures. *Unfallheilkunde* 1982;85:111-115.

32. Durham RM, Mistry BM, Mazuski JE, Shapiro M, Jacobs D: Outcome and utility of scoring systems in the management of the mangled extremity. *Am J Surg* 1996;172:569-574.

33. Gustilo RB: *Management of Open Fractures and Their Complications.* Philadelphia, PA, WB Saunders, 1982.

34. Christian EP, Bosse MJ, Robb G: Reconstruction of large diaphyseal defects, without free fibular transfer, in grade-IIIB tibial fractures. *J Bone Joint Surg Am* 1989;71:994-1004.

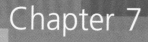

Chapter 7

Wartime Amputee Care

Paul J. Dougherty, MD

Introduction

Amputees represent a small but significant group of combat casualties who require longer hospital stays, more surgical care, and prosthetic fitting compared to the average battle casualty. The wars of the 20th century have found surgeons relearning the principles of amputee care and using the technique of open circular amputation and skin traction as the initial surgical procedure in theater. The techniques and special postoperative care for these patients are not routinely taught in surgical training programs in the United States. Amputees are often the most severely injured patients seen on the battlefield and require priority care at forward surgical echelons.

Conflict can occur without warning and find US military surgeons treating battle casualties with little or no preparation. It is the goal of any military surgeon to be prepared to treat battle casualties and to minimize morbidity and mortality, even with large numbers of patients. Preparedness therefore not only involves the ability to treat battle casualties but also to instruct others on their care.

Amputees have historically been a significant clinical problem for military surgeons because of (1) the severity of injury, (2) high morbidity, and (3) long hospital stays. Very few surgeons have extensive experience caring for amputees in civilian practice, making the study of this type of injury paramount for military surgeons to provide the best care for their patients. There has been a steep learning curve concerning the care of amputees with every conflict during the 20th century.

The latest surgical techniques from civilian practice are often inappropriately applied to patients who must be transported from the combat zone. The goals of initial care must take into account the deleterious effects of evacuation; thus, initial surgery should prepare the patient for the trauma of transportation. In the case of amputees, wound closure is often attempted to provide a residual limb so that a prosthesis may be fitted as soon as possible. As documented in World War I, World War II, and Vietnam, early wound closure in battlefield hospitals has been shown to increase the complication rate.

Over the past several years, the Army Medical Department has assumed responsibility for other missions. Care of refugees and patients who are not US or Allied soldiers, and therefore are not evacuated, has changed the traditional role of military surgeons. These days both initial and definitive care occurs in theater. Patient factors are also variable. The patients may be any age or sex and may have a variety of nutritional and health problems. Prosthetic fitting of the amputated limb is also highly variable and depends on the resources of the international community and the nation itself.

The Civil War
Indications for Amputation

Surgery evolved during the Civil War as did the overall care for the wounded soldier. Early in the war American surgeons relied on accounts from the Napoleonic Wars and from the Crimean War for guidance on indications, techniques, and postoperative care of amputees.

MacLeod[1] reported on amputees during the Crimean War (1853-1856). Amputations were performed in either the primary or secondary periods, depending on how long after injury an amputation occurred. Primary amputations occurred soon after injury, either before or after shock but before sepsis developed. Secondary amputations occurred after sepsis or inflammation had occurred. Indications for primary surgery included open fractures, partial or complete traumatic amputation, and fracture combined with an open joint injury. Secondary surgery was performed when a patient had a clinically infected wound. Primary amputation was preferred because patients with infection were at increased risk of death. MacLeod reported a mortality rate of 37% with primary amputations and 60% with secondary amputations; overall the mortality rate of both groups was 39.8%. His series focused principally on casualties that occurred late in the war.

Two techniques used during the Civil War were (1) a circular technique in which the incisions were made circumferentially around the extremity; and (2) a flap technique in which flaps were made to facilitate closure. MacLeod preferred the circular technique for battle casualties because it preserved residual limb length for prosthetic fitting.

Surgery and anesthesia techniques evolved between 1861 and 1865, and changes were made in the field hospital system, resulting in better care for the wounded soldier in a number of ways. Indications for amputation also evolved. In the Crimea, amputations were performed for gunshot fractures and for mangled limbs. Secondary amputations were performed to treat sepsis.

Gross,[2] writing in 1861, listed the following indications for amputation: crush injury, nerve or blood vessel injury, gunshot fracture with extensive comminution, a major open joint injury accompanied by a fracture, or extensive soft-tissue injury. Hamilton[3] echoed similar indications in the same year and specifically noted that gunshot fractures of the femur were generally an indication for amputation. Surgery was recommended as soon as possible in the primary period of the first day before sepsis had developed.[1-3]

Confederate surgeons published similar recommendations in 1861. Warren[4] advised that amputations be performed as soon as possible and listed partial or complete amputations and comminuted open fractures as indications for primary surgery. After a period of shock but before infection developed, he advised amputation for a partial or complete traumatic amputation, compound or multiple fractures, complicated fractures (ie, major nerve or blood vessel injury), fracture associated with an open joint injury, severe soft-tissue injury, and fracture associated with a severe soft-tissue injury. He stated that "conservatism" with open fractures was not generally indicated in military surgery except in injuries with minimal soft-tissue disruption. Indications for secondary surgery were secondary hemorrhage, rapid drainage, "mortification," decreasing patient strength, "necrosis or malignant disease of bone defying treatment," diseases of joints, and tetanic symptoms. If a patient's condition was such that he could not be transported without deteriorating, amputation was advised.

Early Techniques

Amputations during the Civil War were performed using either the flap or circular techniques. Flaps were constructed in a variety of sizes and shapes to include anterior/posterior, medial/lateral, or single anterior or posterior flap. Advocates claimed that flap amputations provided better soft-tissue coverage and were faster to perform. The circular amputation technique consisted of a circular incision with subsequently more proximal cuts in muscle and bone to produce a concave open residual limb. The circular amputation was thought to preserve residual limb length and was considered safer.[3-8]

Fisher,[9] writing after the battle of Antietam in September 1862, stated that early in the war Confederate surgeons tried to preserve limbs, which often necessitated secondary amputations. Minié balls accounted for 75% of the injuries leading to amputation, followed by grape shot (12.5%) and shell fragments (10.7%).

Letterman[10] who was the medical director of the Army of the Potomac, reported that the incidence of amputation varied widely. In the Battle of Fredericksburg, Virginia, in December 1862, 13.4% of the wounded in the 9th Corps required amputations, whereas the incidence was 3.6% in the 5th Corps. Amputation was the most common operation performed on wounded soldiers.[10,11]

Letterman was also responsible for reorganizing the field hospital system. Initially, regimental surgeons established hospitals for their regiments (approximately 440 men) behind the battle area and operated on soldiers from their units. Letterman transformed various regimental hospitals into aid stations, with one assistant surgeon who provided care and transport to a field hospital at the division level. Medical assets from three to four regiments were used for these division field hospitals. Three surgeons were designated as operators, and others handled records and supply. The conversion to Letterman's system was gradual but in place when the Army of the Potomac fought the Battle of Fredericksburg.[10-13]

By 1863, as surgical techniques evolved and surgeons became more experienced, indications for amputation were becoming more refined. Gunshot fractures of the femur were not always necessarily an indication for amputation. Moses[14] in 1863 reported a 12.9% incidence of amputation associated with long bone fractures for the battles around Chattanooga. Hodgen[15] and Lidell[16] reported good results in treating gunshot fractures of the lower extremity in Hodgen splints. Hodgen himself, who treated survivors of the long evacuation from the battlefield to a large hospital in St. Louis, felt that amputations should be performed only in patients who had injuries to joints, blood vessels, or nerves. Swinburne[5] advocated amputation surgery for a partial or complete traumatic amputation, extensive soft-tissue injury associated with nerve or blood vessel injury and denuded bone, loss of a major blood vessel, or compound fractures of the knee or ankle joint. Most gunshot fractures were treated nonsurgically during the war, and a variety of splints were developed to treat fractures.[13-16]

Later in the war, Hamilton[17] in 1865 recommended that the ideal time to amputate was when shock had subsided but no infection was present. The primary period was ideal but within narrow limits. He advocated the circular technique for the

TABLE 1 Amputation Levels Reported During the Civil War

	Otis and Huntington[18] (%)	Fisher[9] (%)
Shoulder	4.2	7.0
Arm	26.8	35.0
Elbow	0.9	N/A
Below elbow	8.5	7.0
Wrist	N/A	N/A
Hip	0.32	N/A
Thigh	30.0	22.8
Knee disarticulation	0.94	N/A
Leg	26.8	28.0
Foot	0.8	N/A

forearm and leg but flap amputations for the thigh and arm.

Epidemiology

Otis and Huntington[18] recorded the largest collection of information on battlefield casualties from the Civil War. The Army Medical Museum recorded 253,142 casualties in the Civil War; about 20,559 patients (8.1%) had significant amputations (those proximal to the wrist or ankle). In this series, transfemoral amputation was the most common (Table 1). The open circular (or flapless) technique was most commonly used. For transtibial amputees, flaps were used in 1,720 patients (58.8%) and the open circular technique in 1,206 patients (41.2%). The total overall mortality of amputees was 35.7%.

Postamputation Care

Treatment after the amputation varied considerably throughout the course of the war. Jewett,[19] an army surgeon at Gettysburg, wrote of surgeons using dressings, "coal oil," castor oil, water, and other liquids to coat the residual limb. Residual limbs that were initially closed would suppurate and break down, as opposed to wounds left open.

There was no standardized prosthetic fitting or rehabilitation for Civil War amputees. Minor[20] recom-

mended that the artificial limb should be of the same size and shape as the limb replaced; of light, strong, and durable materials; and "well fitting to the residual limb." He felt that the Anglesea and Bly legs were most appropriate because both had an ankle joint. Palmer legs, which had a solid ankle, were also popular. It is not known how many amputees used prostheses because many lower limb amputees walked with ambulatory aids, such as crutches, rather than wearing a prosthesis. Otis and Huntington[18] reported that 40 to 60 patients with knee disarticulations were fitted for a prosthesis.

Amputee care changed during the Civil War as surgeons became more experienced. Use of splints for the treatment of open fractures became more common during the later stages of the war.

World War I

The United States became officially involved late in World War I (1917), whereas the other Allied armies were involved from the beginning. Many American surgeons learned the care of amputees from Allied surgeons who had been involved in the conflict since it began in 1914. Others gained experience by working with voluntary American hospitals (American Ambulance) or with the French and English hospitals prior to American involvement.[21-24]

Early Techniques

Early in World War I, British surgeons performed amputations by constructing flaps and using delayed primary or primary closure. This technique resulted in poor-quality residual limbs and infection, which often necessitated revision surgery to a more proximal level.[25-27]

In 1915 Fitzmaurice-Kelly[27] reported a flapless open amputation in which the level of amputation was at the lowest viable level of tissue. He considered it an emergent procedure that was performed to allow free

drainage of the wound. He also considered the flapless amputation to be a two-staged procedure in which the second procedure was performed at a different time under less urgent circumstances. He described a circumferential skin incision in which the skin and subcutaneous fat were allowed to retract as one layer, and the muscle and bone were divided more proximally. Nerves were tied and cut short to prevent development of neuromas. Blood vessels were also tied and transected. Indications for surgery were gas gangrene, compound comminuted fractures, and multiple wounds (multiple fragment wounds from explosive devices). The advantages of this technique included easy drainage to prevent widespread sepsis, preservation of residual limb length, and decreased risk of secondary hemorrhage. He also recommended skin traction to prevent bone protrusion.

This surgery was often erroneously called a "guillotine" amputation, in which the soft tissues and bone are all transected at one level. Controversy over the terms and the type of amputations to be performed in field hospitals continued for the rest of the war. The construction of flaps that were to be left open until they could be closed was advocated, and the guillotine procedure was condemned because it required a longer healing time and a second, possibly more extensive, operation.[25-27]

Blake[28] in 1914 helped organize what later became known as the American Ambulance, a hospital unit composed of groups from medical schools in the United States. The units were to rotate every 3 months. Lakeside University (Cleveland, Ohio), Harvard University, and the University of Pennsylvania eventually sent units. Blake also helped organize the American Red Cross Military Hospital No. 2 in Paris in 1917; he remained commander in 1918 when the United States became profoundly involved in the war. Over a 4-month period, 55 amputations were performed in this hospital, 70% of which were at

TABLE 2 Amputation Levels Reported During World War I

	Callendar et al[30]	Speed[29]	Blake[23]
Above elbow	31 (20.5%)	27 (22.3%)	3 (5.8%)
Forearm	16 (10.5%)	N/A	2 (3.9%)
Above knee	60 (39.7%)	71 (58.6%)	38 (74.5%)
Below knee	38 (25%)	23 (19%)	N/A
Foot	6 (3.9%)	N/A	N/A

the transfemoral level; overall, 42% were for gas gangrene, 29% for sepsis, and the remainder for trauma. The incidence of admissions for these patients was 1.32%. Blake did not recommend the guillotine or open circular technique because it required a second operation for completion and residual limb fitting[23,24,28] (Table 2).

Crile,[24] who was commander of the Lakeside Unit, did not recommend flaps in patients with a contaminated wound or infection. Rather, he recommended a "flush" amputation that could be revised when the sepsis was quiescent.

Speed,[29] who was with Base Hospital (Chicago Unit) in France in 1918, reported on 121 amputations. Indications for surgery were severe fractures, gas gangrene, sepsis, secondary hemorrhage, and trench foot. The most common level was the transfemoral (58.6%). He recommended an open circular amputation with longitudinal skin slits up the side of the residual limb.

Evacuation Hospital No. 8 reported 151 amputations in 4,714 battle casualties (3.2%) who were admitted from September 13 to November 13, 1918. Of these, 62% were for gangrene, 33.7% for trauma, and 10.5% for sepsis. Again, transfemoral amputations were the most predominant (39%).[30]

Influence of the American Expeditionary Force

In August 1918, the Chief Surgeon of the American Expeditionary Force (AEF) recommended that amputees should be assigned as soon as possible to the orthopaedic service in light of their special needs. If an open circular amputation was performed, the patient could be moved safely 1 week after surgery.[31]

In May 1916, the American Orthopaedic Association meeting voted to appoint a preparedness committee to consider the needs of the United States in the event of American participation in the war. Major Sir Robert Jones of Britain requested in the spring of 1917 that American orthopaedic surgeons augment orthopaedic specialty centers to treat returning wounded British soldiers. At that time, about 65% of the serious battle casualties were extremity wounds and England lacked trained orthopaedic surgeons. Temporary assignment of American orthopaedic surgeons provided them with experience in treating battle casualties prior to their assignment in France with the AEF.[32]

AEF Hospitals

The AEF ran three main types of hospitals: (1) the field hospital, (2) the evacuation hospital, and (3) the base hospital.[31] Field hospitals, which were located 3 to 8 miles from the front lines, provided immediate surgical care for soldiers who could not be transported. These patients would not survive the long evacuation to larger hospitals farther from the front lines. The goal of surgery at these hospitals was to stabilize a patient for further evacuation.

Evacuation hospitals provided the initial surgical care to most patients in France. They were larger (about 1,000 beds), located 9 to 15 miles from the front lines, and provided initial surgery to prevent infection and stabilize patients for evacuation

to a base hospital where more definitive care could be provided.

Base hospitals were established to provide more definitive care to soldiers and prepare them for the long transport by ship back to the United States. A hospital center was established in Savenay, France, with Base Hospital No. 8 as its core unit. An amputation service was established at that hospital to care for amputees returning to the United States. The goals of this service were to provide skin traction, wound care, and physical therapy. A program of early ambulation on a temporary prosthesis, designed based on the experience of Belgian physicians, was also instituted at Savenay, and about 20% of the returning amputees were initially fitted there.[31,33]

Wound closure was performed in certain cases. During quiet times on the front, if a soldier had a localized injury, flaps could be performed followed by primary or delayed primary closure. This procedure was possible only if there were no significant wounds proximal to the amputation site, if the patient was received relatively quickly after injury, and if he could be observed for 10 to 15 days afterward.[31]

Number of Amputations

Of the 550 amputees examined at Savenay, 58% were treated by the open circular technique, 30% by the flap technique with delayed primary closure, and 11% by primary or delayed primary closure alone. Of the residual limbs that were closed, 25% needed to be reopened because of infection.

Kirk[34] reviewed amputee records in the Surgeon General's Office for patients who were operated on in France (Table 3). From these records, he learned that soft-tissue injury with infection as an indication for amputation carried a higher mortality rate than compound fractures. Because the cumulative numbers of amputees in this series exceeded the number of amputees returning to the United States, there is some overlap of

TABLE 3 Amputation Levels and Reported Mortality in the Surgeon General's Office Records

Cause of Amputation	Number	% of Amputations	% Mortality
Compound Fractures			
Tibia/Fibula	1,564	66	17
Femur	770	32.8	29
Knee	8	0.3	37.5
Pelvis	5	0.21	60
Soft-Tissue Injuries			
Leg	664	48.8	23
Thigh	555	40.7	24
Knee	130	9.5	26
Hip	13	9.5	23

TABLE 4 Number of Amputees Returning to the United States in 1918*

Amputation Level	Number	% of Amputations
Above elbow	554	19.1
Elbow	41	1.3
Below elbow	215	7.4
Wrist	26	0.9
Hip	1	0.03
Above knee	1,145	39.6
Knee	97	3.3
Below knee	330	11.4
Ankle	131	4.5
Foot	20	0.7
Partial foot	280	9.6
Multiple sites	50	1.7

*Does not include hand or partial hand amputees.

records. In both categories, the number of transtibial amputations exceeded the number of transfemoral amputations. Kirk does not speculate whether revisions at a higher level were required for these individuals.[34]

The greatest number of casualties in the AEF occurred in 1918, particularly in the fall of that year. The Surgeon General's Office recorded 2,890 amputees returning to the United States (Table 4). This number does not include hand or partial hand amputations. Most of these patients had lower limb amputations, most commonly at the transfemoral level (39.6%).[31]

Care Rendered at US Amputee Centers

Amputee centers were established in the United States to consolidate the specialized care for this group of patients. Walter Reed Army General Hospital had the largest census of these centers; other centers were established at Letterman General Hospital (San Francisco), Ft. Des Moines, Iowa, and Ft. McPherson, Georgia. General Hospital No. 3 in Colonia, New Jersey, was established as an amputee center because of its proximity to harbors where soldiers landed from overseas. By April 1918 the amputee service housed 750 patients. Kirk was assigned to the amputee service at Colonia in 1919 and later went to Walter Reed Army General Hospital.

He later wrote about his experiences at these two hospitals, where he treated about 1,700 patients.[35]

Kirk advocated the guillotine procedure for war casualties because of its simplicity and because it preserved the maximum residual limb length, allowed wide drainage to treat infection, and enabled earlier transport than did other techniques. The guillotine technique was really the open circular technique, which produced a concave residual limb to be maintained in skin traction. Kirk noted that at least 95% of the patients who were received from overseas with guillotine residual limbs needed additional care before prosthetic fitting. Most residual limbs were edematous and had unhealed areas. Other problems included bony protrusion and infection. Organisms most often identified from the residual limbs were *Streptococcus hemolyticus*, staphylococci, *Bacillus proteus*, and Klebs-Löffler bacillus.

Preoperative care of Kirk's patients included skin traction, bed rest, and elevation. Radiographs were obtained on admission to evaluate the bone and to look for foreign bodies. Infection was treated by dressing changes and sodium hypochlorite solution.

Surgery was not performed until the residual limb had been quiescent and radiographs showed no signs of infections, usually after about 6 months. Kirk[35] described three procedures: plastic closure, plastic resection,

and reamputation. Plastic closure was performed when there was enough skin to cover the area, with removal of no more than 1/8 in of bone. Incisions were made through healthy skin only after all scar tissue had been removed. When there was protruding bone covered by granulations, a plastic resection was indicated whereby an incision was made through healthy tissue and dissected back to the saw line through the bone. The bone end and scar mass were then removed as a single piece. A cuff of periosteum was removed from the end and the skin closed. Reamputation of a residual limb was performed either for a residual limb that was too long to be satisfactory or too short to be fitted.

Kirk indicated that ideal residual limb lengths were through the middle third of the leg for transtibial amputees and through the lower and middle third for transfemoral amputees. He did not favor a knee disarticulation because the condyles are a poor weight-bearing surface. Rather, he preferred to cut the bone just above the joint line and use an osteoplastic or tendoplastic closure technique. Upper limb amputations were more forgiving; if the patient healed with skin traction and a terminal scar, a second procedure often was not required. A very short transradial amputation was difficult to fit, and he did not recommend bone shortening with amputations through the proximal third of the forearm or distal third of the arm.

Once the wound on the residual limb was closed, there was a period, usually of several months, before edema would subside. During this time a temporary prosthesis was used. This prosthesis could be mass-produced and required a minimum of fitting. An insert, usually of plaster of Paris, was made, and the patient could then begin gait training (lower limb amputations) or using the upper limbs. At this point, a team of surgeons, limb fitters (prosthetists), and physical therapists (called reconstruction aides at this time) worked together to achieve the best results in the minimum amount of time.[36-38]

Wilson,[33] who was in charge of the amputee service at Savenay where a limited program of early walking had begun for lower limb amputees, believed that if the wound was clean, a patient could begin ambulating after 2 to 3 weeks. At this time, the patient was put into a temporary prosthesis consisting of a socket and frame. The frame could be prefabricated and needed a minimum of fitting, and the socket was generally made from plaster of Paris and molded to relieve wound pressure. He believed that early ambulation promoted wound healing, caused residual limb shrinkage, improved morale, and decreased the time to permanent prostheses.

Care of the AEF amputee was modern in certain aspects. Several innovations considered recent were developed by US Army surgeons during World War I. The team approach, in which a special service of limb fitters, reconstruction aides (physical therapists), and surgeons cared for the patients, was developed at the amputee centers. The open circular technique with postoperative skin traction, a method applied to battle casualties today, originated and was developed during the war. Finally, early walking on a temporary prosthesis was instituted, and then forgotten for many years.[33-41]

World War II
Interwar Years

Advances in the care of amputees between the first and second world wars were principally confined to the improved management of shock and the prevention and treatment of infection. Several authors improved our understanding of the pathophysiology of shock and its treatment.[39-41] The use of sulfonamide compounds in civilian surgery was thought to prevent infection in open fractures, which was the principal cause of amputation during World War I. Penicillin, likewise, was thought to prevent and treat infections in open fractures.[42]

The number of amputees for the US Army during the 1920s and 1930s was not significantly high. Kirk remained in the military with posts in the Philippines and at Walter Reed, Ft. Sam Houston, and Letterman General Hospitals. His report on sites of election for lower limb amputations was published in 1933.[43] The complacency of the 1930s slowly changed to realization that the United States might become involved in World War II. Kirk, sensing the lack of preparedness of the US military, revised his amputation text in 1940 to educate the surgeons expected to care for casualties in this new war. He also wrote about the general treatment of combat casualties in 1940 and 1941[42-44] (AK Willard, personal communication).

Early World War II Experience

British experience in the Western Desert of North Africa revealed problems concerning both field surgery and amputee patients. Armored warfare had become more fluid and mobile than it had been on the western front of World War I, and the medical field service needed to provide initial surgery near the front, as well as evacuation to a hospital in a more stable environment.[45-50]

There were also problems with amputee patients. Those who did not have skin traction after open circular amputations experienced bony protrusion and needed reamputation, with the resultant loss of limb length. Amputations in which the skin had been closed were seldom successful because of infection. A loose closure was recommended to prevent skin retraction and the hazards of a routine closure, with an emphasis on the speed of the initial surgical procedure. Skin traction with the open circular technique was not recommended. After the attack on Pearl Harbor, patients with delayed primary or primary closure became infected and required amputation to a higher level (LT Peterson, unpublished data, 1946).

The lack of success with early closure of wounds led Kirk[51] in 1942 to reemphasize the open circular amputation once again in a technique article he published for those serving or about to serve. The technique at this time was characterized by amputating at the lowest level of viable soft tissue, allowing the skin to retract, and successively cutting layers of muscle and bone more proximally to produce a concave residual limb. The residual limb end allows wide drainage to prevent infection. He recommended the injection of alcohol into the nerves before transecting and double ligation of large vessels with No. 2-0 silk, cotton, or catgut suture. Postoperatively, the patient was to be maintained in continuous skin traction to prevent retraction of the soft tissues. A repair or plastic closure of the residual limb was then performed in patients with an adherent scar. In a later article, Kirk and McKeever[52] emphasized that the open circular technique was a two-staged operation requiring a second surgery for closure of the wound.

The use of this procedure was formalized in April 1943 by Circular Letter No. 91, in which the Office of the Surgeon General outlined the use of the open circular amputation in the-

TABLE 5 Indications for Amputation

Cause of Amputation	WWI (%)	ETO (%)	MTO (%)	RVN (%)
Trauma	25.5	64.3	75.0	89.5
Infection	74.5	14.3	9.5	8.4
Vascular		21.3	14.5	1.9

WWI = World War I

ETO = European Theater of Operations—World War II (Third Army only)

MTO = Mediterranean Theater of Operations—World War II

RVN = Retrospective chart review of patients at Valley Forge Army General Hospital (personal records, P. Dougherty)

ater, allowing the open flap technique only in patients who would not be evacuated and whose wounds would be closed at a later date at the same hospital. Lower limb amputees in the continental United States would be discharged only after they were able to walk on level ground using a temporary prosthesis without ambulatory aids.

Innovations in Initial Management

World War II was characterized by a more mobile form of warfare than World War I, and the medical field service of the US Army, like its British counterpart, evolved to accommodate this new form of warfare. Ideally, initial surgical management of a battle casualty occurred at an evacuation or field hospital, depending on the casualty load and the patient's triage category.[53-55]

The field hospital, which was meant to handle nontransportable patients, collocated with a clearing company in the rear of a division area and was divided into three platoons. One platoon received casualties from the designated clearing company. When this platoon was full, or if the division moved, the platoon stopped taking casualties. When patients could be transported, the unit would move to a new location, set up, and receive casualties. In the meantime, another platoon was receiving new casualties. This system allowed nontransportable patients to be held until stable, yet provided continuous care to an army

on the move. Evacuation hospitals, in contrast, were farther from the front lines and less mobile; these provided initial surgical care for most battle casualties.

Amputee care gradually evolved in North Africa and in the Mediterranean Theater of Operation (MTO). Indications for surgery were severe trauma to the limb, usually a partial or complete traumatic amputation, vascular injury, or uncontrolled or severe sepsis of the limb. The preferred method of amputation was the open circular technique with sulfonamide powder sprinkled on the wound and petroleum jelly gauze placed over the wound. Skin traction was maintained for transportation by an Army half-ring splint.[54]

By August 1944, this policy had been modified to discontinue the sulfonamides and replace the splint with a banjo cast with skin traction. The open circular technique was emphasized as the recommended procedure in theater, with no cuff of periosteum removed from the end of the residual limb. Patients were to be kept in skin traction for about 6 weeks so that an adherent scar could form and then transported to amputee centers in the continental United States. Secondary closures of the upper limb or lower third of the leg were performed through penicillin coverage, if the wound was clean.[54,55]

The European Theater of Operations (ETO) had the largest casualty load for the United States, as about 375,000 of the 600,000 US Army ca-

sualties came from this theater. Battlefield casualties in this theater opened on June 6, 1944, with the Normandy invasion and ended with the surrender of Germany in May 1945. During these 11 months, there was a considerable casualty load and evolution of policy. Some experience was learned from the MTO, but the commands were separate and advances in treatment did not necessarily proceed at the same rate. Before actual combat began in June 1944, guidelines were established outlining the indications and technique of amputations and the care of amputee casualties. Techniques recommended were the open circular technique and a true guillotine in which the skin, subcutaneous fat, fascia, muscle, and bone were all cut at the same level. Sulfonamide powder was to be sprinkled on the wound and then covered with petroleum jelly gauze, a technique already abandoned in the MTO.[56]

In July, these policies were changed. Consultations were now mandatory before an amputation was performed, and the indications were documented in the patient's medical record. Only the open circular technique was recommended. Sulfonamide powder was not to be used, and the patient's wound was to be dressed in fine mesh gauze to allow for drainage, a procedure similar to what was already used in the MTO. Patients were to be placed in a banjo cast for transportation. When amputations were performed for clostridial infection, patients were considered nontransportable for 24 to 48 hours and not placed in skin traction during that time.

By November, no split-thickness skin grafts or secondary closures were to be performed in theater. Patients could be moved to the continental United States after 2 to 3 weeks of skin traction at a general hospital. These later policies remained in effect through the end of the war.[56]

Indications for surgery in the ETO and MTO were primarily the effects of trauma (Table 5), which was in contrast to World War I when infection

TABLE 6 Etiology of Injury Leading to Amputation in the MTO Time Period

Cause of Amputation	1943 (%)	1944-1945 (%)
Fragment	63.7	56.9
Land mine	19.8	37.5
Gunshot	10.1	3.8
Other	6.2	0.85

was the most common cause of amputation. Hampton[55] documented that land mines were increasing in prevalence as wounding agents in the MTO (Table 6). Lower limb amputations predominated, with transtibial amputations the most common, also in contrast to World War I when transfemoral amputations predominated.[55-56] Odom,[57] who was the Third Army surgeon in the ETO, noted that land mines increased the incidence of amputations in the casualty load. He also reported that 9.0% of these patients died of their wounds after reaching medical care alive.

Management in the United States

Once an amputee was ready to be moved to the United States, he was placed in skin traction with a banjo or traction cast to allow for transportation.[58,59]

Once in the United States, the goals of care at these centers varied with the level of amputation.[60-64] Lower limb amputees were to complete their residual limb healing. The open circular technique had been used in most amputations, and the few secondary closures performed in the MTO produced poor-quality residual limbs. Most patients required a second procedure, either plastic closure of the wound or revision. The second procedure could be performed on a residual limb with healthy granulating tissue and no obvious signs of infection. Closure was performed when radiographs showed no sequestrum and were otherwise satisfactory. Follow-up at the amputation centers in the Zone of the Interior was con-

ducted according to the policies that had been established. Amputations had to be performed at as low a level as possible. Wound closure was not to be performed in theater. Heavier skin traction was needed for older amputations, and leaving excess muscle in leg residual limbs was to be avoided.[50,62]

Once healed, the residual limb was to be fitted for a temporary prosthesis so that the patient could learn ambulatory skills. When the edema had subsided and the residual limb had matured, the patient could be fitted with a permanent prosthesis.[60-63]

Upper limb amputations occurred less frequently than lower limb amputations and constituted a different clinical problem with regard to function. The goals of care for upper limb amputees at the amputee centers were residual limb healing, fitting of a prosthesis, and training in activities of daily living. Cosmesis also played a larger role in the care of a patient with an upper limb amputation.[50,62-65]

Mounting casualties and the recognition that they needed specialized care led Rankin, the Surgical Consultant to the US Army Surgeon General, to write Kirk, who in March 1943 had become the commander of Percy Jones Army General Hospital in Battle Creek, Michigan. Rankin wanted to place Kirk in charge of an amputation program and thought he would be the Orthopaedic Consultant to the Surgeon General.

On June 1, 1943, Kirk became the Surgeon General. Five hospitals, Bushnell (Brigham City, Utah), Lawson (Atlanta, Georgia), McCloskey (Temple, Texas), Walter Reed Army General Hospital (Washington, DC) and Percy Jones, had been designated as amputee centers. Problems already identified were the scarcity of surgeons with experience in the care of amputees and the lack of suitable mass-produced prostheses. Planning for amputees included provisions for acquiring suitable temporary prostheses, training personnel, and providing physical therapy.[51,54]

In June 1943, Circular Letter No. 115 outlined the type of temporary prostheses to be used, as well as the procurement and supply of these items at the amputee centers. Circular Letter No. 124, July 15, 1943, outlined the goals of physical therapy before fitting with a prosthesis; these consisted of bandaging to reduce swelling, massage, and stretching exercises to prevent joint contractures.

Peterson,[62] who was the Orthopaedic Consultant to the Surgeon General, documented that 14,912 amputees were received at the US amputee centers. More than 90% of these were received after May 1944, overburdening centers that, on paper, were planned as 500-bed facilities (2,500 total beds). Two other general hospitals became amputee centers, England (Atlantic City, New Jersey) and McGuire (Richmond, Virginia). The bed capacity of these hospitals also expanded to accommodate the casualty load.

The high visibility of amputees, as well as the real and perceived problems of their care, prompted public criticism of the US Army amputee program. As a result, civilian consultants inspected amputee centers in May 1944. The consultants were well-respected academic orthopaedic surgeons who reported on the quality of surgery, of the artificial limbs, and the general care of the amputees. The report was highly commending of the program but did not quell complaints. A second inspection, which occurred in October 1945, was equally commending to the amputee centers.[66-68]

Progress in Prosthetic Management

Prior to World War II, no national research program, either military or civilian, existed to investigate the quality of artificial limbs. Initially, the military believed that this responsibility lay with the Veterans Administration, which had the long-term responsibility for the amputee. The Veterans Administration procured nearly all of its prostheses from commercial manufacturers and therefore lacked its own experienced prosthetists and engineers.

The National Research Council established a Committee on Artificial Limbs at the request of the Surgeon General in February 1945. The committee was chaired by Paul E. Klopsteg of Northwestern University in Evanston, Illinois. The goals of the committee were to assist the Army, Navy, and government in the early procurement of the best prostheses to meet the demands of World War II. Additionally, the committee was to sponsor studies on the mechanical behavior of both normal and artificial limbs, study existing prostheses, and direct research toward improving, simplifying, and standardizing artificial limbs as much as possible. This included investigating potential new materials to manufacture limbs, studying the art of limb fitting, and training the amputee in its use. By August 1945, Kirk noted improvements in upper limb prostheses, the use of plastics, the testing of many different joints, and the use of rubber, fabric, and bonding methods recommended by the National Bureau of Standards.[69-72]

Basic research was conducted at the University of California on gait and the use of muscles to power an upper limb prosthesis; the latter was known as a cineplastic operation. Lower limb studies focused on identifying the elements of normal gait, principles that are still used today. This research, begun in World War II, was ongoing for several years and led to improvements in prostheses.[73-75]

Combat trauma in the Navy and Marine Corps resulted in 1,343 significant amputations, which necessitated the establishment of two additional amputee centers—one at Mare Island, California, and the second in Philadelphia. The clinical experiences of these two centers were published in separate symposia in the US Naval Medical Bulletin in 1945 and 1946.[76-77] The Mare Island experience was unique in that Kessler, an orthopaedic surgeon with an interest in cineplastic amputations, helped improve function in upper limb amputees by use of this technique. Because of his experience and a smaller patient load (758 patients from 1943 to 1945), casualties received at Mare Island received high-quality intensive care that was not possible at other centers.

It is difficult to ascertain how many limbs were amputated after the war because of chronic problems, usually infection, due to battle injuries. Spittler and Taylor[78] documented 150 amputations performed in 1947 and 1948 at Walter Reed Army General Hospital. Most of these patients required amputation because of long-standing osteomyelitis.

Postwar Research and the Korean War

The Committee on Artificial Limbs of the National Research Council sponsored research at various institutions at the instigation of Kirk in an effort to standardize artificial limbs as much as possible. Initial funding in 1945 came from the wartime Office of Scientific Research and Development, and later funding was provided principally by the Veterans Administration.

Initially, no laboratory was specifically established to evaluate amputees. Problems remained in two areas: the ideal reproduction of limb function and the production of materials suitable for artificial limbs. Additional studies were clearly needed to identify the scientific parameters of gait to effectively reproduce them with an artificial limb. In the late 1940s and early 1950s, Saunders and associates,[73] Inman and Ralston,[74] and Levens and associates[75] studied normal and abnormal gait by filming and measuring gait in individuals with and without amputations. Many of their findings are still relevant today.

A suction socket, one in which there is slight negative pressure to maintain contact with the residual limb, was reported by a commission that toured Europe in 1946. This type of socket gained popularity in Germany in the 1930s and was well developed in that country. The socket was tested at the University of California at Berkeley in the late 1940s, and by 1949 this socket was referred to the Veterans Administration hospitals for general use.[68,70,79]

Effects of Cineplastic Techniques

Studies on cineplastic techniques whereby a muscle (pectoralis or biceps brachii) was used to power an upper limb prosthesis were also conducted at the University of California at Berkeley to identify the ideal placement of tunnels and the amount of force generated by the muscles.[74,80] The Army had its own prosthetics research laboratory at the Forest Glen Annex of Walter Reed Army General Hospital. This laboratory was developing and testing upper limb prostheses, including the Army Prosthetics Research Laboratory (APRL) hook. The hook remains open and cable pressure causes it to close, which is the opposite mechanism for all hooks at that time.[80]

Brav and associates[81] at Walter Reed Army General Hospital studied cineplastic techniques beginning in 1948 to determine the true value of the procedure and develop any advantages it might possess. They performed 78 biceps and 29 pectoral cineplastic operations. At the end of 1 year, 73.1% of patients in the biceps group and 31% in the pectoral group were still using their prostheses. The authors concluded that biceps cineplasty was advantageous for transradial amputees because the shoulder harness could be eliminated, and the prosthesis could be used above the patient's head or behind the back. This procedure resulted in increased kinesthetic sense for the patient that was not provided by conventional prostheses. Transhumeral amputees could have more control close to the body while performing multiple tasks without undergoing locking/unlocking procedures. Pectoral cineplasty offered few advantages, except in the case of bilateral shoulder disarticulations in which any extra control was welcome.[81-83]

Patient selection for cineplasty was critical because it involved extensive surgery and training. A team consisting of surgeons, physical therapists, and prosthetists was considered essential for success. Cineplasty is no longer used in the United States because of the advent of myoelectric arms, which require less training, and the fact that surgeons cannot attain the experience necessary to become efficient in this procedure.[81-86]

Korean War

The Korean War found the US Army Medical Department with several orthopaedic surgeons who had World War II service still on active duty.[87] Indications for surgery during this conflict included complete destruction of the blood supply and diffuse clostridial myositis. Consultation with the chief of surgery or senior surgeon, along with documentation in the medical record, was encouraged. Amputations were considered lifesaving procedures and were performed in two stages, the second of which (closure) would be performed in the continental United States. Initial management of battle casualties consisted of the open circular technique at the lowest level of viable soft tissue. Disarticulations were not considered appropriate because of profuse drainage, difficulty with skin traction, and the perceived difficulty in handling the residual limbs. Patients were to be placed in transportation casts for evacuation to Japan and the United States.[87-89]

Late amputations were performed in Japan often more than 2 or 3 days after the wound was incurred in Korea. In LaZerte's[90] report on 104 patients with 108 amputations, indications for late surgery were ischemic gangrene (58% of patients), destructive trauma (35%), and gas gangrene (7%). In another study, of the 1,580 patients listed with amputations resulting from battle wounds, 33.4% died (460 were listed as killed in action and 69 as died of wounds), illustrating the destructive nature of these injuries.[91] Studies of severely injured battle casualties by the Surgical Research Team at the 46th Surgical Hospital reported that the 140 patients admitted with a major amputation during the study period had a hospital mortality rate of 7.85%.[92]

Successful repair of vascular injuries in forward hospitals became possible during the Korean War, which reduced the amputation rate from 50% (in patients with ligated vessels) to 13% (in patients who underwent vascular repair).[93-96]

Howard[97] concluded that the "most massive wounds seen in military surgery were traumatic amputations that occur in land mine warfare" and that "clinical experience clearly indicated that traumatic amputation of the foot at the ankle is not nearly so severe an injury as a traumatic amputation of the mid thigh." He suggested that bilateral transfemoral amputees were in their own special category because they had sustained "the most massive injury seen in battle." On admission, these patients were typically in shock that could not always be explained by blood loss, suggesting other mechanisms for decreased blood pressure.[101,102]

Studies of the severely injured continued into the 1950s at Edgewood Arsenal. Using a goat animal model, Lindsey and associates[98] created bilateral open femur fractures with massive destruction of soft tissues to study what therapy would prolong survival of the animals and what measures could be taken to delay initial surgery. The effectiveness of intravenous fluids, blood, antibiotics, and débridement was tested. Débridement consisted of bilateral hip disarticulations. Compared with controls, all therapeutic measures worked: blood alone, penicillin (preinjury and within 12 hours postinjury), chlortetracycline hydrochloride, chloramphenicol, and bilateral hip disarticulations. The most significant survival rates occurred when all measures were used.[98,99]

Vietnam War

The experience of World War II and Korea was not routinely taught to surgeons prior to deployment to Vietnam. As a consequence, treatment of amputees in forward hospitals was not standardized and occasionally compromised patient care, especially in the earlier stages of the war. As casualties increased, amputee centers in the continental United States slowly began to handle the specialized care required by these patients.

The incidence of amputations at surgical hospitals in Vietnam ranged from 4.5% to 5.6%. Most patients had either partial or complete traumatic amputations as a result of their injuries, necessitating only completion of the residual limb. Trauma was the primary indication for amputation in more than 90% of patients in Vietnam, followed by vascular complications (6%), and infection (3%).[100,101]

Late amputations were performed in cases of infection, either from an open fracture or as the result of a failed vascular repair. Schmitt and Armstrong[102] reported that about 186 (40%) of the 385 patients treated at Clark Air Force Base in the Philippines were in that group. The precise number of late amputations performed because of osteomyelitis is not known. Bagg, cited by Burkhalter,[103] reported that 6.5% of open tibia fractures incurred in Vietnam resulted in amputation when they were evaluated in Japan.

The Wound Data and Munitions Effectiveness Team (WDMET) recorded 98 significant amputations in their series (RF Bellamy, personal communication). Of these, 35 patients died before reaching medical care and one patient died of wounds after reaching medical care alive, a mortality rate similar to that caused by land mine injuries in the Bougainville Campaign.

Valley Forge Army General Hospital Experience

Amputations were caused by land mines and booby traps in 62% of the patients who were examined at Valley Forge Army General Hospital (AM LaNoue, MD, Ft. Leavenworth, KS, unpublished data, 1971). Land mines in Vietnam were unconventional devices made from other ordnance or improvised out of local materials. Transtibial (40%) and transfemoral (27% to 31%) amputations were the most common. Surprisingly, patients who had lost more than one limb comprised 16% of the battlefield casualty amputee admissions at Valley Forge Army General Hospital and 19% of the amputees who were received alive at a medical treatment facility in the WDMET data. It is unknown if this increase was due to improved medical care, which preserved the most severely injured, or if there was a change in the type of weapons used against Americans.

While the recommended technique at this time was an open circular amputation with postoperative skin traction, as in previous wars, this technique was not always used. In his series of 410 amputees received at Valley Forge Army General Hospital between 1969 and 1970, LaNoue reported that 41% of the transtibial amputees had skin closure prior to evacuation and that this group incurred a 56% failure rate due to gross infection. He also found that the time from the date of injury to the date of prosthetic fitting increased from 9 to 11 months when closure was performed before evacuation (AM LaNoue, student paper, US Army C & GS, Ft. Leavenworth, KS).

LaNoue also reported an 88% failure rate in Syme amputations performed in theater, necessitating conversion to amputation at a transtibial level. This failure occurred because the heel pad was partially devascularized by removal of the hindfoot.

Rather, LaNoue recommended that the hindfoot be left intact and that simple wound débridement be performed, leaving the choice of definitive amputation to the receiving physician. The devascularized heel flap did poorly when a patient was transferred to the United States from Vietnam.

LaNoue concluded that initial amputations in theater should follow three principles. First, maximum length should be preserved and definitive procedures ignored until a stable environment could be provided. Second, if a definitive procedure was necessary, the environment must be stabilized and the evacuation deferred. Finally, skin traction needed to be maintained on all residual limbs wherever possible.

Seligson and Baily[104] performed 92 acute combat amputations in 70 casualties between 1970 and 1971. Of these, 24 underwent primary closure and 10 had delayed primary closure. Indications for acute combat amputation included (1) time between injury and surgery of less than 8 hours, (2) closure that did not sacrifice useful bone, (3) no significant trauma proximal to the amputation, and (4) the patient would be held at the hospital for 2 weeks before evacuation. The authors did not report any increase in morbidity with these patients; however, the study was limited to a 2-week follow-up. Wilbur and associates[105] reported that 28% of 300 battle amputees who were admitted to Philadelphia Naval Hospital had undergone wound closure prior to arrival. They also reported that only 44% of all amputees had skin traction before arrival. Both reports show the less than optimal results that occur when a few simple principles are not followed.

Long-Term Follow-Up of Vietnam Amputees

Significant numbers of US Army amputees received treatment at Letterman, Fitzimmons, Walter Reed, Brooke, and Valley Forge Army General Hospitals. Only Valley Forge, however, established an amputee service that combined the skills of the physical therapist, surgeon, and prosthetist onto one team. A staff psychiatrist was added to the team in January 1971. The goals of treatment in these hospitals were to provide residual limb healing, ambulation training (for lower limb amputees) or training in activities of daily living (for upper limb amputees), an initial prosthesis, and a medical board that would allow for medical retirement.[106-107]

By 1969 the number of amputees had become large enough to justify a separate service at Valley Forge Army General Hospital. Patients evacuated from Vietnam were placed with other amputees, evaluated, and started on a program of residual limb healing and physical therapy. Later, patients were fitted with a temporary prosthesis to walk or perform activities of daily living. Because the numbers were significant, these amputees were widely studied. The treatment of amputees generally followed a series of successive stages, consisting of (1) wound healing, (2) preprosthetic training, (3) fitting of provisional prostheses, and (4) fitting of permanent prostheses. Patients generally progressed from one stage to the next in sequential order. Each member of the treatment team was responsible for a specific stage. During wound healing, the surgeon provided most of the care. During preprosthetic training, the therapists worked primarily with the patient. The prosthetist gradually became involved during the provisional and permanent prosthetic stages.[108]

An innovative early ambulation program was initiated at Valley Forge Army General Hospital to shorten the stages of rehabilitation. Patients ambulated earlier, even on open residual limbs, which allowed patients to become upright sooner in an effort to attain an earlier proprioceptive sense. Moreover, weight bearing on lower limb amputations reduced swelling. The hard socket allowed for compression of the residual limb and decreased edema, which was thought to

TABLE 7 Etiology of Injury Leading to Amputation—Valley Forge Army General Hospital

Cause of Amputation	% of Amputations
Land mine/Booby trap	64
Small arms	9.4
Rocket-propelled grenade	6.3
Mortar	5.2
Grenade	4.8
Artillery	3.9
Rocket	3.7

allow earlier prosthetic fitting. Finally, the psychological benefits associated with being upright sooner and earlier independence were well documented. The team approach of the amputee service at Valley Forge Army General Hospital was not always possible on the general orthopaedic service. The entire team on the amputee service followed patients' progress from admission to discharge, providing more comprehensive care to the patient and ultimately better function.

I reviewed the records of 484 battle amputees who were treated at Valley Forge Army General Hospital (hereafter Valley Forge) for level of amputation, indication for initial surgery, and mechanism of injury.[108,109] Groups of amputees were evaluated from time to evacuation to arrival at the hospital, and time to initial (pylon) and permanent prosthetic fitting. Unilateral transtibial amputation was the most common during World War II, and the trend continued. I found a higher proportion of multiple amputees (15.9%) than other studies, probably because Valley Forge was a referral hospital where the more severely wounded patients were concentrated.

Mechanism of injury is shown in Table 7. Sixty-four percent of the patients were injured by land mines or booby traps. Small arms, exploding munitions, and rocket-propelled grenades accounted for the other amputations. Trauma was the cause of amputation in 89.5% of patients,

followed by vascular injury (8.4%) and infection (1.9%).

I also conducted a long-term follow-up of these patients to ascertain the lifetime effects of such injuries.[109] Patients were surveyed regarding their prosthetic history and family life, including the following: marriage and children; number of additional surgeries since their initial amputation; psychiatric history, including membership in Alcoholics Anonymous and marriage counseling; other injuries; and work history.

Transtibial Amputees

Amputation at the transtibial level is the most common in war amputees, representing 37.8% of the amputations in this series.[108] Land mines and booby traps were the most common cause of injury leading to amputation (65.3%), followed by mortar fragments (17%), small arms (8.5%), injuries inside of vehicles (5.5%), and rocket-propelled grenades (3.9%). Indications for surgery were partial or complete traumatic amputation in 82% of patients, infection in 13%, and failed vascular repair in 5%. Evacuation time to Valley Forge averaged 3.5 weeks from the time of injury. Average time to pylon fitting was 5.3 weeks (range, 2 to 16 weeks), and time to permanent prostheses was 6.8 months (range, 1 to 14 months).

Of the 123 patients eligible for the study, 72 (59%) were available for follow-up, and these were divided into two groups. One group had isolated transtibial amputations, and the second had at least one other major injury (polytrauma), defined in this study as a major lower limb long bone fracture, burns over more than 20% of the body surface area, and/or significant head, face, chest, or abdominal wounds. Most of the patients (44) were in the second group. A comparison of employment, marriage, and family factors showed no significant difference between the two groups. However, the reported incidence of psychological care differed significantly ($P < 0.001$) between the two groups, with only 21% of group one

seeking help compared with 50% of group two.

All respondents were presently wearing prostheses, with the first group averaging 15.9 hours per day and the second group, 15.7 hours. Most respondents reported that they had changed prostheses, specifically 78.5% of group one and 72% of group two. The most commonly reported changes were in the foot (22), suspension (20), liner (18), and socket (8). The average number of prostheses used since the first permanent prostheses were fitted was 7.89 (range, 3 to 30) in group one and 8.84 (range, 4 to 30) in group two. Patients reported an average of 1.94 operations since their initial amputation (range, 0 to 13), with 1.36 in group one and 2.32 in group two.

Ertl osteoplasty produces an end-bearing residual limb for transtibial amputees by creating a bony synostosis between the tibia and fibula at the distal end of the residual limb. Deffer and associates,[110] Deffer,[111] and Moll[112] reported that this procedure resulted in a more stable and durable residual limb. Comparison with other transtibial amputees was not documented, however, and the definitive benefits of this level of amputation over the conventional transtibial amputation remain unclear. The Ertl procedure was performed in 42 patients (63%), 19 in group one and 23 in group two.[108] One patient reported having had the bone block removed because of pain. The SF-36 scores for group one were not significantly different ($P < 0.01$) from the controls. Group two patients were significantly different in all areas ($P < 0.01$).

Transfemoral Amputees

The review of records showed that 59% of these patients were injured by land mines and booby traps. Indications for surgery were trauma in 61.8% of patients, failed vascular repair in 29.2%, and infection in 8.7%. The average time to Valley Forge was 4.4 weeks and to pylon was 4 weeks, with permanent prosthetic fitting at an average of 7 months. At follow-up, at an average of 28 years after injury, 51% of those alive and eligible for the study agreed to answer the questionnaire. Of those, 93% are or were married, 91.3% are or have been employed, and 85% have children.[113]

The average number of operations on the residual limb since the initial amputation was 2.4. Six patients (13%) do not presently wear a prosthesis; the others wear theirs an average of 13.5 hours per day and have owned an average of 13.8 prostheses since their initial fitting. Of those who wear a prosthesis, half have changed their prescription since the initial fitting. Twenty-four patients (52%) reported seeking psychological care, including Alcoholics Anonymous and marriage counseling. SF-36 scores were significantly lower ($P < 0.05$) in all categories except mental health.

Bilateral Transfemoral Amputees

Thirty patients (6.2%) were identified as bilateral transfemoral amputees, which is a relatively higher frequency than expected, probably because the more severely injured were referred to Valley Forge.[109] Of these patients, 26 were injured by land mines or booby traps. Other mechanisms of injury included artillery/mortar fire (three patients) and machine gun fire (one patient). Indications for surgery were trauma in 53 (88%) of 60 residual limbs and infection in the remaining seven. The medical records indicated that postoperative skin traction was used in fewer than half the patients. Three patients also sustained an upper limb amputation, with one at the wrist, one above the elbow, and one below the elbow. Documentation of shock and resuscitation attempts was incomplete, but the records of 14 patients indicated that an average of 23.7 units of blood had been transfused.

Patients arrived at Valley Forge an average of 4.5 weeks after injury. Records of 23 patients showed that they were fitted with pylons or stubbies an average of 8.3 weeks after injury (range, 3 to 20 weeks). Records

of 17 patients showed that they were fitted with permanent prostheses an average of 6.5 months after injury (range, 3 to 12 months).

Three patients died since leaving Valley Forge, and 23 of the remaining 27 (85.2%) agreed to answer the questionnaire and SF-36 form. Sixteen of the 23 (69.5%) are employed outside the home even though they have adequate compensation from the Veterans Administration to maintain a modest lifestyle. Twenty-one (91.3%) are or were married, and 20 (87%) had children. Five patients (21.7%) reported the use of mental health services.

Five patients (21.7%) reported that they still wear a prosthesis for an average of 7.7 hours per day. Ten others (43.4%) report using their prostheses an average of 12.8 years after leaving Valley Forge. Five patients report using prostheses today primarily for "going out."

The SF-36 scores of bilateral transfemoral amputees did not significantly differ from those of controls except in the area of physical function. It is not clear why the SF-36 scores for the amputee group were higher than those of the other groups. One explanation might be the small number of patients. Another explanation might be the lower proportion of patients in the other groups that were eligible to participate in the study. Finally, there could be an error in methodology.

Brown[115] studied bilateral lower extremity amputees at Fitzimmons Army General Hospital. These patients had the most severe injuries, most often the result of explosive munitions, and they often had other associated injuries of the trunk, upper limbs, and face. Because these amputees did not have a sound leg available for balance, they needed more time for gait training. These patients were fitted initially with shorter (stubby) prostheses and then advanced to regular prostheses when acceptable gait had been established. Brown emphasized return to recreational activities to help foster confidence, pride, and a

sense of accomplishment in these amputees, all of whom were young and previously athletic. It is unclear how many of them maintained such a high level of function once discharged from the military.

The autobiography of Lewis Puller documents the trauma of a young individual who becomes a multiple amputee.[116] Puller spent approximately 2 years undergoing treatment and rehabilitation after stepping on a booby trap improvised out of a cannon shell. He lost both legs, one at the hip and one at midthigh, and had partial amputations of both hands.

Herndon and associates[117] reported on patients who had femur fractures, in addition to their amputations, and used a cast brace and early ambulation. Patients averaged 22 weeks to healing, had less than 1 cm of shortening, and an average of 75° of knee motion. In another study, Herndon and associates[118] reported three cases of *Mycobacterium fortuitum* infections in the patients who were treated surgically because of resistance to antituberculosis medications.

Philadelphia Naval Hospital and Oakland Naval Hospital were responsible for the treatment of a significant number of Navy and Marine Corps amputees. Golbranson and associates[119] reported on the effectiveness of immediate postoperative fitting and early ambulation. While their discussion focused on older patients with diabetes mellitus and immediate postoperative fitting, the implications for the early fitting of young individuals with amputations due to trauma were significant.

Current Concepts
Mechanisms of Injury

The injury leading to the eventual loss of limb is worth investigating for several reasons. First, war wounds differ from those seen in the civilian community. Second, surgeons need to understand disease processes to better treat the patient.

Land mines are the most common agent of wounding resulting in loss of limb on the battlefield. The US Army classifies land mines as antipersonnel or antimaterial. Antimaterial land mines are designed to destroy or disable vehicles. Antipersonnel land mines are meant to injure individuals. There are four general types of antipersonnel land mines: static, bounding, horizontal spray, and unconventional.

Static land mines are placed above ground or buried and remain in place until detonated by a person who steps on them. They generally have small explosive charges, 100 to 200 grams, and are the most common antipersonnel land mines throughout the world. Surgeons from the former Soviet Union obtained considerable clinical experience with static antipersonnel land mines during the conflict in Afghanistan from 1979 to 1988, which prompted laboratory investigations of the mechanism of injury.[120] They reported that small, static land mines created a very consistent pattern of injury. Closest to the land mine was an area of partial or complete traumatic amputation (avulsion or mangling), usually at the midfoot or distal tibia. Second, there was an area of soft-tissue stripping from the bone or along fascial planes resulting from exploding munition. Tissue in this region, extending up to the knee, may or may not survive. This area is critical in terms of tissue viability and ultimate limb length. More proximally, the effects of the blast itself are limited, though fast translation of the limb may occur. Fragments from the exploding munition, clothing, or debris may injure the contralateral limb or other parts of the body. Factors that influence the injury from a particular land mine include the size and shape of the limb, which part of the foot first touches the land mine, the type of footwear worn, and the amount of debris overlying the land mine.

Bounding mines are land mines that, when tripped, propel a small device such as a grenade vertically to about 1 to 2 m. The device then explodes, causing multiple fragment wounds to persons nearby.

Horizontal spray mines are devices that fire fragments in one direction when detonated. The US Army's Claymore mine, for example, fires about 700 steel balls weighing about 10 grains each in one direction. Patients tend to have multiple small fragment wounds from this injury.

Unconventional devices are land mines or booby traps that are constructed of another piece of ordnance, such as a cannon shell or a grenade. There can also be land mines or booby traps made out of locally available materials. Most amputations performed on US soldiers in Vietnam were caused by these devices. They are also the most common mine seen in Operation Iraqi Freedom.

Issues Affecting Amputation

Indications

Amputations are performed in forward hospitals to save lives, a goal that remains largely unchanged from previous conflicts. Indications are partial or complete traumatic amputations that require only completion of the residual limb, a major vascular injury that cannot be repaired, or overwhelming sepsis.

Limb Salvage Versus Amputation

Every military surgeon should consider whether some limbs amputated in previous conflicts could be salvaged today. To answer this question, the advances made in trauma care over the years must be reviewed, particularly their applicability to severely traumatized limbs. Clearly, the ability to repair a vascular injury has resulted in an overall reduction in the number of amputations because vascular repair was widely attempted during the Korean War. Since Vietnam, the use of free flaps to cover bone defects has prevented infection and improved healing. New designs in external fixation have improved fracture stabiliza-

tion for severe injuries. Most amputations (87%) are partial or complete traumatic amputations, requiring only débridement of the residual limb. Late amputations are the result of infection or failed vascular repair.[108]

Late Amputations

Recent interest has focused on determining which limbs require amputation and which fare best with limb salvage.[121-133] Late amputations (ie, those that occurred after transport) have been analyzed by several authors. Bagg, cited by Burkhalter,[103] reported that 13 of 200 tibia fractures received at the 106th General Hospital in Japan from Vietnam required amputation (10 transtibial and 3 transfemoral). Schmitt and Armstrong[102] found that open fractures with vascular injury were responsible for nearly half (48%) of the late amputations seen in their facility during the Vietnam War, followed by vascular injuries alone (25%), fractures only (17%), and soft-tissue infection (10%).

Open Fractures

Open fractures have been classified since the mid 1970s by the Gustilo and Anderson grading system (grade I, II, and III). This system was later modified to include grades IIIA, B, and C, depending on severity. Grade IIIB fractures are open tibia fractures that require local or free flap coverage of the exposed bone. Grade IIIC fractures have a vascular injury that requires repair. Recently, Brumback and Jones[124] have raised concerns about the interobserver reliability with the classification system.

Caudle and Stern[125] reported on amputation rates associated with 42 type IIIB fractures that required a free flap and 9 type IIIC fractures with repairable vascular injury. Of the patients with IIIB fractures, 17% required amputation, compared with 78% of patients with type IIIC fractures.

Georgiadis and associates[126] evaluated patients with 20 severe tibia fractures that required a free flap for soft-tissue coverage. Of these, only four required amputation. Average follow-up was 35 months. Another 18 patients with severe tibia fractures seen at this facility at the same time required primary amputations. Average follow-up for this group was 44 months. Two patients in the limb salvage group had major vascular injury, whereas 15 of the 18 amputees had vascular injuries. Three patients in the limb salvage group returned to work, compared with 9 of the 18 amputees. Average time to full weight bearing was 13 months for the limb salvage group and 6 months for the amputation group.

Quirke and associates[127] evaluated 35 patients with open tibia fractures and major vascular injuries (Gustilo type IIIC). Of these, 21 underwent primary amputation (60%) and 14 (40%) required vascular repair and fracture stabilization. One underwent late amputation.

Predicting the Need for Amputations

Attempts to predict the need to amputate have resulted in the development of several limb salvage scores. The mangled extremity severity score (MESS), NISSSA (N=Nerve injury, I=Ischemia, S=Soft-tissue injury, S=Skeletal injury, S=Shock, and A=Age), Predictive Salvage Index (PSI), and Limb Salvage Index (LSI) have been evaluated in a few studies characterized by small sample sizes and a wide range of injuries (Gustilo types IIIB and IIIC).[121-123,131]

Bosse and associates[123,131] enrolled 601 patients prospectively in the LEAP (Lower Extremity Assessment Project) study group, which evaluated the MESS, the NISSSA score, the PSI, the Hannover Fracture Scale-97, and the LSI. In this study, there were 55 traumatic amputations, 63 immediate amputations, and 86 delayed amputations. The authors reported that none of the scales was sufficiently predictive in determining when amputation is necessary. Threshold scores were found to have low sensitivity but relatively high specificity and thus could not be recommended as criteria to amputate a limb. Thus far, it appears that no scale can reliability predict the outcome of a severely traumatized limb.

It is not clear, therefore, if the new techniques developed since the Vietnam War will improve limb survival and function for patients injured on the battlefield.

Vascular Repair Failure and Amputation

Vascular repair has been used since the Korean War. Open fractures with associated vascular injury can be treated by fracture stabilization followed by vascular repair. Use of external fixators is indicated to provide access to the vascular structures of the limb. Using local or free flaps for soft-tissue coverage should never be attempted in theater unless the patient is followed through healing by the same surgeon at the same location. Patients who are to be evacuated should not undergo extensive surgery for soft-tissue coverage before evacuation. Attempts at coverage should be performed only when a patient is in a stable environment and will not be moved.[133]

Initial Management
Refugee Care

Recent experience in treating civilian war casualties by the International Committee of the Red Cross (ICRC) has led to guidelines on the care of amputees in strife-torn regions throughout the world. Initial surgical management consists of excising dead tissue, fashioning flaps that can be closed later, and placing the limb in a bulky dressing. The wound is inspected in the operating room a few days later and is closed if the wound condition permits. Patients may be fitted with a prosthesis when the residual limb wound is healed and the edema has subsided. No discussion of early fitting of amputees is presented in ICRC literature.[134-137]

Simper[134] recently reported on the treatment of 111 transtibial amputees in Pakistan, recommending delayed primary closure of the transtibial amputations that result from war wounds. The patients in this series survived a median transport time to the hospital of 14 hours; the more severely injured patients in my series would not have survived that long an evacuation time. In Simper's study, delayed primary closure of the residual limbs was performed a median of 6.4 days from the initial surgery. A total of 13% of the amputations in this series failed. There was no discussion of prosthesis fitting.

The treatment of refugees in a theater of operations or in "nation building" efforts remains dependent on the resources available to the medical staff. Surgeons treating refugees should not plan procedures that require extensive long-term care. Procedures should be planned with the country's resources in mind, not what is possible at a medical center in the United States. In this context, the recommendations by the ICRC are reasonable and can be used to provide the best care for the most people. Patients in this setting can be cared for by the same surgeon and do not have to be evacuated. Fitting of amputees is often problematic because prostheses are expensive and rehabilitation requires additional resources.[134-137]

Care of US or Allied Soldiers

As reported previously, the US Army established an amputee service at Valley Forge Army General Hospital in 1969 to care for the increasing number of amputees during the Vietnam War.[108,109,113] As referenced earlier, LaNoue reported on a group of transtibial amputees who were treated at Valley Forge Army General Hospital and compared those whose wounds were closed in theater to those whose wounds were left open and maintained in skin traction. He examined 230 patients with transtibial residual limbs, some of whom were multiple amputees, and reported that 41% of patients underwent wound closure in theater. Of those closed in theater, 56% experienced failure because of gross infection. Time to permanent prostheses was also longer for patients whose wounds were closed in theater (13 months) compared with those whose residual limb was left open (11 months).

LaNoue indicated that skin traction was essential to prevent complications, especially in patients placed on an airplane to reach the site of definitive care. Skin traction is used to preserve residual limb length and prevent infection.

Recommendations for US or Allied soldiers who must be evacuated from theater are unchanged since the Vietnam War. Surgery should be performed at the lowest viable level of soft tissue with no consideration of the definitive or final level of amputation. The open circular technique, which has since been renamed open length-preserving amputation, should be used with stepwise shortening at levels from the skin to the bone, with the skin the most distal and bone most proximal. All dead or necrotic tissue should be removed. Often with irregular war wounds an oblique wound is created. Wounds should be left open because it is safer for patients evacuated by air. These wounds should be placed in skin traction to prevent bone protrusion and residual limb swelling. Patients should be placed in transportation casts before air evacuation.

Transportation Casts

Transportation casts should be used for patients who are to be removed from combat zone hospitals because these casts provide continuous, portable traction throughout the evacuation chain. Lower limb amputees often can ambulate on crutches if the amputation is an isolated injury, but they should be considered litter patients. Traction can be attached to the litter or a traction splint used; however, neither provides reliable traction that can be maintained throughout the evacuation chain. In addition, no soft-tissue support is provided by these means (AM LaNoue, MD, Ft. Leavenworth, KS, unpublished data, 1971).

Transtibial Amputees Patients with transtibial amputations should be placed in a modified long leg cast. During the last surgery in theater, a dressing should be placed over the wound and then the cast applied. The cast consists of 6-in wide plaster and 6-in cotton padding. The end of the residual limb is cleaned, and an adherent is applied to the skin. Stockinette is applied over the distal end of the residual limb for about the last 10 to 15 cm, and the cast is applied from the end of the residual limb to the proximal thigh. An outrigger, made of a wire (ladder) splint, is used to maintain traction. For transtibial amputees, traction should be from 1 to 2 kg to overcome the elastic recoil of the skin. The cast should be bivalved before air evacuation.[108]

Transfemoral Amputees Transfemoral amputees should be fitted with a hip spica cast, which is best applied during the last surgery in theater. A fracture table can assist the application of the cast. Stockinette is applied to the distal end of the residual limb, similar to transtibial amputees, after a dressing is placed over the wound. The sacrum and anterior superior iliac spine (ASIS) are padded with felt. Six-inch cotton padding is placed from the distal end of the residual limb to the level of the umbilicus, and the contralateral thigh is included. Next, 6-in plaster strips are wrapped, beginning with the involved limb. An outrigger must be incorporated to the distal end to provide traction through the stockinette. The traction should be from 2 to 4 kg, enough to overcome the elastic recoil of the skin. For the last roll, the cotton padding is turned down to the level of the ASIS. In this way, the completed cast leaves the abdomen exposed, which allows respiratory function during transport. The cast should be bivalved before evacuation.[105,113]

Transradial Amputees Transradial amputees are placed in skin traction by applying a dressing over the wound and then stockinette in the manner previously described. A long

arm cast is then applied, using 4-in cotton padding and 4-in wide plaster. An outrigger is applied so that about 1 kg of traction can be maintained. The cast must be bivalved before evacuation.

Transhumeral Amputees Transhumeral amputees can be placed in traction by applying a dressing to the end of the residual limb. Stockinette can be applied over the end of the residual limb only but is usually applied to the entire length of the residual limb. After padding, a wire splint can be fashioned and placed over the distal end of the residual limb. It can then be held in place by plaster of Paris. If the wound is proximal, this technique may not be possible without making a shoulder spica cast (AM LaNoue, MD, Ft. Leavenworth, KS, unpublished data, 1971).

Definitive Management

Upon arrival from overseas, patients should be carefully examined by a team of surgeons, therapists, and nurses. Open residual limbs should be examined and placed in skin traction to prevent bony protrusion. Once examined, lower limb amputees should be fitted with a provisional prosthesis as soon as possible, even if they have open wounds. This prosthesis should be removable to allow access to the wound and skin traction in bed. Clearly, early walking has psychological benefits, improves wound healing, and allows earlier proprioception[108,109,113] (AM LaNoue, MD, Ft. Leavenworth, KS, unpublished data, 1971). Upper limb amputees also require thorough examination and placement in a provisional prosthesis to begin training in activities of daily living. This training should begin daily under the supervision of occupational therapists.[138]

Lower Limb Amputees

Transfemoral amputees received from overseas should be placed in skin traction upon arrival at the hospital in the United States. A provisional prosthesis (pylon) should be fabricated with a plaster socket, a shank, and a foot. Patients should not receive a knee until some gait control and progress in healing are made. A knee may increase the shear forces across the open wound.

As the edema and swelling subside, the patient may be fitted with a knee, and therapy should be directed toward establishing normal gait. Increasing weight bearing decreases edema. As the wound heals, it should be assessed periodically to determine whether additional surgery is indicated. Coverage obtained by skin traction alone often results in a distal scar or adherent tissue to the bone. Myodesis can be considered if the patient's condition is stable in the weeks after injury, if the patient has begun ambulation, and if swelling and edema in the residual limb are decreased. Although there is no "ideal length," limbs less than 10 cm distally from the greater trochanter are more difficult to fit. During the planned second procedure, the adductor and quadriceps may be attached to the distal end of the femur to prevent the potential for abduction contracture.

After the second procedure is complete, the patient may be fitted with a pylon and allowed to ambulate carefully, paying attention to pain and drainage in the residual limb. This pylon should be replaced frequently as the edema and swelling subside. A patient with a well-healed residual limb of a stable size may be fitted with a permanent prosthesis, typically 6 to 8 weeks later in healthy young adults. Unilateral transfemoral amputees treated at Valley Forge Army General Hospital were ready for a permanent prosthesis about 7 months after injury (AM LaNoue, MD, unpublished data, Ft. Leavenworth, KS, 1971). Very short residual limbs can be salvaged using a small pin fixator and lengthening of the bone. The quality of the regenerated bone and skin should be observed.

The Ertl Procedure The Ertl procedure provides a more end-bearing residual limb by creating a bone bridge beween the distal tibia and fibula. This procedure is recommended for young patients who sustain traumatic amputations because it provides a more durable residual limb. Deffer and associates[110] and Deffer[111] reported good results with the use of this technique on Vietnam War transtibial amputees. However, no study compares patients treated with the procedure with those who were not.[108,110,111]

If a secondary procedure is performed, the patient can be fitted on the operating table with a pylon that can be left on for 2 weeks, and gait training can be resumed immediately. The prosthesis can be removed earlier in the event of drainage, pain, or loosening. The pylon is then changed weekly until the edema and swelling have subsided. The patient can then be fitted with a permanent prosthesis.

Syme Ankle Disarticulation
Syme ankle disarticulation is the highest level of amputation a patient can have without wearing a prosthesis for limited ambulation. This procedure should not be performed in theater because the vascular supply to the heel pad can easily be compromised when left open. LaNoue reported that 88% of these procedures performed in theater failed because of sepsis. Forefoot injuries without a compromised heel pad should be débrided, and the patient evacuated from theater. A Syme procedure should be performed only at the site of definitive care (AM LaNoue, MD, Ft. Leavenworth, KS, unpublished data, 1971).

The Syme ankle disarticulation is performed by creating a heel flap and removing the talus and calcaneus. The tendons are cut and allowed to retract. Major vascular structures are ligated and then cut. Because small vessels tend to run with the nerve, they should be ligated and then allowed to retract to prevent neuroma formation. If the procedure is performed in one stage, the malleoli and articular surface of the distal tibia are removed to form the residual limb. The heel flap is brought forward to cover the distal end of the residual limb.

Postoperatively, the patient is placed in a cast with a walking heel to begin ambulation. As ambulation improves and swelling decreases, the cast should be changed. Once the swelling and edema have reached a plateau, the patient can be fitted with a permanent prosthesis. Prosthetic considerations include the use of a foot with limited height so that limb lengthening does not occur, resulting in limb-length discrepancy. A thinner solid ankle-cushion heel (SACH) foot has been the choice for this type of amputation, along with a double-walled prosthesis with an elastic liner.

Upper Limb Amputees

When deemed stable, the patient is placed in skin traction with a transportation cast before evacuation to the United States. Prior to application of the cast, stockinette is applied to the last 15 cm of the skin by means of a skin adherent. For a transradial amputee, the cast consists of a long arm cast with an outrigger made of a ladder wire splint or similar device. Skin traction, sufficient to overcome the elastic recoil of the skin, is applied to the stockinette covering the distal end of the residual limb. The cast must be bivalved before evacuation.[132]

Transhumeral amputees are best served by a shoulder spica cast, which allows an outrigger to be placed to apply traction as indicated above. However, in multiple-trauma patients with chest injuries, a shoulder spica cast may not be possible and should be replaced with a padded coaptation splint with a wire splint such as an outrigger.[137]

Shoulder disarticulation is a rare level of injury. Skin traction may not be possible because of other injuries, but the wounds should be left open during evacuation.

Once at the site of definitive care, patients should be thoroughly examined. All wounds should be uncovered and inspected. The upper limb amputee can be placed in a provisional prosthesis while maintaining skin traction and can begin to learn to perform activities of daily living.

Casts should be changed until the edema and swelling have subsided. At this point, a second procedure may be performed to close the residual limb. Usually, a plastic closure is performed to remove adherent scar and close the wound. Sometimes bone will be shortened to obtain wound closure.

Patients who were injured while holding an explosive device may have bilateral amputations and be partially or completely blind. Of these patients, transradial amputees may benefit from the Krukenberg procedure, which involves separating the radius and ulna to create a pincers mechanism. The pronator teres provides the strongest adduction force in this procedure. This type of amputation does not preclude the use of a standard prosthesis.[130]

Patients with a shoulder disarticulation should undergo skin closure when the soft tissues will tolerate it. They can be fitted with a permanent prosthesis as soon as the wound is healed.

Conclusion

Amputations are the most severe limb injuries seen in war. Care for amputees has been a significant clinical concern for the military in every major conflict in the 20th century. As few surgeons or teams have significant clinical experience in caring for amputees, lapses or inconsistencies occur. Furthermore, the techniques and requirements for patients who are evacuated from overseas hospitals differ from those required by patients treated in civilian hospitals. War surgery for amputations is a two-staged procedure. Initial care to remove the limb to prevent infection and save the patient's life is provided at a forward hospital. Most forward amputations simply complete a partial or complete traumatic amputation. Once stabilized, the patient should be placed in a transportation cast and skin traction for transportation. Unless the surgeon is able to follow a patient for several days postoperatively, the wound must be left open and placed in skin traction to prevent infection and loss of residual limb length.

As was demonstrated in previous conflicts, there is a clear need for amputee centers that specialize in the care of soldiers evacuated from a theater of operations. The main advantages of this consolidation of efforts were described in this chapter; they include maintaining the clinical skills of the nursing staff, prosthetists, therapists, and surgeons to facilitate complete healing of the residual limb; fitting with a provisional prosthesis; rehabilitation; and fitting with a satisfactory permanent prosthesis.

The US military has established an amputee center at Walter Reed Army Medical Center, and clinical experience in treating battle amputees is increasing. Clinical experience can be obtained by working in amputee clinics at Veterans Administration hospitals, but it does not provide experience with the initial care and management of this special group of amputees. Care provided to refugees throughout the world by the ICRC and other organizations provides some experience for the initial care of battle amputees, but there are differences in amputee care because a refugee will not be evacuated out of the country.

References

1. MacLeod GHB: *Notes on the Surgery of the War in the Crimea With Remarks on the Treatment of Gunshot Wounds.* Philadelphia, PA, JB Lippincott, 1862.

2. Gross SD: *A Manual of Military Surgery.* Philadelphia, PA, JB Lippincott, 1861, pp 74-89. (Reprinted by Norman Publishing, San Francisco, CA, 1988.)

3. Hamilton FH: *A Practical Treatise on Military Surgery.* New York, NY, Bailliere Brothers, 1861, pp 165-189. (Reprinted by Norman Publishing, San Francisco, CA, 1989.)

4. Warren E: *An Epitome of Practical Surgery for Field and Hospital.* Richmond, VA, 1863. (Reprinted by Norman Publishing, San Francisco, CA, 1989.)

5. Swinburne J: Amputations. *Am Med Times* 1863;6:149-150.

6. Detmold W: Lectures on military surgery: Lecture VII. *Am Med Times* 1863;6:73-74.

7. Peters DC: Remarks on amputations. *Am Med Times* 1863;6:302-304.

8. Smith DP: Experiences in military surgery. *Am Med Times* 1863;6:110-111.

9. Fisher GJ: Report of fifty-seven cases of amputations in the hospitals near Sharpsburg, MD, after the Battle of Antietam, September 17, 1862. *Am J Med Sci* 1863;XLV:44-51.

10. Letterman J: *Medical Recollections of the Army of the Potomac.* New York, NY, Appleton and Company, 1866.

11. Oblensky FE: Jonathan Letterman. *Mil Med* 1968;133:312-316.

12. Jones GW: The medical history of the Fredericksburg Campaign: Course and significance. *J His Med* 1963;XVIII:241-256.

13. Gibbs OC: Correspondence-Amputations at the Battlefield of Fredericksburg. *Med Surg Report* 1863;9:416-418.

14. Moses I: Surgical notes of cases of gunshot injuries occurring near Chattanooga, Tennessee. *Am J Med Sci* 1863;48:344-366.

15. Hodgen JT: On the treatment of gunshot fractures of the femur and tibia. *Am Med Times* 1863;8:169-170.

16. Lidell JA: Correspondence. *Am Med Times* 1863;8:102-103.

17. Hamilton FH: *A Treatise on Military Surgery.* New York, NY, Bailleire Brothers, 1865, p 420-486.

18. Otis GA, Huntington DC: *The Medical and Surgical History of the War of the Rebellion: Part II.* Washington, DC, Government Printing Office, 1883, vol 2, pp 1-614, 870-871.

19. Jewett CC: After-treatment of amputations and resections in the Third Corps Field Hospital after Gettysburg. *Boston Med Surg J* 1864;70:211-216.

20. Minor JM: Report on artificial limbs. *New York Acad Med* 1861;1:163-180.

21. Goldthwait JE: *The Division of Orthopaedic Surgery in the AEF.* Norwood, MA, Plimpton Press, 1941.

22. Goldthwait JE: The place of orthopedic surgery in the treatment of war casualties. *Mil Surg* 1917;41:450-456.

23. Blake JA: Early experiences in the war. *Mil Surg* 1919;45:626-635.

24. Crile GW: *Notes on Military Surgery.* Cleveland, OH, William Feather, 1924, pp 84-88.

25. Wright GA: Amputation by plane circular section. *Lancet* 1915;2:810-811.

26. Anon: Amputations and amputation residual limbs. *Lancet* 1916;1:870-871.

27. Fitzmaurice-Kelly M: The flapless amputation. *Br J Surg* 1916;3:676-681.

28. Blake JA: Surgical impressions of the World War. *Mil Surg* 1926;58:225-236.

29. Speed K: Base hospital amputations in war. *JAMA* 1918;71:271-274.

30. Callender GR, Coupal JF, Section JF: *Surgery.* Washington, DC, US Government Printing Office, 1929, vol XII, pp 407-461.

31. Weed FW (ed): *Surgery.* Washington, DC, US Government Printing Office, 1927, vol XI, pp 687-712.

32. Orr HW: *An Orthopedic Surgeon's Story of the Great War.* Norfolk, NE, Huse Publishing, 1921.

33. Wilson PD: Early weight-bearing in the treatment of amputations of the lower limbs. *J Bone Joint Surg* 1922;4:224-247.

34. Kirk NT: The development of amputation, in Vasconcelos E (ed): *Modern Methods of Amputation.* New York, NY, Philosophical Library of New York, 1945, pp XI-XXXIV.

35. Kirk NT: *Amputations.* Chicago, IL, WB Conkey, 1924.

36. Garrison FH: Prosthetic appliances in war-time (historical resume). *Mil Surg* 1919;45:507-509.

37. Office of the Surgeon General: Instruments and appliances: Temporary artificial limbs. *Mil Surg* 1918;42:490-498.

38. Office of the Surgeon General: The relation between the amputation and the fitting of the artificial limb. *Mil Surg* 1918;42:154-168.

39. Cannon WB: *Traumatic Shock.* New York, NY, Appleton, 1923, pp 1-149.

40. Blalock A: *Principals of Surgical Care.* St. Louis, MO, CV Mosby, 1940, pp 91-186.

41. Parsons EB, Phemister DB: Hemorrhage and "shock" in traumatized limbs. *Surg Gyn Obstet* 1930;51:196-207.

42. Churchill ED: *Surgeon to Soldiers.* Philadelphia, PA, JB Lippincott, 1972, pp 36-58.

43. Kirk NT: Amputation residual limbs of the lower extremity. *J Bone Joint Surg* 1933;15:101-111.

44. Kirk NT: Organization for evacuation and treatment of war casualties. *Ann Surg* 1941;113:1020-1033.

45. Gordon-Taylor G: On amputations. *Lancet* 1942;262:619.

46. Mitchell GAG, Logie NJ, Handley RS: Casualties from the western desert and Libya. *Lancet* 1941;260:713-716.

47. Anon: With the Eighth Army. *Lancet* 1942;263:15-16.

48. Logie NJ: Surgical gleanings from the Middle East. *Lancet* 1943;265:658-662.

49. Harris RI: Amputations. *J Bone Joint Surg* 1944;26:626-634.

50. McFarlane JA: Wounds in modern war. *J Bone Joint Surg* 1942;24:739-752.

51. Kirk NT: Amputations in war. *JAMA* 1942;120:13-16.

52. Kirk NT, McKeever FM: The guillotine amputation. *JAMA* 1944;124:1027-1030.

53. Churchill ED: The surgical management of the wounded in the Mediterranean Theater at the time of the fall of Rome. *Ann Surg* 1944;120:268-283.

54. Snyder HE: Fifth US Army, in Carter NB (ed): *Surgery in World War II: The Activities of the Surgical Consultants.* Washington, DC, US Government Printing Office, 1962, vol 1, pp 333-464.

55. Hampton OP: Amputations, in Cleveland M (ed): *Surgery in World War II: Orthopedic Surgery in the Mediterranean Theater of Operations.* Washington, DC, US Government Printing Office, 1957, pp 245-270.

56. Cleveland M (ed): Amputations, in *Surgery in World War II: Orthopedic Surgery in the European Theater of Operations.* Washington, DC, US Government Printing Office, 1956, pp 155-167.

57. Odom CB: Causes of amputations in battle casualties with emphasis on vascular injuries. *Surgery* 1946;20:562-569.

58. Barnett HE, Weinstein L: Use of the traction cast in guillotine amputations. *Bull US Army Med Dept* 1944;2:83-87.

59. Macgrath JL: Traction of soft tissues: A new method following amputation. *Mil Surg* 1944;93:373-374.

60. Thompson VP: The amputation residual limb from the prosthetic point of view. *JAMA* 1944;124:1036-1040.

61. Thompson TC: Temporary prostheses. *JAMA* 1944;124:1041-1047.

62. Peterson LT: The Army amputation program. *J Bone Joint Surg* 1944;26:635-638.

63. McKeever FM: A discussion of controversial points in amputation surgery. *Surg Gyn Obs* 1946;82:495-511.

64. McKeever FB: Upper-extremity amputations and prostheses. *J Bone Joint Surg* 1944;26:660-671.

65. Steindler A: Artificial limbs. *Mil Surg* 1940;86:560-564.

66. Phalen JM: Editorial: On the subject of amputations. *Mil Surg* 1944;94:377.

67. Klopsteg PE: The functions and activities of the Committee on Artificial Limbs of the National Research Council. *J Bone Joint Surg* 1947;29:538-540 .

68. Conn H, Magnuson PS, Wilson PD: Report of Civilian Consultants Committee on Army Amputation Services. *Mil Surg* 1946;98:52-57.

69. Anon: Improved artificial hand. *Bull US Army Med Dept* 1947;VII:338-340.

70. Brodbeck JA: Experiment with the suction socket for transfemoral amputees. *Bull US Army Med Dept* 1947;VII:408-411.

71. Kissane MM: A light-weight end bearing thigh bucket. *Bull US Army Med Dept* 1947;VII:406-407.

72. Thomas A: Anatomical and physiological considerations in the alignment and fitting of amputation prostheses for the lower extremity. *J Bone Joint Surg* 1944;26:645-659.

73. Saunders JB, Inman VT, Eberhart HD: The major determinants in normal and pathological gait. *J Bone Joint Surg Am* 1953;35:543-558.

74. Inman VT, Ralston HJ: The mechanics of voluntary muscle, in Klopsteg PE, et al (eds): *Human Limbs and Their Substitutes.* New York, NY, McGraw Hill, 1954, pp 296-317.

75. Levens AS, Inman VT, Blosser JA: Transverse rotation of the segments of the lower extremity in locomotion. *J Bone Joint Surg Am* 1948;30:859-872.

76. Kessler HH: The cineplastic amputation. *Surg Gyn Obs* 1939;68:554-563.

77. Kessler HH: Cineplastic amputations. *Surg Clin* 1944;24:453-466.

78. Spittler AW, Taylor LW: Causes for amputations performed at Walter

Reed General Hospital during 1947 and 1948. *J Bone Joint Surg Am* 1949; 31:800-804.

79. Eberhart HD, McKennon JC: The suction socket suspension, in Klopsteg PE, et al (eds): *Human Limbs and Their Substitutes*. New York, NY, McGraw Hill, 1954, pp 653-675.

80. Taylor CL: Control design and prosthetic application of biceps and pectoral cineplasty, in Klopsteg PE, et al (eds): *Human Limbs and Their Substitutes*. New York, NY, McGraw Hill, 1954, pp 318-358.

81. Brav EA, Spittler AW, Luscombe HB, et al: Cineplasty: An end-result study. *J Bone Joint Surg Am* 1957;39:59-76.

82. Alldredge RH: The cineplastic method in upper extremity amputations. *J Bone Joint Surg Am* 1948;30:359-372.

83. Brav EA, MacDonald WF, Woodard GH: Follow-up notes on articles previously published in the journal. *J Bone Joint Surg Am* 1964;46:1137-1138.

84. Mazet R: Cineplasty. *J Bone Joint Surg Am* 1958;40:1389-1400.

85. Spittler AW, Rosen IE: Cineplastic muscle motors for prostheses of arm amputees. *J Bone Joint Surg Am* 1951; 33:601-611.

86. Canty TJ: New cineplastic prosthesis. *J Bone Joint Surg Am* 1951;33:612-617.

87. Cleveland M, Manning JG, Stewart WJ: Care of battle casualties and injuries involving bones and joints. *J Bone Joint Surg* 1951;33:517-521.

88. Bowers WF, Merchant FT, Judy KH: The present story on battle casualties from Korea. *Surg Gyn Obs* 1951;93: 529-542.

89. Canty TJ: Amputations and recent developments in artificial limbs. *Armed Forces Med Jour* 1952;3:1147-1152.

90. LaZerte GD: Extremities amputated because of war wounds sustained in Korea. *US Army Med Bull* 1953;1:118-123.

91. Reister F: *Battle Casualties and Medical Statistics: U.S. Army Experience in the Korean War*. Washington, DC, Government Printing Office, 1973.

92. Sako Y: A survey of evacuation, resuscitation and mortality in a forward surgical hospital, in Howard JM (ed): *Battle Casualties in Korea: The Battle Wound. Clinical Experiences*. Washington, DC, Walter Reed Army Medical Center, 1955, vol III, pp 9-21.

93. Jahnke EJ, Seely SF: Acute vascular injuries in the Korean conflict, in Howard JM (ed): *Battle Casualties in Korea: The Battle Wound. Clinical Experiences*. Washington, DC, Walter Reed Army Medical Center, 1955, vol III, pp 91-112.

94. Hughes CW: The primary repair of wounds of major arteries, in Howard JM (ed): *Battle Casualties in Korea: The Battle Wound. Clinical Experiences*. Washington, DC, Walter Reed Army Medical Center, 1955, vol III, pp 122-131.

95. Hughes CW: Acute vascular trauma in Korean War casualties: An analysis of 180 cases, in Howard JM (ed): *Battle Casualties in Korea: The Battle Wound. Clinical Experiences*. Washington, DC, Walter Reed Army Medical Center, 1955, vol III, pp 132-147.

96. Inui FK, Shannon J, Howard JM: Arterial injuries in Korea: Experience with 111 cases, in Howard JM (ed): *Battle Casualties in Korea: The Battle Wound. Clinical Experiences*. Washington, DC, Walter Reed Army Medical Center, 1955, vol III, pp 113-121.

97. Howard JM: Resucitation of the battle casualty. A resume, in Howard JM (ed): *Battle Casualties in Korea: The Battle Wound. Clinical Experiences*. Washington, DC, Walter Reed Army Medical Center, 1955, vol III, pp 72-87.

98. Lindsey D, Wise HM, Knecht AT, Noyes HE: The role of clostridia in mortality following an experimental wound in the goat. *Surgery* 1959;45: 602-611.

99. Mansberger AR: A new preparation for the study of experimental shock from massive wounds. *Surgery* 1958; 43:708-720.

100. Byerely WG, Pendse PD: War surgery in a forward surgical hospital in Vietnam: A continuing report. *Mil Med* 1971;134:221-226.

101. Jones EL, Peters AF, Gasior RM: Early management of battle casualties in Vietnam. *Arch Surg* 1968;97:1-15.

102. Schmitt HJ, Armstrong RG: Wounds causing loss of limb. *Surg Gyn Obs* 1970;130:682-684.

103. Burkhalter WE (ed): Penetrating wounds of the leg, in *Surgery in Vietnam: Orthopedic Surgery*. Washington, DC, US Government Printing Office, 1994, pp 39-53.

104. Seligson D, Baily R: Traumatic amputations. *Clin Orthop* 1976;114:304-306.

105. Wilbur MC, Willett LV, Buono F: Combat amputees. *Clin Orthop* 1970; 68:10-13.

106. Frank JL: The amputee war casualty in a military hospital: Observations on psychological management. *Int J Psychiatry Med* 1973;4:1-16.

107. Mayfield GW: Vietnam war amputees, in Burkhalter WE (ed): *Surgery in Vietnam: Orthopedic Surgery*. Washington, DC, US Government Printing Office, 1994, pp 131-153.

108. Dougherty PJ: Transtibial amputees from the Vietnam War. *J Bone Joint Surg Am* 2001;83:383-389.

109. Dougherty PJ: Long-term follow-up study of bilateral-above-the-knee amputees from the Vietnam War. *J Bone Joint Surg Am* 1999;81:1384-1389.

110. Deffer PA, Moll JH, LaNoue AM: the Ertl osteoplastic transtibial amputation (Proceedings). *J Bone Joint Surg Am* 1971;53:1028.

111. Deffer PA: Ertl osteoplasty at Valley Forge General Hospital. *Amputee Clinics* 1969;1:1-2.

112. Moll JA: More on the Ertl osteoplasty. *Amputee Clinics* 1970;2:6.

113. Dougherty PJ: Long term follow up of unilateral transfemoral amputees from the Vietnam War. *Trauma* 2003; 54:718-723.

114. Burkhalter WE (ed): *Surgery in Vietnam: Orthopedic Surgery*. Washington, DC, US Government Printing Office, 1994, pp 189-209.

115. Brown PW: Rehabilitation of bilateral lower extremity amputees. *J Bone Joint Surg Am* 1970;52:687-700.

116. Puller LB: *Fortunate Son*. New York, NY, Bantam Books, 1993.

117. Herndon JA, Tolo VT, LaNoue AM, Deffer PA: Management of fractured femora in acute amputees: Results of early ambulation in a cast-brace and pylon. *J Bone Joint Surg Am* 1973;55: 1600-1613.

118. Herndon JH, Dantzker DR, LaNoue AM: Mycobaterium fortuitum infections involving the extremities. *J Bone Joint Surg Am* 1972;54:1279-1282.

119. Golbranson FL, Asbelle C, Strand D: Immediate postsurgical fitting and

early ambulation: A new concept in amputee rehabilitation. *Clin Orthop* 1968;56:119-131.

120. Nechaev EA, Grisanov AI, Fomin NF, Minnullin IP: *Mine Blast Trauma: Experience from the War in Afghanistan.* Stockholm, Sweden, Falths Tryckeri, 1995 [In Russian].

121. Bondurant FJ, Cotler HB, Buckle R, et al: The medical and economic impact of severely injured lower extremities. *J Trauma* 1988;28:1270-1273.

122. Bonanni F, Rhodes M, Lucke JF: The futility of predictive scoring of mangled lower extremities. *J Trauma* 1993;34:99-104.

123. Bosse MJ, MacKenzie E, Kellam JF, et al: A prospective evaluation of the clinical utility of the lower-extremity injury-severity scores. *J Bone Joint Surg Am* 2001;83:3-14.

124. Brumback RJ, Jones AL: Interobserver agreement in the classification of open fractures of the tibia. *J Bone Joint Surg Am* 1994;76:1162-1166.

125. Caudle RJ, Stern PJ: Severe open fractures of the tibia. *J Bone Joint Surg Am* 1987;69:801-806.

126. Georgiadis GA, Behrens FF, Joyce MJ, Earle AS, Simmons AL: Open tibial fractures with severe soft-tissue loss. *J Bone Joint Surg Am* 1993;75:1431-1441.

127. Quirke TE, Sharma PK, Boss WK, Oppenheim WC, Rauscher GE: Are type IIIC lower extremity injuries an indication for primary amputation? *J Trauma* 1996;40:992-996.

128. Lange RH, Bach AW, Hansen ST Jr, et al: Open tibia fractures with associated vascular injuries: Prognosis for limb salvage. *J Trauma* 1985;25:203-208.

129. Helfet DL, Howey T, Sanders R, Johansen K: Limb salvage versus amputation. *Clin Orthop* 1990;256:80-86.

130. Lerner RK, Esterhai JL, Polomano RC, Cheatle MD, Heppenstall RB: Quality of life assessment of patients with posttraumatic fracture nonunion, chronic refractory osteomyelitis, and lower-extremity amputation. *Clin Orthop* 1993;295:28-36.

131. Bosse MJ, MacKenzie EJ, Kellam JF, et al: An analysis of outcomes of reconstruction or amputation of leg-threatening injuries. *N Engl J Med* 2002;347:1924-1931.

132. McNamara MG, Heckman JD, Corley FG: Severe open fractures of the lower extremity: A retrospective evaluation of the Mangled Extremity Severity Score (MESS). *J Orthop Trauma* 1994;8:81-87.

133. McNamara JJ, Brief DK, Beasley W, Wright JK: Vascular injury in Vietnam combat casualties. *Ann Surg* 1973;178:143-147.

134. Simper LB: Transtibial amputation in war surgery: A review of 111 amputations with delayed primary closure. *J Trauma* 1993;34:96-98.

135. Coupland RM: *Amputations for War Wounds.* Geneva, Switzerland, International Committee of the Red Cross, 1992.

136. Atesalp AS, Erler K, Gur E, Solakoglu C: Below-knee amputations as a result of land-mine injuries: Comparison of primary closure versus delayed primary closure. *J Trauma* 1999;47:724-727.

137. Traverso LW, Johnson DE, Fleming A, Wongrukmitr B: Combat casualties in Northern Thailand: Emphasis on land mine injuries and levels of amputation. *Mil Med* 1981;146:682-685.

138. Burkhalter WE, Mayfield G, Carmona LS: The upper extremity amputee. *J Bone Joint Surg Am* 1976;58:46-51.

Section II

The Upper Limb

Kinesiology and Functional Characteristics of the Upper Limb

Brian J. Hartigan, MD
Shahan K. Sarrafian, MD

Introduction

The functional capacity of the upper limb is determined by the shoulder complex, elbow, wrist, and hand developing multiple integrated spheres of action. In normally proportioned limb segments, this capacity is limited in relation to the surrounding space. For example, in the standing position, the upper limb field of motion reaches the midthigh region. Any more distal point on the lower limb or on the ground is reached through mobility provided by the hip, knee, ankle, and trunk (Figure 1). More distant points in space come within the reach of the upper limb action when functionally integrated with gait.

A maximum arcuate field or envelope of action termed E_1 (Figure 2) is traced by the most distal point of the upper limb through the motion of the shoulder complex, all other joints being held in extension. Within this envelope, the elbow, wrist, and fingers have their own fields of motion, E_2, E_3, and E_4, respectively. These contained capabilities enrich the functional performance of the upper limb.

Shoulder Complex
Motion in the Coronal (Frontal) Plane

When the arm and forearm are held in the neutral position, the upper limb sweeps a circular surface in the coronal plane. The very distal point of

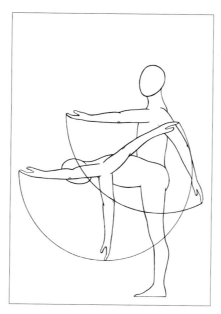

Figure 1 The field of motion of the upper limb is a circle, with the length of the limb the radius. Any point more distant in space or distal to the midthigh is reached through associated hip, knee, ankle, and trunk motion.

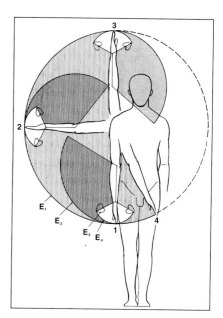

Figure 2 Elevation of an externally rotated upper limb in the coronal plane. Complete exploration of the outer half of a circle is possible through the envelope of action E_1. The elbow allows sweeping of space E_2. The wrist develops motion field E_3. The spiral envelope of motion E_4 is determined by finger motion.

the limb traces an envelope of action E_1 (Figure 3).

The shoulder is in neutral rotation in position 1, and the limb can be elevated in the outer half of the circle to positions 2 and 3. The elbow does not contribute to functional exploration in this segment of the arc of motion. If the wrist is initially held in neutral rotation, the hand sweeps the space

E_3, and the fingers explore the interior of this space through E_4. Beyond position 3, the shoulder rotates externally and complete elevation is achieved at position 4. In this second arc of motion, the elbow explores the segment of the space through its action envelope E_2. The sweeping of the inner half of the coronal circle is possible from position 4 to 5 through in-

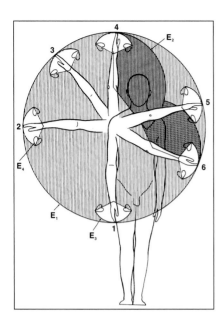

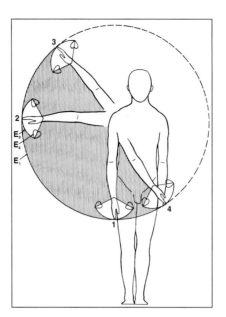

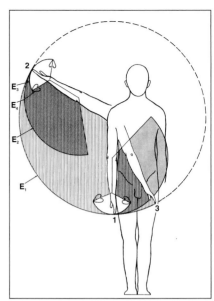

Figure 3 Motion in the coronal plane, starting with the neutral position of the upper limb, position 1. It is possible to explore space from position 1 to 2 without associated external rotation. No elbow action is possible then. The limb is elevated from position 3 to 4 through association of external rotation. Descent from position 4 to 5 involves internal rotation. From position 5 to 6 and 1, the limb derotates to reach a neutral position.

Figure 4 Motion in the coronal plane with the upper limb in neutral rotation. No elbow action is present in this plane.

Figure 5 Motion in the coronal plane with the upper limb in complete internal rotation. The field of motion E_1 is limited, but elbow motion is possible by exploring space E_2. The wrist and digits are continuously functional.

ternal rotation of the shoulder, and the elbow action dissipates. The shoulder rotates externally from position 5 to 6, and elbow function reappears, whereas with further external rotation from position 6 to 1, the elbow action dissipates again.

When the upper limb is maintained in neutral rotation at the shoulder, motion is quite restricted (Figure 4), and no elbow action is possible in this plane. Maintaining the limb in complete external rotation permits easy exploration of the outer half of the coronal circle, whereas any functional motion in the inner half is very restricted. The elbow envelope of action is clearly visible now in all positions (Figure 2).

Placement of the limb in complete internal rotation significantly restricts the field of motion (Figure 5), but elbow action is possible from position 1 to 2. The coronal plane is also explored posteriorly in the inner half space (Figure 6). With a position of

internal rotation at the shoulder, the limb traces a small arc of displacement that allows the elbow, wrist, and hand to sweep the surface corresponding to the gluteal area and up to the opposite scapular region. From position 3, the elbow envelope of action scans the posterior aspect of the back and shoulder.

During elevation of the upper limb in the coronal plane, motion is determined by the glenohumeral joint and scapulothoracic upward rotation (Figure 7). Scapular rotation not only contributes to overall elevation but also is important for maintaining constant fiber length of the deltoid, allowing deltoid motion over a variety of arm positions. The acromioclavicular and sternoclavicular joints also participate in a synchronized manner, producing clavicular rotation and elevation. Humeral external rotation accompanies the elevation for the performance of a smooth motion (Figure 8). Beyond 90° of elevation, this external rotation is necessary to free the greater tuberosity from the coracoacromial arch. Additionally, external rotation of the humerus relaxes the inferior glenohumeral ligaments, releasing the inferior checkrein effect.[1]

From 0° to 30° of elevation (Figure 7), a variably greater amount of motion occurs at the glenohumeral joint compared with the scapulothoracic joint. The precise ratio has been debated and is subject to individual variation. During the last 60° of elevation, the glenohumeral and scapulothoracic joints contribute equally. Through the entire arc of elevation, the overall ratio of glenohumeral joint motion to scapulothoracic joint motion is 2:1.

During upper limb elevation, the clavicle does not remain still. It elevates 30° to 40° at the sternoclavicular joint, with the maximum at about 130° of elevation[2] (Figure 9). The clavicle also rotates on its long axis beyond 90° of arm elevation. Approximately 40° of clavicular rotation occurs with respect to the sternum. However, less rotation occurs with respect to the acromion because of the concomitant synchronous rotation of the scapula during elevation of the arm. A combined acromioclavicular motion of 20° occurs during the initial and terminal phases of elevation (Figure 7).

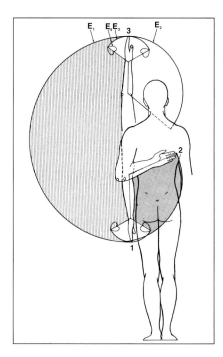

Figure 6 Motion in the coronal plane posterior to the body. The gluteal area and mid and lower portions of the back are within reach of the internally rotated upper limb, position 1, combined with the elbow field of motion, position 2. The posterior aspect of the neck and shoulders is reached by external rotation, position 3, combined with the elbow field of motion E_2.

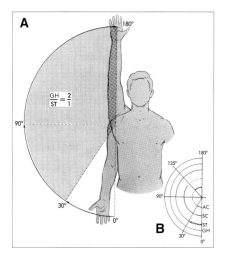

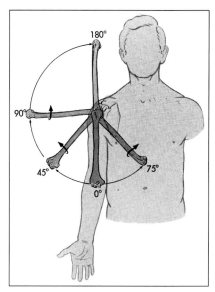

Figure 7 A, Elevation of the upper limb from 0° to 180°. From 0° to 30°, the motion is mostly glenohumeral (GH), with scapulothoracic (ST) motion occurring to a variable degree. Overall, the ratio between glenohumeral and scapulothoracic motion GH:ST is 2:1. **B,** Sternoclavicular (SC) motion occurs during the initial 130° of arm elevation. Acromioclavicular (AC) motion occurs from 0° to 30° and then from 135° to 180°, with a range of motion of 20°.

Figure 8 Natural elevation of the upper limb in the coronal plane involves 90° of external rotation. Elevation in the lower and inner segment of a circle involves internal rotation.

The motor units responsible for glenohumeral elevation are the middle segment of the deltoid muscle and the muscles of the rotator cuff: the supraspinatus, infraspinatus, teres minor, and subscapularis muscles (Figure 10). Electromyography (EMG) and selective nerve blocks, used to study the contributions of these muscles, have shown that the deltoid and all four rotator cuff muscles are active throughout the full range of motion in both flexion and abduction.[2,3] The deltoid and supraspinatus act synergistically to produce glenohumeral elevation, while the infraspinatus, teres minor, and subscapularis muscles stabilize the humeral head to prevent cephalic migration. Although the exact contributions of the deltoid and supraspinatus have been debated, it appears that the deltoid becomes progressively more effective with increas-

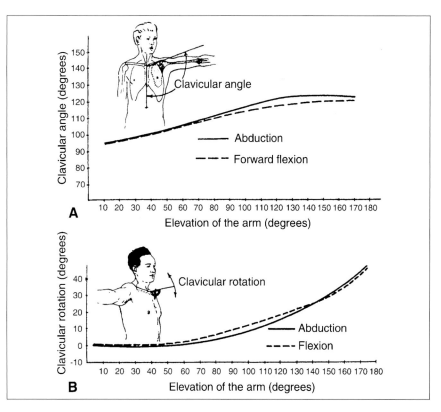

Figure 9 Clavicular elevation and rotation. **A,** Sternoclavicular motion in the form of clavicular elevation of 40° occurs, primarily during the initial 130°. **B,** Beyond 90°, clavicular rotation occurs on the long axis. *(Reproduced with permission from Inman VT, Saunders M, Abbott LC: Observations on the function of the shoulder joint.* J Bone Joint Surg *1944;26:1-30.)*

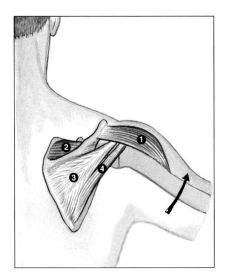

Figure 10 Elevators at the scapulo-humeral joint in the coronal plane. 1 = middle deltoid, 2 = supraspinatus, 3 = infraspinatus, 4 = teres minor. The subscapularis, which lies anteriorly and cannot be seen on this view, is also an elevator.

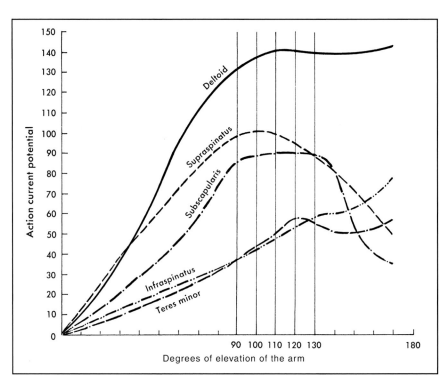

Figure 11 EMG activity of the elevators at the scapulohumeral joint in the coronal plane. All five muscles are active from 0° to 90°. Beyond 110°, the deltoid holds a maximum level of activity. The supraspinatus decreases in activity after 100°. The infraspinatus and teres minor maintain high levels of activity during the second half of elevation to ensure necessary external rotation of the shoulder. *(Reproduced with permission from Inman VT, Saunders M, Abbott LC: Observations on the function of the shoulder joint. J Bone Joint Surg 1944;26:1-30.)*

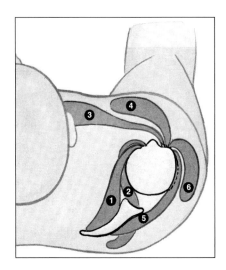

Figure 12 Rotators at the scapulo-humeral joint. Internal rotators: 1 = subscapularis, 2 = latissimus dorsi and teres major, 3 = pectoralis major, 4 = anterior deltoid. External rotators: 5 = infraspinatus and teres minor, 6 = posterior deltoid.

ing elevation, most likely the result of the improved moment arm.

EMG studies (Figure 11) show that the deltoid action potential increases steadily with elevation, reaches a maximum at 110°, and maintains a plateau level of activity with a final peak at full elevation. The supraspinatus reaches a peak at 100°,

and beyond this point its activity diminishes and traces a sine wave. The subscapularis reaches a peak at 90°, maintains a plateau level up to 130°, and diminishes rapidly in action. The teres minor reaches the maximum at 120° and maintains a high level of activity, whereas the infraspinatus increases steadily in activity from the initial position to that of full elevation. The action of the teres minor and infraspinatus is necessary to continue the external rotation of the humerus during the last stage of elevation. The posterior segment of the deltoid also participates as an external rotator (Figure 12).

Upward rotation of the scapula is achieved by the upper trapezius, levator scapulae, and upper portion of the serratus anterior contracting concomitantly with the lower trapezius and lower serratus anterior to act on the scapula as a force couple (Figure 13). When the upper limb moves in the

lower and inner quadrant of the envelope of action E_1, it is adducted and internally rotated. The internal rotation is brought about by the subscapularis, pectoralis major, and anterior segments of the deltoid (Figure 12). Adduction is determined by the latter two muscles, supplemented by the action of the coracobrachialis (Figure 14). During the anterior adduction-internal rotation, the scapula is abducted or protracted. This motion is controlled by the serratus anterior and the pectoralis minor (Figure 15). When the upper limb moves in a similar lower and inner quadrant but posterior to the body, the limb is once more adducted and internally rotated. Posterior adduction is brought about by the latissimus dorsi, teres major, long head of the triceps, and posterior segment of the deltoid (Figure 14). The latissimus dorsi and teres major also determine the associated internal rotation (Figure 12). During this

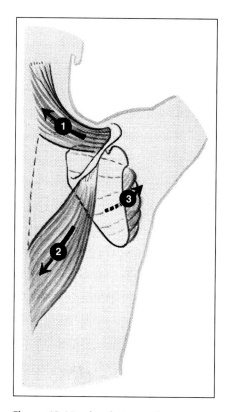

Figure 13 Muscles that contribute to up-ward rotation of the scapula. 1 = upper trapezius, 2 = lower trapezius, 3 = serra-tus anterior.

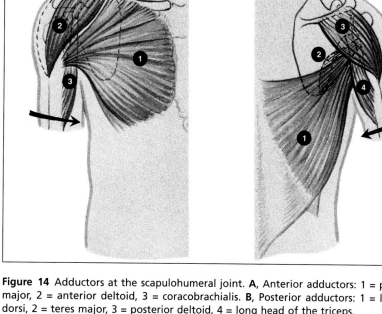

Figure 14 Adductors at the scapulohumeral joint. **A,** Anterior adductors: 1 = pectoralis major, 2 = anterior deltoid, 3 = coracobrachialis. **B,** Posterior adductors: 1 = latissimus dorsi, 2 = teres major, 3 = posterior deltoid, 4 = long head of the triceps.

same motion, the scapula is adducted or retracted by the middle segment of the trapezius and the combined action of the rhomboidei and latissimus dorsi (Figure 16).

When the upper limb is in a maximum position of elevation and is brought down in the coronal plane in the outer half circle, the scapula makes a downward rotation. This is determined by the combined action of the latissimus dorsi, the lower segment of the pectoralis major (the pectoralis minor acting as the lower component for a force couple), and the levator scapulae, with the rhomboidei acting as the upper component of the rotational couple (Figure 17). Downward stabilization of the limb in the coronal plane is functionally important in activities such as crutch walking or parallel bar exercising. Depressors of the shoulder complex responsible for this function include the latissimus dorsi, the lower segment of the trapezius, the lower seg-

ment of the pectoralis major, the pectoralis minor, and the subclavius (Figure 18).

Upward stabilization in the coronal plane is also necessary for functional purposes, as in carrying heavy loads on the shoulders. This is controlled by the elevators of the scapula: the levator scapulae, upper segment of the trapezius, and rhomboidei (Figure 19).

Motion in the Sagittal and Transverse (Horizontal) Planes

From a neutral rotational position, the upper limb moves in the sagittal plane and sweeps the surface from position 1 to 3 (Figure 20). The elbow, wrist, and hand are capable of functioning in this plane through their envelopes of action E_2, E_3, and E_4, respectively.

In position 3, the elbow action extends farther posteriorly, with the hand reaching the posterior aspect of

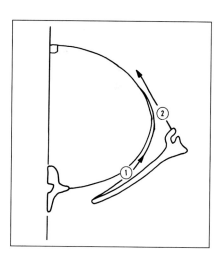

Figure 15 Abductors or protractors of the scapula. 1 = serratus anterior, 2 = pectoralis minor.

the shoulder. Further movement in the posterior half of the field is possible through the internal rotation of the shoulder, followed by gradual external rotation to bring the limb to its neutral initial position (Figure 21). Elevation of the upper limb, or flexion

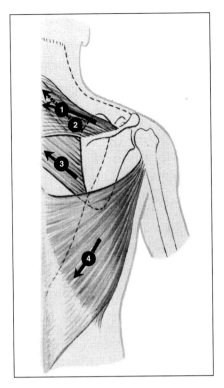

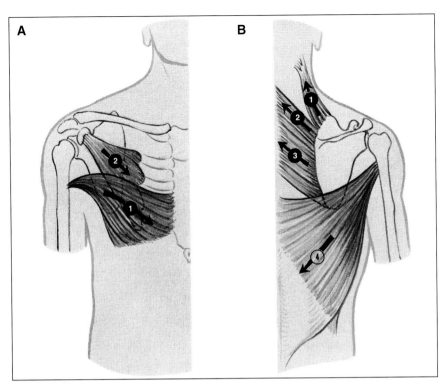

Figure 16 Adductors or retractors of the scapula. 1 = middle trapezius, 2 = rhomboideus minor, 3 = rhomboideus major, 4 = latissimus dorsi.

Figure 17 Muscles that contribute to downward rotation of the scapula. **A,** Anterior view. 1 = lower segment of the pectoralis major, 2 = pectoralis minor. **B,** Posterior view. 1 = levator scapulae, 2 = rhomboideus minor, 3 = rhomboideus major, 4 = latissimus dorsi.

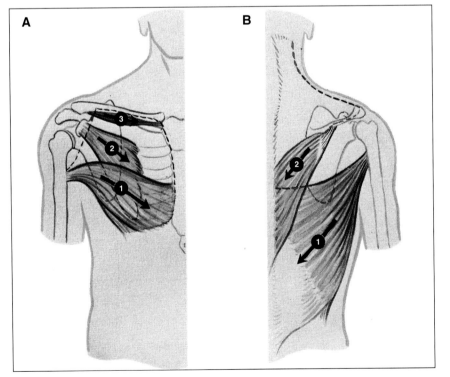

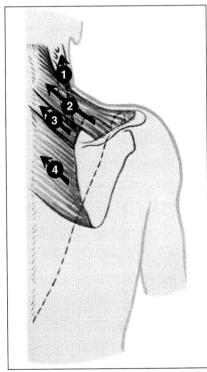

Figure 18 Depressors of the scapula. **A,** Anterior view. 1 = lower segment of the pectoralis major, 2 = pectoralis minor, 3 = subclavius. **B,** Posterior view. 1 = latissimus dorsi, 2 = lower segment of the trapezius.

Figure 19 Elevators of the scapula. 1 = levator scapulae, 2 = upper segment of the trapezius; 3 = rhomboideus minor, 4 = rhomboideus major.

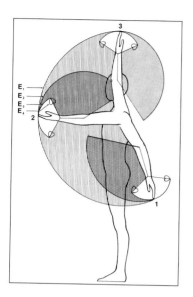

Figure 20 Elevation in the sagittal plane. Exploration of space from position 1 to 3 is possible in the neutral rotational position of the shoulder. Elbow action E₂ is present in the plane. In position 3, the posterior segment of space is reached through elbow action.

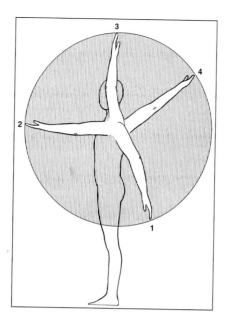

Figure 21 Motion in the sagittal plane. A posterior arc of motion from position 3 to 4 is possible through internal rotation. From position 4 to 1, the limb derotates to reach the neutral position.

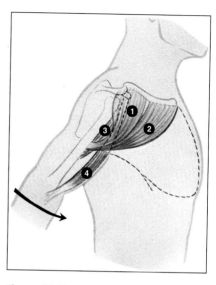

Figure 22 Flexors at the scapulohumeral joint. 1 = anterior segment of the deltoid, 2 = clavicular segment of the pectoralis major, 3 = coracobrachialis, 4 = biceps. The arrow indicates flexion.

from position 1 to 3, is determined by the anterior segment of the deltoid, biceps, coracobrachialis, and clavicular head of the pectoralis major (Figure 22). The rotator cuff is also active in stabilizing the humeral head. The scapulothoracic mechanism participates in the motion through upward scapular rotation at a glenohumeral/scapulothoracic ratio of 2:1.[2] From the elevated position 3, the upper limb is brought down by the posterior segment of the deltoid, long head of the triceps, latissimus dorsi, and pectoralis major (Figure 23). Beyond neutral, the motion continues as extension. Motor units responsible for extension include the posterior deltoid, middle deltoid, and subscapularis. As the degree of extension increases, the supraspinatus becomes more active. Throughout extension, the subscapularis and supraspinatus act as prime stabilizers of the humeral head, with a range of extension of 60°[4,5] (Figure 24). When the upper limb is elevated to 90° in the coronal plane, the distal point of the limb scans the horizontal plane and traces an arc of 185°[5] (Figure 25). The flex-

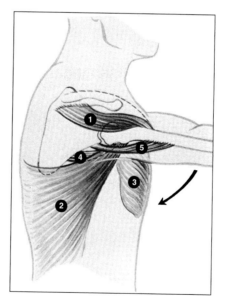

Figure 23 Extensors at the scapulohumeral joint. 1 = posterior deltoid, 2 = latissimus dorsi, 3 = pectoralis major, 4 = teres major, 5 = long head of the triceps.

ors and extensors of the glenohumeral joint control the motion.

Rotary Capability of the Shoulder Complex

When the upper limb is held in neutral rotation at the shoulder and the

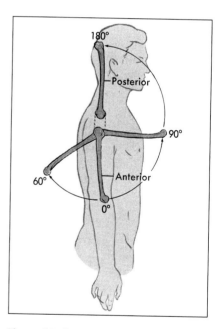

Figure 24 Flexion at the scapulohumeral joint is 180°, and no combined rotation is necessary. Extension is 60°.

elbow is flexed at 90°, the distal point traces an arc of internal rotation of 70° and an arc of external rotation of 100°. With the shoulder elevated 90° in the coronal plane, this rotary capability changes to 90° of external rotation and 70° of internal rotation[4,5] (Figure 26).

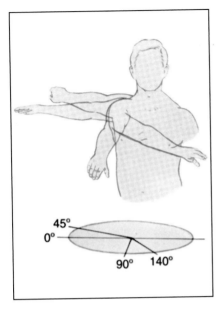

Figure 25 In the horizontal plane, the arm can achieve 140° of flexion and 45° of extension.

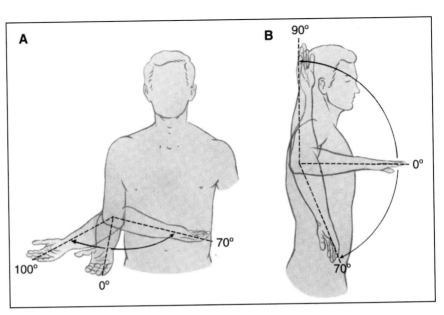

Figure 26 Rotation at the scapulohumeral joint. **A**, With the arm in neutral elevation, external rotation of 100° and internal rotation of 70° is possible. **B**, With the arm elevated 90°, external rotation of 90° and internal rotation of 70° is possible.

	1	2	3	4
Brachialis	+ +	+ +	+ +	+ + +
Biceps	+ +	+ +	+	+ + +
Brachioradialis	+	+	+	+ +

Figure 27 Muscle activity during elbow flexion. (1) Flexion in supination without resistance; (2) Flexion in neutral without resistance; (3) Flexion in pronation without resistance; (4) Flexion in supination with resistance. The brachialis is the baseline flexor. The biceps is the reserve flexor. Its action is decreased in pronation but increased when the forearm is supine, especially when resistance is encountered. Its action is decreased in pronation. The brachioradialis is more active against resistance. +++ = maximum activity, ++ = mild activity, + = minimal activity.

The infraspinatus is responsible primarily for external rotation of the humerus (Figure 12), with varying degrees of assistance provided by the teres minor and posterior deltoid depending on the position of the arm. As the arm is abducted, the posterior deltoid becomes more important, accounting for 60% of the strength in 90° of abduction.[6]

Internal rotation of the humerus is produced by the combined action of the pectoralis major, latissimus dorsi, teres major, and subscapularis (Figure 12). As abduction of the arm increases from 0° to 90°, activity of the subscapularis, pectoralis major, and latissimus dorsi tends to decrease, whereas activity of the deltoid increases.[6]

Elbow

The elbow joint determines an arc of motion, E_2, with a range from 0° to 150°. The orientation of the plane of action is closely influenced by the rotational position of the shoulder joint. For example, when the arm is elevated in the coronal plane, the envelope of action E_2 of the elbow is located in this plane if the shoulder is in external or internal rotation.

Although the motion of the elbow has been classified as a hinge joint, its motion is better described as a loose hinge. The instant center of rotation varies throughout the arc of flexion-extension. Because this variation occurs over a small area, it is considered a single axis of rotation, passing through the center of the arcs formed by the trochlear sulcus and the capitellum. Using external landmarks, this corresponds to a line passing through the inferior aspect of the medial epicondyle and the center of the lateral epicondyle.[7]

The main flexors of the elbow are the brachialis, biceps, and brachioradialis. Intricate interactions and a wide range of participation are accomplished by the elbow flexors depending on the position of the fore-

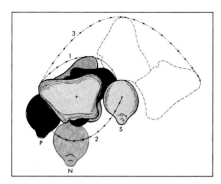

Figure 28 Rotation at the distal radio-ulnar joint. In habitual rotation, the axis passes through the middle of the distal end of the radius (+). From supination to pronation, the radial styloid traces curve 1 and the head of the ulna traces curve 2. From supination (S) to neutral (N), the head of the ulna is extended and laterally displaced. From neutral (N) to pronation (P), it is flexed and further laterally displaced. When the axis of motion passes through the center of the ulnar head, the latter stays still during rotation, whereas the radial styloid traces a very large curve (3). The location of the axis of rotation is determined by a peripheral point of fixation.

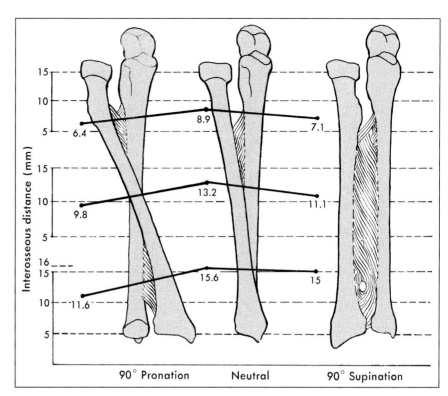

Figure 29 Radiohumeral interosseous distance in pronation, neutral, and supination. The distance is maximal in neutral and minimal in pronation. *(Adapted with permission from Christensen JB, Adams JP, Cho KO, et al: A study of the interosseous distance between the radius and ulna during rotation of the forearm. Anat Rec 1968;160:261-271.)*

arm, degree of elbow flexion, and the applied load.[8,9] The brachialis is the "workhorse" flexor and is active at any rotational position of the forearm, any degree of elbow flexion, and with or without load applied to the flexing forearm (Figure 27). Because of the insertion of the brachialis on the ulna, there is no influence on activity with forearm rotation. The biceps is also active throughout a full range of elbow flexion; however, its activity decreases during forearm pronation. The greatest biceps activity occurs with the forearm in a neutral position and whenever any resistance is encountered. The brachioradialis is active throughout elbow flexion, and like the brachialis, its activity is essentially independent of forearm rotation.

The main extensors of the elbow include the triceps and the aconeus. Their activity is not influenced by forearm rotation because of the insertion site on the ulna. However, activity is heightened with increasing elbow flexion as well as with an in-

creased load. Contrary to previous studies,[10] the different heads of the triceps generally are active in a similar manner throughout motion.

Forearm

Forearm rotation occurs about the proximal and distal radioulnar joints, with the radius rotating around the ulna. Rotation of the ulna with respect to the humerus is also coupled with forearm rotation. External rotation of the ulna occurs with supination, and internal rotation occurs with pronation. When measured at the wrist, forearm rotation averages about 75° of pronation to 85° of supination.[5] Approximately 17° of additional pronation and supination is seen when measured at the hand because of contributions from the radiocarpal and midcarpal joints.

The axis of pronation-supination is variable in location and dependent on the distal point of fixation[11] (Fig-

ure 28). Proximally, the axis passes through the capitellum and the concave center of the radial head. Distally, it passes somewhere between the radial and ulnar styloids. When the ulna is fixed in position, such as when the forearm and hand are resting on their ulnar border, the longitudinal axis of pronation-supination passes through the concave center of the radial head proximally and near the fovea of the distal ulna distally.[12] This axis is oblique to the longitudinal axis of both the radius and the ulna and is independent of elbow flexion-extension. The hand makes a circumferential transposition with the radial styloid tracing a large arc of motion. However, in the average habitual motion, the axis of rotation passes through the distal end of the radius and not the ulnar head.[13] During this rotatory motion, the distal radius and the ulnar head trace arcs of motion that are comparable in size. Starting from the position of supination, the

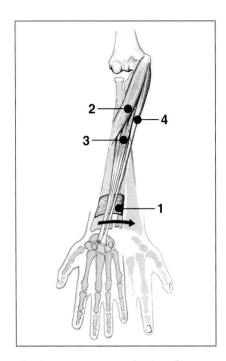

Figure 30 Pronators of the forearm. (1) pronator quadratus, main pronator; (2) pronator teres, reserve pronator; (3) flexor carpi radialis, an accessory pronator; (4) palmaris longus, an accessory pronator.

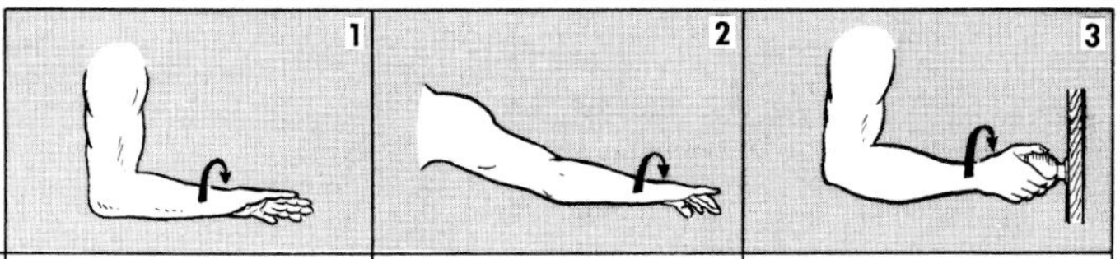

	1	2	3
Pronator teres	+	+	+ + +
Pronator quadratus	+ +	+ +	+ + +

Figure 31 Pronation of the forearm. (1) Pronation with the elbow flexed without resistance; (2) pronation with the elbow extended without resistance; (3) pronation against resistance. The pronator quadratus is the main pronator active at all positions of the elbow. The pronator teres increases in activity only against resistance or when speed is required. +++ = maximum activity, ++ = mild activity, + = minimal activity.

head of the ulna is extended and laterally translated in the neutral position. In pronation, the ulnar head is flexed and further displaced laterally.

It is important to note that motion at the distal radioulnar joint is not purely rotational. Because of the differing radii of curvature between the sigmoid notch of the distal radius and the ulnar head as well as some inherent ligamentous laxity, translation in the dorsal-volar direction occurs with forearm rotation. Furthermore, in the pronated position, the obliquity of the radius makes it relatively shorter than the ulna, producing a more positive ulnar variance.

The interosseous membrane that unites the radius and ulna relaxes or tenses during pronation-supination. The interosseous distance measured in the distal, middle, and proximal thirds of the forearm is largest in the neutral position and smallest in full pronation[14] (Figure 29). Therefore, the tension in the membrane is minimal in full pronation. During a fall on the outstretched pronated hand, the

interosseous membrane is not the main element of pressure transmission to the elbow through the ulna. When load is applied to the forearm from a distoproximal direction, the radius transmits 57% of the load directly to the humerus and 43% to the ulna.[15]

The forearm is pronated primarily by the pronator quadratus and the pronator teres (Figure 30). The main pronator is the pronator quadratus; the action of the muscle is independent of the position of the elbow. The pronator teres is a reserve pronator that reinforces power when speed is required or resistance is applied to the motion[16] (Figure 31). The relative contributions of the accessory pronators, the flexor carpi radialis and palmaris longus, to pronation is debatable. The forearm is supinated primarily by the supinator muscle (Figure 32). The biceps is the reserve supinator and reinforces the action when fast supination is required or resistance is encountered (Figure 33). The extensor carpi radialis longus and brevis may be accessory supinators.

Wrist

The wrist, which acts as a universal joint, has principal planes of motion in the sagittal plane (flexion/extension) and in the coronal plane (radial-ulnar deviation). It also contributes minimally to pronation-

supination in the transverse plane. In isolated flexion-extension, the wrist develops a spheroid type of motion envelope E_3 (Figure 34) that permits the hand to move without digital motion.[12] However, most activities require a combination of wrist motions. The combination of wrist extension and pronation-supination permits the hand to explore the outer half of a circle. The flexed wrist, when rotated, permits the hand to explore the inner half of a circle. This latter motion allows functional activities related to the body. Functionally, the hand is used more frequently with the wrist extended and radially deviated or with flexion combined with ulnar deviation.

The carpus consists of the distal carpal row, which includes the trapezium, trapezoid, capitate, and hamate, and the proximal carpal row, which is made up of the scaphoid, lunate, and triquetrum. The pisiform is not functionally part of the proximal carpal row because it lies within the flexor carpi ulnaris and acts as a sesamoid bone through its articulation with the triquetrum. Although there is some angular intercarpal rotation between the bones within a row, the bones of each row move synergistically and can be considered a functional unit with most wrist motion occurring at the radiocarpal and midcarpal joints. In both flexion-extension and radial-

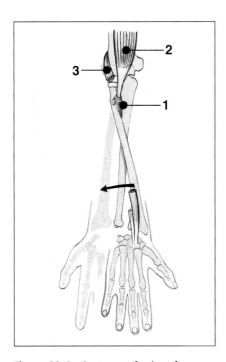

Figure 32 Supinators of the forearm. (1) Supinator, main supinator; (2) biceps, reserve supinator; (3) extensor carpi radialis longus and brevis, questionable accessory supinators. The arrow indicates supination.

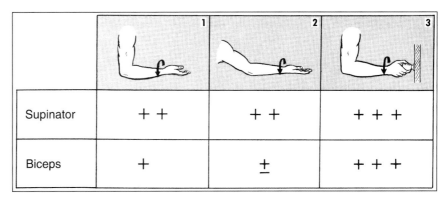

	1	2	3
Supinator	+ +	+ +	+ + +
Biceps	+	±	+ + +

Figure 33 Supination of the forearm. (1) Supination with the elbow flexed without resistance; (2) supination with the elbow extended without resistance; (3) supination against resistance. +++ = maximum activity, ++ = mild activity, + = minimal activity, - = no activity. The supinator is the main supinator. The biceps is the reserve supinator, functioning best with the elbow flexed 90° or when speed or power is required.

ulnar deviation, the center of rotation is in the head of the capitate.

Overall, the average range of wrist flexion and extension is 75° to 90°. Through the flexion-extension arc, the proximal and distal rows move in similar directions. Wrist flexion, which produces flexion and ulnar deviation of both rows, and extension, which produces extension and radial deviation, generates an overall coupled wrist motion of flexion-ulnar deviation and extension-radial deviation. Flexion-extension is motored by the pull of the extrinsic flexor and extensor muscles on the metacarpal bases. The distal carpal row is pulled in a similar direction because of the secure association of the metacarpal bases to the distal carpal at the second through fifth carpometacarpal joints. The proximal carpal row follows because of articular contact and ligamentous attachments to the distal row. Overall, the midcarpal joint contributes 60% of the arc of flexion and the radiocarpal joint contributes 40%. In extension, the midcarpal contrib-

utes 34%, with the remaining 66% contributed by the radiocarpal joint[17] (Figure 35).

The wrist flexors are the flexor carpi radialis and ulnaris and the palmaris longus. The long digital flexors are accessory flexors at the wrist. The wrist extensors are the extensor carpi radialis longus and brevis and the extensor carpi ulnaris. The digital extensors are the accessory extensors of the wrist.

Lateral motion at the wrist averages 15° to 25° of radial deviation and 25° to 40° of ulnar deviation. With radial-ulnar deviation, the two carpal rows demonstrate reciprocating motion with the proximal carpal row sliding in the direction opposite of hand movement. During radial deviation, motion occurs primarily at the midcarpal joint, with the distal row extending, deviating radially, and translating from a dorsal to palmar direction. The proximal row flexes and displaces to a less pronounced degree in an ulnar direction. During ulnar deviation, motion occurs at both the intercarpal and radiocarpal joints. The distal row flexes and deviates ulnarly whereas the proximal row extends and moves radially at the radiocarpal joint.

The radial deviators of the wrist are the extensor carpi radialis longus and brevis, flexor carpi radialis, abductor pollicis longus, and extensor

pollicis brevis. The ulnar deviators are the extensor carpi ulnaris and flexor carpi ulnaris, with the extensor carpi ulnar is becoming more effective with forearm pronation.

The degree of participation of the digital motors determines recruitment of the wrist motors. When the wrist is in extension and the fingers make a soft fist, the following wrist motors are active in descending order: extensor carpi radialis brevis, extensor carpi ulnaris, and extensor carpi radialis longus. With a tight fist, all three extensors are maximally active[18] (Figure 36). When the fingers are gently extended and the wrist is held in extension, the extensor carpi ulnaris and flexor carpi ulnaris are active. The forceful opening of the fingers brings into action, in descending order, the following additional wrist motors: extensor carpi radialis brevis, palmaris longus, extensor carpi radialis longus, and flexor carpi radialis[18] (Figure 37). Grip strength is maximal with the wrist in 35° of extension and 7° of ulnar deviation and is significantly reduced when the wrist deviates from this position.[13]

Hand
Fingers

Located at the end of a multisegmented system, the hand functions within the action envelope E_3 of the

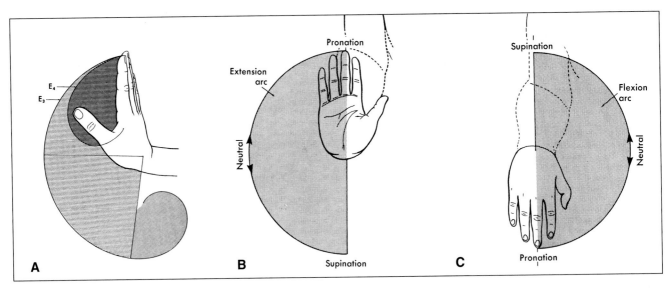

Figure 34 A, Field of motion of the wrist and hand, where E_3 is the action envelope of the wrist and E_4 is the action envelope of the finger tracing an equiangular spiral. The field of motion of the finger is within E_3 when the wrist is extended and projects proximally when the wrist is flexed. **B,** The extended wrist, when rotated, explores the outer half of a circle that is the base of spheroid E_3. **C,** The flexed wrist, when rotated, explores the inner half of a circle that is the base of spheroid E_3.

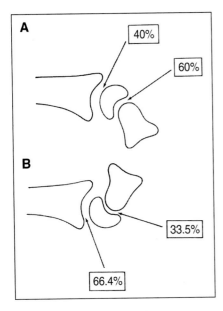

Figure 35 Contribution of the radiocarpal and midcarpal joints to flexion-extension. **A,** For flexion, 60% is midcarpal and 40% is radiocarpal. **B,** For extension, 33.5% is midcarpal and 66.4% is radiocarpal. *(Reproduced with permission from Sarrafian SK, Melamed JL, Goshgarian GM: Study of wrist motion in flexion and extension.* Clin Orthop *1977; 126:153-159.)*

wrist. The flexing finger traces an action envelope, E_4, that is an equiangular spiral[19] (Figure 34). When the wrist is extended, the field of motion of the fingers is within the wrist envelope E_3. With wrist flexion, the action envelope E_4 of the fingers extends beyond the field of motion of the wrist (Figure 34).

With prehension of the fingers, the interphalangeal and metacarpophalangeal joints must flex in a coordinated fashion to permit wrapping of the digital palmar surface over the surface of the object. Separately, the distal joint is flexed by the flexor profundus, the middle joint by the flexor superficialis, and the metacarpophalangeal joint by the intrinsic muscles. The coordination of flexion at the interphalangeal and the metacarpophalangeal joints is brought about by the instantaneous participation of the extrinsic-intrinsic motors commanded by the motor cortex as well as through passive restraints. This passive restraint is primarily the result of the oblique retinacular ligament that arises from the palmar aspect of the proximal phalanx and adjacent flexor sheath, passing volar to the proximal interphalangeal joint, lateral to the middle phalanx, and dorsal to the distal interphalangeal joint, inserting into the distal extensor hood. This ligament coordinates flexion and extension at the proximal interphalangeal and distal interphalangeal joints.

A fine mechanism of coordination is present locally in the fingers at the level of the interphalangeal joints as initially presented by Landsmeer[20] (Figure 38). Finger flexion is initiated at the level of the distal interphalangeal joint by the flexor digitorum profundus. As the distal interphalangeal joint flexes, the terminal tendon is displaced distally, causing distal movement of the extensor trifurcation through pull of the lateral slips, resulting in relaxation of the central slip. Simultaneously, the oblique retinacular ligament attached to the terminal tendon also increases in tension and, passing volar to the axis of the proximal interphalangeal joint, automatically flexes the middle phalanx. This is a passive mechanism of interphalangeal joint motion. When the proximal interphalangeal joint is flexed approximately 70°, the previously relaxed central slip develops tension, pulling the extensor trifurcation farther distally, relaxing the lateral slips, lateral conjoined tendon, and terminal tendon. This unloading of the terminal tendon allows for complete flexion of the distal interphalangeal joint without encountering resistance from the extensor tendon. Any break in this system of activation and coordination interferes with the function of prehension.

The absence of intrinsic muscle action not only breaks the contour of the longitudinal arch of the finger but also creates an abnormal pattern of function. The three joints flex successively from a distoproximal direction rather than simultaneously, and this pattern of flexion prevents the palmar skin from making the necessary surface contact with the object.

In the absence of resistance, the flexor digitorum profundus is the primary finger flexor. However, when resistance is encountered, the flexor digitorum superficialis becomes activated to assist in proximal interphalangeal flexion and the interossei become more responsible for metacarpophalangeal flexion.

The opening of the fingers is an essential prerequisite for the act of prehension. As in finger flexion, extension occurs through a complex interaction of active and passive forces. Extension of the metacarpophalangeal joint is controlled by the long extensor. Although a direct connection between the extensor tendon and the proximal phalanx is usually present, action at the metacarpophalangeal joint occurs primarily through two indirect mechanisms. First, an indirect action is exerted in conjunction with the flexor digitorum superficialis.[6] With the metacarpophalangeal and proximal interphalangeal joints in full flexion, the initial pull of the extensor acts on the middle phalanx via the central slip. This force is transmitted through the proximal interphalangeal joint to the head of the proximal phalanx, producing extension at the metacarpophalangeal joint. The flexor digitorum superficialis is necessary in this action to prevent initial proximal interphalangeal extension. Second, as the metacarpophalangeal joint extends, the sagittal bands migrate proximally, over the metacarpophalangeal joint, allowing the pull of the extensor hood to act through the sagittal bands on the proximal phalanx, producing further extension at the metacarpophalangeal joint.

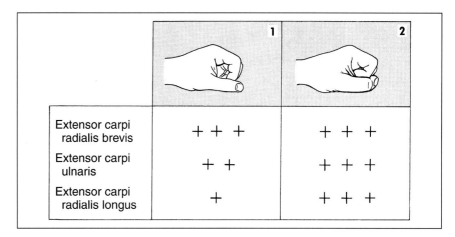

Figure 36 Participation of the wrist motors in wrist extension (1) when making a soft fist and (2) when making a tight fist. +++ = maximum activity, ++ = mild activity, + = minimal activity.

	1	2
Extensor carpi radialis brevis	+ + +	+ + +
Extensor carpi ulnaris	+ +	+ + +
Extensor carpi radialis longus	+	+ + +

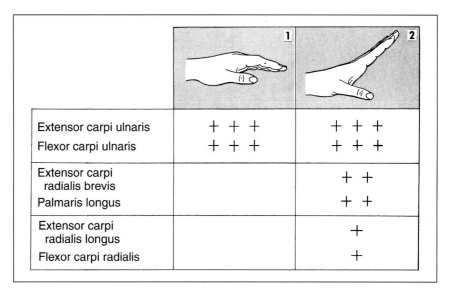

Figure 37 Participation of the wrist motors in wrist extension (1) when opening the fingers gently and (2) when opening the fingers forcefully. +++ = maximum activity, ++ = mild activity, + = minimal activity.

	1	2
Extensor carpi ulnaris	+ + +	+ + +
Flexor carpi ulnaris	+ + +	+ + +
Extensor carpi radialis brevis		+ +
Palmaris longus		+ +
Extensor carpi radialis longus		+
Flexor carpi radialis		+

The proximal interphalangeal joint is extended by the active force of the lumbricals and central slip of the long extensor. When the proximal interphalangeal joint extends actively, the oblique retinacular is subjected to tension and automatically extends the distal joint.[20] This is another mechanism of coordination on the extensor side of the finger. Additionally, the distal joint is extended by the terminal tendon, which is formed by the long extensor lateral slip but also receives a contribution from the corresponding intrinsic tendons (Figure 39).

Lateral motion and rotation of the fingers are determined by the intrinsic muscles. The dorsal interossei abduct or spread the fingers, whereas the volar interossei adduct the fingers relative to a functional axis passing through the third metacarpal. There is more abduction to the finger in extension and less in flexion because of the relative laxity of the collateral ligaments in extension. A final passive mechanism of flexion-extension of the finger is present through a tenodesis effect: wrist extension flexes the fingers, and wrist flexion extends them.

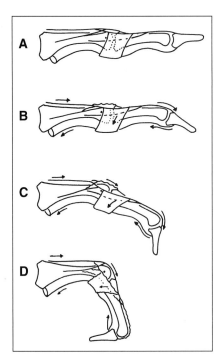

Figure 38 Landsmeer's concept of coordination of interphalangeal joint flexion. **A,** Finger in extension. **B,** Active flexion at the distal interphalangeal joint increases tension in the terminal extensor tendon and oblique retinacular ligament. Extensor trifurcation advances distally, extensor central slip relaxes, and the middle joint flexes automatically to the same degree. **C** and **D,** As flexion continues, the middle slip increases in tension. Trifurcation advances more distally, relaxing the lateral tendons and terminal tendon, including the oblique retinacular ligament. The distal joint then flexes without encountering extensor resistance.

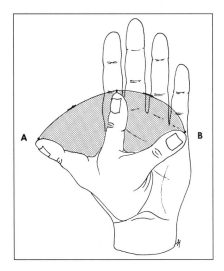

Figure 41 The thumb traces an equiangular spiral when sweeping the palmar surface from A to B.

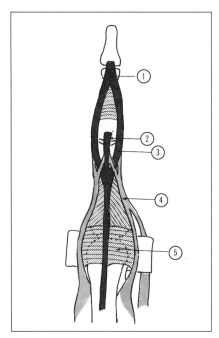

Figure 39 Extensor system for the distal interphalangeal joint. 1 = terminal tendon, 2 = middle slip, 3 = lateral slip, 4 = intrinsic tendon, 5 = quadrilateral lamina.

Thumb

Motion of the thumb occurs through the trapeziometacarpal, metacarpophalangeal, and interphalangeal joints. Flexion-extension motion occurs in the plane parallel to the palm with flexion being across the palm, toward the hypothenar eminence, and extension being away from the palm. Extension has also been referred to as radial abduction. Abduction-adduction of the thumb occurs in the plane perpendicular to the palm.

The thumb sweeps a conoid surface[21] through circumduction. This curved surface is flattened on the palmar aspect (Figure 40). All functional activities of the thumb occur within this envelope. Through flexion-adduction, the thumb traces the segment of the base of the cone along the palmar surface. The curve traced during this motion is an equiangular spiral[21] (Figure 41). Through extension-abduction, the ray returns to its initial position.

A fundamental function of the thumb is opposition with the fingers

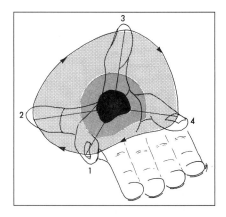

Figure 40 Field of motion of the thumb. The basic motions are: 1 to 2, extension and abduction in the palmar plane; 2 to 3, abduction in the plane perpendicular to the palm with pronation; 3 to 4, flexion, adduction, and further pronation; 4 to 1, extension and palmar abduction with supination; 1 to 4, flexion, adduction, and pronation.

that occurs as the pad of the thumb is set against the pad of a corresponding finger. To bring about opposition, the thumb is abducted in a plane perpendicular to the palm and flexed and rotated (pronated) on its long axis (Figure 42). The thumb and the pad of the finger make contact along the equiangular spiral curve of the finger. This action involves motion at all three articulations of the thumb, with the carpometacarpal joint being the most important. Overall, the carpometacarpal joint allows approximately 50° to 60° of flexion-extension, 40° to 45° of abduction-adduction, and 10° to 20° of axial rotation.[22]

Opposition occurs in multiple stages (Figure 42). First, the thumb is extended and supinated to open the first web space. This is motored by the abductor pollicis longus, extensor pollicis brevis, and abductor pollicis brevis. Additionally, the extensor pollicis longus acts to extend (and hyperextend) the interphalangeal joint, bringing the thumb tip farther from the palm. The thumb is then sequentially abducted, flexed, and pronated to position the tip against the pad of a corresponding finger. This action is determined by the abductor pollicis brevis, opponens pollicis, and the flexor pollicis brevis. In weak opposition, the action of the opponens pollicis predominates.[23] As the force of opposition increases, flexor pollicis brevis activity increases and exceeds the opponens pollicis (Figure 43). In forceful opposition to the ulnar digits, the opponens pollicis becomes more predominant and the adductor pollicis becomes involved. Additionally, as resistance increases, the extrinsic muscles are recruited.

Functional Activities

The functional activities of the hand are extensive but can be grouped into nonprehensile and prehensile activities. The former includes touching, feeling, pressing down with the fingers, tapping, vibrating the cord of a musical instrument, lifting or pushing with the hand, etc. Prehensile activities are grouped into precision and power grips.[23] Precision grip involves participation of the radial side of the hand with the thumb, index, and middle fingers to form a three-jaw chuck. When the pads of these digits come into contact, the grip is described as palmar, whereas for very precise work, contact with the tip of the same digits creates a tip type of grip. A lateral, or key, grip involves contact of the pad of the thumb with the lateral aspect of the corresponding finger in its distal segment.

A power grip predominantly involves the ulnar aspect of the hand with involvement of the little and ring fingers. The radial three digits also participate actively either in a pure power pattern form or by adding an element of precision to the power grip. The power grip can be divided into three subtypes: cylindrical, spherical, and hook. Despite the many functions of the hand, any prehensile act, when arrested instantaneously, might fit in one of these patterns in a pure or combined form.

In a cylindrical grip, all fingers are flexed maximally, such as around the handle of a tool, and the counterpressure to the flexing fingers is provided

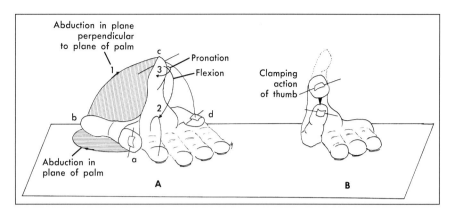

Figure 42 Opposition of the thumb. **A,** Initially, the first web space is opened by extension and supination of the thumb (a to b). The thumb is then abducted through curve 1 (b to c), bringing it perpendicular to the palm. Flexion (curve 2) and pronation (curve 3) complete the motion, positioning the thumb tip against the tip of a corresponding finger (c to d). **B,** In full opposition, the thumb tip is fully pronated, with the two nails nearly parallel and opposite one another.

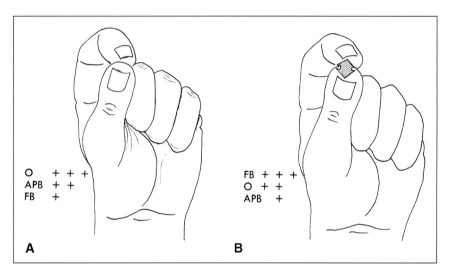

Figure 43 Muscle activity during **A,** weak opposition, and **B,** strong opposition. O = opponens pollicis; APB = abductor pollicis brevis; FB = flexor pollicis brevis. +++ = maximum activity, ++ = mild activity, + = minimum activity.

by the thenar eminence. More power is provided to this grip when the thumb wraps around the flexed fingers. If an element of precision is necessary, the thumb will adopt a longitudinal position of adduction that allows for small adjustments of posture. In general, the pattern of the grip during prehension is determined by the intention and not necessarily by the shape of the object.[24] Finger flexion is primarily powered by the flexor digitorum profundus. The flexor digitorum superficialis and the interossei become involved if more power is necessary. The thumb brings

its contribution with the thenar muscles and the flexor pollicis longus.

The spherical grip is used to hold objects such as a ball. It is similar to a cylindrical grip in terms of motor force, although the interossei are more active as a result of the abduction of the metacarpophalangeal joints. When a large object is held, a power grip is used with minimal flexion of the fingers, which are abducted and rotated, and the thumb participates at the opposite pole by stabilizing the object and providing the necessary counterpressure. With a smaller spherical object, the fingers are adducted and the thumb is in opposition; this pattern of prehension is of the precision type.

The hook power grip involves flexion of both interphalangeal joints, especially the proximal interphalangeal joint, and minimal participation of the metacarpophalangeal joint. The flexor digitorum profundus and flexor digitorum superficialis are both involved. This pattern is used in carrying a suitcase and can be maintained for a prolonged period of time.

References

1. Morrey BF, Itoi E, An KN: Biomechanics of the shoulder, in Rockwood CA Jr, Matsen FA III, Wirth MA, Harryman DT (eds): *The Shoulder,* ed 2. Philadelphia, PA, WB Saunders, 1998, pp 233-276.

2. Inman VT, Saunders JR, Abbott LC: Observations on the function of the shoulder joint. *J Bone Joint Surg* 1944; 26:1-30.

3. Howell SM, Imobersteg AM, Seger DH, Marone PJ: Clarification of the role of the supraspinatus muscle in shoulder function. *J Bone Joint Surg Am* 1986;68:398-404.

4. American Academy of Orthopaedic Surgeons: *Joint Motion: Method of Measuring and Recording.* Chicago, IL, American Academy of Orthopaedic Surgeons, 1965.

5. Boone DC, Azen SP: Normal range of motion of joints in male subjects. *J Bone Joint Surg Am* 1979;61:756-759.

6. Simon SR, Alaranta H, An KN, et al: Kinesiology, in Buckwalter JA, Einhorn TA, Simon SR (eds): *Orthopaedic Basic Science: Biology and Biomechanics of the Musculoskeletal System,* ed 2. Rosemont, IL, American Academy of Orthopaedic Surgeons, 2000, pp 731-827.

7. Morrey BF, Chao EY: Passive motion of the elbow joint. *J Bone Joint Surg Am* 1976;58:501-508.

8. Long C II, Conrad PW, Hall EA, Furler SL: Intrinsic-extrinsic muscle control of the hand in power grip and precision handling: An electromyographic study. *J Bone Joint Surg Am* 1970;52: 853-867.

9. Funk DA, An KN, Morrey BF, Daube JR: Electromyographic analysis of muscles across the elbow joint. *J Orthop Res* 1987;5:529-538.

10. Travill AA: Electromyographic study of the extensor apparatus of the forearm. *Anat Rec* 1962;144:373-376.

11. Capener N: The hand in surgery. *J Bone Joint Surg Br* 1956;38:128-151.

12. Hollister AM, Gellman H, Waters RL: The relationship of the interosseous membrane to the axis of rotation of the forearm. *Clin Orthop* 1994;298: 272-276.

13. O'Driscoll SW, Horii E, Ness R, Cahalan TD, Richards RR, An KN: The relationship between wrist position, grasp size, and grip strength. *J Hand Surg Am* 1992;17:169-177.

14. Christensen JB, Adams JP, Cho KO, Miller L: A study of the interosseous distance between the radius and ulna during rotation of the forearm. *Anat Rec* 1968;160:261-271.

15. Halls AA, Travill A: Transmission of pressures across the elbow joint. *Anat Rec* 1964;150:243-247.

16. MacConaill MA, Basmajian JV (eds): *Muscles and Movements: A Basis for Human Kinesiology.* Baltimore, MD, Williams & Wilkins, 1969.

17. Sarrafian SK, Melamed JL, Goshgarian GM: Study of wrist motion in flexion and extension. *Clin Orthop* 1977;126: 153-159.

18. Radonjic D, Long C II: Kinesiology of the wrist. *Am J Phys Med* 1971;50: 57-71.

19. Littler JW: On the adaptability of man's hand: With reference to the equiangular curve. *Hand* 1973;5:187-191.

20. Landsmeer JMF: The anatomy of the dorsal aponeurosis of the human finger and its functional significance. *Anat Rec* 1949;104:31-44.

21. Littler JW: Hand structure and function, in Littler JW, Cramer LM, Smith JW (eds): *Symposium on Reconstructive Hand Surgery.* St Louis, MO, CV Mosby, 1974, pp 3-12.

22. Cooney WP III, Lucca MJ, Chao EY, Linscheid RL: The kinesiology of the thumb trapeziometacarpal joint. *J Bone Joint Surg Am* 1981;63:1371-1381.

23. Forrest WJ, Basmajian JV: Functions of human thenar and hypothenar muscles: An electromyographic study of twenty-five hands. *J Bone Joint Surg Am* 1965;47:1585-1594.

24. Napier JR: The prehensile movements of the human hand. *J Bone Joint Surg Br* 1956;38:902-913.

Chapter 9

Body-Powered Components

Charles M. Fryer, MS
Gerald E. Stark Jr, CP
John W. Michael, MEd, CPO

Introduction

Body-powered components have been used in upper limb prostheses for centuries and are still commonly prescribed today. Body-powered control indicates that an upper limb prosthesis uses body movements, harnessed with control straps and cables, to operate the various prosthetic components or controls.

When body power is insufficient or undesirable, externally powered components may be used. External power is derived from a source outside the body. Although contemporary versions are battery-powered electronic devices, pneumatic, hydraulic, and other power sources have been used in the past.

Body-powered cable systems, developed from common bicycle controls, offer the advantages of low cost, light weight, and high reliability because of their mechanical simplicity. Their widespread use throughout the world underscores the practical advantages of these components.

Body-powered control systems also have significant disadvantages. The harness required to transmit muscle forces inevitably restricts the amputee's work envelope and encumbers the unaffected side. The amputee must often exert significant effort and grossly exaggerate body movements to generate sufficient force and excursion to operate the component. Higher-level amputees may be physically unable to generate sufficient

motion or force because of the limited leverage of short bony remnants. Finally, the robot-like appearance of some body-powered components can be disconcerting to the general public as well as to the amputee.

Terminal Devices

The most distal component of an upper limb prosthesis is called the terminal device. Terminal devices can be classified as passive or active prehensile devices. Because passive devices do not require moving parts, cables, or batteries for operation, they are typically light in weight and reliable.

Passive Terminal Devices

The most commonly prescribed passive terminal device is the passive hand (Figure 1). Many passive hands have bendable or spring-loaded fingers that can provide a static grasp for objects. The more natural appearance of the terminal device provides increased social acceptance. Partial hand or finger prostheses can provide opposition for remaining fingers or a mobile thumb.

Some passive terminal devices resemble children's mittens and hence they are called "mitts" (Figure 2). The passive mitt has a soft and flexible shape similar to the cupped human hand. Mitts are often recommended as the first terminal device for infants as they learn to sit up, crawl, walk,

and develop bimanual skills. Passive mitts are also used in sport activities, especially where physical contact with more rigid terminal devices could cause injury to the wearer or other participants. Some passive devices have specialized shapes to facilitate particular recreational activities.

Passive terminal devices that function primarily as specialized tools are also available. Some are shaped for specific tasks whereas others have adapters that allow direct attachment of various standard tools to the prosthetic wrist (Figure 3). These terminal devices provide a wide array of tool options for carpentry, gardening, domestic chores, and mechanic work. Virtually any tool can be adapted by the custom addition of an attachment with a spring-operated ball. The tool can then be quickly inserted into the device and positioned in pronation or supination in 90° increments. Some partial hand amputees use a soft wrist-hand orthosis to attach such tools to the palmar area for intermittent use.

Active Prehensile Devices

Prehensors offering active grasp may be classified according to their mode of operation. Voluntary-opening devices are normally held closed by a spring or rubber band mechanism and opened when the control cable is pulled. The object is then grasped with the pinch force proportional to

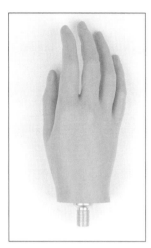

Figure 1 Passive hands with bendable fingers are valued for their cosmetic appeal, light weight, and basic function. A stock production or custom cosmetic glove is pulled over the hand to provide the outer covering. (*Courtesy of Hosmer Dorrance Corp, Campbell, CA*)

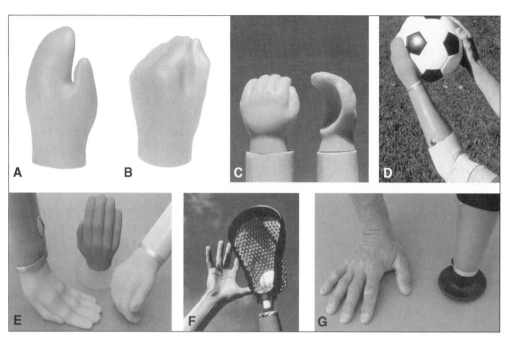

Figure 2 Flexible passive mitts are available in a variety of designs, sizes, and skin tones. **A,** Infant mitt. **B,** Closed crawling mitt. **C,** Child mitt. **D,** Sport mitt. **E,** Flexibility and skin tone options. **F,** Passive catching terminal device. **G,** Passive "mushroom" gymnastic terminal device. (*A and B Courtesy of Hosmer Dorrance Corp, Campbell, CA. C through G courtesy of Therapeutic Recreation Systems, Boulder, CO*)

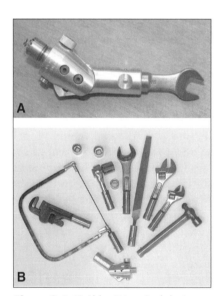

Figure 3 A, N-Abler II terminal device with adjustable flexion wrist for use with task-specific interchangeable tools. **B,** Small sample of interchangeable hand tools. (*Courtesy of Texas Assistive Devices, LLC, Brazoria, TX*)

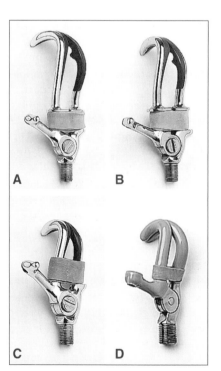

Figure 4 Voluntary-opening hook-type terminal device. **A,** Model 5X adult terminal device. **B,** Model 88X small adult terminal device. **C,** Model 10 children's terminal device. **D,** Model 12P infant's terminal device. (*Courtesy of Hosmer Dorrance Corp, Campbell, CA*)

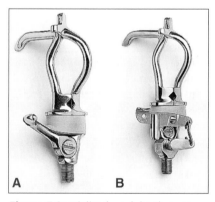

Figure 5 Specialized work hook–type terminal device. **A,** Model 7 farmer's hook. **B,** Model 6 farmer's hook with back-lock feature. (*Courtesy of Hosmer Dorrance Corp, Campbell, CA*)

the number of rubber bands or springs used when cable tension is released. The object can then be held passively until the user applies force to the control cable to release the object. Inversely, voluntary-closing devices are normally held open and close when the control cable is pulled. Pinch is regulated by the amount of force the user applies to the control cable. Prehensors may also be subdivided into hand-like and utilitarian shapes. The traditional utilitarian shape is the split hook.

Voluntary-Opening Hooks

Many voluntary-opening hook terminal devices are fairly similar in function and shape and differ primarily in size and material. The original split-hook design was created in 1912 by D.J. Dorrance, an upper limb amputee, to provide active prehension (the traditional C-shaped hook used in the days of pirates was a passive device). Because of its versatility and reliability, the voluntary-opening hook with canted fingers is the most commonly prescribed terminal device in North America (Figure 4). European manufacturers also offer voluntary-opening hooks, and many offer alternative grip-force springs and finger geometries that differ from the more familiar American designs.

A numbering system developed by the major American producer of hooks is commonly used to identify the type of hook being prescribed. Each number and letter denotes the size, shape, or type of hook. The series 5 hooks are the standard adult size with canted fingers. The term "canted" refers to the slanted configuration of the hook fingertips, which facilitates visual feedback during fine motor tasks. Because no prehensor yet offers sensation, the amputee must rely on vision to confirm that grasp has been successful. The letter X indicates the addition of nitrile rubber finger linings to improve friction and grasp, especially on metal objects like doorknobs. The letter A indicates aluminum alloy, which reduces the weight of a steel hook by 50% and is

satisfactory for all but the most rugged of users. Originally all hooks were stainless steel, but this material is now usually reserved for heavy-duty users with more rugged demands, particularly those with transradial amputations. For transhumeral and higher levels of loss, aluminum alloy hooks are generally preferred because of the ease of elbow flexion facilitated by the reduced terminal weight compared with steel devices. The series 8 hooks are slightly smaller and intended for women or teens; the series 10 is for children, and the series 12 is an infant's hook. Addition of the letter P indicates that the hook has been coated with plastisol, a soft rubber material available in a variety of skin tones. This soft coating provides a moderate amount of protection for the user and siblings.

A second characteristic shape is the work hook, identified by the number 7. This device has a large opening between the two fingers that is designed to grasp shovel handles and similar objects (Figure 5, *A*). This heavy-duty stainless steel device is commonly prescribed for adult male amputees who perform manual labor. The specialized fingers also have a number of subtle contours that facilitate holding, grasping, and carrying such items as buckets, chisels, knives, nails, and carpentry tools. Although sometimes referred to as a "farmer's hook," the device has value for anyone engaged in manual tasks, including workshop activities. Another variation, termed "LO," has a larger opening between the finger tines to better grasp large-diameter handles and brooms. The series 6 has the same finger shape as the 7 but includes a back-lock feature that prevents the hook from opening inadvertently when lifting a heavy load (Figure 5, *B*.

Some hook fingers offer a symmetric shape that facilitates grasp of cylindrical objects such as bottles more easily than canted fingers (Figure 6). The "two-load" hook has lyre-shaped fingers for this purpose. As the name suggests, a small switch at the base of the thumb permits the amputee to

engage either one spring (1.6 kg) or two springs (3.2 kg) to vary the pinch force. Because the fingers are hollow alloy, they are not suitable for heavy-duty use. The 555 hook is an aluminum alloy hook with more rugged solid fingers in the same lyre shape; the 555-SS model offers the same design in stainless steel (Figure 7).

Because most amputees find the canted approach satisfactory, the lyre shape is more commonly prescribed for use by bilateral upper limb amputees on the nondominant side to provide an alternative prehension pattern that is optimized for cylindrical objects. The combination of a canted hook with a lyre-shaped hook offers individuals with bilateral upper limb loss ready access to different gripping geometries.

The CAPP terminal device, originally developed at the Child Amputee Prosthetics Project at UCLA, offers voluntary opening function with a unique shape that is neither hook nor hand like (Figure 8). Clever use of contours and rubber materials provides a reasonably secure grasp despite the limited pinch force that a child can generate. Children frequently refer to this device as their "alligator" or "helper." This terminal device is popular for children because initially the caregiver can place objects in its grip, but the device does not require much body-powered force for the child to open it to release the object. The shape is neutral, for left or right side use, and can be cabled by the prosthetist to offer either an external or internal exit for the cable pull.

Voluntary-Closing Hooks

Voluntary-closing hooks normally open when the amputee is relaxed, are closed by pulling the control cable, resulting in a direct gradient of pinch force, depending on the force applied. The pinch force at the fingers can be very light or extremely strong because it is not limited by the number of rubber bands or springs, as is the case with voluntary-opening devices. Most voluntary-closing hooks do not have an inherent locking mechanism, so

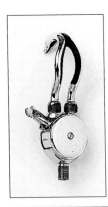

Figure 6 Two-load hook. (*Courtesy of Hosmer Dorrance Corp, Campbell, CA*)

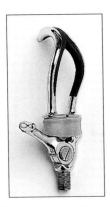

Figure 7 Model 555-SS, lyre-shaped hook in stainless steel. (*Courtesy of Hosmer Dorrance Corp, Campbell, CA*)

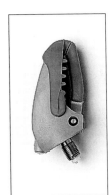

Figure 8 The CAPP terminal device, referred to by children as their "alligator" or "helper," provides a unique set of gripping surfaces. (*Courtesy of Hosmer Dorrance Corp, Campbell, CA*)

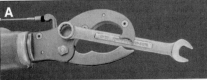

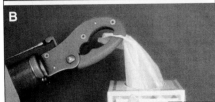

Figure 9 A, The TRS Grip voluntary-closing terminal device has multiple gripping geometries and is available in steel, aluminum alloy, or titanium. **B,** Plastic coating is also available. (*Courtesy of Therapeutic Recreation Systems, Boulder, CO*)

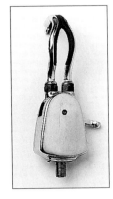

Figure 10 APRL voluntary-closing hook. (*Courtesy of Hosmer Dorrance Corp, Campbell, CA*)

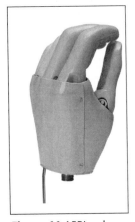

Figure 11 APRL voluntary-closing hand. (*Courtesy of Hosmer Dorrance Corp, Campbell, CA*)

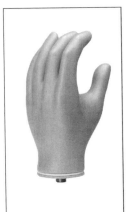

Figure 12 Soft voluntary-closing hand. (*Courtesy of Hosmer Dorrance Corp, Campbell, CA*)

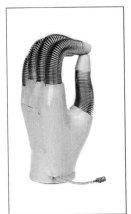

Figure 13 Becker Lock-Grip hand. (*Courtesy of Hosmer Dorrance Corp, Campbell, CA*)

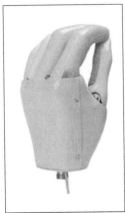

Figure 14 Sierra voluntary-opening hand. (*Courtesy of Hosmer Dorrance Corp, Campbell, CA*)

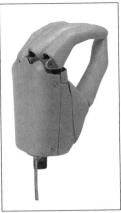

Figure 15 Dorrance voluntary-opening hand. (*Courtesy of Hosmer Dorrance Corp, Campbell, CA*)

the amputee must apply continuous force on the cable to maintain the grasp on an object. Although this is physiologically normal, some patients find this requirement objectionable and prefer other terminal devices. Acceptance of voluntary-closing terminal devices has been greatest for children and unilateral transradial amputees, particularly those with long residual limbs. Although

voluntary-closing terminal devices may be used for transhumeral and higher levels of amputation, the harness design requires special attention to conserve cable excursion.

The most popular group of voluntary-closing devices is the TRS Grip and Adept series (Therapeutic Recreational Systems, Boulder, CO) (Figure 9). These unique terminal devices are available for adults and children in aluminum, steel, and titanium, with and without urethane coatings. These terminal devices feature multiple cylindrical gripping surfaces within the fingers for gross motor prehension; fine prehension is provided by the fingertips. To maintain grasp, a ball cleat assembly can be attached to the forearm that engages a ball on the cable; alternatively, the terminal device can be modified so that a pin inserted proximally keeps the thumb in the closed position. Client acceptance has been particularly strong among children and athletic adults because the uncoated versions are very rugged and durable.

The APRL hook was developed by the Army Prosthetics Research Laboratory after World War II using biceps cineplasty as the source for body power (Figure 10). This voluntary-opening device has replaceable lyre-shaped hook fingers with a mechanism that allows two different finger openings and a gripping back-lock feature enabling the user to passively hold an object. The back-lock feature can be turned off for a "freewheeling" mode. The device is unique among hooks in that the operating lever or thumb is located on the ulnar side of the device. Like other voluntary-closing terminal devices, the APRL hook provides graded prehension, ie, the pinch force is as gentle or strong as the force generated by the amputee. This capability is believed to improve proprioception, particularly with cineplasty actuation. Unfortunately, the mechanical complexity of this device renders it both costly to manufacture and prone to breakdown. Although the graded prehension is of particular value to selected bilateral upper limb amputees, the hollow aluminum lyre-shaped fingers it shares with the two-load hook are somewhat fragile. Given the small remaining population of amputees with cineplasties, the APRL hook is currently prescribed primarily for satisfied previous wearers.

Voluntary-Closing Hands

Although voluntary-closing hands theoretically offer the same advantage of graded prehension as hooks, the frictional losses in the mechanism are much greater. The rubber-like cosmetic glove that covers the hand further impedes motion, and the thick fingers often block visual feedback from the fingertips. Functional voluntary-closing hands are now available that reduce the frictional losses by eliminating the glove and simplifying the internal mechanisms. Originally developed for pediatric use, these designs employ a soft polymer hand-like exterior with the thumb and first two fingers providing three-jaw chuck-grip prehension. These hands come in a variety of adult, child, and infant sizes. The APRL hand (Figure 11), available only in an adult male size, has features similar to the APRL hook—an automatic back-lock feature for holding objects and two grip openings.

Body-powered hands are also available with the same finger assemblies and external appearance (when the cosmetic glove is applied) as electronic hands (Figure 12). These hands are also available in a voluntary-opening configuration.

Voluntary-Opening Hands

Although a number of voluntary-opening hands are available, few are used as active terminal devices. In addition to the problems of frictional loss, restricted motion by the glove, and contours that block visual inspection, all voluntary-opening devices offer only limited pinch force. These factors significantly limit their usefulness for grasp and release tasks.

Many amputees want an interchangeable hand for social occasions in addition to a utility hook device for general use; this is the most common indication for prescribing a body-powered hand. Voluntary-opening hands are rarely appropriate for bilateral upper limb amputees because of their grip limitations. Externally powered hands offer far greater pinch force and much better grasp and release function and are consequently often preferred over body-powered hands.

Lock-Grip and Imperial Hands

The Lock-Grip (Figure 13) and Imperial hands (Becker Mechanical Hand Corp, St. Paul, MN) are voluntary-opening hands with control cable tension that causes all five fingers to open in spherical and cylindrical prehension. The Lock-Grip model contains a mechanism that locks the fingers in the closed position. Fingers can be opened from the fully closed position only when tension is applied to the control cable by the amputee. Lock-Grip hands are available in multiple sizes. The Imperial model, available in a large adult size only, permits easy adjustment of finger prehension force with a screwdriver.

Sierra Voluntary-Opening Hand

The Sierra voluntary-opening hand (Hosmer Dorrance, Campbell, CA), like the APRL hand, has a two-position stationary thumb (Figure 14). From the fully closed position, control cable tension causes the first two fingers to move away from the thumb. As tension on the control cable is relaxed, springs cause the fingers to move back toward the thumb. A back-lock feature operates in all finger positions, enabling the amputee to hold heavy objects securely. Finger opening and release of the back-lock mechanism are operated simultaneously through a single control cable. The Sierra voluntary-opening hand is available in a large adult size only.

Dorrance Functional Hands

Dorrance voluntary-opening hands (Hosmer Dorrance, Campbell, CA) allow the prosthetist to adjust finger prehension by installing different tension springs (Figure 15). They are available in a range of adult sizes.

Soft Voluntary-Opening Hand

Soft voluntary-opening hands have internal aluminum or nylon frames covered by a soft plastic shell. Some also have an adjustable pinch force from 1 to 6 lbs with a back-lock mechanism when the hand is closed. They are offered with a dorsal or palmar cable exit in a range of adult sizes (Figure 16).

CAPP Voluntary-Opening Hand

This voluntary-opening hand for children uses the same "alligator" mechanism found in the CAPP terminal device in a gloveless urethane configuration that resembles a hand (Hosmer Dorrance, Campbell, CA) (Figure 17). This creates an easy-to-operate voluntary-opening device that looks more natural than either the CAPP terminal device or a hook.

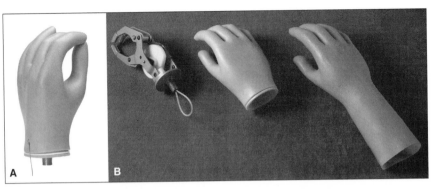
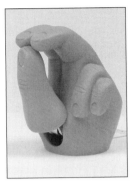

Figure 16 A, Soft voluntary-opening hand. (*Courtesy of Hosmer Dorrance Corp, Campbell, CA*) **B,** Components of soft voluntary-opening hand–inner mechanism, inner hand shell, and outer cosmetic glove. (*Courtesy of Otto Bock Healthcare-USA, Minneapolis, MN*)

Figure 17 CAPP voluntary-opening hand. (*Courtesy of Hosmer Dorrance Corp, Campbell, CA*)

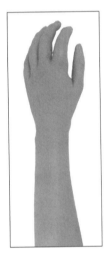

Figure 18 Custom production glove. (*Courtesy of Hosmer Dorrance Corp, Campbell, CA*)

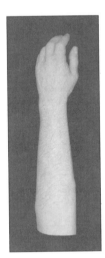

Figure 19 Custom-sculpted glove. (*Courtesy of Aesthetic Concern, Middletown, NY*)

Cosmetic Gloves

The cosmetic glove is a rubberized covering that protects the hand mechanism from contamination and also modifies the external appearance of the prosthesis. The glove is applied over the shell of a passive hand or over the mechanism of an active prehensor and must be replaced at regular intervals when it deteriorates from the wear and tear of normal use.

Three different levels of cosmetic appearance can be provided. A stock production glove, the least costly and most commonly prescribed covering, is ordered by the prosthetist on the basis of approximate hand size and skin tone. Most come in generic male, female, adolescent, and child contours in roughly two dozen shades of pink to brown skin tones. The mannequin-like appearance of a stock glove can be improved by subtle painting of veins and other structural details, or the application of fingernail polish.

A custom production glove is manufactured from a donor mold of a hand similar in shape to the amputee's. The prosthetist sends a precise mold of the partial hand amputation to the factory so that the best match can be selected. A wider selection of skin tones is available than for the stock glove, and realism can be enhanced by artistic painting and fingernail polish (Figure 18).

The custom-sculpted glove offers the most natural appearance. The glove is handmade from a sculptured reverse copy of the remaining hand. The skin tones and color are matched using a calibrated photograph of the unaffected side. These artistic restora-

tions are usually made of a special silicone elastomer that is more stain resistant than the polyvinyl chloride plastic commonly used in the less expensive gloves. Some prosthetists refer the amputee directly to a cosmetic restorationist, who creates a custom-sculpted glove that precisely matches the amputee's appearance and fits perfectly over the completed prosthesis (Figure 19). Custom-sculpted gloves can be fashioned to fit over both passive and active prosthetic hands, including myoelectrically controlled devices.

Wrist Units

Prosthetic wrist units attach the terminal device to the prosthesis and provide active or passive pronation and supination of the terminal device. With most body-powered systems, the terminal device is simply screwed into the wrist, which is permanently anchored into the forearm section.

The amputee must be provided with a full range of pronation and supination so that the terminal device can be positioned in the most functional attitude for specific tasks. The degree of voluntary pronation and supination retained depends primarily on the length of the remaining radius and ulna. When more than half the forearm bones have been lost to amputation, little or no voluntary pronation and supination can be captured by the socket. Even at the very

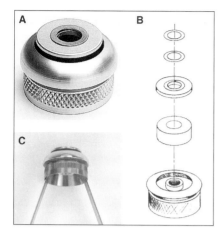

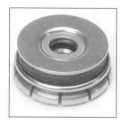

Figure 21 Low-profile friction wrist for wrist disarticulation prostheses. (*Courtesy of Hosmer Dorrance Corp, Campbell, CA*)

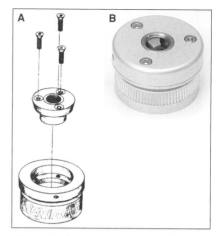

Figure 20 A, "Economy" friction wrist model. B, Inner rubber washer provides friction. C, Heavy-duty version with steel or titanium straps. (*Courtesy of Hosmer Dorrance Corp, Campbell, CA*)

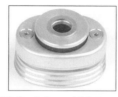

Figure 22 Oval-shaped friction wrist unit. (*Courtesy of Hosmer Dorrance Corp, Campbell, CA*)

Figure 23 A, Inner friction unit for constant-friction wrist with nylon ring. B, Mechanical-type constant-friction wrist. (*Courtesy of Hosmer Dorrance Corp, Campbell, CA*)

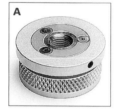 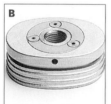 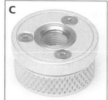 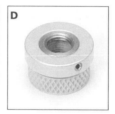 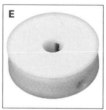 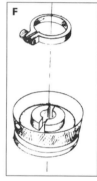

Figure 24 A, Large, round constant-friction wrist. B, Oval shape. C, Medium size, round shape. D, Infant size. E, Lightweight and simple Delrin wrist. F, Simple collar-type friction for Delrin Wrist. (*Courtesy of Hosmer Dorrance Corp, Campbell, CA*)

long transradial levels of amputation, pronation and supination can be restricted by some self-suspending supracondylar socket designs that effectively block all pronation and supination by extending proximally above the elbow joint.

Friction Wrist Units

Friction wrist units are the most commonly prescribed wrist option. A set screw or spacer washers are adjusted so that sufficient friction is applied to prevent terminal device rotation under load, yet not so much that the amputee cannot manually rotate the terminal device with the sound hand (Figure 20). Bilateral amputees usually preposition their terminal devices by striking one against the other, or by gripping a stable object such as a table edge and then rotating the terminal

device into the desired position. Friction wrist units are available in aluminum or stainless steel and in a full range of infant, child, and adult sizes. Special friction wrist units designed for wrist disarticulation prostheses are made as thin as possible to minimize the length of the prosthetic forearm beyond the residual limb (Figure 21).

Oval-shaped friction wrist units are available in adult and medium sizes and provide a smoother transition to the socket contours for long transradial levels of amputation (Figure 22). Because many prosthetic hands have an oval base, the oval-shaped wrist unit also provides a smoother transition from the prosthetic hand to the prosthetic forearm. When the prosthetic hand is rotated into pronation or supination, however, there will be a noticeable prominence at the wrist be-

cause the hand and wrist contours are no longer congruent.

Friction wrist units are durable and economical but do not provide a constant resistance to pronation and supination. With these older designs, a rubber washer is compressed to create friction as the terminal device stud is screwed into the wrist unit. As the terminal device is unscrewed, friction is reduced; consequently, the stabilizing force varies with the pronation or supination position of the terminal device.

Constant-Friction Wrist Units

Constant-friction wrist units are generally preferred because they are designed to provide constant friction throughout the range of rotation of

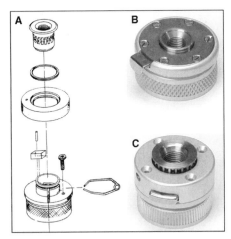

Figure 25 A, Quick-change wrist. Disconnect mechanism with insert nut (far right). **B,** Pushbutton-type. **C,** Medium size. (*Courtesy of Hosmer Dorrance Corp, Campbell, CA*)

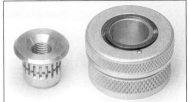

Figure 26 Ring-type quick-change wrist unit. (*Courtesy of Hosmer Dorrance Corp, Campbell, CA*)

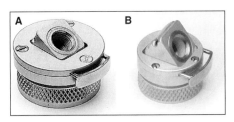

Figure 27 Flexion wrist. **A,** Adult version. **B,** Smaller medium size. (*Courtesy of Hosmer Dorrance Corp, Campbell, CA*)

the terminal device. Most constant-friction units employ a nylon-threaded insert (Figure 23). When a small set-screw in the body of the wrist is turned, the nylon thread is deformed against the stud of the terminal device, creating constant friction. When the threads wear out, the insert can be replaced, returning the wrist to like-new condition. Some versions use a mechanical wedge that presses on the terminal device stud. This design resists wear and thermal breakdown better than the nylon wrists, yet has equally smooth friction resistance. Constant-friction wrist units are available in both round and oval configurations (Figure 24). In the round configuration, infant through adult sizes are available. In the oval configuration, only adult and medium sizes are manufactured.

Quick-Disconnect Wrist Units

Quick-disconnect wrist units are designed to facilitate rapid interchange of different terminal devices (Figure 25). All commercially available quick-disconnect wrist units allow the amputee to exchange different terminal devices and to lock them down in the desired attitude of supination or pronation.

Most quick-disconnect units employ an adapter, which is screwed tightly on the threaded stud of the various terminal devices to be interchanged. In these units, light downward pressure on the activating lever by the amputee unlocks the terminal device but does not cause its ejection. With the terminal device unlocked, the amputee manually rotates the device to the desired attitude of pronation or supination. Application of a proximally directed axial force with the sound hand will then lock the terminal device in the new position. Heavy downward pressure on the activating lever causes ejection of the adapter and attached terminal device. This option is popular when using the device through a cosmetic glove. Another control option uses a ring that is rotated in one direction for pronation and supination positioning and in the other direction for disconnection (Figure 26). Quick-disconnect units are available in an adult or medium size with a round or oval configuration in either aluminum or steel.

Wrist Flexion Units

Wrist flexion is particularly useful for activities at the midline—toileting, eating, shaving, dressing, etc. Such activities are generally performed more easily with the sound hand than with a prosthesis. For this reason, prosthetic wrist flexion is seldom necessary for unilateral amputees unless range of motion is restricted in the more proximal joints. However, wrist flexion capability is very important for the bilateral upper limb amputee who must perform all daily activities

with prostheses. Because the mechanism adds weight near the termination of the prosthesis, it is sometimes prescribed only for the dominant side. Two types of mechanism can provide wrist flexion.

The flexion wrist replaces the common constant-friction wrist and allows manual prepositioning of the terminal device in neutral, 30° of volar flexion, or 50° of volar flexion (Figure 27). The terminal device can also rotate about its mounting stud in any of the positions.

The wrist flexion unit is used in conjunction with the friction wrist (Figure 28). This dome-shaped device also has three locking positions—0°, 25°, and 50° of volar flexion. Because the entire unit can rotate where it mounts to the wrist, the terminal device covers a wider work envelope than the flexion wrist. This can be advantageous for the bilateral amputee struggling to perform midline activities. However, this unit is significantly heavier and longer than the flexion wrist because it must be coupled in addition to a wrist.

Another wrist option offers passive wrist extension for pediatric use when the prosthesis is used for crawling. This wrist uses a wedge of soft foam that can compress when the passive mitt terminal device is extended. Passive wrist extension also facilitates such activities as holding the handlebars of a bicycle.

Rotational Wrists

Friction wrist units described earlier in this chapter may present difficulties for amputees who engage in work or avocational activities that exert

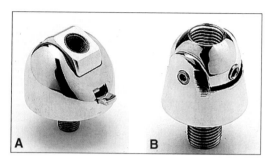

Figure 28 Wrist flexion unit, **A,** Adult size. **B,** Child size. (*Courtesy of Hosmer Dorrance Corp, Campbell, CA*)

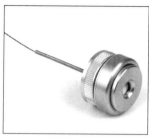

Figure 29 Rotational wrist unit. (*Courtesy of Hosmer Dorrance Corp, Campbell, CA*)

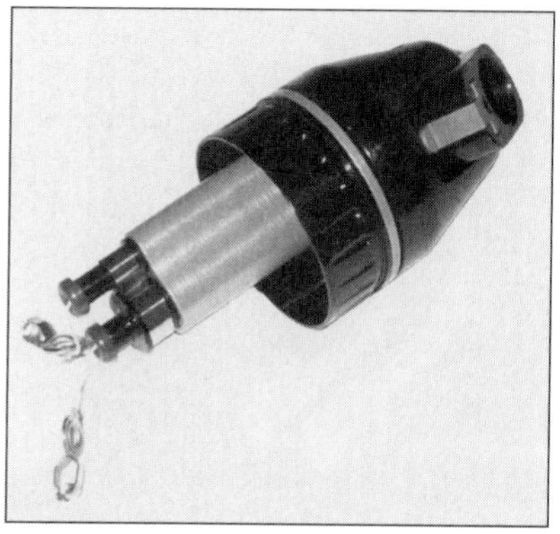

Figure 30 Four-function wrist allowing flexion, extension, pronation, and supination. (*Courtesy of Texas Assistive Devices, LLC, Brazoria, TX*)

high rotational loads on the terminal device. Friction and constant-friction wrist units tend to permit unwanted rotation when subjected to very high torsional loading.

Rotational wrist units are cable-controlled, positive-locking mechanisms (Figure 29). In the unlocked mode, these units permit manual prepositioning of the terminal device in almost any attitude of supination or pronation throughout a 360° range. Once locked in position, these units provide much greater resistance to rotation than friction units do.

The bilateral amputee may find that rotational wrist units better facilitate prepositioning of the terminal devices. With the wrist unit unlocked and the terminal devices fully supinated or pronated, tension on the terminal device control cable causes the terminal device to rotate back to the neutral position.

Another wrist variation, called the four-function wrist, combines the rotational wrist with a flexion wrist. The name refers to the four wrist functions of flexion, extension, pronation, and supination. A rotational wrist is spring loaded to move into a pronated position when unlocked. With a pull of the control cable, it is brought into proper position and locked with a reciprocating mechanism. A rubber band attached to the wrist brings the wrist into flexion when unlocked and is positioned in the same manner. This type of wrist can be adapted from existing componentry or pur-chased as an off-the-shelf device (Figure 30).

Elbow Units
Elbow Units for Transradial Amputees
Flexible Hinges

With amputation through the distal third of the forearm, the amputee retains a limited amount of active supination and pronation. Flexible hinges permit active use of residual forearm rotation, minimizing the requirement for manual prepositioning of the terminal device by the amputee. Although flexible hinges of metal cable or leather are commercially available, custom-made hinges of Dacron webbing are most commonly used. They attach proximally to the triceps pad and distally to the prosthetic forearm and should allow prosthesis rotation of at least 50% that of the anatomic residual forearm rotation (Figure 31).

Rigid Hinges

Amputations at or above the midforearm level basically eliminate the possibility of transmitting active supination or pronation to the terminal device. At these levels of amputation, the amputee must resort to manual prepositioning of the terminal device; consequently, the use of rigid hinges does not restrict voluntary pronation or supination. The primary advantage of rigid hinges is that they protect the residual limb against torque loads.

They are typically available in adult, medium, and child sizes.

Single-Axis Hinges

Single-axis hinges are designed to provide axial (rotational) stability between the prosthetic socket and residual forearm during active prosthesis use (Figure 32). Correctly aligned single-axis hinges should not restrict the normal flexion-extension range of motion of the anatomic elbow joint. The joints should be set in a certain amount of preflexion to load the stops of the joint when carrying heavy objects. This helps unweight the shorter residual limb and prevents hyperextension.

Polycentric Hinges

Short transradial levels of amputation require that the anteroproximal trim line of the prosthetic socket be close to the elbow joint. With a high anterior socket wall, complete elbow flexion tends to be restricted by the bunching of soft tissue in the antecubital region. Polycentric hinges reduce this tendency for bunching by providing more room in the cubital area as the elbow is flexed, thereby increasing the range of motion at this joint (Figure 33).

Step-Up Hinges

Amputations immediately distal to the elbow joint require a prosthetic socket with extremely high trim lines

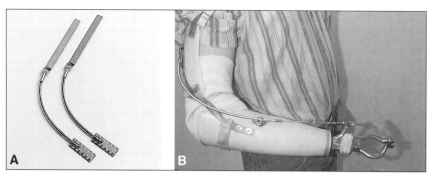

Figure 31 A, Cable-type flexible hinges. **B,** Transradial prosthesis with Dacron flexible hinges. *(Courtesy of Hosmer Dorrance Corp, Campbell, CA)*

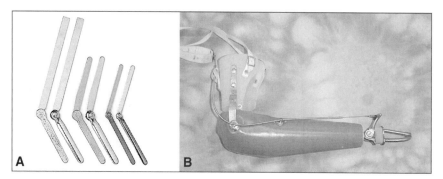

Figure 32 A, Three sizes of single-axis hinges. **B,** Transradial prosthesis with single-axis hinges. *(Courtesy of Hosmer Dorrance Corp, Campbell, CA)*

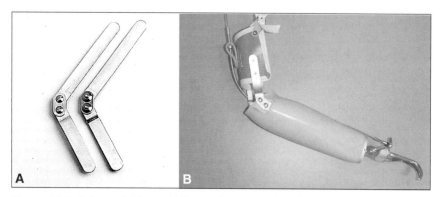

Figure 33 A, Polycentric hinges. **B,** Transradial prosthesis with polycentric hinges. *(Courtesy of Hosmer Dorrance Corp, Campbell, CA)*

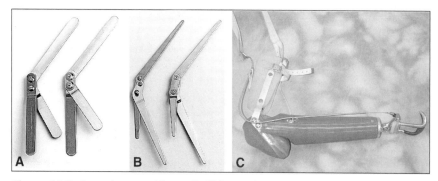

Figure 34 A, Geared step-up hinges. **B,** Sliding action step-up hinges. **C,** Transradial prosthesis with step-up hinges demonstrates the split-socket configuration. *(Courtesy of Hosmer Dorrance Corp, Campbell, CA)*

to provide adequate stability. Consequently, flexion of the anatomic elbow joint is often restricted to 90° or less. In situations in which full range of elbow flexion has been compromised as a result of trauma or disease, step-up hinges may be used to enhance remaining flexion to ensure greater overall function.

The use of step-up hinges requires that the prosthetic forearm and socket be separated (Figure 34). Thus, prostheses using step-up hinges are frequently referred to as split-socket prostheses. Step-up hinges amplify the excursion of anatomic elbow joint motion by a ratio of approximately 2:1; thus, 60° of flexion of the anatomic elbow joint causes the prosthetic forearm (and terminal device) to move through a range of approximately 120° of motion. The increased range of motion requires that the amputee exert twice as much force to flex the step-up hinge.

There are two types of step-up hinges, sliding action and geared joints. The sliding action step-up hinges sometimes tear clothing and require a split-housing cable system. Geared step-up hinges are more fully enclosed and may use a standard Bowden cable system. Both versions require special fixtures to align properly.

Residual Limb–Activated Locking Hinge

Amputees with very high transradial levels of amputation are often unable to operate a conventional transradial prosthesis due to inadequate strength, range, or load surface on the residual limb. With residual limb–activated locking hinges, the transradial prosthesis is controlled as if it were an elbow disarticulation prosthesis with outside locking hinges (Figure 35). Because there is no forearm to functionally use for elbow flexion, a split-housing dual-control cable system must be provided in which glenohumeral flexion causes elbow flexion. A split socket is created so that the short residual limb can lock and unlock the mechanical elbow joint. Residual limb–activated locking hinges are available in two sizes, adult and small.

Elbow Units for Elbow, Transhumeral, and Below-Shoulder Disarticulation Amputees

Replacement of the anatomic elbow joint requires a body-powered substitute that permits flexion and extension control through a range of approximately 135°. In addition, the unit must permit the amputee to lock and unlock the elbow at various points throughout the 135° range of motion.

Outside-Locking Hinges

Elbow disarticulation and transcondylar levels of amputation usually require the use of outside-locking hinges. Standard prosthetic elbow units would result in an excessively long humeral section and shortened forearm segment, creating an unnatural appearance. Significant elbow center discrepancies may also make table-top activities more difficult.

Outside-locking hinges are available in standard and heavy-duty models (Figure 36). The standard units provide seven different locking positions throughout the range of flexion and come in adult, medium, and child sizes. The heavy-duty model provides five locking positions and is variable only in the adult size.

Inside-Locking Elbow Units

Amputations through the humerus approximately 5 cm proximal to the elbow joint provide adequate space to accommodate inside-locking elbow mechanisms. Inside-locking units permit the amputee to lock the elbow in any of 11 positions of flexion (Figure 37). Heavy-duty versions are available that reduce the number of locking positions to eight. All inside-locking units incorporate a friction-held turntable that permits manual prepositioning of the prosthetic forearm to substitute for the loss of active external and internal humeral rotation.

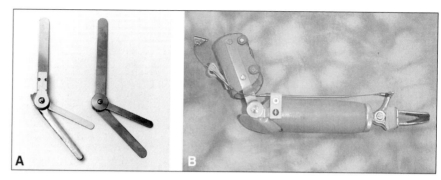

Figure 35 A, Residual limb–activated locking hinge. **B,** Transradial prosthesis with residual limb–activated locking hinge. *(Courtesy of Hosmer Dorrance Corp, Campbell, CA)*

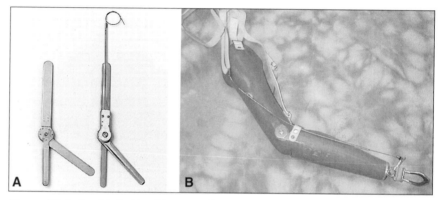

Figure 36 A, Outside-locking hinge. **B,** Elbow disarticulation prosthesis with outside-locking hinges. *(Courtesy of Hosmer Dorrance Corp, Campbell, CA)*

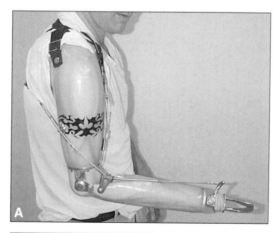

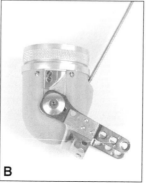
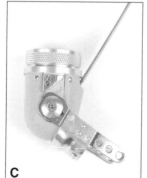
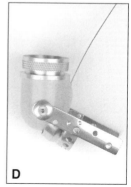

Figure 37 A, Transhumeral patient using inside-locking elbow. **B,** Adult size inside-locking elbow. **C,** Medium size elbow. **D,** Small size elbow. *(Courtesy of Hosmer Dorrance Corp, Campbell, CA)*

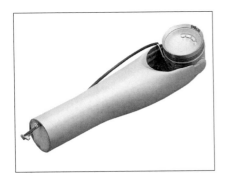

Figure 38 Automatic Forearm Balance (AFB) elbow. *(Courtesy of Otto Bock Healthcare-USA, Minneapolis, MN)*

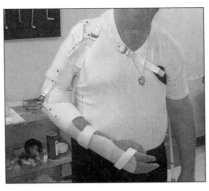

Figure 39 Flail-arm hinge "prosthosis" for patient with brachial plexus injury.

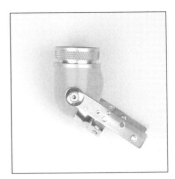

Figure 40 Small passive friction elbow. *(Courtesy of Hosmer Dorrance Corp, Campbell, CA)*

Otto Bock developed a body-powered elbow that has been optimized to work with an externally powered terminal device. It can lock and release in an infinite number of positions because of its friction clutch design. This locking mechanism also allows a unique "slip-stop" function. Pulling the control cable a few millimeters fully locks or unlocks the elbow. Pulling the cable very slightly "slips" the clutch so that gravity gently lowers the forearm. When the forearm reaches the desired position, the amputee simply relaxes the cable tension, and the elbow immediately locks the forearm in that position. These body-powered elbows are also well suited for use with proximal electronic or myoelectric connections that are prerouted inside the forearm-turntable assembly, with distal connections for the hand and battery (Figure 38).

Other elbows have been designed with reciprocal flexion locking action that also includes a humeral rotation unit. This is operated by twisting the ring at the base of the turntable to unlock transverse rotation, which then has an adjustable friction control. An opposite twist again locks the elbow rotation into place. The attachment ring comes in five configurations, with the adult-size diameter at 70 mm.

Flail-Arm Hinges

Flail-arm hinges are intended for postbrachial plexus injury "prosthoses" and contain an oversized clock-spring mechanism to partially counterbalance the weight of the forearm (Figure 39). They may be used singly or in pairs depending on the degree of counterbalance desired. They may also be combined with a single free joint or a single locking joint as necessary.

Another type of brachial plexus hinge uses the same action as a beach lounge chair; the elbow is ratcheted into position and released with full flexion. This version uses one small medially mounted upright to support the arm.

Friction Units

Friction elbows are very lightweight and simple to operate but require passive positioning of the forearm (Figure 40). For this reason, they are often appropriate for cosmetic restorations, pediatric applications, congenital anomalies, and situations in which brachial plexus injury or other factors preclude active elbow function.

Elbow Flexion Assists

The spring-lift assist is a clock-spring unit, similar to the flail-arm hinge, that can be added to a body-powered elbow. The function of the spring-lift assist is to partially counterbalance the weight of the prosthetic forearm and reduce the force necessary for elbow flexion. Reduced force requirements may permit subtle harnessing adjustments so that the amputee will require less excursion. Although optional, elbow flexion assists are routinely prescribed, particularly for use with heavier terminal devices or hand prehensors (Figure 41).

Otto Bock has developed a spring-loaded cam mechanism mounted within the forearm that can be adjusted to completely counterbalance the weight of the forearm-wrist-terminal device assembly during elbow flexion (Figure 38). While the Automatic Forearm Balance unit works well with a body-powered cable that actively flexes the elbow, it can also be adjusted so that the amputee can simply swing the forearm into position by throwing the prosthesis forward and then activate the clutch lock to stabilize it.

Shoulder Units

Shoulder mechanisms may be classified according to the degree of motion allowed. The simplest design is called a bulkhead because the humeral segment is directly connected to the socket and no motion can occur. Many unilateral amputees find this acceptable and appreciate the lower prosthesis weight that results from omitting this joint.

Passively moveable friction-loaded shoulder joints are available and provide some assistance with dressing and desktop activities. Single-axis units permit only abduction; double-axis units allow abduction and flexion (Figure 42); and triple-axis (Figure

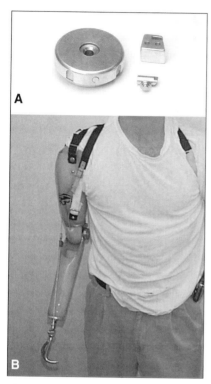

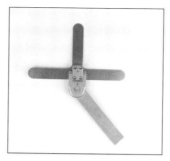

Figure 42 Flexion abduction joint with passive friction control for shoulder motion. *(Courtesy of Hosmer Dorrance Corp, Campbell, CA)*

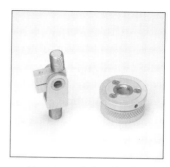

Figure 43 Universal shoulder joint uses a friction wrist proximally and distally to allow glenohumeral rotation. *(Courtesy of Hosmer Dorrance Corp, Campbell, CA)*

Figure 41 A, Spring-lift assist device with internal clock-spring unit. **B,** Patient with lift assist mounted medially on elbow axis. *(Courtesy of Hosmer Dorrance Corp, Campbell, CA)*

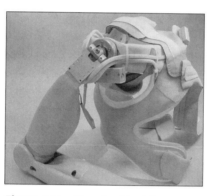

Figure 44 Locking shoulder joint. *(Courtesy of Liberating Technologies, Inc, Holliston, MA)*

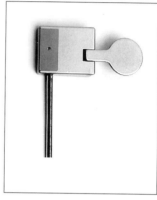

Figure 45 Nudge control unit can be used as a control alternative to lock and unlock the elbow or shoulder joint. *(Courtesy of Hosmer Dorrance Corp, Campbell, CA)*

43) and ball-and-socket configurations permit universal passive motion. Most are available in small, medium, and large sizes.

A locking shoulder joint is currently available that can stabilize the shoulder in 36 different flexion positions. This is beneficial for those who wish to use the body-powered or externally powered terminal device for upper quadrant activities such as reaching items on a high shelf. This shoulder can be locked and unlocked manually or by using an electronic switch option. A second hinge with friction control is integrated into this unit to provide abduction/adduction stabilization (Figure 44).

Nudge Control Unit

The nudge control unit is a paddle-shaped lever that can be pushed by the chin or phocomelic digit or against environmental objects to provide a small amount of cable excur-

sion. It is usually prescribed when other body motions are not available. Although originally designed to provide elbow locking and unlocking, it can also be adapted to operate other components, including flexion and rotation wrist units (Figure 45).

Endoskeletal Upper Limb Prostheses

Two different endoskeletal upper limb prosthetic systems are currently available in the United States. The systems consist of tubular humeral and forearm elements, and the components allow for encasement in cosmetic foam covers. After final shaping and covering with a skin-colored stockinette, the completed prosthesis affords a high degree of cosmetic acceptability (Figure 46). In addition to

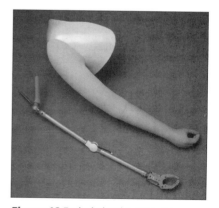

Figure 46 Endoskeletal construction, showing ball-and-socket shoulder joint with foam cover. *(Courtesy of Otto Bock Healthcare-USA, Minneapolis, MN)*

improved cosmesis and softness, modular prostheses are lighter weight than conventional artificial limbs.

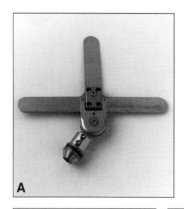

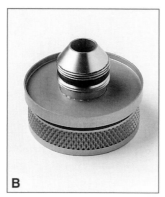

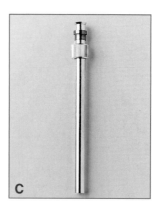

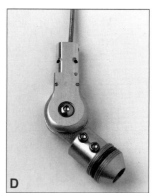

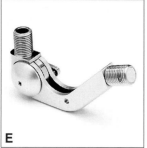

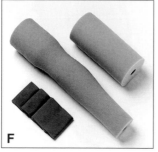

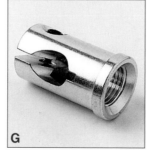

Figure 47 Endoskeletal system components. **A,** Shoulder joint, **B,** Turntable attachment. **C,** Endoskeletal pylon **D,** Reciprocating elbow. **E,** Pushbutton unlock elbow. **F,** Foam cover before shaping. **G,** Endoskeletal wrist. *(Courtesy of Hosmer Dorrance Corp, Campbell, CA)*

One endoskeletal design permits passive or cable-operated elbow flexion with manual locking. Passive prepositioning of the humeral segment in internal or external rotation and the forearm in supination or pronation is achieved by the use of rotation adapters. The hands provide a wide variety of terminal device options—cable-controlled, voluntary-opening or voluntary-closing units, and a passive hand unit with a spring-activated thumb and fingers. For the shoulder disarticulation level,

this endoskeletal prosthesis offers two friction-loaded, passively positionable shoulder units, a ball-and-socket joint, and a flexion-extension, abduction-adduction hinge.

Another system includes components for transradial, transhumeral, and shoulder disarticulation levels of amputation (Figure 47). Socket attachment turntables permit passive rotation of the humeral and forearm segments. All terminal devices with the standard ½-in-20 thread can be used, but usually a cosmetic passive

hand is chosen. A separate wrist unit that fits within the tubular construction allows for manual prepositioning of the terminal device in flexion.

Three elbow units are available for either cable-controlled or manual operation—a constant-friction elbow, an elbow with manual lock, and an elbow joint with a cable-controlled locking mechanism. For the shoulder disarticulation level, a flexion-extension, abduction-adduction hinge that can be positioned manually is available.

Chapter 10

Harnessing and Controls for Body-Powered Devices

Charles M. Fryer, MS
John W. Michael, MEd, CPO

Introduction

In body-powered upper limb prosthetic applications, the main functions of control and suspension are closely interrelated. The prosthesis is suspended on the residual limb by the intimacy of the socket fit and by a system of nonelastic straps collectively referred to as a harness. In a well-designed harness, the straps are strategically positioned in relation to the shoulder girdle and/or thorax so that the amputee can control the prosthetic components with a minimum of exertion and body motion. To understand the two main functions of a prosthetic harness, it is first necessary to examine the mechanical operating principles of prosthetic control systems.

Mechanics of the Transradial Control System

The transradial prosthetic control system is a one-cable, or "single-control," system. A stainless steel control cable is firmly attached at its proximal end to one of the nonelastic straps of the harness (Figure 1). Distally, the cable terminates at some type of prehension device.

Prehension devices, usually referred to as terminal devices, typically consist of either prosthetic hands with one or more movable fingers or two-fingered devices with a hook-type configuration. The amputee uses shoulder motion on the amputated side to apply tension to the control cable. The cable tension is transmitted to the operating lever, or "thumb," of the terminal device and causes one finger of the hook to move away from the other stationary finger (Figure 2, A). When cable tension is relaxed, the movable finger closes on the stationary finger (Figure 2, B). With this type of device, the force of prehension is determined by the number of rubber bands located at the bases of the hook fingers. As a general rule, each rubber band produces approximately 0.45 kg

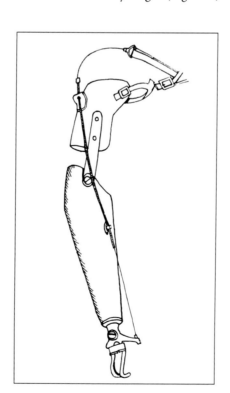

Figure 1 Transradial prosthetic control system. *(Reproduced with permission from* Below and Above Elbow Harness and Control System. *Evanston, IL, Northwestern University Prosthetic-Orthotic Center, 1966.)*

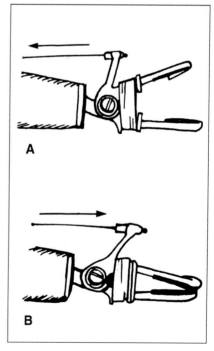

Figure 2 Prehension device with the cable tensed **(A)** and with the cable relaxed **(B)**. *(Reproduced with permission from* Below and Above Elbow Harness and Control System. *Evanston, IL, Northwestern University Prosthetic-Orthotic Center, 1966.)*

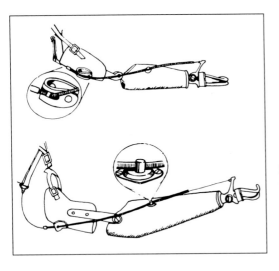

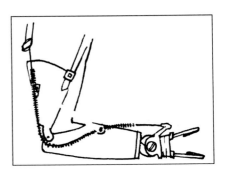

Figure 3 Control cable housing. *(Reproduced with permission from* Below and Above Elbow Harness and Control System. *Evanston, IL, Northwestern University Prosthetic-Orthotic Center, 1966.)*

Figure 4 The length of the control cable remains constant. *(Reproduced with permission from* Below and Above Elbow Harness and Control System. *Evanston, IL, Northwestern University Prosthetic-Orthotic Center, 1966.)*

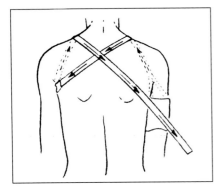

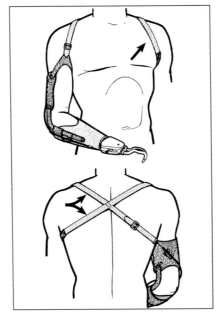

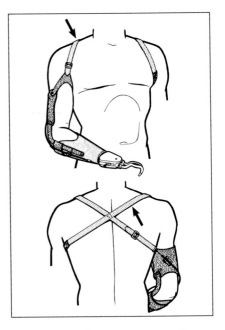

Figure 5 Figure-of-8 configuration of a standard transradial harness. *(Reproduced with permission from Santschi WR (ed):* Manual of Upper Extremity Prosthetics, ed 2. *Los Angeles, CA, University of California Department of Engineering, 1958.)*

Figure 6 Axilla loop. *(Reproduced from Pursley RJ: Harness patterns for upper-extremity prostheses, in* Orthopaedic Appliances Atlas. *Chicago, IL, American Academy of Orthopaedic Surgeons, 1960.)*

Figure 7 Anterior support strap. *(Reproduced from Pursley RJ: Harness patterns for upper-extremity prostheses, in* Orthopaedic Appliances Atlas. *Chicago, IL, American Academy of Orthopaedic Surgeons, 1960.)*

(1 lb) of prehensile force between the hook fingers.

Most of the control cable is encased in a flexible stainless steel housing (Figure 3). At its upper end, the housing through which the control cable passes is attached to the triceps pad of the prosthesis by a fixture called a crossbar assembly. A base plate and retainer serve to anchor the distal end of the cable housing at approximately the midforearm level of the prosthesis.

The cable housing is an integral part of the transradial single-control system. In effect, the housing maintains a constant length of the control cable regardless of the angular attitude of the anatomic elbow joint. The

amount of body motion used to operate the terminal device remains essentially the same whether the elbow is flexed to 135° or is completely extended (Figure 4).

Figure-of-8 Transradial Harness

The standard transradial harness for the adult unilateral amputee is composed of 2.5- cm-wide nonelastic web-

bing. The webbing is arranged to form a horizontally oriented figure-of-8 pattern (Figure 5). The axilla loop, which serves as the primary anchor from which two other straps originate, encircles the shoulder girdle on the nonamputated side (Figure 6).

The second component of the transradial harness is the anterior support strap or, as it is sometimes called, "the inverted Y suspensor." The

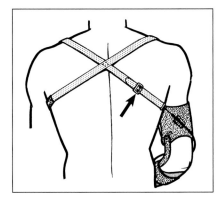

Figure 8 Control attachment strap. *(Reproduced from Pursley RJ: Harness patterns for upper-extremity prostheses, in* Orthopaedic Appliances Atlas. *Chicago, IL, American Academy of Orthopaedic Surgeons, 1960.)*

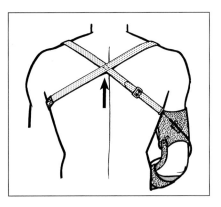

Figure 9 Cross point of a harness sewn together. *(Reproduced from Pursley RJ: Harness patterns for upper-extremity prostheses, in* Orthopaedic Appliances Atlas. *Chicago, IL, American Academy of Orthopaedic Surgeons, 1960.)*

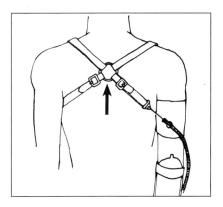

Figure 10 Cross point of a harness connected by a stainless steel ring. *(Reproduced with permission from* Below and Above Elbow Harness and Control System. *Evanston, IL, Northwestern University Prosthetic-Orthotic Center, 1966.)*

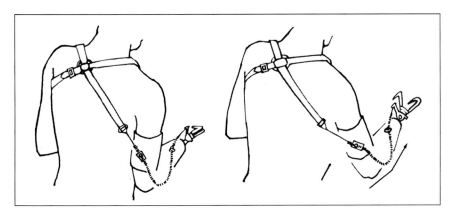

Figure 11 Glenohumeral joint flexion for operating a terminal device. *(Reproduced with permission from* Below and Above Elbow Harness and Control System. *Evanston, IL, Northwestern University Prosthetic-Orthotic Center, 1966.)*

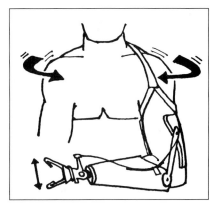

Figure 12 Biscapular abduction for terminal device operation.

anterior support strap originates at the axilla loop, passes over the shoulder on the amputated side, and attaches to the anteroproximal margins of the triceps pad of the prosthesis (Figure 7). The primary function of the anterior support strap is to resist displacement of the socket on the residual limb when the prosthesis is subjected to heavy loading.

The control attachment strap originates at the axilla loop and terminates at the proximal end of the prosthetic control cable (Figure 8). Anchored by the axilla loop, the control attachment strap acts as an extension of the control cable. Located between the spine and the inferior angle of the scapula, the control attachment strap permits scapular abduction and shoulder flexion on the amputated side for operation of the terminal device.

The posterior junction of the axilla loop, where the anterior support and control attachment straps cross, may be either sewn together (Figure 9) or connected by a stainless steel ring (Figure 10). In the latter case, the harness is referred to as a transradial, ring-type harness. Because they are less restrictive, ring-type harnesses enjoy a high degree of acceptability by most transradial amputees. Whether the harness straps are sewn together or attached to the axilla loop by a steel ring, mechanical efficiency is enhanced if the cross point is located below the spinous process of C7 and slightly toward the nonamputated side. When sufficient excursion is available, most amputees prefer a slightly looser harness with the cross point located at the midline.

The primary body control motion for operating the terminal device of a transradial prosthesis is flexion of the glenohumeral joint (Figure 11), which enables excellent generation of force and provides sufficient cable travel for full terminal device operation. When terminal device operation in a fixed position or close to the midline of the body is required, such as when buttoning a shirt, the standard transradial harness permits the amputee to use biscapular abduction for terminal device operation (Figure 12).

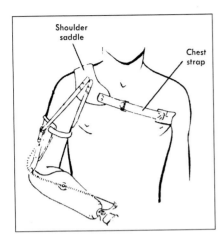

Figure 13 Shoulder saddle harness. *(Reproduced with permission from Santschi WR (ed): Manual of Upper Extremity Prosthetics, ed 2. Los Angeles, CA, University of California Department of Engineering, 1958.)*

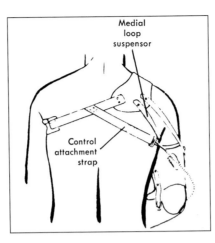

Figure 14 Location of the control attachment strap on a shoulder saddle harness. *(Reproduced with permission from Santschi WR (ed): Manual of Upper Extremity Prosthetics, ed 2. Los Angeles, CA, University of California Department of Engineering, 1958.)*

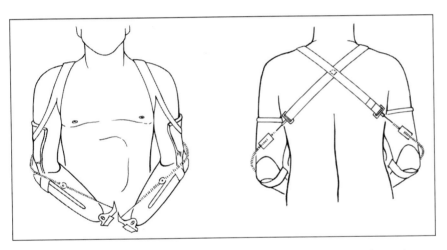

Figure 15 Bilateral transradial harness. Note the location of the control attachment strap in the back view. *(Reproduced with permission from Santschi WR (ed): Manual of Upper Extremity Prosthetics, ed 2. Los Angeles, CA, University of California Department of Engineering, 1958.)*

the prosthesis is distributed over the shoulder on the amputated side rather than being transmitted to the axilla on the nonamputated side. This redistribution of loading is accomplished by fitting a fairly wide flexible shoulder saddle on the amputated side. Two support straps extend from the posterior portion of the shoulder saddle through D-rings located on the medial and lateral surfaces of the triceps pad and terminate on the anterior surface of the saddle. The shoulder saddle is anchored in place with a chest strap. Because the control attachment strap is located in essentially the same place as in the figure-of-8 harness, the midscapular level, the amputee uses glenohumeral flexion and/or scapular abduction for terminal device operation (Figures 13 and 14).

Bilateral Transradial Harness

The harness pattern for the bilateral transradial amputee differs only slightly in that the axilla loops are omitted. Viewed from the rear, the control attachment strap for operation of the right terminal device extends obliquely upward across the back and terminates as the anterior support strap for the left prosthesis (Figure 15). Conversely, the control attachment strap for operation of the left terminal device becomes the anterior support strap for the right prosthesis. As in the case of the standard unilateral harness, the posterior cross point may be sewn together or connected by a stainless steel ring. The bilateral transradial amputee uses the same body control motions, glenohumeral flexion and/or biscapular abduction, for terminal device operation as does the unilateral transradial amputee.

Transradial Harness Modifications

For amputees with a short transradial amputation, step-up hinges may be

Heavy-Duty Transradial Harness

A major disadvantage of the standard figure-of-8 harness for transradial amputees relates to the axilla loop. The axillary portion of the loop should always be padded and worn on top of an undergarment. However, when significant tension is applied to the anterior support and control attachment straps, the loop is driven vertically upward into the axilla on the nonamputated side. Over a period

of time, this excessive pressure in the axillary area may cause skin irritation and can produce neurotrophic changes from brachial plexus pressure. When it is anticipated that the transradial amputee will engage in very strenuous activities, particularly the repeated lifting of heavy objects, it is recommended that a different transradial harness system be considered.

One alternative transradial harness is generally referred to as a "heavy-duty" or "shoulder-saddle" harness. With this harness, tension loading on

used with a split socket to provide a 2:1 ratio of elbow flexion to socket motion, but this configuration requires the amputee to use approximately twice as much force to flex the prosthetic forearm. Because split sockets are used only at very short transradial levels of amputation, the extra force required may cause considerable discomfort on the volar or radial surfaces of the remaining portion of the forearm. For these amputees, a relatively simple control system modification may be used to minimize discomfort and facilitate elbow flexion.

The modification consists of splitting the cable housing into proximal and distal segments similar to those used for the transhumeral prosthesis. The proximal piece of housing is attached to the triceps pad and the distal piece to the prosthetic forearm. The control cable is now exposed as it passes anterior to the elbow joint. Tension applied to the control cable by glenohumeral flexion on the amputated side assists in elbow flexion (Figure 16).

In some instances, the unilateral transradial amputee can be fit with a socket that obviates the need for the suspensory function of a harness. Such self-suspending prostheses are held on the residual limb by the intimacy of the socket fit proximal to the olecranon and humeral epicondyles and in the antecubital fossa, or through the use of a roll-on liner. Because these fittings eliminate the need for a triceps pad and anterior support strap, the harness consists of a simple axilla loop around the shoulder on the nonamputated side. Extending obliquely downward across the amputee's back, the control attachment strap runs from the axilla loop to the terminal device control cable (Figure 17). As in the case of the figure-of-8 harness, shoulder flexion and/or scapular abduction on the amputated side are the control motions for terminal device operation. The disadvantage of this type of harnessing is that long-sleeved clothing is difficult to wear.

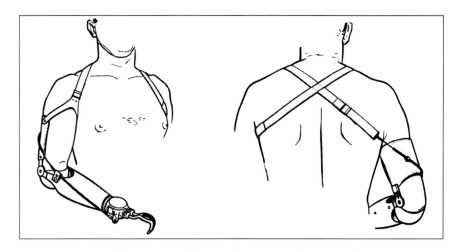

Figure 16 Modification of the cable housing in a transradial harness. *(Reproduced from Bechtol CO: Anatomic and physiologic considerations in the clinical application of upper-extremity prosthesis, in Edwards JW (ed):* Orthopaedic Appliances Atlas. *Ann Arbor, MI, American Academy of Orthopaedic Surgeons, 1960.)*

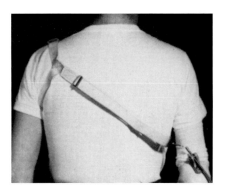

Figure 17 Modified harness to a self-suspending socket.

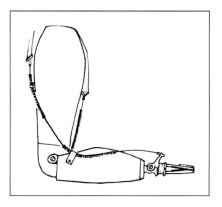

Figure 18 Transhumeral control system. Note the use of two cables. *(Reproduced with permission from* Below and Above Elbow Harness and Control System. *Evanston, IL, Northwestern University Prosthetic-Orthotic Center, 1966.)*

Mechanics of the Transhumeral Control System

Transhumeral prostheses are usually operated by two distinctly separate control cables (Figure 18). One cable flexes the prosthetic elbow joint and operates the terminal device, and the second cable permits the amputee to lock and unlock the prosthetic elbow.

Elbow Flexion/Terminal Device Control Cable

The housing through which the elbow flexion/terminal device cable passes is split into two separate parts (Figure 19). The proximal portion of the split housing (A) is attached to the poste-

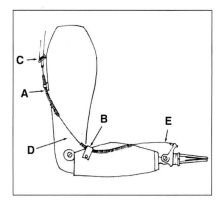

Figure 19 Split housing for cable in an elbow flexion/terminal device. *(Reproduced with permission from* Below and Above Elbow Harness and Control System. *Evanston, IL, Northwestern University Prosthetic-Orthotic Center, 1966.)*

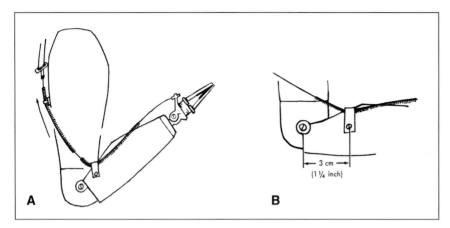

Figure 20 A, Prosthetic elbow flexed using a split cable housing. **B**, Placing the elbow flexion attachment 3 cm distal to the elbow axis usually is satisfactory, but the exact location should be determined on an individual basis. *(Reproduced with permission from Below and Above Elbow Harness and Control System. Evanston, IL, Northwestern University Prosthetic-Orthotic Center, 1966.)*

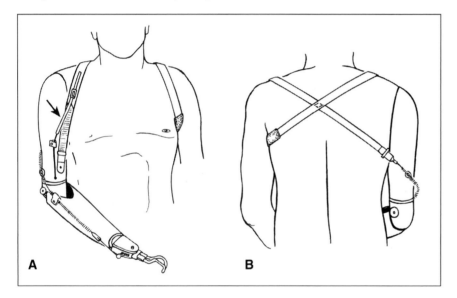

Figure 21 Elbow lock control cable. *(Reproduced from Pursley RJ: Harness patterns for upper-extremity prostheses, in Orthopaedic Appliances Atlas. Chicago, IL, American Academy of Orthopaedic Surgeons, 1960.)*

The ease with which the amputee can operate the elbow unit and terminal device depends, to a considerable extent, on the location of the elbow flexion attachment. Greater force and less cable excursion are required when the elbow flexion attachment is closest to the elbow axis. Conversely, a more distal placement of the attachment requires less force but greater cable excursion.

Generally, the longer the residual limb, the farther the elbow flexion attachment may be placed from the elbow axis. Higher transhumeral levels of amputation require a more proximal placement of the attachment to minimize the excursion required. Although initial placement of the elbow flexion attachment 3 cm distal to the elbow axis usually is satisfactory, in most instances, its precise location should be determined on an individual basis (Figure 20).

Elbow Lock Control Cable

The proximal end of the elbow lock control cable originates at the anterior suspension strap (Figure 21). Passing down the anteromedial surface of the humeral section of the prosthesis, the distal end of the cable engages the elbow locking mechanism. The elbow lock works on an alternator principle: pull and release to lock, pull and release to unlock. An excursion of approximately 1.3 cm and a force of approximately 0.9 kg (2 lb) are necessary to cycle the elbow unit.

In summary, the operating sequence of the two cable systems used with most transhumeral prostheses is as follows: (1) tension applied to the elbow flexion/terminal device control cable causes the elbow to flex; (2) when the desired angle of elbow flexion is achieved, the rapid sequential application and release of tension on the elbow lock control cable locks the elbow; and (3) with the elbow locked, the reapplication of tension on the elbow flexion/terminal device control cable permits operation of the terminal device (Figure 22).

rior surface of the humeral section of the prosthesis. The distal portion of the split housing (B) is fixed to the prosthetic forearm by a device called an elbow flexion attachment.

As shown in Figure 19, the elbow flexion/terminal device control cable originates at the control attachment strap of the harness (point C). Passing through the proximal portion of the split housing, the control cable is exposed anterior to the mechanical elbow axis (point D). The elbow flexion/terminal device control cable continues through the distal portion of the split housing and terminates with its attachment at the terminal device (point E). Because the housing is in two separate pieces and the control cable passes in front of the elbow axis, tension applied to the cable causes the prosthetic elbow to flex. The flexion is limited to the gap between the two cable housings.

Split housing systems provide sequential control because cable excursion results first in elbow flexion. Once the elbow unit is locked, further cable excursion operates the terminal device.

Figure-of-8 Transhumeral Harness

Although the full operation of the terminal device of a transradial prosthesis requires only 5 cm of cable excursion, more than twice that amount of excursion is required for full elbow and terminal device operation of a transhumeral prosthesis. Consequently, great attention must be paid to the details of fitting the transhumeral harness. Precision in the location of the harness and control system components is essential for achieving satisfactory comfort and function.

Like the standard transradial harness, the transhumeral harness typically consists of a system of interconnected nonelastic and elastic straps laid up in a figure-of-8 pattern. The common elements of the standard transhumeral harness are the axilla loop, anterior and lateral support straps, control attachment strap, and elbow lock control strap. The axilla loop acts as the fixed anchor from which other harness components originate. Some of the straps originating at the axilla loop serve to suspend the prosthesis on the residual limb, while others provide the amputee with volitional control of the prosthetic components.

Anterior Support Strap

The anterior support strap, sometimes referred to as the elastic suspensor, originates at the axilla loop (Figure 21, A). Passing over the shoulder on the amputated side, the strap continues down the anteromedial surface of the humeral section of the prosthesis. The anterior support strap terminates with its attachment on the anterior surface of the prosthetic socket slightly proximal to the mechanical elbow joint (Figure 21, B). When viewed from the front, it should be noted that the distal two thirds of the anterior support strap consists of elastic webbing.

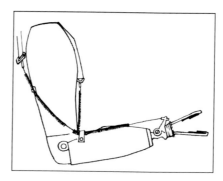

Figure 22 Reapplication of tension on the elbow flexion/terminal device control cable permits operation of the terminal device. *(Reproduced with permission from* Below and Above Elbow Harness and Control System. *Evanston, IL, Northwestern University Prosthetic-Orthotic Center, 1966.)*

The anterior support strap serves several functions in the transhumeral harness system. Anchored to the axilla loop posteriorly and to the humeral section anteriorly, the strap helps to suspend the prosthesis against axial loading. However, because the anterodistal two thirds of the strap consists of elastic webbing, suspensory function is limited.

A second function of the anterior support strap is to help prevent rotation of the prosthetic socket on the residual limb during prosthetic use. The transhumeral amputee uses glenohumeral flexion on the amputated side to flex the prosthetic elbow and/or operate the terminal device. Because the proximal control cable housing is attached on the posterolateral surface of the humeral section of the prosthesis, glenohumeral flexion tends to result in external rotation of the socket on the residual limb. The anterior support strap running downward mediolaterally resists this rotation.

Axilla Loop

Working as a key element of the entire harness, the axilla loop should encircle and fit the shoulder on the nonamputated side as securely as possible. A small, snug axilla loop, one that does not compromise amputee comfort excessively, provides the

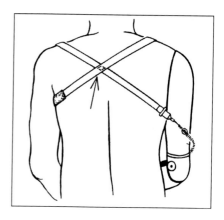

Figure 23 The posterior intersection of the harness straps (arrow) should ideally be positioned toward the nonamputated side of the body. *(Reproduced from Pursley RJ: Harness patterns for upper-extremity prostheses, in* Orthopaedic Appliances Atlas. *Chicago, IL, American Academy of Orthopaedic Surgeons, 1960.)*

best prosthetic suspension and control. To maintain a fairly snug axilla loop, the posterior intersection of the harness straps should be positioned slightly toward the nonamputated side of the body (Figure 23).

Lateral Support Strap

The lateral support strap shown in Figure 24 is the primary suspensory element of the harness. Originating posteriorly from the upper portion of the axilla loop, the strap is directed horizontally and stitched to the anterior support strap at the points marked A and B. The lateral end of the strap passes just anterior to the acromion and is attached close to the proximal trim line of the prosthetic socket at the point marked C. In addition to its suspensory function, the strap helps to prevent external rotation of the socket on the limb when tension is applied to the elbow flexion/terminal device control cable.

Control Attachment Strap

The control attachment strap originates at the posterior intersection of the axilla loop. Running obliquely downward across the amputee's back, the control attachemnt strap termi-

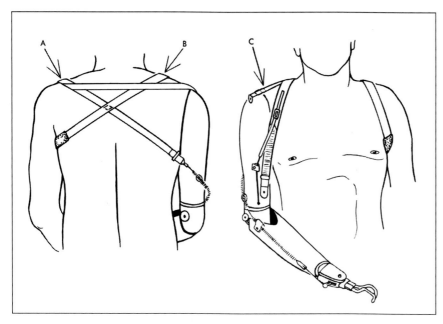

Figure 24 Location of the lateral support strap in a figure-of-8 transhumeral harness. *(Reproduced from Pursley RJ: Harness patterns for upper-extremity prostheses, in Orthopaedic Appliances Atlas. Chicago, IL, American Academy of Orthopaedic Surgeons, 1960.)*

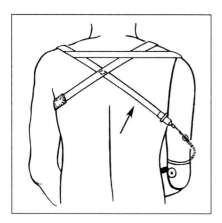

Figure 25 Location of the control attachment strap in a figure-of-8 transhumeral harness. *(Reproduced from Pursley RJ: Harness patterns for upper-extremity prostheses, in Orthopaedic Appliances Atlas. Chicago, IL, American Academy of Orthopaedic Surgeons, 1960.)*

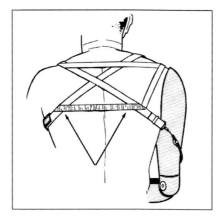

Figure 26 Cross-back strap (arrows) used as an adjunct to a standard transhumeral harness. *(Reproduced from Pursley RJ: Harness patterns for upper-extremity prostheses, in Orthopaedic Appliances Atlas. Chicago, IL, American Academy of Orthopaedic Surgeons, 1960.)*

nates with its direct attachment to the elbow flexion/terminal device control cable (Figure 25). With the control attachment strap firmly fixed at its proximal end by the axilla loop, it is easy to visualize how shoulder flexion on the amputated side creates both the cable tension and cable excursion required for elbow flexion and terminal device operation.

The proper location of the control attachment strap as it passes from the axilla loop to the elbow flexion/terminal device control cable is important. If the control attachment strap lies too high on the amputee's back, shoulder flexion will not produce sufficient cable excursion for full operation of the mechanical elbow and terminal device. Too low a strap

position requires the amputee to use unnecessarily forceful shoulder flexion for full operation. With the control attachment strap located at approximately the midscapular level, midway between the spine and inferior angle, the amputee usually will be able to achieve full operation of the components using a moderate amount of force.

Cross-Back Strap

A cross-back strap is sometimes used as an adjunct to the figure-of-8 transhumeral harness (Figure 26). Originating at the axilla loop close to the posterior axillary fold, the cross-back strap passes horizontally across the amputee's back and terminates at the distal end of the control attachment strap. Indications for the use of this strap relate primarily to amputee comfort and ease of prosthetic operation.

At midhumeral and higher levels of transhumeral amputation, it becomes increasingly important that the harness be fitted as intimately as possible. Because a snug harness fit requires a relatively small axilla loop, the loop may cause axillary discomfort on the nonamputated side. This discomfort is caused by vertical compression of the pectoral, teres major, and latissimus dorsi tendons by the axilla loop during strenuous prosthetic usage. The use of a cross-back strap in such instances helps to reduce the magnitude of the vertically directed force created by a snug axilla loop.

Another indication for the addition of a cross-back strap is when the posterior intersection of the harness rides too high on the amputee's back. With the posterior intersection of the harness on or superior to the spinous process of C7, the amputee is uncomfortable, and the work efficiency of the entire harness and control system is diminished. The cross-back strap helps to maintain the posterior intersection of the harness below the spinous process of C7.

As noted earlier in this chapter, the split housing transhumeral prosthetic control system requires approximately 11.3 cm of cable excursion for full elbow and terminal device operation. Whether or not the amputee is able to generate this much cable excursion depends to a great extent on the path of the control attachment strap as it crosses the amputee's back. Ideally, the path of the strap should run between the spine and inferior angle of the scapula. Cable excursion, normally produced by glenohumeral flexion on the amputated side, diminishes as the path of the control attachment strap moves closer to the shoulder joint. The addition of a cross-back strap helps to keep the path of the control attachment strap positioned lower on the back.

Cross-back straps may be made of either elastic or nonelastic webbing. The nonelastic strap provides the amputee with more positive control of the prosthetic components and overall tautness of the harness. An elastic strap provides less positive control but greater degrees of comfort and mobility of the shoulder girdle.

Elbow Lock Control Strap

The elbow lock control strap originates at the upper, nonelastic portion of the anterior support strap and is attached at its distal end to the elbow lock control cable (Figure 27). To either lock or unlock the prosthetic elbow, the amputee must first apply tension and then, in rapid sequence, relax tension on the elbow lock control cable. Although the cable excursion requirement for prosthetic elbow operation is small, approximately 1.3 cm, the body motion is somewhat complex. The amputee applies tension to the elbow lock control strap and cable by slight extension and abduction of the glenohumeral joint, combined with equally slight shoulder depression on the amputated side. This motion, in addition to exerting tension on the elbow lock control strap and cable, also stretches the elastic portion of the anterior support strap. With the rapid return of the prosthesis to the starting position, the elastic tension of the anterior support

strap serves to complete the lock/unlock cycle.

Special Considerations

The ring-type harness does not offer the same degree of function in transhumeral harnessing as it does at the transradial level. At midhumeral and higher levels of amputation, it becomes increasingly important that the harness fit as snug as possible. Ring-type harnesses do not permit the same degree of tautness in the straps of the system as do stitched harnesses. Consequently, at the higher transhumeral levels, the ring-type harness does not provide a very high degree of positive control of the prosthetic components unless the straps are sewn in place after adjustment.

The standard figure-of-8 harness is suitable for and acceptable to most unilateral transhumeral amputees. However, the unilateral transhumeral amputee who engages in unusually strenuous physical activity on a regular basis may find the standard harness uncomfortable. During periods of heavy work, the relatively narrow straps tend to subject the soft tissues over which they pass to inordinately high unit pressures. Particularly vulnerable are the skin, tendons, and neurovascular structures of the axilla on the nonamputated side. The problem is further compounded at the transhumeral level because maximal control of the components of the prosthesis requires the use of a small, snug axilla loop.

Alleviation of axillary discomfort for the transhumeral amputee may sometimes be achieved through the use of a shoulder saddle harness. The transhumeral shoulder saddle harness distributes tension loading on the prosthesis to the shoulder on the amputated side. Because the control attachment and elbow lock control straps run along the same paths as they do in the standard harness, the body control motions for prosthetic operation remain essentially unchanged (Figure 28).

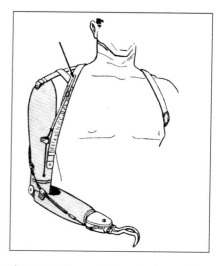

Figure 27 Elbow lock control strap (arrow) on a transhumeral harness. *(Reproduced from Pursley RJ: Harness patterns for upper-extremity prostheses, in* Orthopaedic Appliances Atlas. *Chicago, IL, American Academy of Orthopaedic Surgeons, 1960.)*

The harness for the bilateral transhumeral amputee consists of two figure-of-8 harnesses without axilla loops (Figure 29). The control attachment strap for the right prosthesis passes over the amputee's left shoulder and becomes the anterior support strap for the left prosthesis. Likewise, the left control attachment strap becomes the right anterior support strap. At their intersection in the midline of the amputee's back, the two straps are sewn together. As in the unilateral harness system, the elbow lock control straps of the bilateral harness originate on the nonelastic portion of the anterior support strap. The lateral support straps consist of a continuous piece of nonelastic webbing attached close to the proximal trimlines of both sockets and pass slightly anterior to the acromion processes. Posteriorly, the lateral support straps are stitched to the anterior support straps. Whereas a cross-back strap is considered optional in the standard unilateral transhumeral harness, it is an essential component in the bilateral harness. As seen in Figure 29, the cross-back strap runs horizontally between the two control attachment straps. The over-the-shoulder

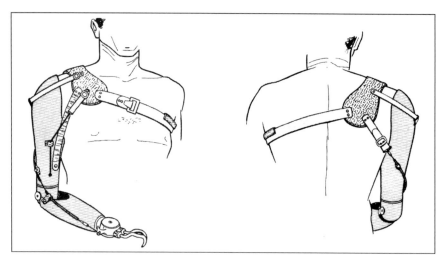

Figure 28 Transhumeral shoulder saddle harness. *(Reproduced from Pursley RJ: Harness patterns for upper-extremity prostheses, in* Orthopaedic Appliances Atlas. *Chicago, IL, American Academy of Orthopaedic Surgeons, 1960.)*

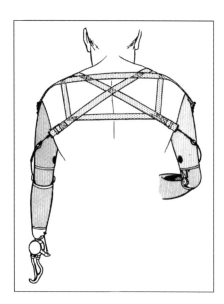

Figure 29 Harness for a bilateral transhumeral amputee (posterior view). *(Reproduced from Pursley RJ: Harness patterns for upper-extremity prostheses, in* Orthopaedic Appliances Atlas. *Chicago, IL, American Academy of Orthopaedic Surgeons, 1960.)*

Figure 30 Harness for a bilateral transhumeral amputee (anterior view). *(Reproduced from Pursley RJ: Harness patterns for upper-extremity prostheses, in* Orthopaedic Appliances Atlas. *Chicago, IL, American Academy of Orthopaedic Surgeons, 1960.)*

straps complete the figure-of-8 harness for the bilateral transhumeral amputee.

At their posterior origins, the over-the-shoulder straps are sewn to the control attachment straps. The straps are also stitched to the lateral support straps at a point before they pass over

the amputee's shoulder. The over-the-shoulder straps terminate anteriorly by attachment to the nonelastic portions of the anterior support straps (Figure 30).

The bilateral transhumeral harness permits the amputee to use glenohumeral flexion and/or scapular ab-

duction for elbow flexion and terminal device operation. Elbow lock control is achieved with slight glenohumeral extension and abduction combined with shoulder depression. Two major problems confront the bilateral amputee with this type of harness. First, the amputee will encounter some difficulty in operating both prostheses simultaneously. Tension applied to both elbow flexion/terminal device cables permits opening (or closing) of both terminal devices, but both terminal devices cannot be operated to effect simultaneous opening and closing on opposite sides without relaxing tension on one of the cables. Consequently, the possibility of active bimanual manipulation of objects is minimal. A second major deficiency of this harness system is that it does not permit the amputee to lift any significant amount of weight in the terminal device of either prosthesis.

One approach to overcome some of these limitations may be to provide an externally powered prosthesis on one side and a body-powered device on the other. Providing prostheses with differing control systems usually permits independent operation of one or both artificial arms.

Shoulder Disarticulation Harness

At the shoulder disarticulation level of amputation, the absence of glenohumeral flexion as a control source requires the use of other body motions for prosthetic operation. Biscapular abduction is, at least for most adult male amputees, the best available body motion for generating sufficient cable tension to flex the elbow and operate the terminal device of the prosthesis. It should be noted, however, that many people with high-level amputations cannot generate sufficient excursion or strength to operate a fully body-powered system. Therefore, the use of externally powered components is often required and frequently preferable.

The force generated by active biscapular abduction is best harnessed through use of a chest strap (Figure 31, A). Composed of 3.8-cm-wide nonelastic webbing, the chest strap originates with a buckle on the anterior surface of the shoulder cap of the socket. Running horizontally across the amputee's thorax, the strap passes immediately inferior to the axilla on the nonamputated side. The chest strap terminates posteriorly with its attachment to the proximal end of the elbow flexion/terminal device control cable.

Vertical suspension of the chest strap and prosthetic socket is augmented by the use of an elastic suspensor strap. The anterior suspensor originates posteriorly on the chest strap (Figure 31, B). Passing over the shoulder on the amputated side along a diagonal path, the suspensor terminates with its attachment to the proximal surface of the shoulder cap. In addition to assisting with vertical support, the anterior suspensor prevents external rotation of the socket on the shoulder during use of the prosthesis.

Biscapular abduction is usually strong enough to produce sufficient cable tension for fully operating the elbow and terminal device of a shoulder disarticulation prosthesis. Abduction of the scapulae is, however, a poor body motion for generating adequate cable excursion. Very few shoulder disarticulation amputees are capable, through biscapular abduction, of generating enough cable excursion to permit complete elbow and terminal device operation.

Because biscapular abduction is a good source for generating cable tension but a poor source of cable excursion, an excursion amplifier is sometimes provided (Figure 32). A simple excursion amplifier consists of a small pulley attached near the posterior end of the chest strap of the harness. The proximal end of the elbow flexion/terminal device cable passes through the pulley and is attached to the posterior surface of the prosthetic shoul-

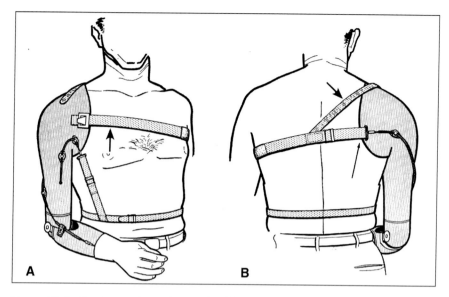

Figure 31 A, Chest strap (arrow) on a shoulder disarticulation harness. **B,** Elastic anterior suspensor chest strap (arrow) on a shoulder disarticulation harness. *(Reproduced with permission from Pursley RJ: Orthop Prosthet Appl J 1955;9:15.)*

der cap. With this type of amplifier, each 2.5 cm of cable excursion generated by biscapular abduction causes the elbow flexion/terminal device control cable to move through an excursion of 5 cm. Consequently, 5.6 cm of chest expansion produces the 11.3 cm of cable excursion required for full elbow and terminal device operation.

It should be noted that although the incorporation of a pulley in the harness system doubles the cable excursion, it also doubles the input force required for elbow flexion and/or terminal device operation. Because biscapular abduction is a good source of force generation, this increased force requirement does not pose a major problem for some adult shoulder disarticulation amputees, but others do better with externally powered components.

Depending on factors such as body build, adequate range of scapulothoracic motion, and the neuromuscular coordination of the amputee, locking and unlocking of the elbow unit of a shoulder disarticulation prosthesis can be performed in one of several different ways. The preferred body-powered method involves the incorporation of the elbow lock control

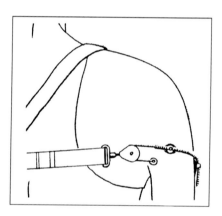

Figure 32 Excursion amplifier on a shoulder disarticulation strap. *(Reproduced with permission from Santschi WR (ed): Manual of Upper Extremity Prosthetics, ed 2. Los Angeles, CA, University of California Department of Engineering, 1958.)*

strap as an anterior extension of the chest strap.

In this method, the anterior attachment of the chest strap is bifurcated (Figure 33). The upper leg of the split strap consists of nonelastic webbing. The lower leg is nonelastic at its extremities—its origin on the chest strap and attachment on the socket—but has a segment of elastic webbing at its center. A nonelastic elbow lock control strap originates at the chest strap, passes laterally be-

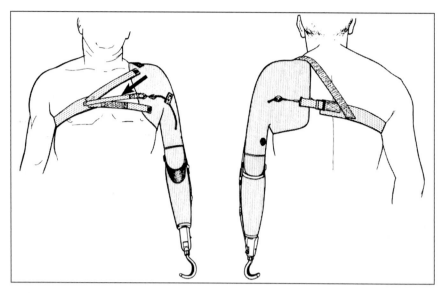

Figure 33 Elbow lock control strap (arrow) incorporated as an anterior extension of the chest strap on a shoulder disarticulation prosthesis. *(Reproduced from Pursley RJ: Harness patterns for upper-extremity prostheses, in* Orthopaedic Appliances Atlas. *Chicago, IL, American Academy of Orthopaedic Surgeons, 1960.)*

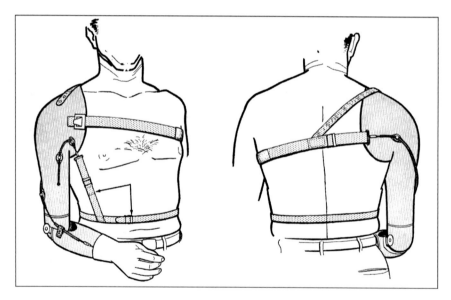

Figure 34 Waist belt on a shoulder disarticulation prosthesis as an alternative elbow lock control. *(Reproduced with permission from Pursley RJ:* Orthop Prosthet Appl J *1955; 9:15.)*

tween the two legs of the split strap, and attaches directly to the proximal end of the elbow lock control cable. With this harness arrangement, cable tension for locking and unlocking the elbow is created by scapular adduction on the amputated side. Incorporation of the elbow lock control strap with the chest strap makes it easier to don the prosthesis but requires a fairly high level of neuromuscular coordination for successful operation.

An alternative arrangement for elbow lock control requires the use of a waist belt (Figure 34). The waist belt serves to anchor the distal end of the elbow lock control strap. From its anchor on the waist strap, the control strap runs obliquely upward where it attaches to the proximal end of the el-

bow lock control cable. With the waist belt system, the primary body control motion for cycling the elbow unit is shoulder elevation on the amputated side.

A third option for achieving body-powered elbow lock control requires the use of a nudge control mounted on the anteroproximal surface of the prosthetic shoulder cap (Figure 35). The nudge control for locking and unlocking the elbow is operated by force exerted by the amputee's chin. Nudge control is usually reserved for severely disabled persons such as bilateral shoulder disarticulation amputees. Realistically, the functional expectations for persons with bilateral shoulder disarticulation amputations are extremely limited. With the help of adaptive equipment, environmental modifications, and modifications of clothing, it may be possible to achieve a reasonable degree of partial independence in the basic functions of personal hygiene, dressing, and eating. Fitting with prostheses is difficult and may not add much more practical function.

There is no such thing as a "standard" harness for bilateral shoulder disarticulation amputees. The specifics of the prosthesis and control system are best left to the experience and ingenuity of the prosthetist, therapist, physician, patient, and members of the patient's family.

The unilateral prosthesis may be provided and should permit active operation and passive prepositioning of a lightweight terminal device, active or passive flexion of the wrist unit, active flexion and locking of the elbow unit, passive external and internal rotation of the humeral section, and passive prepositioning of the shoulder joint in flexion and abduction.

Absence of the humeral heads narrows the girth of the shoulder girdle and reduces the effectiveness of biscapular abduction as a work source. A small, well-padded plastic cap covering the apex of the acromion on the side opposite the prosthesis enhances

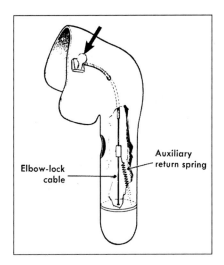

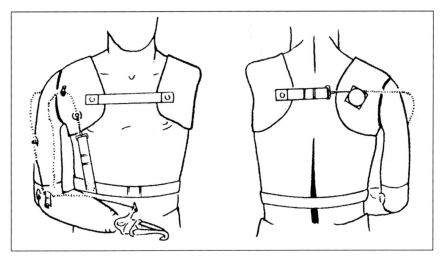

Figure 35 Nudge control (arrow) is an alternative elbow lock control on a shoulder disarticulation prosthesis. *(Reproduced with permission from Santschi WR (ed): Manual of Upper Extremity Prosthetics, ed 2. Los Angeles, CA, University of California Department of Engineering, 1958.)*

Figure 36 A small, well-padded plastic cap covers the apex of the acromion on the side opposite the prosthesis. *(Reproduced with permission from Santschi WR (ed): Manual of Upper Extremity Prosthetics, ed 2. Los Angeles, CA, University of California Department of Engineering, 1958.)*

the available range of biscapular motion, thereby preserving the important control source (Figure 36).

Biscapular abduction and the use of an excursion amplifier may permit adequate cable excursion for producing a reasonable degree of elbow flexion and terminal device operation. Shoulder elevation on the amputated side may be used for elbow lock control.

Harnessing patterns for scapulothoracic amputation do not differ significantly from those used in the shoulder disarticulation, except that the efficiency of operation is less. Most persons with high-level amputations benefit from the use of externally powered componentry.

Harnessing for Switch Control of Externally Powered Components

Many of the harnesses described in this chapter can be modified to operate a microswitch or force sensor to control electrically powered elbow, wrist, or hand components. For this application, there are two important requirements that differ from harness configurations that directly operate a body-powered device: (1) minimizing the excursion generated, and (2) protecting the microswitch or force sensor from force overloads.

Because it takes less than 10 mm of movement to operate most microswitch or force sensors, there is no need to generate additional excursion. One of the easiest ways to reduce excursion is to loosen the control strap, which also increases amputee comfort. However, care must be taken to avoid making the harness so loose that gross body movements are required to actuate the switch. Another way to minimize the excursion is to route the control cable through or near a joint. For example, routing the control cable near the glenohumeral joint will minimize the excursion generated by forward humeral flexion for transhumeral applications. Control motions with less inherent excursion, such as shoulder elevation, are particularly suitable for switch control.

There are two principal methods to protect the switch from overloads. The first method incorporates a segment of nonelastic webbing that bridges the switch and limits the total excursion. If the pull switch has a total operating range of 0 to 5 mm, then the webbing bridge is attached with just enough slack that limits the harness pull to a maximum of 6 mm. This does not interfere with full voluntary operation but prevents excessive motion from damaging the switch. The second method incorporates a segment of elastic webbing in the control strap, often in combination with the nonelastic webbing bridge previously discussed. During extreme movements, the elastic segment stretches and reduces the stress on the switch. If the elastic strap is too easy to stretch, the amputee is then forced to make a greater movement to operate the control device. This usually is considered undesirable but can sometimes be an advantage if the patient is having difficulty distinguishing between small switch movements.

Conclusion

A well-designed harness provides suspension, rotational control, switch operation, or activation of a body-powered component. To facilitate patient acceptance, it should also be comfortable for the amputee to wear and simple to don and doff.

Chapter 11

Components for Electric-Powered Systems

Craig W. Heckathorne, MSc

Introduction

Since the publication of the second edition of the *Atlas* in 1992, the use of prostheses with electric-powered components has continued to grow. Four factors were identified in the 1992 edition to explain the increase in the number of successful electric-powered fittings over the previous decade. These factors, which still exert a strong influence on the expanding use of electric-powered systems, are (1) technologic advances in actuators, materials, and controllers (generally outside the field of prosthetics); (2) conceptual advances leading to designs with improved performance characteristics; (3) a growing body of experience guiding successive clinical fittings; and (4) the willingness of a diverse community of prosthetists, engineers, therapists, designers, physicians, allied health workers, and exemplary users to share their knowledge and experience.

This chapter provides an overview of upper limb electric-powered components for adults, emphasizing the design aspects that influence their performance and use. The devices that are described are limited to components that are commercially available and readily obtained in North America.

The chapter is organized into five sections—prehension mechanisms, wrist mechanisms, enhancements to body-powered elbows, elbow mechanisms, and enhancement of a manual shoulder joint. Each section begins with a general description of the components to be covered. Common characteristics and features are described, and if data are available, comparisons are drawn between the device and its physiologic counterpart. Detailed descriptions of available components follow, covering construction and mechanical specifications for each device, performance characteristics, control systems offered by the manufacturer, and (if applicable) compatible control systems offered by other suppliers.

In the discussions of control options, a common control terminology is used to identify the number of distinct control sources and distinct device functions. For example, a myoelectric controller might be described as providing two-site, two-function control. This indicates that two separate and independent muscle sites are required to operate the controller and that two functions (eg, "open" and "close") can be controlled voluntarily. The "off" condition is generally assumed unless noted otherwise because it is not practical for a battery-powered device to remain on continuously in the absence of a control signal. In the case of control by means other than muscle signals, or when myoelectric control is one of several options, the more general term *source* is used rather than *site*. In discussing myoelectric controllers, *myoelectrode* is used to denote an as-sembly that has electronics, generally the preamplifier and filters, along with the metal electrodes used to pick up the surface muscle signals.

This chapter is intended to be a component review; therefore, techniques for incorporating components into prosthetic systems and fabricating prostheses are not covered. Technical manuals and courses are available from the various manufacturers for this purpose. Techniques for integrating multiple systems into a single prosthesis and for designing hybrid systems combining body-powered and electric-powered componentry are also not discussed; these areas of specialization would warrant separate and detailed treatment. However, integrated systems that are provided by a manufacturer as a specific option are described.

Prehension Mechanisms

Electric-powered prehension devices are available in a variety of forms, not all of which resemble the anatomic hand. Despite differing appearances, all commercially available electric-powered prehension devices function in much the same way—with a single degree of freedom of motion that brings two (or three) surfaces in op-position, allowing for the grasping of objects. None of the devices offers independent movement of individual fingers, and all have fixed prehension patterns.

Early development of electric-powered prehension devices emphasized preservation of an anatomic appearance.[1-3] This preference grew out of two broad, mutually reinforcing considerations. One was a sensitivity to the sociologic, symbolic, and aesthetic qualities associated with the human hand, qualities that can be powerful shapers of individual perceptions.[4,5] The second consideration was a general expectation that in an environment of objects manufactured to be handled by human hands, a device with hand-like characteristics would offer the best prehension function. This expectation was taken literally, with the adoption of shape as a principal characteristic.[6]

These considerations carry just as much validity today as in the early years. Although quality of appearance can vary considerably, the cosmetic function of a prehensor with a hand-like shape has been shown to be a strong determinant of personal acceptance.[7-10] In addition, the broad contact surfaces of the electric-powered hand and frictional properties of the cosmetic glove offer good grasp and retention of held objects. The other significant factors cited for the acceptance of hand-like prehensors—higher prehension force, reduced operating effort, increased comfort associated with the absence of control harnessing in myoelectrically controlled prehensors, and prehension control independent of the position of the prehensor with respect to the body—are equally applicable to electric-powered prehensors not shaped like hands.

Electric hand prehensors have not, however, proved to be the ideal prosthetic solution that early developments seemed to promise. Almost four decades of experience with commercial electric hands have underscored the technologic limitations of the designs and the deficiencies in our understanding of the physiology of the human hand, especially with regard to control. Fidelity to an anatomic shape entails engineering compromises that diminish not only the prehensile function but also the overall mechanical function of electric prehensors.[10,11] The hand-like shape and fixed orientation of the fingers make precise tasks difficult to perform; although a special consideration with bilateral amputations, this shortcoming is also cited by persons with unilateral amputations. The ability to reorient the electric hand is significantly limited because of the associated loss of the physiologic wrist in most upper limb amputations, and this cannot be compensated by changing the orientation of the fingers. The size and shape of the electric hand can obstruct the view of the object being grasped or the work area in general. Shape constraints have also limited the form and arrangement of structural frames and finger armatures; these parts can be damaged by heavy use. The polyvinyl chloride material from which most cosmetic gloves are made is more durable than silicone alternatives, but it is susceptible to staining from common dyes, inks, and other substances. Power is lost in compressing and stretching the cosmetic plastic forms and gloves enclosing the mechanisms, contributing to the degradation of overall performance.

These observations have led to increasing recognition that prehension devices shaped like hands are most useful if supplemented with other prosthetic devices that have characteristics not constrained by fidelity to an anatomic shape.[3,10-12] Use of body-powered prostheses with hook-type prehensors is frequently cited in association with use of electric-powered prostheses. Adaptors and tools that can be held within the electric hand and mechanical tools that can be interchanged with the hand prehensor are now available. Several electric-powered prehensors that do not have a hand-like shape are commercially available for use with (or in place of) electric hands.

General Characteristics of Commercial Electric Prehensors

Prehension devices shaped like hands are made for the European and North American markets by Otto Bock Health Care, CentriAB, Motion Control, Inc, and RSLSteeper (Table 1). Electric prehensors with nonanatomic shapes are made by Otto Bock, Hosmer Dorrance Corporation, Motion Control, and RSLSteeper. Specific characteristics of these devices are provided in Table 2 (hand-like devices) and Table 3 (non–hand-like devices).

All of the prehensors shaped like hands are configured for palmar prehension, the opposition of the distal palmar pad of the thumb with the distal palmar pads of the index and middle fingers. Of the prehension patterns identified by Schlesinger,[13] Keller and associates[14] determined that palmar prehension predominated in the holding of objects for use by the dominant hand. The predominance of palmar prehension has also been demonstrated for grasping by the nondominant hand.[15] The persistence of this configuration in prosthetic hand designs and its general acceptance over the years supports these observations.

To achieve the palmar prehension pattern, the fingers of electric-powered hands are fixed in slight flexion at positions approximating the interphalangeal joints. The resulting finger shape also creates a concave inner prehension surface that is useful for cylindrical grasp. Additionally, the frictional properties of the entire surface of the cosmetic glove of the electric hand facilitate fixation and stabilization of objects against surfaces or against the body.[16] The prehension patterns of prehensors that do not have a hand-like shape (Table 3) are discussed later, in the detailed device descriptions.

Among the mechanical characteristics listed in Tables 2 and 3 are maximum prehension force, maximum width of opening, and speed of move-

TABLE 1 Manufacturer Contact Information

Centri AB
Datavägen 6
S-175 43 Järfälla
Sweden

phone: +46 8 580 311 65
fax: +46 8 580 811 28
email: centri@centri.se
website: http://www.centri.se/main.htm

Hosmer Dorrance Corporation
561 Division Street
Campbell, CA 95008
USA

phone: 1-408-379-5151
fax: 1-408-379-5263
email: customerservice@hosmer.com
website: http://www.hosmer.com/

Liberating Technologies, Inc
325 Hopping Brook Road, Suite A
Holliston, MA 01746-1456
USA

phone: 1-508-893-6363
orders: 1-800-437-0024
fax: 1-508-893-9966
email: info@liberatingtech.com
website: http:// www.liberatingtech.com

Motion Control, Inc
2401 South 1070 West, Suite B
Salt Lake City, UT 84119-1555
USA

phone: 1-888-696-2767
fax: 1-801-978-0848
email: info@utaharm.com
website: http://www.utaharm.com

Otto Bock HealthCare
Two Carlson Parkway, Suite 100
Minneapolis, MN 55447-4467
USA

phone: 1-800-328-4058
fax: 1-800-962-2549
email: info@ottobockus.com
website: http://www.ottobockus.com

RSLSteeper
Queen Mary's University Hospital
Roehampton
Roehampton Lane
London
SW15 5PL
United Kingdom

phone: 0208 788 8165
fax: 0208 788 0137
email: sales@rehab.co.uk
website: http://www.rslsteeper.com

ment of the fingers. These characteristics merit additional discussion because of their significant impact on the prehensile function of the devices.

Prehension Force

Force, a relatively easy characteristic to quantify, is often cited as a "figure of merit" for a prehension device. However, little is known about how prehension force capacity, frictional properties of the surfaces in contact, and conformability to surface features contribute to adequate grip. Because changes in either of the latter two characteristics can significantly alter the effectiveness of the applied force, force should not be considered in isolation from the other prehensile characteristics when comparing particular devices.

Rationales for force requirements of prosthetic prehensors are typically based on physiologic performance. One study of human prehension force indicated that adult men could produce maximum mean forces of 95.6 N for palmar prehension, 103 N for lateral prehension, 93.4 N for tip prehension, and 400 N for cylindrical grasp.[17] More recent reports of larger populations have produced slightly different means but generally support the earlier study.[18,19]

Another investigation indicated that prehension forces to a maximum of 66.7 N were necessary to carry out a variety of activities of daily living.[20] Peizer and associates[1] proposed that this be a minimum standard for the maximum prehension force of an electric prehensor, reasoning that higher forces could only improve the prehensile utility of a prosthetic prehensor.

All of the devices listed in Tables 2 and 3 have specified maximum prehension forces, some of them approaching or exceeding physiologic levels and most exceeding the minimum standard proposed by Peizer and associates.[1] However, devices capable of achieving high prehension force do not necessarily apply that force as effectively or more effectively than a device with a lower maximum

prehension force. The frictional properties of the materials lining the prehension surfaces and the ability of these materials to conform to the surfaces of held objects will also influence the effectiveness of the applied grip force.

Regulation of the applied force (below the maximum) is a function of the control system of the particular device and is discussed later, in the detailed device descriptions. No commercial electronic system provides direct sensory feedback of applied force. Gripping force must be estimated indirectly through its effect on the object being grasped, the response of the prehensor as force increases, or some relationship between the magnitude of the user's control signal and the force applied by the mechanism.

All of the electric prehensors include some mechanism for maintaining grip force in the absence of a control signal and without additional power to the motor, similar to the function of a vise. This is an important feature, essential to the overall performance of a prehensor. Without this feature the motor would need to be powered while it is not moving, a condition of stall. A motor draws high currents during stall, which would deplete a battery supply within a relatively short time.

The same mechanism that maintains the applied force also prevents the fingers from being pried open by external forces while an object is grasped. This feature is certainly helpful when using tools and other implements held in the prehensor. To prevent damage, most prehensors incorporate some method (such as a clutch) that allows the fingers to open under excessive external forces. This method can also be used to force the fingers open in the event that the prehensor does not respond to an opening control signal and the user wants to release a held object.

Width of Opening

Studying the handling of common objects, Keller and associates[14] deter-

TABLE 2 Characteristics of Adult Electric-Powered Prehensors: Hand-like Devices

Device	DMC Plus System Electric Hand	Centri Electric Hand	Motion Control Hand	MultiControl Plus Electric Hand
Manufacturer	Otto Bock	CentriAB	Motion Control	RSLSteeper
Adult sizes available (circumference at knuckles, in inches)	7¼, 7¾, 8¼	7 ¼, 7¾	7 ¼, 7¾, 8¼	7¼, 7½, 7¾
Width across knuckles (in cm)	7.6, 8.0, 8.9	N/A	7.6, 8.1, 9.1	7.0, 7.6, 8.3
Circumference at knuckles (in cm)	18.4, 19.7, 21.0	18.4, 19.7	19.0, 19.5, 21.4	19.1, 20.3, 21.6
Length *	≈ 14 cm	≈ 7.5 (size 7 ¾)	13.7 cm (size 7¾)	13.7 cm (all sizes)
Weight	440 g (size 7¼) [‡]	250 g (size 7¾)	433 g (size 7¾) [‡]	370 g (size 7¾)
Maximum grip force [†]	90 N	68 N (size 7¼) 81 N (size 7¾)	98.1 N (at 7.2 V)	55 N to 65 N
Maximum opening width	10.0 cm	7.6 cm (size 7¾)	10.0 cm (size 7¾)	7.0 cm
Average maximum speed	13.0 cm/s	10.0 cm/s (size 7¾)	≈ 10.7 cm/s at 7.2 V (size 7¾)	8.75 cm/s
Operating voltage	6 to 7.2 V	6 to 9 V	6 to 18 V	6 V

*Length is measured from thumb tip to proximal base plate of mechanism (at junction of wrist).

†Grip force is measured at fingertips in palmar prehension pattern.

‡Weight is for mechanism and inner hand shell, no glove.

TABLE 3 Characteristics of Adult Electric-Powered Prehensors: Non–hand-like Devices

Device	System Electric Greifer	NU-VA Synergetic Prehensor	ETD	Multicontrol Powered Gripper
Manufacturer	Otto Bock	Hosmer-Dorrance	Motion Control	RSLSteeper
Length*	17.1 cm	19.0 cm	16.2 cm	≈ 16 cm
Weight [†]	540 g	≈ 435 g	408 g	500 g
Maximum grip force [‡]	160 N	111 N	111 N	50 N
Maximum opening width	9.5 cm	60° or 10.2 cm[§]	78° or 13 cm[§]	8.0 cm
Average maximum speed	18.0 cm/s	170°/s or 29.1 cm/s	15.7 cm/s at 6 V 41.9 cm/s at 14 V	10 cm/s
Operating voltage	6 to 7.2 V	9 V	6 to 14 V	6 V

* Length is measured from the most distal aspect of the prehensor "fingers" to the proximal base plate of the mechanism (at junction of wrist).

† Weight is with Otto Bock–style quick-disconnect wrist. Some prehensors are offered with other types of wrist adapters.

‡ Grip force is measured at tips of prehensor "fingers."

§ Angular displacement is a measure of the arc traversed by the finger(s). Linear measurement is the approximate distance between the two fingers at their most distal extent.

mined that 5.1 cm of prehensile opening was needed most of the time, but an 8.2-cm opening was needed occasionally. Peizer and associates[1] suggested the 8.2-cm opening as a minimum opening. This recommendation was adopted by the Panel on Upper-Extremity Prosthetics of the National Research Council. Persons who had experience with prosthetic prehensors having an opening of 11.43 cm indicated a preference for the wider opening, although it was not used often.[2] The maximum openings of the prehensors in Tables 2 and 3 are close to or exceed the minimum of 8.2 cm recommended by Peizer and associates.[1]

Speed of Movement

Based on a study of users' experiences with electric prehensors available at the time, Peizer and associates[1] recommended a minimum closure rate of 8.25 cm/s measured at the fingertip. This minimum standard, considered a high standard in 1969, is ex-

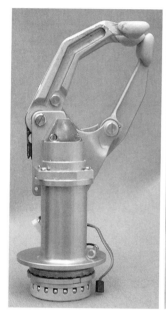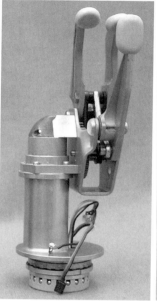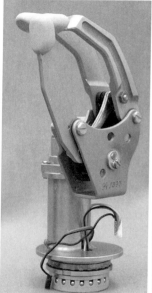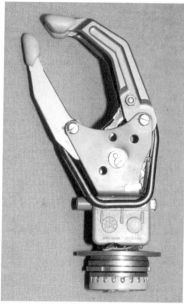

Figure 1 Otto Bock System Electric Hand. The three images on the left are without electronics. The fourth image (far right) shows the on/off switch and control electronics mounted between the finger chassis and the base plate of the hand. *(Courtesy of the Northwestern University Rehabilitation Engineering Research Program.)*

ceeded by all of the prehensors in Tables 2 and 3.

Unpublished data (G. Glickman, Northwestern University, 1978) on physiologic finger speeds indicate maximum human finger velocities of approximately 40 radians/s (2,290°/s) for movements through a range of 75°. Assuming a finger length from the metacarpophalangeal joint to the tip of 10 cm, the maximum velocity at the fingertip would be 400 cm/s. These data provide an appreciation for the upper limit on physiologic finger speed, which is far in excess of the speeds attainable by any of the prosthetic prehensors.

In the same study, finger velocities were measured for an untimed pick-and-place task involving blocks of various sizes. Average finger velocities in this functional activity were considerably less than the maximum and were on the order of 3.0 radians/s (172°/s). Only the Hosmer Synergetic Prehensor and the Motion Control ETD (Table 3) achieve or exceed this speed. The maximum speeds of electric hands in Table 2 are less than half the average physiologic finger speed. The usefulness of having prosthetic finger speeds on the order of func-

tional physiologic speeds is greatly dependent on the control scheme with which the prehensor is operated. For devices capable of higher speeds, a proportional relationship between the magnitude of the control signal and the response of the prehensor appears necessary to achieve confident and acceptable operation.

Electric Hand-like Devices
Otto Bock System Electric Hands

Otto Bock Health Care manufactures several different models of their System Electric Hands—the Digital Twin Hand, the DMC (Dynamic Mode Control) Plus Hand (see Table 2 for specifications), the SensorHand, the Transcarpal Hand, and a System Electric Hand (with no electronics, for use with other manufacturers' electronic controllers). These hands all have different features but also have several common characteristics. All System Electric Hands are available in the same three adult sizes, denoted by the circumferential dimension (in inches) at the knuckles—7¼, 7¾, and 8¼. The hands are composed of three separate parts: the inner mechanism, a plastic hand-like form, and a cos-

metic glove.[3] The plastic form fits over the mechanism, giving the device the general hand-like shape and dimensions. The glove, made of polyvinyl chloride, is pulled over the plastic form and provides gender-related characteristics and cosmetic coloration.

The mechanism is similar in configuration in all models and includes the electric motor, an automatic gear transmission, a support structure, and the finger assembly (Figures 1 and 2). Except in the Transcarpal Hand, the electric motor is mounted between the finger assembly and the wrist at a right angle to the axes of rotation of the fingers and thumb, in line with the long axis of the forearm. In the Transcarpal Hand, the motor assembly is at a right angle with respect to the axes of the thumb and fingers, but it is shorter and rotated into the distal palmar region of the hand to shorten the length of the hand. In all hands, only the thumb, index, and middle fingers are part of the mechanism's finger assembly. The thumb and fingers are oriented to provide palmar prehension. The fingers, which are coupled as one unit, are driven simultaneously with the thumb in a plane

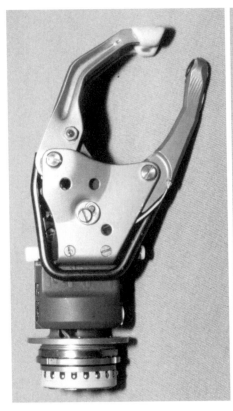
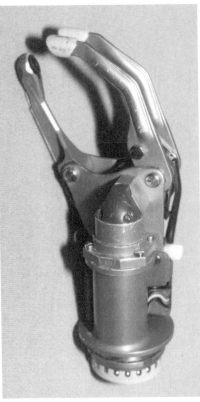

Figure 2 Otto Bock SensorHand. The slip sensor is the small disklike part on the end of the palmar surface of the thumb. *(Courtesy of the Northwestern University Rehabilitation Engineering Research Program.)*

perpendicular to the axis of the finger joints. The plastic form added over the mechanism incorporates the smaller two fingers. A wire frame within the form links these fingers to the middle finger so that the smaller fingers move somewhat in concert with the mechanized fingers.

When the fingers are in motion (that is, not gripping an object), the transmission is in high gear, which allows the fingers and thumb to move at a speed up to the maximum noted in Table 2. When an object is grasped, the transmission remains in high gear until the prehension force reaches 10 N, at which point it will automatically downshift to drive the fingers slower but at higher torque, to a maximum prehension force of about 90 N. Without this automatic transmission, it would not be possible to achieve both the speed and maximum prehension force of the Otto Bock Hand with a single-motor design. In general, single-motor drive units are limited by a trade-off between speed and torque (the higher the speed, the lower the torque). When an object is gripped tightly, it cannot be released immediately because the transmission must reduce the prehension force while in low gear until it reaches the transition grip force, at which point it can shift to high gear and open the fingers. The delay in opening response is generally not noticeable to users if the gripping force is low to moderate.

The drive mechanism also includes a back-lock feature to maintain the prehension force when the motor is off and to prevent the fingers from opening. It is possible to override the effect of the back lock, if necessary, by levering the hand to create very high forces at the fingertips that exceed the torque setting of the hand's slip clutch. Operation of the slip clutch does not damage the mechanism, and the fingers can be closed manually (for appearance) until the control problem is corrected.

The primary prehension pattern of the System Electric Hand is palmar prehension. The mechanical arrangement of the thumb and fingers also provides cylindrical grasp for objects of moderate dimensions. For very wide objects (near the limit of the hand opening), the fingers are not able to encircle the object to secure it; however, the plastic of the cosmetic glove provides friction that maintains a reasonably effective grasp. The use of a pliable hand form over the mechanism also improves the grasp because the inner surfaces of the hand are able to accommodate the shape of objects, thus providing many points of contact between the prehension surfaces and the object being grasped.

Several options are available from Otto Bock to supplement the prehension features of the System Electric Hands. A pincers or tweezers that is keyed to fit the fingers of the hand prehensor can provide tip prehension for handling small objects. If the prehensor is equipped with a quick-disconnect wrist, it can be removed and one of a variety of work tools can be connected to the wrist of the forearm for special functions. These tools are not electrically powered, however. One could also exchange the hand prehensor for a System Electric Greifer or other electric prehensor with a compatible wrist connector and electronics.

The Digital Twin Hand, the DMC Plus Hand, and the SensorHand differ primarily in the manner in which the hand responds to control signals. The Digital Twin Hand provides control at constant speed or constant rate of change of torque. When a user generates a myoelectric signal that exceeds a minimum threshold, a control signal is generated to open or close the prehensor. For the time that the amplitude of the myoelectric signal is above the threshold, the prehensor will continue to operate; however, the degree to which the signal exceeds the threshold does not alter the action of the mechanism. Regardless of the strength of the contraction generating the signal, the prehensor will move at only one speed or generate grip force (in low gear) at only one rate. In effect, the myoelectric signal is activating an electronic switch, and for this reason, this type of control has been termed "myoswitch control."[21] An alternative to myoelectric control for this hand is the use of electromechanical switches. Otto Bock provides several types of switches, including a cable pull switch, a harness pull switch, and a rocker switch. All switches provide operational positions for both opening and closing the prehensor.

Although the hand moves at constant speed, the user can control the amount of opening or closing of the fingers by the length of time the control signal is maintained. To improve control of the opening and closing, the Digital Twin Hand moves at 11.0 cm/s, slower than the maximum speed of 13.0 cm/s for the DMC Plus Hand and the SensorHand. Grip force is also controlled by the length of time the control signal is maintained. The rate of change of grip force is constant; therefore, the longer the person maintains the control signal, the more the grip force will change. When gripping objects, the user can grip with a low force by keeping the control signal on for a short period of time. A higher grip force can be reached by keeping the control signal on for a longer period. The maximum grip force of the Digital Twin Hand is 90 N, the same as that of the DMC Plus Hand.

The Digital Twin Hand can be operated in a two-site, two-function mode with either myoelectrodes or switches, or in a single-site, two-function mode with a single myoelectrode. In the single-site control mode, the initial rate of change of the myoelectric signal determines if the hand will open or close. For example, if the user produces a moderate, slowly increasing contraction, the hand will close. A stronger, rapidly increasing contraction will cause the hand to open.

The DMC Plus Hand provides for proportional control of the speed of the hand and the force of gripping. Control is accomplished with myoelectrodes, using a two-site, two-function scheme. When the hand is moving in space, the magnitude of the myoelectric signal controls the speed of the movement. A low amplitude signal (light muscle contraction) produces slow movement; a higher amplitude signal (moderate to strong muscle contraction) produces faster movement. When gripping, the magnitude of the signal controls the force applied by the fingers. A low amplitude signal will produce a light gripping force, regardless of how long the signal is maintained. With the Digital Twin Hand, a low amplitude myoelectric signal would cause the force to change slowly, but the force would eventually reach the maximum possible for the hand if the low signal was maintained long enough. Although the user cannot directly feel the force being applied to an object, the DMC Plus Hand enables the user to gauge the grip force by sensing how hard the controlling muscle is being contracted.

The SensorHand (Figure 2) offers a variety of control modes using one or two myoelectrodes or electromechanical switches. The key difference between the SensorHand and the other Bock System Electric Hands is the ability of the hand to monitor the slip of a held object and automatically increase the grip force to stop the slipping.[22] This feature is achieved with a sensor that is built into the palmar surface at the end of the thumb (Figure 2). The sensor uses a force-sensitive conductive plastic overlaid with an array of electrical contacts to measure the three-dimensional force applied to the thumb tip when an object is grasped between the thumb and fingers. The force at the thumb has two components. One component is the normal force, which is the force applied perpendicular to the face of the slip sensor. This force is approximately equal to the grip force produced by the SensorHand. The other

force component is the tangential force. This is the force (such as that produced by gravity) parallel to the surface of the slip sensor that might cause an object to slide over the face of the sensor, or to slip. For an object not to slip, the ratio of the tangential force to the normal force must be in a specific range, dependent on the frictional properties of the surfaces in contact. Whenever the thumb sensor detects that the ratio of tangential force to normal force exceeds the allowed range, the control electronics activate the hand motor to increase the grip force until the ratio is brought back into the desired range.

A second force transducer, a strain gauge in the linkage between the thumb and fingers, measures the grip force in situations in which the grasped object is positioned in the hand in such a way that it is not pressing against the thumb sensor. The strain gauge transducer allows the user to maintain proportional control of grip force; however, the hand will not respond automatically if the held object begins to slip. The automatic response to slip can only be active when the held object is pressing against the thumb sensor.

The SensorHand has weight and maximum speed specifications similar to those of the DMC Plus Hand listed in Table 2. The maximum grip force is higher—100 N, compared to 90 N for the DMC Plus Hand.

A fourth System Electric Hand model is the Transcarpal Hand (Figure 3), a reworking of the standard configuration of the Bock mechanism to shorten the length of the hand. This model will fit users with longer residual limbs, such as those with carpal bones or very short segments of the metacarpals, and not produce a limb-length discrepancy.[23] The shortening is achieved by reducing the length of the drive unit and rotating it into the distal portion of the palmar region of the hand and the proximal phalanx of the ring finger. With this modification, the base of the hand is essentially the base of the finger chassis. Although it is not the shortest

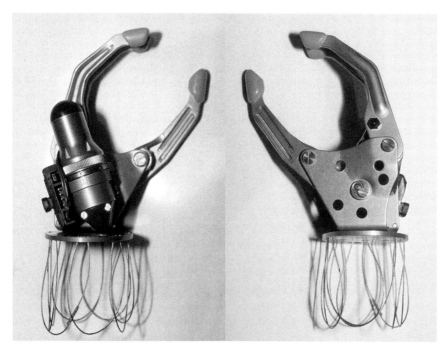

Figure 3 The mechanism for the Otto Bock Transcarpal Hand. Note the different arrangement of the drive unit and position of the base plate compared with the Sensor-Hand in Figure 2. The loops of wire beneath the base plate secure the mechanism into the socket lamination. *(Courtesy of the Northwestern University Rehabilitation Engineering Research Program.)*

electric hand, the Transcarpal Hand is 3.7 cm shorter than the wrist disarticulation versions of the other Bock System Electric Hands.

The Transcarpal Hand is also lighter than the DMC Plus Hand by about 120 g. The size 7¼ Transcarpal Hand weighs only 320 g. Other than the length and weight, the Transcarpal Hand has performance specifications similar to those of the DMC Plus Hand (Table 2). It has the same average maximum speed and the same maximum grip force. The Transcarpal Hand is available with DMC Plus control or Digital Twin control.

The fifth System Electric Hand model is a version with no electronics; it can be used with electronic controllers from other manufacturers. The electrical connection to this hand is directly to the motor leads through the on/off switch. Performance characteristics will depend on the particular electronics driving the hand and the voltage of the battery. The other System Electric Hands are designed for a 6.0-V nickel-cadmium or 7.2-V lithium ion battery.

An important feature of the electronics of the Otto Bock System Electric Hands is a current cut-off circuit. This circuit senses the motor current and automatically cuts off power to the motor to avoid a stall condition. Stall occurs when the drive unit has reached its maximum output torque and the motor stops rotating. Powering a stalled motor draws high current that will quickly deplete the battery capacity. All System Electric Hand models have a current cut-off circuit except the model designed to be used with controllers from other manufacturers, which has no electronics. When using this model, existence of a current cut-off feature (sometimes referred to as an energy-saving feature) in the controller should be determined because the presence or absence of this feature will affect overall performance.

Centri Electric Hands

The Centri Electric Hands are available in two adult sizes, 7¼ and 7¾. As with all hands described in this section, these sizes approximate the cir-

cumferential dimension at the knuckles in inches. The Centri hand design includes the articulated mechanism (Figure 4), a hand-shaped inner form that fits over the mechanism, and a cosmetic glove that is pulled over the form.

The Centri Hand mechanism incorporates a two-motor design. One motor drives the fingers open and shut against a stationary thumb, and a second motor locks the fingers (to maintain grip force) when there is no drive signal. The locking motor is not powered when the fingers are locked in place.

The mechanism includes all four fingers. The first and second fingers (index and middle) are linked to the motor drive train and apply the grip force in opposition to the thumb. The third and fourth fingers are linked to the first and second so that they move with the first and second fingers as they open and close. The hand mechanism is configured to reproduce the palmar prehension grasp pattern; however, the mechanism moves at two axes of rotation. The overall appearance of the motion of the hand as it closes on an object is that of a tenodesis type of motion (Figure 5). The base of the hand extends with respect to the forearm as the fingers close, and it flexes as the fingers open. This pattern of hand motion may give the hand a more physiologic appearance. The biaxial motion pattern is unique to the Centri Electric Hands.

The Centri Electric Hands are particularly notable because they are the lightest and shortest electric hands (Table 2). The size 7¾ Centri Electric Hand is about 2.5 cm shorter than the Bock Transcarpal Hand and weighs 250 g versus 320 g for the size 7¼ Bock Transcarpal Hand. The maximum grip force, maximum opening width, and average maximum speed of the Centri Electric Hands are lower than the Otto Bock DMC Plus Hand (Table 2).

The Centri electronic hand controller is a separate unit not built into the hand. This factor should be considered in the design of any prosthesis

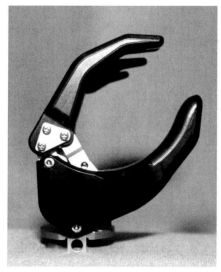 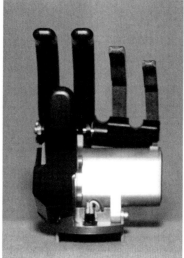 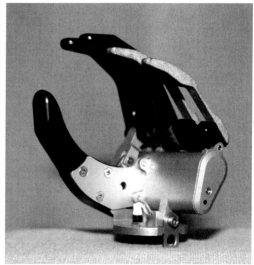

Figure 4 Centri Electric Hand. All four fingers are incorporated into the mechanism. *(Courtesy of the Northwestern University Rehabilitation Engineering Research Program.)*

incorporating the Centri Electric Hand. It can be operated with myoelectrodes or Force Sensing Resistors and provides proportional control of speed and rate of change of grip force.

Motion Control Hands

Motion Control produces only adult-sized electric hands in sizes 7¼, 7 ¾, and 8¼. The hands are available in four versions—standard, short, with a flexion wrist, and with a built-in controller. Table 2 lists the features of the standard version. Like the Otto Bock and Centri hands, the Motion Control Hands are made up of three parts: the mechanism, a hand-shaped inner form that fits over the mechanism, and the outer cosmetic glove (Figure 6).

The mechanism of the Motion Control Hand has a transverse-mounted motor and automatic gear transmission driving the thumb and first two fingers (index and middle) in opposition. The two fingers are linked together to move as a single unit, and both the fingers and the thumb move as the hand opens and closes. The on/off switch, mounted below the finger assembly, incorporates a third position that acts as a safety release. When the switch is pushed all the way in from the back of the hand, the fingers are disengaged

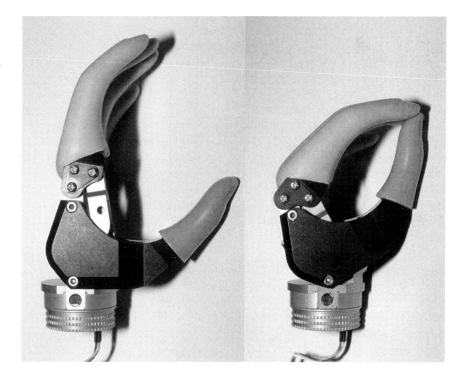

Figure 5 The Centri Electric Hand has two axes of motion during opening and closing. As the fingers close, the base of the mechanism extends with respect to the forearm. As the fingers open, the base flexes. The pattern of hand motion, similar to a tenodesis type of gripping motion, is believed by some users to give the hand a more physiologic appearance. *(Courtesy of the Northwestern University Rehabilitation Engineering Research Program.)*

from the gear train and can be opened manually with little force. This is the only electric hand that offers this feature.

The automatic transmission provides the Motion Control Hand with fast speed in high gear, when the fingers are moving freely, and high torque in low gear, when the fingers are closed on an object. The Motion Control Hand has the highest prehension force of the four hands listed

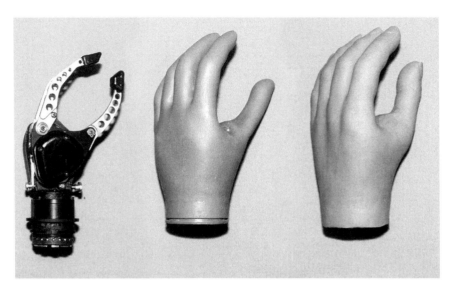

Figure 6 Motion Control Electric Hand. Shown from left to right are the mechanism, the hand-shaped inner form, and the cosmetic glove. *(Courtesy of the Northwestern University Rehabilitation Engineering Research Program.)*

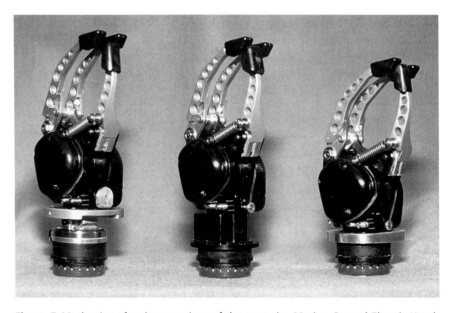

Figure 7 Mechanisms for three versions of the same size Motion Control Electric Hand. Shown from left to right are the model with the flexion wrist option, the standard version, and the short version. *(Courtesy of the Northwestern University Rehabilitation Engineering Research Program.)*

in Table 2. Its average maximum speed, lower than that of the Bock DMC Plus Hand, can be increased by powering the hand at a voltage greater than 7.2 V, up to 18 V. Higher battery voltage will increase the speed of the hand but will not significantly affect the maximum prehension force. The maximum force is limited to 98.1 N by the current cut-off circuit.

The short hand version of the Motion Control Hand reduces the length of the standard size 7¾ hand by 1.3 cm (Figure 7). The amount of shortening is slightly less for the size 7¼ hand and slightly more for the size 8¼ hand.

Unique among electric hands, the Motion Control Hand is available with a flexion wrist (Figure 7). The flexion mechanism is built into the hand between the drive assembly and the wrist connector, adding slightly more than 0.3 cm to the length of the size 7¾ hand and increasing the weight by 48 g over that of the standard size 7¾ hand. With the flexion mechanism, the hand can be locked in three positions: 30° of flexion, neutral, and 30° of extension. The lock is released manually by a spring-loaded push plate on the back of the hand near the base. The short hand and the hand with flexion wrist option have the same specifications for maximum grip force, maximum opening width, and average maximum speed, as shown in Table 2 for the standard Motion Control Hand.

The fourth version of the Motion Control Hand has the ProControl 2 electronic controller built into the hand. This version, the ProHand, requires only connection of battery and myoelectrodes at the wrist connector. The ProControl 2, also available as a separate control module, is manufactured by Motion Control and provides proportional myoelectric control of speed and rate of change of grip force. Versions of the Motion Control Hand other than the ProHand require an external control module. All versions of the hand incorporate a current cut-off circuit to prevent the motor from being powered in stall.

RSLSteeper Electric Hands

RSLSteeper manufactures the Multi-Control Plus Electric Hand in three sizes: 7¼, 7½, and 7¾. The hand includes the mechanism with thumb and index and middle fingers, a hand-shaped shell that encircles the mechanism proximal to the fingers, and a cosmetic glove (Figure 8). The thumb and the index and middle fingers are molded of hard plastic directly over the armature of the finger assembly and are separate from the shell. The ring and little fingers are molded of pliable plastic and attached to the plastic shell. The ends of the thumb and index and middle fingers are lined with a soft elastomeric material

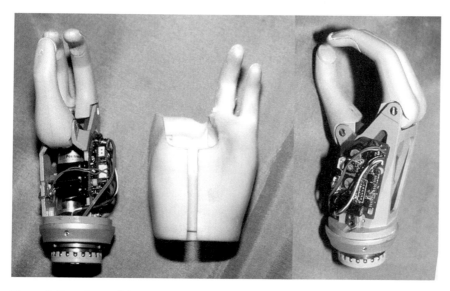

Figure 8 Two views of the mechanism and electronic controller for the RSLSteeper MultiControl Plus Electric Hand. In the center is the hand-shaped shell that protects the electronics and gives the device its overall shape. *(Courtesy of the Northwestern University Rehabilitation Engineering Research Program.)*

on the palmar surfaces that deforms and shapes itself to the contact surfaces of held objects.

The mechanism incorporates a single motor with gear reducer, drive screw, and nut actuator, all held within a support structure. The first two fingers (as one unit) and thumb are linked to the nut and to the stationary support structure. As the nut travels along the screw, the fingers and thumb pivot and move in the palmar prehension pattern. On initial closing, the MultiControl Plus Electric Hand can achieve a maximum grip force of 55 N. Once that force is reached, the user can boost the maximum grip force to 65 N with an additional closing command. This higher grip force is less than the minimum proposed by Peizer and associates,[1] and is the lowest maximum grip force of the four electric hands in Table 2. In addition to the lowest grip force, the RSLSteeper hands also have the smallest maximum opening width and the lowest average maximum speed.

The electronic controller for the MultiControl Plus Electric Hand is built into the hand. Five control options are provided and can be selected with a rotary switch mounted to the controller circuit board. Three control options are available for single-site, two-function control. The three options differ primarily in the manner in which the user controls closing of the hand: (1) close automatically whenever the opening signal is gone; (2) close at constant speed under direct control of the user; or (3) close at a speed proportional to the magnitude of the user's control signal. The fourth and fifth options provide two-site, two-function control using two independent control sources. The two-site options differ in control of movement—either at a constant speed or at a speed proportional to the magnitude of the control signal. The RSLSteeper controller can accept inputs from myoelectrodes or switches, but only myoelectrodes are compatible with the proportional control options. The built-in electronics also provide for energy saving through a motor cut-off circuit.

Nonhand Prehension Devices

The driving force for the design of all nonhand prehensors is the desire to overcome the various functional deficiencies of electric hands that result from designs constrained by a hand-like shape and appearance.[11] For the most part, the nonhand prehensors are used in special situations to complement the function provided by electric hands. However, some individuals, particularly those with bilateral amputations, might choose to use nonhand prehensors exclusively.

Four nonhand prehensors are described below: the Otto Bock System Electric Greifer, the Hosmer NU-VA Synergetic Prehensor, the Motion Control ETD, and the RSLSteeper MultiControl Powered Gripper. A summary of device characteristics appears in Table 3. A fifth device, the Hosmer NY Prehension Actuator, is a mechanism to power cable-actuated split hooks. This Hosmer device is described at the end of this section on nonhand prehensors, but it is not listed in Table 3.

Otto Bock System Electric Greifer

The Otto Bock System Electric Greifer (Figure 9) was developed by Otto Bock as an alternative to the System Electric Hand for work situations that require higher prehension force or that might damage the mechanism of the hand prehensor or damage or discolor the cosmetic glove.[3] It can be easily interchanged for the hand prehensor when used with the Otto Bock quick-disconnect wrist unit. The Greifer is available in one size, which can be either a right or left unit. The mechanism is encased in a multiple-piece shell made of a durable hard plastic and is available with or without rubber pads lining the prehension surfaces of the fingers.

The two fingers of the Greifer are broad-surfaced and arranged to move symmetrically in opposition. They are articulated so that as they move, the distal prehension surfaces remain parallel to one another. The shape and articulation of the fingers provide lateral prehension and, for objects of moderate size, cylindrical prehension. Adjustable tips, with or without rubber lining, provide tip prehension for handling smaller objects. The tips can be replaced with optional blanks ma-

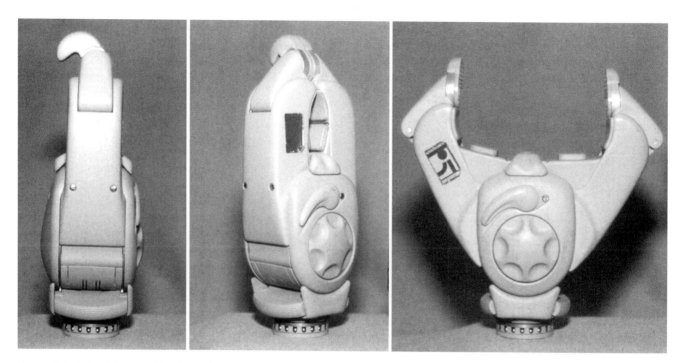

Figure 9 Otto Bock System Electric Greifer. The right panel shows the Greifer with the fingers fully opened. The center view shows the wheel that rotates as the fingers move; this wheel can be turned to open or close the fingers manually. The lever just above the wheel disengages the fingers from the gear train, allowing them to be opened freely. *(Courtesy of the Northwestern University Rehabilitation Engineering Research Program.)*

chined for specific applications. A screwdriver is required to adjust the position of the tips or to interchange them.

In comparison to the System Electric Hand, the Greifer is longer by 3 cm and is about 100 g heavier, making it the heaviest electric prehensor. It has approximately the same maximum width of finger opening as the System Electric Hand. In terms of mechanical performance, the Greifer is faster and can develop significantly higher prehension force, about 75% greater than that of the DMC Plus System Electric Hand. At a maximum grip force of 160 N, the Greifer has the highest maximum grip force of any electric prehensor.

The Greifer also incorporates an automatic transmission to enable the fingers to move relatively fast through space yet exert high forces when closed on an object. When the Greifer first closes on an object, it will grip up to a maximum force of 10 N, after which the transmission will downshift for gripping at higher forces. There is a short delay before the transmission downshifts, which en-

ables users to grasp lighter and more delicate objects at the lower force and stop the closing signal before higher forces are applied. The transmission of the Greifer differs from that of the System Electric Hand in that there is very little delay between an "open" command and movement of the fingers, even after high prehension forces have been applied.

As with the System Electric Hand, a back-lock mechanism prevents the fingers of the Greifer from opening when power is not applied. For safety, this feature can be circumvented in one of two ways if the Greifer is not responding to an "open" command. First, an external control wheel, in line with the motor, can be turned manually to drive the fingers open. This control wheel also provides visual feedback of the action of the drive mechanism during normal operation. Second, a lever near the base of the fingers disengages the fingers from the drive transmission, enabling them to be moved freely. Neither method damages the Greifer in any way.

In addition to the same wrist rotation capability of the System Electric

Hand, the Greifer also has built-in wrist flexion. The plane of flexion is perpendicular to the prehension surfaces of the fingers.

Otto Bock control options for the Greifer include the DMC Plus and the Digital Twin options. These controllers are built into the Greifer and work in the same manner as they do for the System Electric Hands, facilitating interchange between the Greifer and a System Electric Hand. A model of the Greifer without electronics is also available for use with other manufacturers' controllers.

Hosmer NU-VA Synergetic Prehensor

The NU-VA Synergetic Prehensor (Figure 10) was designed as an alternative to a hand prehensor, with speed and force characteristics approaching those of the physiologic hand. It was developed by the Prosthetics Research Laboratory of Northwestern University with the support of the Department of Veterans Affairs and is manufactured by the Hosmer Dorrance Corporation. The performance objectives of the prehensor are

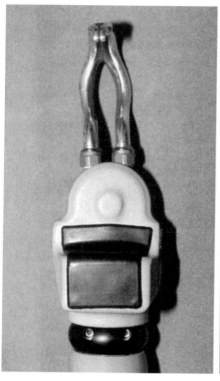
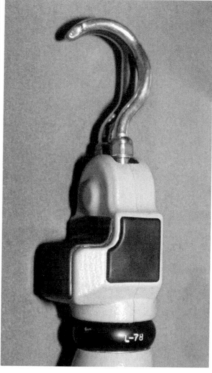

Figure 10 Hosmer NU-VA Synergetic Prehensor. Note the lyre-shaped finger opening of the APRL voluntary-closing hook. The black pads on the case are a high-friction material for nongrasping functions such as holding one object against another or pushing an object over a surface. *(Courtesy of the Northwestern University Rehabilitation Engineering Research Program.)*

achieved with a two-motor design using the concept of synergy.[24]

Separate motors and gear trains are used to drive the two opposing fingers. One finger is driven at high speed but low torque, and the other finger is driven at low speed but high torque. In grasping an object, therefore, the fast finger can quickly close on the object, and the high-torque finger applies the force necessary to secure the object. The synergetic design also permits immediate release of objects when an "open" signal is generated because the high-torque and high-speed fingers are driven simultaneously. The maximum speed of movement of the fast finger of the Synergetic Prehensor is approximately that of the average speed of functional physiologic finger movements, and the maximum prehension force applied at the tip of the high-torque finger is approximately that measured for palmar prehension in adult men.

The mechanism and support structure of the prehensor are encased in a two-piece plastic shell, and the fingers of the Synergetic Prehensor are the same removable hook-shaped fingers as developed for the body-powered Army Prosthetics Research Laboratory (APRL) voluntary-closing hook. The hook-shaped fingers provide powered lateral and tip prehension as well as passive hook prehension. For objects of moderate diameter with respect to the size of the prehensor, the lyre-shaped contour of the opening between the fingers provides for cylindrical grasp. The fingers are lined with neoprene to achieve higher contact friction during grasping. Neoprene pads are also arrayed on the case to facilitate activities in which the prehensor body is used to hold objects in place against other objects or to exert pushing forces on objects.

The drive train of the fast finger incorporates a back-lock mechanism,

which prevents the high-torque finger from pushing the faster, lower torque finger back as objects are grasped. As with other prehensor designs, the back-lock also enables objects to be held without continued operation of the motors. Should the prehensor not respond to an "open" signal when closed on an object, the fingers can be opened by a safety breakaway when external forces on the fingers exceed 133 N. This mechanism can be manually reset, and its operation does not damage the prehensor.

In addition to near-physiologic speed and force, the synergetic design is also energy efficient. Once the fast finger closes on an object and ceases to move, its motor is electronically cut off; therefore, it does not run in stall during the application of force by the high-torque finger. To close on an object and grasp it with a force (at the fingertips) of 75 N, the prehensor draws an average of 138 mA, or about 1.2 W.[25] Using a 100-mAh rechargeable 9-V transistor-type battery, the prehensor can perform approximately 1,300 cycles of opening and then closing to a prehension force of 75 N on a single battery charge. Therefore, it is possible to use these small, readily available batteries for a full day's use of the Synergetic Prehensor.

Control of the Synergetic Prehensor is best achieved with a proportional system because of the speed of response of the device. A two-site, two-function proportional myoelectric controller is available from Hosmer Dorrance. This controller differs somewhat from other proportional myoelectric controllers in that the myoelectric signal is not smoothed by filtering but rather is used to generate full-voltage pulses that increase in width and number in proportion to the amplitude of the myoelectric signal.[26] By processing the muscle signal in this manner and using the mechanical smoothing inherent in the drive system, the time delay associated with electronic filtering is eliminated and the stiction of the mechanism (the resistance to moving when initially powered) is overcome. These

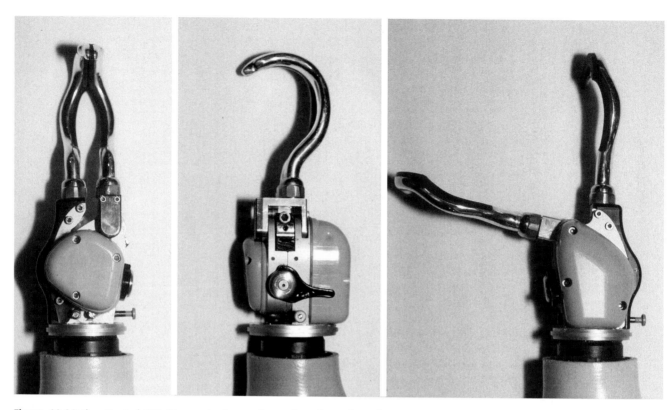

Figure 11 Motion Control ETD. The center image shows the safety release lever that disengages the fingers from the gear train. The view on the right shows the moving finger in its fully opened position; the other finger is stationary. *(Courtesy of the Northwestern University Rehabilitation Engineering Research Program.)*

two factors contribute to the almost instantaneous response of the Synergetic Prehensor and the ability to have good control even at low signal levels.

Motion Control ETD

The newest nonhand prehension device is the Motion Control Electric Terminal Device (ETD), which was released in mid 2003 (Figure 11). The mechanism of the ETD uses a motor and gear transmission similar to that of the Motion Control Hand. The mechanism is encased in water-resistant housings, allowing the user to expose the ETD to water and non-corrosive liquids without damaging the mechanism. The fingers are the same as those of the body-powered APRL Voluntary Closing Hook and the Hosmer Synergetic Prehensor; therefore, it offers the same advantageous prehension patterns—active lateral and tip prehension, active cylindrical grasp for objects of moderate diameter, and passive hook prehension. Unlike the fingers and thumb of the Motion Control Hand,

only one of the two hook-shaped fingers of the ETD is driven; the other is stationary. As with the Motion Control Hand, the ETD incorporates a safety release that disengages the moving finger from the gear train. The ETD is available in left and right models because of the moving and stationary finger arrangement.

The ETD is the lightest nonhand prehension device and offers the widest maximum opening width of any electric-powered prehensor. It can be operated at voltages from 6 to 14 V. Above 10 V, the speed of the ETD exceeds that of the Hosmer Synergetic Prehensor.

The ETD is available in three versions: standard, with flexion wrist, and with the built-in ProHand electronic controller. The standard version requires an external controller, such as Motion Control's ProControl 2. The flexion wrist option increases the length beyond that of the standard version. As with the Motion Control Hand, the flexion wrist option for the ETD provides three

locked positions—30° of flexion, neutral, and 30° of extension. All versions of the ETD include an energy-saver circuit to prevent the motor from being powered in a stalled condition.

RSLSteeper MultiControl Powered Gripper

The current MultiControl Powered Gripper from RSLSteeper (Figure 12) is essentially a complete reworking of the original Powered Gripper described by Kemp.[11] Except for the angular hook-shaped fingers, little remains of the early version. The device now has a single motor drive unit that powers both fingers to open and close simultaneously. The MultiControl Powered Gripper has the lowest maximum grip force, the smallest maximum opening width, and the slowest average maximum speed of any of the nonhand prehension devices (Table 3).

The body and fingers of the Powered Gripper are metal castings. The fingers are contoured to provide pas-

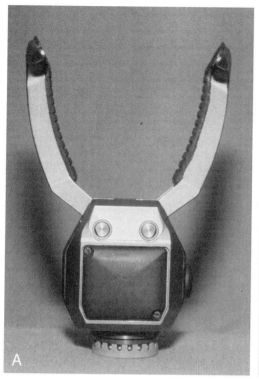
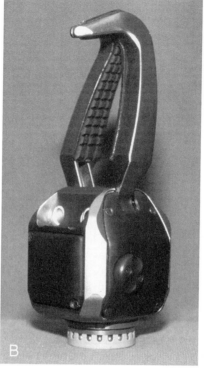
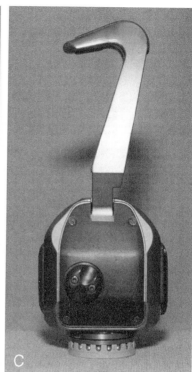

Figure 12 RSLSteeper MultiControl Powered Gripper. **A,** Fingers in fully opened position. **B,** Grooved lining on the prehension surface of the fingers. **C,** External wheel that can be turned manually to open or close the fingers when the Powered Gripper is not responding. *(Courtesy of the Northwestern University Rehabilitation Engineering Research Program.)*

sive hook prehension and have flattened opposing surfaces for powered lateral and tip prehension. The opening between the fingers is also contoured to accommodate cylindrical objects. The prehension force of the Powered Gripper is enhanced by the use of relatively soft frictional rubber pads to line the fingers. The pads are grooved over their surfaces. The grooves allow the pads to deform and mold to the shapes of held objects, distributing the prehension force over a broader contact area.

An external wheel on one side of the MultiControl Powered Gripper is connected to the drive train of the fingers. If the device fails to open, the user can turn the wheel to open the fingers manually.

The same control schemes used for the RSLSteeper MultiControl Plus Electric Hand are available with the Powered Gripper. A special version of the Powered Gripper without electronics is available for use with other manufacturers' controllers.

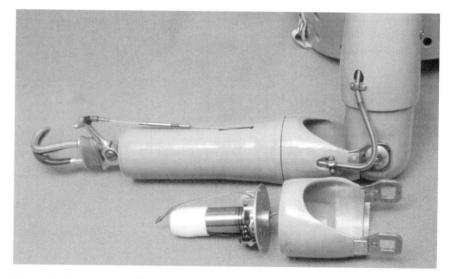

Figure 13 Hosmer NY Prehension Actuator. The complete forearm assembly is shown attached to the Hosmer NY Electric Elbow. The mechanism of the Prehension Actuator (with the forearm shell removed) and the forearm saddle assembly with forearm rotation joint are shown next to the completed assembly. *(Courtesy of the Northwestern University Rehabilitation Engineering Research Program.)*

Hosmer NY Prehension Actuator

Because the NY Prehension Actuator (PA) is not a true prehension device, its characteristics are not included in Table 3. The PA is a forearm assembly (Figure 13) containing a motorized winch that provides electric-powered operation of a cable-actuated, voluntary-opening split hook.[27] The device was originally designed by William Lembeck of New York University as a complete forearm setup for use with the Hosmer E-200 and E-400 mechanical elbows or the Hosmer NY Electric Elbows. In that configuration, the mechanism occupies the distal 10.8 cm of the forearm with a rotation joint proximal to the mechanism. The forearm segment proximal to the rotation joint contains the forearm saddle assembly for the elbow and, because of the saddle's dimensions, has a minimum length from the elbow axis of 9.5 cm. The complete forearm setup has a minimum length from the elbow axis to the distal face of the wrist of 20.3 cm. Longer forearms are provided by lengthening the distal forearm segment, thus keeping the weight of the mechanism (about 218 g) as proximal as possible. Rotation to orient the split hook is done proximal to the PA to maintain an efficient alignment between the cable attachment post of the split hook and the cable leading from the actuator mechanism.

The PA is typically powered by a 6-V battery pack, and at that voltage it can open a split hook with three rubber bands. The time required to open the hook to its limit is approximately 1 second, though it is dependent on the number of bands used with the hook.

Controlled activation of the PA causes it to pull the split hook open. If the control signal stops before the PA pulls the hook to full opening, the hook is closed by the rubber bands. If the control signal is maintained after the hook reaches full opening, the PA is electrically cut off so that it does not draw motor current and the motor is dynamically braked. The dynamic braking, which is maintained as long as the control signal is present, allows the split hook to close but at a slow speed. This action gives the user time to adjust the position of the split hook relative to the object being grasped. When the control signal is withdrawn, the braking is removed and the split hook closes freely.

Commentary on Electric Prehensors

The interplay of psychological and social aspects associated with the shape of the human hand and the need for prehension function and independent capability are complex. Generalizations favoring one type of prehensor over any other are limiting, and there is little consensus among users of prosthetic prehensors as to which device is best suited as a replacement for the physiologic hand. Even the similarity to the anatomic hand that is possible with modern electric hand-like prehensors is not universally desired. Some individuals, particularly those with bilateral amputations, are appreciative of the prehension and performance advantages of prehensors that do not have a hand-like shape. Others find the apparent cosmesis of electric hands insufficient and are repelled by it, preferring a device that has a form truer to its gripping function. Until a more versatile anthropomorphic prehension device is developed, the need for a variety of options will remain.

Wrist Mechanisms

Studies of hand use in performing various common activities and occupational tasks have shown that forearm rotation and wrist motions are used to a significant extent in these actions.[17,28-31] Most of the activities studied revealed that the joint moved through a range of motion during the course of an activity versus assuming a variety of fixed positions across the activities. In studies incorporating many different activities, the total range of motion spanned was found to be approximately 100° for forearm rotation, 80° for wrist flexion and extension, and 60° for radial and ulnar deviation of the wrist.[17,29] For the specific task of eating, the total range of motion was about 100° for forearm rotation, 30° for wrist flexion and extension, and 30° for radial and ulnar deviation of the wrist.[31]

With the exception of the Otto Bock Electric Wrist Rotator, all commercial prosthetic wrist components are manually positioned or body powered. Many factors complicate the development of electric-powered wrist components. From a component design viewpoint, size and weight constraints are imposed by the location of the joint. The device must fit within a cylinder about 5 cm in diameter and occupy as little length as possible, to accommodate a variety of residual limb lengths.

The component must also be relatively lightweight to minimize counterforces exerted on the residual limb (for a transradial fitting) and minimize countertorque, which would reduce the lift capacity of a prosthetic elbow in higher level fittings. And though lightweight, the structure must be robust enough to withstand the forces that are exerted on the prehensor and transferred back to the residual limb through the wrist joint. Another consideration with respect to weight is the requirement for relatively low power consumption to eliminate the need for an additional battery if used in conjunction with other electric components.

The key functional question is which joint motions should be provided. The anatomic forearm and wrist joints can be approximated by a triaxial joint with the axes of rotation, flexion, and deviation (roll, pitch, and yaw) having a point of intersection near the base of the prehensor. All three motions have been shown to contribute to functional activities.

At least one additional control source would be needed for each powered joint of wrist motion unless the control system operates in a sequential manner. Even sequential control would require at least two control sources—one for selection and one for movement control.

Finally, the performance of the component must be far superior to the alternatives for the user to be attracted to its operation. For an individual with a unilateral amputation, the primary alternative is the intact

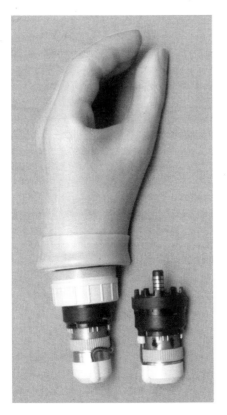

Figure 14 Otto Bock Electric Wrist Rotator. The rotator (shown below by itself) interfaces mechanically and electrically with the Otto Bock–style quick-disconnect wrist adaptor. *(Courtesy of the Northwestern University Rehabilitation Engineering Research Program.)*

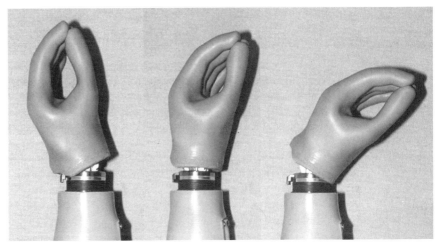

Figure 15 Wrist flexion option for the Motion Control Electric Hand. Pictured from left to right are 30° of extension, neutral position, and 30° of flexion. The plate extending from the left at the base of the hand is the spring-loaded lock release. *(Courtesy of the Northwestern University Rehabilitation Engineering Research Program.)*

limb, which can be used preferentially for activities involving significant forearm and wrist motion. On the prosthetic side, the person could use compensatory motions of proximal physiologic joints and have manually positioned mechanical wrist components that would offer adjustable fixed orientations of the prehensor. Although operation of these components typically involves the physiologic hand, the operation is relatively quick and straightforward. The fact that this technique is so widespread underscores the remarkable qualities of the physiologic wrist. Persons using this technique do so without giving much thought to what they are doing with their intact wrist and hand while using them to position the prosthetic wrist.

For individuals with bilateral arm amputations, there are alternative methods for actuating and positioning mechanical wrist components that do not necessarily require the contralateral limb. However, these components normally cannot be operated to perform work, such as turning a handle. Nor can they typically be adjusted dynamically during a motion, such as adjusting the wrist attitude while raising a utensil to the mouth. Although these deficiencies have inspired many designers to attempt to fashion a more versatile electric-powered wrist, advances have been slow and no multiaxial components are commercially available.

Otto Bock Electric Wrist Rotator

The Electric Wrist Rotator developed by Otto Bock addresses many of the difficulties outlined in the preceding paragraphs to provide the functional analog of forearm rotation (Figure 14). The drive unit is a single motor and gear reducer with a rotation axis in line with the longitudinal axis of the forearm. The rotator is structurally supported within the lamination collar of the Bock quick-disconnect wrist and can fit any of the three sizes of wrist lamination collars, which have diameters of 4.0, 4.5, and 5.0 cm. Its length is 6.7 cm from the distal edge of the lamination collar to the proximal surface of the motor housing.

The rotator is relatively lightweight at 96 g, approximately 20% of the weight of an Otto Bock System Electric Hand. It is also relatively energy efficient, drawing a no-load current of 150 mA; the stall current is 1,000 mA. The power requirements are such that it is feasible to operate an Otto Bock System Electric Hand or Greifer along with the Electric Wrist Rotator from a single 6- or 7.2-V Otto Bock battery. Whether one battery will last an entire day depends on the extent to which the devices are used.

The rotator mechanism is also protected from external forces through its attachment to the wrist lamination collar. Side forces and axial forces exerted on the prehensor are transferred to the lamination collar and prosthetic forearm rather than to the rotator mechanism. Excessive torque on the prehensor will cause the ratchet of the prehensor's portion of the quick-disconnect wrist to slip rather than backdrive the wrist mechanism.

The coaxial electrical coupling of the Bock quick-disconnect wrist allows the rotator to turn an electric prehensor continuously in either direction. In general, however, the performance characteristics of the rotator have been compromised to

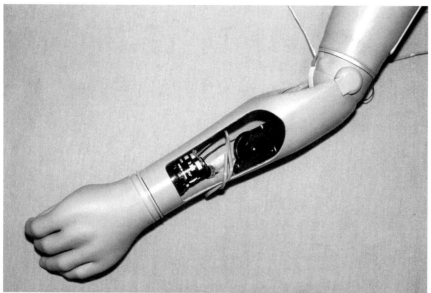

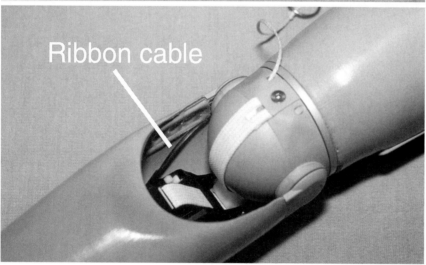

Ribbon cable

Figure 16 Otto Bock ErgoArm Hybrid Plus. The upper image is a demonstrator transhumeral prosthesis with a forearm cutaway to show the wrist rotator and the Automatic Forearm Balance device. The lower photograph shows one of the two ribbon cables that pass through the elbow to transfer control signals and power to the distal components. *(Courtesy of the Northwestern University Rehabilitation Engineering Research Program.)*

accommodate the size, weight, and power requirements. The rotator does not generate high torque and is therefore not recommended for work such as turning valves or door handles unless the resistance is minimal. The rotation is primarily for prepositioning and changing the orientation of the prehensor before an action or while the prehensor is holding a lightweight implement, such as a utensil with food or a cup of liquid. The speed of the rotator is 13.5 rpm

(1.41 radians/s or 81°/s). Physiologic forearm rotation can achieve time-averaged maximum velocities in excess of 14 radians/s (800°/s) for pronation and 20 radians/s (1,150°/s) for supination.[32]

Electronic controllers from Otto Bock, Motion Control, and Liberating Technologies provide two-source, four-function sequential control of the rotator and an electric-powered prehension device. Controllers for direct, independent control of the rota-

tor are available from Hosmer Dorrance and Liberating Technologies. Specifics on the control options and requirements can be obtained from the manufacturers. Contact information for all the manufacturers mentioned in this chapter is provided in Table 1.

Wrist Flexion Units

Although no commercial components provide electric-powered wrist flexion, this is an important function for individuals with bilateral arm amputations and for some with unilateral amputations. Accordingly, it is useful to know how this function can be provided in prosthetic fittings involving electric prehensors.

The Otto Bock System Electric Greifer and the Motion Control Electric Hand and ETD have wrist flexion options built into the prehensors. The flexion joint for the Otto Bock System Electric Greifer is a manually positioned friction joint that can be adjusted for more or less friction. The range of motion is from +45° to -45° and occurs in a plane perpendicular to the prehension surfaces of the fingers. The flexion joint for the Motion Control prehensors provides three locked positions at 30° of extension, neutral, and 30° of flexion (Figure 15). For the Motion Control Electric Hand, the flexion occurs in a plane perpendicular to the prehension surfaces of the finger. For the Motion Control ETD, the flexion is in a plane parallel to the prehension surfaces of the fingers.

For other electric prehensors, engineers and prosthetists have devised a variety of techniques for adapting commercially available mechanical flexion components for use with electric prehensors. The Sierra Wrist Flexion Unit and the Hosmer Flexion-Friction Wrist have both been used in clinical electric-powered fittings. Modifications to both the wrist component and the wrist coupling of the prehensor may be required, depending on what specific components are being used together. It is important to provide a pathway for the electrical

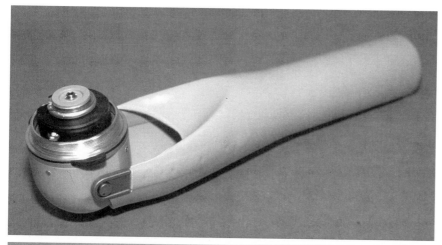

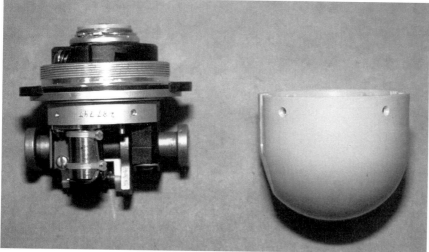

Figure 17 RSLSteeper Electric Elbow Lock. Shown above is the complete elbow-forearm assembly. The lower panel shows the posterior aspect of the elbow mechanism with the elbow cap off. The vertical cylinder-shaped part to the left of center in front of the elbow axle is the lock motor. *(Courtesy of the Northwestern University Rehabilitation Engineering Research Program.)*

wires through the wrist unit to the prehensor and to limit any rotation joint crossed by the wires with a mechanical stop so that the wires will not be damaged by unrestricted continuous rotation in one direction.

Commentary on Wrist Components

The significant role of forearm and wrist motions in the fine orientation and positioning of the human hand is well documented. The need for this capability in a prosthetic limb is just as great. The prosthetic wrist may actually hold more significance than its physiologic counterpart in the context of the total prosthesis. Prosthetic

fingers cannot be repositioned within the prehensor to accommodate orientation requirements the same way physiologic fingers can be repositioned to augment the anatomic wrist position. In addition, compensatory motions of proximal physiologic joints may be restricted by the suspension of the prosthesis or the harnessing for control actions. For individuals with bilateral amputations, particularly those with amputation levels above the elbow, the need for assisted wrist function on at least one side becomes even more demanding. The technologic obstacles and control problems are major. However, the potential functional advantages of better

wrist components will likely continue to drive development efforts.

Enhancements to Body-Powered Elbows

This section covers body-powered elbows that have been enhanced to support the fitting of electric-powered prehension devices or that incorporate electric locks.

Otto Bock ErgoArm Hybrid Plus

The Bock ErgoArm Hybrid Plus is an elbow-forearm assembly with an internal mechanical lock. The elbow joint can be positioned by body motion using a cable and harness or by ballistic motion and can be locked in any position within its range of motion. The forearm includes the Automatic Forearm Balance unit, a cam and spring assembly that can be set to provide a countertorque to the effect of gravity on the mass of the forearm and prehension components. The countertorque reduces the actuating force needed to position the elbow.

To facilitate the fitting of electric-powered components for prehension and rotation, the ErgoArm Hybrid Plus has an internal feed-through wiring harness (Figure 16). Connectors in the proximal cover of the elbow can receive myoelectrodes, switches, and a battery. From the connectors, internal ribbon cables lead into the forearm within the joint side straps. The cables end in connectors compatible with the Otto Bock Wrist Rotator or wrist coaxial connector to provide power and control of an electric prehension device.

Otto Bock ErgoArm Electronic Plus

The Electronic Plus elbow-forearm assembly is identical to the ErgoArm Hybrid Plus except that the elbow lock is motorized. As with the body-powered elbow lock, each operation of the electric lock changes its state, from locked to unlocked or from un-

TABLE 4 Characteristics of Adult Electric Elbows

Device	NY Electric Elbow (large model)	Boston Digital Arm System	Utah Arm 2 (elbow only)
Manufacturer	Hosmer Dorrance	Liberating Technologies	Motion Control
Turntable diameter	7.1 cm	7.0 cm	7.0 cm
Humeral dimension*	10.8 cm	10.5 cm	13.0 cm
Minimum forearm dimension†	No required forearm componentry	20.3 cm	24.8 cm
Weight	0.55 to 0.62 kg (depending on battery used and without forearm)	1.02 kg (with standard forearm shell)	0.91 kg (with standard length forearm shell)
Maximum live-lift capacity	3.4 N·m	≈ 14.2 N·m	4.3 N·m (estimated)
Passive (locked) lift capacity	24.4 to 27.1 N·m	68 N·m	68 N·m
Range of motion	5° to 135°	0° to 135°	15° to 150°
Speed	100°/s, no load 56.5 °/s, with countertorque of 1.7 N·m	123°/s, no load 113°/s, with countertorque of 1.6 N·m	112.5°/s, with weight of Otto Bock System Electric Hand countertorque ≈ 1.44 N·m
Battery type‡ (all rechargeable)	5 or 6.25 V; nonremovable	12 V; removable, but remains in arm during recharging	12 V; removable

*With the elbow flexed 90°, the humeral dimension is from the proximal edge of the turntable lamination collar to the distal aspect of the elbow cap.

†For both the Boston Digital Arm System and the Utah Arm 2, length is measured from the posterior aspect of the elbow, flexed 90°, to the most distal aspect of an Otto Bock quick-disconnect wrist lamination collar.

‡*Nonremovable* and *removable* refer to the procedure used for recharging.

locked to locked. It can be actuated with a switch or with a two-site, two-function myoelectrode setup using cocontraction of the muscle sites. A mechanical override allows for operation of the lock if the battery is depleted or an electronic problem occurs.

RSLSteeper Electric Elbow Lock

The RSLSteeper Electric Elbow Lock (Figure 17) was the first to be incorporated into a body-powered elbow. The electric lock is a major advantage for individuals who can benefit from a cable-actuated mechanical elbow but have difficulty producing the control motions or forces required by the body-powered lock. The lock motor is operated by an electromechanical switch or by single-site myoswitch control. There is no mechanical override in the RSLSteeper unit.

Elbow Mechanisms

Three electric elbows are available for adults: the Hosmer NY Electric El-

bow, the Liberating Technologies Boston Digital Arm System, and the Motion Control Utah Arm 2. These elbows differ from one another in mechanical configuration, drive mechanism, and control options. Table 4 summarizes characteristics of these devices, and each of the elbows is described below.

In addition to the powered elbow joint, all of the elbows incorporate a friction joint or turntable for manual humeral rotation. With the Hosmer NY Electric Elbow, the friction is adjusted by a crown nut on a threaded stud centered in the proximal surface of the elbow enclosure. Access to this nut must be provided in the fabrication of the humeral shell. The Boston Digital Arm System uses a split compression ring, and the Utah Arm 2 has an external split collar for friction adjustment of the humeral rotation joint. No special accommodation must be made in the fabrication of the humeral shell for these two elbows for access to the adjustment.

Elbows are generally used to position the prehension device, then kept in place while performing some ac-

tivity. However, lifting capacity is an important characteristic, especially for individuals with bilateral amputations. The three elbows have maximum live-lift (lifting by powering the elbow) capacities ranging from 3.4 N·m to 14.2 N·m (Table 4). At a distance of 30 cm from the elbow axis, the Hosmer NY Electric Elbow can lift a maximum weight of 1.1 kg; the Boston Digital Arm System can lift a maximum weight of 4.7 kg. The weight of the materials of the forearm, wrist component, and prehension device must be subtracted from these values to estimate the maximum weight of an object that can be held and lifted. An adult electric hand-like prehensor weighs roughly 0.45 kg. Assuming a distance of 30 cm from elbow axis to palm, this type of prehensor would reduce the maximum weight of an object that can be lifted to approximately 0.65 kg for the Hosmer NY Electric Elbow and 4.25 kg for the Boston Digital Arm System. Subtracting the weight of the forearm and wrist componentry would further reduce these values.

In comparison, the lifting capacity of the physiologic elbow can exceed 25 kg for an adult man at low speeds of flexion[33] and can exceed 13 kg at flexion speeds of about 57°/s.[34] Clearly, the same types of activities cannot be performed with an electric elbow as with the physiologic elbow, particularly those involving the active lifting of moderate to heavy loads.

Heavier loads can be lifted by a prosthesis with an electric elbow, but in a passive manner—by locking the elbow in place after prepositioning it, using body movement and posture to orient the prehensor to grasp the object, and then straightening the body without actively moving the elbow joint. In this way, objects that exceed the live-lift capacity of the elbow can still be lifted. However, even this technique is limited by the breakaway device or slip clutches incorporated into the elbow mechanisms to protect them against mechanical overload. This overload protection also serves to protect the user, to a degree, from excessive forces transferred through the socket during accidents such as falls. The elbow would give way if the person fell onto the prosthesis. Both the Boston Digital Arm System and the Utah Arm 2 have passive lift capacities of 68 N·m, and the Hosmer NY Electric Elbow has a capacity between 24.4 N·m and 27.1 N·m. With an electric prehensor and distance to the elbow axis of 30 cm, the Boston Digital Arm System and Utah Arm 2 can be used to passively lift an object weighing up to 23 kg; the Hosmer NY Electric Elbow will passively lift 8.1 to 9.1 kg.

As with lift capacity, the speed of elbow motion is often cited as a significant feature in comparisons of prosthetic elbows. However, important perspective can be gained by considering speeds of electric elbows in comparison to physiologic performance. The average maximum speed of physiologic elbow flexion for adult men has been measured at about 600°/s for movements through a 120° range,[32] with peak speeds in excess of 900°/s.[32,35] Clearly, the maximum

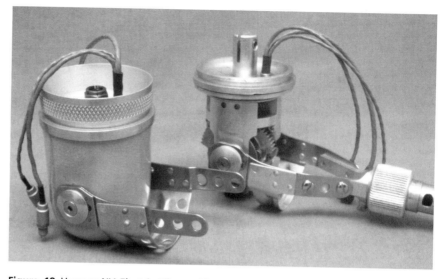

Figure 18 Hosmer NY Electric Elbows. The exoskeletal model in the foreground has a humeral turntable and a forearm saddle for lamination. The endoskeletal model on the right has attachments for humeral and forearm pylons. The cables coming from the tops of both models are connections for the controller and battery pack.

speeds of adult electric elbows (Table 4) are far less than these values. However, maximum speeds of elbow flexion are probably rarely attained in daily functional activities. Peak physiologic elbow speeds more typical of those that might be seen in common functional activities have been found to be correlated to the amplitude of the movement with the following approximate relationship: speed (°/s) = (2.9°/s/°) × (angular distance in °).[32] For a movement over a 10° range, the peak velocity during the movement would be about 29°/s. For a greater angular movement of 90°, the peak velocity would be about 261°/s. Therefore, it would appear that all of the electric elbows can approach functional physiologic speeds over short distance movements but are significantly slower than the physiologic elbow over larger angular movements.

Perhaps more important than the measured speed of an electric elbow is how it is controlled in relation to its speed of response. For an extreme example, it would be difficult to position a fast elbow using switch control that actuated the elbow at full speed in flexion and in extension. The user would have a tendency to overshoot the target position and would likely not be able to make small changes in

position. Accordingly, as electric elbows have become faster, the use of proportional velocity control has grown. In this type of control, the magnitude of the input signal, which the user is presumed to be able to regulate, determines in direct proportion the speed of motion. By creating a higher amplitude signal, the user directs the elbow to move faster, up to the limits of the mechanism; by producing lower level signals, the user drives the elbow at slower speed.

Hosmer NY Electric Elbow

The Hosmer NY Electric Elbow was designed at New York University by William Lembeck under the direction of Sidney Fishman.[27] The prototype of this mechanism was originally conceived for use by children and was evaluated in the 1970s. Subsequent modification of the prototype design and the involvement of the Hosmer Dorrance Corporation led to the commercialization of large- and medium-sized versions, introduced in 1983. The two sizes are equivalent to the E-400 and E-200 Hosmer Dorrance body-powered elbows, which can be alternatively fit to prostheses originally configured with the electric elbow. Hosmer Dorrance also introduced versions of the elbows for exo-

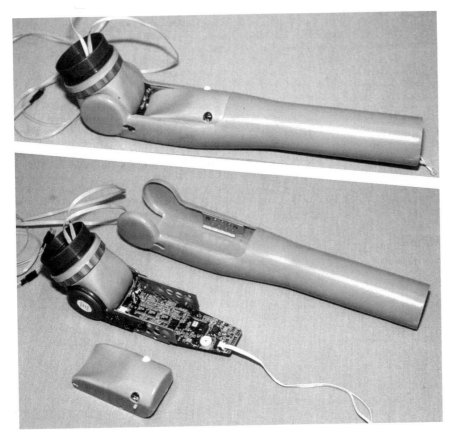

Figure 19 Liberating Technologies Boston Digital Arm System. Shown above is the complete elbow-forearm assembly. The lower photograph shows the forearm support frame and the programmable controller circuit board after the 12-V battery pack (bottom left) and forearm shell are removed. *(Courtesy of the Northwestern University Rehabilitation Engineering Research Program.)*

skeletal and endoskeletal applications (Figure 18).

The same motor and drive mechanism, which is contained in the elbow cap, is used for all versions of the elbow; therefore, mechanical performance characteristics are the same for all models. External dimensions, the turntable, and the forearm saddle attachments vary by model. The absence of fixed componentry in the forearm and the use of a forearm saddle provide considerable freedom in the length and customized shaping of the forearm section.

The elbow is powered by a separate battery pack, available in four and five AA-cell configurations, which can be positioned within the prosthesis as appropriate. Placement in the humeral section is preferable to placement in the forearm because additional weight in the forearm will

reduce the functional lift capacity, the maximum weight of an object that can be lifted by the elbow.

A pawl-type locking mechanism, placed in an early stage of the drive train, locks the elbow virtually anywhere through its 130° range. Locking is automatic whenever the control signal ceases. The elbow can also be made to swing freely by driving it to its fully extended position, at which point the free swing automatically engages. Once engaged, the elbow can be swung or pushed unpowered anywhere within its full range of motion. Free swing is disengaged by activation of the flexion control. Elbows can be equipped with or without the free swing feature, and elbows without free swing can be retrofit to incorporate it.

Two control options are available from Hosmer Dorrance: switch con-

trol using two-function electromechanical switches; and two-site, two-function myoswitch control. A variety of electromechanical switches are available from the manufacturer, including cable and harness pull switches and one-site and two-site push switches. Other switch configurations are also possible. Both the switch control and the myoswitch control operate the elbow at one speed. This speed cannot be adjusted and is determined by the battery voltage, the load on the elbow, and the direction of movement (the elbow is faster extending with gravity than lifting against gravity). The elbow can be used with controllers from other manufacturers, such as the VariGrip Controller from Liberating Technologies. This controller provides proportional control of the elbow and allows for a greater variety of input transducers.

Numerous configurations are possible using the electric elbow in conjunction with wrist and prehension components that have control sources separate from the source (or sources) operating the elbow. Hosmer Dorrance does not offer methods for integrating control of the elbow with other electric components, except its Hosmer NY PA. In configuration with the PA (Figure 13), the elbow can be operated by a three-function cable pull switch. The first two functions operate the elbow in flexion and extension, and the third function (with the switch control cable fully extended) operates the opening of the PA. The relatively light weight of the PA in combination with an aluminum split hook (compared with the weight of electric-powered prehensors in Tables 2 and 3) and the more proximal location of its center of mass help maximize the effective lift capacity of the NY Electric Elbow.

Liberating Technologies Boston Digital Arm System

The Boston Digital Arm System (Figure 19) is the third commercial model of the device originally known as the

Boston Elbow. The origins of this elbow date back to the 1960s in a cooperative research and development venture of the Liberty Mutual Insurance Company, the Liberty Mutual Research Center, the Massachusetts Institute of Technology, the Harvard University Medical School, and Massachusetts General Hospital.[36,37] The first prototypes were encouraging, but considerable development by the Liberty Mutual Research Center during the first half of the 1970s was necessary to produce a version that could be commercialized. Robert Jerard redesigned the original prototype, proving that a commercial version was feasible, and T. Walley Williams III implemented the commercialization and directed subsequent design alterations. Trials with the commercial elbow were begun in 1975, and the first Boston Elbows were made available in 1979. Since its introduction, the elbow system has undergone two major redesigns. In its present form as the Boston Digital Arm System, the system integrates a high-performance direct-drive electric elbow with a microprocessor-based controller capable of accepting a variety of input transducers and controlling up to five devices.

The electric elbow portion of the Boston Digital Arm System is available in one size and is configured with the motor and gearing within the elbow cap and the battery and electronics supported in a metal forearm frame. A prefabricated plastic forearm shell encloses and protects the forearm componentry and provides the wrist connection.

The drive mechanism includes a three-phase brushless motor with direct-drive gearing and a wave generator to achieve efficient gear reduction. Although a three-phase brushless motor requires additional control electronics, this type of motor offers higher overall performance (Table 4). The maximum live-lift capacity of the Boston Digital Arm System is more than three times that of the Utah Arm 2 with comparable average maximum speed characteristics.

A bidirectional, reverse locking clutch holds the position of the elbow whenever it is unpowered. The elbow can be locked in any position within its range of 135°. A free swing range of 45° of flexion from the stopped position of the elbow can be engaged and disengaged by manual operation of a mechanical slide bar.

Of the three adult electric elbows, the Boston Digital Arm System offers the greatest range of control options, including multicomponent control, through the programmability of its controller. The system can accept inputs from myoelectrodes, force-sensitive resistors, linear resistors, and switches. Depending on the number of physiologic control sources available from the user, the system can be configured to control the elbow, an electric prehension device, an electric wrist rotator, and two other electric components. Although it is preferable to use separate and independent control sources for each component, sequential control can be used when there are fewer control sources available to the user than components to be controlled. Proportional control schemes are preferable to take full advantage of the Boston Digital Arm System's electric elbow and high-performance prehension devices. However, when switch control is necessary, the Boston Digital Arm System can be programmed to limit the performance of devices to enable effective control by switches.

Control schemes for the Boston Digital Arm System continue to evolve in response to clinical fittings. Specific information on available control options is available from the manufacturer (Table 1).

Motion Control Utah Arm 2

The original Utah Artificial Arm was developed at the University of Utah in the latter half of the 1970s by a team led by Stephen Jacobsen, PhD. In its first clinical fitting in 1980, the system included the electric elbow mechanism and the control electronics developed by the Utah team and a body-powered voluntary-opening split-hook prehensor.[38] In 1982, Motion Control, Inc, the company formed to manufacture and market the Utah Arm, introduced a proportional myoelectric controller that allowed the elbow to be used in conjunction with an electric prehensor.[39,40] An additional control option, the force-actuated ServoPro, was introduced in the 1990s. During that decade, the electronics for the elbow and hand underwent major revision; the Utah Arm 2 was introduced in 1998 (Figure 20).

As it is presently configured, the Utah Arm 2 includes a motorized elbow mechanism, a friction-type humeral turntable, a forearm shell, and electronics for both the elbow and an optional electric prehension device. The prehensor control electronics can also operate a wrist rotator alternately with the prehensor.

The Utah Arm 2 is available in one size. The battery pack and elbow electronics are contained within the stationary (with respect to the humeral section) enclosure distal to the turntable. The motor, mechanical transmission, and prehensor electronics are located in the forearm section. The forearm shell is a finished injection-molded plastic enclosure that can be cut to a shorter length or lengthened by addition of an extension. Elbow rotation occurs about an axis through the anterior aspect of the joint. This placement allows flexion to approximately 150°, bringing the prehensor nearer to the face with less shoulder flexion than is possible with other elbow designs. Modularity of the electrical and mechanical assemblies is a hallmark of the Utah Arm 2, facilitating access for troubleshooting and replacement of subunits.

Two control options are available. The first is a two-site proportional myoelectric control. Switch control is not feasible because of the relatively high speed of the elbow, which is faster than 100°/s with an electric prehension device (Table 4). Nonlinear filtering of the myoelectric signals provides for quick response of the elbow to sudden high-amplitude

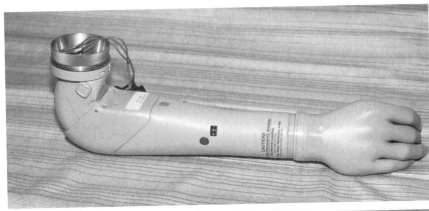

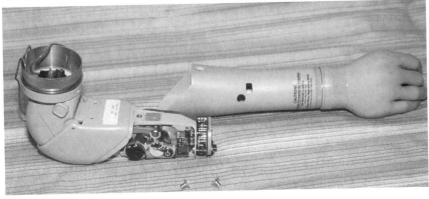

Figure 20 Motion Control Utah Arm 2. Shown above is the complete elbow-forearm assembly. In the lower photograph, the forearm cover has been removed, revealing the drive mechanism and the electronic prehensor controller (at the distal end of the drive assembly). The 12-V battery pack is in the elbow cap below the humeral turntable. *(Courtesy of the Northwestern University Rehabilitation Engineering Research Program.)*

changes in the control signals to achieve fast movements, yet smoother response for slower-changing lower amplitude signals used in more precise movements.

Locking of the elbow is engaged whenever it is held stationary for a set period of time (the length of which can be adjusted) or when a momentary switch is actuated. The elbow has 22 locked positions throughout its range of motion. Unlocking can be effected in several ways: by rapid co-contraction of the controlling muscles (rate control), by a slower contraction of at least one muscle (threshold control), or by actuation of the same momentary switch that can be used for locking. Lock control by the switch is always available. Rate control or threshold control of unlocking are mutually exclusive and are determined by an adjustment in the electronics.

Whenever the elbow is locked, the same myoelectric sources used to control the elbow are automatically channeled to proportionally control opening and closing of an electric prehension device. Unlocking the elbow by rate control returns control to the elbow without inadvertent operation of the prehensor. If an electric wrist rotator is used, an additional control switch is required to switch control between the prehensor and rotator while the elbow is locked. When the elbow is unlocked, neither the prehensor nor the rotator can be activated. This control scheme is referred to as sequential control because the same myoelectric sites control each of the devices and control is sequenced, under the direction of the user, from one device to another.

The second control option is the ServoPro controller. This control configuration uses a strain-gauge transducer fastened in line with a user's control harness. Pulling on the harness with forward flexion of the arm at the shoulder, in the case of a transhumeral fitting, or scapular abduction for a shoulder disarticulation fitting exerts a force on the transducer that is converted to a control signal. When in elbow control, the magnitude of the force on the transducer directly controls the angular position of the elbow. As with myoelectric control, the elbow is locked by holding it stationary for a short period of time. When locked, force on the transducer controls opening and closing of an electric prehensor. Unlocking and return to elbow control is effected by a quick hard pull on the transducer.

When the elbow is unlocked and no control signals are present, the elbow is in a powered free swing mode. The free swing is powered (unlike the free swing modes of the Boston Digital Arm System and the Hosmer NY Electric Elbow) because the drive transmission of the Utah elbow remains engaged during free swing. To overcome the electromechanical inertia of the drive mechanism, the motor actively flexes and extends the elbow, thus drawing battery current, as the arm is swung. The action of the motor is controlled by the response of a load cell transducer to the torque exerted on the forearm during body movements.

Commentary on Electric Elbows

Although the design and performance characteristics of electric elbows have been improved, the performance level remains below that of the physiologic elbow. Although it is not yet possible to truly restore elbow function with these prosthetic components, electric elbows can provide valuable function. There are significant differences among the elbows available. Consequently, the many attributes of each type—including factors such as weight and size, control options, integration into a complete prosthesis,

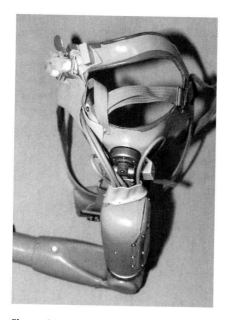

Figure 21 LTI-Collier Locking Shoulder Joint implemented in a left shoulder disarticulation prosthesis. *(Courtesy of the Northwestern University Rehabilitation Engineering Research Program.)*

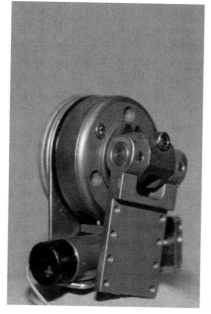
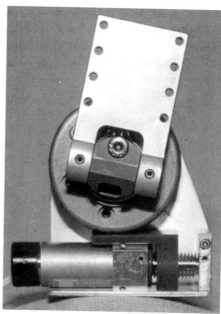

Figure 22 Liberating Technologies Motor-Drive Lock/Unlock Actuator and LTI-Collier Locking Shoulder Joint. On the right, the humeral attachment plate is abducted to show the motor and drive screw of the actuator. *(Courtesy of the Northwestern University Rehabilitation Engineering Research Program.)*

and capacity for being finished in a cosmetically acceptable form—should be considered in the decision to incorporate one in a fitting.

Enhancement of a Manual Shoulder Joint

No electric-powered mechanisms for positioning a prosthetic shoulder joint are commercially available. However, one locking shoulder joint, the LTI-Collier Locking Shoulder Joint, manufactured by Liberating Technologies, can be fit with an electric lock actuator. This is a two-degree-of-freedom shoulder joint (Figure 21). The adduction-abduction axis is hingelike with adjustable friction; however, the flexion-extension axis can be locked in 10° intervals.

In manual operation, the flexion-extension lock is spring-loaded to remain locked. Actuating a nudge control connected to a lock release lever disengages the lock, allowing the joint to swing relatively freely. While the joint is held unlocked, the user can flex the shoulder joint by simply leaning over so that gravity pulls the arm into flexion with respect to the body. When the nudge control is released, the lock reengages and the shoulder remains flexed as the user stands upright.

When the user cannot manually operate a nudge control or prefers an alternative way of controlling the lock, the nudge control and cable can be replaced by the Liberating Technologies Motor-Drive Lock/Unlock Actuator (Figure 22). The actuator can be operated with a switch or with a myoelectrode or force-sensitive resistor through an electronic controller. If the prosthesis includes the Boston Digital Arm System, the actuator can be controlled through this system with an appropriate input transducer.

Summary

Significant changes have occurred in the types and characteristics of electric-powered upper limb components since the publication of the second edition of the *Altas of Limb Prosthetics* in 1992. More device options, improved performance characteristics, and greater versatility in the implementation of control strategies are providing additional benefit to individuals with upper limb amputations. However, much remains to be done to develop prosthetic devices and control schemes that parallel physiologic performance and restore function. Although advances have been made, new developments are by no means inevitable. Many factors beyond technologic and conceptual breakthroughs must be integrated to create an environment that supports and encourages innovation and provides for the transfer of innovation into clinical practice. The speed with which this chapter is transformed from a state-of-the-art review to a historical footnote will be a measure not only of the technologic advances in our culture but also of the vitality and earnestness of the community working to improve the capabilities of persons who use upper limb prostheses.

References

1. Peizer E, Wright DW, Mason C, Pirello T Jr: Guidelines for standards for externally powered hands. *Bull Prosthet Res* 1969;10-12:118-155.

2. Childress DS: Artificial hand mecha-

nisms, in *Proceedings of the Mechanisms Conference and International Symposium on Gearing and Transmissions.* Fairfield, NJ, American Society of Mechanical Engineers, 1972, pp 1-11.

3. Näder M: The artificial substitution of missing hands with myoelectrical prostheses. *Clin Orthop* 1990;258:9-17.

4. Alpenfels EJ: The anthropology and social significance of the human hand. *Artif Limbs* 1955;2:4-21.

5. Simpson DC: The functioning hand, the human advantage. *J R Coll Surg Edinb* 1976;21:329-340.

6. Simpson DC: Functional requirements and systems of control for powered prostheses. *Biomed Eng* 1966;1:250-256.

7. Northmore-Ball MD, Heger H, Hunter G: The below-elbow myo-electric prosthesis: A comparison of the Otto Bock myo-electric prosthesis with the hook and functional hand. *J Bone Joint Surg Br* 1980;62:363-367.

8. Chan KM, Lee SY, Leung KK, Leung PC: A medical-social study of upper limb amputees in Hong Kong: A preliminary report. *Orthot Prosthet* 1984;37:43-48.

9. Billock JN: Upper limb prosthetic terminal devices: Hands versus hooks. *Clin Prosthet Orthot* 1986;10:57-65.

10. Millstein SG, Heger H, Hunter GA: Prosthetic use in adult upper limb amputees: A comparison of the body powered and electrically powered prostheses. *Prosthet Orthot Int* 1986;10:27-34.

11. Kemp MC: Design and development of an electrically powered prosthetic gripper, in *Proceedings of the First International Workshop on Robotic Applications in Medical and Health Care.* Ottawa, Canada, National Research Council Canada, 1988, pp 19.1-19.5.

12. Datta D, Kingston J, Ronald J: Myoelectric prostheses for below-elbow amputees: The Trent experience. *Int Disabil Stud* 1989;11:167-170.

13. Schlesinger G: Der Mechanische Aufbau der künstlichen Glieder, in *Ersatzglieder und Arbeitshilfen, Part 2.* Berlin, Germany, Springer-Verlag, 1919.

14. Keller AD, Taylor CL, Zahm V: *Studies to Determine the Functional Requirements for Hand and Arm Prostheses.* Los Angeles, CA, University of California, Department of Engineering, 1947.

15. Toth PJ: *Hand Function Differentiation.* Evanston, IL, Northwestern University, 1991. Thesis.

16. van Lunteren A, van Lunteren-Gerritsen GHM, Stassen HG, Zuithoff MJ: A field evaluation of arm prostheses for unilateral amputees. *Prosthet Orthot Int* 1983;7:141-151.

17. Taylor CL: The biomechanics of the normal and of the amputated upper extremity, in Klopsteg PE, Wilson PD (eds): *Human Limbs and Their Substitutes.* New York, NY, McGraw-Hill International Book Co, 1954.

18. Mathiowetz V, Kashman N, Volland G, Weber K, Dowe M, Rogers S: Grip and pinch strength: Normative data for adults. *Arch Phys Med Rehabil* 1985;66:69-74.

19. Imrhan SN: Trends in finger pinch strength in children, adults, and the elderly. *Hum Factors* 1989;31:689-701.

20. Taylor CL: Control design and prosthetic adaptations to biceps and pectoral cineplasty, in Klopsteg PE, Wilson PD (eds): *Human Limbs and Their Substitutes.* New York, NY, McGraw-Hill International Book Co, 1954.

21. Michael JW: Upper limb powered components and controls: Current concepts. *Clin Prosthet Orthot* 1986;10:66-77.

22. Puchhammer G: The tactile slip sensor: Integration of a miniaturized sensory device on a myoelectric hand. *Orthop-Tech Quarterly* 2000;7-12.

23. Dietl H, Gröpel W: Versorgung nach Teilhandamputationen mit myoelektrischen Komponenten. *Orthop-Tech* 2001;1:21-23.

24. Childress DS: An approach to powered grasp, in Gavrilovic M, Wilson AB Jr (eds): *Proceedings of the Fourth International Symposium on Advances in External Control of Human Extremities.* Dubrovnik, Yugoslavia, Yugoslav Committee for Electronics and Automation, 1972, pp 159-167.

25. Childress DS, Grahn EC: Development of a powered prehensor, in *Proceedings of the 38th Annual Conference of Engineering in Medicine and Biology.* Chicago, IL, The Alliance for Engineering in Medicine and Biology, 1985, p 50.

26. Childress DS, Strysik JS: Controller for a high-performance prehensor, in *Proceedings of the 23rd Annual Rocky Mountain Bioengineering Symposium.* Columbia, MO, Instrument Society of America, 1986, pp 65-67.

27. Prout W: The New York Electric Elbow, the New York Prehension Actuator, and the NU-VA Synergetic Prehensor, in Atkins DJ, Meier RH (eds): *Comprehensive Management of the Upper-Limb Amputee.* New York, NY, Springer-Verlag, 1989.

28. Engen TJ, Spencer WA: *Development of Externally Powered Upper Extremity Orthotics, Final Report.* Houston, TX, Texas Institute for Rehabilitation and Research, 1969.

29. Morrey BF, Askew LJ, An KN, Chao EY: A biomechanical study of normal functional elbow motion. *J Bone Joint Surg Am* 1981;63:872-877.

30. Palmer AK, Werner FW, Murphy D, Glisson R: Functional wrist motion: A biomechanical study. *J Hand Surg Am* 1985;10:39-46.

31. Safaee-Rad R, Shwedyk E, Quanbury AO, Cooper JE: Normal functional range of motion of upper limb joints during performance of three feeding activities. *Arch Phys Med Rehabil* 1990;71:505-509.

32. Doubler JA: *An Analysis of Extended Physiological Proprioception as a Control Technique for Upper-Extremity Prostheses.* Evanston, IL, Northwestern University, 1982. Dissertation.

33. Komi PV: Relationship between muscle tension, EMG and velocity of contraction under concentric and eccentric work, in Desmedt JE (ed): *New Developments in Electromyography and Clinical Neurophysiology, Vol 1.* Basel, Switzerland, S Karger AG, 1973.

34. Jørgensen K, Bankov S: Maximum strength of elbow flexors with pronated and supinated forearm, in *Medicine and Sport, Vol 6, Biomechanics II.* Basel, Switzerland, S Karger AG, 1971.

35. Pertuzon E, Bouisset S: Maximum velocity of movement and maximum velocity of muscle shortening, in *Medicine and Sport, Vol 6, Biomechanics II.* Basel, Switzerland, S Karger AG, 1971.

36. Tanenbaum SJ: *The Boston Elbow—Health Technology Case Study 29.* Report OTA-HCS-29. Washington, DC, U.S. Congress, Office of Technology Assessment, 1984.

37. Williams TW: Use of the Boston elbow for high-level amputees, in Atkins DJ,

Meier RH (eds): *Comprehensive Management of the Upper-Limb Amputee.* New York, NY, Springer-Verlag, 1989.

38. Jacobsen SC, Knutti DF, Johnson RT, Sears HH: Development of the Utah artificial arm. *IEEE Trans Biomed Eng* 1982;29:249-269.

39. Sears HH, Andrew JT, Jacobsen SC: Clinical experience with the Utah Artificial Arm, in *The Canadian Association of Prosthetists and Orthotists Yearbook.* 1984, pp 30-33.

40. Sears HH, Andrew JT, Jacobsen SC: Experience with the Utah Arm, hand, and terminal device, in Atkins DJ, Meier RH (eds): *Comprehensive Management of the Upper-Limb Amputee.* New York, NY, Springer-Verlag, 1989.

Chapter 12

Control of Limb Prostheses

Dudley S. Childress, PhD
Richard F. ff. Weir, PhD

Introduction

This chapter deals primarily with control of externally powered (electric-powered) prostheses. Prostheses that are entirely cable-actuated and body-powered are covered in chapter 9, as are the various control schemes of cable-operated prostheses. Nevertheless, cable-operated systems will also be considered in this discussion because of the many ways they can be used in conjunction with externally powered components. Particularly with prostheses for high-level unilateral and bilateral limb loss, the systems of choice often use hybrid control (cable, myoelectric, switches, or some combination of these or other methods) and hybrid power (electric- and body-powered). Additionally, powered systems can be set up to emulate cable systems as a form of boosted control. For individuals with high-level bilateral limb loss, we often recommend fitting one arm with body power and the opposite limb with electric power.[1] Consequently, any general discussion of control systems for individuals with arm loss should include both body power and cable control.

Until fairly recently, discussions of limb prosthesis control generally focused on upper limb prostheses. Only rarely was control of lower limbs the topic (an exception was emphasis on extension of the thigh to control extension of a knee mechanism in transfemoral prostheses). With lower limbs, discussion centered primarily on interface loads, suspension, and alignment because the lower limb must bear significant loads and its activity is highly repetitive and stylized. However, recent success using microprocessors in artificial knee joints has heightened the consideration given to the control of lower limbs.

Microprocessor control of a knee prosthesis is often a reflex control that is more or less automatic. By monitoring the state of the knee in stance phase (how much it is bent, which direction it is bending, and how fast it is bending) and by monitoring the location of the ground-reaction force with respect to the knee, a properly programmed microprocessor can adjust knee stiffness to keep the user from falling or to facilitate the walking cycle. The same can be done during swing phase. Microprocessor control at the knee provides a type of artificial reflex control that occurs automatically. The user is not aware of the control decisions that are constantly being made. Artificial reflex control can be particularly advantageous in the control of knee stiffness during walking. Artificial reflex control can also be effective in upper limb control systems. The automatic control of prehension force in the Otto Bock SensorHand (Otto Bock, Duderstadt, Germany) is one example of artificial reflex control in upper limb components. The gripping force of this hand is increased automatically if a sensor detects that the object being held is slipping out of the grip.

Reflex action in a prosthesis (upper or lower limb) can reduce the mental load on the user by removing the user from the control loop while improving performance of the artificial limb. Figure 1 shows how feedback occurs in human-prosthesis systems. With control interface feedback, the operator receives feedback via the same channel through which the prosthesis is controlled (eg, the control cable of a body-powered prosthesis). Because control interface feedback is usually in a form easily interpreted by the user, it can be interpreted at a subconscious level, reducing the mental burden on the user. Artificial reflexes are closed loops within the controller/prosthesis mechanism itself that seek to remove the operator from the control loop altogether, and hence also relieve the mental load. Such systems use onboard intelligence to automatically respond to some external sensor input. Incorporation of artificial reflexes in many kinds of prosthetic limbs will likely increase over the next decade. Most powered upper limb prostheses receive feedback primarily through visual feedback with some assistance from incidental feedback (feedback that is incidental rather than by design, such as motor whine, prosthesis

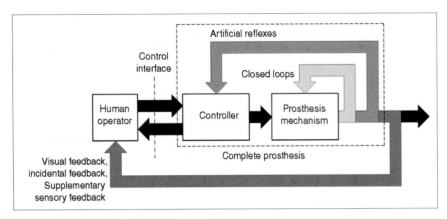

Figure 1 Feedback in human-prosthesis systems.

vibration, socket forces, etc). Supplementary sensory feedback may be provided through the use of vibrations to the skin, pressure to the skin, electrical stimulation of the skin, by auditory cues, and by other means. Because these methods are supplementary to normal sensory feedback paths, however, the feedback is not presented in a physiologically useful manner. Closed loops are feedback pathways to improve the performance of the mechanism itself, such as position or velocity control. Microprocessors are relatively inexpensive and can run on low power in many prosthetic applications. A key issue for the success of these types of automatic control systems is user confidence. Users will not relinquish control unless they have high confidence in the system. The mechanisms must also be fail-safe so that limbs will not collapse in the event of electronic controller failure.

Several similarities exist between upper limb prosthesis control and lower limb control. An individual with a transtibial prosthesis, for example, has awareness (mostly via the intact knee joint) of where the artificial limb is in space, how fast the shank is moving, and what forces are acting on the limb. The transradial cosmetic prosthesis (or myoelectric prosthesis) acts in a similar fashion. The intact elbow joint informs the user of the position of the arm in space and its angular velocity and provides information concerning forces acting on the limb. The trans-

tibial prosthesis with a foot and the transradial prosthesis with a cosmetic hand are essentially similar in structure. Both have passive terminal devices, one a passive foot and the other a passive hand. However, if the passive hand is replaced by an active hand—perhaps one controlled myoelectrically—the focus of attention is usually the control of opening and closing the hand. Hence, myoelectric control can divert attention from the fact that the elbow joint is largely responsible for the somewhat natural control of the transradial prosthesis, just as the knee is the source of the natural control of the transtibial prosthesis. The next decade of transtibial prostheses may well have electronic controls of the ankle and foot, which may similarly divert attention from the importance of the knee joint in providing natural control of the transtibial prosthesis.

Goals for Limb Prosthesis Control

Several highly desirable attributes of control systems for limb prostheses merit discussion. Although some may be difficult if not impossible to achieve in practice, keeping these ideals in mind is important to stimulate continued improvement and development of control systems. These attributes are (1) low mental loading or subconscious control, (2) user-friendliness, (3) independence in multifunctional control, (4) simulta-

neous and coordinated control of multiple functions, (5) near-instantaneous response, (6) noninterference with the individual's remaining functional abilities, and (7) a natural appearance and quiet movement.

First, the system should have low mental loading or subconscious control; that is, the prosthesis can be used without much thought by the user. Successful control systems enable individuals to engage their artificial limbs almost subconsciously, the way people commonly use their limbs. The prosthesis should serve rather than dominate the user. The user should be able to think about other things while using the prosthesis. This kind of control will require proprioceptive and sensory feedback of the right modality, which often can be obtained simply by making the limb an extension of the most distal remaining joint of the body, as is the case with transtibial and transradial prostheses. Artificial reflex actions, such as those of the SensorHand, will also help improve subconscious control by transferring the effort involved in monitoring the device from the user to the device controller.

Second, the control should be user-friendly, or simple to learn to use. Learning to control the prosthesis should be intuitive and natural. This kind of control should enable people to learn quickly and easily how to use the prosthesis. This is one reason why myoelectric control for the person with a transradial amputation has been so successful. Physiologically and intuitively appropriate control actions are used to control the artificial hand because the extrinsic muscles of the hand reside in the forearm. This concept of appropriate control sites is at the heart of the surgical procedure advanced by Kuiken and associates[2] to reinnervate a section of muscle tissue with nerves that control the forearm musculature.

Third, independent control of a function should be provided without activating or interfering with other control systems of a multifunctional prosthesis. For example, a person with prostheses on both arms should be able to use each limb independently. Operation of one prosthesis should not cause unintended activity of the prosthesis on the opposite side. A common example of failure of independent action is in typical cable-operated, body-powered transhumeral prostheses with a voluntary opening hook. If the user attempts to lift a heavy load, the hook tends to open during the lifting process. In bilateral cable-operated prostheses, flexion of one arm can generate unintended flexion in the other arm as well.

Fourth, coordinated, simultaneous control of multiple functions in effective and meaningful ways, without excessive mental effort, is one of the amazing aspects of control of the human hand and arm. This capability, which is currently not available in practical prostheses, subsumes many of the other desirable attributes.

Fifth, prosthetic systems should respond quickly to inputs so that time delays between input and output are not noticeable to the user. All functions should be directly accessible to the user, without perceived time delays. Delays greater than 100 ms are readily perceptible. Simultaneous action of various joints may require even quicker actions in a prosthesis; 50 ms is a desirable objective.

Sixth, a control system should not sacrifice the user's remaining functional abilities. Control systems should never encumber any natural movements that can be applied to useful purposes. In general, it is unwise to sacrifice any useful natural body function for the control of a prosthesis. The prosthesis should be used to supplement, not limit, available functional ability.

Last, the control system should have a natural appearance and quiet movement. A control system should not detract from the appearance of the limb, either statically or dynamically. Aesthetically pleasing movements affect prosthesis appearance just as size, shape, and color do. De-sirable movements are compliant, silent, and do not appear mechanical.

Although this list of desirable control attributes for prostheses can certainly be extended, many are difficult to achieve with current technology and knowledge of human-machine control. In reality, these attributes are essentially control attributes exhibited by the human hand/arm system. The ideal system would be biomimetic, but because such a system is not feasible at this time from an engineering standpoint, prosthetists and designers must decide where to focus their efforts.

Design Considerations

What should be controlled by prosthesis control systems depends heavily on the philosophic approach taken to artificial limb design. If the objective is to design an artificial arm that emulates a human arm as closely as possible, a designer/developer might want to control joint compliance[3,4] and other variables in an attempt to make the prosthetic limb exhibit several characteristics of the human arm/hand system. However, if at this stage of arm/hand prosthesis development good biomimetic designs are not clinically viable, then other approaches need to be considered, at least for the near future. If designers of prostheses truly want to help people with limb loss over the next several decades, they should take a clinical approach and design prostheses that effectively are tools that assist with activities of daily living.[5] It may be desirable for the tool to look like an arm/hand as well as function like one, but appearance and function sometimes conflict.

Practical issues of prosthesis design also support the "tool" approach to arm prostheses. When an individual stands erect and holds a heavy object in the hand with the elbow bent at 90°, for example, muscular action and expenditure of energy is required at the elbow. If an electric-powered arm prosthesis were used in this way, the battery would be depleted rather quickly even though no external work is being performed. A design compromise such as a mechanically locking elbow would be appropriate. Although this control choice of a lockable joint is not biomimetic, it is practical.

This chapter concentrates on controls and systems that enable people to use prostheses primarily as assistive tools. The goal is to help those with upper limb loss at least regain basic functions such as reaching, grasping, and holding.

Control Variables

Joints of a prosthesis need to move freely so that the limb can be maneuvered easily into the desired position for operation. It may also be advantageous to control the rate of movement (velocity) to the desired position. Once the limb is in position, prehension force can be controlled. And when a desirable position is reached, it may be advantageous to lock specific joints, perhaps all of them. Thus, the variables to be controlled in arm prostheses include position, velocity, prehension force, and joint status (locked or free).

In many situations (eg, pushing), it is advantageous for a prosthetic arm to be completely rigid (all joints positively locked). In other instances, such as walking, the joints of an upper limb prosthesis need to be free so that the artificial limb(s) can swing somewhat naturally with the gait cycle.

Control of upper limbs usually brings to mind functions such as positioning (reaching), grasping/releasing, and lifting/holding. However, the ability to make joints rigid or free is also an important function to be controlled in practical arm prostheses. In the future, continuous control of the stiffness of joints from the free state to the locked state may be possible. At the present time, however, only the free (ie, very low friction) and locked (ie, extremely high friction) conditions are practical to

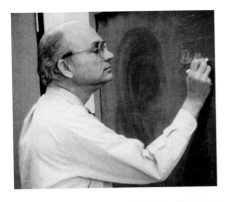

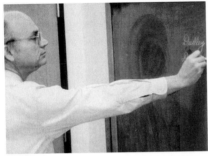

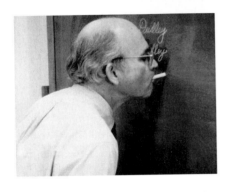

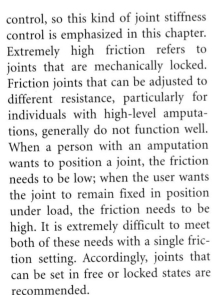

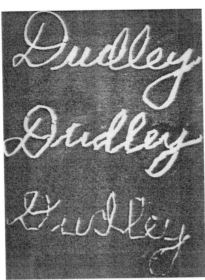

Figure 2 Different sets of muscles can be used to achieve similar results, illustrating a principle described by Bernstein[6] in 1967. The upper signature was written using primarily muscles of the hand. In the center photograph, the corresponding signature was generated primarily with muscles of the shoulder. The bottom photograph demonstrates creation of the lower signature with primarily leg and torso movements transmitted to the chalkboard by the semirigid connection of chalk, teeth, and neck. The lower signature could also have been written using neck motions. This signature is not as smoothly written because of the friction between the chalk and the board and lack of a mouthpiece to stabilize the chalk in the mouth.

or attached in some way to the head, arms, or hands. Simpson[7] called this approach extended physiological proprioception (EPP). This principle is used in transtibial prostheses, in the walking cane, in the long cane (for vision impairment), in mouthsticks, and, of course, by anyone who plays tennis, squash, baseball, or golf, or who uses hammers or screwdrivers. This powerful principle provides a practical guide for building and controlling limb prostheses. The approach is also useful in designing and developing aids for individuals to cope with various disabling conditions. New York artist Chuck Close, who became paralyzed at the height of his career, was told by his therapist that he didn't paint with his hands, he painted with his brain. Some observers believe that Close paints even better without control of his hands.

Sources of Body Inputs to Prosthesis Controllers

The human body generates a variety of control signals that can be used to operate prostheses.[8] Inputs typically come from muscular activity—directly, indirectly through joints, and indirectly through by-products of muscular contraction (eg, myoelectricity, myoacoustics, muscle bulge, tendon tightening, changes in muscle hardness/softness with contraction, or changes in the electrical impedance of muscle mass with contraction). Signals also can be obtained from brain waves (electroencephalograms), voice, feet, eyes, and tongue; however, very few of these sources of control have proved practical in daily applications with artificial limbs. The most common control options (Table 1) are classified as two types, biomechanical and bioelectric/acoustic.

The biomechanical sources listed in Table 1 have been used extensively with good results for control of body-powered prostheses. This kind of control is somewhat similar to that used by a pilot in a stunt plane. Through a

control, so this kind of joint stiffness control is emphasized in this chapter. Extremely high friction refers to joints that are mechanically locked. Friction joints that can be adjusted to different resistance, particularly for individuals with high-level amputations, generally do not function well. When a person with an amputation wants to position a joint, the friction needs to be low; when the user wants the joint to remain fixed in position under load, the friction needs to be high. It is extremely difficult to meet both of these needs with a single friction setting. Accordingly, joints that can be set in free or locked states are recommended.

If the elbow and wrist of a transhumeral prosthesis are locked and the grasp is secure, the user can easily hammer nails or push heavy objects with the prosthesis, provided the limb is fairly rigid with respect to the torso. Torso motion can be used quite naturally to strike objects such as nails with a prosthesis that is rigid and firmly attached to the torso. Similarly, if the joints of a shoulder disarticulation prosthesis are locked, the natural motion of the torso can be extended through the prosthesis to produce rather natural control (assuming secure grasp). Figure 2 illustrates the principle described by Bernstein[6] that similar results can be achieved by different sets of muscles. Holding the chalk rigidly, the author can write his name by moving the torso with the legs. It is well known that some painters paint extremely well using stick extensions (brushes) in their mouth

control stick and cables, the pilot can easily control flight surfaces of the aircraft. The cables provide feedback on the position, velocity, and force associated with the flight surfaces. The controller enables the airplane and pilot to be somewhat united. Another illustration of this kind of control through cables is the hand brakes of a bicycle.

The same kind of inputs can be used with some powered prostheses (boosted control). In fact, increased flexibility can be obtained for these inputs with powered prostheses because force/excursion requirements can often be relaxed considerably when using powered components (eg, with power steering in automobiles).

Biomechanical inputs can be interfaced with prostheses in many ways other than using Bowden cables; however, not all of these methods provide the level of feedback that Bowden cables produce. Basically, a force or movement of a body part (eg, residual limb, chin/head, etc) is used to move a mechanical lever to operate an electric switch, activate an electronic switch, push on a pressure-sensitive transducer, or otherwise operate some kind of position, force, or touch/proximity transducer.

Transducers

Many types of transducers can detect biomechanical signals (force or excursion) and turn them into electrical signals for control purposes. These types include mechanical switches, which require both force and excursion to turn on or off, sensitive transducers, which change their resistance when force is applied yet have essentially no excursion (isometric); and excursion transducers, which measure distance but require essentially no force. Some of these transducers are described in greater detail in chapter 11.

Switches

Electrical switches are applicable to many prosthetic systems and can often be used interchangeably. However, care must be exercised when attempting to use transducers, and sometimes even simple switches, with control systems for which they were not designed or are not compatible. Specifications for voltage amplitude, voltage polarity, electrical impedance, and wiring connections must be met before transducers can be inserted into control systems for which they may not originally have been designed.

Rocker and push-button switches can be operated easily by pressing against them with a body movement. Switches are easy to use, simple, and inexpensive. In addition, their assembly into a whole prosthesis is fairly intuitive. Unfortunately, switch control is not always sufficient to achieve good prosthesis control.

Switches also can provide multiple functions from one source. One frequently used push-button switch produces one function when pushed part way and another function when pushed in completely. In this manner, the two functions of a powered prosthetic joint or prehensor can be controlled with a switch mechanism that is activated by only one control source. Switch inputs can be arranged with electronics so that codes can be used to produce certain prosthetic functions. A wide variety of control schemes are possible with simple switches and electronics though not all are practical.

TABLE 1 Control Options

Biomechanical Sources
Movement/force from a body joint or multiple joints (position, force/pressure)
- Chin and head force/movement
- Glenohumeral flexion/extension
- Glenohumeral abduction/adduction
- Biscapular and scapular abduction
- Shoulder elevation/depression
- Chest expansion
- Elbow or wrist movement

Direct force/motion from muscle
- Force/motion from muscle with a tunnel cineplasty
- Force/motion from skin that is adherent to underlying muscle
- Krukenberg surgical procedure (long transradial amputation)

Bioelectric/Acoustic Sources
Myoelectric potentials (muscle electricity)
Myoacoustic (muscle sounds)
Neuroelectric potentials (neuron and nerve signals)

Integrated Versus Modular Prosthetics Systems

One way to approach prosthetic limb control systems is to break down upper limb prosthetics systems into joints (powered and nonpowered components), control systems, transducers, and other parts rather than considering the system as a whole. A key advantage of the modular approach is flexibility in system design. Modularity is practical because different parts can be substituted as a client's needs change. However, the modular approach may not attain the highest functional goals. Only systems designed from an integrated standpoint can truly be optimized. Systems that use force input from the user to the controller, for example, need powered components with very low backlash and very low static friction if they are to work well without exhibiting limit cycle behavior.[9]

Myoelectric Control

Myoelectric control is the control of a prosthesis or other system through the use of "muscle electricity." The control source is a small electrical potential from an active muscle. This electrical potential is electronically processed to activate a switch controller or a proportional controller of power to an electric motor, which in turn drives the prosthetic system (eg,

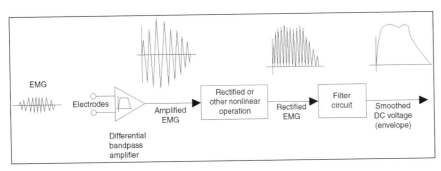

Figure 3 Diagram of myoelectric signal (EMG) processing in a typical myoelectric control system. Three "dry" metal electrodes are always associated with each differential amplifier. The small AC potential from the muscle is amplified, band limited, and changed into a DC potential by full-wave rectification, squaring, root mean squaring, or some other appropriate nonlinear processing. In a typical circuit, this DC potential is commonly smoothed with a low-pass filter to obtain the envelope of the EMG signal. The smoothed DC voltage can be compared in a logic circuit with a threshold voltage. If the smoothed DC voltage is greater than the threshold voltage, power is supplied to the prosthesis motor; if not, the motor remains off.

hand or elbow). Muscle electricity is a by-product of muscle action, just as mechanical noise is a by-product of an internal combustion engine. The electrical signal may be picked up with electrodes on the surface of the body as well as internal wire/needle electrodes or telemetry implants. Surface electrodes are currently the only practical way to receive myoelectric signals for prosthesis control because the electrodes are used for long periods of time every day and hence must be benign to skin and tissues. The surface method of detection of muscle activity is aptly illustrated in the standard electrocardiogram (ECG), which is the electromyogram (EMG) of the heart muscle. A gel-type electrolyte is usually applied to the skin during ECG procedures to lower the electrical resistance of the skin. With prosthesis control, however, gel electrolyte is not recommended because of possible skin irritation with long-term use. Consequently, inert metal electrodes such as stainless steel are usually used in myoelectric prostheses. Although they are often called "dry" electrodes because of the absence of electrode paste (conductive gel), they are not truly dry because the body's own perspiration serves as a reasonably good electrolyte for the electrodes, eliminating the need for conductive pastes.

Just as with an ECG, with a myoelectric prosthesis, special care must be taken to reduce the influence of environmental electrical signals such as broadcast waves, fluorescent lights, motor arcing, and power lines that may cause the prosthesis to operate inadvertently. These interference signals may be many times larger than the myoelectric signal itself. A typical surface EMG may have a peak-to-peak amplitude of around 100 µV, whereas noise signals may be a thousand times greater. The electrical noise can be eliminated for the most part by good electronic circuitry that features differential amplification, filtering, and thresholding, and by good electrode positioning and design techniques. To reduce electrical noise pick-up, the electronic amplifiers are often packaged together with the metal electrodes so that the connecting wires between the electrodes and the amplifiers are extremely short (Figure 3). When the electronic amplifier or the amplifier and processor electronics are put into a single package with the metal electrodes on the outside, the whole package is often called an electrode; however, only the metal parts that interface with the user's skin are the actual electrodes.

The characteristics of myoelectric signals and the processing of myoelectric signals for use in prosthesis control have been described exten-

sively in the literature. Good technical sources for information in this area are the review of myoelectric control by Parker and Scott[10] and the discussion of myoelectric signals by Basmajian and DeLuca.[11] Scott[12] authored an elementary introduction to myoelectric prostheses, including control, and a comprehensive bibliography concerning myoelectric control of limb prostheses was prepared by Scott and Childress.[13]

The use of myoelectric control in arm prostheses has increased dramatically during the last two decades. Although some may consider this technique a result of space-age electronics and integrated circuits, in reality the first myoelectric control system was built in Germany in the 1940s.[14] The concept is thus 60 years old, much older than the solid-state electronics that made the method ultimately practical. The early German system and an early British system[15] were designed with vacuum-tube electronic technology. British scientists[16,17] were instrumental in advancing the concepts of myoelectric control early on and constructed some novel circuitry. Soviet scientists were the first to design a transistorized myoelectric system that could be carried on the body.[18] Collaboration between a German company, Otto Bock, and an Austrian hearing aid company, Viennatone, led to the first transradial myoelectric system commercially available in the United States. Many other commercial myoelectric systems have followed (see chapter 11).

Because no control inputs within our common daily experience are analogous to those of myoelectric control, it will be described more fully here than the more intuitive biomechanical control approaches. Electricity from skeletal muscles appears with voluntary muscle contraction. This voluntary control is one of the excellent attributes of myoelectric control. A myoelectrically controlled system will work only when the person with an amputation generates voluntary muscle action. Such a system is immune to influence from external forces, prosthesis location, or body position/motion. Similarly, myoelectric prostheses should be unaffected by external electrical interference (noise) except for very exceptional environmental circumstances.

The myoelectric signal itself is a somewhat randomly shaped signal that comes from the spatial and temporal summation of the asynchronous firing of single motor units within the muscle. It is a kind of electrical interference pattern that results from the electrical depolarization of thousands of muscle fibers (perhaps several hundred per motor unit for typical forearm muscle action) when they are activated by motoneurons. This electric wave can only be described statistically because its amplitude and frequency are constantly varying, even when an individual holds muscle action as constant as possible. However, the general range of amplitude and the dominant frequency of a typical surface signal are both 100 (100 µV for peak-to-peak amplitude and 100 Hz for the approximate frequency of maximum energy). The voltage of a typical surface EMG is roughly one million times less than that of electrical wiring in a typical home in the United States. This voltage can be amplified by increased muscle action or reduced all the way to zero when the muscle is inactive. There is very little energy in a surface EMG greater than about 400 Hz.

In electronic design, amplification of the voltage of the surface EMG up to a level of from 1 to 10 V is frequently desirable. An amplification of 10,000 to 100,000 (1.0/0.0001 or 10.0/0.0001) is needed to accomplish this increase. To avoid noise amplification as much as possible, bandpass differential amplifiers are used so that voltages common to the two inputs (common-mode voltages) are rejected and so that amplification is most effective for frequencies around 100 Hz. No amplification is necessary greater than about 400 Hz for control purposes because the signal above this frequency is relatively low. Frequen-cies less than about 10 Hz are often not amplified to any extent so that slow polarization voltage changes that may occur over time at the electrode-skin interface are not amplified; this may be of special importance with "dry" electrodes.

A myoelectrically controlled prosthesis can only function in its normal fashion when all the electrodes are positioned properly on the body. All electrodes should remain in contact with the skin at all times during prosthesis use. If electrodes lose contact with the skin, lack of control and/or electrical interference may occur. For this reason, the prosthetist should fabricate a diagnostic prosthesis with a clear plastic socket that allows observation of the electrodes while the prosthesis is used in different positions and under various loading conditions. The socket should be designed so that the electrodes maintain contact with the skin for all reasonable external load applications, prosthesis positions, and movement velocities.

The body acts as an antenna, picking up electrical noise from the environment. Consequently, "tipping" (touching the exposed electrodes with the fingers) introduces electrical noise through the fingers to the electrodes and into the electronics. There are no myoelectric signals in the fingertips because there are no muscles in the fingers. The "tipping" response should not be interpreted to mean that the electrode is a touch sensor or a pressure sensor in regular use; it is not. When touched, the myoelectric system responds to the stray electrical noise present on the body coming from radio and television broadcasting, fluorescent lights, electric motors, etc. Tipping is often used to demonstrate the general action of the prosthesis when it is not on the body; however, an expected response to touching the electrodes does not necessarily mean that the myoelectric system is completely functional. Malfunctioning amplifiers may respond to tipping even when they no longer function correctly as differential am-plifiers. Although a correct tipping response is necessary, it is not a sufficient test to determine if a myoelectric prosthesis is functioning properly.

In a myoelectric system, amplification is followed by electronic processing that usually turns the myoelectric signal, an AC potential, into a DC potential of a given polarity (in Figure 3, the DC potential is positive). The envelope of this DC potential goes up and down as the myoelectric signal increases or decreases in amplitude, that is, as the muscle action increases or decreases. Electronic logic circuitry can be designed so that if the DC potential is greater than some threshold voltage (such as 1.0 V), then the circuit will turn on an electronic switch that allows electric power to flow to the prosthesis motor. The result of contracting a muscle to a certain level thus results in power delivery to the driving motor of the hand or arm. If the DC potential falls below the threshold, the power to the motor is turned off.

In myoelectric control, power to the motor is provided by the voltage and current from the battery, not the electricity from muscles. The myoelectric signal is used only for control purposes. In actuality, the electronics of myoelectric control systems vary with each manufacturer. Some have circuits that enable the power to be applied to the motor in a manner proportional to the myoelectric signal amplitude. Some can turn the motor on and also reverse its direction of action (polarity/rotation) while using only one myoelectric control site. Others use two or more myoelectric control sites to effect action of a motor or motors. The system depicted in Figure 4 is a typical transradial myoelectric prosthesis with a generic design for a two-site, two-function myoelectric control system.

In two-site or multisite EMG systems, after the EMG has been amplified, band-limited, and "enveloped," a decision block is needed to determine which EMG signal should be used for control so that the appropriate mo-

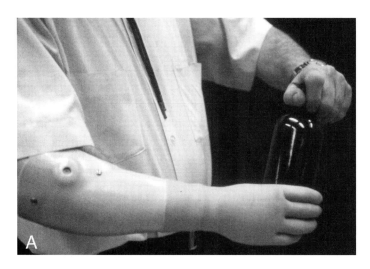

Figure 4 A, Use of a transradial myoelectric prosthesis. The system uses two myoelectric sites on the residual limb. **B,** Diagram of signal flow in a typical two-site, two-function myoelectric hand prosthesis. A two-site system must have a method of determining which of the two incoming signals to use to drive the motor. One method is to use a drive signal proportional to the magnitude of the difference between the two incoming signals and send it to the motor—the "most-on" method. An alternative is the "first-on," or lockout method. With the first-on method, the first signal to cross an "on" threshold is sent to the motor; any other signal is ignored, (locked out) until the "on" signal level drops below a second "off" threshold. Both on-off (digital) and proportional control of hands are possible.

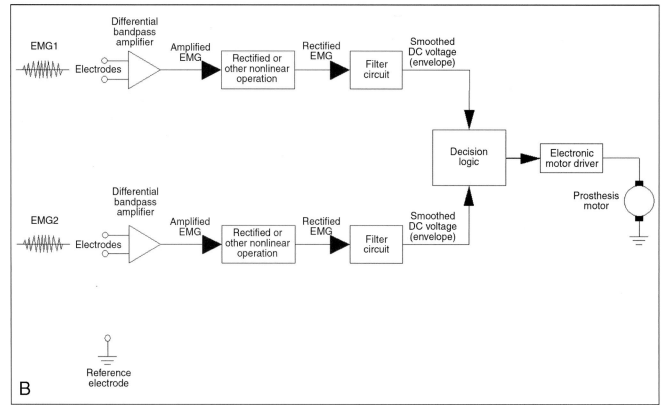

tors in the prosthesis can be actuated. Traditionally, one of three methods is used: a "crisp threshold" strategy, a "most-on" or "difference" strategy, or a "first-on" or "lockout" strategy. With a crisp threshold, any signal with amplitude greater than a given threshold value is determined to be "on" and remains "on" until it drops below this threshold. In a proportional system, the amount of amplitude greater than the "on" threshold determines how "on" the motor should be.

With a "first-on" or "lockout" strategy, the first signal to cross a preset "on" threshold (hence the term "first on") is the signal that is used to control the motor(s), and all other signals are ignored, or "locked out," even if they cross the threshold voltage, until the first "on" signal has crossed back below a second "off" threshold. The Hosmer Dorrance Corporation's (Campbell, CA) myopulse modulation EMG system[19] and Otto Bock Corporation's (Minneapolis, MN)

standard two-site systems (personal communication, with Pat Prigge, Otto Bock Health Care, Minneapolis, MN, 2003) both use this approach in their decision logic.

With a "most-on" or "difference" strategy, the largest amplitude EMG signal relative to an "on" threshold is the signal used to control the motor(s). This method works on a sample-by-sample basis: no signals are locked out, even after one has crossed the threshold. The Utah Arm

(Motion Control Inc, Salt Lake City, UT) uses this approach for its decision block (unpublished data, Motion Control Inc, Salt Lake City, UT, 1998).

In all these methods, the "on" threshold and the "off" threshold do not have to be the same. Different "on" and "off" thresholds provide hysteresis for the signal, which can make the system more stable in the face of noise or conflicting inputs.

Myoelectric control of a hand or other type of prehensor is particularly applicable to transradial amputation levels because individuals with acquired amputations usually have a phantom sensation of the missing hand. When the person with an amputation thinks of moving the phantom hand, the muscles remaining in the residual limb are activated naturally. Therefore, it is possible to relate original finger extensor muscles with opening of the prosthetic hand by placing electrodes on the skin near these muscles, for example, the extensor digitorum. The original finger flexor muscles can likewise be used, usually in conjunction with wrist flexor muscles, for the signal site to close the prosthetic hand. As a consequence, a rather natural relationship can exist between thinking about operating the phantom limb and actual operation of the hand prosthesis. In addition, the individual with a transradial prosthesis is able to have proprioception from the elbow joint concerning where the prosthesis is with respect to the body, how fast it is moving through space, and what external forces are acting upon it. Consequently, transradial myoelectric prostheses foster good control because much of the movement and function is somewhat natural.

Myoacoustic Signals

Myoacoustic signals (auditory sounds when muscles are active) were first observed long ago but only recently have been reinvestigated in depth for their potential in the control of prostheses.[20] Myoacoustic control systems are very similar in structure to myoelectric systems. At this time, there is

no compelling reason to move from myoelectric control to myoacoustic control. The primary advantage of myoacoustic control over myoelectric control may be that the acoustic sensor does not have to be in direct contact with the skin. Its main disadvantage is the difficulty with elimination of extraneous mechanical noises. When a prosthesis strikes an object or rubs against something in the environment, large mechanical vibrations can be created that may activate the prosthesis inadvertently. Elimination of this unwanted acoustic noise from the system appears to be quite challenging.

Prosthesis Control Using Muscle Bulge or Tendon Movement

Tendon or residual muscle movement has been used to actuate pneumatic sensors interposed between a prosthetic socket and the superficial tendons and/or muscle. These sensors can be used for prosthesis control. The Vaduz hand, developed by a German team headed by Dr. Edmund Wilms in Vaduz, Liechtenstein, following World War II, used muscle bulge to increase pneumatic pressure to operate a switch-controlled voluntary-closing position-servo hand (ie, hand position was proportional to the amount of pneumatic pressure).

Simpson[21] used muscle bulge to provide a control signal for the proportional control of an Otto Bock gas-operated hand. The width of opening of the hand was proportional to the force applied by the bulge of the muscle. Because the bulging muscle had to exert significant pressure to ensure sufficient force for control valve operation, a subconscious feedback path existed through the pressure sensors of the skin. This device was a precursor to Simpson's concept of extended physiologic proprioception.[7]

In 1999, the Rutgers University multifunctional hand received considerable media attention after reports of a multifunctional controller

that allowed individuals with amputations to play the piano in a laboratory setting.[22] This controller incorporated multiple pneumatic sensors that were actuated by the movement of the superficial extrinsic tendons associated with individual finger flexors. For this hand to be clinically viable, the developers need to resolve some of the issues that led to the failure of previous attempts to use pressure/muscle hardness transducers. A key issue is inability of the system to differentiate between actual control signals from a tendon and external pressures or impact from objects in the environment. In activities of daily living, a prosthesis wearer will exert forces and moments on the socket that may actuate the pressure sensors and issue commands to the drive system of the prosthesis.

In the 1970s, Otto Bock developed a control system that used muscle hardness to control an electronic prosthesis.[23] Advantages of the system were its immunity to electrical and magnetic fields, imperviousness to changes in skin impedance, and freedom from a quiescent current drain. This system was used to provide on-off and proportional control. Although the system was commercially available for several years, its use was never widespread.

Implants and Neuroelectric Control

The allure of neuroelectric control, in which implanted microelectrodes interface directly with nerves and possibly with neurons, is its potential to provide multiple-channel control and multiple-channel sensing. This is because many motor and sensory neurons are associated with each nerve. Neuroelectric control, however, remains a control possibility of the future. This method of control requires indwelling components of some kind (eg, telemetry implants) because neuroelectric signals are generally too weak to be picked up on the surface of the skin.

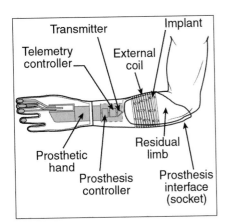

Figure 5 Planned implantable myoelectric sensor system. The external coil is laminated directly into the prosthetic interface during socket fabrication and the telemetry controller is incorporated along with the prosthesis controller in the body of the prosthesis. Signals from the implants in the arm, linked through the external coil, control the prosthesis via reverse telemetry. Implant power is supplied through the external coil using forward telemetry.

A good deal of research concerning prosthesis connections with nerves and neurons has been conducted,[24-26] but the practicality of human-machine interconnections of this kind is still problematic. Nervous tissue is sensitive to mechanical stresses; in addition, this form of control also requires implanted devices. Edell[24] attempted to use nerve cuffs to generate motor control signals. Kovacs and associates[25] tried to encourage nerve fibers to grow through arrays of holes in silicon integrated circuits that had been coated with nerve growth factor. Andrews and associates[26] reported on their progress in developing a multipoint microelectrode peripheral nerve implant. They used a 100×100 grid array of silicon microelectrodes that they inserted into a peripheral nerve bundle with a pulse of air. Although these authors are still working with animal models, they can identify individual neuron action potentials and claim good long-term results at this point. Concerns about the permanence of electrode array fixation have yet to be addressed.

Brain-machine interfaces are a variation of peripheral neural interfaces that use electroencephalogram signals (EEGs) for control purposes. EEGs are electric signals that are detected on the surface of the skull as a by-product of the natural functioning of the brain. Researchers at Duke University implanted an electrode array into the cerebellum of a monkey; using appropriate pattern recognition software, the monkey controlled a remote manipulator at a distance of more than 1,000 km via the Internet.[27] One of the goals of this research was to enable patients with quadriplegia to interact with their environment. Wolpaw and associates[28] reported on the use of an implanted electrode array to control a robot arm, and Kennedy and associates[29] documented the use of implanted cortical electrode arrays to enable patients with shut-in syndrome to control a computer cursor. Reger and associates[30] demonstrated a hybrid neurorobotic system based on two-way communication between the brain of a lamprey and a small mobile robot. The lamprey brain was kept alive in vitro and was used to send and receive motor control and sensory signals. This research illustrated a bidirectional interface between nervous tissue and a machine. Although a long way from practical application in prosthetics, this work reflects important advances in the area of human-machine prosthesis interfaces.

The development of BIONs[31] (Alfred Mann Foundation, CA) for functional electrical stimulation is a promising new implant technology that may have a far more immediate effect on prosthesis control. These devices are hermetically encapsulated, leadless electrical devices that are small enough (2 mm in diameter and 15 mm in length) to be injected percutaneously into muscles. They receive power, digital addressing, and command signals from an external transmitter coil worn by the patient. The attraction of this technology for use in control of multifunctional devices is that these devices can be implanted by

injection without surgery. In addition, the hermetically sealed capsule and electrodes necessary for long-term survival in the body have already been approved for use in humans by the US Food and Drug Administration in functional electrical stimulation systems. BIONs thus represent an enabling technology for a prosthesis control system based on implanted myoelectric sensors. Whereas three or four independent EMG sites can be located on the surface of a residual limb, many more independent EMG sites could likely be created in the same residual limb using implanted sensors. Intramuscular EMG signals from multiple residual muscles offer a way to provide simultaneous control of multiple degrees of freedom in a multifunction prosthesis. At the very least, seamless sequential control should be possible; that is, sequential control without intermediate steps such as muscle cocontraction or actuation of locking mechanisms. R.E. Reilly, developer of one of the earliest implantable myoelectric sensor (IMES) systems said, "The appeal of implanted electrodes for EMG control seems obvious: there is good reason to believe that by localizing the points at which EMG is picked up, these points can be treated as relatively independent control sites. Therefore, the number of degrees of freedom that can be simultaneously controlled and coordinated in an externally powered prosthesis is expected to be greater in comparison with surface EMG or mechanical control sites. Not only do superficial muscles become more distinguishable, but it becomes possible to consider using deeper muscles as additional control sites, and also control by single motor units."[32]

Weir and associates[33] are currently involved in an effort to revisit the idea of implantable myoelectric sensors for multichannel/multifunction prosthesis control. IMESs will be built that will be transcutaneously coupled through a magnetic link to an external exciter/data telemetry reader. Each IMES will be packaged in a BION II hermetic ceramic capsule.[34] These capsules are small enough to permit injection through a 12-gauge hypodermic needle. The external exciter/data telemetry reader will consist of an antenna coil laminated into a prosthetic interface so that when the prosthetic socket is donned, this coil will encircle the IMES and be in an optimal geometry to inductively couple with these electrodes. No percutaneous wires will cross the skin. The prosthesis controller will take the output of an exciter/data telemetry reader and use this output to decipher user intent (Figure 5).

Multifunctional Mechanisms and Control

Many attempts have been made to design fully articulated arms and hands to recreate the full function of the hand. Taylor[35] remarked that all such attempts had been complete failures.

Myoelectric control, once considered to be the cutting edge of technology, was advanced as a natural approach for the control of prostheses because it allowed individuals with amputation to use the same mental processes to control their prostheses as they had used in controlling their physiologic limb.[36,37] However, current state-of-the-art electronic prosthetic hands are generally single-degree-of-freedom (opening and closing) devices usually implemented with myoelectric control. Current prosthetic arms requiring multiple-degree-of-freedom control most often use sequential control. Locking mechanisms and/or special switch signals are used to change control from one degree of freedom to another. As currently implemented, sequential control of multiple motions is slow; consequently, transradial prostheses are generally limited to just opening and closing of the hand, greatly limiting the function of these devices. Individuals with recent hand amputations expect modern hand prostheses to be like hands. Because these devices fail to meet some users' expectations, they may be underutilized or rejected. The major factor limiting the development of more sophisticated hand/arm prostheses is the difficulty in finding sufficient control sources to control the many degrees of freedom required to replace a physiologic hand and/or arm.

The decade from 1965 to 1975 was one of unprecedented research on the control of artificial limbs. The research, particularly that conducted in Europe, was stimulated by limb absences at birth that resulted from use of the drug Thalidomide during pregnancy. That period of activity and research was also marked by excitement resulting from the practical introduction of myoelectric control during the mid 1960s. The Swedish Board for Technical Development sponsored a workshop on control of prostheses and orthoses in 1971, and the proceedings of that meeting represent a landmark publication on prosthesis control research.[38] Worldwide, many new government initiatives were established during this period. Developments included the Edinburgh Arm,[39] the Boston Arm,[37,40] the Philadelphia Arm,[41,42] the Wasada Hand,[43] the Belgrade Hand,[44,45] the Sven Hand,[46] and the Utah Arm.[47]

Although many ideas were tried and tested during this period, only a few devices ever made it from the laboratory into everyday clinical practice. The Edinburgh Arm, which was pneumatically powered, saw some clinical usage but was complex and lacked the robustness necessary for everyday use. This arm is not available today, but it was important as an implementation of Simpson's ideas on extended physiologic proprioception (EPP). The Boston Arm, developed at Massachusetts Institute of Technology (MIT), had the first myoelectrically controlled elbow. This elbow was extensively redesigned for commercial production.[48] The current version is the Boston Elbow III (Liberating Technologies, Holliston, MA). The Utah Arm, which was influenced by the MIT research, is commercially available through Motion Control Inc.[49]

The Sven Hand never experienced widespread clinical use, even though it was employed extensively in multifunction control research using pattern recognition of myoelectric signals.[50,51] The pattern recognition system they used was based on multiple EMG signals, which were processed using adaptive-weighted filters. The weighting values of these filters were adjusted to tailor the system to the individual. Henry Lymark, director of the Handikappinstitutet of Stockholm, Sweden, later created a simplified version of the Sven Hand called the ES Hand in an attempt to produce a more robust, and hence more clinically viable, version of the Sven Hand. The ES Hand possessed an adaptive grip and a passive two-position thumb. It was powered by a single motor with differential drives to the fingers. Unfortunately, Lymark died soon after the initial development of this hand and the project was never continued.

Like the Sven Hand, the Philadelphia Arm[41,42] was used in research on multifunction control using weighted filters for the pattern recognition problem and achieved good results. The Belgrade Hand was likewise never used clinically but has ended up in the robotics field in the form of the Belgrade/USC robotic hand.[52]

A more recent offering is the multifunctional hand designed by Yves Lozac'h.[53] This hand was a single-degree-of-freedom hand (opening and closing); however, because the hand had articulated fingers that could move independently of each other, it was capable of forming an adaptive grip for grasping objects. An adaptive grip requires lower forces than conventional prosthetic hands to hold objects because the object to be grasped can be encircled. Operating under the assumption that a practical prosthetic hand can have only one axis of rotation for the thumb, Lozac'h[54] performed a series of experiments to determine if there was a preferred working plane for a single-degree-of-freedom active thumb. He concluded that the preferred working plane of the thumb lay between 45° and 55°. In our opinion, the Lozac'h hand looked impressive at a demonstration in 1992, but it did not have enough torque to operate within a conventional cosmetic glove.

Complex time, frequency, and time-frequency identification techniques have subsequently been used to extract features from myoelectric signals for multifunction prosthesis control, thanks to the advent of high-speed digital electronics that can handle algorithms of high computational complexity in close to real time. Graupe and associates[55] conducted a stochastic time series analysis of EMG signals. Other teams used neural networks to perform the pattern recognition and feature extraction,[56-58] whereas Farry and associates[59] used genetic algorithms. The features described by Hudgins and associates[57] are the most widely used. They proposed extracting several parameters out of the first 200 ms of EMG and developed an approach for the classification of four different motions or muscle contractions. Their classification scheme used five different features (mean absolute value, mean absolute value slope, zero crossings, slope sign changes, and waveform length) from several time segments of each signal. A multilayer neural network with back propagation classified myoelectric patterns using these features.

Farry and associates[58] used the five features above as well as a few of their own with genetic programming algorithms instead of neural networks for classification. Chan and associates[60] used fuzzy logic with the Hudgins group features. Engelhart's team[61] combined wavelet analysis with maximum likelihood estimation. The processing time required for these complex algorithms is nontrivial. Any delay greater than about 100 ms in the response of the output to a change in the input is perceptible as a sluggish response. Parker and Scott[10] suggest that delays between input and output should not exceed 200 ms; even this can be unacceptable for high-performance prosthetic components. Based on our experience, we believe that designers should try to achieve an update rate of no more than 50 ms.

Although few clinically available devices use these control approaches, the work of Hudgins and associates[57] and the earlier effort of Herberts and associates[62] demonstrate that some form of pattern recognition of myoelectric signals (adaptive filtering techniques, neural networks, genetic algorithms, fuzzy logic, etc) may have merit as a means of controlling multifunction devices. With a pattern recognition type of controller, the user must first train the controller to recognize specific patterns of EMG signals. These EMG signals are generated by the user's residual limb in response to the user's visualization of his or her phantom limb performing a specific function. The controller records the resulting EMG signals generated by the residual musculature during the training trial. This training process is repeated several times for each function. The recorded EMGs associated with each function are then analyzed offline to extract either the relevant features (using a neural network in the case of the Hudgins team[57]) or the appropriate filter weights (for the adaptive filter of the Herberts group[62]). The resultant feature parameters or filter weights are then stored in the controller and used by the controller to recognize similar patterns in future combinations of myoelectric signals.

Some alternatives to myoelectric pattern recognition, such as the system Kyberd and Chappell[63] call "hierarchical artificial reflexes," have been used to automate the control process in an effort to reduce the mental burden placed on the user. Kyberd and Chappell's device is basically a multifunctional hand; however, they take the operator out of the loop and use onboard processing and sensors in the hand to tell the hand which pattern to adopt. The operator provides a conventional single-degree-of-freedom "open" or "close" EMG signal. By allowing the processor to take control, the mental load on the operator is reduced.

In 2002, Ajiboye and associates[64] presented a multifunctional controller based on fuzzy logic techniques with an update rate of 50 ms. This controller is based on three or four myoelectric sites (the maximum number of sites that could be isolated without cross talk becoming unacceptable) and uses fuzzy logic techniques to detect EMG onset and classify user intent. The controller is being developed as part of a project to build a new multifunctional hand prosthesis.[65] Three to four independent EMG sites will be used to control three or four degrees of freedom in the prosthetic hand. Membership functions for each myoelectric channel are based on training data, and the four sites are located with standard clinical techniques. Rules defining the different EMG levels associated with a particular function are generated automatically based on the recorded training data.

Most multifunctional prosthesis designs are doomed by practicality, long before control interface becomes an issue. Prosthesis users are not gentle with their devices; they expect them to work in all sorts of situations never dreamed of by their designers. Most mechanisms fail because of insufficient durability, poor performance, and complicated control. No device will be clinically successful if it breaks down frequently. A multifunctional design by its very nature is more complex than a design with a single degree of freedom. From a maintenance standpoint, the device will have more components with a greater potential to fail. Articulated joints on fingers are more likely to fail than monocoque (solid-finger) designs. To achieve the increased function possible with a multiple-degree-of-freedom hand, however, some of the robustness and simplicity of a single-degree device must be sacrificed.

Another practical consideration is performance. The hand must be able to generate enough torque and speed and also have sufficient width of opening to be useful. Many laboratory designs have performed well until a cosmetic glove was added. A cosmetic glove is standard for prosthetic hands. Unless a mechanism is designed specifically for use without a glove, the effect of the glove on performance must be taken into consideration. The ES Hand was designed to work in its own cover, while the Belgrade Hand needed an additional cover. The pinch force of a multifunctional hand does not need to be as high as that of single-degree-of-freedom hands because the adaptive nature of the grip enables the hand to encompass objects. Multifunctional hands should still be capable of high speeds of opening, however, and have a pinch force of at least 68 N.[66] An in-depth review of the practical issues related to the design of prosthetic hand and arm components was prepared by Weir.[67]

The Role of Surgery in the Creation of Control Sites/Sources

Amputation surgery plays a critical role in the clinical outcomes of prosthesis fittings and can significantly affect control of limb prostheses. Unfortunately, the number of surgeons with an active interest in amputation and amputation issues has declined appreciably, particularly compared with the years immediately following World War II. If the control of limb prostheses is to advance along a broad front, advancements in surgery and surgical techniques are just as necessary as technical progress. Technological advancements and surgical advancements in prosthetics should be integrated, synergistic activities. Techniques in orthopaedic surgery, vascular surgery, plastic surgery, and neurosurgery have advanced rapidly over the past 30 years. Unfortunately, the impact of many of the new tech-

niques on prosthesis control would be far greater if surgeons, prosthetists, and engineers had consistently worked together on limb control problems. Surgical procedures are covered elsewhere in this book, but the impact of surgical techniques, objectives, and decisions on control sites and function is discussed in this chapter.

Bones and Joints

Preservation of joints and bone length consistent with good medical practice generally leads to improved prosthesis control. With transradial amputations, the limb should be as long as possible. Wrist disarticulations conserve natural supination-pronation of the forearm, provide contours for prosthesis suspension, and create a force-tolerant distal end for the limb. The elbow joint should be saved whenever possible because it greatly enhances prosthesis control, just as an intact knee enhances lower limb prosthesis control. Bone lengthening might be considered for increasing the length of very short limbs when practical. If all fingers have been amputated, decisions about saving the wrist joint must be made on an individual basis. Persons with partial hand amputations now have access to improved finger components that are short enough so that the fitting does not make the limb too long. A functional human wrist joint is highly desirable because of its freedom of movement to position an artificial prehension component. In the past, fitting options were limited to passive/cosmetic prostheses and opposition posts. Current fitting options are discussed in chapter 14. Otto Bock now has a shorter hand prosthesis; an even shorter partial hand mechanism is under development through the Veterans Administration Rehabilitation Research and Development Service[68] of the US Department of Veterans Affairs. If functional wrist movements can be conserved using flexible sockets, truly exceptional prostheses for this long-neglected amputation level may result.

Angle Osteotomies

From a control standpoint, transhumeral amputations follow guidelines similar to those for transradial amputations. Elbow disarticulations conserve humeral rotation, can be used to aid prosthesis suspension, and provide a force-tolerant distal end. Long transhumeral limbs often achieve good control of prosthetic elbow flexion using glenohumeral flexion. If a disarticulation is not possible, the length should usually be shortened enough to accommodate elbow mechanisms without compromising function. Marquardt[69] has used angle osteotomies of the distal humerus to improve mechanical coupling between the humerus and the prosthesis so that humeral rotation of the prosthesis is readily controlled by natural humeral rotation.

For optimum control, the surgeon should attempt to save a short humerus if it will be voluntarily mobile because a mobile short humeral neck can be used to activate control switches or to push against pressure-sensitive pads. Muscles attached to it may also be used for myoelectric control purposes. If amputation above the elbow is performed after brachial plexus injury, it is often helpful to have the flail humerus fused with the scapula at the glenohumeral joint so that the humeral section can be controlled to some extent by action of the scapula.

Soft-Tissue Conservation and Reconstruction

When possible, surgeons should conserve residual muscles that might be used for myoelectric or other control sources. Myoplasty and/or myodesis procedures ensure the ability to develop tension when muscles are voluntarily contracted. Myoplasty procedures that connect antagonist-agonist muscle groups at the distal end of the residual limb are often used to keep the muscles in a dynamic, somewhat natural working relationship. This can preserve muscle tone and increase the potential for good two-site myoelec-

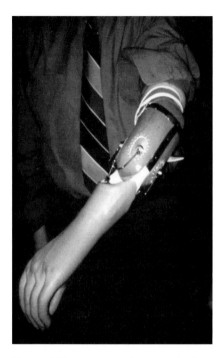

Figure 6 Forearm muscle tunnel cineplasty in the German style of prosthesis. These were seldom used in the United States because of the limited force and excursion available from forearm muscles.

tric control from these muscles. In myodesis, the residual muscle is stitched to the bone. Single muscles that may have no functional purpose after amputation yet can be voluntarily activated should be attached to a reaction point and saved for possible use as a myoelectric control site. Preservation of muscle tone, length, and excursion are of paramount importance for the success of future surgical procedures in creating novel physical muscle-prosthesis interfaces. Myoplasty could be performed on the superficial residual muscles, and myodesis could be used on the deep residual muscles.

Cineplasty

Surgical procedures such as the Vanghetti-Sauerbruch-Lebsche muscle tunnel cineplasty or the tendon exteriorization cineplasty,[70] which externalize the force and excursion of a muscle or tendon, can provide good control interfaces. The Vanghetti-Sauerbruch-Lebsche muscle tunnel cineplasty is an evolution of the tendon "loops" and "clubs" of Vanghetti,[71-73] the muscle tunnel cine-

plasties of Sauerbruch,[74] and their later modification during World War II by Lebsche.[75] The surgical procedure to create a Vanghetti-Sauerbruch-Lebsche muscle tunnel cineplasty was most recently described by Brückner.[76]

This control technique was revived in Europe in the 1980s.[76-78] Brückner and Thomas[79] documented their experiences with the functional value of the Sauerbruch-Lebsche procedure. They created a total of 20 tunnels in 16 patients over a period starting in 1988; all but one of these tunnels were considered successful. They noted that the functional outcome (use of the prosthesis), however, depended on the motivation and mental well-being of the patient. Others agreed that this was critical to the success of the procedure.[80,81] With the exception of Brückner and Thomas[79] and Beasley,[70] few surgeons since Sauerbruch and Lebsche have systematically examined new ways to externalize the force of muscles for control. A muscle tunnel cineplasty is shown in Figure 6.

Although tunnel cineplasties have been rare in the United States since the 1970s, they offer a unique way for surgeons to create control sources. New surgical techniques and the wide availability of powered prostheses may lead to a revival of this procedure. Leal and Malone[82] successfully fitted a person with a transradial amputation who had a standard biceps tunnel cineplasty with an electric hand that was switch-controlled from the cineplasty site. Lücke and associates[83] discussed the use of cineplasty in connection with modern electronic prosthesis technology. Beasley's[70] tendon exteriorization cineplasty procedure shows promise. Tendon exteriorization does not traumatize the muscle itself and therefore is thought to have minimal influence on a muscle's circulation and neurologic mechanisms. This procedure illustrates the potential for surgical creation of several such control sources on the forearm; these could enable individuals with a long transradial amputation to

gain coordinated control of individually powered prosthetic fingers in the future. We recently reported the fitting of a proof-of-concept prosthesis using tendon exteriorization cineplasties as control inputs to powered prosthesis controllers.[84]

Surgical creation of several new miniature tunnel cineplasty control sources on the torso may be particularly desirable for individuals with high-level bilateral limb loss who need multifunctional control yet have limited control sites. Marquardt[85] described the use of a pectoral cineplasty to actuate a three-position pull switch to provide sequential switch control of an electromechanical hand and wrist rotator. Direct muscle control through tunnel cineplasties is particularly attractive because of the proprioception they naturally provide to the user. This feature accomplishes one of the key goals of limb prosthesis control, obtaining good control of multiple prosthetic functions without too much mental exertion given over to the control process by the user. Powered prostheses make the use of tunnel cineplasty control sources possible even when they can develop only small forces or excursions. The combination of powered prostheses and electronic position control systems, in conjunction with new surgical techniques and procedures such as multiple miniature tunnel cineplasties, may open up a new era of control based on the older yet still vital ideas of muscle cineplasty.

Adherence of the skin to underlying muscle is a less direct method of using a muscle as a control source. Skin adherence generates skin motion when muscle contraction causes movement. This method of control was presented by Seamone and associates.[86]

Other surgical reconstructions incorporate phalangization of the remaining bones, such as those of the forearm in the Krukenberg procedure.[87] The Krukenberg method originated in Germany in 1917 and received much impetus in Germany and Russia throughout World War II.

Swanson and Swanson[88] explained the use of the Krukenberg procedure in children; Mathur and associates[89] documented experiences with the procedure in India; and Baumgartner and Asey[90] of Germany presented an overview of 19 individuals with bilateral amputations who had Krukenberg hands for an average of 45 years. Although excellent functional results can be obtained with this procedure, it is not widely used because of poor cosmesis.

The Krukenberg procedure remains a viable method to enable direct prehension control. Older surgical procedures such as the Krukenberg procedure can effectively complement modern surgical procedures. The patient in Figure 7 had a modern toe transplant procedure on the right side and a Krukenberg procedure on the left. Because the patient was blind, retention of tactile sensation for interaction with the environment was of primary importance. A Krukenberg procedure can also be used for control of powered transradial prostheses. Some users choose to use their Krukenberg limbs in the privacy of their homes because of the excellent sensory and motor qualities, but prefer to use prostheses over their arms when they are in public venues. Although this procedure has been used primarily with blind individuals with bilateral hand amputations, the procedure may have application for sighted individuals and individuals with unilateral amputations in certain circumstances.[91] Activation of pressure-sensitive transducers by the Krukenberg limb is one application for control of a hand; myoelectric control is another option.

Neuromuscular Reorganization

Kuiken and associates[2] suggest a promising new surgical technique, the use of neuromuscular reorganization to improve the control of artificial arms. Although the limb is lost in an amputation, the control signals to the limb remain in the residual peripheral

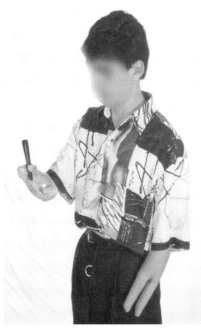

Figure 7 An older surgical procedure (Krukenberg) complements a modern surgical procedure (toe transplant) to restore function to a blind patient. The toe transplant to the right arm restored fine grasping function to the right side, while surgical revision of the left arm to enable the radius and ulna to be used as large fingers (Krukenberg procedure) restored gross prehensile ability to the left side. In both instances, tactile sensation is preserved. Preservation of tactile sensation is of particular importance for the restoration of function in blind individuals. Both procedures were performed in 1995 by a hand surgeon at Northwestern Memorial Hospital in Chicago, Illinois.

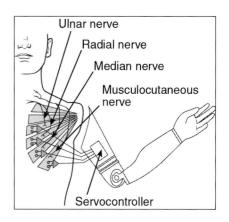

Figure 8 Neuromuscular reorganization. Diagram illustrates how reinnervation of the pectoralis muscle with the major nerves of the arm might be used to create physiologically correct myoelectric control sites for prosthetic arm control.

nerves of the amputated limb. The potential to tap into these lost control signals may be realized using nerve-muscle grafts. As first suggested by Hoffer and Loeb,[92] it may be possible to denervate expendable regions of muscle in or near an amputated limb and graft the residual peripheral nerve stumps to these muscles. The peripheral nerves would then reinnervate the muscles and these nerve-muscle grafts would provide additional control signals for an externally powered prosthesis (Figure 8).

The concept is to denervate a muscle that is not functionally critical and reinnervate it at multiple places with nerves that formerly went to the hand

and forearm. After reinnervation, the muscle may be a good source of multiple myoelectric sites or provide other kinds of input for prosthesis control. The primary advantage of a nerve-graft system is the potential for a greater number of discrete control signals that relate directly to the original function of the limb. In the case of the person with a high-level amputation, the median, ulnar, radial, and musculocutaneous nerves are usually still present. The musculocutaneous nerve controls elbow flexion, while the radial nerve controls extension. Pronation of the forearm is directed by the median nerve, and supination is directed by the radial and musculocutaneous nerves. Extension of the hand is governed by the radial nerve, and flexion by the median and ulnar nerves. Because each of these nerves innervate muscles that control the motion about different degrees of freedom, they should theoretically supply at least four independent control signals. The nerves would be controlling functions in the prosthesis that were directly related to their normal anatomic function. Furthermore, existing myoelectric technologies could be applied to make the additional control signals accessible without the use of implanted nerve cuffs, implanted transmitter-receiver systems, or percutaneous devices. IMESs placed at the time of initial surgery might complement this procedure nicely. Another advantage is that the shoulder would be free to control other functions, such as an artificial shoulder. This new approach has been successfully applied in one patient with bilateral, high-level amputations to control a shoulder disarticulation prosthesis. Each of the residual brachial plexus nerves was grafted to a different region of deinnervated pectoralis muscle. Kuiken and associates[2] are presently considering using this technique with unilateral amputations at the transhumeral level, grafting nerves to different regions of deinnervated biceps brachii.

Instead of myoelectric sites, miniature tunnel cineplasties could be created in the reinnervated muscle. In conjunction with miniature tunnel cineplasties, the work of Kuiken's group[2] presents interesting possibilities for future long-term research. They demonstrated that a section of muscle could be denervated and then hyperreinnervated with a different nerve. Thus, it might be possible to reinnervate a piece of previously denervated sound muscle with a rerouted nerve from the residual limb. A miniature tunnel cineplasty performed on this newly reinnervated muscle could create a source of prosthesis control. In theory, the amputee would not need to relearn how to control the reinnervated muscle; physiologically correct control could be maintained and sensory feedback would be available through the cineplasty.

Osseointegration

Another surgical intervention is the pioneering work in the area of direct skeletal attachment (osseointegration) conducted by Brånemark[93] and his associates[94] in Sweden, which is described in more detail in chapter 54. These orthopaedic surgeons and engineers have created interfaces for direct skeletal attachment systems for upper and lower limb amputations. With osseointegration, a prosthesis is attached directly to the skeleton via a titanium abutment that protrudes through the skin from the cut end of the bone. Brånemark's techniques appear to have greatly diminished the infection problem that persisted in earlier efforts.[95] Direct extensions of fingers or thumb bones are good examples of EPP. Should direct skeletal attachment prove viable, it could revolutionize the prosthetic fitting of some amputation levels. The prosthesis of the future might be a multifunctional device that is mounted into the skeleton using osseointegration and controlled with neuromuscular reorganized multiple miniature muscle cineplasties.

Control of Prostheses for Unilateral Limb Loss

Although fittings of individuals with unilateral amputations are technically much simpler than bilateral fittings, many individuals with unilateral limb loss do not wear the prosthesis, particularly those with transhumeral and higher level limb loss. The person with a unilateral amputation has a physiologic arm and hand that can accomplish most tasks. Therefore, the prosthesis at best serves only in an assistive mode. Some individuals with an amputation may want a prosthesis primarily for appearance. Some may incorporate it extensively into their activities and body image, while others may use it only for specific functions (such as work or sport activities). Many individuals with unilateral amputations decide not to wear a prosthesis. Professionals associated with prosthesis fittings need to support the patients' decisions about using prostheses. Nonetheless, they must also inform the patient about what kind of fitting might best serve his or her goals. Prosthetic fitting of individuals with an upper limb amputation is partially an iterative process because these individuals cannot know what problems they will face until they actually use a prosthesis in their natural environment. In addition, their true feelings and desires may take time to mature and to emerge. An amputation often leads to job changes and other changes that require time to be sorted out. The prosthesis exists amid many life changes and this makes the initial prescription difficult. Accordingly, diagnostic and temporary prostheses can be very useful for early fittings.

Unilateral Transradial Prostheses

Transradial prostheses may be controlled successfully in several ways. Cable-controlled voluntary-opening and voluntary-closing prehensors (nonanthropomorphic) work well with individuals with transradial amputations, although cable-controlled mechanical hands are generally inefficient. When myoelectric control first became available, it was thought to have more important applications for higher level amputations than transradial amputations. However, myoelectric control has performed admirably at this level; in fact, its application for the person with a transradial amputation is the most common (Figure 4). Use of two myoelectric sites is preferred to control the two functions (closing/opening) of the hand because this gives the operator direct control of each function. This kind of control can become subconscious in nature for some individuals. The prehensor can be various electronic hands or other nonanthropomorphic electronic prehensors.

Single-site, two-function control is quite acceptable for individuals with an amputation who do not have two good myoelectric sites. It has been used effectively with both children, in the New Brunswick system, and adults. Combination of the single-site, single-function myocontroller of hand opening with automatic-powered closing (the St. Anthony control circuit, or "cookie crusher" system) has been effective with very young children born with limb absences.

A pair of single-site, two-function controllers can be used to control four functions of powered hand opening/closing and powered pronation/supination by the person with a short transradial amputation. In general, supination/pronation is not necessary for most individuals with a unilateral amputation unless a particular vocation or hobby demands it. Powered supination/pronation adds weight distally and also adds complexity. Sockets and apparatus that allow natural supination/pronation powered by residual movements of the amputated limb are recommended whenever possible.

Sears and Shaperman[96] demonstrated the effectiveness of proportional control in 1991. However, if powered prostheses have slow dynamic responses (ie, hands open or close at slow rates), then proportional control is not necessary for effective control; on-off control is sufficient. Rapidly moving prostheses with maximum angular velocities greater than 2.0 to 3.0 rad/s (~115°/s to 172°/s) require proportional control.

Control of Unilateral Transhumeral Prostheses

As with transradial prostheses, transhumeral prostheses can function well with totally cable-operated body-powered prostheses when relatively long limbs remain. Several other approaches are common.

For individuals with a transhumeral amputation with long residual limbs, the hybrid approach of a cable-operated, body-powered elbow combined with myoelectric control from the biceps (closing) and triceps (opening) of a powered prehensor (hand or nonhand) is a very functional fitting approach. This approach has been used effectively in Europe for more than 30 years. Billock[97] has used this technique effectively with many people. It is a relatively simple approach, technically comparable to a transradial myoelectric fitting (Figure 9). The hybrid control/power approach has reasonable proprioceptive qualities and allows simultaneous coordinated control of elbow and prehensor function. Opening of the prehensor during forearm lifting against a load is avoided, which is a problem with a cable-operated elbow if the cable is also used to operate a voluntary-opening (spring-return) prehensor. We believe that myoelectric control of prehension, in this case from the biceps and triceps, is somewhat natural because gripping objects strongly often involves contraction of muscles quite distant from the hand. The relationship between prehension and muscle contraction has been called the myoprehension concept.[98]

RSL Steeper (London, England) offers a body-powered elbow that is designed for a hybrid control approach to transhumeral fittings. The elbow encompasses an electrical switch that is connected with the elbow locking mechanism. When the elbow is unlocked, the electrical switch is open; when locked, the switch is closed. This allows a single cable to operate their servo-controlled hand, and also the elbow, without interaction. When the cable is pulled to operate the unlocked elbow, the electrical connection to the hand is turned off. When the elbow is locked, the connection to the hand is on; pulling on the cable operates the hand through the position servo-control system. Another way to use this elbow design is to place a two-position switch in series with the cable that controls the elbow. When the elbow is unlocked, cable operation is normal. When the elbow is locked, pulling the cable lightly will activate the first position of the switch and close the hand. Pulling the cable with greater force will activate the second position on the switch and open the hand. In both cases, the concept is to reduce the number of control sources needed. However, simultaneous control of both functions is impossible with this control approach.

An alternate but similar approach is to use a powered elbow instead of the body-powered elbow yet control it in a similar fashion, using the cable to operate a position servomechanism controlling the elbow. This approach is a type of boosted cable control. Be-

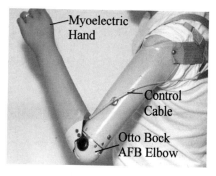

Figure 9 Hybrid unilateral transhumeral fitting consisting of a body-powered elbow and myoelectrically controlled hand. The elbow is controlled in the usual fashion by glenohumeral flexion assisted by a counterbalancing elbow (Otto Bock Automatic Forearm Balance [AFB] Elbow, Otto Bock). This type of elbow is used because myoelectric hands tend to be heavy. The myoelectric hand is closed by activation of the biceps brachii and opened by action of the triceps.

cause the cable is connected directly to the output position of the elbow, the position of the body cannot get ahead of the corresponding position of the elbow and forearm. This kind of controller is similar in operation to automobile power steering. The approach is based on Simpson's principles of EPP.[7] Heckathorne and associates[99] have reported on this technique for a clinical fitting. The advantages are that proprioception is maintained even while using a powered elbow, and the force and excursion necessary to operate the elbow can be matched to the user's force and excursion capabilities. This particular control approach has been described in detail by Doubler and Childress[100,101] and is reviewed in some depth by Weir.[102]

If individuals with transhumeral amputations cannot operate a body-powered elbow well for reasons such as difficulty with the locking and unlocking function, a powered elbow can be used. The elbow is often myoelectrically controlled, with flexion by the biceps and extension by the triceps. The prehensor can be cable-controlled and body-powered. This can be an effective prosthesis in a work environment if a total cable-driven system cannot be used. This

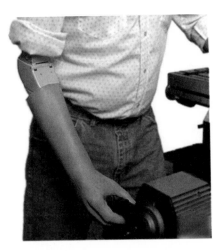

Figure 10 Myoelectrically controlled Utah Arm (Motion Control Inc). Elbow flexion and extension are controlled proportionally by myoelectric signals from the biceps brachii and the triceps, a natural kind of elbow control. After the forearm remains in one position for a set period of time, the elbow locks mechanically and control is transferred automatically to the hand (myoprehension). A rapid co-contraction of both muscles is used to transfer control back to the elbow. (*Photograph courtesy of Motion Control, Salt Lake City, Utah.*)

approach has been promoted for use with the electronic elbow from Liberating Technologies.

For individuals with transhumeral amputations who do not want to use the harness of cable control or cannot tolerate a harness (because of skin grafts, for example), or for individuals with a relatively short limb (weak glenohumeral leverage), the controls can be completely myoelectric. A two-site myoelectric control system that can be used to control the elbow proportionally in a Utah Arm is shown in Figure 10. If the elbow is held stationary for a short period of time, the elbow automatically locks and this action transfers the myoelectric proportional control to the hand. A quick co-contraction of the biceps and triceps muscles is used to transfer control back to the elbow. This is a form of two-site, four-function control in which all functions are not directly accessible. Control can be alternated between the hand and the elbow.

Unilateral Shoulder Disarticulation Prostheses

Individuals with unilateral shoulder disarticulation often choose not to wear prostheses. Some prefer to wear a lightweight passive prosthesis that swings comfortably during walking and can be positioned for placement of the cosmetic hand in their lap when they sit. Light, passive grasp by the cosmetic hand may provide some utility. Body-powered prostheses are marginally effective at this level of amputation, when the contralateral limb is fully functional. The user often has somewhat limited force and excursion, compared with the person with a mid- to long transhumeral amputation, and a body-powered system may be difficult to operate. A powered prosthesis (eg, electric elbow with electric hand or other powered prehensor) may also be undesirable at this level of amputation because of the marginal functional gains when the opposite limb is fully capable. Powered limbs also add weight, a negative factor in this kind of fitting.

Control of Prostheses for Bilateral Limb Loss

Fitting problems become dramatically different when both arms are missing. Because of the numerous combinations of bilateral limb loss that exist when amputation level, long versus short variations, associated movement limitations, and pathologies of limb segments are considered, only a few conditions will be addressed in this section. The focus is on general principles for the fittings rather than specific details.

Bilateral Long Transradial Amputations

Individuals with long bilateral limb loss can effectively control a wide range of prostheses, from cable-controlled voluntary-opening hooks to bilateral myoelectric hands. A key goal is to preserve the physiologic pronation-supination remaining, on both sides. Although bilateral powered hands and myoelectric control are often used, we believe that these individuals frequently benefit from at least one cable-controlled hook-like prosthesis. Passive (friction or locking) wrist flexion will be useful, at least on the dominant side. Conventional cable-controlled hooks on both sides are also very functional; this approach provides the precision capabilities of hook prehensors along with good proprioception from the cable-operated control systems and the long residual limbs. The option finally selected will be highly dependent on the needs and preferences of the user. Powered hand prostheses may be used bilaterally for aesthetic concerns; however, there are functional disadvantages. Hands are usually limited to one prehension pattern (palmar prehension), and their bulk adds difficulty in constricted spaces and often blocks sightlines to objects.

Bilateral Transradial Amputations With One Long Limb and One Short Limb

Individuals with one long limb and one short limb may be fitted with cable control or myoelectric control on both sides. Hybrid control may be useful; the long (dominant) side can be provided a cable-controlled hook with wrist flexion and the short side fitted with a myoelectrically controlled hand (perhaps with an electric wrist rotator). A wide range of fitting possibilities is possible. A completely cable-controlled system with hooks also can be very effective, as demonstrated by so many individuals with an amputation who have developed exceptional arm/prehensor skills.

Transhumeral and Transradial Amputations

Individuals with both transhumeral and transradial amputations also can be fitted well with body-powered, cable-controlled systems. The functional dexterity that many of these in-

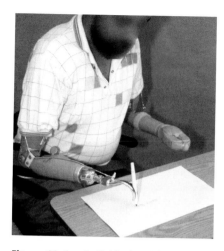

Figure 11 An individual with bilateral transhumeral amputations fitted with a body-powered system on the right side with single-cable, four-function control through which he can control the elbow, wrist flexion, wrist rotation, and prehension. The left side is fitted with a body-powered elbow; single-site, two-function myoelectric control of the Otto Bock Greifer prehensor (Otto Bock) from the biceps brachii; and a passive wrist rotator that can be rotated by rubbing the crepe rubber band encircling it against the body.

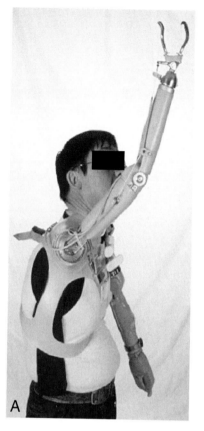
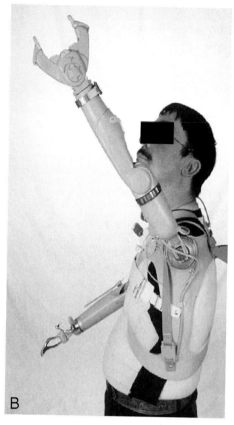

Figure 12 Man with bilateral shoulder disarticulations who has been fitted with prostheses on both sides. **A,** The right side is fitted with a single-cable, four-function, body-powered system and Liberty-Collier locking shoulder joint (Liberating Technologies Inc). Chin levers are used to lock and unlock the shoulder, elbow, and wrist rotator. A lever on the wrist unlocks and locks the wrist flexion unit. **B,** The left side is fitted with a Liberty-Collier locking shoulder joint, powered elbow (Liberty Mutual), powered wrist rotator (Otto Bock), and powered prehensor (Otto Bock Greifer; Otto Bock). A mechanical chin lever is used to lock and unlock the shoulder. Chin movement against rocker switches controls the elbow, wrist, and prehensor. The two arm systems are mechanically decoupled because one is entirely body-powered and the other is entirely electronic, except for the passive joints. The body-powered prosthesis is used as the dominant arm, with the electronic limb assisting. These prostheses enable this individual to be highly functional.

dividuals develop with this kind of control is extraordinary. The transradial side is normally considered the dominant side for fitting. If the transhumeral amputation is reasonably long, cable control can be used on the transradial side with a cable-controlled, body-powered elbow on the transhumeral side, in conjunction with myoelectric control of an electronic prehensor. When the transhumeral amputation is short, a powered elbow should be considered.

Bilateral Transhumeral Amputations

Individuals with bilateral transhumeral amputations frequently use external power on one side or the other, but totally body-powered, cable-controlled systems can be functional at this level. We believe these individuals should be fitted with a body-powered, cable-controlled system on one side—usually the side with the longest residual limb but possibly the side of original hand dominance if the residual limb is long enough. Single-cable control of four body-powered functions has been found to be very functional. This is a technique pioneered by George Robinson at Robin Aids Prosthetics (Vallejo, CA) and applied there by James Caywood. Their system has been redesigned so that its fabrication is more modular and easier to apply.[103] The single-cable, four-function control approach allows a person with bilateral transhumeral amputations to independently position joints of the arm and lock them into position. One cable can be used to flex the elbow, open the terminal device, rotate the wrist, and flex the wrist. Controls are added to lock and unlock the wrist rotator, the wrist flexor, and the elbow, which allows the limb to be rigid or free. This four-function mechanism is described in greater detail by Heckathorne and associates.[104]

A body-powered elbow and myoelectrically controlled prehensor can be fitted to the nondominant side if the residual limb is fairly long. An electric elbow may be useful if the limb is short, using myoelectric or rocker-switch control (Figure 11).

Short Transhumeral and Bilateral Shoulder Disarticulation Amputations

Bilateral shoulder disarticulations are handled like the transhumeral amputations. We use a four-function body-powered cable-controlled system on the dominant side (Figure 12). The nondominant side is fitted with a powered elbow, a powered prehensor, and a powered wrist rotator. The wrist rotator and the powered prehensor are controlled by chin movement against rocker switches. The elbow is controlled by a two-position pull switch that is activated by shoulder elevation. Heckathorne and associates[1] described the complementary function of bilateral hybrid prostheses of this type. The user can don and doff the prostheses independently, and he uses them effectively in activities of daily living. Nevertheless, modification of the home environment was necessary to simplify function.

Use of a totally body-powered system on one side and an electric system on the other allows the two systems to be effectively decoupled from a control standpoint. Forces and motions to activate the body-powered side do not activate the electric system on the opposite side. Likewise, operation of the electric prosthesis does not activate the body-controlled system. This automatic decoupling allows the individual to concentrate on the prosthesis being operated without having to consider both simultaneously. All joints have positive locks so that the user does not have to worry about joint movement due to external loads. The MICA shoulder joints (Liberating Technologies Inc) have positive locking, enabling the user to position the limb well above the shoulders. This is accomplished by placing the limb on a table surface with the shoulder free. If the user bends the torso toward the table surface and then locks the shoulder joint with that orientation, the arm will be positioned above the shoulders when the torso is brought back to vertical (Figure 12).

Summary

The loss of a hand or arm is a major disability. Unfortunately, today's prosthetic components and interface techniques are still a long way from realizing fully functioning artificial arm or hand replacements with physiologic speeds of response and strength that can be controlled almost without thought. Heckathorne (personal communication, 2003) believes the perception of prosthetics research is not like that of research in the physical sciences. In the physical sciences, the goal is generally abstract and the details are obscure to the layperson. In prosthetics research, every person with a traumatic amputation or unilateral congenital limb deficiency knows the goal on a very personal level. Every advancement in limb prosthetics is compared to recreation of the physiologic limb and the experience with the artificial limb. Although many people use prostheses and thus appear to accept the state of the art, they are generally not satisfied with it. Prosthetics research is driven by dissatisfaction.

Acknowledgments

We thank the Veterans Administration Rehabilitation Research and Development Service and the National Institute on Disability and Rehabilitation Research for their sustaining support that facilitated development of this chapter. We are also grateful to Craig Heckathorne and Edward Grahn for their valuable assistance and significant influence.

References

1. Heckathorne CW, Krick H, Uellendahl J, Wu Y, Childress DS: Achieving complementary manipulative function with bilateral hybrid upper-limb prostheses. *Arch Phys Med Rehabil* 1990;71:773.

2. Kuiken TA, Rymer WZ, Childress DS: The hyper-reinnervation of rat skeletal muscle. *Brain Res* 1995;676:113-123.

3. Abul-Haj CJ, Hogan N: Functional assessment of control systems for cybernetic elbow prostheses. Part I: Description of the technique. *IEEE Trans Biomed Eng* 1990;37:1025-1036.

4. Abul-Haj CJ, Hogan N: Functional assessment of control systems for cybernetic elbow prostheses. Part II: Application of the technique. *IEEE Trans Biomed Eng* 1990;37:1037-1047.

5. Michael JW: Upper limb powered components and controls: Current concepts. *Clin Prosthet Orthot* 1986;10:66-77.

6. Bernstein N: *The Co-ordination and Regulation of Movements*, London, England, Pergamon Press, 1967.

7. Simpson DC: The choice of control system for the multimovement prosthesis: Extended physiological proprioception, in Herberts P, Kadefors R, Magnusson RI, Petersen I (eds): *The Control of Upper-Extremity Prostheses and Orthoses*. Springfield, IL, Charles C Thomas Publishers, 1974, pp 146-150.

8. Childress DS: Powered limb prostheses: Their clinical significance. *IEEE Trans Biomed Eng* 1973;20:200-207.

9. Farrell T: *The Effect of Non-Linearities on Extended Physiological Proprioception (EPP) Control of a Powered Prosthesis*. Evanston, IL, Northwestern University, 2003. Thesis.

10. Parker PA, Scott RN: Myoelectric control of prostheses. *Crit Rev Biomed Eng* 1986;13:283-310.

11. Basmajian J, DeLuca C: *Muscles Alive*, ed 5. Baltimore, MD, Williams & Wilkins, 1985.

12. Scott RN: An introduction to myoelectric prostheses, in *U.N.B. Monographs on Myoelectric Prostheses*. Fredericton, Canada. University of New Brunswick Bio-Engineering Institute, 1984.

13. Scott RN, Childress DS: A bibliography on myoelectric control of prostheses, in *U.N.B. Monographs on Myoelectric Prostheses*. Fredericton, Canada. University of New Brunswick Bio-Engineering Institute, 1989.

14. Reiter R: Eine neue Elektrokunsthand. *Grenzgebiete Med* 1948;1:133-135.

15. Battye CK, Nightingale A, Whillis J: The use of myoelectric currents in the

operation of prostheses. *J Bone Joint Surg Br* 1955;37:506-510.

16. Bottomley AH, Kinnier Wilson AB, Nightingale A: Muscle substitutes and myoelectric control. *J Br Inst Radio Eng* 1963;26:439-448.

17. Bottomley AH: Myo-electric control of powered prostheses. *J Bone Joint Surg Br* 1965;47:411-415.

18. Popov B: The bio-electrically controlled prosthesis. *J Bone Joint Surg Br* 1965;47:421-424.

19. Childress DS: An approach to powered grasp, in Gavrilovic MM, Wilson AB Jr (eds): *Proceedings of the Fourth International Symposium on External Control of Human Extremities: Advances in External Control of Human Extremities, August 28–September 2, 1972.* Belgrade, Yugoslavia, Yugoslav Committee for Electronics and Automation (ETAN), 1973, pp 159-167.

20. Barry DT, Cole NM: Muscle sounds are emitted at the resonant frequencies of skeletal muscle. *IEEE Trans Biomed Eng* 1990;37:525-531.

21. Simpson DC: Powered hand controlled by "muscle bulge." *J Sci Instrum* 1966;43:521-522.

22. Abboudi RL, Glass CA, Newby NA, Flint JA, Craelius W: A biomimetic controller for a multifinger prosthesis. *IEEE Trans Rehabil Eng* 1999;4:121-129.

23. Näder M: Erfahrungen und Beobachtungen mit Myobock I, Derzeitiger Stand der Entwicklung der Otto Bock Myostat Systems. *Orthop Technik* 1970; 22:337-340.

24. Edell DJ: A peripheral nerve information transducer for amputees: Long-term multichannel recordings from rabbit peripheral nerves. *IEEE Trans Biomed Eng* 1986;33:203-214.

25. Kovacs GT, Storment CW, Jemes B, et al: Design and implementation of two-dimensional neural interfaces. *Proceedings of the 10th Annual Conferences of the IEEE Engineering in Medicine and Biology Society.* New Orleans, LA, 1988, pp 1649-1650.

26. Andrews B, Warwick K, Jamous A, Gasson M, Harwin W, Kyberd P: Development of an implanted neural control interface for artificial limbs. *Proceedings of the 10th World Congress of the International Society for Prosthetics and Orthotics.* Copenhagen, Den-

mark, ISPO Publications, 2001, pp TO8.6.

27. Wessburg J, Stambaugh CR, Kralik JD, et al: Real-time prediction of hand trajectory by ensembles of cortical neurons in primates. *Nature* 2000;408: 361-365.

28. Wolpaw JR, Birbaumer N, Heetderks WJ, et al: Brain-computer interface technology: A review of the first international meeting. *IEEE Trans Rehabil Eng* 2000;8:164-173.

29. Kennedy PR, Bakay RA, Moore MM, Adams K, Goldwithe J: Direct control of a computer from the human central nervous system. *IEEE Trans Rehabil Eng* 2000;8:198-202.

30. Reger BD, Fleming KM, Sanquineti V, Alford S, Mussa-Ivaldi FA: Connecting brains to robots: The development of a hybrid system for the study of learning in neural tissues. *Artif Life* 2000;6: 307-324.

31. Loeb GE, Richmond FR, Olney S, et al: Bionic neurons for functional and therapeutic electrical stimulation. *IEEE Eng Med Biol Mag* 1998;20:2305-2309.

32. Reilly RE: Implantable devices for myoelectric control, in Herberts P, Kadefors R, Magnusson RI, Petersén I (eds): *Proceedings of the Conference on the Control of Upper-Extremity Prostheses and Orthoses.* Springfield, IL, Charles C. Thomas, 1973, pp 23-33.

33. Weir RF *ff*, Troyk PR, DeMichele G, Kuiken T: Implantable myoelectric sensors (IMES) for upper-extremity prosthesis control. Preliminary work. *Proceedings of the 25th Silver Anniversary International Conference of the IEEE Engineering in Medicine and Biology Society (EMBS).* Cancun, Mexico, September 17-21, 2003.

34. Arcos I, David R, Fey K, et al: Second-generation microstimulator. *Artif Organs* 2002;26:228-231.

35. Taylor CL: The biomechanics of the normal and of the amputated upper extremity, in *Human Limbs and Their Substitutes.* New York, NY, McGraw-Hill, 1954, p 176.

36. Hogan NJ: *Myoelectric Prosthesis Control: Optimal Estimation Applied to EMG and Cybernetic Considerations for Its Use in a Man-Machine Interface.* Boston, MA, Massachusetts Institute of Technology, 1976. Dissertation.

37. Mann RW: Efferent and afferent control of an electromyographic proportional rate, force sensing artificial elbow with cutaneous display of joint angle. *Proceedings of the Symposium on the Basic Problems of Prehension, Movement, and Control of Artificial Limbs.* London, England, Institution of Mechanical Engineers, 1968, pp 86-92.

38. Herberts P, Magnusson R, Kadefors R, et al (eds): *The Control of Upper-Extremity Prostheses and Orthoses.* Springfield, IL, Charles C Thomas Publishers, 1974.

39. Simpson DC: An externally powered prosthesis for the complete arm. *Biomed Eng* 1969;4:106-110.

40. Mann RW, Reimers SD: Kinesthetic sensing for the EMG controlled "Boston arm." *IEEE Transactions on Man-Machine Systems* 1970;11:110-115.

41. Wirta RW, Taylor DR Jr: Development of a multiple-axis myoelectrically controlled prosthetic arm, in Advances in external control of human extremities. *Proceedings of the Third International Symposium on External Control of Human Extremities.* Dubrovnik, Yugoslavia, Yugoslav Committee for Electronics and Automation (ETAN), 1970.

42. Taylor DR, Finley FR: Multiple-axis prosthesis control by muscle synergies. The control of upper-extremity prostheses and orthoses, in Herberts P, Kadefors R, Magnusson RI, Petersén I (eds): *Proceedings of the Conference on the Control of Upper-Extremity Prostheses and Orthoses.* Springfield, IL, Charles C Thomas, 1974, pp 181-189.

43. Kato I, Yamakawa S, Ichikawa K, Sano M: Multifunctional myoelectric hand prosthesis with pressure sensory feedback system Waseda hand 4P, in Advances in external control of human extremities. *Proceedings of the Third International Symposium on External Control of Human Extremities.* Dubrovnik, Yugoslavia, Yugoslav Committee for Electronics and Automation (ETAN), 1970, pp 155-170.

44. Razic D: Kinematics design of a multifunctional hand prosthesis, in Advances in external control of human extremities, in Gavrilovic MM, Wilson AB Jr (eds): *Proceedings of the Fourth International Symposium on External Control of Human Extremities.* Dubrovnik, Yugoslavia, Yugoslav Com-

mittee for Electronics and Automation (ETAN), 1973, pp 177-183.

45. Stojiljkovic ZV, Saletic DZ: Tactile pattern recognition by Belgrade hand prosthesis, in Advances in external control of human extremities. *Proceedings of the Fifth International Symposium on External Control of Human Extremities.* Dubrovnik, Yugoslavia, Yugoslav Committee for Electronics and Automation (ETAN), 1975.

46. Herberts P, Almström C, Caine K: Clinical application study of multifunctional prosthetic hands. *J Bone Joint Surg Br* 1978;60:552-560.

47. Jacobsen SC, Knutti DF, Johnson RT, Sears HH: Development of the Utah artificial arm. *IEEE Trans Biomed Eng* 1982;29:249-269.

48. Williams TW: Use of the Boston elbow for high-level amputees, in Atkins DJ, Meier RH (eds): *Comprehensive Management of the Upper-Limb Amputee.* New York, NY, Springer-Verlag, 1989, pp 211-220.

49. Sears HH, Andrew JT, Jacobsen SC: Experience with the Utah arm, hand, and terminal device, in Atkins DJ, Meier RH (eds): *Comprehensive Management of the Upper-Limb Amputee,* New York, NY, Springer-Verlag, 1989, pp 194-210.

50. Lawrence PD, Kadefors R: Classification of myoelectric patterns for the control of a prosthesis, in the control of upper-extremity prostheses and orthoses, in Herberts P, Kadefors R, Magnusson RI, Petersén I (eds): *Proceedings of the Conference on the Control of Upper-Extremity Prostheses and Orthoses.* Springfield, IL, Charles C Thomas, 1974, pp 190-200.

51. Almstrom C, Herberts P, Korner L: Experience with Swedish multifunctional prosthetic hands controlled by pattern recognition of multiple myoelectric signals. *Int Orthop* 1981;5:15-21.

52. Beattie D, Iberall T, Sukhatme GS, Bekey GA: EMG control for a robot hand used as a prosthesis, in Bacon DC, Rahmin T, Harwin WS (eds): *Proceedings of the Fourth International Conference on Rehabilitation Robotics (ICORR).* Wilmington, DE, Applied Science & Engineering Laboratories, University of Delaware, A.I. duPont Institute, 1994, pp 67-72.

53. Vinet R, Lozac'h Y, Beaudry N, Drouin G: Design methodology for a multifunctional hand prosthesis. *J Rehabil Res Dev* 1995;32:316-324.

54. Lozac'h Y: The preferred working plane for an active thumb. *Proceedings of the 2nd International Conference on Rehabilitation Engineering (RESNA 84).* Washington, DC, RESNA Press, 1984, pp 24-25.

55. Graupe D, Salahi J, Zhang DS: Stochastic analysis of myoelectric temporal signatures for multifunctional single-site activation of prostheses and orthoses. *J Biomed Eng* 1985;7:18-29.

56. Kelly MF, Parker PA, Scott RN: The application of neural networks to myoelectric signal analysis: A preliminary study. *IEEE Trans Biomed Eng* 1990;37:221-230.

57. Hudgins BS, Parker PA, Scott RN: A new strategy for multifunction myoelectric control. *IEEE Trans Biomed Eng* 1993;40:82-94.

58. Farry KA, Walker ID, Sendonaris A: Teleoperation of a multifingered robotic hand with myoelectrics. *Proceedings of Myo-Electric Control Symposium '93 (MEC'93).* New Brunswick, Canada, University of New Brunswick, 1993, pp 115-122.

59. Farry KA, Fernandez MS, Abramczyk ME, Novy BS, Atkins D: Applying genetic programming to control of an artificial arm. *Proceedings of Myo-Electric Control Symposium '97 (MEC'97).* New Brunswick, Canada, University of New Brunswick, 1997, pp 50-55.

60. Chan FH, Yang YS, Lam FK, Zhang YT, Parker PA: Fuzzy EMG classification for prosthesis control. *IEEE Trans Rehabil Eng* 2000;8:305-311.

61. Engelhart K, Hudgins B, Parker PA: A wavelet-based continuous classification scheme for multifunction myoelectric control. *IEEE Trans Biomed Eng* 2001;48:302-311.

62. Herberts P, Almström C, Kadefors R, Lawrence P: Hand prosthesis control via myoelectric patterns. *Acta Orthop Scand* 1973;44:389-409.

63. Kyberd PJ, Chappell PH: The Southampton hand: An intelligent myoelectric prosthesis. *J Rehabil Res Dev* 1994;31:326-334.

64. Ajiboye AB, Weir RF, Heckathorne CW, Childress DS: Neurofuzzy logic as a control algorithm for an externally powered multifunctional hand prosthesis. *Proceedings of the Myoelectric Controls Conference (MEC2002).* New Brunswick, Canada, University of New Brunswick, 2002, pp 126-130.

65. Weir RF: Design of a clinically viable multifunctional prosthetic hand. *Proceedings of the Myoelectric Controls Conference (MEC2002).* New Brunswick, Canada, University of New Brunswick, 2002, pp 2-5.

66. Peizer E, Wright DW, Mason C, et al: Guidelines for standards for externally powered hands. *Bull Prosthet Res* 1969; 10:118-155.

67. Weir RF: Design of artificial arms and hands for prosthetic applications, in Myer Kutz (ed): *Standard Handbook of Biomedical Engineering & Design.* New York, NY, McGraw-Hill, 2003, pp 32.1–32.61.

68. Weir RF, Grahn EC, Duff SJ: A new externally-powered, myoelectrically controlled prosthesis for persons with partial hand amputations at the metacarpals. *J Prosthet Orthot* 2001;12:26-31.

69. Marquardt E: The operative treatment of congenital limb malformation: Part I. *Prosthet Orthot Int* 1980;4:135-144.

70. Beasley RW: The tendon exteriorization cineplasty. *Inter-Clin Info Bull* 1966;5:6-8.

71. Vanghetti G: Plastica dei Monconi a Scopo di Protesi Cinematica. *Arch Ortop* 1899a;16:305-324.

72. Vanghetti G: Plastica dei Monconi a Scopo di Protesi Cinematica. *Arch Ortop* 1899b;16:385-410.

73. Vanghetti G: Plastica dei Monconi ed Amputazioni Transitore. *Arch Ortop* 1900;17:305-329.

74. Sauerbruch F: *Die Willkürlich Bewegbare Künstliche Hand. Eine Anleitung für Chirurgen und Techniker.* Berlin, Germany, Julius Springer-Verlag, 1916.

75. Lebsche M: Ohnhänder: Aus dem Caritasspital Schloß Fürstenried. *Langenbecks Arch Surg* 1950;265:292-295.

76. Brückner L: Sauerbruch-Lebsche-Vanghetti cineplasty: The surgical procedure. *Orthop Traumatol* 1992;1:90-99.

77. Biedermann WG: Ist der Sauerbrucharm noch aktuell? *Orthop Technik* 1981;32:156-161.

78. Baumgartner R: Möglichkeiten und Grenzen der Prothesenversorgung der oberen Extremität. *Biomed Technik* 1985;30:340-344.

79. Brückner L, Thomas M: Der funktionelle Wert des Sauerbruch-Armes. *Z Orthop* 1994;132:185-192.

80. Brav EA, MacDonald WF, Woodard GH, Leonard F: Follow-up notes on articles previously published in the journal: Cineplasty–ten years later. *J Bone Joint Surg Am* 1964;46:1137-1138.

81. Brav EA, Fletcher MJ, Kuitert JH, et al: Cineplasty, an end-result study. *J Bone Joint Surg Am* 1957;39:59-76.

82. Leal JM, Malone JM: VA/USMC electric hand with below elbow cineplasty. *Bull Prosthet Res* 1981;10:52-56.

83. Lücke R, Marquardt E, Carstens C: Abstract: Kineplasty according to Sauerbruch: The fresh indication for the pectoralis canal in amputations in the region of the shoulder girdle. *Proceedings of the Sixth World Congress of the International Society for Prosthetics and Orthotics (ISPO), November 12-17, 1989.* Copenhagen, Denmark, ISPO Publications, Kobe, Japan, p 200.

84. Weir RF, Heckathorne CW, Childress DS: Cineplasty as a control input for externally powered prosthetic components. *J Rehabil Res Dev* 2001;38:357-363.

85. Marquardt E: Come-back of the pectoral cineplasty. *J Assoc Child Prosthet Orthot Clin* 1987;22:32.

86. Seamone W, Schmeisser G, Hoshall H: A powered cable drive for prosthetic-orthotic systems, in Gavrilov M, Wilson AB Jr (eds): *Proceedings of the Fourth International Symposium on Advances in External Control of Human Extremities.* Dubrovnik, Yugoslavia, Yugoslav Committee for Electronics and Automation, 1973, pp 736-755.

87. Krukenberg H: *Über Plastische Umwertung von Armamputationsstümpfen.* Stuttgart, Germany, 1917.

88. Swanson AB, Swanson GD: The Krukenberg procedure in the juvenile amputee. *Clin Orthop* 1980;148:55-61.

89. Mathur BP, Narang IC, Piplani CL, Majid MA: Rehabilitation of the bilateral below-elbow amputee by the Krukenberg procedure. *Prosthet Orthot Int* 1981;5:135-140.

90. Baumgartner RF, Asey CH: The Krukenberg hand: Late results and todays indications. *Proceedings of the 7th World Congress of the International Society for Prosthetics and Orthotics (ISPO).* Chicago, IL, 1992, p 205.

91. Ryder RA: Occupational therapy for a patient with a bilateral Krukenberg amputation. *Am J Occup Ther* 1989;43:689-691.

92. Hoffer JA, Loeb GE: Implantable electrical and mechanical interfaces with nerve and muscle. *Ann Biomed Eng* 1980;8:351-360.

93. Brånemark PI: Osseointegration: Biotechnological perspective and clinical modality, in Brånemark PI, Rydevik BL, Skalak R (eds): *Osseointegration in Skeletal Reconstruction and Joint Replacement.* Chicago, IL, Quintessence Publishing Co Inc, 1997, pp 1-24.

94. Brånemark R, Brånemark PI, Rydevik B, Myers RR: Osseointegration in skeletal reconstruction and rehabilitation: A review. *J Rehabil Res Dev* 2001;38:175-182.

95. Hall CW, Rostoker W: Permanently attached artificial limbs. *Bull Prosthet Res* 1980;10:98-100.

96. Sears HH, Shaperman J: Proportional myoelectric hand control: An evaluation. *Am J Phys Med Rehabil* 1991;70:20-28.

97. Billock J: Upper limb prosthetic management: Hybrid design approaches. *Clin Prosthet Orthot* 1985;9:23-25.

98. Childress DS: Biological mechanisms as potential sources of feedback and control in prostheses: Possible applications, in Murdoch G, Donovan R (eds): *Amputation Surgery & Lower Limb Prosthetics.* New York, NY, Blackwell Scientific Publications, 1988, pp 197-203.

99. Heckathorne CW, Strysik J, Grahn EG: Design of a modular extended physiological proprioception controller for clinical applications in prosthesis control. *Proceedings of the 12th Annual Conference on Rehabilitation Engineering Technology (RESNA).* New Orleans, LA, 1989, pp 226-227.

100. Doubler JA, Childress DS: An analysis of extended physiological proprioception as a control technique. *J Rehabil Res Dev* 1984;21:5-18.

101. Doubler JA, Childress DS: Design and evaluation of a prosthesis control system based on the concept of extended physiological proprioception. *J Rehabil Res Dev* 1984;21:19-31.

102. Weir RF ff: *Direct Muscle Attachment as a Control Input for a Position Servo Prosthesis Controller.* Evanston, IL, Northwestern University, 1995. Dissertation.

103. Childress DS, Krick H, Heckathorne CW, Uellendahl J: Positive-locking components and hybrid fitting concepts for persons with high level bilateral arm amputations. *Proceedings of the 12th Annual Conference on Rehabilitation Engineering Technology (RESNA),* New Orleans, LA 1989, pp 296-297.

104. Heckathorne CW, Duff S, Uellendahl J, Childress D: The trans-humeral four-function forearm set-up. *Proceedings of the Ninth World Congress of the International Society for Prosthetics and Orthotics, Amsterdam, The Netherlands, June 28-July 3, 1998.* Copenhagen, Denmark, ISPO Publications, 1998, pp 601-603.

Chapter 13

Partial Hand Amputation: Surgical Management

E. Ouellette, MD, MBA

Introduction

The primary goals of amputation surgery are preservation of length and useful sensibility, prevention of symptomatic neuromas and adjacent joint contracture, early prosthetic fitting where applicable, and prompt return of the patient to work or play.[1] When the amputation is for a malignant tumor, the primary goal is to restore the best function possible while preserving life. Evidence exists that after amputation of a limb, the brain reorganizes in both the motor and sensory cortices.[2] The opposite motor and sensory cortices increase activity. This plasticity has been demonstrated in both animals and humans by monitoring activity via transcranial magnetic stimulation. In Macaque monkeys, the somatotopic map for the residuum of a finger that has been amputated occupies the same area that once represented the entire finger.[3] This plastic adaptation of the brain may provide opportunities to enhance the amputee's rehabilitation.

Hand Function

The primary objective of hand surgery is to restore function to an injured hand, so the surgeon should understand basic hand function and how to evaluate it before undertaking repair or reconstruction. The method of evaluating function must adequately assess the extent of the injury and predict the outcome of reconstruction.[4-8]

A number of standard tests are now used to evaluate the musculoskeletal components, sensation, and functional capacity of the hand. The musculoskeletal assessments include measurement of muscle strength and joint range of motion, and sensory function is evaluated through tactile sensitivity.[9-11] Functional capacity is determined by direct observation of a patient's ability to manipulate objects and otherwise use the hand.[12-14] How to assess functional impairment resulting from lost range of motion is well outlined in several sources, including the American Medical Association's *Guides to the Evaluation of Permanent Impairment.*[7,15-17]

Prehensile activities involve power and precision grips and are evaluated by grip strength measurement and, in the case of precision grips, by a movement profile as well.[18,19] The hand dynamometer provides the most consistent measure of power grip strength, assessed by averaging three separate trials.[20] Three types of precision grip involve the thumb and index and middle fingers: tip pinch, three-jaw chuck pinch, and lateral pinch. Tip pinch between the thumb and the index finger is used to pick up objects such as paper clips; the three-jaw chuck pinch uses all three digits to grasp objects more firmly; and lateral pinch, which, like tip pinch, is between the thumb and the index finger, is used to hold a key. These grip mea-

surements are also most accurate when three trials are averaged.

Evaluating tactile sensitivity includes assessing discrimination thresholds for pressure, temperature, vibration, and two-point discrimination.[21,22] Normal, static two-point discrimination at the fingertips is approximately 6 mm.[11,23] Moving two-point discrimination can also be used to test the mechanoreceptors in the hand.[24,25] Normal values for moving two-point discrimination are slightly lower (4 mm) than those for static two-point discrimination measured in the same person.

Pressure sensitivity can be evaluated by Semmes-Weinstein monofilaments,[26] which are a series of nylon filaments of decreasing diameters such that the force required to bend each filament after skin contact is less for each successive filament. These are applied in succession until the patient is unable to feel the pressure. Pressure sensitivity does not correlate with two-point discrimination.

Point localization, tactile object recognition, and sudomotor function are also important in evaluating sensory deficits. Point localization is tested by touching the skin with a probe in one or two separate locations and asking the patient to identify those locations.[15,27] Tactile object recognition, also known as tactile gnosis or stereognosis, is the ability to recognize an object placed in the

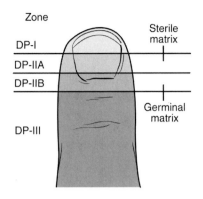

Figure 1 The Hirase classification of fingertip amputation zones based on surgical treatment.

hand. The time the patient takes to identify the object is also recorded. Sudomotor function is evaluated by the Ninhydrin sweat test[5,24] or the wrinkle test.[28] When a peripheral nerve is cut, innervation of the sweat glands is lost, and the skin becomes dry. The return of sudomotor function closely follows the return of tactile sensibility.[5,27] The sudomotor test is valued as a confirmation of nerve return. The wrinkle test is performed by placing the hand in warm water (42°C) for 20 to 30 minutes. If the skin is denervated, it will not wrinkle because the sympathetic nerve fibers that supply the sweat glands are absent.

To more fully evaluate functional activities of the hand, a number of tests have been devised that involve manipulating small objects or performing activities of daily living. The only objective measurement is the time it takes to perform the tasks.[5,29,30] These tests are important because they require a combination of functions measured by all the previous methods, thus measuring the ability to execute certain tasks by the hand. At present, these are the best instruments to evaluate hand function as a whole.

Fingertip Injuries

Fingertip injuries are very common among industrial workers and also in children. A common scenario is when an industrial worker, usually working with a circular saw, accidentally amputates the finger at the midnail area. Children sustain fingertip amputations when a door is forcefully slammed on the digit. The treatment depends on whether the clean, amputated tissue is available. In adults, the best treatment is to apply a full-thickness defatted skin graft taken from the part. If there are losses in the nail bed on the remaining digit, a full-thickness graft of nail matrix can be taken from the amputated part to restore the matrix of the remaining digit. In children, no defatting is done, and the clean amputated part is accurately replaced with as few sutures as possible in a circular manner so that revascularization may occur. If the amputated part is not brought in or is dirty and therefore unusable, reconstruction is the only option.

Fingertip injuries have benefited from microsurgical techniques, which add to the variety of treatment choices. A new understanding of what can be revascularized successfully has led to a new classification developed by Hirase[31] that divides the distal phalanx (DP) into several zones based on the anastomotic level of the digital artery and the surgical treatment for replantation (Figure 1). The anastomotic level is defined as the location at which arterial repair in a replantation has been performed. This classification allows treatment decisions to be made based on the level of injury. The recommended surgical procedure for zone DP-I amputations is a composite graft and ice-water cooling. Zone II is divided into parts A and B. The recommended surgical procedure for both zones DP-IIA and DP-IIB is arterial anastomosis, without using Kirschner wires (K-wires) for bone fixation, if possible. There is no need to perform treatment for venous return in zone DP-IIA. Zone DP-IIB should be treated with a partial nail resection and the use of heparin gauze or medical leeches. The digital nerve should be sutured if possible. The recommended surgical treatment for zone DP-III is to perform arterial and venous anastomosis, to use K-wires for bone fixation, and to suture the digital nerves bilaterally.[31] A free vascularized nail graft from the toe to the fingertip can provide satisfactory functional as well as aesthetic results. By transferring an osteoonychocutaneous flap from the toe, it is possible to restore the fingertip and any associated nail involvement.[32] Brown and associates[33] have described an alternative technique to restore the fingertip and nail bed using local or regional flaps.

Pocketing has also become a useful method for fingertip replantation. This technique uses a deep abdominal fascia pocket surrounding a de-epithelialized finger pulp. Kim and associates[34] and Lee and associates[35] believe that pocketing improves survival of the replanted fingertip because of the vascularity within the fascia. To be successful, the procedure must be performed soon after the injury, before necrosis occurs. The pocketing procedure is performed after all other treatments available have failed. There are also four classic modes of reconstructing the fingertip to avoid amputating the distal phalanx. These are fat advancement and split- or full-thickness skin grafting, V-Y plasty, cross-finger flaps, and distant flaps. These are well described in standard texts[36] (Figures 2 and 3).

Replantation

Since the first report of successful reattachment of an amputated thumb by Komatsu and Tamai[37] in 1968, advances in microsurgical technique and increased experience have made replantation routinely possible in microsurgical centers. In the hand, there is little or no muscle tissue to sustain anoxic damage, and successful replantation following cold ischemic times of more than 30 hours has been reported.[1] Virtually every person in the continental United States can therefore be considered to be within range of a microsurgical center and thus a potential candidate for replantation. Although there are preoperative

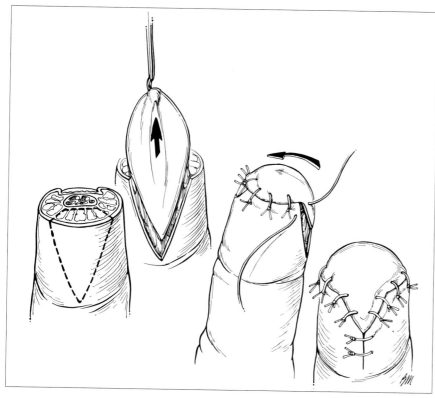

Figure 2 The Atasoy-Kleinert volar V-Y technique. This is useful in distal fingertip injuries with bone exposed where there is sufficient volar tissue. With volar pad tissue loss, there is usually insufficient skin for this technique to be used. *(Adapted with permission from Louis DS: Amputations, in Green D (ed): Surgery of the Hand, ed 2. New York, NY, Churchill Livingstone, 1988. Illustration by Elizabeth Roselius, © 1988.)*

guidelines for replantation, the ultimate decision must often be made in the operating room. The referring physician must take care not to commit the replantation team to too much or too little in preoperative discussions with the patient and family.

Indications

Generally accepted indications for replantation include amputations of multiple digits or those through the palm or near the wrist.[38,39] In addition, virtually any amputation in a child should be replanted. Although vascular repair is technically more difficult in children and success rates lower than in adults, the superior neurologic recovery in children, particularly in young children, makes this effort worthwhile.[40] Most patients report excellent levels of satisfaction with replanted thumbs. Significant stiffness at the interphalangeal (IP) and metacarpophalangeal (MCP) joints does not hamper the thumb

with an intact carpometacarpal articulation.[39] Perhaps the most important reason for acceptable function of the replanted thumb is that no completely satisfactory substitute for its function is available. This not only guarantees that the patient will use the replanted thumb, but also that the usual activities of daily living will maximize restoration of motion.

The same considerations also apply to replanting multiple fingers. Although the function of each digit may not be better than that achieved in single-digit replantation, these digits may contribute significantly to overall hand function when few or no remaining normal digits are available for substitution.[39,41] In these cases, each additional digit, unless it is severely impaired, can add significantly to the width and strength of the hand.

Indications for replantation of a single digit, except the thumb, are more controversial.[39] Replantations distal to the flexor superficialis inser-

tion (ie, the middle phalanx) usually do well. They exhibit significantly better range of motion (approximately 80° of proximal IP joint motion) than do replants proximal to the flexor superficialis insertion, which have an average proximal IP joint motion of approximately 35°. Scott and associates[42] found the total active motion of replants through the proximal phalanx to be poor (averaging 120°) in 84% of their patients. Joint stiffness combined with limited sensibility may seriously limit the use of a replanted digit when three normal digits are available for substitution. Even worse, the impaired function of the replanted finger may seriously jeopardize use of the entire hand. Causes of limited use may include decreased sensibility, pain, cold intolerance, and quadriga. Quadriga is the loss of full excursion in one profundus tendon that causes decreased motion in others because of their anatomic interconnections. For these reasons, many authors no longer recommend proximal replantation of single digits, except in the occasional patient for whom a full complement of digits is a professional necessity (eg, a musician) or perhaps in children.[43]

The management of one particular type of single-digit amputation, ring finger avulsion injuries, has been the subject of debate.[43] Although complete amputations by this mechanism have not been recommended for replantation in the past,[44] it has since been demonstrated that the level of experience of the surgical team and liberal use of vein grafts are of far greater significance than the mechanisms of injury in predicting success.[45]

Contraindications

Relative contraindications to replantation include associated life-threatening injury or the presence of systemic disease, particularly any that would affect the patient's vasculature or ability to withstand a prolonged surgical procedure. Factors pertaining to the injury itself, including severe

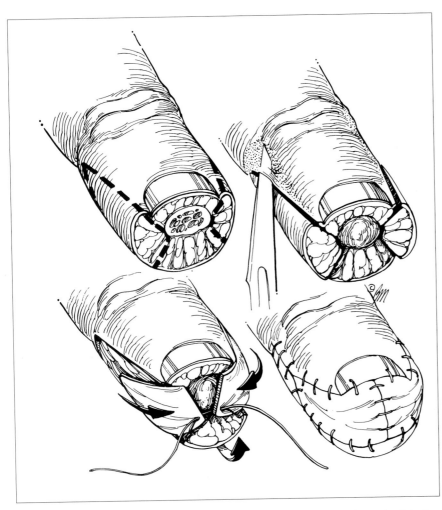

Figure 3 The Kutler lateral V-Y technique for closure of distal fingertip injuries. *(Adapted with permission from Louis DS: Amputations, in Green DP (ed):* Surgery of the Hand, *ed 2. New York, NY, Churchill Livingstone, 1988. Illustration by Elizabeth Roselius, © 1988.)*

crush or avulsion, gross contamination, the presence of injury at multiple levels, or excessive delay in treatment, may also make attempts at replantation inadvisable.[41]

The ultimate question to be answered is whether the replanted part will function in a manner that will surpass amputation. Although the strictly medical issues involved in making such a decision are complex enough, the surgeon must also consider and discuss with the patient the psychological and economic implications of the available options.[38] The surgeon must remember that the functional results of digit salvage are not enhanced by the ability to reestablish circulation when other tissues at the same level are injured.

Results

Once the decision for replantation has been made, survival rates in most recent series approach 80% to 90% or greater at all levels.[38,41-43,46] The major factors influencing survival are the age of the patient and experience of the surgeon.[43] Early complications requiring reoperation are related to vascular occlusion in up to 40% of cases.[47,48] Slightly less than half of the digits requiring early reoperation are salvageable.[48] Fortunately, infection following replantation in the hand is rare.[41,46,47] The incidence of postoperative hemorrhage reported in various series ranges from rare to nearly 50% of cases.[41,47] The severity of this complication is difficult to quantify, and the incidence of bleeding significant enough to require reoperation has not been reported. Postoperative heparinization seems to be associated with higher rates of hemorrhagic complications, and today, most surgeons routinely administer heparin only to those patients with severe crush or avulsion injuries in whom the risk of thrombosis is greatest.[47] Leeches may also be of benefit if there is difficulty with venous drainage.

Recovery of sensation following replantation is slightly poorer than that after digital neurorrhaphy for lacerations of the digits. If nerve repair is delayed or requires the use of grafts, recovery of sensation is not as good as with primary repair. Virtually all patients develop protective sensation, and the two middle fingers regain measurable two-point discrimination. Approximately one half will exhibit two-point discrimination of 10 mm or less.[38,41,42] Gelberman and associates[29] have shown a quantitative correlation between the return of sensation and restoration of digital vascularity.

Other late complications include bony malunion or nonunion, with an incidence of less than 5% in most series,[40,45,46] and the almost universal presence of cold intolerance.[38,42] Urbaniak and associates[43] state that this problem usually resolves spontaneously in the year or two following replantation, although it may remain indefinitely as a minor problem in colder climates.

Secondary operations are performed on 15% to almost 50% of patients, with tenolysis and release of joint contracture being the most common procedures.[48] Very few patients require late secondary reamputation.[45] Virtually all patients say they are satisfied with replantation, with few stating that they would have preferred amputation.[38,41-43]

It is difficult to appreciate how patients integrate the function of the replanted digit or digits with that of the remainder of the hand and even more difficult to quantify. Data regarding return to work do give some indication of fairly normal functional use, and the ability to do so is of obvious economic, social, and personal significance to the patient. Early return to work should be considered a priority of rehabilitation.[42,43]

Thumb Amputation

The thumb is required for both power and precision grip. To achieve this, the thumb must have adequate length, sensation, and stability as well as the ability to oppose the fingers.

Loss of the thumb at the level of the MCP joint constitutes a 40% loss of hand function and a 36% loss of function of the entire upper limb.[16] There is still controversy over exactly how much length must be lost before impairment is significant. For example, disarticulation through the IP joint of the thumb is rated as a 20% impairment of the hand.[16] Whatever the amputation level, the patient must have an adequate residuum to maintain pinch and grip.

Once length is considered adequate, sensation must be considered, including tactile perception and two-point stereognosis. Without these, it is difficult to recognize an object or localize its position in the hand. In addition, a functional thumb must have at least protective sensation.[49]

Active opposition of the thumb and index finger is necessary for grasping and pinching, with motion occurring at the carpometacarpal joint of the thumb. If this joint is destroyed or unstable, it can be fused with the thumb in a fully opposed position in which it serves as a post. This position enables the fingers to brace objects against the immobile thumb. Motion at the IP or MCP joint is not an absolute necessity for normal thumb function.

Restoration of thumb function by replantation should be considered first after thumb amputation. Replantation has become a reliable and well-documented surgical procedure as microvascular surgical techniques have improved.[49] Only after replantation is not successful or found to be not feasible should other reconstructive procedures be considered.

Thumb reconstruction requires assessment of the patient's age, sex, occupation, hand dominance, and the remaining structure and function of the injured hand. The level of amputation in the thumb determines which procedures should be considered.

Amputation of the Distal Phalanx of the Thumb

The functional impairment of amputation at this level is minimal. Primary goals are skeletal stability and adequate pain-free skin coverage with good sensation. There are numerous techniques that will maintain length and provide sensation.

For losses of soft tissue dorsally with minimal loss of length from the distal phalanx, healing by secondary intention or skin grafting is possible. If these methods do not provide adequate coverage, lateral triangular advancement flaps or pedicle flaps may be used.

When the soft-tissue loss is greater and there is digital nerve damage, other procedures may be necessary to preserve length and maintain good sensation. These include palmar advancement flaps, cross-finger flaps, and neurovascular island flaps.

Amputation Through the Mid-distal Phalanx and Midproximal Phalanx

At these levels of amputation, loss of length, which affects pinch and grip strength, causes the functional impairment. The carpometacarpal joint is usually not involved, thus preserving good rotation and mobility. The goals are restoration of length and sensibility.

A free toe transfer satisfies all the requirements of reconstruction at this level.[50,51] If this is unacceptable to the patient, other reconstructive procedures can be used, such as "phalangization" of the first metacarpal, which deepens the first web space to improve grip and pinch.

The web space procedures available include both simple and four-flap Z-plasties and dorsal rotational or remote pedicle flaps. These are most easily performed when the underlying soft tissues are minimally scarred and there is good joint mobility. When there are contractures of the muscles and scarring with loss of mobility, a pedicle flap from uninjured tissue must be used. This can be accomplished by placing a cross-arm flap, free flap, or reverse radial artery flap into the web space. By deepening the web space and releasing contracted tissue, the thumb is effectively lengthened.

Disarticulation at the Metacarpophalangeal Joint

At this level, no normal thumb function remains. Restoration of length, stability, sensation, and mobility is required. Lengthening the residuum by as little as 2 cm may improve function dramatically.

Procedures that have been used to gain length and sensibility at this level are pollicization, including transfer replantation of salvaged injured digits to the thumb position, or toe-to-hand transfers, metacarpal lengthening, bone grafting with tubed pedicle flaps, and composite radial forearm island flaps.[49]

Sensation must be achieved for these techniques to restore useful function. For this reason, bone grafting with flap coverage is a less satisfactory alternative. For metacarpal lengthening, two thirds of the first metacarpal with good skin coverage must be present. Pollicization and transfer of free tissue offer the best chances of restoring thumb function.

Amputation Through the Proximal Third of the First Metacarpal

This injury represents a complete functional loss of the thumb and subtotal or total loss of the first metacarpal with resultant loss of mobility

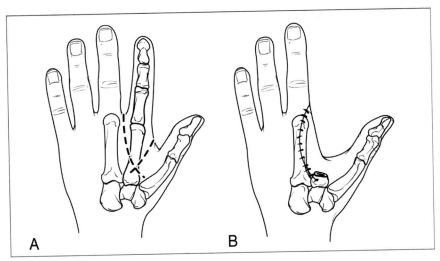

Figure 4 Technique of index ray amputation. The index metacarpal is transected at the metaphyseal flare. **A,** Racquet incision. **B,** Following index ray amputation. *(Adapted with permission from Louis DS: Amputations, in Green DP (ed): Surgery of the Hand, ed 2. New York, NY, Churchill Livingstone, 1988.)*

through the carpometacarpal joint. Reconstructive options are essentially limited to pollicization and island, or free finger, transfers. If the carpometacarpal joint is intact with a residual portion of metacarpal, a finger transfer to the thumb can be performed with minimal loss of mobility. If the entire first metacarpal is absent, the finger should be transferred with its MCP joint to preserve some motion.

Toe-to-thumb transfer is best when other fingers are mutilated. This is the only technique currently capable of restoring function when only metacarpals remain.

Ray Amputations

Ray amputations are rarely performed emergently. They are usually part of the reconstruction of a hand in which an amputation is necessary for trauma, tumor, infection, or failed replantation. If function of a digit is severely impaired or if its presence adversely affects the function of adjacent digits, removal of the entire ray should be considered to improve function of the hand as a whole.[36]

In amputation, considerations for preventing complications such as painful neuromas, closing the gap created between rays, and minimizing

cosmetic deformities are different for each ray. Index ray resection (Figure 4) has two potential associated complications to be averted. The first is debilitating pain resulting from excessive mobilization of the radial digital nerve during surgery. Pain appears in the first 8 weeks following surgery, and reoperation is not usually successful. The second complication is an intrinsic plus deformity of the middle finger resulting from transfer of the first dorsal interosseous muscle to act as the second dorsal interosseous muscle in an attempt to improve the pinch strength of the middle finger. This procedure is not necessary, and the resultant deformity will further hinder hand function.[52]

In a middle ray resection, it may be difficult to close the space between the ring and index rays (Figure 5). A soft-tissue closure of the gap using the deep intervolar plate ligaments can be performed with minimal rotational deformity of the fingers as a result (Figure 5, A). Transferring the index finger metacarpal to the base of the middle finger metacarpal is another acceptable method of reducing the gap, giving an excellent functional and cosmetic result (Figure 5, B).

Ring ray resections are similar to those of the middle ray except that the remaining gap can usually be

closed more easily. If it is difficult to reduce the space, the fifth metacarpal base can be allowed to slide spontaneously radially if the entire base of the fourth metacarpal is excised. The fifth metacarpal can also be transposed to the base of the remaining fourth metacarpal after amputation, but this is rarely necessary.

Fifth ray resections require that the base of the fifth metacarpal be retained because of the insertion of the extensor carpi ulnaris (Figure 6). The hypothenar muscles are used to provide padding over the base but are not reattached to the fourth interosseous muscle tendon because this, too, can cause an intrinsic plus deformity and loss of function.

Finger Amputations

By definition, finger amputations involve bone of the fingers. Function can be preserved by shortening or maintaining length, depending on the anatomic situation. Flap coverage similar to the type used in fingertip injuries may be used to preserve length. If this is unnecessary, then bone can be trimmed and the primary wound closed.

It is not necessary to remove articular cartilage in disarticulations through the IP joints. In fact, there is evidence that the inflammatory response to amputation is less when the cartilage is left intact. The condyles, however, should be trimmed so that they are not prominent. Both the tendon and the digital nerves should be found and transected so that clean ends may retract proximally. The flexor and extensor tendons should not be sewn to each other because the excursion of these tendons would be limited, thus limiting range of motion of the amputated and adjacent fingers.

The most significant complication of amputation at the distal IP joint is the lumbrical plus finger. This is caused by the flexor digitorum profundus retracting proximally after transection. As it retracts, the lumbrical muscle is pulled taut. When the

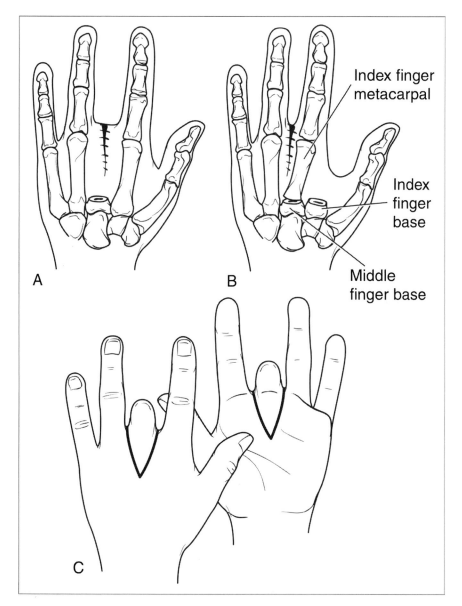

Figure 5 Middle ray resection with and without translocation of the index finger. **A,** Simple middle ray resection. **B,** Middle ray resection with translocation of the index finger metacarpal. **C,** Consider ray resection to improve function in middle and/or ring finger amputations.

patient attempts to flex the MCP and proximal IP joints while making a fist, the involved finger's proximal phalangeal joint extends paradoxically. Tension of the unrestrained flexor digitorum profundus tendon is transmitted through the lumbrical muscle to the dorsal hood mechanism to produce this effect. This can be alleviated by releasing the lumbrical muscle from its origin on the flexor digitorum profundus tendon in the palm. It is unnecessary to perform this at the time of the amputation because

this complication develops in few fingers amputated at the distal IP joint.

An amputation through the middle phalanx distal to the insertion of the flexor digitorum sublimis tendon is very functional. If resection is proximal to this, flexion control of the remaining middle phalanx is lost, and disarticulation at the proximal IP joint is recommended. The proximal IP joint should be approached in a fashion similar to the distal IP joint.

When amputation through the proximal phalanx occurs in the mid-

dle or ring fingers, a ray resection should be considered to improve function. The space left in the center of the hand cannot be compensated for except by closing the gap with a ray resection or with a prosthesis (Figure 5, *C*).

Amputations in children are special situations; replantations and revascularizations are always attempted. Saies and associates[53] studied the rate of survival of these and found that, like adults, children do better when the amputation occurred by sharp laceration without crushing. Replantations have a 72% survival rate after lacerations but have only a 53% survival rate after crush or avulsion injuries. When amputation is incomplete and revascularization is performed, the rate of survival is 100% after lacerations but only 75% after crush or avulsion injuries. In children younger than 9 years, the younger the child, the greater the chance of survival for a replanted finger. This age relationship does not hold true for revascularization.[53]

The reconstructive operations currently used for children who have lost fingers range from great-toe transfers for thumb restoration, other toe transfers for traumatic digital amputations, pollicization of fingers, and modified toe and great-toe transfer techniques.[54-58] These techniques are also used in adults for similar reconstructions to improve hand or limb function. Severe crush injuries resulting in loss of the entire hand are possible indications for a toe transfer to the forearm. The transferred toe can control a specially designed multiple-degree-of-freedom electronic prosthetic hand after rehabilitation and adaptation training.[59] Brain plasticity facilitates this growing trend of marrying reconstructive surgery with prosthetic design.

Hand Reconstruction

When replantation is not feasible after single- or multiple-finger amputations, the surgeon should focus on reconstructing the remaining hand so

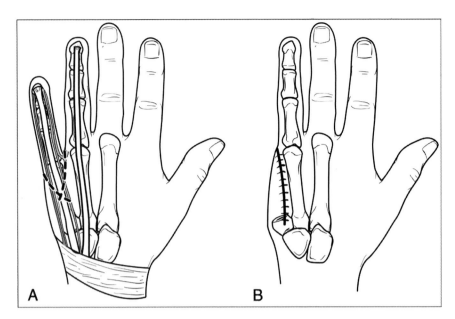

Figure 6 Ray amputation of the little finger is accomplished by transecting the metacarpal at its base and preserving the hypothenar muscles to serve as an ulnar pad for the hand. **A,** Racquet incision. **B,** Following little finger amputation.

that the patient can wear a prosthesis. Preserving the general function of the hand is fundamental to reconstruction.

When the patient has retained a "basic" hand including the thumb and at least one finger, the surgeon must consider the space between the fingers. Is that space adequate or excessive? Is there a painful neuroma in the midpalmar area that would inhibit function? Is there adequate skin coverage? Is there good sensation?

If a contracture exists, that area should be released and reconstructed with a long-lasting, soft piece of skin, ideally a distant free flap with sensation.

If the patient presents with a thumb and no other digit, reconstructing an opposing finger is a priority. A toe with its neurovascular bundle may be transferred to provide an opposing finger. The ideal timing of this procedure is at least 6 months after the original injury so that there is time for scars to mature and significant contractures to develop, allowing the surgeon to include more skin with the transferred toe, if needed after contracture release.

When coverage must provide subcutaneous tissue and sensation, potential donor procedures are a free lateral arm flap or a radial artery fasciocutaneous flap. The free lateral arm flap has a very good cushion of fat and fascia as well as a sensory nerve that can be sutured to the recipient nerve. This is also true for the radial artery flap, where the superficial radial nerve can provide innervation. These flaps are capable of withstanding prosthesis use very nicely. Other donor sites are available but do not provide as good a sensory component as these flaps.

Complications

Numerous complications can occur after amputation in the hand. Although much has been written concerning solutions to these problems, particularly the painful neuroma, few authors have attempted to examine the true nature and prevalence of these complications. The incidence of complications varies considerably in the literature, depending somewhat on how diligently the complications are reported. The reported need for

reoperation following amputation ranges from 2% to 25%.[60-62]

Most complications involve pain[60] and are therefore at least partially subjective. The patient's attempt to come to terms with an amputation involves a complex and interrelated series of physical, psychological, emotional, aesthetic, economic, and cultural adaptations. To say that well-motivated amputees do better may be trite, but it is also quite true. A review of patients who underwent amputations involving the hand revealed few of these complications, a high level of acceptance, and an almost universal return to preamputation activities.[63]

Pain after amputation may be caused by inadequate soft-tissue coverage of the residuum, an entrapped neuroma, or pain syndromes such as reflex sympathetic dystrophy. Painful amputations because of adherent or excessive scarring, poor padding, or protuberant bone are much more common in the digits than at the metacarpal level. These usually result from an injudicious attempt to save length at all costs. Although maintaining length is a concern, such residua seriously jeopardize function of the entire hand. Tension-free closure with appropriate shortening or tissue transposition should be performed initially.[60] Late treatment of such a problem is usually best managed by more proximal amputation, although occasionally local flap coverage may be considered for specific indications.[64-66]

The incidence of painful neuroma following amputation in the hand has been reported to range from less than 1% to 25% or greater.[52,61] The number of treatments proposed to prevent or manage a painful neuroma is large.[67] Occasionally, nonsurgical methods such as desensitization, transcutaneous nerve stimulation, or neural blockade may prove to be curative, but an established painful neuroma often requires a surgical solution.[65,68,69] Tupper and Booth[70] reported a 71% overall success rate with simple excision of the neuroma when the nerve end was allowed to retract under cover of more proximal, unscarred, and well-padded tissue. Other authors have had significantly less success with this technique. Transposition of the intact neuroma to a better padded, preferably dorsal location seems to provide the most consistent and significant long-term relief of pain.[30,66] The most promising new technique that may be considered when local soft tissue for transposition is inadequate is centrocentral nerve union, whereby two proximal nerve ends are joined with intervening graft.[71]

Nail deformity following amputation at or near the level of the germinal matrix is generally best treated by ablating the remaining perionychium and germinal matrix and covering the defect with a skin graft. Deformity more distal in the nail may be treated similarly; however, reconstruction with a sterile matrix graft, a germinal matrix graft, or a combination of both may be considered. The hooked nail resulting from the loss of distal phalangeal support is exceptionally difficult to treat, with resorption of distally located bone grafts and recurrence of deformity being the norm.

Quadriga (profundus tendon blockage) may limit motion of adjacent unaffected fingers after amputation. The three ulnar profundus tendons arise from a common muscle belly and are further interconnected in the palm by the bipeniform origins of the two ulnar lumbricals. Scarring of these tendons within the amputated finger or in the palm may limit excursion of the adjacent fingers. Early and full active motion of the intact fingers postoperatively usually prevents this complication.[72] Once scarring occurs, surgical correction by release of the adherent profundus tendon is quite successful.

Paradoxical extension of the proximal IP joint during attempted flexion because of retraction of the divided profundus tendon and its associated lumbrical origin is rare. Interconnections of the profundus tendons in the palm and the relatively greater strength of the flexor system make this lumbrical plus deformity uncommon. When it does occur, dividing the lumbrical tendon cures it. Median nerve compression after retraction of the profundus tendon and its lumbrical into the carpal tunnel is another rare complication.[73]

Cold intolerance after amputation is common, although this usually resolves over time without treatment. The dysvascular residuum, which is painful, nonfunctional, and prone to repeated trauma and ulceration, is generally best treated by more proximal amputation. Occasionally, pharmacologic treatment or local sympathectomy by excision of vessel adventitia may prove effective, although long-term benefits are uncertain.[73]

Summary

When a hand surgeon is faced with the decision to perform a partial hand amputation, the primary goal is to restore function. Aesthetics of the hand should be a secondary consideration. To restore the best postamputation function possible, a solid understanding of basic hand function is necessary. A thorough evaluation of the remaining function of a severely injured or diseased hand, coupled with an in-depth patient interview in which the specific requirements of hand function are assessed, will lead to an educated decision on amputation, replantation, and/or prosthetics.

A crucial part of restoring maximum hand function postamputation with replantation or prosthesis is a rigorous therapy program. The patient's inherent brain plasticity should be tapped through biofeedback. The patient needs constant motivation and encouragement from the treating physician and the therapy team. In some cases, sessions with a psychologist may be indicated to overcome barriers in dealing with this new life situation. Overall, a patient stands a good chance to return to a functional and fulfilling life.

References

1. May JW: Letter: Digit replantation with full survival after 28 hours of cold ischemia. *Plast Reconstr Surg* 1981;67:566.

2. Schwenkreis P, Witscher K, Janssen F, et al: Changes of cortical excitability in patients with upper limb amputation. *Neurosci Lett* 2000;293:143-146.

3. Manger PR, Woods TM, Jones EG: Plasticity of the somatosensory cortical map in Macaque monkeys after chronic partial amputation of a digit. *Proc R Soc Lond B Biol Sci* 1996;263:933-939.

4. Aulicino PL, DuPuy TE: Clinical examination of the hand, in Hunter JM, Schneider LH, Mackin EJ, Callahan AD (eds): *Rehabilitation of the Hand*, ed 2. St. Louis, MO, CV Mosby, 1984, pp 25-48.

5. Bell J: Sensibility testing: State of the art, in Hunter JM, Schneider LH, Mackin EJ, Callahan AD (eds): *Rehabilitation of the Hand*, ed 2. St. Louis, MO, CV Mosby, 1984, pp 390-398.

6. Brand PW (ed): *Clinical Mechanics of the Hand*. St. Louis, MO, Mosby-Year Book, 1985, pp 61-191.

7. Dellon AL (ed): *Evaluation of Sensibility and Re-education of Sensation in the Hand*. Baltimore, MD, Williams & Wilkins, 1981, pp 95-139.

8. Smith HB: Hand function evaluation. *Am J Occup Ther* 1973;27:244-251.

9. Gellis M, Pool R: Two-point discrimination distances in the normal hand and forearm: Application to various methods of fingertip reconstruction. *Plast Reconstr Surg* 1977;59:57-63.

10. Greenseid DZ, McCormack RM: Functional hand testing: A profile evaluation. *Plast Reconstr Surg* 1968;42:567-571.

11. Hallin RG, Wiesenfeld Z, Liundblom U: Neurophysiological studies on patients with sutured median nerves: Faulty sensory localization after nerve regeneration and its physiological correlates. *Exp Neurol* 1981;73:90-106.

12. Jebsen RH, Taylor N, Trieschmann RB, Trotter MJ, Howard LA: An objective and standardized test of hand function. *Arch Phys Med Rehabil* 1969;50:311-319.

13. Jones LA: The assessment of hand function: A critical review of tech-

niques. *J Hand Surg Am* 1989;14:221-228.

14. Levin S, Pearsall G, Ruderman RJ: Von Frey's method of measuring pressure sensitivity in the hand: An engineering analysis of the Weinstein-Semmes pressure aesthesiometer. *J Hand Surg Am* 1978;3:211-216.

15. Dellon LA: The moving two-point discrimination test: Clinical evaluation of the quickly adapting fiber/receptor system. *J Hand Surg Am* 1978;3:474-481.

16. Engelberg A (ed): *Guides to the Evaluation of Permanent Impairment,* ed 3. Chicago, IL, American Medical Association, 1988, pp 20-21.

17. Fess EE: The need for reliability and validity in hand assessment instruments. *J Hand Surg Am* 1986;11:621-623.

18. McPhee SD: Functional hand evaluations: A review. *Am J Occup Ther* 1987;41:158-163.

19. Mattiowetz V, Kashman N, Volland G, et al: Grip and pinch strength: Normative data for adults. *Arch Phys Med Rehabil* 1985;66:69-74.

20. Schmidt RT, Toews JV: Grip strength as measured by the Jamar dynamometer. *Arch Phys Med Rehabil* 1970;51:321-327.

21. Owen GE Jr: Sensibility testing, in Owen GE Jr, Spinner M (eds): *Management of Peripheral Nerve Problems.* Philadelphia, PA, WB Saunders, 1980, pp 3-15.

22. Parry CB: Peripheral nerve injuries: Sensation. *J Bone Joint Surg Br* 1986;68:15-19.

23. Onne L: Recovery of sensibility and sudomotor activity in the hand after nerve suture. *Acta Chir Scand Suppl* 1962;300:1-69.

24. Moberg H: Objective methods for determining the functional value of sensitivity in the hand. *J Bone Joint Surg Br* 1958;40:454-476.

25. Poppen NK, McCarroll HR Jr, Doyle JR, Niebauer JJ: Recovery of sensitivity after suture of digital nerves. *J Hand Surg Am* 1979;4:212-225.

26. Semmes J, Weinstein S, Ghent L, Teuber HL (eds): *Somatosensory Changes After Penetrating Brain Wounds in Man: Normative Study.* Cambridge, MA, Harvard University Press, 1960, pp 4-11.

27. Weinstein S: Intensive and extensive aspects of tactile sensitivity as a function of body part, sex, and laterality, in Kenshalo DR (ed): *The Skin Senses.* Springfield, IL, Charles C Thomas, 1968, pp 195-222.

28. O'Riain S: New and simple test of nerve function in the hand. *Br Med J* 1973;3:615-616.

29. Gelberman RH, Urbaniak JR, Bright DS, Levin LS: Digital sensibility following replantation. *J Hand Surg Am* 1978;3:313-319.

30. Herndon JH, Eaton RG, Littler JW: Management of painful neuromas in the hand. *J Bone Joint Surg Am* 1976;58:369-373.

31. Hirase Y: Salvage of fingertip amputated at nail level: New surgical principles and treatments. *Ann Plast Surg* 1997;38:151-157.

32. Hirase Y, Kojima T, Matsui M: Aesthetic fingertip reconstruction with a free vascularized nail graft: A review of 60 flaps involving partial toe transfers. *Plast Reconstr Surg* 1997;99:774-784.

33. Brown RE, Zook EG, Russell RC: Fingertip reconstruction with flaps and nail bed grafts. *J Hand Surg Am* 1999;24:345-351.

34. Kim KS, Eo SR, Kim DY, Lee Sy, Cho BH: A new strategy of fingertip reattachment: Sequential use of microsurgical technique and pocketing of composite graft. *Plast Reconstr Surg* 2001;107:73-79.

35. Lee PK, Ahn ST, Lim P: Replantation of fingertip amputation by using the pocket principle in adults. *Plast Reconstr Surg* 1999;103:1428-1435.

36. Louis DS: Amputations, in Green DP (ed): *Operative Hand Surgery,* ed 2. New York, NY, Churchill Livingstone, 1988, pp 61-119.

37. Komatsu S, Tamai S: Successful replantation of a completely cut-off thumb: Case report. *Plast Reconstr Surg* 1968;42:374-377.

38. Glas K, Biemer E, Duspiva KP, Werber K, Stock W, Hernald E: Long-term follow-up results of 97 finger replantations. *Arch Orthop Trauma Surg* 1982;100:95-98.

39. Strickland JW: A rationale for digital salvage, in Strickland JW, Steichen JB (eds): *Difficult Problems in Hand Surgery.* St. Louis, MO, CV Mosby, 1982, pp 243-252.

40. McC O'Brien B, Franklin JD, Morrison WA, MacLeod AM: Replantation and revascularisation surgery in children. *Hand* 1980;12:12-24.

41. Morrison WA, O'Brien BM, Macleod AM: Evaluation of digital replantation: A review of 100 cases. *Orthop Clin North Am* 1977;8:295-308.

42. Scott FA, Howar JW, Boswick JA Jr: Recovery of function following replantation and revascularization of amputated hand parts. *J Trauma* 1981;21:204-214.

43. Urbaniak JR, Roth JH, Nunley JA, Goldner RD, Koman LA: The results of replantation after amputation of a single finger. *J Bone Joint Surg Am* 1985;67:611-619.

44. Urbaniak JR, Evans JP, Bright DS: Microvascular management of ring avulsion injuries. *J Hand Surg Am* 1981;6:25-30.

45. Kay S, Werntz J, Wolff TW: Ring avulsion injuries: Classification and prognosis. *J Hand Surg Am* 1989;14:204-213.

46. Tamai S: Digit replantation: Analysis of 163 replantations in an 11 year period. *Clin Plast Surg* 1978;5:195-209.

47. Leung PC: An analysis of complications in digital replantations. *Hand* 1980;12:25-32.

48. Scott FA: Complications following replantation and revascularization, in Boswick JA (ed): *Complications in Hand Surgery.* Philadelphia, PA, WB Saunders, 1986, pp 205-214.

49. Strickland J: Thumb reconstruction, in Green DP (ed): *Operative Hand Surgery,* ed 2. New York, NY, Churchill Livingstone, 1988, pp 2175-2261.

50. May JW Jr, Rohrich RJ: Microneurovascular great toe-to-hand transfer for thumb reconstruction, in Green DP (ed): *Operative Hand Surgery,* ed 2. New York, NY, Churchill Livingstone, 1988, pp 1295-1309.

51. Urbaniak JR: Other microvascular reconstruction of the thumb, in Green DP (ed): *Operative Hand Surgery,* ed 2. New York, NY, Churchill Livingstone, 1988, pp 1311-1330.

52. Murray JF, Carman W, MacKenzie JK: Transmetacarpal amputation of the index finger: A clinical assessment of hand strength and complications. *J Hand Surg Am* 1977;2:471-481.

53. Saies AD, Urbaniak JR, Nunley JA,

Taras JS, Goldner RD, Fitch RD: Results after replantation and revascularization in the upper extremity in children. *J Bone Joint Surg Am* 1994;76: 1766-1776.

54. Weinzweig N, Chen L, Chen ZW: Pollicization of the mutilated hand by transposition of middle and ring finger remnants. *Ann Plast Surg* 1995;34: 523-529.

55. Wei FC, el-Gammal TA, Chen HC, Chuang DC, Chiang YC, Chen SH: Toe-to-hand transfer for traumatic digital amputations in children and adolescents. *Plast Reconstr Surg* 1997; 100:605-609.

56. Tomaino MM: Restoration of functional prehension after radial hemi-hand amputation in a three-year-old child: Rationale for and long-term result after great toe transfer. *J Hand Surg Am* 2001;26:617-622.

57. Foucher G, Chabaud M: The bipolar lengthening technique: A modified partial toe transfer for thumb reconstruction. *Plast Reconstr Surg* 1998;102: 1981-1987.

58. Koshima I, Kawada S, Etoh H, Saisho H, Moriguchi T: Free combined thin wrap-around flap with a second toe proximal interphalangeal joint transfer for reconstruction of the thumb. *Plast Reconstr Surg* 1995;96:1205-1210.

59. Chen Z, Hu TP: A reconstructed digit by transplantation of a second toe for control of an electromechanical prosthetic hand. *Microsurgery* 2002;22: 5-10.

60. Conolly WB, Goulston E: Problems of digital amputations: A clinical review of 260 patients and 301 amputations. *Aust N Z J Surg* 1973;43:118-123.

61. Fisher GT, Boswick JA Jr: Neuroma formation following digital amputations. *J Trauma* 1983;23:136-142.

62. Harvey FJ, Harvey PM: A critical review of the results of primary finger and thumb amputations. *Hand* 1974; 6:157-162.

63. Brown PW: Less than ten: Surgeons with amputated fingers. *J Hand Surg Am* 1982;7:31-37.

64. Brown PW: Complications following amputations of parts of the hand, in Boswick JA (ed): *Complications in Hand Surgery*. Philadelphia, PA, WB Saunders, 1986, pp 197-204.

65. Grant GH: Methods of treatment of neuromata of the hand. *J Bone Joint Surg Am* 1951;33:841-848.

66. Laborde KJ, Kalisman M, Tsai TM: Results of surgical treatment of painful neuromas of the hand. *J Hand Surg Am* 1982;7:190-193.

67. Whipple RR, Unsell RS: Treatment of painful neuromas. *Orthop Clin North Am* 1988;19:175-185.

68. Omer GE: The painful neuroma, in Strickland JW, Steichen JB (eds): *Difficult Problems in Hand Surgery*. St. Louis, MO, CV Mosby-Year Book, 1982, pp 319-323.

69. Smith JR, Gomez NH: Local injection therapy of neuromata of the hand with triamcinolone acetonide: A preliminary study of twenty-two patients. *J Bone Joint Surg Am* 1970;52:71-83.

70. Tupper JW, Booth DM: Treatment of painful neuromas of sensory nerves in the hand: A comparison of traditional and newer methods. *J Hand Surg Am* 1976;1:144-151.

71. Gorkisch K, Boese-Landgraf J, Vaubel E: Treatment and prevention of amputation neuromas in hand surgery. *Plast Reconstr Surg* 1984;73:293-299.

72. Neu BR, Murray JF, MacKenzie JK: Profundus tendon blockage: Quadriga in finger amputations. *J Hand Surg Am* 1985;10:878-883.

73. Barton NJ: Another cause of median nerve compression by a lumbrical muscle in the carpal tunnel. *J Hand Surg Am* 1979;4:189-190.

Chapter 14

Partial Hand Amputation: Prosthetic Management

Chris Lake, CPO

Introduction

Amputation distal to the wrist is one of the most common upper limb deficiencies[1] and is difficult to treat successfully with a prosthesis. Reasons for poor results include functional limitations of prosthetic technology, discomfort at the prosthetic interface, unsatisfactory appearance, and absence of tactile sensation.[2] Until the late 1990s, treatment with a prosthesis was limited by the lack of both acceptable electronic prostheses and precise treatment parameters. As Michael[3] noted, physicians and prosthetists were challenged by the need to identify a prosthesis that would "add a measure of function to diminish the substantial loss faced by the partial-hand amputee."

By the beginning of the 21st century, however, the situation had changed. Advances in upper limb prostheses once found only in the research laboratory had begun to become commercially available. The availability of these new prostheses creates a challenge for the treating prosthetist. Because many patients with limb deficiencies distal to the wrist have declined prosthetic intervention in the past,[3] the prosthetist may have limited experience with partial hand amputations.

Patient Evaluation

Evaluation of the person with an upper limb deficiency varies greatly from that of the individual with a lower limb deficiency. The significance of the physical deficit becomes apparent when the physiologic complexity of lower limb ambulation is compared with that of upper limb bimanual manipulation. Each person experiences the amputation through a unique perceptual filter, which depends on that person's life history, personality style, stage of life, social support network, and other factors.[3] Therefore, the evaluation will be enhanced by the active participation of an occupational therapist and a psychologist, whose expertise will help in the development of a successful, comprehensive rehabilitation plan.

The cause of most lower limb amputations is vascular, but approximately 90% of upper limb amputations involve trauma.[4] Traumatic amputations require careful evaluation of scar tissue, range of motion, and tissue density (Figure 1).

Sensation in the residual limb should be evaluated thoroughly, with loss of protective sensation warranting the same careful management as does hypersensitivity. Although pain is most common in phalangeal-level amputations, pain also may occur in more proximal level amputations. Pain at these other levels may result from the surgeon's attempt to save as much length as possible. Maintenance of length is of concern; however, keeping tissue that should have been removed can seriously jeopardize the function of the entire hand.[5]

A myoelectric test of the residual musculature provides the information needed for consideration of myoelectric prostheses and a means of comparing muscle characteristics. Particular sites to be considered include the most distal aspects of the wrist flexors and extensors, as well as the intrinsic musculature found about the thenar and hyperthenar eminences. The prosthetist should observe the prospective sites throughout the range of motion of the wrist to detect the likelihood of inadvertent myoelectric signals.

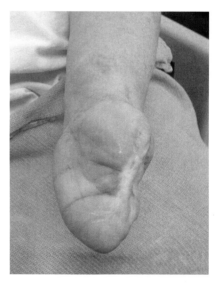

Figure 1 Traumatic transmetacarpal-level amputation with significant adherent scarring along the palmar surface.

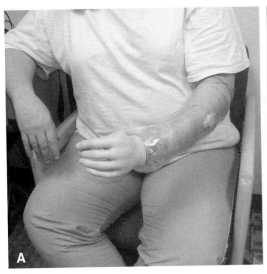
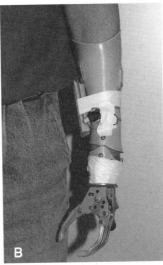

Figure 2 A, Nonarticulated design immobilizing the wrist. **B,** Articulated design preserves voluntary wrist flexion and extension. (Courtesy of Otto Bock, USA.)

Finally, limb dominance should be observed because it can dictate a particular physiologic use pattern relative to gross and fine motor skills in which dominance may indicate a propensity for fine pinch.[6] The rehabilitation team should consider the individual's vocational and other interests when formulating short- and long-term goals.

Goals of Prosthetic Management

Protection of the residual limb is the first goal of prosthetic management. Because many partial hand amputations are the result of trauma that damages the soft tissues and vascular structure of the hand, the residual limb can be significantly compromised by pressures exerted by the prosthetic components in any type of grasping pattern unless it is protected. Socket biomechanics that allow optimal stabilization of the prosthetic socket about the residual limb must be considered for residual limb protection. Optimal stabilization can be achieved by several methods, including custom silicone restoration using a suction fit, non–wrist-encapsulating or articulated wrist design that suspends over the residual anatomy and suction-type interfaces that extend

proximal to and encapsulate the wrist (Figure 2).

The second goal, bimanual stability, is to enable the patient to effectively manipulate an object or perform a task using both the contralateral and affected hands. This goal is directly related to the third goal, restoration of prehension patterns, with regard to a common problem in partial hand amputees, contralateral overuse syndrome. Results of studies of individuals with partial hand amputations have pointed out a high incidence of this syndrome. Prosthetic studies have indicated a 50% likelihood that individuals with a unilateral amputation will experience problems in the contralateral side.[7] Similar results are seen in stroke patients with only one functioning upper limb.[8] Contralateral overuse syndrome leads to a decrease in hand function that often is associated with pain and discomfort, and it can necessitate surgical treatment if conditions that exacerbate the syndrome are not addressed effectively. The syndrome can be alleviated only through bimanual stability and the restoration of prehension patterns.

The last goal of prosthetic management is to provide acceptable cosmesis and durability given the location of the amputation. Achievement of func-

tional and aesthetically pleasing results often requires fitting the client with more than one prosthesis.[3] The functional capacity of the normal human hand can be compared with that of a well-equipped toolbox. Therefore, the person with an upper limb deficiency requires the use of different prostheses to perform the many and varied activities of daily living, just as the completion of a large project requires the use of several different tools. Aesthetic restoration can be critical to the amputee's acceptance of the prosthesis, but it is virtually impossible to maximize both function and appearance in a single prosthesis. The prosthetist can achieve a more successful result by fitting two different prostheses for the same patient.

Amputation Levels and Prosthetic Options

Partial hand amputation can involve various levels of longitudinal and transverse loss that dictate different treatment options. The person with a partial hand deficiency has five fundamental prosthetic options: (1) no prosthetic intervention, (2) a passive prosthesis, (3) a body-powered prosthesis, (4) an externally powered prosthesis, and (5) multiple task-specific prostheses.

No Prosthetic Intervention

Any of a host of factors can lead a patient to decline prosthetic management. When the individual can maintain bimanual function with the residual limb, there may be no need for a prosthesis (Figure 3). Also, the residual limb shape may be so unnatural that the patient rejects prosthetic fitting because the limb cannot be fit in a manner that is cosmetically acceptable when compared with the opposite limb.

Passive Prosthesis

For the individual with a partial hand deficiency, a passive type of prosthesis that provides no active movement of

the fingers can offer the restoration of several grasp patterns.[9,10] A recent study has shown that individuals with passive prostheses actively use their prostheses as frequently as do individuals with functional prostheses[11] (Figure 4). Even though passive prostheses do not offer active grasp and release, they can be used to stabilize objects, to push against items, and to perform other functional tasks. This type of prosthesis usually incorporates a secure socket that is stabilized about the residual limb by means of a total contact suction fit. This type of socket provides the foundation for moldable fingers or an opposition post that can be used to manipulate objects. When residual fingers are present, they can oppose the prosthetic fingers or post and provide active grasp and release. Passive prostheses have been used successfully for most levels of partial hand loss, as shown in Figures 5 through 7.

Body-Powered Prostheses

Body-powered prostheses for partial hand deficiencies can be divided into two categories: cable-driven and wrist- or finger-driven devices. Cable-driven partial hand prostheses have the same inherent advantages and disadvantages as do cable-driven prostheses for amputations at higher levels. Disadvantages include limited grip force, discomfort from the required harness, and reduction of the functional envelope secondary to harness and cable movement. Wrist- or finger-driven devices can provide active grip or pinch force, but actuation may sometimes inadvertently position the fingers in a less functional position.

Externally Powered Prostheses

Until recently, no commercially available electronic terminal devices suitable for use with partial hand amputations were available, although some efforts to modify wrist disarticulation components were reported in the literature.[12] However, in 2001, Dietl and Hell (unpublished data) reported that

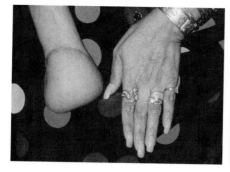 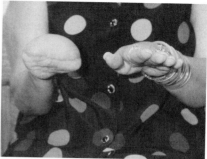

Figure 3 Situation in which the patient may decline a prosthesis. The bulbous shape of the residual limb precludes a cosmetic final result.

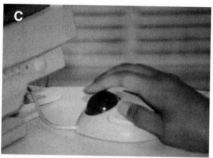 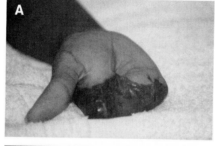 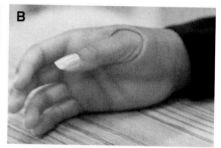 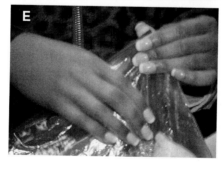 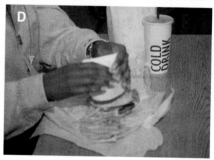

Figure 4 Passive prosthesis use. **A,** Traumatic transmetacarpal-level amputation. **B,** Appearance of the passive prosthesis. **C** through **E,** Examples of how the amputee can use the passive prosthesis.

a new electrically powered hand prosthesis approximately 3 cm shorter than prior options had been used successfully by selected patients with partial hand amputations (Figure 8).

Task-Specific Prostheses

Task-specific prostheses are available for both vocational and avocational activities. These prostheses usually involve some degree of customization to effectively meet the needs of the individual. Minimizing the overall length of the prosthesis is always a concern, but many specialized terminal devices can be modified for use by partial hand amputees, as illustrated in Figure 9.

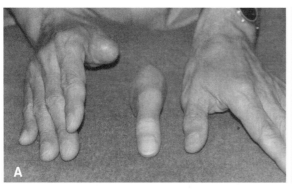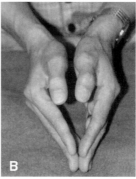

Figure 5 A, Silicone passive prosthesis for a traumatic thumb amputation. B, The appearance of the prosthesis in place. (Courtesy of Life Like Laboratories, Dallas, TX.)

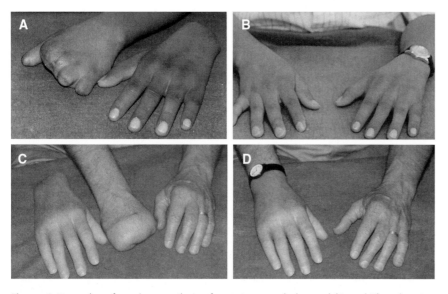

Figure 6 Examples of passive prostheses for metacarpophalangeal (A and B) and metacarpal (C and D) traumatic amputations. (Courtesy of Life Like Laboratories, Dallas, TX.)

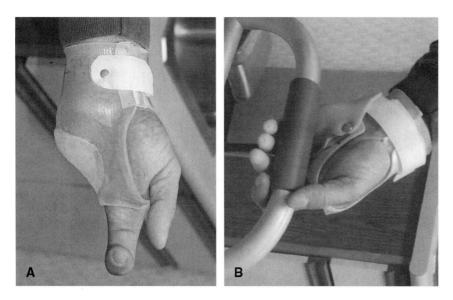

Figure 7 A and B, Opposition post for absent middle, ring, and little fingers.

Staging of Care

For the person with a partial hand amputation, three distinct stages of care can be defined: preprosthetic, preparatory prosthesis and interim therapy, and definitive prosthesis and therapy. Occupational therapy should be incorporated throughout all phases of care.

The preprosthetic phase is characterized by therapy designed to prepare the residual limb for fitting. This phase may involve many techniques and procedures designed to reduce edema, preserve and enhance range of motion, strengthen musculature, and desensitize the residual limb. The prosthetist should evaluate the individual at this time, discuss all the prosthetic options, and formulate the prosthetic plan in conjunction with a comprehensive therapy program.

The preparatory prosthesis and interim therapy stage ideally is completed as soon as possible after the injury, thereby allowing rapid return to function (Figure 10). It is generally believed that early return to function leads to optimal prosthetic function, and patients who return to work sooner also report increased self-esteem.[13] During this phase, the prosthetist and therapist work together to address the functional limitations of both the amputation level and prosthetic options. If an opposition post device is indicated, a skilled therapist can quickly form a temporary device from low-temperature thermoplastics. Preliminary prosthetic designs can also be evaluated in the therapy environment, where input from the rehabilitation team can be obtained. This input can provide a valuable assessment tool for the prosthetist before definitive prosthetic fabrication.

After a thorough assessment, which can last from several days to several weeks depending on the complexity of the fitting, the definitive prosthesis can be provided. At this stage, the prosthetist and therapist focus on encouraging the patient to use the prosthesis in a wider range of activities.

Socket Design

Socket designs for partial hand prostheses can permit active pronation, supination, wrist flexion, and wrist extension. For heavy lifting and similar tasks, however, it often is necessary to extend the socket up onto the forearm to stabilize the prosthesis sufficiently, and this longer socket design can interfere with these movements.

One common approach is the use of dental alginate, rather than plaster bandages, because the resulting model is a very accurate representation of the three-dimensional contours of the bony residual limb that is typical for this level of loss. The semiflexible consistency of alginate makes these molds well suited for irregularly shaped residual limbs in which some distal areas are more bulbous than proximal ones (Figure 11). Trimlines and socket contours are generally dictated by the geometry of the remaining portions of the hand and fingers. Because of the intimate fitting required, as well as the limited surface area distal to the wrist joint, the use of multiple test sockets is almost always necessary. In the typical case, the prosthetist will use local heat to reform the clear thermoplastic test socket as necessary, often modifying repeatedly the positive plaster model and molding a new test socket for further fitting trials. Once the socket fits comfortably and range of motion is unrestricted, the desired articulations and components can be added and their alignment checked and modified as necessary.

Suspension

Suspension is unique to the configuration of the specific residual limb. Methods include suction liners, roll-on liners, and anatomically contoured designs that suspend over the residual anatomy. The greater the loads to be carried with the prosthesis, the more difficult it is to provide comfortable suspension without interfering with residual wrist motion.

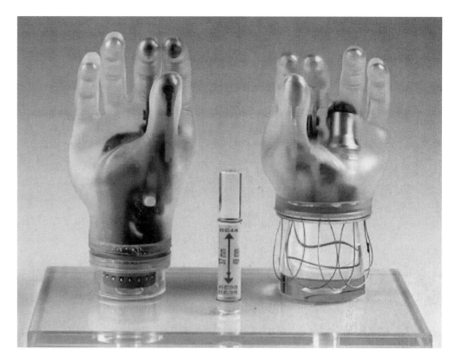

Figure 8 Transcarpal electronic hand (right) (Otto Bock, Duderstat, Germany) compared with a standard Otto Bock electronic hand (left). (Courtesy of Otto Bock, USA.)

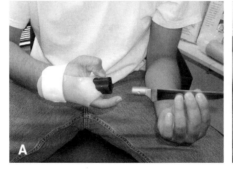

Figure 9 Task-specific option for the partial hand amputee using the remnant thumb to actuate a quick-disconnect wrist (Texas Assistive Devices, Brazoria, TX).

Components
Passive Prosthesis

The passive prosthesis generally is composed of flexible plastic or silicone material. Polyvinyl chloride is less expensive, but it stains easily. Silicone restorations are usually created by specialized anaplastic prosthetists, who can fashion devices that appear very lifelike. The prosthetist can sometimes modify a standard passive hand, attaching it to the socket and blending in the contours so that the entire assembly can be covered by the same low-cost prefabricated glove

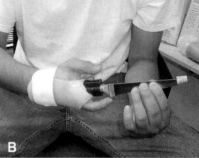

Figure 10 Fitting a fully functional interim prosthesis encourages continued use of the involved limb for bimanual activities.

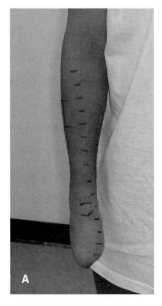

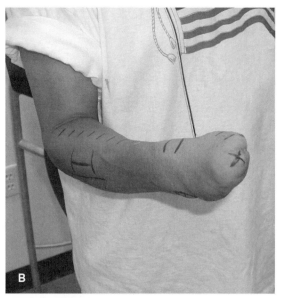

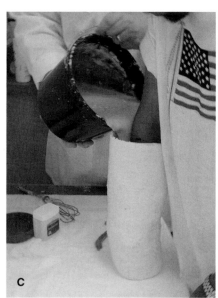

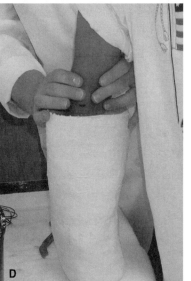

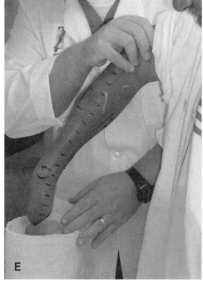

Figure 11 Alginate impression technique. **A** and **B,** Significant anatomic landmarks, prospective electrode placement, and medial-lateral and anterior-posterior dimensions are delineated at 2-cm intervals from the most distal aspect of the residual limb proximally to the cubital fold. **C,** Alginate is poured into the cylinder as the patient maintains position of the residual limb approximately 2 to 3 cm from the bottom of the cylinder. **D,** The limb must be supported because any movement will distort the negative mold. **E,** The patient is instructed to relax the residual limb as the limb is guided directly out of the cylinder. Pouring water into the top of the cylinder before removing the residual limb will help minimize suction.

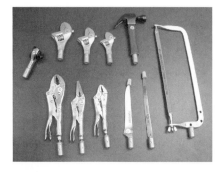

Figure 12 Modified tools that can be interchanged according to the specific task being performed (Texas Assistive Devices, Brazoria, TX).

used for wrist disarticulations and higher level amputations.

Body-Powered Prosthesis

A limited number of commercial components are available to create a body-powered or externally powered partial hand prosthesis (Figure 12). These terminal devices can be interchanged between passive task-specific prostheses and body-powered cable-driven prosthetic limbs.

Externally Powered Prosthesis

Selected partial hand amputees can use a special electronic hand operated by electrodes that are intrinsic or extrinsic to the hand. Force Sensing Resistors can also be used at this level. These input devices consist of a Force Sensing Resistor matrix that the user activates by means of a phocomelic finger or mobile metacarpal.

Biomechanics of Control and Alignment

Biomechanical considerations regarding control and alignment include the use of orthotic principles such as tenodesis action to actuate prehension

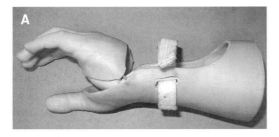

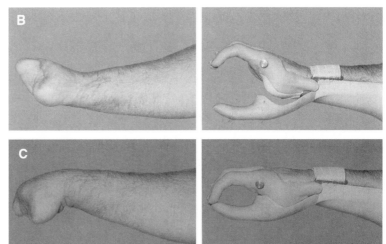

Figure 13 Wrist-driven partial hand prosthesis **(A)** allows for varied grip force and enhanced proprioception. **B** and **C**, Extension of the wrist opens the prosthesis. **D** and **E**, Flexion of the wrist closes the prosthesis. (**B** through **E** are reproduced with permission from Nader M (ed): *Otto Bock Prosthetic Compendium: Upper Extremity Prostheses. Berlin, Germany, Schiele & Schon, 1990.*

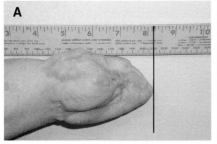

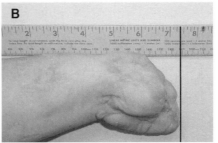

Figure 14 The effect of residual limb alignment on residual limb length. By investigating different positions of the residual limb, the prosthetist can adjust the overall length of the prosthesis, allowing for optimal bilateral symmetry.

Figure 15 Freedom of motion in the articulated design, seen in the preliminary fitting stage.

(Figure 13) and harnessing principles similar to those used for higher level losses.

Alignment often is dictated by the unique contours of the hand remnants, although this can sometimes be compensated for by adjusting the position of the residual limb. Figure 14 illustrates one example in which placing the residual limb in a certain position reduced the overall length enough to significantly improve the symmetry of the final prosthesis. If wrist flexion and extension are retained, this should be captured in the prosthesis whenever feasible (Figure 15).

Case Studies
Case Study 1

A 34-year-old woman (Figure 16) with a transmetacarpal-level amputation of the left hand secondary to industrial saw trauma was evaluated ap-

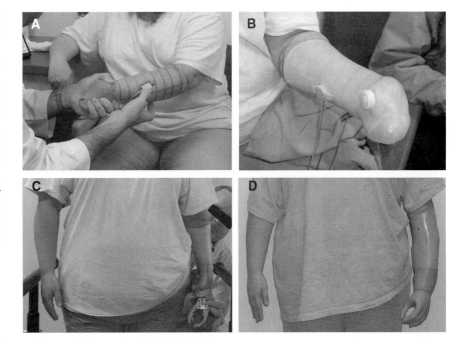

Figure 16 A 34-year-old woman with a transmetacarpal-level amputation of the left hand. **A**, Myoelectric testing before impression. The measurement levels are delineated circumferentially. **B**, Diagnostic socket. **C**, Aligning the hand while referencing a mirror so that the patient can provide feedback. **D**, Finished prosthesis.

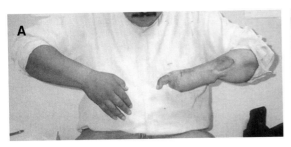
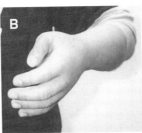
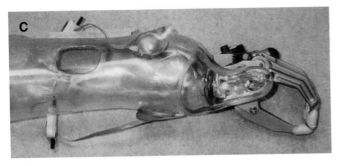
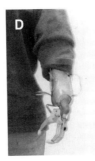
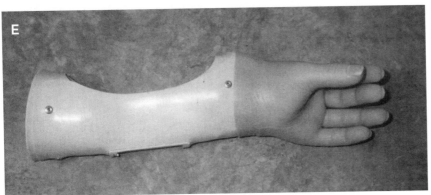
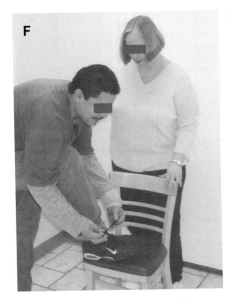
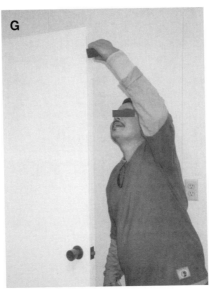

Figure 17 A 30-year-old man with a transverse amputation involving the left hand, wrist complex, and forearm. **A,** Initial presentation. **B,** Malrotation of the thumb preventing effective opposition of the passive fingers with the prior prosthesis. **C,** Preliminary prosthesis. **D,** Preliminary prosthesis. **E,** Definitive prosthesis. **F** and **G,** Occupational therapy training.

proximately 1 year posttrauma. By this time, she had undergone six separate surgeries involving failed replantation, vein and skin grafting, and management of a bone spur. Residual limb evaluation revealed significant scarring and adhesions, and the soft tissues had a medium to firm consistency. Comprehensive evaluation and treatment included the provision of both a myoelectric prosthesis for everyday activities and a passive silicone restoration for activities such as jet skiing and other water-related activities that would damage the myoelectric prosthesis.

The condition of the residual limb indicated the need for an encapsulated design to protect tissue integrity and increase the weight-bearing surface area. The rehabilitation team will evaluate the patient's progress in using this design and the tissue integrity of the residual limb at regular intervals before initiating the transition to a nonencapsulated design that allows wrist flexion and extension.

Case Study 2

A 30-year-old man with a transverse amputation involving the left hand, wrist complex, and forearm secondary to industrial punch press trauma was evaluated approximately 2 years posttrauma (Figure 17). By this time, he had undergone more than 10 surgeries to address painful range of motion. Malrotation of the thumb, diminished range of motion, and muscle strength test results indicating less than 1 lb of pinch force limited the patient's success with his current passive prosthesis. Following comprehensive evaluation, a myoelectric prosthesis was prescribed for everyday activities and a task-specific prosthesis was prescribed for vocational activities such as jewelry making.

Summary

Prosthetic options for partial hand loss have increased in recent decades to better meet the patient's needs, and patient acceptance has improved as a result. Research is underway to develop smaller, lighter, and more sophisticated electronic terminal devices for partial hand amputees.[14] Improvements in materials and available components have allowed the prosthetist to create specialized devices that meet the numerous challenges presented by the widely varying geometry of partial hand amputations.

Acknowledgment

I am grateful to Julie Lake for literary review and editing.

References

1. Dietl H, Gröpel W: Versorgung nach Teilhandamputationen mit myoelektrischen Komponenten. *Orthop Technik* 2001;1:21-23.

2. Wedderburn A, Caldwell RR, Sanderson ER, et al: A wrist-powered prosthesis for the partial hand. *J Assoc Child Prosthet Orthot Clin* 1986;21: 42-45.

3. Michael JW: Prosthetic and orthotic management, in Bowker JH, Michael JW (eds): *Atlas of Limb Prosthetics: Surgical, Prosthetic, and Rehabilitation Principles*, ed 2. Rosemont, IL, American Academy of Orthopaedic Surgeons, 2002, pp 217-226. (Originally published by Mosby-Year Book, 1992.)

4. Baumgartner R: Upper extremity amputations, in *Surgical Techniques in Orthopaedics and Traumatology*. Philadelphia, PA, Elsevier, 2001, vol 4.

5. Ouellette EA, McAuliffe JA, Carneiro R: Partial-hand amputations: Surgical principles, in Bowker JH, Michael JW (eds:) *Atlas of Limb Prosthetics: Surgical, Prosthetic, and Rehabilitation Principles*, ed 2. Rosemont, IL, American Academy of Orthopaedic Surgeons, 2002, pp 199-216. (Originally published by Mosby-Year Book, 1992.)

6. Swanson AB, de Groot Swanson G, Goran-Hagert C: Evaluation of impairment of hand function, in Hunter JM, Schneider LH, Mackin EJ, Callahan AD (eds): *Rehabilitation of the Hand: Surgery and Therapy*, ed 3. St. Louis, MO, CV Mosby, 1990, pp 109-138.

7. Jones LE, Davidson JH: Save that arm: A study of problems in the remaining arm of unilateral upper limb amputees. *Prosthet Orthot Int* 1999;23:55-58.

8. Sato Y, Kaji M, Tsuru T, Oizumi K: Carpal tunnel syndrome involving unaffected limbs of stroke patients. *Stroke* 1999;30:414-418.

9. Muilenburg AL, LeBlanc MA: Body-powered upper-limb components, in Atkins DJ, Meier RH III (eds): *Comprehensive Management of the Upper-Limb Amputee*. New York, NY, Springer-Verlag, 1989, pp 28-38.

10. Roeschlein RA, Domholdt E: Factors related to successful upper extremity prosthetic use. *Prosthet Orthot Int* 1989;13:14-18.

11. Fraser CM: An evaluation of the use made of cosmetic and functional prostheses by unilateral upper limb amputees. *Prosthet Orthot Int* 1998;22:216-223.

12. Putzi R: Myoelectric partial-hand prosthesis. *J Prosthet Orthot* 1992;4: 103-108.

13. Malone JM, Fleming LL, Roberson J, et al: Immediate, early, and late postsurgical management of upper-limb amputation. *J Rehabil Res Dev* 1984;21: 33-41.

14. Weir RF, Grahn EC, Duff SJ: A new externally powered, myoelectrically controlled prosthesis for persons with partial-hand amputations at the metacarpals. *J Prosthet Orthot* 2001;13:26-31.

Chapter 15

Wrist Disarticulation and Transradial Amputation: Surgical Management

Patrick Owens, MD

E. Anne Ouellette, MD, MBA

Introduction

Trauma is the cause of 90% of amputations in the upper limb. Individuals age 20 to 40 years are most commonly affected, with men sustaining four times as many amputations as women;[1,2] the right and left limbs are affected equally. The remaining causes of amputation include burns, peripheral vascular disease, neurologic disorders, infections, malignant tumors, contractures, and congenital deformities.[3]

With improvements in limb salvage techniques, a malignant tumor in a limb no longer automatically necessitates amputation. Microvascular surgical procedures have also aided in the salvage of limbs after trauma. Despite these advances, certain situations still require amputation.

General Surgical Considerations

The goal of amputation surgery is a functional, pain-free residual limb. The amputation level is chosen based on the level of injury or extent of the disease process. In the case of trauma, all nonviable tissue and foreign material must be removed prior to wound closure. Because this may require several débridements, primary wound closure is often contraindicated. Greater residual limb length can often be preserved by covering the wound with split-thickness skin grafts, free flaps, or groin flaps.[4] Patients rarely require or request revision surgery for shortening of the bone.

High-voltage electrical burns of the upper limb are a special consideration because necrosis of the deep compartment muscles is often severe, whereas the superficial muscles may remain viable. The deep muscles should be explored early and débrided by extensive fasciotomy. Primary amputations are often required, but a longer residual limb is possible if the superficial muscles are viable and are used to enclose the radius and ulna.[5]

Amputation Through the Carpus

Amputation through the carpus has advantages over amputation at more proximal levels (Figure 1). With preservation of the carpus, wrist flexion and extension and forearm pronation and supination are maintained. The surgical technique is similar to other amputations in the upper limb. The palmar-to-dorsal skin flap ratio should be 2:1; this allows the carpus to be covered with durable palmar skin. Wrist motor strength is increased by attachment of the wrist flexors and extensors to the remaining carpal bones. A mobile carpal segment covered with sensate skin allows the patient to perform bimanual activities without using a prosthesis. Prostheses can be fashioned with either a body-powered or a myoelectric terminal device and a socket that extends no farther than the elbow. If the socket is hinged at the wrist, the am-

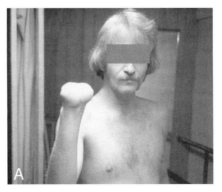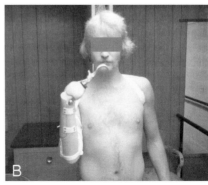

Figure 1 Patient with an amputation through the carpus. **A,** The residual limb is covered with sensate skin, allowing limited bimanual function without a prosthesis. **B,** The prosthesis is articulated at the radiocarpal joint, allowing easy positioning of the terminal device.

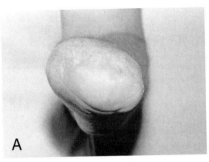
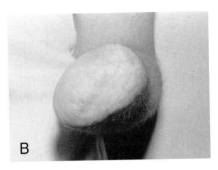
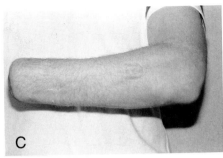

Figure 2 Disarticulation of the left wrist. Active pronation **(A)** and active supination **(B)** following wrist disarticulation. **C,** Lateral view of the residual limb following wrist disarticulation. Note the smooth distal contours and the impression from a myoelectric limb electrode over the extensor muscle mass.

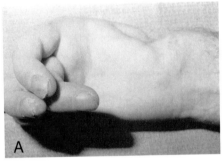
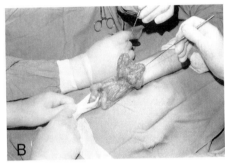
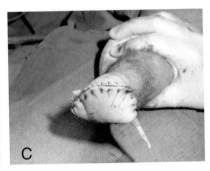

Figure 3 Wrist disarticulation following a severe crush injury. **A,** The hand was painful and totally functionless, and the patient requested amputation. **B,** A full-thickness palmar flap is raised. Note the rigidity of the proximal interphalangeal joints. **C,** Closure of the wound, demonstrating distal coverage with a thick palmar flap. *(C is courtesy of J.H. Bowker, MD.)*

putee can easily position the terminal device by radiocarpal flexion. Despite the functional advantage of an articulated socket, some amputees prefer a more cosmetically pleasing nonarticulated socket.

Wrist Disarticulation

Amputation through the radiocarpal joint allows the patient to retain virtually full forearm pronation and supination. It also provides a long lever arm, which facilitates lifting of the terminal device and its load (Figure 2).

In wrist disarticulation, the patient is positioned supine on the operating table. A tourniquet is applied to allow clear visualization of the tissues and minimize blood loss. Prior to applying the tourniquet, the limb may be exsanguinated with an elastic bandage or, in the case of tumor or infection, by elevation alone. Regional anesthesia should be used when possible. Contraindications to regional anes-

thesia include infection at the anesthesia injection site, coagulopathy, lack of patient cooperation, and lack of patient responsiveness. As with elective amputations through the carpus, such as for severe brachial plexus injuries, vasculopathies, and severe deformities in certain patients, palmar and dorsal flaps are created in a 2:1 ratio to provide adequate tissue for closure (Figure 3). The flaps should include the deep fascia to ensure an adequately padded residual limb.[1] In acute traumatic situations, where standard flaps may not be possible, nonstandard skin flaps should be used to salvage residual limb length.

The radial, ulnar, and anterior and posterior interosseous arteries, as well as the larger veins, must be isolated and ligated or coagulated. After identification of the median, ulnar, posterior interosseous, and superficial radial nerves, they are drawn distally under moderate tension and

transected, then allowed to retract proximally into the soft tissues to prevent entrapment of neuromas in the incisional scar. Specifically, the transected end of the superficial radial nerve should lie beneath the belly of the brachioradialis muscle. Alternatively, a second, more proximal incision can be made in the forearm to transect the nerves even farther from the distal end of the residual limb.

The carpus is carefully separated from the radius by division of the radiocarpal capsular and ligamentous structures under traction. If the triangular fibrocartilage complex and distal radioulnar joint are damaged, painful rotation (pronation/supination) and instability of the radioulnar joint may result. If reconstruction of the distal radioulnar joint complex is not possible, amputation at the long transradial level should be considered. The radial and ulnar styloids should be shaped to create a smooth, symmetric contour to facilitate prosthetic fitting; however, to

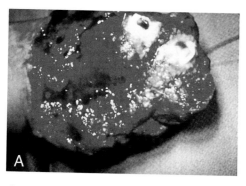
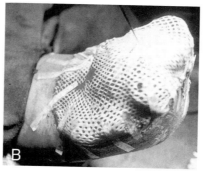
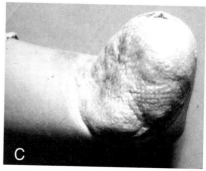

Figure 4 Use of skin grafting and myoplasty to maintain maximum residual limb length following traumatic transradial amputation. **A,** Although no skin remained on the anterior aspect of the residual limb, enough muscle tissue was salvageable to cover all but the tips of the radius and the ulna. **B,** Intraoperative photograph of complete split-thickness skin coverage. **C,** The elbow joint was salvaged by myoplasty and skin grafting. This made it possible to successfully fit the amputee with a prosthesis at the transradial level. *(Courtesy of J.H. Bowker, MD.)*

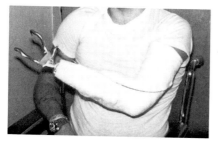

Figure 5 Patient fitted with immediate postoperative prosthesis following wrist disarticulation. The elbow was immobilized for 1 week postoperatively to prevent painful stress on the incision. Note the figure-of-9 harnessing to the opposite shoulder, which activates the terminal device.

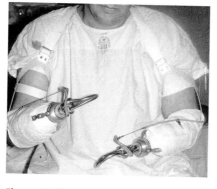

Figure 6 Bilateral transradial amputee fitted with a second set of temporary prostheses. The elbows are free, and the conjoined harnessing system allows activation of the terminal devices singly or together. With this fitting, the amputee is partially independent in activities of daily living.

avoid damage to the triangular fibrocartilage complex, only the tip of the ulnar styloid should be removed. The dorsal and palmar tendons are transected and stabilized under physiologic tension. The tourniquet is deflated prior to wound closure to allow for hemostasis. The wound is then closed in layers, and a bulky compressive dressing is applied.

Transradial Amputation

Maximum possible residual limb length should be preserved in amputations through the forearm to maintain a stronger lever arm and retain maximum pronation and supination. A very short residual limb may have difficulty tolerating the weight of a

myoelectric prosthesis. The length of the prosthesis will be more cosmetically appealing, however, when the amputation is performed no less than 2 cm proximal to the wrist, thus leaving sufficient space for the prosthetic components.

The surgical principles of wrist disarticulation apply to transradial amputations. Equal dorsal and palmar flaps are created distal to the intended level of bone amputation. The periosteum is incised sharply, the bones are cut, and the ends are smoothed carefully. The nerves are transected as described above and allowed to retract beneath the muscle bellies. Myodesis or myoplasty is performed to create a stabilized muscle

mass, which is especially helpful in later myoelectric fitting. To obtain the most functional result, the surgeon should restabilize the distal muscle insertion and thereby avoid a mobile sling of muscle moving over the bone. The deep layers should be stabilized with myodesis or tenodesis directly to bone or periosteum. The more superficial layers are secured with myoplasty to the fascia of the deeper layers.

With very proximal amputations, it may be necessary to detach the biceps tendon from the radius and reattach it proximally on the ulna. Reattachment of the biceps tendon too distally, however, can result in a flexion contracture. The radius should then be removed entirely. Only 4 to 5 cm of ulnar length is required for prosthesis fitting with retention of elbow flexion. To provide a longer forearm segment in certain cases, Ilizarov bone lengthening techniques have been used, sometimes in combination with free flap coverage.[6] When one forearm bone is significantly longer than the other, and the longer one can be covered adequately with soft tissue, it is preferable to maintain the maximum residual limb length rather than to shorten the longer bone. This can be accomplished by fusing the two bones in a neutral position, creating a one-bone forearm.

Coverage is best achieved with local skin flaps, taking care to prevent adherence of the skin to underlying bone. If insufficient skin is available, skin grafts, abdominal flaps, or free flaps can be used for coverage. Skin grafts may require additional care initially but usually do well with maturation (Figure 4). When inadequate soft tissue remains for closure at a desirable level, free latissimus dorsi flaps or even innervated free flaps from amputated parts may be used.

Nearly one third of transradial amputees require revision surgery. This mainly occurs when there has been severe swelling that has receded, leaving a bulbous or flabby residual limb, or when too much soft tissue was saved at the initial amputation. Every effort should be made to maintain even a short transradial level as long as a useful range of motion of the elbow can be preserved.

Significant flexion or extension contractures of the elbow, resulting in loss of function, may develop in some patients with transradial amputations. Longer residual limbs may benefit from contracture release. In shorter residual limbs, elbow contractures can be managed by an elbow arthrodesis at 90° of flexion rather than by an elbow disarticulation or transhumeral amputation.[1]

Prosthesis Fitting

The most important variable in the successful prosthetic rehabilitation of the upper limb is early fitting. Training with a temporary prosthesis should begin during the immediate postoperative period; this can be accomplished by adding prosthetic prehension and suspension components to a rigid dressing. The patient can begin using this immediate postoperative prosthesis within 1 to 2 days, preserving two-handed grasping patterns and decreasing prosthesis rejection rates[3,7,8] (Figures 5 and 6). Rigid dressings also allow better control of postoperative edema and protect the wound from external trauma.

Some surgeons, however, advocate the use of compressive elastic dressings postoperatively, combined with early elbow range of motion. Early prosthetic fitting remains equally important in these patients.

References

1. Baumgartner R: Upper extremity amputations, in DuParc (ed): *Surgical Techniques in Orthopaedics and Traumatology,* Orlando, FL, Harcourt International, 2003, vol 4.

2. Atroshi I, Rosberg HE: Epidemiology of amputations and severe injuries of the hand. *Hand Clin* 2001;17:343-350.

3. Burkhalter WE, Mayfield GE, Carmona LS: The upper extremity amputee: Early and immediate post-surgical prosthetic fitting. *J Bone Joint Surg Am* 1976;58:46.

4. Rohrich RJ, Erlichman RJ, May JW Jr: Sensate palm of hand free flap for forearm length preservation in nonreplantable forearm amputation: Long term follow-up. *Ann Plast Surg* 1991;26:469-473.

5. d'Amato TA, Kaplan IB, Britt LD: High-voltage electrical injury: A role for mandatory exploration of deep muscle compartments. *J Natl Med Assoc* 1994;86:535-537.

6. Kour AK, Seo JS, Pho RW: Combined free flap, Ilizarov lengthening and prosthetic fitting in the reconstruction of a proximal forearm amputation: A case report. *Ann Acad Med Singapore* 1995;24:135.

7. Tooms RE: Amputations of the upper extremity, in Crenshaw A (ed): *Campbell's Operative Orthopaedics,* ed 8. St. Louis, MO, Mosby-Year Book, 1992, vol 2, pp 711-721.

8. Sarmiento A, McCollough NC, Williams EM, et al: Immediate post surgical prosthetic fitting in the management of upper extremity amputees. *Artif Limbs* 1968;12:14-16.

Chapter 16

Wrist Disarticulation and Transradial Amputation: Prosthetic Management

Carl D. Brenner, CPO

Introduction

Several facts relevant to helping upper limb amputees reach their optimum rehabilitation potential are addressed in this chapter. These facts are: (1) only a very small portion of prosthetic clinical practice involves the upper limb amputee; (2) early prosthetic intervention is crucial to achieving successful outcomes; (3) the patient and health care team should consider carefully the implications amputation level has for prosthesis use; (4) consideration of the five categories of upper limb prostheses can effectively identify and meet the needs of upper limb amputees; and (5) electronic limb banking helps reduce costs while enhancing care.

Trends in Upper Limb Prosthetics

Overall, most upper limb prosthetic cases involve wrist disarticulations and transradial amputations. Upper limb prosthetic fittings are declining, especially as a percentage of total prosthetic fittings. In 1964, Glattly[1] reported that of all prostheses prescribed, 1 in 7 were fitted for upper limb patients; 10 years later, Kay and Newman[2] reported that upper limb fittings represented only 1 in 12 prostheses. In 2001, the American Orthotic and Prosthetic Association reported that only 1 in 15 fittings was for an upper limb prosthesis.[3]

This trend may be caused by several factors that are converging. First, the number of lower limb amputations is increasing as the population ages; this may accelerate even more as the baby boom generation reaches its sixth decade. Second, the number of upper limb amputations may have decreased since the successful implementation of federal safety regulations under the Occupational Safety and Health Act of 1970, which resulted in a much safer workplace. In addition, there have been advancements in surgical and rehabilitative techniques related to upper limb salvage and reconstruction procedures. At the same time, the number of board certified prosthetists has increased more than threefold since 1971,[4,5] resulting in a further drop in the number of upper limb fittings completed by the average prosthetist in general practice.

In response to these trends, the American Academy of Orthotists and Prosthetists formed the Upper Limb Prosthetics Society in 1991 to provide a forum for education and communication among the practitioners of this specialty. The realization that upper limb prosthetic fitting and care require special expertise on the part of both the prosthetist and the occupational therapist will result in improved care for all upper limb amputees.

Advantages of Early Intervention

Of the many developments since the 1980s regarding management of upper limb amputees, early prosthetic intervention has had the single largest impact. Early intervention, in this context, is defined as the application of some form of upper limb prosthesis within the first 30 days after amputation.[6] The traditional approach, which delayed prosthetic fitting for 5 to 10 months,[7] or until full healing had been achieved, yielded a rejection rate of at least 50%.[8-10] However, the application of a prosthesis within the first 30 days of amputation has dramatically improved long-range outcomes, with some centers reporting rates of prosthetic use and acceptance of 90% and higher.[6,9] This improvement is believed to be the result of effective preservation of bimanual functional patterns resulting from early prosthetic training.[9,11]

The use of an immediate or early postoperative prosthesis has been shown to be effective in achieving the goals of early intervention, which include decreased edema, decreased postoperative pain and phantom pain, increased prosthetic use, improved proprioceptive/prosthetic transfer, and improved psychological adaptation to the amputation.[6,9,11] Although this procedure has been used widely in lower limb applications since

TABLE 1 Ideal Prosthesis Fitting Timetable for Wrist Disarticulations and Transradial Level Amputations

Type of Prosthesis	Postoperative Application
Immediate or early postoperative prosthesis	24 hours to 14 days
Preparatory/training body-powered prosthesis	2 to 4 weeks
Definitive body-powered prosthesis	6 to 12 weeks
Preparatory/training electronic prosthesis	6 to 12 weeks
Definitive electronic prosthesis	4 to 6 months

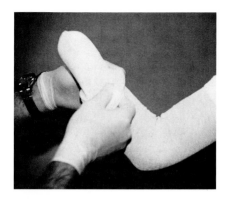

Figure 1 A second layer of stockinette is applied over the dressing of a wrist disarticulation to facilitate easy removal and application of the postoperative prosthesis.

the late 1960s, it has remained underutilized in upper limb applications despite the fact that it does not jeopardize wound healing in the upper limb, as is sometimes the case in weight-bearing lower limb situations.[9,11]

Wrist Disarticulation Versus Transradial Amputation: Prosthetic Implications

The long-standing principle in amputation surgery is to "save all length." The advantages of disarticulation surgery through the wrist over a higher level amputation have been understood for decades. However, two major issues are limb length and residual pronation and supination. With a wrist disarticulation, the use of a prosthesis will frequently result in a length discrepancy that is cosmetically unacceptable to the patient.[10] This is particularly true when a quick-disconnect wrist is employed to provide easy interchangeability between a hook terminal device and an electronic hand. In addition, if adequate residual pronation and supination are absent, disarticulation surgery is usually contraindicated because the amputee will have active wrist rotation only if there is sufficient room for an electronically controlled wrist rotation module. If skin grafting would be necessary to preserve the viability of a disarticulation surgical level, a higher level amputation just proximal to the graft site may prove to be a more appropriate decision to avoid delays in

the fitting process. A shorter residual limb is especially advantageous if the amputee will alternate between an electronic prosthesis and a body-powered prosthesis.

For the amputee to receive all the potential benefits of wrist disarticulation, the residual limb must retain a large percentage of normal pronation and supination after surgery and must be covered with durable skin and soft tissues that will tolerate suspension forces applied just proximal to the styloids. Although specialized terminal devices are available for wrist disarticulation applications, the choice of components is much more limited when compared with those available for transradial amputations. The patient should be aware of the trade-offs in appearance and options that a wrist disarticulation requires and should feel that the benefits of added leverage, voluntary pronation and supination, and distal suspension outweigh the limitations.

Types of Prostheses Used in Upper Limb Rehabilitation

Five distinctly different types of prostheses make up the armamentarium necessary to provide optimum and comprehensive management for the upper limb amputee. They are (1) immediate/early postoperative, (2) preparatory/training body-powered, (3) definitive body-powered, (4) preparatory/training electronic, and (5) definitive electronic prostheses. The fitting timetable for the use of these prostheses is shown in Table 1.

Immediate and Early Postoperative Prostheses

The first early intervention decision to be considered is whether to provide an immediate or early postoperative prosthesis. An immediate postoperative prosthesis is applied in the operating room at the time of final surgical closure, whereas an early postoperative prosthesis is applied any time between surgery and suture removal. There appears to be no significant difference in long-range outcomes between immediate and early postoperative application in the upper limb; however, immediate application can provide additional psychological benefits to the patient and the patient's family.[6,9]

Essentially, the same technique is used for both procedures. First, two separate layers of stockinette are applied directly over the dressing (Figure 1), followed by distal padding that consists of lamb's wool, sterile fluffs, or a reticulated urethane foam pad. The padding is then covered with a thin cast/socket fabricated of plaster or fiberglass casting tape (Figure 2). This socket extends to the level of the epicondyles but leaves the elbow free. A thermoplastic frame with a lightweight terminal device is then taped in place with a good-quality linen adhesive tape (Figure 3), followed by a similar application of tape to affix the flexible elbow hinges that are connected to the triceps pad. A standard Bowden cable assembly is applied, and either a shoulder saddle harness or, more typically, a figure-of-8 harness is employed for suspension and terminal device control. When all of the components have been taped to the cast/socket, a final covering of a self-adhering elastic bandage is applied to reinforce the fixation of the components (Figure 4). No synthetic casting tape or plaster should be used to attach the components to the inner socket, thereby ensuring easy removal of the components when changing the cast/socket. The two stockinette socks applied at the beginning of the procedure allow easy removal and application of the postoperative prosthesis, which facilitates wound inspection and management.[9] However, the patient and the nursing staff should be advised that removal should be done for only very short periods of time to minimize edema. Occupational therapy with this prosthesis generally can be started as soon as the patient is alert and able to follow directions.[9,11]

Preparatory/Training Body-Powered Prostheses

The second type of prosthesis used in the management of upper limb amputees is the preparatory/training body-powered prosthesis. This prosthesis is applied when the wound has healed and the immediate postoperative edema has resolved. The preparatory/training prosthesis differs from the postoperative prosthesis in that the preparatory socket is made over a plaster model of the patient's residual limb, the prosthesis is fabricated from more durable materials, and its design allows for the easy interchangeability of various components during the evaluation process (Figure 5). To achieve a successful outcome, a preparatory/training prosthesis should be designed and fitted with the same care as a definitive system, including the use of test sockets when necessary.

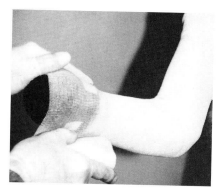

Figure 2 Fiberglass casting tape is rolled over the distal pad of reticulated foam. The cast is terminated just distal to the epicondyles to allow free elbow flexion.

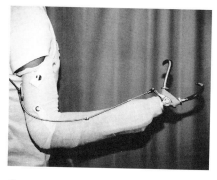

Figure 4 A final covering of a self-adhering elastic bandage is used to reinforce the fixation of the components. This early postoperative wrist disarticulation prosthesis is shown with a figure-of-8 harness, triceps cuff, and flexible elbow hinges.

The goals of the preparatory/training prosthesis are preparation of the limb for prosthesis use, evaluation, and training. In terms of preparation, the prosthesis provides continued edema control, a reduction in patient pain and anxiety, and conditioning of the tissues to accept the forces exerted by a prosthetic socket. As an evaluation tool, the prosthesis helps the clinic team and the patient determine which components provide the greatest benefit, aids the rehabilitation team in assessing the patient's level of motivation and compliance, and allows the patient to become familiar with the functional value and limitations of a body-powered prosthesis. With regard to training, the preparatory prosthesis helps the patient preserve two-handed function

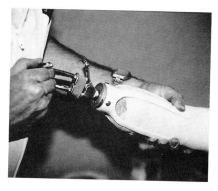

Figure 3 A thermoplastic frame is positioned to hold a lightweight terminal device, in this case an aluminum model 5XA hook and friction wrist, in place.

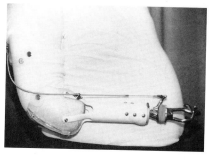

Figure 5 This preparatory/training body-powered short transradial prosthesis is shown with a thermoplastic socket, single-axis elbow joint, Bowden cable assembly, and an interchangeable quick-disconnect locking wrist with a stainless steel model 7 work hook.

and allows the amputee to practice using a body-powered prosthesis for the normal activities of daily living.

Definitive Body-Powered Prostheses

Once the patient has worn a postoperative prosthesis until the wound is healed, followed by a preparatory body-powered prosthesis until the limb volume has stabilized, the formulation of definitive prosthetic prescription specifications is relatively straightforward. If the two previous prostheses accomplished the goals of providing a comprehensive evaluation of the socket design and the harnessing system and of determining which wrist and elbow components proved most functional, then most elements of an appropriate prescription become evident based on the patient's

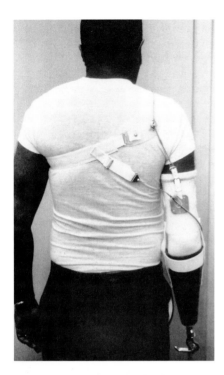

Figure 6 A definitive body-powered transradial prosthesis with triceps cuff, flexible elbow hinges, laminated socket, and shoulder saddle harness with Bowden cable control.

actual experience. However, several additional factors should be considered when developing definitive specifications, including the socket design, the elbow joint, the wrist component, and the harness design.

Socket Designs

Sockets designed for use with body-powered prostheses are either harness-suspended or self-suspended. As a general rule, the longer the residual limb, the lower the proximal trim line of the socket can be. When the patient retains a significant amount of natural pronation and supination after surgery, the proximal trim line of the socket should be cut low enough to preserve at least 50% of the active pronation and supination. Although several self-suspended sockets are now available for wrist disarticulations and long transradial level amputations, most designs require some form of suspension/control harness and so significantly restrict range of motion.

Elbow Joints

The flexible elbow hinge is the most common type of elbow joint used with a wrist disarticulation or transradial amputation. It can be made of either triple-thickness Dacron webbing or flexible metal cable. When socket rotation around the residual limb becomes a problem secondary to a very short bone length, a single-axis elbow joint is the most effective way to provide stability. In those rare instances in which the patient has very limited elbow flexion and it is crucial to reach the face with the prosthesis, as in the case of the bilateral amputee, step-up hinges may prove beneficial.

Wrist Components

The four most commonly used wrist units are the standard friction wrist, the quick-disconnect/locking wrist, the flexion wrist, and the multidirectional ball-and-socket wrist. For adult unilateral amputees who use more than one terminal device or routinely perform activities that require the elimination of any unwanted wrist rotation during functional performance, the quick-disconnect/locking wrist has proved to be most useful. When normal functional performance of the contralateral upper extremity has been compromised, or for bilateral amputees, a flexion wrist may be appropriate to add an additional measure of function. A standard friction wrist is the most popular and economical component that provides passive wrist rotation. A multidirectional ball-and-socket wrist unit provides not only wrist flexion but also wrist extension as well as radial and ulnar deviation.

Harness Designs

The three basic harness designs are the figure-of-9, the figure-of-8, and the shoulder saddle harness with a chest strap. The figure-of-9 harness is used primarily with a self-suspended socket that requires a harness only to provide terminal device operation. The most popular harness, the figure-of-8, can be fitted with either a sewn

cross point or a ring to provide adjustable posterior fixation for all the straps. The shoulder saddle harness is beneficial for amputees who do an unusual amount of heavy lifting (Figure 6). It also provides relief from some of the pressure on the axilla exerted by a figure-of-9 or figure-of-8 harness. However, the shoulder saddle harness is frequently rejected by patients who prefer to wear an open V-necked shirt or blouse that would expose the chest strap.

Advantages and Disadvantages

Among the advantages of the body-powered prosthesis are the freedom to operate in an unencumbered manner within most physical environments and the ability to achieve a high level of accuracy and speed during functional performance.[10,12,13] The primary disadvantages of the body-powered prosthesis are the discomfort caused by the shoulder harness and the appearance of the hook terminal device, which can generate negative attention.[10,13]

Preparatory/Training Electronic Prostheses

Since the 1980s, electronic and microprocessor technology has made significant contributions to the field of prosthetics, leading to increasing complexity and a much broader array of options for the upper limb amputee. Although this has led to improved electronic prostheses, it has also complicated the decision-making process for the prosthetist. Fortunately, the use of a temporary electronic prosthesis allows the clinician and the patient the opportunity to evaluate and experience many different design and component options before coming to a final conclusion.[14-16] Therefore, the preparatory/training electronic prosthesis should be considered a separate and distinct procedure in the total evaluation process of the upper limb amputee's needs.

Fitting and Controls

The fitting of a preparatory electronic prosthesis should be conducted with the same care as the fitting of any definitive prosthesis. However, the less expensive fabrication process and components provide a very cost-effective way of analyzing the patient's needs.

Careful fitting of the temporary prosthesis ensures that the experience of the patient while wearing the prosthesis will be very close to the experience of wearing a more costly definitive electronic limb. The same techniques are used for taking the negative plaster mold of the residual limb and subsequent modification as with a definitive fitting. A transparent test socket is then made over the modified plaster model, and this is used to evaluate the suspension and stability of the socket design and establish electrode sites. The test socket is then used to create the final positive master model over which the preparatory electronic socket will be fabricated. Once the socket has been fabricated, it is attached to a removable fitting frame that connects to the electronic components and protects the wiring and electronic circuits. Finally, a standard protective outer glove is applied over the prosthesis to cover the inner shell of the electronic hand (Figure 7). It is very important that the patient receive preprosthetic myoelectric signal training prior to the start of prosthetic fabrication and fitting. Following the fitting, the patient should continue with occupational therapy that stresses the specific activities that relate to the patient's daily routine, both on and off the job.

Although most electronic prostheses primarily use myoelectric signals to command the prosthesis, three other electronic control modes can be used in a preparatory or a definitive electronic prosthesis. These are electronic servo controls, electronic switch controls, and electronic touch controls.[14,17,18] A prosthesis can have a combination of one or more electronic controls in addition to one or more body-powered controls, in which case it is called a hybrid system.[14] Although hybrid systems are used primarily in amputation levels above the elbow, they may also be indicated for a patient with marginal elbow function. Such situations may require step-up body-powered elbow hinges in conjunction with either a switch controlled or myoelectrically controlled terminal device and/or wrist rotator.

Goals of the Preparatory/Training Electronic Prosthesis

As with the preparatory/training body-powered prosthesis, the goals of the preparatory/training electronic prosthesis are preparation of the residual limb for prosthesis use, evaluation, and training. By way of preparation, the prosthesis helps establish ideal definitive myoelectric signal sites, provides the opportunity to improve marginal myoelectric signals, and helps condition the tissues contained within a self-suspended socket. In terms of evaluation, the prosthesis has four specific objectives: (1) validation of the socket design and selected electronic components, (2) assessment of the patient's motivation and commitment to derive maximum benefit from an electronic prosthesis, (3) provision of the patient with the opportunity to determine the actual functional value of the electronic prosthesis when compared with other options, and (4) the development of clinical evidence to substantiate a cost-benefit analysis of various alternatives. The training objectives of a temporary electronic prosthesis include refinement of the patient's overall prosthetic control and the opportunity to practice activities of daily living with an appropriate electronic limb.

Definitive Electronic Prostheses

After proceeding through the four types of prostheses, the amputee and the clinic team are now positioned to determine the specifications for the definitive prosthesis. Because no consensus exists regarding the respective advantages of body-powered and electronic prostheses, providing the amputee an opportunity to personally experience the actual benefits and limitations of each of these systems allows the final choice to be made with some assurance that no major oversights have occurred. In today's health care environment, resources and funding are limited; therefore, effective methods for evaluating expensive technology should be used whenever possible. Because work-related injuries are one of the prime sources of upper limb loss, the ability of amputees to return to work has proved to be a useful measure of a successful outcome. Most amputees treated with the comprehensive methods presented here have returned to work.[6,9,13]

Socket Designs

One important decision is the choice of socket design. Ideally, the patient will have had the opportunity to try more than one type of socket suspension at the time the test sockets were

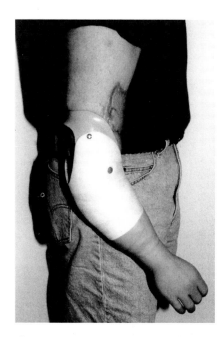

Figure 7 A preparatory/training electronic transradial prosthesis with Northwestern supracondylar socket with olecranon cut-out and removable fitting frame.

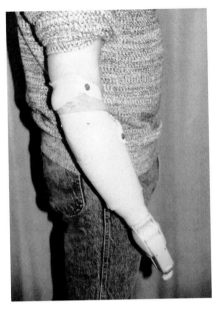

Figure 8 A definitive electronic wrist disarticulation prosthesis with a myoelectric greifer, quick-disconnect wrist, and floating brim suspension.

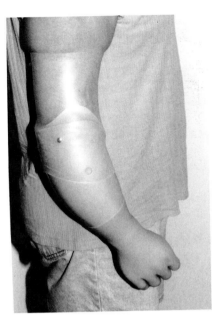

Figure 9 A definitive electronic transradial prosthesis with external silicone suspension sleeve and myoelectric hand.

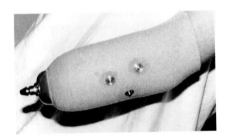

Figure 10 An internal roll-on locking liner with distal shuttle-lock pin and integrated snap-on electrodes.

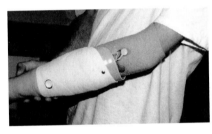

Figure 11 A preparatory/training myoelectric transradial prosthesis with internal roll-on suction liner, shuttle-lock system, and snap-on electrode wire harness.

being evaluated. This is particularly important with wrist disarticulations or long transradial amputations. Socket designs fall into four basic categories: (1) supracondylar brims that capture the humeral epicondyles and the posterior olecranon, (2) external suspension sleeves that use either atmospheric pressure or skin traction to maintain suspension, (3) suprastyloid suspensions for wrist disarticulation amputees with prominent styloids, and (4) internal roll-on locking liners.[19]

Four basic types of supracondylar designs are reported in the literature: the Muenster socket for short transradial amputations,[10] the Northwestern supracondylar socket for midlength transradial amputations,[20] the modified supracondylar brim with an olecranon cut-out for long transradial amputations,[21] and the floating brim suspension for long transradial amputations and wrist disarticulations (Figure 8). The external sleeve suspension techniques include latex rubber or silicone sleeves, which rely on atmospheric pressure suspension (Figure 9); neoprene sleeves, which rely on a combination of atmospheric pressure and skin traction; and elastic sleeves, which provide skin traction suspension, relying only on the grip of a breathable elastic sleeve on the skin. Because these designs extend beyond the elbow joint, they prevent the amputee from using residual voluntary pronation and supination.

Suspension designs that involve suprastyloid purchase use three types of suspension. These designs include silicone bladder suspension, window/door suspension with elasticized closure, and soft removable inserts that grip the styloids.

The last category of socket designs are those that use internal roll-on locking liners. These designs use either a shuttle-lock system for short and midlength transradial level amputations (Figures 10 and 11) or a lanyard locking system for long transradial amputations and wrist disarticulations.[22-24]

The latter two suspension methods can be combined with abbreviated trim lines that terminate well distal to the epicondyles. This permits the amputee to use residual pronation and supination to position the terminal device precisely.

The specific suspension method selected for the definitive prosthesis is based on how effective and comfortable prior suspension methods have proved to be for the patient's customary activities. Ease of application and removal are also important factors for consideration.

Cost and Maintenance

When considering the viability of selecting electronic prostheses, the issues of cost and maintenance should be addressed. Although cost has long been a major obstacle in providing advanced technology to amputees, in the past decade, most amputees have been found to have sufficient health care insurance to cover the cost of these procedures.[16,25] In addition, many upper limb losses occur in job-related situations and are covered by workers' compensation programs. As a result, funding no longer presents insurmountable obstacles for most patients.

The recent formation of electronic limb banks and leasing programs has made a favorable impact on the cost and complexities of providing sophisticated electronic limbs.[16,25] Electronic limb banks collect a variety of electronic components, including electronic hands, electrodes and electronic switching mechanisms, batteries, and battery chargers. All of these components can be leased to the patient on a trial basis for a modest charge. For a fraction of the purchase cost of new electronic hardware, the patient can obtain the necessary electronics in a preparatory/training prosthesis. There are three types of limb banks, with the most common being a private limb bank that is generally organized and funded by an individual prosthetic laboratory. The second type is a commercial limb bank sponsored by a manufacturer of electronic limb components, and the third type is an institutional limb bank that is generally organized and supported by either a hospital or a charitable organization.[16,25]

A secondary concern is the maintenance and corresponding downtime that may be associated with the continuous operation of a sophisticated electronic system. For the most part, electronic prostheses have been found to require maintenance at approximately as often as do body-powered prostheses. However, because repairs of electronic prostheses tend to take longer, the downtime required for maintenance can be a major stumbling block unless the services are provided by a specialty center that has a service delivery system that efficiently deals with the unique problems of repairing electronic prostheses.[16,26] Electronic limb banks have proved to be the best solution to the problem of downtime. Such limb banks provide a replacement component that can be installed when immediate repair of the prosthesis is not possible.[16,25] The solution that appears to be forthcoming is the development of regional specialty centers that can provide immediate service for electronic prostheses.[26]

Advantages and Disadvantages

For most adult amputees, the biggest advantage of an electronic prosthesis is the freedom from a control/suspension harness through the use of a self-suspended socket that provides a maximum degree of comfort.[10] Other amputees report that the ability to function with a prosthesis that has a close resemblance to a normal human hand is most important.[14,27]

Reported disadvantages include that although the electronic terminal device generally provides a much stronger grip force, it may be somewhat slower in operation than a body-powered hook.[13,27] Second, the lack of freedom to use the electronic prosthesis in hostile environments where dirt, water, dust, grease, and solvents are in frequent contact with the prosthesis has proved to be a major drawback.[10,14,16] However, the problem of a hostile environment has been partially remedied by the availability of various electronic hook terminal devices. As a result, many amputees have found that the best solution is to have both a body-powered and an electronic prosthesis available to use at their discretion, depending on the situation.[14,28]

Summary

Each of the five types of prostheses used in upper limb rehabilitation has a very specific role in the comprehensive care of upper limb amputees. Each system can provide information to guide decisions that lead to the best outcome for each individual amputee. Although circumstances may not permit or necessitate the use of all five systems for every patient, the use of two or three of these techniques is almost always possible and indicated. Following this model assures the patients, the patients' families, clinicians, caregivers, and third-party payers that the highest quality and most cost-effective methods have been used to help upper limb amputees reach their maximum rehabilitation potential.

References

1. Glattly HW: A statistical study of 12,000 new amputees. *South Med J* 1964;57:1373-1378.

2. Kay HW, Newman JD: Amputee survey, 1973-74: Preliminary findings and comparisons. *Orthot Prosthet* 1974;28: 27-32.

3. *2000 Orthotics and Prosthetics Business and Salary Survey Report.* American Orthotic & Prosthetic Association.

4. *1971 Registry.* American Board for Certification in Orthotics and Prosthetics.

5. *2001 Registry and Reference Guide.* American Board for Certification in Orthotics and Prosthetics.

6. Malone JM, Fleming LL, Roberson J, et al: Immediate, early, and late postsurgical management of upper-limb amputation. *J Rehabil Res Dev* 1984;21: 33-41.

7. Davies EJ, Friz BR, Clippinger FW: Amputees and their prostheses. *Artif Limbs* 1970;14:19-48.

8. LeBlanc MA: Patient population and other estimates of prosthetics and orthotics in the U.S.A. *Orthot Prosthet* 1973;27:38-44.

9. Malone JH, Childers SJ, Underwood J, Leal JH: Immediate postsurgical management of upper-extremity amputation: Conventional, electric and myoelectric prosthesis. *Orthot Prosthet* 1981;35:1-9.

10. Northmore-Ball MD, Heger H, Hunter GA: The below-elbow myoelectric prosthesis: A comparison of the Otto Bock myoelectric prosthesis with the hook and functional hand. *J Bone Joint Surg Br* 1980;62:363-367.

11. Burkhalter WE, Mayfield G, Carmona LS: The upper-extremity amputee: Early and immediate post-surgical prosthetic fitting. *J Bone Joint Surg Am* 1976;58:46-51.

12. Billock JN: The Northwestern University supracondylar suspension technique for below-elbow amputations. *Orthot Prosthet* 1972;26:16-23.

13. Kritter AE: Myoelectric prostheses. *J Bone Joint Surg Am* 1985;67:654-657.

14. Millstein SG, Heger H, Hunter GA: Prosthetic use in adult upper limb amputees: A comparison of the body powered and electrically powered prostheses. *Prosthet Orthot Int* 1986; 10:27-34.

15. Billock JN: Upper limb prosthetic management: Hybrid design approaches. *Clin Prosthet Orthot* 1985; 9:23-25.

16. Brenner CD: Electronic limbs for infants and pre-school children. *J Prosthet Orthot* 1992;4:24-30.

17. Supan TJ: Transparent preparatory prostheses for upper limb amputation. *Clin Prosthet Orthot* 1987;11:45-48.

18. Michael JW: Upper limb powered components and controls: Current concepts. *Clin Prosthet Orthot* 1986;10:66-77.

19. Nichol WR: Electronic touch controls for prostheses. *J Assoc Child Prosthet Orthot Clin* 1986;21:33.

20. Gaber TA, Gardner CM, Kirker SG: Silicone roll-on suspension for upper limb prostheses: Users' views. *Prosthet Orthot Int* 2001;25:113-118.

21. Sauter WF: Three-quarter-type Muenster socket. *J Assoc Child Prosthet Orthot Clin* 1985;20:34.

22. Daly W: Clinical application of roll-on sleeves for myoelectrically controlled transradial and transhumeral prostheses. *J Prosthet Orthot* 2000;12:88-91.

23. Heim M, Wershavski M, Zwas ST, Siev-Ner I, Nadvorna H, Azaria M: Silicone suspension of external prostheses: A new era in artificial limb usage. *J Bone Joint Surg Br* 1997;79:638-640.

24. Salam Y: The use of silicone suspension sleeves with myoelectric fittings. *J Prosthet Orthot* 1994;6:119-120.

25. Epps CH Jr: Editorial: Externally powered prostheses for children-1984. *Clin Prosthet Orthot* 1985;9:17-18.

26. Brenner CD: Demographic and logistical considerations for pediatric electronic limb applications. *Journal of Proceedings,* AAOP 19th Annual Meeting and Scientific Symposium, 1993, p 11.

27. Stein RB, Walley M: Functional comparison of upper extremity amputees using myoelectric and conventional prostheses. *Arch Phys Med Rehabil* 1983;64:243-248.

28. de Bear P: Functional use of myoelectric and cable-driven prostheses. *J Assoc Child Prosthet Orthot Clin* 1988;23:60-61.

Chapter 17

The Krukenberg Procedure

Pradip D. Poonekar, MD

Introduction

The human hand represents a major milestone in human evolution because of its highly specialized structure and function. Even the most sophisticated prosthetic terminal device is a woefully inadequate substitute for the hand, with its extraordinary dexterity and versatility. By virtue of its sensory feedback, the hand can assess the physical properties of an object such as its shape, size, surface texture, consistency, compressibility, and weight. In darkness, the hand can partially substitute for the eyes and can also provide a form of nonverbal communication. Thus, in addition to enabling an individual to perform the essential activities of daily living, the hand may also serve as "eyes" for the blind and "tongue" for the mute.

Amputation of one hand is a major impairment but one to which an individual can readily adapt, provided that the remaining upper limb is intact. Bilateral upper limb amputation is a significantly greater loss, however. And if bilateral amputation is accompanied by blindness, the situation is initially overwhelming. The blind bilateral upper limb amputee will be dependent on others for even the most basic activities of daily living.

In 1916, Hermann Krukenberg,[1-3] a German army surgeon during World War I, introduced his reconstructive procedure for transradial amputees, which was used extensively for both wounded soldiers and civil-ians. This operation reshapes the forearm of the transradial amputee into muscle-powered sensate radial and ulnar rays that effectively function as forceps,[4-6] chopsticks,[7-9] or pincers.[10-12] This reconstruction, however, results in a rather uncosmetic appearance and thus is rarely performed in most Western countries in spite of the excellent results achieved in selected patients.[13-15] A well-trained amputee who has had the Krukenberg procedure can typically perform most activities of daily living without a prosthesis. Even after the procedure, the amputee retains the same choices for prostheses as any other transradial amputee. Vocational, social, or cosmetic reasons may affect the decision to use a prosthesis.

Indications and Contraindications

The Krukenberg procedure can be performed on transradial residual limbs that result from amputations from many causes. The most common traumatic causes of transradial amputation include crush injuries that occur in traffic accidents, cutting or crushing injuries caused by unprotected machinery, frostbite, electrical burns, and injuries caused by explosive devices. The Krukenberg operation is often used to address the types of injuries inflicted by war.[9,12]

In patients with congenital upper limb deficiency, the operation is advocated beginning at 2 years of age with consideration for the associated developmental milestones.[5,16-18] A digit associated with a transradial deficiency should be preserved because it may assist in grip function.

The classic indication for the Krukenberg procedure is in a person with a bilateral transradial amputation who was blinded in the same incident, usually the premature detonation of an explosive device such as a hand grenade. The procedure often results in excellent restoration of a powerful and sensitive grip,[19-24] but despite these undisputed functional advantages, recommending the operation for every transradial amputee may be unrealistic because of the resulting unnatural appearance. The Krukenberg operation should, therefore, be undertaken only in a select group of highly motivated individuals. Candidates for the procedure may have either bilateral or unilateral transradial amputation, and they should be informed of the advantages and limitations of the procedure.[25-29] In the unilateral transradial amputee, the reconstructed limb will greatly augment the function of the normal limb by acting as an assistive "hand."

The Krukenberg procedure is of particular importance in countries where prosthetic services are nonexistent and/or the cost of a prosthesis

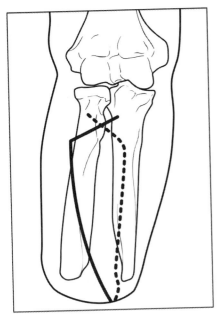

Figure 1 Orientation of the fasciocutaneous flaps for the Krukenberg procedure. The solid line depicts the anterior offset L-shaped incision, and the dotted line depicts the reversed posterior incision.

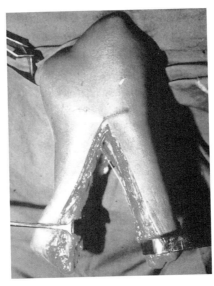

Figure 2 Intraoperative photograph showing myodesis attachment of extensor and flexor groups. The L arm of the incision has been drawn on the skin but has not been incised at this stage of the procedure. Note the wide passive separation of the radius and ulna required for functional pincer grasp.

is prohibitive. This combination of circumstances was seen during the civil war in Sierra Leone, where the rebels chopped off the hands of captured combatants and noncombatants alike. These persons were sent back to their villages unable to care for themselves. The rehabilitation team surgeons working with these victims opted for the Krukenberg procedure as the long-term solution.[12,30] After a series of successful Krukenberg operations in the 1980s, Bangladesh issued a commemorative postal stamp showing an individual who had been treated with bilateral Krukenberg procedures, writing with his residual limbs.

The Krukenberg procedure is contraindicated in transradial amputees younger than 2 years of age, in the extremely old who are otherwise dependent on others, and in individuals who cannot accept the appearance of the modified residual limb. The operation is also contraindicated when there is a severe elbow joint contracture or when the residual limb will be too short for effective pincer function (ie, less than 10 cm in adults).[9]

Preoperative Care

Because of the unique cosmetic aspects of the Krukenberg procedure, sighted candidates, in particular, should have the opportunity to meet a successful Krukenberg amputee to assess the dexterity and versatility of the prehensile rays for various tasks. At the same time, the candidate can discuss issues pertaining to the appearance of the limb(s) with an experienced user.[31-36] If a Krukenberg amputee is not locally available, various forms of electronic media can be used so that the candidate can meet a "virtual" Krukenberg user.

Careful preoperative consideration of these issues by the surgical candidate should lead to easier acceptance of the final appearance of the limb. Preoperative care should also include exercises to improve the range of motion and strength of both the reconstructed and intact upper limbs.

Surgical Technique

The Krukenberg operation is basically the conversion of a transradial resid-

ual limb into sensate, muscle-powered radial and ulnar pincers, thus creating a unique form of prehension.

Skin Incision

Under tourniquet control, the anterior skin incision begins at a point 8 cm distal to the elbow crease and 2.5 to 3.0 cm lateral to the midaxial line. A short extension is made proximally and medially at an angle of 45° for 2.5 cm. Returning to the starting point, the incision is continued distally to the midaxial point at the end of the residual limb. This offset L-shaped incision results in an ulnar flap that is larger than the radial flap. A similar but reversed posterior forearm incision is then made, resulting in a larger offset radial flap (Figure 1). Both flaps are raised with their underlying fascia.

Muscle Management

The forearm muscles that power the wrist and fingers are bluntly dissected into radial and ulnar groups, beginning proximally and continuing to the end of the residual limb. Muscles that insert onto the radius and ulna, such as the pronator teres and anconeus, are not disturbed. Separation of the muscle groups exposes both the anterior and posterior surfaces of the interosseous membrane. The membrane is divided along its ulnar attachment, taking care to preserve the interosseous vascular bundle. This incision is extended proximally to an extent that provides 12 cm of passive separation between the tips of the radius and ulna during the surgical procedure (Figure 2).

Nerve Management

The median nerve, under slight traction, is ligated and divided where it emerges from the pronator teres. The ulnar nerve is similarly divided under traction so that its end retracts into the proximal muscle mass.

Vessel Management

Radial, ulnar, and interosseous vessels are separately ligated just proximal to the proposed site of bone division.

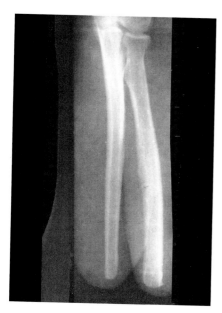

Figure 3 Radiograph showing ideal uniform muscular envelope covering radial and ulnar rays, which was achieved with complete primary skin closure.

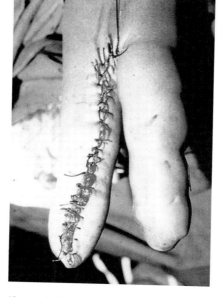

Figure 4 Intraoperative photograph of complete coverage of both rays with opposing sensate skin, which was achieved without muscle debulking.

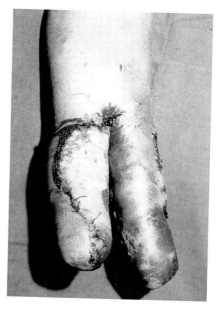

Figure 5 Intraoperative photograph showing a split-thickness skin graft covering the muscle mass when complete primary closure is not possible without muscle debulking.

Bone Management

To create effective pincers, the radius and ulna must be of equal length. The bones are marked at a point 18 to 20 cm distal to the elbow crease. The periosteum is incised circumferentially 2 cm distal to this mark and elevated as a sleeve to the proposed level of bone division. The bones are cut, the edges are filed smooth, and the periosteal tubes are snugly closed over the bone ends. The previously separated muscle groups are sewn securely to the periosteal sleeves at the tips of their respective rays. This myodesis is essential for the functional stability of these muscles and should result in a uniform muscle envelope enclosing each bone (Figure 3).

Skin Closure

After releasing the tourniquet and ensuring hemostasis, the skin is closed, beginning at the proximal end of the wound. Because the incisions began 8 cm distal to the elbow crease, a proximal web of soft tissue is maintained. The L-shaped skin flaps can be passed between the radius and ulna over the pronator teres and sutured over the web. This technique not only covers the web of the pincer with normal skin but also prevents future scarring between the rays. The offset incisions result in normally sensate opposing skin in the distal one third of the radial and ulnar rays, which is crucial for optimal utility of the pincers (Figure 4). The wound is closed with a drain at the web of the newly formed pincers. A number of variations in skin closure have been advocated to achieve complete primary coverage of the radial and ulnar rays with sensate skin. Krukenberg advocated the use of a U-shaped midline incision.[1,37] Methods that replaced this approach were derived from the principles of plastic surgery. These include an offset incision with either a proximal V- or L-shaped extension, which helps to cover the newly formed web of the forceps, or an S-shaped incision.[12,17,29,38-41] Some have advocated a special inverted L-shaped incision at the distal end to ensure normally sensate skin in opposition at the tips.[11,29,42,43] To facilitate primary coverage of the rays and to avoid the need for a split-thickness skin graft, muscle debulking has been advocated, even to the extent of retaining only the pronator teres, supinator, flexor carpi ulnaris, and brachioradialis, resulting in an almost subcutaneous radius and ulna.[6,22,44] Based on experience at the Artificial Limb Centre at Pune, India, with more than 500 Krukenberg procedures during the past 50 years, a split-thickness graft is recommended rather than muscle debulking because of the potential for skin necrosis or bone necrosis when enveloping muscles are excised. If primary skin closure on the radial or ulnar ray is not possible, a split-thickness skin graft is used to cover the exposed muscle mass (Figure 5).

Special Considerations

Other newer variations of the Krukenberg procedure include the adjuvant use of wire fixators such as the Ilizarov ring mechanism or Joshi's external stabilization system (JESS) axial fixator to lengthen a very short transradial residual limb. A fixator may also be used to keep the radius and ulna distracted during the postoperative period. Skin coverage for

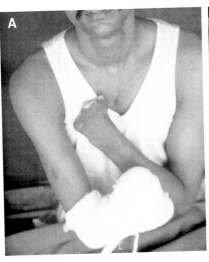

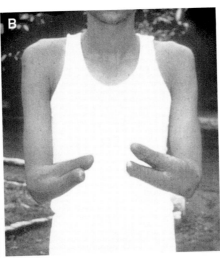

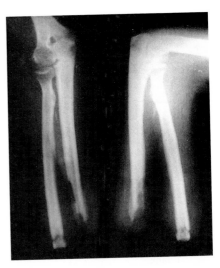

Figure 6 A, The postoperative dressing after a Krukenberg procedure (right residual limb). The radial and ulnar rays are dressed individually and separated as widely as possible with bulky wool or gauze. In this photo, the patient was preoperative for a left Krukenberg procedure. **B,** Postoperative photograph of a similar patient with healed residual limbs after the Krukenberg procedure.

Figure 7 AP and lateral radiographs showing distal bone necrosis of both the radius and ulna after extensive muscle debulking to achieve primary closure.

the lengthened bones can be achieved by the staged use of tissue expanders, which provides primary closure with sensate skin without the use of a split-thickness graft.[45]

The Krukenberg procedure can be undertaken in children as young as 2 years of age. Care is taken to avoid any injury to the distal physes, if present, for young patients with congenital limb deficiency because major upper limb growth occurs at the wrist. In adults with a shorter transradial residual limb, the length of the base of the pincers can be reduced to 6 cm instead of the ideal 8 cm. Another option is to reduce the length from the web to the distal end to 8 to 10 cm, instead of the ideal 12 cm.

Immediate Postoperative Management

An important part of immediate postoperative management is the separate dressing of the radial and ulnar rays with care to keep them as widely distracted as possible, using wool or gauze as a spacer (Figure 6). The first dressing change is done 4 or 5 days postoperatively; subsequent dressing changes at intervals of 2 to 3 days are

recommended, depending on the condition of the rays. Sutures are generally removed 12 to 14 days postoperatively. The drain from the base of the pincers is removed after 48 hours without disturbing the main dressing.

Postoperative Complications

As with any other amputation, intraoperative damage to vessels or skin closure under tension may result in flap necrosis. Subsequent management depends on the degree of necrosis. If the necrosis is superficial and small in area, débridement may suffice. If a large area is necrotic, a split-thickness graft may be necessary. If necrosis of a bone tip occurs, waiting for 2 to 3 weeks is recommended to allow demarcation of the sequestrum, which can then be excised (Figure 7). A length disparity of more than 2 cm between the radial and ulnar rays requires reshaping to equalize length. If the muscles slip off the tip of the rays, the function of the pincers will be seriously compromised. This complication results from either insecure anchoring of the periosteal tube over the radial and ulnar tips, or from an unbalanced, poorly anchored myode-

sis. Reanchoring the muscle sling over the bone tips corrects this problem.

Rehabilitation

Immediately after removal of the sutures 12 to 14 days postoperatively, physical training of the forearm muscles is initiated. The amputee is taught to open and close the newly bifid forearm to function as a pair of pincers. The muscles that facilitate opening of the pincers are those aligned on the lateral side of the radius (brachioradialis, extensor carpi radialis longus and brevis, radial portion of the extensor digitorum communis, and biceps) and those on the medial side of the ulna (flexor carpi ulnaris, the ulnar part of the digitorum sublimis, the brachialis, and the anconeus). The muscles that facilitate closing of the pincers are on the medial side of the radius (pronator teres, supinator, flexor carpi radialis, the radial aspect of the flexor digitorum sublimis, and palmaris longus) and those on the lateral side of the ulna (extensor carpi ulnaris, ulnar part of the extensor digitorum communis, and triceps). Evaluations, including the use of electromyography, have been used to describe the de-

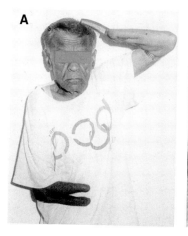
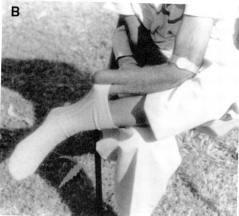
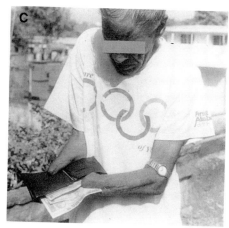

Figure 8 Functional independence in self-care achieved by a bilateral Krukenberg amputee. **A,** Combing hair. **B,** Donning sock. **C,** Removing bank notes from a wallet.

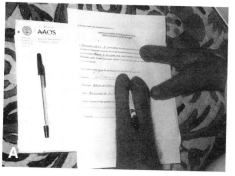
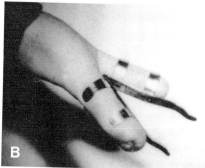
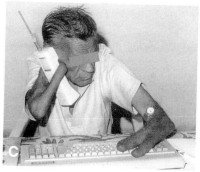

Figure 9 Functional independence in work-related activities. **A,** Signing a document. **B,** An adaptive device for fine prehension. **C,** Using a computer keyboard and telephone.

tailed muscle action in residual limbs after the Krukenberg procedure.[5,9,29,44]

Initiation of early physical training of the forearm muscles is important because of the somatosensory plasticity of the brain.[46] Initially, training focuses on passive movement of the rays. Active exercises are gradually introduced. Throughout the rehabilitation program, the opening and closing action should be performed only in the sagittal plane to avoid any pronation and supination so that precision in grasping is encouraged from the beginning.[6,28,47,48] Electrical stimulation of muscles can also be quite useful in rehabilitating the muscles.

The action of opening and closing is gradually enhanced by increasing the amount of opening between the tips and by strengthening the relevant muscle groups. An improved ability to open and close the bifid forearm allows the patient to reproduce many functions of the hand (Figure 8). The end result is an individual who can be totally independent, even when performing precision work such as threading a needle or participating in vocational activities, including handling a phone or computer (Figure 9). Individuals who are blind can learn the Braille alphabet.[49]

Summary

The loss of one hand is a major impairment, but independence is much more difficult to achieve with the loss of both hands, especially when associated with blindness. The Krukenberg procedure converts the transradial residual limb to a pair of pincers, which functions as an efficient, sensate grasping organ. This in turn trans-

lates into an opportunity for independent living with renewed vocational options. The Krukenberg procedure need not be limited to use in blind, bilateral transradial amputees. This procedure can be undertaken in any well-motivated, normally sighted bilateral or even unilateral transradial amputee with excellent results. The resultant bifid forearm may not be cosmetically acceptable to some amputees, which is a relative contraindication despite its functional utility. The procedure is an important option for transradial amputees residing in a country that has rudimentary or nonexistent services to provide prostheses.

A Krukenberg procedure does not alter the amputee's choice of a prosthesis. Prostheses can be prescribed as for any other transradial amputee, ranging from a cosmetic prosthesis to a conventional transradial prosthesis or a myoelectric prosthesis, depending on the intended use.[18,50-53] If a prosthesis is used, additional rehabilitative training under the guidance of an occupational therapist can be helpful, depending on which prosthesis is available and/or required.

References

1. Krukenberg H: Über die plastische Umwertung von Amputationsstümpfen. Stuttgart, Germany, *Enke-Verlag,* 1917.

2. Marquardt E: Die Krukenberg-Plastik: Originalmethode und Modifikation für blinde Ohnhänder. *Beschäftigungstherapie und Rehab* 1978;17:221-225.

3. Baumgartner R: Indikationsstellungen für die Krukenberg-Greifhand aufgrund von Langzeitergebnissen. *Z Orthop* 1944;132:180-184.

4. Henry AK: An operation for making the forearm prehensile after loss of a hand. *Br J Surg* 1928;16:188-197.

5. Swanson AB: The Krukenberg procedure in the juvenile amputee. *J Bone Joint Surg Am* 1964;46:1540-1548.

6. Gu YD, Zhang LY, Zheng YL: Introduction of a modified Krukenberg operation. *Plast Reconstr Surg* 1996;97: 222-226.

7. Editorial: Krukenberg's chopsticks. *BMJ* 1978;1:129.

8. Powell HD: Letter: Krukenberg's chopsticks. *BMJ* 1978;1:511.

9. Garst RJ: The Krukenberg hand. *J Bone Joint Surg Br* 1991;73:385-388.

10. Colp R, Ransohoff NS: The Krukenberg stump. *J Bone Joint Surg* 1933;15: 439-443.

11. Tubiana R: Krukenberg's operation. *Orthop Clin North Am* 1981;12:819-826.

12. Irmay F, Merzouga B, Vettorel D: The Krukenberg procedure: A surgical option for the treatment of double hand amputees in Sierra Leone. *Lancet* 2000; 356:1072-1075.

13. Kallio KE: Recent advances in Krukenberg's operation. *Acta Chir Scand* 1948; 97:165-168.

14. Ritsila V, Kivilaakso R: Modification of Krukenberg's kineplastic operation. *Ann Chir Gynaecol* 1976;65:338-341.

15. Egloff DV, Cantero J: Reconstruction of a pinch through transfer of a single toe: Survey on five cases. *Ann Chir Main* 1989;8:207-216.

16. Harrison SH, Mayou B: Bilateral Krukenberg operations in a young child. *Br J Plast Surg* 1977;30:171-173.

17. Swanson AB, Swanson GD: The Krukenberg procedure in the juvenile amputee. *Clin Orthop* 1980;148:55-61.

18. Marquardt E: The multiple limb-deficient child, in Bowker JH, Michael JW (eds): *Atlas of Limb Prosthetics: Surgical, Prosthetic, and Rehabilitation Principles,* ed 2. Rosemont, IL, American Academy of Orthopaedic Surgeons, 2002, pp 839-884. (Originally published by Mosby-Year Book, 1992.)

19. Colp R: Abstract: Krukenberg amputation. *Ann Surg* 1933;97:277-279.

20. Bauer KH: Zum Problem der Ohnhänderversorgung und zur Frage der operativen Behandlung insbesondere des Krukenberg-Armes. *Verh Dtsch Orthop Ges Beilage Z Orthop* 1948;78:51-53.

21. Buck-Gramcko D: Hat sich die Krukenberg-Operation bewährt und ist sie im Hinblick auf die modernen Handprothesen noch indiziert? *Ztschr-Orthop* 1954;85:460-484.

22. Nathan PA, Trung NB: The Krukenberg operation: A modified technique avoiding skin grafts. *J Hand Surg Am* 1977;2:127-130.

23. Mathur BP, Narang IC, Piplani CL, Majid MA: Rehabilitation of the bilateral below-elbow amputee by the Krukenberg procedure. *Prosthet Orthot Int* 1981;5:135-140.

24. Sinaki M, Dobyns JH, Kinnunen JM: Krukenberg's kineplasty and rehabilitation in a blind, bilateral full-hand amputee. *Clin Orthop* 1982;169:163-166.

25. Bunnell S: Contractures of the hand from infections and injuries. *J Bone Joint Surg* 1932;14:27-46.

26. Alldredge RH: The cineplastic method in upper-extremity amputations. *J Bone Joint Surg Am* 1948;30:359-373.

27. De Santolo AR: A new approach to the use of the Krukenberg procedure in unilateral wrist amputations: An original functional-cosmetic prosthesis. *Bull Hosp Jt Dis Orthop Inst* 1984;44: 177-187.

28. Vilkki SK: Free toe transfer to the forearm stump following wrist amputation: A current alternative to the Krukenberg operation. *Handchir Mikrochir Plast Chir* 1985;17:92-97.

29. Marquardt E, Martini AK: Krukenberg-plasty in the E. Marquardt modification. *Handchir Mikrochir Plast Chir* 1985;17:117-121.

30. De Smet L: Are there still indications for the Krukenberg kineplasty? Report of two patients. *Chir Main* 1999;18: 132-135.

31. Kreuz L: Die Herrichtung des Unterarmstümpfes zum natürlichen Greifarm nach dem Verfahren von Krukenbergs. *Zentralbl Chir* 1944;71:1170-1175.

32. Thomsen W: Diskussionsbeitrag zum Thema Krukenberg-Plastik. *Verh Dstch Orthop Ges* 1948;78:60-61.

33. Lischenewsky SM: Effectivität der operativen plastichen Spaltung von Unterarmstümpfen. *Orthop Tech* 1978;29: 114-116.

34. Lescoeur JE (ed): *Amputés Des Membres Supérieurs: Leurs Vrais Problemes: Chirurgie, Appareillage, Reeducation, Avenir.* Paris, France, Maloine, 1979.

35. Frantz CH, Aitken GT: Management of the juvenile amputee. *Clin Orthop* 1959;14:30-49.

36. Song R: Experiences with the Krukenberg plastic operation. *Clin Plast Surg* 1982;9:79-84.

37. Krukenberg H: Erfahrungen mit der Krukenberg-Hand. *Arch Klin Chir* 1931;165:191-201.

38. Squires BT: Note on two cases of Krukenberg's operation. *Br J Surg* 1937;25:464-466.

39. Simon P: Modalitäten des wieder eingetretenen Hautgefühlesauf Bauchhautplastiken von Krukenberg-Greifarmen. *Monatsschr Unfallheilkd* 1961;46A:1540-1549.

40. Gosset J, Langlais F: Digitization of the forearm: Indications, technique, long term results. *Ann Chir* 1975;29: 1073-1078.

41. Loosli-Guignard RM, Verdan C: Krukenberg's operation: Indications and limitations. *Ann Chir Main* 1983; 2:154-159.

42. Marquardt E, Martini AK: Amputation surgery of the upper extremities. *Z Orthop Ihre Grenzgeb* 1979;117:622-631.

43. Martini AK: The Krukenberg plasty and the provision of additional pros-

theses and technical aids. *Z Orthop Ihre Grenzgeb* 1983;121:196-202.

44. Zanoli R: Krukenberg-Putti amputation-plasty. *J Bone Joint Surg Br* 1957;39:230-232.

45. Stober R, Traub S: Modified Krukenberg-plasty with callus distraction of the stump and complete skin closure of both forearm branches. *Handchir Mikrochir Plast Chir* 1998;30: 325-329.

46. Borsook D, Becerra L, Fishman S, et al: Acute plasticity in the human somatosensory cortex following amputation. *Neuroreport* 1998;9:1013-1017.

47. Heyne S: Ergotherapie bei blinden Ohnhändern mit Krukenberg-Plastik. *Beschäftigungstherapie und Rehab* 1978; 17:227-234.

48. Ryder RA: Occupational therapy for a patient with a bilateral Krukenberg amputation. *Am J Occup Ther* 1989;43: 689-691.

49. Lob A: Krukenberg's plastic operation in peacetime. *Hefte Unfallheilkd* 1970; 105:1-48.

50. Moberg E: Hand surgery and the development of hand prostheses. *Scand J Plast Reconstr Surg* 1975;9:227-230.

51. Visuthikosol V, Wongbusarakum S, Navykam T, Kruavit A: The Krukenberg procedure in the bilateral amputee after electrical burn. *Ann Plast Surg* 1991;27:56-60.

52. Heger H, Millstein S, Hunter GA: Electrically powered prostheses for the adult with an upper limb amputation. *J Bone Joint Surg Br* 1985;67:278-281.

53. Dalsey R, Gomez W, Seitz WH Jr, Dick HM, Hutnick G, Akdeniz R: Myoelectric prosthetic replacement in the upper-extremity amputee. *Orthop Rev* 1989;18:697-702.

Chapter 18

Elbow Disarticulation and Transhumeral Amputation: Surgical Management

Patrick Owens, MD
E. Anne Ouellette, MD, MBA

Introduction

The etiology of 90% of upper limb amputations is trauma. Men sustain four times as many amputations as women, with most injuries occurring in individuals age 20 to 40 years.[1] Functional rehabilitation is especially important in these young patients. Other causes of amputations include burns, malignant tumors, neurologic disorders, infections, congenital deformities, and peripheral vascular disease. In the upper limb, vascular etiologies of amputation are as common in children as in adults because of conditions such as fulminating meningococcemia and disseminated intravascular coagulation. Although amputation rates for malignant tumors in the upper limb have decreased with advances in limb salvage techniques, amputation is still sometimes required for tumor control. Amputation may also be necessary in patients with severe, nonreconstructable brachial plexus injuries.

General Surgical Considerations

Replantation

Because of advances in microvascular techniques, replantation has been a viable option in traumatic upper limb amputations since the first successful upper limb replantation in 1962. Children are candidates for replantation at nearly any level of amputation because of better long-term functional outcomes.[2] In adults, however, less than 25% of patients regain functional use of the limb,[3] and some require revision to a transradial amputation to maximize functional use of the limb. Major replantation above the level of the wrist carries significant metabolic risks to the patient because of the volume of involved muscle.[4] However, patients with sensation and some residual function in the replanted limb have better functional outcomes than amputees with prostheses.[3]

Level of Amputation

Amputation should be performed at the most distal level possible that allows for control of the disease or is consistent with the zone of injury. Wound coverage is best achieved with local skin flaps that allow for adequate padding and closure.[1] Greater residual limb length can often be preserved by covering the wound with skin grafts, free or abdominal flaps, or flaps from the amputated parts.[5] Ilizarov bone lengthening techniques have been described[6] but are rarely indicated with use of modern prosthetic sockets.[1]

Controversy exists over whether to perform a long transhumeral amputation or an elbow disarticulation. The disarticulation allows enhanced suspension and rotational control of the prosthesis. In adults, however, retention of full humeral length precludes the use of a prosthetic elbow. In addition, the external hinge elbow mechanisms that are available for disarticulation are less pleasing cosmetically.

In children, transhumeral amputation results in a high incidence of bony overgrowth that requires revision; therefore, elbow disarticulation is the level of choice.[7] The slowed humeral growth that occurs after elbow disarticulation will result in a humeral length at maturity that allows use of a prosthetic elbow while retaining the suspension and rotational control benefits of an elbow disarticulation.[8]

Several issues arise with more proximal amputations. For effective control of the shoulder, the insertion of the deltoid must be retained. High proximal transhumeral amputation is preferable to shoulder disarticulation cosmetically because it retains the shoulder contour, but functionally, the two levels are similar. When amputations are performed at the level of the surgical neck, abduction contractures can occur; therefore, primary shoulder arthrodesis can be considered at this level.[1] Prosthetic suspension is more easily accomplished with retention of the proximal humerus, and function is somewhat improved for both the myoelectric and body-powered prostheses.

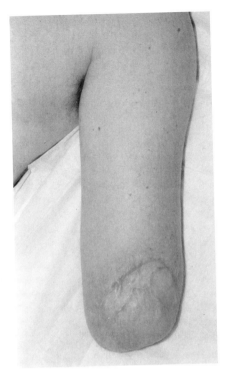

Figure 1 Mature traumatic elbow disarticulation allowed successful prosthetic fitting. *(Courtesy of John H. Bowker, MD.)*

Technique

The use of a pneumatic tourniquet is recommended for more distal amputations to aid in visualization of major neurovascular structures. Exsanguination is accomplished by elevation of the limb for 2 to 3 minutes. Double ligation of the major arteries should be performed along with ligation of the larger collateral vessels. The tourniquet should always be deflated prior to wound closure to ensure hemostasis.

The median, ulnar, radial, and medial and lateral antebrachial cutaneous nerves should be identified, transected under modest tension, and allowed to retract under proximal soft tissue several centimeters proximal to the bone ends. This increases the likelihood that any neuroma formation will occur in a well-protected area.[9] The posterior flap should be longer than the anterior flap if possible; this allows closure of the wound away from the distal end of the residual limb. Alternatively, equal anterior and posterior flaps can be used.

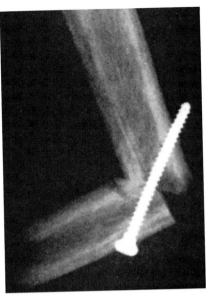

Figure 2 Marquardt angulation osteotomy of transhumeral amputation showing flexion of the distal fragment over the anterior cortical fulcrum. An incomplete posterior osteotomy was performed to minimize further loss of length. The prosthesis socket can be fitted around the anterior bony prominence to enhance suspension and rotational control of the prosthesis. *(Reproduced with permission from Marquardt E, Neff G: The angulation osteotomy of above-elbow stumps. Clin Orthop 1974;104:232-238.)*

Elbow Disarticulation

After the skin flaps are created, the flexor and extensor muscle origins are removed sharply from the epicondyles. The nerves and blood vessels are isolated and treated as described above. The biceps, brachialis, and triceps tendons should be transected, followed by division of the capsular and ligamentous attachments. An oscillating saw may be used to remove the prominences of the medial and lateral epicondyles and the distal humerus. This maintains the expanded end of the humerus and facilitates better rotational control of the prosthesis while reducing the chance of skin pressure ulcers related to the prominent epicondyles. The biceps and triceps should be attached at physiologic tension to the distal portion of the residual limb (Figure 1).

Transhumeral Amputation

Every attempt should be made to retain maximum possible residual limb length. The principles of transhumeral amputation are the same as for elbow disarticulation. The periosteum should be incised sharply to reduce the risk of overgrowth, and the long posterior flap should include the triceps muscle. At the time of wound closure, the triceps and the biceps should be secured to the humerus using transosseous sutures (myodesis). This will ensure adequate padding for the distal bone end and stable muscles for myoelectric sensors. For amputations through the surgical neck, shoulder arthrodesis should be performed primarily.

For patients with long or midlength humeral segments, an angulation osteotomy, as described by Marquardt and Neff,[10] facilitates the fitting and function of the prosthesis by providing both better suspension and rotational control. The unique abbreviated socket suspended from the angled humeral segment frees the shoulder joint, facilitating overhead reaching and the substitution of shoulder rotation for wrist rotation. A 70° angle with respect to the humeral shaft, apex dorsal, is desirable. Neusel and associates[11] reported straightening of the humerus within 2 years following the osteotomy in nearly two thirds of children. In contrast, the adults showed no loss of angulation.

In children, the osteotomy is made approximately at the junction of the middle and distal thirds of the humerus. An anterior closing wedge osteotomy is performed, leaving the posterior periosteum intact. The bone fragments are secured with a Kirschner wire. If removal of a wedge results in unacceptable shortening, an incomplete posterior osteotomy is performed, and the bone is flexed over the anterior cortical fulcrum to the desired angulation and fixed (Figure 2). Local periosteal flaps are used to cover the posterior bony defect, and a cast is worn for 5 to 6 weeks postoperatively.

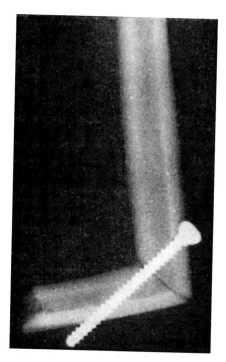

Figure 3 Marquardt angulation achieved by anterior closing wedge osteotomy. *(Reproduced with permission from Marquardt E, Neff G: The angulation osteotomy of above-elbow stumps. Clin Orthop 1974;104:232-238.)*

In adults, an anterior closing wedge osteotomy is made 5 to 7 cm proximal to the bone ends (Figure 3). Osteosynthesis is obtained with a lag screw. With good fixation, casting generally is not required for immobilization, although it can be used to control postoperative swelling.

References

1. Baumgartner R: Upper extremity amputations, in DuParc (ed): *Surgical Techniques in Orthopaedics and Traumatology.* Orlando, FL, Harcourt International, 2003, vol 4.

2. Jaeger SH, Tsai TM, Kleinert HE: Upper extremity replantation in children. *Orthop Clin North Am* 1981;12:897-907.

3. Graham B, Adkins P, Tsai TM, Firrell J, Breidenbach WC: Major replantation versus revision amputation and prosthetic fitting in the upper extremity: A late functional outcomes study. *J Hand Surg Am* 1998;23:783-791.

4. Wood MB, Cooney WP III: Above elbow limb replantation: Functional results. *J Hand Surg Am* 1986;11:682-687.

5. Weinberg MJ, Al-Qattan MM, Mahoney J: "Spare part" forearm free flaps harvested from the amputated limb for coverage of amputation stumps. *J Hand Surg Br* 1997;22:615-619.

6. Mertens P, Lammens J: Short amputation stump lengthening with the Ilizarov method: Risks versus benefits. *Acta Orthop Belg* 2001;67:274-278.

7. Aitken GT: Surgical amputation in children. *J Bone Joint Surg Am* 1963;45:1735-1741.

8. Abraham E, Pellicore RJ, Hamilton RC, Hallman BW, Ghosh L: Stump overgrowth in juvenile amputees. *J Pediatr Orthop* 1986;6:66-71.

9. Whipple RR, Unsell RS: Treatment of painful neuromas. *Orthop Clin North Am* 1988;19:175-185.

10. Marquardt E, Neff G: The angulation osteotomy of above-elbow stumps. *Clin Orthop* 1974;104:232-238.

11. Neusel E, Traub M, Blasius K, Marquardt E: Results of humeral stump angulation osteotomy. *Arch Orthop Trauma Surg* 1997;116:263-265.

Chapter 19

Elbow Disarticulation and Transhumeral Amputation: Prosthetic Management

Wayne K. Daly, CPO, LPO

Introduction

Successful patient rehabilitation and effective functional use of a transhumeral or elbow disarticulation prosthesis depend on many factors. Key elements that influence prosthetic outcome include (1) the lever arm length of the remaining bone, (2) the quality and nature of the skin and soft-tissue coverage of the limb and torso, (3) muscle function and tone in the residual limb, (4) pain control in the residual limb, (5) joint range of motion and strength of the residual limb and upper body, and (6) rehabilitation support, ie, the availability and skill of psychological, rehabilitation therapy, and prosthetic practitioners. All of these elements must be considered carefully to achieve the best possible prosthetic outcome. Most studies have shown a long-term rate of prosthetic wear for transhumeral and elbow disarticulation amputees of less than 50%.[1] Although there may be many reasons for these findings, these levels of loss clearly present a significant rehabilitation challenge. Careful surgery, evaluation, prosthetic fitting, and therapy are all crucial to successful outcome and optimal prosthetic function. Each of these factors and appropriate prosthetic options are discussed in this chapter.

Patient Evaluation

The patient should be evaluated carefully to assess the numerous elements noted above that influence the successful use of the prosthesis. A careful analysis of the patient's physical capability and appropriate prosthetic options will reduce the long-term cost of care while increasing the functional use of the prosthesis. Although a prosthesis is not absolutely necessary for an amputee to function and many activities can be accomplished with one hand in the case of a unilateral loss, there are solid reasons for considering a suitable prosthesis. Clinical experience and recent studies suggest that overuse problems with the remaining hand and arm may develop in as many as 50% of upper limb amputees.[2,3] Active use of a prosthesis is believed to reduce this risk. A prosthesis also facilitates the many tasks requiring bimanual capabilities.

Bone Length

The length of the remaining bone is crucial to prosthesis design and function. Although trauma situations may limit the surgical options, the best possible residual limb should be provided for future rehabilitation. In the case of elective or revision surgery, extra care in planning for the most functional residual limb can facilitate the best possible outcome.[4] The length of the bone is a primary consideration in the biomechanics of the artificial arm. In general, a longer humeral segment will provide more le-

verage to control the prosthesis. Residual limb length will also affect the choice of elbow components. In adults, humeral transection 10 cm above the olecranon tip enables use of all available prosthetic components, including externally powered alternatives. Excess residual limb length from redundant tissue is functionally useless and serves only to complicate the prosthetic fitting. Copious redundant tissue makes donning the prosthesis much more difficult, often compromises cosmesis, and may preclude the use of typical elbow components.

Soft-tissue coverage also affects prosthetic function because a painful residual limb will limit the force that the amputee can comfortably generate to control the prosthesis. Adherent, scarred distal tissue shortens the effective lever arm available to generate control forces nearly as much as if the bone was transected at a higher level.

Amputation proximal to the deltoid insertion will render active placement of the prosthesis in space impossible for the amputee. Biomechanically, patients with very short humeral remnants function as if they have a shoulder disarticulation. Lengthenings using the Ilizarov technique or fibular bone grafts have proven successful in improving prosthetic function in some amputees.[5,6] The elbow disarticulation level offers several functional advantages that are especially valuable for the bilateral

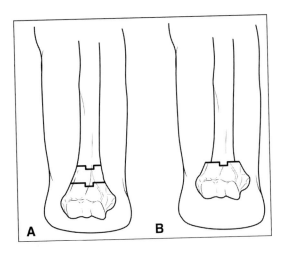

Figure 1 Osteotomy procedure used by de Luccia and Marino[7] to reduce the humeral length of an elbow disarticulation by 3 cm. **A,** Location of cut lines on the humerus. **B,** Reduced length with removal of the bone segment.

upper limb amputee who must use the residual limb for self-care. The humeral condyles can provide body-controlled, active humeral rotation of the prosthesis. This significantly increases the active work envelope of the prosthesis compared with the passive humeral rotation offered by the typical prosthetic elbow mechanism used for transhumeral and higher levels. An elbow disarticulation also may be useful in children because the epiphysis is preserved, thus preventing bony overgrowth and maintaining growth potential. The elbow disarticulation level requires the use of small locking joints located adjacent to the humeral epicondyles, external to the socket, reducing the durability and cosmesis of the prosthesis. Some attempts have been made to reduce the length problem of this level by using a length osteotomy to shorten the humerus while maintaining the epicondyles for rotation control and suspension[7] (Figure 1). This technique permits the use of standard prosthetic components while maintaining the functional advantages of the elbow disarticulation. In essence, this method creates a foreshortened residual limb, substantially improving cosmesis. The final result is analogous to the reduced final growth length of a pediatric elbow disarticulation. Because voluntary control of humeral rotation is so helpful in achieving independence, an angulation osteotomy has been proposed for bilateral amputees to provide active humeral rotation without the bulk of the elbow disarticulation epicondyles.[8,9]

Quality of Skin and Soft Tissue

The quality of the skin and soft-tissue coverage of the bone are important for both the function and comfort of the prosthesis. If the bone is not well protected, it will be difficult for the amputee to maintain the precise fit necessary to prevent excessive pressure and pain in the residual limb. Scar tissue and skin grafts should be placed away from the cut end of the bone and away from the axilla whenever possible. In a prosthesis, the anterior, lateral, and axillary surfaces of the residual limb are major pressure- and force-bearing areas; any painful or severely scarred tissue in these areas will complicate prosthetic fitting. Burns and scar tissue on the torso will also complicate the harness design and may require a self-suspending, externally powered prosthesis to prevent recurrent skin damage.

Muscle Strength and Tone

Muscle function and strength ultimately determine how functional the prosthesis will be. Muscles that have been surgically stabilized with myodesis provide superior control of the prosthesis, optimize myoelectric signals, and are believed to prevent the pain and marked atrophy that may develop over time with unstabilized muscle. Brachial plexus injuries may benefit from a shoulder fusion to eliminate subluxation, extend the scapular lever arm, and eliminate the need to cover much of the torso to stabilize the prosthesis. Careful consideration of the fusion angle and humeral length facilitate a prosthetic fitting of the brachial plexus amputee.[10]

Joint Range of Motion

Joint range of motion is significant to prosthetic function because restriction of motion will reduce the capability of the prosthesis. Restricted motion of either shoulder will reduce available body control motions and may require externally powered components to provide adequate function. Although full joint range is not always required for prosthetic use, biscapular motion and humeral range of motion on the amputated side are especially critical to the function of the prosthesis. Frozen shoulder syndrome and subluxation must be prevented whenever possible and treated aggressively when present.

Rehabilitation Support

Psychological counseling is often overlooked in the care of the amputee, but it can be very helpful with pain control and emotional adjustment. A well-trained multidisciplinary team facilitates successful prosthetic rehabilitation, especially in bilateral amputees. Peer visitation and support groups may also be helpful during the post-amputation adjustment period. Other important considerations include prompt prosthetic fitting; care in designing and creating the prosthesis; and structured follow-up, training, and therapy.

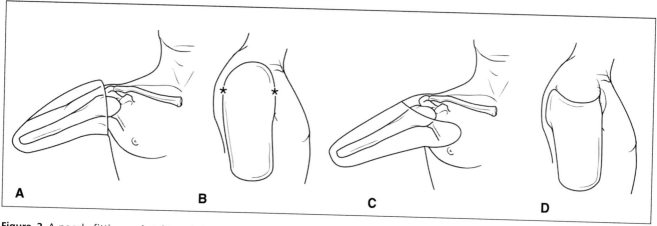

Figure 2 A poorly fitting socket (**A** and **B**) tends to gap when the arm is abducted or flexed. A more intimately contoured socket (**C** and **D**) offers better contact and control.

Prosthesis Design
Socket Design

The socket design will vary with the length of the residual limb and the suspension method chosen. The most common transhumeral socket designs are rigid fiber-reinforced plastic lamination or a flexible thermoplastic socket with rigid open frame. Special care in shaping the proximal trimlines is necessary to provide rotational stability and suspension, particularly as the residual limb becomes shorter (Figure 2). Flexible open-frame sockets provide a softer interface for the skin and are reported to be cooler and more comfortable for the amputee[11] (Figure 3).

When fully formed condyles are present, the width and length of these structures must be accommodated in the socket. Three common designs include the fenestrated, screw-in, and flexible wall socket types discussed below. With elbow disarticulations, the socket provides rotational control and suspension from the oval shape at the end of the limb.

Suspension Systems

The prosthesis can be suspended by a harness, suction, a roll-on liner, anatomic contouring, or any combination of these methods. The traditional figure-of-8, chest strap, and shoulder saddle harnesses provide suspension as well as control of the body-powered components. The major drawback of any harness is the inevitable restriction in range of motion, chafing from the straps, and the potential for pressure on the contralateral axilla, which can lead to nerve damage in the opposite arm over time.[2]

The suction socket provides excellent suspension and control but requires very stable limb volume and sufficient skill to apply the prosthesis with a "pull-in" sock. Suction suspension is often used in conjunction with externally powered components to eliminate or reduce the amount of harnessing necessary.

The roll-on liner can also be used to suspend the prosthesis and will accommodate mild to moderate volume changes in the limb. This system has proved successful with both body-powered and externally powered components.[12-14]

Elbow disarticulation prostheses typically rely on the epicondyles for suspension, provided they are well-shaped and not tender. The widest portion of the condyles must pass into the socket and then somehow be "locked" in place. Windowed or flexible wall sockets are often used to provide entry and suspension at this level (Figure 4). Some practitioners use a spiral groove or cut-out in the socket to "screw" the epicondyles into the end of the socket (Figure 5). The shape and pressure tolerance of the

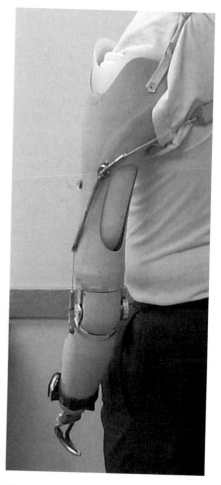

Figure 3 Posterior view of a flexible socket, rigid-frame transhumeral prosthesis with body-powered elbow.

epicondyles will determine the best design for the elbow disarticulation level.

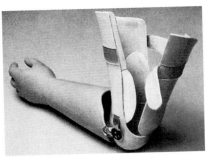

Figure 4 Elbow disarticulation prosthesis with a removable door for donning and suspension. *(Reproduced with permission from Otto Bock Prostesen-Kompendium: Prostesen für die obere Extremität. Berlin, Germany, Schide & Schoen, 1976.)*

Stages of Care
Immediate/Early Management

The cited advantages of immediate and early postsurgical prosthetic fitting for lower limb amputees include control of edema and a reduction in postamputation pain by containing the residual limb in a rigid dressing. These same factors apply to upper limb loss.[15] The practical difficulty in postoperative fitting of patients with transhumeral amputation has been maintaining suspension of the cast as residual limb volume decreases. This has limited the use of postoperative dressings for this group. There may be a psychological benefit to early fitting; some evidence exists that successful prosthetic use is higher when the fitting is completed within a "golden period" of 30 days after surgery.[15]

Once primary healing has occurred, the limb must be shaped and desensitized to prepare for the prosthetic fitting. Shrinkers or elastic bandage wraps are helpful to shape the soft tissue and reduce the size of the limb in preparation for fitting (Figure 6). Active joint range-of-motion exercise and pain control are necessary during this time. Prosthetic evaluation and counseling should begin as soon as possible, both to answer patient questions and to develop a clear plan of care. Part of the plan will be determining funding sources (eg, insurance plans) and any restrictions that they

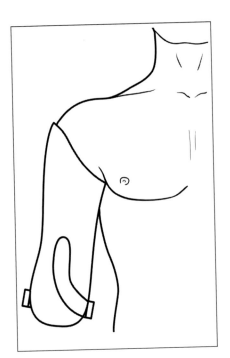

Figure 5 Elbow disarticulation socket using a spiral slot for donning and suspension by screwing the epicondyles into place. *(Adapted with permission from Bray JJ: Prosthetic Principles: Upper Extremity Amputations (Fabrication and Fitting Principles). Los Angeles, CA, Prosthetics Orthotics Education Program, University of California Press.)*

might pose. In selective cases, a preparatory prosthesis will provide function while early limb atrophy takes place. Actively managed early care is the foundation for later success, not simply a time to wait for healing.

Provision of the Prosthesis

The prosthesis should be provided in a timely manner, ideally within 30 to 60 days after surgery, to increase the likelihood of use. An evaluation prosthesis is often helpful to refine the design and desired functional performance of the prosthesis, particularly for more complex cases such as bilateral loss or high-level amputation.

Specialized training of amputees to improve skill in using a prosthesis is important if they are to receive the full benefit of prosthetic use. This training can be part of the physical and occupational therapy of the early healing phase, but special focus on the use of the prosthesis is also

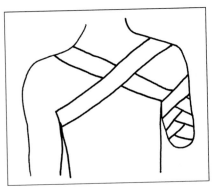

Figure 6 Back view of one method for wrapping the transhumeral residual limb in an elastic bandage.

needed later in rehabilitation. An emphasis on bimanual activity will increase the amputee's confidence and capability with the prosthesis.

After the prosthesis is delivered, there should be a follow-up plan to maintain and refine long-term function. Modification of the harness or socket is common to accommodate changes in the residual limb and to improve function by relocating cable reaction points. Ongoing follow-up ensures that continued improvement to the prosthetic design will occur as the amputee becomes more proficient and contributes to attainment of the best possible functional outcome.

Components

The selection of components will vary depending on the character of the residual limb and the individual needs of the amputee. Harness design will depend in large part on the body shape and functional capabilities of the amputee. The figure-of-8 harness provides the greatest available excursion but tends to create pressure problems on the contralateral axilla. The shoulder saddle and chest strap design reduces axilla forces and provides better lifting capability but does not harness shoulder excursion of the contralateral side.

The traditional body-powered locking elbow with harness-controlled lock is generally preferred if the patient can operate it well. Lift assists or forearm-balancing designs should be added in most cases to re-

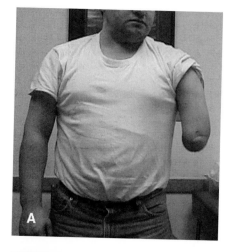
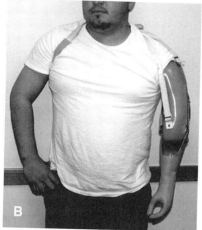
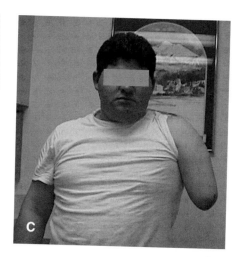

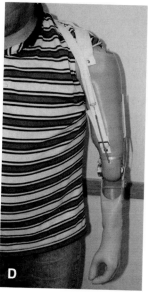
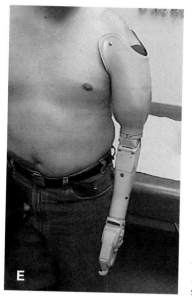

Figure 7 Patient described in case study 1. **A,** Initial amputation with excessive distal redundant tissue and length. **B,** Fitted as an elbow disarticulation because of the length of the redundant tissue. **C,** After revision to remove excess tissue and stabilize the muscles. **D,** Fitted transhumeral prosthesis and figure-of-8 harness, roll-on suspension sleeve, and body-powered elbow. **E,** Fitted with a roll-on sleeve, self-suspending, myoelectrically controlled prosthesis.

duce the force required for elbow flexion. A quick-disconnect wrist allows the patient to exchange terminal devices (TDs) more easily; otherwise, a lightweight constant-friction wrist will suffice. Many patients prefer to have both a hook and a hand TD because they have different but complementary functions. If the available excursion is not sufficient to control a fully body-powered prosthesis effectively, then external power is required. As a general rule, the shorter the residual limb, the more limited the excursion available. Endoskeletal systems for upper limb prostheses are not as durable as an exoskeletal design, but they can restore body symmetry while minimizing weight and are well suited for passive prostheses.

Biomechanics of Control

The function of a body-powered prosthesis is completely dependent on the amount of cable excursion created by the patient. A rough measure of available cable excursion can be made by placing a tape measure around the sound axilla to the midpoint of the residual limb. The difference in tape length from shoulders at neutral position to full bilateral shoulder protraction and 45° of humeral flexion will approximate the maximum potential excursion. For full body-powered control of the elbow and TD, roughly 11.5 cm of cable excursion is needed.

If force or excursion is inadequate for full body power, then external power is essential if the patient is to actively control the prosthesis. Myo-electric or servo controls are now available that can provide proportional speed and force control for both elbows and TDs. It is quite common to use a body-powered elbow with a switch- or myoelectric-controlled TD. This arrangement simplifies harnessing while providing quick elbow flexion plus force feedback through the harness. An electronic elbow and body-powered TD offer similar advantages, except that elbow motion is slower while TD speed is more rapid. A prosthesis with two or more powered components will be heavier and more costly than a hybrid system that includes at least one body-powered component. Switch and servo controls require only a light harness to activate the controls

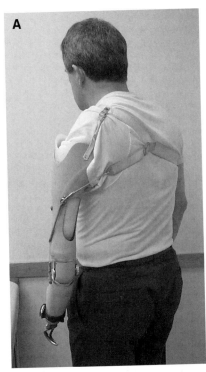
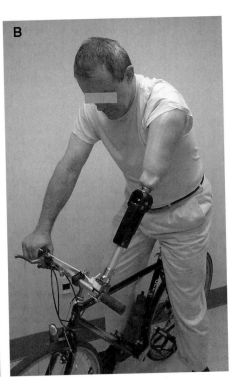

Figure 8 Patient described in case study 2. **A,** Patient wearing a flexible wall socket with chest strap suspension and body-powered elbow and hook. **B,** Patient wearing a special-purpose prosthesis with roll-on sleeve suspension, nylon transfemoral knee unit used as an elbow, and quick-disconnect wrist used for bicycling.

and can be considered if reliable myoelectric control is not available.

Case Studies
Case Study 1

A 24-year-old male laborer was injured in a conveyer belt accident on the job. He sustained a severe crush injury to his left arm that resulted in a transhumeral amputation. The limb was surgically closed but there was significant distal redundant tissue and scarring from the skin trauma (Figure 7, *A*). Glenohumeral and scapular range of motion was good and shoulder strength was very good, but the residual limb measured 2.5 cm longer than the opposite epicondyle length because of the redundant tissue. The patient was first seen for prosthetic care 8 weeks after amputation, at which time the residual limb was not yet completely healed because of the amount of skin trauma. The patient was provided with elastic shrinkers to facilitate limb shaping and support

the distal tissues, which were painful when unsupported. Because of funding delays, fitting could not begin until 10 weeks postoperatively, at which time the residual limb was well healed but the patient still had moderate pain.

The prosthesis (Figure 7, *B*) included a total-contact laminated socket with outside locking hinges (to accommodate the excessive residual limb length), a figure-of-8 harness, and a voluntary opening hand and interchangeable voluntary opening aluminum split hook. After training with a therapist, the patient could use the prosthesis, but the pain in the residual limb from neuromas and scar tissue failed to resolve. Months later, the patient elected to undergo revision surgery to reduce the excessive distal tissue, stabilize the muscles, remove the scar tissue, and resect the painful neuromas. The surgeon removed 7.5 cm of excess soft tissue from the distal end of the limb and performed a myoplasty to stabilize the muscles (Figure

7, *C*). Two months later, the patient received a new prosthesis with a body-powered locking elbow and chest strap to reduce harness pressure on the opposite axilla. This prosthesis also included a roll-on suspension liner to further reduce the harness forces (Figure 7, *D*). Eleven months after the injury, a new prosthesis was prescribed to eliminate the continued irritation from the harness and provide a more powerful grip than the body-powered device permitted. Because the myoplasty resulted in good control of the residual limb muscles, the patient received a myoelectrically controlled prosthesis with powered elbow, hand, and hook (Figure 7, *E*). He now wears a prosthesis full time, interchanging body-powered and externally powered prostheses depending on the activities being performed. The patient underwent one additional neuroma excision since this fitting, reducing his pain sufficiently that he was able to work full time while using the prosthesis.

This case study illustrates that with ongoing follow up, and revision surgery when necessary, an initially marginal situation can be improved and the functional capability of the patient greatly increased. Prosthetic follow-up care should be a continuing process to provide the best possible long-term functional outcome.

Case Study 2

A 54-year-old man who was injured in military action at age 21 years underwent a left transhumeral amputation. He had been fitted with many different prostheses over the decades but now wears a flexible socket, rigid-frame prosthesis with a chest strap harness. This configuration offers good function and frees up the contralateral shoulder for work activities (Figure 8, *A*). He also has a prosthesis for cycling. This activity-specific prosthesis includes a roll-on suction suspension sleeve, a nylon prosthetic knee unit that serves as the elbow, and a quick-disconnect wrist for safety (Figure 8, *B*). This design allows him to steer a bicycle while absorbing much of the vibration from the handlebars.

Many upper limb amputees benefit from special-purpose designs. The creative challenge for the prosthetist is to adapt components intended for other uses to create workable solutions for specific needs.

Summary

Many factors influence the successful use of prostheses by elbow disarticulation and transhumeral amputees. In view of the historically low wearing rates at this level, the rehabilitation process must be optimized for amputees. Careful surgical intervention can preserve useful length and enhance the amputee's functional capabilities. In addition, providing a well-fitted prosthesis with appropriate components, training, and ongoing follow up will improve prosthetic use and quality of function. As the patient's needs and abilities change over time, the prosthesis must likewise evolve if it is to continue to provide optimal function.

References

1. Pinzur MS, Angelats J, Light TR, Izuierdo R, Pluth T: Functional outcome following traumatic upper limb amputation and prosthetic limb fitting. *J Hand Surg Am* 1994;19:836-839.

2. Jones LE, Davidson JH: Save that arm: A study of problems in the remaining arm of unilateral upper limb amputees. *Prosthet Orthot Int* 1999;23:55-58.

3. Reddy MP: Nerve entrapment syndromes in the upper extremity contralateral to amputation. *Arch Phys Med Rehabil* 1984;65:24-26.

4. Wood MR, Hunter GA, Millstein SG: The value of revision surgery after initial amputation of an upper or lower limb. *Prosthet Orthot Int* 1987;11:17-20.

5. Ilizarov GA: The possibilities offered by our method for lengthening various segments in upper and lower limbs. *Basic Life Sci* 1988;48:323-324.

6. Andrew JT: Elbow disarticulation and transhumeral amputations: Prosthetic principles, in Bowker JH, Michael JW (eds): *Atlas of Limb Prosthetics: Surgical, Prosthetic, and Rehabilitation Principles*, ed 2. Rosemont, IL, American Academy of Orthopaedic Surgeons, 2002, pp 255-264. (Originally published by Mosby-Year Book, 1992.)

7. de Luccia N, Marino HL: Fitting of electronic elbow on an elbow disarticulated patient by means of a new surgical technique. *Prosthet Orthot Int* 2000;24:247-251.

8. Barcome DF, Eickman L: Prosthetic management of high bilateral upper-limb amputees: A case report. *Orthot Prosthet* 1980;34:3.

9. Marquardt VE: The multiple limb-deficient child, in *Atlas of Limb Prosthetics: Surgical, Prosthetic, and Rehabilitation Principles*, ed 2. Rosemont, IL, American Academy of Orthopaedic Surgeons, 2002, pp 608-612. (Originally published by Mosby-Year Book, 1992.)

10. Malone JM, Leal JM, Underwood J, Childers SJ: Brachial plexus injury management through upper limb amputation with immediate postoperative prosthesis. *Arch Phys Med Rehabil* 1982;63:89-91.

11. Fishman S, Berger N, Edelstein J: ISNY flexible sockets for upper-limb amputees. *J Assoc Child Prosthet Orthot Clin* 1989;24:8.

12. Daly W: Clinical application of roll-on sleeves for myoelectrically controlled transradial and transhumeral prostheses. *J Prosthet Orthot* 2000;12:88-91.

13. Salam Y: The use of silicone suspension sleeves with myoelectric fittings. *J Prosthet Orthot* 1994;6:119-120.

14. Ross J, Radocy B: Preliminary experiences in applying silicone suction socket (3S) prostheses to upper-extremity amputees. *J Assoc Child Prosthet Orthot Clin* 1990;25:27.

15. Malone JM, Fleming LL, Roberson J, et al: Immediate, early, and late postsurgical management of upper-limb amputation. *J Rehabil Res Dev* 1984;21:33-41.

Chapter 20

Amputations About the Shoulder: Surgical Management

Douglas G. Smith, MD

Introduction

Fortunately, amputations about the shoulder are rare, accounting for only a small percentage of all amputations.[1,2] Because surgeons may have little practical experience with the variety of shoulder-level amputations, it becomes imperative for surgeons who may have to perform these procedures to understand the complex anatomy and reconstructive goals of these difficult amputations. Shoulder-level amputations are most commonly considered for tumors, trauma, infection, and congenital abnormalities. For patients with congenital limb deficiencies in the shoulder region, the need for surgical revision is rare and usually best avoided.

Although the techniques described in this chapter are based on generally accepted principles and anatomic approaches,[3] there are many occasions when tissues required for standard amputation techniques are simply not available for reconstruction and closure of a shoulder amputation site.[4-8] This is especially true for cases involving malignant tumors, severe trauma, or necrotizing fasciitis, for which the surgeon will almost always need to individualize the surgical approach and reconstructive plan based on which tissues are involved and which are salvageable. Considerable surgical ingenuity can be required.

Amputations at the shoulder involve a variety of levels and techniques. It is best to consider amputa-

tions at the ultrashort transhumeral level to be modified shoulder disarticulations because both the surgical closure and rehabilitation goals more closely match this level. Retaining the proximal portion of the humerus preserves a more normal shoulder contour, allowing shirts and coats to drape more naturally. Depending on the reason for the amputation, a true shoulder disarticulation can occasionally be performed with reasonable reshaping of the shoulder contour using the deltoid and pectoralis major for muscle reconstruction. Occasionally, no healthy soft tissue or muscle for plastic reconstruction of this area is available.

The scapulothoracic amputation, formerly referred to as the "forequarter amputation," removes the upper limb between the scapula and thoracic wall, including the lateral clavicle. Unfortunately, this amputation is quite disfiguring because the lateral neck structures slope directly onto the rib cage. Local soft tissue for reconstruction of a more normal shoulder contour is not available because the loss of the shoulder musculature typically necessitates this level of amputation. Free-tissue transfer for later reconstruction of both the scapulothoracic amputation and shoulder disarticulation has been described and is technically possible, but almost always as a later, staged procedure. The risks, benefits, and timing of this

extensive reconstruction must be balanced carefully.[9,10]

There are also internal amputations, or en bloc resections, that retain some distal limb function, such as the claviculectomy, scapulectomy, and the intercalary shoulder resection, as described by Tikhor[11] and Linberg.[12] Typically, these procedures are performed for osteomyelitis or primary bone tumors. Preserving the neural and vascular supply to the distal limb is essential to retain near-normal function of the hand, wrist, and elbow. Regrettably, without the important positioning function of the shoulder girdle, the patient loses the ability to use the hand in its normally large sphere of activity, limiting function to a much smaller zone of activity in front of the body, as if the upper limb were bound to the chest wall. Because of the loss of stability and strength at the shoulder girdle, these procedures greatly compromise general strength of the upper limb, although grip strength can be retained.

Postoperative management for all the various shoulder-level amputations typically consists of careful reconstructive closure, suction drainage to help manage the dead space, and a soft dressing with compressive elastic wrapping around the thorax. Rigid dressings are often uncomfortable and unnecessarily cumbersome in the shoulder area and do not provide the same benefits for wound management

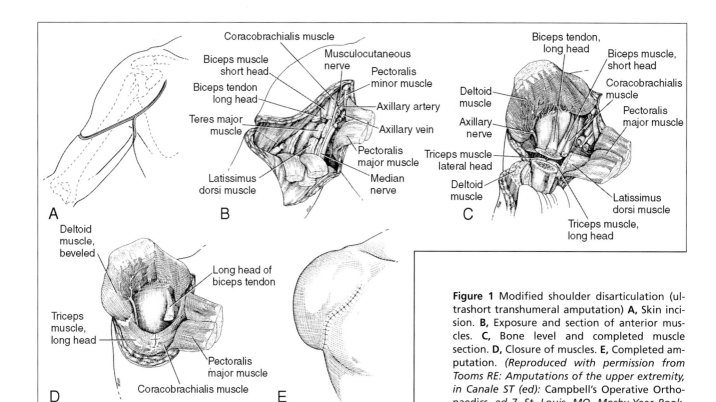

Figure 1 Modified shoulder disarticulation (ultrashort transhumeral amputation) **A,** Skin incision. **B,** Exposure and section of anterior muscles. **C,** Bone level and completed muscle section. **D,** Closure of muscles. **E,** Completed amputation. *(Reproduced with permission from Tooms RE: Amputations of the upper extremity, in Canale ST (ed):* Campbell's Operative Orthopaedics, *ed 7. St. Louis, MO, Mosby-Year Book, 1987.)*

and pain control. Nevertheless, early postoperative prosthetic techniques are available and have been described and used successfully by Burkhalter and associates[13] and Malone and associates.[14]

Amputation Levels and Techniques
Modified Shoulder Disarticulation

The ultrashort transhumeral amputation can be considered a modified shoulder disarticulation because there is no intent to create a residual limb. A small portion of the proximal humerus is retained to improve the contour of the shoulder region and assist in the fitting of shirts and other clothing. Equally important, even a small humeral remnant can allow the prosthetist to use voluntary motion to actuate an externally powered gripper via miniature touch pads or similar microswitches. When the deltoid muscle is carefully reattached, some amputees can differentiate myoelec-

tric signals from the anterior, medial, and posterior portions of the deltoid muscle. This offers three independent and proportional control signals to actuate the prosthesis. When body-powered components are used, the added bony width from the humeral remnant is an advantage because it increases the available excursion.

The typical flap coverage is based on the deltoid myofasciocutaneous flap, which is advanced distally over the axillary area (Figure 1). The incisions follow the anterior and posterior borders of the deltoid muscle, except that the flap is not tapered distally. The distal portion of the incision should remove all or most of the axillary skin that is prone to sweating and hair growth. When the deltoid flap is not available for coverage, then anterior, posterior, or axillary skin may be required for closure. The interval between the anterior deltoid and the pectoralis major muscles provides a direct approach to the humerus and the shoulder region. Following ligature of the cephalic vein, the deltoid is gently elevated from its

humeral attachment. Because the humerus is transected just above the insertion of the pectoralis major muscle, this insertion is dissected off the humeral shaft for later reattachment to the residual humeral head. The latissimus dorsi muscle is also detached from the humerus and tagged for later reattachment. The subscapularis tendon and the rest of the rotator cuff are left undisturbed and attached to the humeral head.

The brachial vessels are identified, divided, and doubly ligated with care to avoid ligation of the brachial plexus nerves with the vessels. The nerves are separated and individually transected under gentle traction, which allows retraction away from vessel ends and away from exposed areas that can be locations of pressure or scarring. With an oscillating saw, the humerus is cut through the surgical neck. The remaining proximal humerus will go into unopposed abduction because of the unopposed action of the rotator cuff. The edges of the bone should be gently rounded to remove sharp edges, especially on the lateral and anterior surfaces. The residual humerus should then be balanced with reattachment of the pectoralis major and the latissimus dorsi muscles. If muscle rebalancing is not technically possible, then excessive abduction can occur over time, and this complicates prosthetic fitting and cosmesis. Baumgartner[15] suggests that, for slightly longer humeral segments, a primary arthrodesis in a neutral position should be considered. Because the small portion of humerus does help retain a more normal shoulder contour, there is no need for osteotomy or reshaping of the acromion or coracoid process.

The deltoid myofasciocutaneous flap is advanced distally over the rebalanced humeral head, with the bulk of this muscle providing the final contour of the shoulder and axillary portion of the incision. Typically, deep suction drainage is placed under the deltoid muscle. The flap is inset with a deep fascial closure, and the subcutaneous tissue and skin are closed with gentle techniques.

True Shoulder Disarticulation

As with the modified procedure described above, the ideal coverage for a true shoulder disarticulation is based on the deltoid myofasciocutaneous flap, which is advanced distally over the axillary area (Figure 2). The incisions follow the anterior and posterior borders of the deltoid muscle, except the flap is not tapered distally. The distal portion of the incision should remove the axillary skin that is prone to sweating and hair growth. When the deltoid flap is not available for coverage, the anterior, posterior, or axillary skin may be required for closure. The interval between the anterior deltoid and the pectoralis major muscles provides a direct approach to the proximal humerus and the shoulder region. Following ligation of the cephalic vein, the deltoid muscle is gently elevated off of its humeral attachment. The pectoralis major insertion is then dissected off the

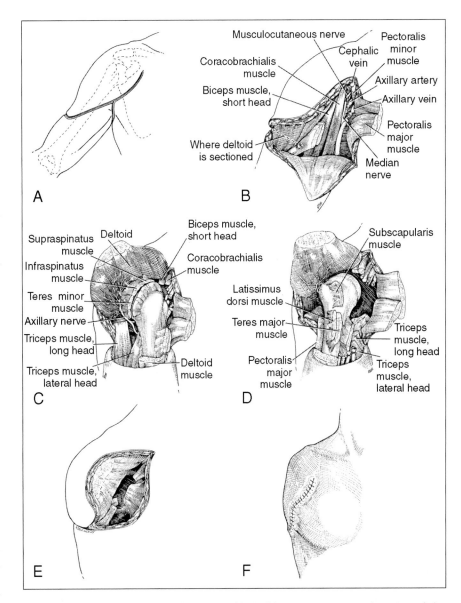

Figure 2 True shoulder disarticulation. **A,** Skin incision. **B,** Exposure and section of the neurovascular bundle. **C,** The deltoid muscle is reflected; the arm is placed in internal rotation, and the supraspinatus, infraspinatus, and teres minor tendons and the posterior capsule are sectioned; the coracobrachialis and biceps muscles are sectioned at the coracoid. **D,** The arm is placed in external rotation, and the subscapularis muscle and anterior capsule are sectioned. **E,** The muscles in the glenoid fossa are sutured. **F,** Completed amputation. *(Reproduced with permission from Tooms RE: Amputations of the upper extremity, in Canale ST (ed):* Campbell's Operative Orthopaedics, *ed 7. St. Louis, MO, Mosby-Year Book, 1987.)*

humerus for use in closure and coverage of the glenoid area. The latissimus dorsi muscle is also removed from the humerus for later reattachment into the glenoid fossa.

In the true shoulder disarticulation, following detachment of the rotator cuff, the capsule is divided first superiorly and anteriorly, then inferiorly, and finally posteriorly. The bra-

chial vessels are identified, divided, and doubly ligated. As with the modified shoulder disarticulation, care is taken to avoid entrapment of the brachial plexus nerves with the vessels.

If adequate muscle tissue remains, there is no need to do any contouring or reshaping of the glenoid fossa, the acromion, or the coracoid process. The pectoralis major and the latissi-

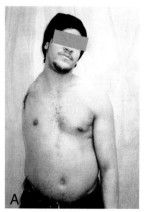 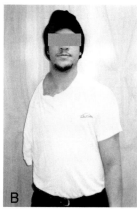 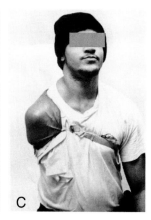

Figure 3 A, Appearance following scapulothoracic amputation. **B,** Clothing drapes in an awkward fashion. **C,** A simple shoulder cap can improve the contour of the chest and shoulder area. *(Courtesy of Prosthetics Research Study, Seattle, WA.)*

mus dorsi muscles can be sutured to remnants of capsule and to the rotator cuff tendons to fill the glenoid fossa. The attachment of the muscle to the capsule or the edge of the glenoid fossa is important to avoid a mobile muscle sling that can slide back and forth over the glenoid, creating a bursal area and a potential source of grinding and pain. The deltoid myofasciocutaneous flap is advanced distally for coverage and final contouring of the shoulder and axillary portion of the incision. Suction drainage is typically placed deep to the deltoid muscle. As noted previously, if the deltoid muscle insertion is sufficiently stabilized, the amputee may have three independent myoelectric control sites.

If the deltoid muscle is not available to pad the shoulder region, reducing the prominence of the anterior acromion and coracoid process should be considered. Most commonly, the anterior third of the acromion is removed and smoothed and the coracoid process shortened to minimize abrupt changes in bony contour under the fasciocutaneous closure.

Scapulothoracic Amputation

This radical procedure surgically removes the entire upper limb, including the scapula and most of the clavicle off of the thoracic wall. The primary indications are malignant tumors, severe proximal necrotizing fasciitis, or severe trauma.[16-18] With necrotizing fasciitis in the shoulder girdle, patients are typically near death, and the procedure becomes emergent, as the last hope to save the patient's life. The amputation is unfortunately quite disfiguring because the lateral neck structures slope directly onto the rib cage, resulting in a significant cosmetic deformity (Figure 3).

The surgery is extensive but not especially complicated when performed using standard techniques that have been developed over the last century.[19-27] There are two main approaches to the scapulothoracic amputation, depending on whether the subclavian vessels are approached and managed from the anterior or the posterior side. The anterior approach starts by preliminary exposure and osteotomy of the clavicle to visualize the vessels. The posterior approach begins with detachment of the muscles from the medial and superior scapula, allowing mobilization of the arm and scapula laterally to allow the vessels to be visualized from underneath the scapula. Several reports indicate that blood loss may be less with the posterior approach, but no direct comparative studies have been published.

Because tissue involvement with neoplasm or infection can be extensive, careful planning is required to obtain adequate skin and soft-tissue coverage.[17,18,28,29] Malignant tumors often invade regional lymph nodes as well as the chest wall, a situation that can complicate the extent of the operation.[30-32] Not infrequently, primary closure is impossible. Achieving wound closure may require a staged procedure with initial open wound management and later coverage with skin or composite grafts. Several recent articles, including those by Cordeiro and associates[9] and Zachary and associates,[10] highlight the use of free-tissue transfer in which tissue is occasionally obtained from the distal aspect of the amputated limb to obtain closure following radial tumor resections.

Anterior Approach

In most situations in which a scapulothoracic amputation is required, the deltoid muscle and overlying tissues are absent, infected, or involved with the malignancy and, therefore, are not available for reconstruction. In the standard anterior approach, a fasciocutaneous flap is created from the superior aspect of the shoulder and neck with an incision that starts near the medial clavicle and passes laterally along the anterior-inferior aspect of the clavicle as far laterally as the morbid tissue safely permits.[33] The incision then proceeds up and over the shoulder near the acromion to the spine of the scapula and then toward the posterior midline, dropping inferiorly to the spine of the scapula and then distally along the medial border of the scapula. Elevating this fasciocutaneous flap exposes the clavicle and superior scapular area. The inferior portion of the incision starts near the middle of the clavicle, then proceeds toward the coracoid process, along the deltopectoral groove to the anterior axillary fold, across the axilla to the posterior axillary fold, and finally traverses the scapula to join the superior incision near the distal angle of the scapular body (Figure 4).

The clavicle is exposed and divided near the lateral margin of the sternocleidomastoid muscle. If not involved with diseased tissue, the medial 2 to

3 cm of clavicle can be left intact. If necessary, it can be removed by careful dissection through the sternoclavicular joint. The external jugular vein is located just above the medial clavicle at the lateral border of the sternocleidomastoid muscle and should be protected and preserved if possible. The lateral portion of the clavicle can be mobilized or removed at the acromion to visualize the subclavian vessels. Exposure of the vessels is improved by releasing the pectoralis major from the humerus and the pectoralis minor from the coracoid process. More proximal exposure of the subclavian vessels is obtained by first dividing the axillary fascia, then the costocoracoid membrane that lies between the pectoralis minor and the subclavius, and finally elevating the periosteum from the deep surface of the clavicle. The subclavian artery and vein are identified and carefully ligated separately. Care must be taken to avoid ligating any of the brachial plexus nerves with the vessels. The brachial plexus is dissected from around the vessels, and each trunk is separately transected and allowed to retract.

Sectioning the latissimus dorsi muscle allows the arm to fall posteriorly away from the chest wall, improving access for the deep dissection. Later, by positioning the arm forward across the chest, the posterior incision can be carried along the scapular spine to release the insertion of the trapezius and along the medial border of the scapula to release the omohyoid, levator scapulae, rhomboideus major and minor, and the serratus anterior muscles. The final soft-tissue attachments in the axillary area are divided, and the limb is removed.

Reconstruction with the remaining muscles occurs after removal of the underlying morbid tissue. Typically, the pectoralis major muscle is sutured to the trapezius muscle, and the remaining muscles are closed in layers over the lateral chest wall. The skin flaps are brought together and tailored for accurate approximation. Suction drainage is placed, and the wound is closed with interrupted sutures. Sup-

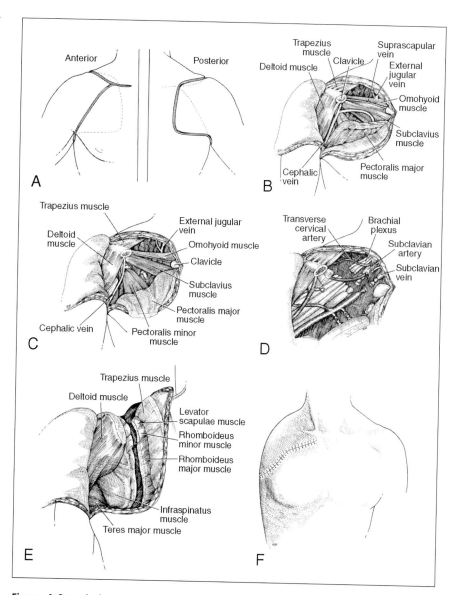

Figure 4 Scapulothoracic amputation through an anterior approach. **A,** Skin incision. **B,** Resection of the clavicle. **C,** Lifting of the pectoralis major muscle. **D,** Section of the vessels and nerves after incision through the axillary fascia and insertion of the pectoralis minor, the costocoracoid membrane, and the subclavius. **E,** Section of supporting muscles of the scapula. **F,** Completed amputation. *(Reproduced with permission from Tooms RE: Amputations of the upper extremity, in Canale ST (ed): Campbell's Operative Orthopaedics, ed 7. St. Louis, MO, Mosby-Year Book, 1987.)*

portive dressings are applied with gentle pressure, achieved by secure wrapping around the chest wall.

Posterior Approach

In 1922, Littlewood[34] described a technique for scapulothoracic amputation approaching the shoulder area initially from the posterior aspect (Figure 5). Some consider this approach to be technically easier than the anterior approach.[5,35] Although the incisions are

referred to as "posterior" and "anterior," in actuality they might be best described as "superior/posterior" and "inferior/anterior." The patient is positioned on the uninvolved side near the edge of the operating table. Two incisions are required—one posterior (cervicoscapular) and one anterior (pectoroaxillary). Later, the anterior incision passes through the axillary area to join the posterior incision and allow removal of the limb. The poste-

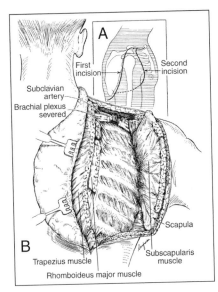

Figure 5 Scapulothoracic amputation through a posterior approach (the Littlewood technique). **A,** Skin incision. **B,** Exposure of the vessels after exposure of the muscles holding the scapula to the chest wall and section along the scapular border. *(Reproduced with permission from Tooms RE: Amputations of the upper extremity, in Canale ST (ed): Campbell's Operative Orthopaedics, ed 7. St. Louis, MO, Mosby-Year Book, 1987.)*

rior incision is made first. Beginning at the medial end of the clavicle, the incision extends laterally just superior to the clavicle along the entire length of the bone. The incision proceeds up over the acromion process to the posterior axillary fold and then continues along the axillary border of the scapula to a point inferior to the distal scapular angle. Finally, the posterior incision curves medially to end 2 inches from the midline of the back. A large full-thickness flap of skin, subcutaneous tissue, and fascia (if not diseased) is elevated medially off the scapular muscles to a point just medial to the vertebral border of the scapula.

Next, the muscles holding the scapula to the chest wall are divided along the scapular border. The trapezius, latissimus dorsi, levator scapulae, rhomboideus major and minor, serratus anterior, and omohyoid muscles are all identified and divided parallel with the scapula. The main vessels that supply this part of the shoulder re-

gion, the branches of the transverse cervical and transverse scapular arteries, are identified and ligated. The soft tissues are then freed from the clavicle, and the bone is divided at its medial end. The subclavius muscle is also divided.

The limb is then mobilized anteriorly and laterally so that the surgical approach can continue beneath the scapula. As the limb is mobilized laterally, the subclavian vessels and the brachial plexus are placed under tension, making their identification easier. The subclavian artery and vein are identified, separated, and carefully doubly ligated. Care must be taken to avoid ligating any of the brachial plexus nerves with the vessels. The brachial plexus is identified from around the vessels, and each trunk is separated, transected, and allowed to retract.

The anterior incision is then begun at the middle of the clavicle. It curves inferiorly just lateral, but parallel, to the deltopectoral groove, extends across the anterior axillary fold, and is finally carried inferiorly and posteriorly to join the posterior axillary incision at the lower third of the axillary border of the scapula. The pectoralis major and minor muscles are divided, completing removal of the limb. Muscle closure is done in layers with retained muscles as allowed by the pathology. The skin flaps are trimmed to fit and closed with interrupted sutures. Typically, suction drainage in conjunction with a firm pressure dressing to the chest wall are used to facilitate wound management.

Internal Amputations, or En Bloc Resections

Internal amputations, or en bloc resections, are performed in an attempt to retain some distal limb function. These procedures include claviculectomy, scapulectomy, and intercalary shoulder resection, as described by Tikhor[11] and Linberg.[12] Typically, these procedures are performed for primary bone tumors and commonly used adjuvant radiation or chemotherapy to improve local tumor con-

trol.[30,36] Preserving the neural and vascular supply to the distal limb is essential to retain near-normal function of the hand, wrist, and elbow. Regrettably, without the important positioning function of the shoulder girdle, the placement of the hand in its normally large sphere of activity is lost, limiting its function to a much smaller zone of activity in front of the body, as if the upper limb were bound to the chest wall. Although grip strength can be retained, overall upper limb strength is greatly compromised in these procedures because of the lack of stability and strength at the shoulder girdle.[37]

Claviculectomy

Resection of all or some of the clavicle, although rarely indicated, has occasionally been recommended to treat localized malignancy or chronic osteomyelitis.[38-42] The amount of resection is determined by the nature, extent, and location of the disease. The surgical approach is along the anterior aspect of the clavicle and typically extends the length of the bone, from the sternoclavicular joint to the acromioclavicular joint. Biopsy sites, if present, are widely excised.

The deltoid muscle insertion is elevated first to expose the distal clavicle. The conoid and trapezoid ligaments and the capsule of the acromioclavicular joint are divided. Moving toward the midline, the sternocleidomastoid muscle is carefully sectioned, protecting the external jugular vein. Medially, a portion of the pectoralis major must be incised. The subclavicular muscle is excised in cases of tumor as the clavicle is lifted from its bed, but the muscle is often retained in patients with osteomyelitis. In some cases, the medial clavicle can be retained, and in others, the medial sternoclavicular capsule, sternohyoid muscle insertion, and costoclavicular ligament are divided to allow removal of the entire clavicle.

Closure is performed in layers to minimize dead space. Suction drainage is placed, and compression dressings and a sling are applied. The shoulder and the arm are mobilized after initial wound healing has begun. Technical variations, based on the site and nature of the disease, require that each surgery be individualized. Reported series usually include only a few patients, and there are few data on the functional limitations following clavicular resection.[39-43]

Scapulectomy

Scapulectomy is used primarily for isolated neoplasms of the scapula, a condition only rarely seen. Excision of the scapula for primary bone tumors was first described in 1864, by James Syme, professor of surgery at the University of Edinburgh.[44] When scapulectomy is performed following a biopsy, wide resection of the biopsy site is required. The surgical description presented here can serve as a general guideline, but variations are often needed, as determined by the extent of the disease.[45-49]

This surgery is most often performed with the patient prone, a support placed under the affected shoulder, and the arm draped to allow access to the entire scapular region and free movement of both the humerus and scapula. The procedure can also be performed with the patient in a lateral position if necessary. Typically, the incision begins at the tip of the acromion and extends medially along the scapular spine to its midportion, then curves distally to the inferior angle of the scapular body. Muscles both deep and superficial to the scapula are resected, as dictated by the type and extent of the neoplasm.

The latissimus dorsi muscle is detached from the inferior angle, allowing the scapula to be tilted upward and outward. The vertebral border of the scapula is dissected free, and the remaining insertions of the inferior and middle trapezius muscles are detached from the scapular spine. The rhomboids are exposed beneath this interval and then divided. The dissection continues along the subscapular space. The scapula is mobilized up-

ward and outward to allow access to the subscapular space. The superior trapezius is divided from the scapular spine, the acromion, and the distal clavicle, followed by sectioning of the levator scapulae muscle. The superficial cervical and descending scapular vessels are isolated and ligated. The suprascapular vessels and nerves are exposed, and as the scapula is lifted further laterally from the thorax, the brachial plexus and axillary vessels come into view.

The supraspinatus, infraspinatus, and serratus anterior muscles are removed along with the scapula. The nature and extent of the pathologic process will dictate whether it is possible to preserve the acromion and the continuity of the superior trapezius-deltoid suspensory system. The deltoid muscle is freed from the spine of the scapula and the acromion. The teres major and the long head of the triceps muscles are transected. The subscapular artery is visualized and ligated as it comes off the axillary artery. The underlying axillary and radial nerves are preserved.

Disarticulation of the acromioclavicular joint and detachment of the coracoclavicular ligaments allow further mobilization of the scapula. Finally, the pectoralis minor, coracobrachialis, and the short head of the biceps muscles are detached from the coracoid process, and the rotator cuff is transected during external and internal rotation of the humerus, completely freeing the scapula. A portion of the residual rotator cuff insertion can be used to stabilize the clavicle, suspend the humerus, and preserve a more normal shoulder contour. The wound is closed in layers over a suction drain. Compression dressings are applied, and the arm is supported in a Velpeau's bandage.

Internal or Intercalary Shoulder Resection (Tikhoff-Linberg Procedure)

The technique of removing most of the muscles and bones of the shoulder region, while preserving the necessary neurologic and vascular struc-

tures for limited elbow, wrist, and hand function, was first advanced by Tikhor[11] and Linberg.[12] The surgical goal is to suspend the remaining humerus to the remaining clavicle or chest wall to minimize excessive drooping.[50-54] Many individuals use an orthotic device to strap or stabilize the upper arm to the chest wall to take advantage of the retained elbow, wrist, and hand function. Although the sphere of hand function is limited to activities near the midline of the body, many patients appreciate having a sensate, functioning hand to assist in performing the activities of daily living. In a review of 19 patients with an average follow-up of more than 6 years, Voggenreiter and associates[55] concluded that despite a 74% complication rate, the Tikhoff-Linberg procedure had a functional outcome superior to scapulothoracic amputation.

For this procedure, patients are positioned in a full lateral position, lying on the uninvolved side. The arm, shoulder, and shoulder girdle are draped free for manipulation and positioning during surgery. The incision resembles a tennis racquet with the "handle" starting along the clavicle and extending laterally out toward the arm. The racquet-shaped portion of the incision extends distally along the deltopectoral groove to the midpoint of the medial edge of the biceps, curves laterally across the deltoid insertion, and then proceeds posteriorly onto the back toward the inferior angle of the scapula. Finally, the incision curves upward to join the original clavicular incision near the acromioclavicular joint.

Deeper dissection is performed from both the anterior and posterior aspects and, in a sense, combines the classic anterior technique of scapulothoracic amputation with the posterior approach. The brachial plexus and major vessels are preserved. After the scapulothoracic muscles are detached and the deltoid, biceps, and triceps muscles are sectioned, the humerus is transected at or below the surgical neck, as determined by the extent of disease. The proximal humerus, scapula, and most of the clavicle are resected en bloc. The biceps, triceps, and deltoid muscles are attached to the thoracic wall, while the trapezius suspends the arm as firmly as possible without compromising neurovascular integrity. The tissues are closed to minimize dead space, and suction drainage is placed. Soft compression dressings and a Velpeau's bandage are used postoperatively.

The arm requires support with a sling or an orthosis for at least several months during the healing process, and many patients require long-term stabilization of the upper arm to the chest wall to maximize distal function by overcoming the absent shoulder stability. Rehabilitation training concentrates on strengthening the muscles of the neck and trunk and of the arm distal to the site of amputation of the humerus. With this approach, no attempt is made to restore a semblance of shoulder function, but an adequate degree of hand, wrist, forearm, and elbow function can be achieved. The defect in the shoulder girdle and shoulder contour can be concealed with a light shoulder padding to provide a more normal contour of the shoulder area under clothing.

Amputation for Severe Brachial Plexus Injury

Modern management of severe brachial plexus injuries is directed much more aggressively at repairing and grafting the damaged nerve segments than in the past. The tremendous number of different injury patterns, the unpredictable nature of recovery, and the complex emotional issues mandate that management decisions be individualized. Although amputation of all or part of the dysfunctional limb can be considered when reconstructive efforts have failed, I believe it is not appropriate to encourage amputation at an early stage. Patients need time to adapt to the injury, allow for recovery, and learn about reconstructive options. Even if a complete

brachial plexus injury leaves patients with no motor or sensory function, they need to be advised about the advantages and disadvantages of retaining a nonfunctional arm. Patients need time to come to terms with the hope versus the practical reality of neurologic recovery. Education, support, and visitor programs with other brachial plexus injury patients tend to be most helpful. This process simply cannot be rushed.

Amputation is considered most often to unload the nonfunctional weight of the paralyzed upper limb from the shoulder and scapulothoracic joints and to remove a part that hinders function because it simply gets in the way. Discussing the specific goals for function, cosmesis, and prosthetic use before the surgery can be very helpful for both the patient and the surgeon. The most common amputation plan is for either a transhumeral amputation or a shoulder disarticulation to manage a totally dysfunctional arm after a complete brachial plexus avulsion. Some patients use part of the flail arm to stabilize objects, especially when working at a desk. In these cases, a midlength transhumeral amputation retains enough of the arm to serve that role, but it removes enough to improve the problem of "dead" weight and some of the cumbersomeness of a flail arm. This level of amputation also retains enough upper arm to accommodate attempts at prosthetic fitting. Other patients find that the remaining flail upper arm remains a significant hindrance and prefer a shoulder disarticulation.

If a transhumeral amputation is planned, a concomitant or secondary shoulder arthrodesis can be considered, but the decision remains controversial and should be individualized. One clinical series reported a slightly better rate of return to work in a group of patients with transhumeral amputation without shoulder arthrodesis.[56] In my opinion, if there is no glenohumeral joint motor control, but there is active scapulothoracic motion, shoulder arthrodesis can be

beneficial as an adjunct to the transhumeral amputation. This is particularly true if prosthetic fitting is to be attempted because the patient can generate significant range of motion as well as stabilize the prosthesis using the scapular muscles (Figure 6). If both joints are flail, arthrodesis is probably not beneficial, and prosthetic fitting will be more difficult and require a more extensive socket to stabilize the prosthesis by encompassing more of the chest and back. Conversely, if both joints have motor control, arthrodesis is not needed.

Prosthetic expectations in these patients should be very conservative. Prosthetic fitting adds weight to a dysfunctional shoulder girdle, often defeating one of the original goals of the amputation by stressing the neck and shoulder region. More recent designs that stabilize the prosthesis on the torso are often preferable to earlier approaches that primarily load the humeral remnant. Although most patients who decide to proceed with amputation hope that the prosthesis will restore their function, most ultimately choose to not wear an active prosthesis or use it in a limited way for very specific tasks. Surgeons consulted for assistance in the decision-making process need to understand the underlying dream and also the eventual realities. Occasionally, a very lightweight, cosmetic prosthesis is desired and indicated to help restore body image. Some patients who initially use an active prosthesis ultimately conclude that a biomechanically simpler passive artificial arm is sufficient for their needs.

Postural Abnormalities Following Shoulder-Level Amputation

The normal symmetry and balance around the shoulders and upper body is altered following high-level upper limb amputation or brachial plexus

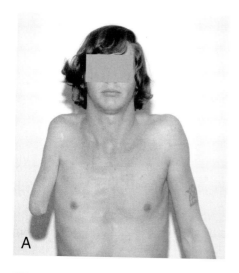

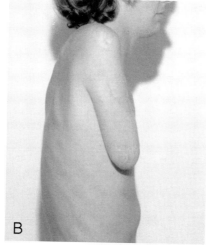

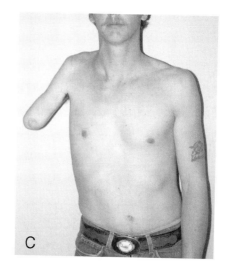

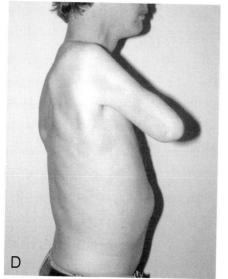

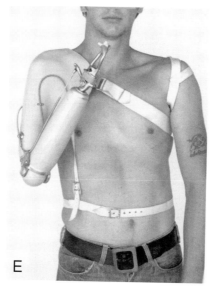

Figure 6 A patient with a brachial plexus injury required amputation after a severe burn injury to the asensate hand. Attempted abduction **(A)** and forward flexion **(B)** before glenohumeral arthrodesis results in scapulothoracic motion only because of a flail glenohumeral joint. After glenohumeral arthrodesis, the patient can successfully abduct **(C)** and forward flex **(D)** to approximately 30°. **E,** Prosthetic fitting with traditional body-powered device was successful with an extended socket to better manage the weight of the prosthesis. (Courtesy of John Bowker, MD, Miami, FL.)

injury. The normal posture and shoulder position is maintained through a balance of the muscular forces and the weight of the arm. After upper limb amputation, the muscles that elevate the shoulder girdle are no longer balanced by the weight of the arm and the muscles depressing the shoulder. The result is an upward elevation described as a hiking of the shoulder. This "high shoulder" tends to accentuate the cosmetic loss and is very noticeable and disconcerting to many patients. Unfortunately, although wearing a full prosthetic limb can be helpful by adding weight to the shoulder, it does not completely eliminate the high shoulder. Corrective exercises begun very soon after the amputation can be helpful in minimizing this postural tendency. In most circumstances, the shoulder girdle elevation is inevitable, but it can be minimized by appropriate physical therapy.

For some individuals with shoulder-level amputation, the spine can assume a postural scoliosis during standing (Figure 7). Muscle imbalance is again considered to be the primary cause, coupled with the change in dependent weight. Although it can be seen in adults, it is more often seen in younger, skeletally immature amputees. The combined postural deformities of high thoracic scoliosis and elevation of the shoulder girdle produce asymmetry of the head and neck, with the head appearing to be placed asymmetrically as the person stands.

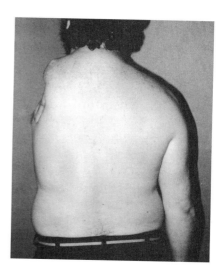

Figure 7 Posterior view of a man with postural scoliosis and elevation of the shoulder area following left shoulder disarticulation.

In general, no corrective splinting or orthotic device successfully counteracts these postural changes associated with shoulder-level amputation. Neck and shoulder girdle exercises offer the most effective prophylaxis and treatment.

References

1. Anderson-Ranberg F, Ebskov B: Major upper extremity amputation in Denmark. *Acta Orthop Scand* 1988;59:321-322.

2. Chappell PH: Arm amputation statistics for England 1958-88: An exploratory statistical analysis. *Int J Rehabil Res* 1992;15:57-62.

3. Harty M, Joyce JJ: Surgical approaches to the shoulder. *Orthop Clin North Am* 1975;6:553-564.

4. Bauman PK: Resection of the upper extremity in the region of the shoulder joint. *Khirurg Arkh Velyaminova* 1914;30:145-149.

5. Burgess EM: Sites of amputation election according to modern practice. *Clin Orthop* 1964;37:17-22.

6. Burton DS, Nagel DA: Surgical treatment of malignant soft-tissue tumors of the extremities in the adult. *Clin Orthop* 1972;84:144-148.

7. Grimes OF, Bell HG: Shoulder girdle amputation. *Surg Gynecol Obstet* 1950;91:201.

8. Jall CB, Bechtol CO: Modern amputation technique in the upper extremity. *J Bone Joint Surg Am* 1963;45:1717-1722.

9. Cordeiro PG, Cohen S, Burt M, Brennan MF: The total volar forearm musculocutaneous free flap for reconstruction of extended forequarter amputations. *Ann Plast Surg* 1998;40:388-396.

10. Zachary LS, Gottlieb LJ, Simon M, et al: Forequarter amputation wound coverage with an ipsilateral, lymphedematous, circumferential forearm fasciocutaneous free flap in patients undergoing palliative shoulder-girdle tumor resection. *J Reconstr Microsurg* 1993;9:103-107.

11. Tikhor PT: *Tumor Studies.* Russia, 1900.

12. Linberg BE: Interscapulothoracic resection for malignant tumors of the shoulder joint region. *J Bone Joint Surg* 1928;10:344-349.

13. Burkhalter WE, Mayfield G, Carmona LS: The upper-extremity amputee. Early and immediate post-surgical prosthetic fitting. *J Bone Joint Surg Am* 1976;58:46-51.

14. Malone JM, Fleming LL, Roberson J, et al: Immediate, early, and late postsurgical management of upper-limb amputation. *J Rehabil Res Dev* 1984;21:33-41.

15. Baumgartner R: Upper extremity amputations, in *Surgical techniques in Orthopaedics and Traumatology.* Paris, France, Elsevier, 2001, p 14.

16. Fanous N, Didolkar MS, Holyoke ED, Elias EG: Evaluation of forequarter amputation in malignant diseases. *Surg Gynecol Obstet* 1976;142:381-384.

17. Pack GT: Major exarticulations for malignant neoplasms of the extremities: Interscapulothoracic amputation, hip joint disarticulations and interilio-abdominal amputation: A report of end results in 228 cases. *J Bone Joint Surg Am* 1956;38:249-262.

18. Roth JA, Sugarbaker PH, Baker AR: Radical forequarter amputation with chest wall resection. *Ann Thorac Surg* 1984;37:432-437.

19. Bogacki W, Spyt T: Interscapular-thoracic amputation of the arm. *Nowotwory* 1980;30:261-264.

20. Haggart GE: The technique of interscapulothoracic amputation. *Lahey Clin Bull* 1940;2:16.

21. Ham SJ, Hoekstra HJ, Schraffordt KH, et al: The interscapulothoracic amputation in the treatment of malignant diseases of the upper extremity with a review of the literature. *Eur J Surg Oncol* 1993;19:543-548.

22. Hardin CA: Interscapulothoracic amputations for sarcomas of the upper extremity. *Surgery* 1961;49:355-358.

23. Levinthal DH, Grossman A: Interscapulothoracic amputations for malignant tumors of the shoulder region. *Surg Gynecol Obstet* 1939;69:234.

24. Moseley HF: *The Forequarter Amputation.* Edinburgh, Scotland, E and S Livingstone, 1957, p 49.

25. Nadler SH, Phelan JT: A technique of interscapulo-thoracic amputation. *Surg Gynecol Obstet* 1966;122:359-364.

26. Sperling P, Rloding H: Interthoraco-scapular amputation (forequarter amputation). *Zentralbl Chir* 1981;106:340-343.

27. Zancolli E, Mitre HJ, Bick M, et al: Interscapulo-cleidothoracic disarticulation: Indications and technique. *Prensa Med Argent* 1965;52:1122-1126.

28. Mansour KA, Powell RW: Modified technique for radical transmediastinal forequarter amputation and chest wall resection. *J Thorac Cardiovasc Surg* 1978;76:358-363.

29. Trishkin VA, Saakian AM, Stoliarov VI, Kochnev VA: Interscapulothoracic amputation in treating malignant tumors of the upper extremity and shoulder girdle. *Vestn Khir Im I Grek* 1980;124:75-78.

30. Marcove RC: Neoplasms of the shoulder girdle. *Orthop Clin North Am* 1975;6:541-552.

31. Pack GT, Ehrlich HE, Gentil F: Radical amputations of the extremities in the treatment of cancer. *Surg Gynecol Obstet* 1947;84:1105-1116.

32. Pack GT, McNeer G, Coley BL: Interscapulo-thoracic amputations for malignant tumors of the upper extremity: A report of thirty-one consecutive cases. *Surg Gynecol Obstet* 1942;74:161.

33. Tooms RE: Amputation surgery in the upper extremity. *Orthop Clin North Am* 1972;3:383-395.

34. Littlewood H: Amputations at the shoulder and at the hip. *BMJ* 1922;1:381.

35. Knaggs RL: Mr. Littlewood's method of performing the interscapulo-thoracic amputation (Letter to the editor). *Lancet* 1910;1:1298.

36. Salzer M, Knahr K: Resection of malignant bone tumors. *Recent Results Cancer Res* 1976;54:239-256.

37. Kneisl JS: Function after amputation, arthrodesis, or arthroplasty for tumors about the shoulder. *J South Orthop Assoc* 1995;4:228-236.

38. Abbott LC, Lucas DB: The function of the clavicle: Its surgical significance. *Ann Surg* 1954;140:583-599.

39. Copland SM: Total resection of the clavicle. *Am J Surg* 1946;72:280.

40. Kochhar CL, Strivastava LK: Anatomical and functional considerations in total claviculectomy. *Clin Orthop* 1976;118:199.

41. Lewis MM, Ballet FL, Kroll PG, Bloom N: En bloc clavicular resection, operative procedure and postoperative test-

ing of function. *Clin Orthop* 1985;193:214.

42. Spar I: Total claviculectomy for pathological fractures. *Clin Orthop* 1977;129:236-237.

43. McLaughlin J: Solitary myeloma of the clavicle with long survival after total excision: Report of a case. *J Bone Joint Surg Br* 1973;55:357-358.

44. Syme J: *Excision of the Scapula.* Edinburgh, Scotland, Edmonton and Douglas, 1864.

45. DeNancrede CBG: End-results of total excision of the scapula for sarcoma. *Ann Surg* 1909;50:1-22.

46. DePalma AF: Scapulectomy and a method of preserving normal configuration of the shoulder. *Clin Orthop* 1954;4:217-224.

47. Nakamura S, Kusuzaki K, Murata H, et al: Clinical outcome of total scapulectomy in 10 patients with primary malignant bone and soft-tissue tumors. *J Surg Oncol* 1999;72:130-135.

48. Rodriguez JA, Craven JE, Heinrich S, Wilson S, Levine EA: Current role of scapulectomy. *Am Surg* 1999;65:1167-1170.

49. Turnbull A, Blumencranz P, Fortner J: Scapulectomy for soft tissue sarcoma. *Can J Surg* 1981;24:37-38.

50. Pack GT, Baldwin JC: The Tikhor-Linberg resection of shoulder girdle. *Surgery* 1955;38:753-757.

51. Pack GT, Crampton RS: The Tikhor-Linberg resection of the shoulder girdle: Indications for its substitution for interscapulothoracic amputation: Recent data on end-results of the forequarter amputation. *Clin Orthop* 1961;19:148.

52. Guerra A, Capanna R, Biagini R, et al: Extra-articular resection of the shoulder (Tikhoff-Linberg). *Ital J Orthop Traumatol* 1985;11:151-157.

53. Janecki CJ, Nelson CL: En bloc resection of the shoulder girdle: Technique and indications. *J Bone Joint Surg Am* 1972;54:1754-1758.

54. Ye Q, Zhao H, Shen J: Modified en bloc resection procedure for malignant tumor of the shoulder girdle. *Acta Academiae Medicinae Sinicae* 1994;16:378-382.

55. Voggenreiter G, Assenmacher S, Schmit-Neurburg KP: Tikhoff-Linberg procedure for bone and soft tissue tumors of the shoulder girdle. *Arch Surg* 1999;134:252-257.

56. Rorabeck CH: The management of the flail upper extremity in brachial plexus injuries. *J Trauma* 1980;20:491-493.

Chapter 21

Amputations About the Shoulder: Prosthetic Management

John M. Miguelez, CP
Michelle D. Miguelez, JD
Randall D. Alley, CP

Introduction

The prosthetic rehabilitation of an individual with a humeral neck, glenohumeral, or interscapulothoracic level of absence has traditionally been a significant challenge to the rehabilitation team, often resulting in poor success rates. Each of these levels is anatomically unique, but the overall approach to the prosthetic management is similar (Figure 1). This chapter describes the three phases of prosthetic management that are critical to long-term prosthesis use and patient satisfaction: (1) the preprosthetic phase, during which the prosthetic rehabilitation plan is formulated; (2) the interim phase, during which the diagnostic prosthesis, which evolves into the definitive prosthesis, is created; and (3) the postprosthetic phase, during which the focus is on prosthetic refinement and training. The systematic method of care described in this chapter can maximize the patient's prosthetic rehabilitation potential.

Preprosthetic Phase

The preprosthetic phase includes the physical assessment of the patient, a thorough consideration of prosthetic design criteria, a discussion of prosthetic options and components, and, finally, the formulation of the prosthetic rehabilitation plan. The physical assessment of the individual with upper limb absence is one of the most crucial aspects of the rehabilitation process, because this is when information is gathered, both clinically and through open dialogue, that serves as the basis for subsequent rehabilitation. Failure to devote sufficient time and focus to the preprosthetic phase has directly contributed to the historically suboptimal prosthetic success rates for individuals with limb absence or amputation at the glenohumeral and associated levels.

Assessment

Initially, the practitioner should record not only the level(s) and side(s) of involvement but also whether or not a loss of dominance occurred. An overall health assessment should be made, and particular attention should be paid to cardiac and associated circulatory health because such proximal levels of limb loss require the user to expend considerable effort during operation of a body-powered or hybrid prosthesis. Ipsilateral considerations include the cause of absence, the date and extent of injury if applicable, tissue condition, range of motion and strength (for gross movement as well as the myoelectric signal), and any associated discomfort or sensitivity related to the region, whether from contact pressure, potential weight bearing, or motions required for operation of the prosthesis. All of these elements are vitally important when considering not only the socket design but also the control strategy. The extent of contralateral limb loss, deficiency or other involvement, and the degree of function present should be noted. All the considerations that apply to the ipsilateral remnant are relevant to the contralateral limb, as harnessing design and control strategies must incorporate contralateral involvement. Lower limb deficiencies also play a significant role in balance, donning and doffing, and general upper limb component selection. For example, the prosthesis for an individual with an upper limb deficiency who uses a cane or a walker should have sufficient prehensile grip to withstand the forces applied to these balance aids.

Myotesting is important to determine the feasibility of using myoelectric control. The information myotesting provides is also important as a feedback tool for teaching and training and is a quantifiable assessment of patient progress. The interaction of the myoelectric signals during agonistic and antagonistic contractions in each relevant muscle or muscle group must be assessed, not simply the amplitude of a single channel in isolation. (*Agonist* and *antagonist* are loosely defined here as they relate to prosthetic function, which may or may not differ from physiologic function, depending on the muscle or muscle groups involved.) Finally, the practitioner must define the optimal

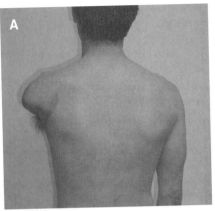
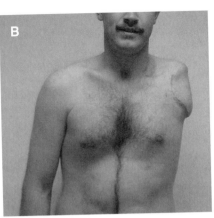
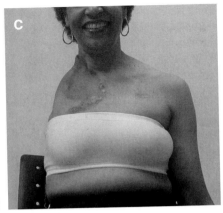

Figure 1 Typical clinical presentation of residual limb at the humeral neck **(A)**, shoulder disarticulation **(B)**, and interscapulothoracic levels **(C)**.

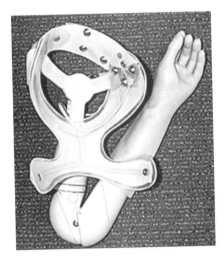

Figure 2 Infraclavicular socket showing electrode placement.

placement of electrodes within socket confines, taking into consideration comfort from electrode contact pressure and the consistency of contact under varying conditions (Figure 2). This is discussed more fully later in this chapter.

The prosthetist should discuss the limitations of terminal devices and other components to help the patient develop a realistic set of expectations. The tendency to become "one-handed" and overuse the unimpaired limb should be discussed during the assessment. Important prosthetic design considerations include whether donning and doffing will be assisted or unassisted and whether any movements are to be avoided during this process. The availability of assistance

from family, friends, or others should be considered. Any prior prosthetic experiences, such as the option used, the socket design, and the patient's perception of its effectiveness, comfort, and ease of use should be discussed and noted.

The patient's level of cognitive ability may also limit the options appropriate for successful prosthetic use. Therefore, another goal of the evaluation is to understand the various control schemes and their cognitive demands on the user.

The vocational and avocational pursuits and personal desires of the individual must be discussed thoroughly during the patient assessment. Individuals with similar levels of limb absence may require completely different strategies to attain a successful result. In addition to the obvious physical issues of choosing suitable components, psychological and psychosocial elements must be considered carefully when designing the appropriate prosthesis.[1] The loss or absence of a limb at any level, whether from an acquired amputation or congenital deficiency, dramatically affects an individual's body image and self-esteem, and this psychological impact should be a primary focus of the evaluator.

Therapeutic intervention during the preprosthetic, interim, and postprosthetic phases is critical to the prosthetic rehabilitation of the individual with absence at the gleno-

humeral or associated level. The presence of an occupational therapist during the assessment is very helpful in the psychological, physical, and psychosocial preparation of the individual. Preprosthetic therapy should include strength training of the ipsilateral side, the contralateral upper limb, and the lower limbs; maintenance and enhancement of range of motion; desensitization techniques; edema control; and, if necessary, wound care.

Unfortunately, patient information on the various aspects of upper limb prosthetics is limited. Therefore, the practitioner should spend considerable time educating the patient about the basics of casting, fabrication, delivery, postprosthetic procedures, available technology, and potential functional gains and other attributes for each option.

Components

Regardless of the prosthetic option or control strategy selected, prostheses for these levels require components at the shoulder, elbow, and wrist as well as a terminal device. The three basic shoulder joint options are nonarticulated, friction, and locking. In some situations, such as for children or for the patient requiring an activity-specific prosthesis, a nonarticulated shoulder is preferred because this minimizes the added weight, bulk, and complexity of this portion of the artificial limb. A friction shoulder joint (Figure 3) allows the patient to position the arm in space, which is helpful for eating, self care, and other tasks. The friction shoulder joint is the simplest articulated joint, but it has the disadvantage that the contralateral limb must be used to assist with positioning. A locking shoulder joint allows the patient to position and then lock the humeral section in space, permitting bimanual activities. The locking mechanism can be activated by using a nudge control with the chin. Biscapular abduction, shoulder elevation, and humeral remnant motion including flexion, extension, and abduction can be captured through a harness system to activate a pull switch. The nudge lever and the pull switch are offered in either mechanical or electric locking versions. The latter requires significantly less excursion and force but is heavier and more complex.

Far more excursion and force are required to activate a body-powered elbow than an electric-powered one. At these high levels, the skeletal lever arm is sufficiently compromised that many patients find it difficult, if not impossible, to produce sufficient excursion to fully flex and lock a body-powered elbow. Without the use of a multiposition elbow, the amputee cannot effectively position the terminal device in space to accomplish activities of daily living. In the past, an excursion amplifier was sometimes used to compensate for the reduced excursion available at these levels. The improved excursion required the user to generate increased force, however, which many found objectionable. In recent decades, electric-powered elbows have been more widely used for such high-level fittings because they require far less effort to operate than does a body-powered component, with or without an excursion amplifier.

The four basic wrist units are friction, locking, flexion, and quick-disconnect. A wrist unit allows the user to position the terminal device using the contralateral hand or compensatory gross body movements, expanding the user's functional enve-lope. The selection of a wrist unit is based on the functional requirements of the patient, not the level of amputation or deficiency.

Hooks generally have been considered more functional than body-powered hands. The prehension pattern was considered superior for activities of daily living that involve precision. In addition, patients and rehabilitation professionals preferred hooks because of their more rugged design and usefulness for heavy-duty activities. The preference for hooks is especially pronounced with body-powered prostheses because body-powered hands provide less grip force and require significantly greater excursion and force to operate. Therefore, patients with these high levels of absence often find body-powered hands difficult to operate because of the inherently short lever arm of the residuum at these levels. Because electric-powered hands offer increased grip force yet require less gross body motion to operate, they have been used more widely during the past several decades for individuals with amputations and deficiencies at these levels.

Prosthetic Options

It is imperative to discuss the prosthetic options available to facilitate the patient's participation in the rehabilitation process. Primary prosthetic options include independence without a prosthesis, use of a passive prosthesis, or use of an active prosthesis. Active prostheses can be further classified by the control method provided: body-powered, externally powered, or a hybrid system combining both body- and externally powered components. Some patients prefer an activity-specific prosthesis optimized for one task. These devices may incorporate active or passive terminal devices.

Independence Without a Prosthesis

The choice not to wear a prosthesis is an important option. Individuals who

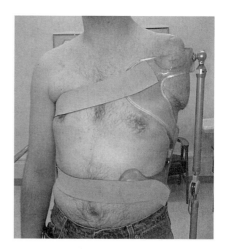

Figure 3 Infraclavicular socket with passive ball-and-socket friction shoulder joint.

have experienced complete loss of the arm or who were born with such high-level absence may find the discomfort of high-level prostheses too great an obstacle to overcome. The loss of tactile sensation caused by wearing a socket can be another reason for rejection of a prosthesis. Many high-level amputees find that an active prosthesis offers only limited functional advantages.

Passive Prostheses

Many types of passive prostheses are designed for individuals with high levels of limb absence (Figure 4), including shoulder caps, which are often used as cosmetic restorations at the shoulder disarticulation and interscapulothoracic (ISO term: forequarter) levels. The most common reasons an individual with a high-level loss opts for a passive prosthesis over an active one are reduced weight, improved cosmesis, and reduced energy and cognitive requirements. Initial, maintenance, and repair costs are typically lower than for other types of prostheses, although a high-definition silicone restoration may be more expensive than a simple mechanical prosthesis. The passive prosthesis offers little or no pinch force. Some passive prostheses have embedded wires in the hand component that allow prepositioning of the prosthetic digits by shaping the fingers manually.

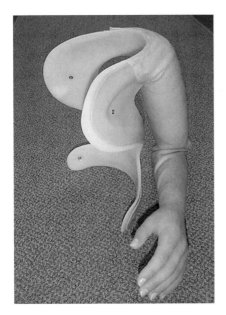

Figure 4 Example of a passive prosthesis; harness for suspension is not pictured.

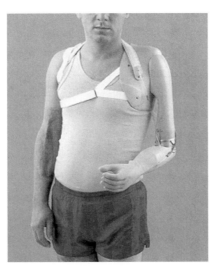

Figure 5 Example of a body-powered prosthesis with cable-operated elbow and hand. The shoulder and wrist are passive friction joints.

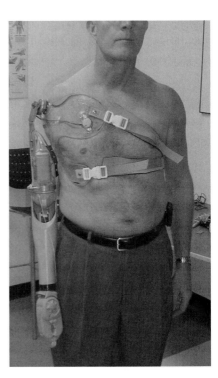

Figure 6 Example of a hybrid prosthesis with locking shoulder joint, body-powered elbow, and externally powered wrist and terminal device.

(Active) Body-Powered Prostheses

Operating body-powered prostheses at the humeral neck, glenohumeral, and interscapulothoracic levels presents a daunting challenge: generating enough force and excursion to activate the body-powered elbow, wrist, and hand components (Figure 5). Because of the absence of the skeletal lever arm and limited available excursion, the functional envelope is significantly reduced. Maximum elbow flexion is often difficult to achieve, as is any amount of abduction, because of the absence or limited length of the humerus.

The harness that is used at this level must provide maximum efficiency and hence is often fairly restrictive. Users may find it uncomfortable, especially in the contralateral axilla, which is often used as an anchor point. Compression of the nerve bundle in this region can result in nerve entrapment syndrome, in which anesthesia can occur if a sensory nerve is affected, and paralysis if a motor nerve is involved.[2]

Significant energy expenditure is also required to operate a body-powered prosthesis at these proximal levels of limb absence. This can be a contraindication for individuals whose capacity has been diminished as a result of disease or medications, for those who have contralateral involvement, or for the elderly, who may simply not possess enough strength for adequate function.[3] In addition, cosmetic appearance is limited, at best, and the gross body movements required for actuation call attention to the artificial limb.

One of the most significant advantages of a cable and harness system is the inherent feedback. The commonly used hook terminal device allows for greater visibility when acquiring, manipulating, or grasping objects. Body-powered prostheses are more durable than are electric-powered prostheses. Body-powered prostheses weigh less, and this weight is distributed more optimally than it is in most hybrid and electric-powered designs. Body-powered elbows can be flexed more rapidly than electronic elbows, although at extremely high levels the lack of sufficient excursion may negate this potential advantage.

Harness and cable systems do not require battery charging, installation, or removal, or the dexterity and the cognitive ability required to perform these operations. Finally, the initial, maintenance, repair, and replacement costs for body-powered prostheses are almost invariably less than for their electric-powered counterparts.

(Active) Hybrid Prostheses

A hybrid prosthesis has both body-powered and electronic components. The most common configuration incorporates a body-powered elbow and electric-powered terminal device (Figure 6). Hybrid prostheses offer the advantages of both body-powered and electric-powered prostheses while minimizing their disadvantages. Hybrid prostheses are a viable option even for patients with amputations at the humeral neck and higher when adequate strength and excursion remain.

Combining the two types of control has several potential advantages. The use of an electronic terminal device reduces the harnessing needed because body-powered motion is required only to flex the elbow. The functional envelope is enlarged in many instances, particularly when myoelectric control is feasible. Pinch force is also much greater with an electronic device than is possible with body-powered, voluntary-opening terminal devices. Also, an electronic terminal device usually provides both voluntary opening and voluntary closing, a more natural reproduction of human hand movement. Operating the terminal device via myoelectric control is believed to improve muscle tone and reduce disuse atrophy. Advantages of the body-powered elbow are that it provides more rapid flexion/extension movements, gives the user important sensory feedback from the harness forces, and reduces the overall weight of the prosthesis. Also, the initial, maintenance, and repair costs of the system are less because an electronic elbow is not needed. Finally, a hybrid control system can encourage simultaneous operation of the elbow and terminal device.

(Active) Externally Powered Prostheses

Electric-powered components minimize the energy expenditure and discomfort associated with a control cable and harness (Figure 7). Both static and dynamic cosmesis are improved when a control cable is not required for either terminal device or elbow operation. Like hybrid systems, a myoelectric system offers increased pinch force, voluntary opening and closing, and, although a prosthetic shoulder joint permits only passive positioning, the potential for an even greater functional envelope.

A myoelectric elbow has the disadvantage of lacking the direct feedback offered by a harness and cable system, although indirect feedback is still available based on input effort, duration of supplied signal, elbow vibration, and sound. The weight of a fully electronic system is considerable, and care must be taken to ensure that the socket provides at least partial suspension to minimize the weight borne by sensitive areas. In addition, every externally powered prosthesis has battery installation, removal, and

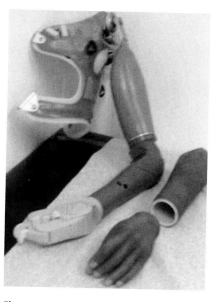

Figure 7 Example of an externally powered prosthesis with locking shoulder joint plus myoelectric elbow, wrist, hand, and interchangeable electronic lock terminal device.

maintenance requirements, and operation of the primary and secondary electronic controls can impose a substantial cognitive demand on the user. Despite these disadvantages, many individuals with glenohumeral-level absences do well with completely electronic prostheses.

Activity-Specific Prostheses

Activity-specific devices include recreational prostheses and those designed to facilitate work tasks or activities of daily living. Activity-specific prostheses are very effective in accomplishing the specific tasks for which they are designed. Because these prostheses usually require only simple controls and minimal components, they are often less costly than more complex designs (Figure 8). The chief disadvantage of an activity-specific prosthesis is that it has limited utility. Interchangeable activity-specific prostheses can help to address this limitation.

Design Considerations

The foundation for successful prosthesis use is the socket. Unless the socket is comfortable and securely suspended, the prosthesis will not be

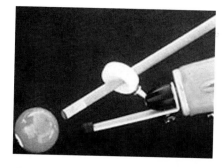

Figure 8 Activity-specific terminal device for playing billiards. *(Courtesy of Bob Radocy.)*

worn on a sustained basis. At the glenohumeral level, the key to achieving stability is an intimately fitted socket that provides rigidity in load-bearing areas and serves as a secure platform for anchoring components.[4]

Individuals with amputations and absences at the glenohumeral and associated levels have reported many problems with long-term prosthesis use. Frequently mentioned issues include the weight of the prosthesis, heat buildup within the socket, lack of stability, reduced control of the terminal device in certain planes and body positions, and difficulty in independent donning. The socket design must distribute the load primarily over areas with sufficient tissue padding while eliminating excessive pressure on skeletal protuberances. Heat buildup while wearing a prosthesis is directly related to the amount of skin covered by the socket and the resulting lack of heat dissipation. Therefore, reducing the surface area of the socket can greatly improve comfort and patient acceptance. Lack of stability and reduced control of the terminal device in certain planes and body positions are both results of a socket that changes position during movement. Without a stable socket, the efficiency of the harness system is greatly reduced. Consequently, the wearer must produce more gross body movement to operate the prosthesis, resulting in increased fatigue and frustration. With improved socket stability, a less complex harness system may be sufficient, which facilitates the donning process.

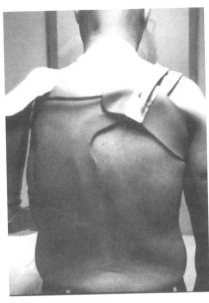

Figure 9 Early body-powered socket design demonstrating extensive coverage of the ipsilateral torso.

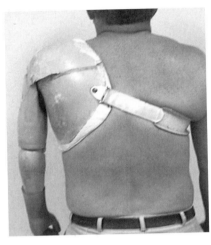

Figure 10 Body-powered socket design covering less of the torso surface area than did early designs.

To create an effective prosthesis, the prosthetist must be able to assess the many design criteria both individually and as they relate to one another. The harness system must be determined during the preprosthetic phase, as this will influence the socket design. The harness is especially critical in bilateral deficiencies or when significant areas of scarring or skin graft are present. With amputations at the humeral neck (see Case Study 2), the remnant humerus can often be used for primary or secondary control strategies, which may affect component selection and socket design. Finally, it is important to clarify the patient's cosmetic expectations for the prosthesis because these considerations may also affect component selection, socket design, control strategies, and long-term acceptance. The optimal socket is the one that balances these interrelated goals to meet the needs of the individual amputee.

Formulation of the Rehabilitation Plan

The preprosthetic phase culminates with the formulation of a detailed prosthetic rehabilitation plan. Comprehensive evaluations by the other members of the rehabilitation team, including the physician, the physical and occupational therapists, the psychologist, and the rehabilitation coordinator, should be concurrent with the prosthetic assessment. Interaction and communication among rehabilitation team members is critical to success at these levels. Once all members of the rehabilitation team have offered their recommendations, a final rehabilitation plan can be formulated. The recommendations must take into account the patient's physical capacity and willingness to commit to what is often a rigorous fitting and training schedule.[5] A patient who has a sense of control and active participation in the formulation of the rehabilitation plan is more likely to put forth the effort necessary to execute the plan successfully.

The rehabilitation plan integrates the patient's prosthetic, therapeutic, psychological, and medical needs based on short- and long-term goals. Prosthetic options affect occupational therapy, physical therapy, and psychological counseling.[6] One of the greatest challenges is orchestrating the interaction of the various services. When treatment team schedules are not coordinated in advance, lapses in care can delay the rehabilitation process and lead to patient frustration and discouragement. Progress evaluations should be scheduled regularly, during which the status and the evolving goals of the patient are discussed and the plan modified as necessary.

Interim Prosthetic Phase

After a thorough prosthetic and therapeutic rehabilitation plan has been formulated, the interim prosthetic phase starts. During this phase, the prosthesis is created and therapy transitions from general residual limb preparation to specific prosthetic training. Therapy could include electromyographic (EMG) site selection and specific muscle differentiation for a myoelectric prosthesis or further shoulder complex strengthening for body-powered components. This phase also includes the cast impression, creation of a diagnostic prosthesis, and the assessment of functional use of the diagnostic prosthesis, and it concludes with fabrication and delivery of a definitive prosthesis. The diagnostic prosthesis ensures that optimal socket fit and comfort and prosthesis control/function, alignment, and definitive fabrication specifications have been achieved.

The type of prosthesis control chosen influences socket design and should therefore occur before an impression of the patient's residual limb is taken. Regardless of which prosthetic option is selected, all glenohumeral and associated level prostheses require a stable and comfortable socket to support the prosthetic shoulder, elbow, wrist unit, and terminal device components.

Socket Design

Despite differences in anatomy, socket designs for humeral neck amputations, glenohumeral disarticulations, and interscapulothoracic-level amputations are similar and have gradually evolved to cover less of the torso. Early socket styles, which contained all of the shoulder girdle and covered much of the trunk, were bulky and hot and sometimes impinged on the clavicle or acromion[7,8] (Figure 9). These early designs were replaced by sockets with more abbreviated trimlines that reduced weight and heat buildup[9] (Figure 10). More extensive harnessing was often required to stabilize the prosthesis, however, despite the smaller surface area of the socket.

Simpson and Sauter are credited with the next evolution in socket design, the Perimeter Frame.[10] Made of lightweight aluminum, this socket included large windows, or "cutouts," in the anterior, posterior, and acromioclavicular regions (Figure 11). By moving the acromioclavicular area or humeral neck inside the socket, the amputee could activate switches controlling electronic devices with good results. Myoelectrodes in the Perimeter Frame had limited success, however, because it was difficult to maintain skin-to-electrode contact.[11]

In the 1980s, infraclavicular designs were developed.[12] The infraclavicular design differs from its predecessors because it does not enclose the shoulder complex to support the weight of the prosthesis. Instead, it relies on compression of the deltopectoral muscle group anteriorly and the scapular region posteriorly.[13] Intimate anatomic contouring of these load-bearing areas stabilizes the socket on the torso (Figure 12), enabling the wearer to effectively position the terminal device in space. Infraclavicular sockets are also less noticeable under clothing than are other designs. Because the acromioclavicular complex is not encased in this design, it is free to move independently of the socket. This movement can be used to activate secondary control inputs to control wrist rotation, shoulder or elbow locks, etc.[14,15]

Diagnostic Assessment

The diagnostic socket with the harness affixed should be assessed both statically and dynamically while the patient is standing, sitting, and bending forward and to the side. It is important to evaluate the load-bearing surfaces and ensure that forces are evenly distributed so that excessive

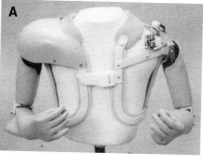

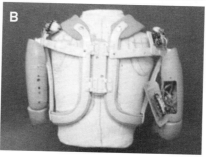

Figure 11 Perimeter Frame–type socket. **A,** Anterior view. **B,** Posterior view.

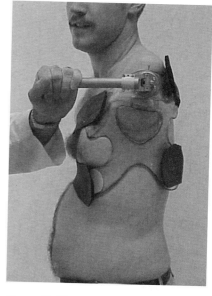

Figure 12 The prosthetist applies downward force to the humeral segment, demonstrating the stability achieved with this infraclavicular socket design.

pressure is not applied to any single area.

Diagnostic assessment also focuses on the identification and verification of sufficient EMG signal recognition for myoelectric control, sufficient capture of excursion for body-powered control, or both for hybrid control. An experienced therapist is extremely valuable in assisting the patient and practitioner with locating and strengthening specific muscle groups. When myoelectric control is selected, the diagnostic socket should be carefully examined for consistent skin contact, especially during contraction of the desired control muscles.[16] Some myoelectric systems require the patient to quickly cocontract antagonistic muscles to control functions such as unlocking the elbow or transferring control from the terminal device to an electric wrist rotator.[17] Some patients have difficulty contracting both targeted control muscles simultaneously and will require either therapy training or a different control scheme. When body-powered control is provided, the socket should be evaluated for maximum range of motion to determine optimal excursion. At the gleno-

humeral and associated levels, range of motion and associated excursion are often insufficient for effective control of a fully body-powered prosthesis. This is even more problematic for children and for people of slight build or with narrow shoulders.

Once the controls have been confirmed, the components can be mounted and aligned. The location and angles of abduction/adduction and internal rotation of the shoulder joint should mirror the center of the contralateral shoulder. With humeral neck–level amputations, the mechanical shoulder joint location may not be anatomic, to avoid creating a prosthesis with obvious shoulder asymmetry. For patients with cosmetic concerns, one solution is to mount the shoulder joint inferior to the distal aspect of the humeral neck (Figure 13).

After all components have been attached and aligned, reliable control of the shoulder, elbow, wrist, and terminal device should be verified. Secondary control options, including a remote on/off, shoulder lock, elbow unlock, and wrist rotation, require analysis of gross body movement and selection of appropriate input options, often push- or pull-type

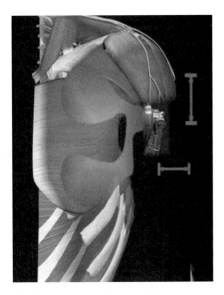

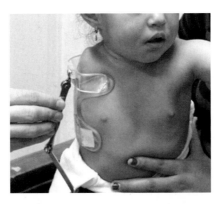

Figure 14 Child with high-level congenital deficiency. Note the contour of the affected side compared with the contralateral shoulder.

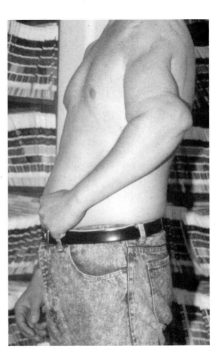

Figure 13 Diagnostic prosthesis with the shoulder joint located inferior to the humeral neck.

Figure 15 Surgical removal of the proximal humerus results in a sensate arm with functioning musculature that hangs at the patient's side. Firing the biceps results in telescoping of the humeral soft tissues but not in elbow flexion.

switches. Push switches can be activated with the chin, with elevation of the acromial complex, or with movement of the humeral neck. Pull switches are attached to the harness and are activated by excursion of the harness. Verifying control isolation (after each control option is added) ensures that inadvertent activation of a particular function does not occur.

Before creating the definitive prosthesis, the prosthetist must determine the socket material and thickness, frame color and composition, trimlines, and mounting locations for secondary control inputs. This is best accomplished while the patient is wearing the diagnostic prosthesis. The prosthesis is ready for final fabrication when all issues of comfort, control, function, cosmesis, and fabrication have been thoroughly addressed. By following this protocol, few unanticipated issues will arise during the delivery of the definitive prosthesis, and alterations should be minimal.

Postprosthetic Phase

Prosthetic delivery is the culmination of much hard work by the patient and the rehabilitation team and can be quite gratifying. Once the prosthesis is donned, the fit, function, and range of motion should be assessed carefully to ensure that accurate duplication of the diagnostic prosthesis has been achieved. Controls and adjustments should be verified to optimize function. This could include snugging the harness of a body-powered component or fine-tuning the electronics for a myoelectric device.

The patient's perceptions are critical to the process. A prosthesis that may appear to fit and function well from the rehabilitation team's perspective will still not be successful if it does not meet the patient's requirements. For example, the harness may seem too tight or the patient may feel that too much effort is required or that cosmetic issues have not been adequately addressed. Responding to such concerns with specific changes and involving the patient in the decision-making process gives a sense of empowerment and increases the likelihood of a positive long-term outcome.

Another important responsibility of the rehabilitation team is to help the patient develop realistic expectations. When the definitive prosthesis is delivered, the patient must confront the limitations of a prosthesis. Even the best-designed prosthesis cannot replace the function of a human arm. This can often be an emotional time, and access to a support network that includes a psychologist or counselor

is beneficial. This is especially true for the glenohumeral-level amputee because the loss at this level is so significant.

Occupational therapy becomes the focal point of the postprosthetic phase. The goal of postprosthetic therapy should be the integration of the prosthesis into the patient's lifestyle. The therapist begins with specific controls training: flexing and positioning the elbow, opening and closing the terminal device, and supinating and pronating the wrist. With guidance and practice, the patient will master these skills and then translate them into task-specific activities. During this process, it is important that the therapist and prosthetist maintain consistent communication to ensure seamless rehabilitation. Often the prosthesis requires minor adjustments as new tasks are undertaken or to address residual limb volume changes. Care and maintenance of the prosthesis, including cleaning the prosthesis and personal hygiene,

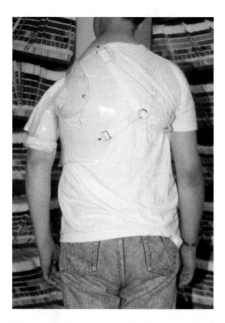

Figure 16 Clear test socket has a perimeter socket that is stabilized on the torso. The posterior humeral shell is articulated near the glenohumeral joint region, permitting the patient to passively abduct the arm for sitting at a desk or table.

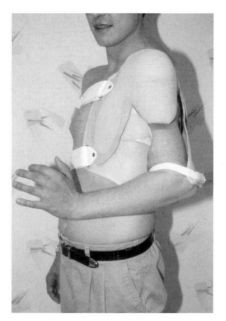

Figure 17 The finished "prosthosis" allows the patient to actively flex and extend the elbow for desktop activities. The lightweight padded shell restores shoulder symmetry under clothing.

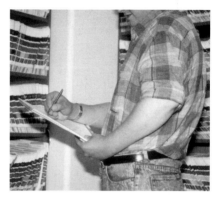

Figure 18 Although active flexion beyond 90° is impossible, the left hand can assist the unimpaired limb in light tasks, despite the absence of the humerus.

should also be discussed. Finally, a specific plan for long-term follow-up care and component maintenance should be formulated.

Special Considerations
Congenital Absence

Acquired amputations and congenital absences at the glenohumeral level have distinct clinical presentations that affect prosthetic management differently. With congenital absence (Figure 14), the clavicle and scapula are often misshapen and may be fused. They are usually foreshortened, and the lateral aspects are swept upward, creating a prominent and usually very mobile bony spur.[18] The rest of the shoulder area is often fleshy and has the potential for weight support, but the lack of bony structures often results in problems with stability. The shoulder profile drops away quite sharply from the bony point of the glenoid area, and a prosthetic shoulder joint can be incorporated without cosmetic or technical difficulty.[19]

Intercalary Amputations

Intercalary amputations, which are rarely encountered, are extremely challenging for the prosthetist-orthotist to manage. One example is the Tikhoff-Linberg resection, where much of the humerus is removed but the balance of the upper limb remains sensate with intact musculature. It is tempting to consider these patients as having a loss similar to a brachial plexus injury, but prosthetic solutions that are successful for brachial plexus injuries often fail with this population. The overwhelming functional deficit is the complete loss of internal skeletal stability. As a consequence, when the patient fires the elbow flexors, the arm shortens but the forearm does not reach a horizontal position, as shown in Figure 15. Because the forces generated by the upper arm musculature are considerable, it is virtually impossible to create an external "prosthesis" that will prevent such telescoping from occurring.[20] In addition, it is impossible to carry even very light objects in the hand because the entire arm is connected to the torso only by soft tissues.

A locking elbow orthosis is not of much use because the skeletal loss makes the humeral section unstable. Biomechanically, it is necessary to create a prosthetic socket-like structure on the chest to stabilize the arm support, and many patients reject devices that extend from the torso to the wrist. In some instances, a posterior humeral trough connected to a torso platform can provide sufficient counterforce to permit the patient to voluntarily flex and extend the arm for desktop activities (Figures 16 through 18). Articulated devices, whether body-powered or electric-powered, are not always successful for this population because the intact forearm and hand weigh much more than would a hollow prosthetic forearm segment.

Case Studies
Case Study 1

A 22-year-old man incurred a brachial plexus injury secondary to a water skiing accident, resulting in a flail arm. Eight years after the injury, after multiple surgeries to attempt neural reconstruction, the patient elected to undergo a shoulder disarticulation. The residual limb/shoulder girdle had healthy skin without scar or graft tissue. However, the pectoralis muscle was significantly atrophied secondary to the brachial plexus injury and produced a 13-μV maximum EMG signal. The range of scapular motion was

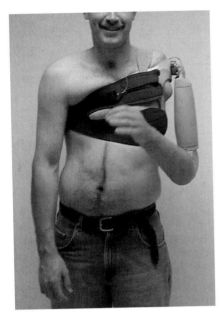

Figure 19 Definitive myoelectric prosthesis for an individual with shoulder-level brachial plexus injury.

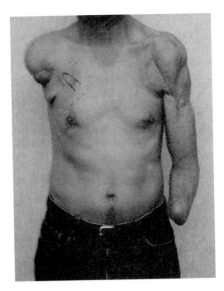

Figure 20 Individual with bilateral amputations, at the humeral neck and at the transradial level.

Case Study 2

A 39-year-old man presented 5 years postinjury with bilateral amputations (left side, transradial level; right side, humeral neck–level) secondary to an electrical burn (Figure 20). The right residual limb/shoulder girdle exhibited minimal scar and graft tissue and good range of motion and strength of the humeral neck. However, the left side (transradial level) had extensive scar and graft tissue in the areas of the scapula, pectoralis, deltoid, and axilla, which limited the ability to anchor the control/suspension harness for the humeral neck–level prosthesis through the axilla region. The patient had adequate EMG signals on both residual limbs, in excess of 80 µV. The team's focus was on obtaining patient independence, reducing prosthesis weight and heat buildup, increasing grip force, enlarging the functional envelope, and limiting shear forces on the scar and graft tissue.

On the right side (humeral neck–level), the patient was fitted with a hybrid prosthesis that used myoelectric control of electronic work hooks and wrist rotators, plus cable-operated control of an elbow with a forearm balancing unit (Figure 21). The cable-operated elbow significantly reduced the overall weight of the prosthesis.

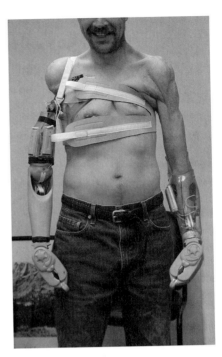

Figure 21 Definitive hybrid prosthesis for an individual with bilateral amputations, at the humeral neck and transradial level. Note the position of the shoulder joint

extremely limited. The infraspinatus muscle produced an EMG signal in excess of 70 µV. The patient reported overuse of his surviving hand and wrist and had a strong interest in maximum function with a good cosmetic appearance.

The patient was fitted with an infraclavicular socket using myoelectric control to operate an electric elbow, hand, and wrist rotator, plus switch control of an electric locking shoulder joint. The infraspinatus muscle site was used to proportionally control elbow flexion and terminal device closing, allowing precise positioning of the elbow and fingers. The weaker pectoralis muscle was used to provide single-speed control of terminal device opening. To decrease the weight of the prosthesis and reduce heat buildup, the socket trimlines were abbreviated and a window was cut inferior to the axilla. The resulting prosthesis allowed the patient to perform bimanual activities with a grip force in excess of 20 lb. The forearm and hand were covered with a custom silicone synthetic skin to closely resemble the contralateral limb and to address the patient's concerns regarding body image (Figure 19).

The patient used ballistic body movements to flex the prosthetic elbow and humeral neck abduction/flexion to control the elbow locking mechanism, eliminating the need to route harness straps for elbow flexion across the fragile axilla region. The infraclavicular socket permitted independent locking of the cable-operated elbow because the humeral neck was not contained within the socket.

The left side (transradial level) was fitted with a self-suspending myoelectric prosthesis with an electronic work hook and wrist rotator control. Myoelectric control offered enhanced grip force and enlarged the functional envelope compared with the patient's previous body-powered prosthesis. By using a special donning aid incorporating a weighted, extra-long lanyard, the patient learned to don the transradial prosthesis independently by using his legs and feet to manipulate the lanyard. He then could use the transradial myoelectric prosthesis to don the prosthesis on the opposite side. The increased grip force, larger functional work envelope, and independent donning characteristics of these prostheses have allowed this patient to live independently in the community.

Summary

Recent improvements in components and control options have achieved successful prosthetic fitting of many amputees with glenohumeral and associated levels of loss. When body-powered components were the only available option, prosthetic fitting was not as successful. A comprehensive and systematic approach, coordinated by an experienced rehabilitation team consisting of a physician, physical and occupational therapists, a psychologist, a rehabilitation coordinator, and a prosthetist can improve long-term success rates with these prostheses. The outcome is best when the patient has a sense of control and active participation throughout the rehabilitation process. Verifying optimal fit and function of the diagnostic prosthesis before fabrication of the definitive device has proved to be an effective method to avoid costly modifications that can result in loss of confidence for the patient.

Acknowledgment

The authors would like to thank John W. Michael, MEd, CPO, for contributing the section on fitting intercalary amputations.

References

1. Alley RD: The prosthetist's evaluation and planning process with the upper extremity amputee, in Atkins DJ, Meier RH (eds): *Functional Restoration of Adults and Children With Upper Extremity Amputation.* New York, NY, Demos, 2004, pp 125-126.

2. Reddy M: Nerve entrapment syndrome in upper extremity contralateral to amputation. *Arch Phys Med Rehabil* 1984;65:24-26.

3. Mckenzie DS: Powered prosthesis for children: Clinical considerations. *Prosthet Int* 1967;3(2/3):5-7.

4. Alley RD, Miguelez JM: Prosthetic rehabilitation of glenohumeral level deficiencies, in Atkins DJ, Meier RH (eds): *Functional Restoration of Adults and Children With Upper Extremity Amputation.* New York, NY, Demos, 2004, pp 244-250.

5. Atkins D: Adult upper-limb prosthetic training, in Atkins DJ, Meier RH (eds): *Comprehensive Management of the Upper Limb Amputee.* New York, NY, Springer-Verlag, 1989, p 58.

6. Canelon MF: Training for a patient with shoulder disarticulation. *Am J Occup Ther* 1993;47:174-178.

7. Brooks MA, Dennis JF: Shoulder disarticulation type prostheses for bilateral upper extremity amputees. *Inter Clin Info Bull* 1963;2:1-7.

8. Neff GG: Prosthetic principles in shoulder disarticulation for bilateral amelia. *Prosthet Orthot Int* 1978;2:143-147.

9. Wright TW, Hagen AD, Wood MB: Prosthetic usage in upper extremity amputations. *J Hand Surg Am* 1995;20:619-622.

10. Neff G: Prosthetic principles in bilateral shoulder disarticulation or bilateral amelia. *Prosthet Orthot Int* 1978;2:143-147.

11. Mongeau M, Madon S: Abstract: Evaluation prosthetic fitting of 13 shoulder disarticulation clients since 2 years. *J Assoc Child Prosthet Orthot Clin* 1990;25:26.

12. Sears HH, Andrew JT, Jacobsen SC: Experience with the Utah arm, hand, and terminal device, in Atkins DJ, Meier RH (eds): *Comprehensive Management of the Upper Limb Amputee.* New York, NY, Springer-Verlag, 1989, pp 200-201

13. Alley RD, Sears HH: Powered upper limb prosthetics in adults, in Muzumdar A (ed): *Powered Upper Limb Prostheses.* Berlin, Springer-Verlag, 2004, pp 133-138.

14. Miguelez J, Miguelez M: The Micro-Frame: The next generation of interface design for glenohumeral disarticulation and associated levels of limb deficiency. *J Prosthet Orthotics* 2003;15:66-71.

15. Daly W: Upper extremity socket designs. *Phys Med Rehabil Clin North Am* 2000;11:627-638.

16. Heger H, Millstein S, Hunter G: Electrically-powered prostheses for the adult with an upper limb amputation. *J Bone Joint Surg Br* 1985;67:278-281.

17. Stern P, Lauko T: A myoelectrically controlled prosthesis using remote muscle sites. *Inter Clin Info Bull* 1973;12:1-4.

18. Hall C, Bechtol CO: Modern amputation technique in the upper extremity. *J Bone Joint Surg* 1963;450:1717-1722.

19. Cooper R: Prosthetic principles, in Bowker JD, Michael JW: *Atlas of Limb Prosthetics: Surgical, Prosthetic, and Rehabilitation Principles.* Rosemont, IL, American Academy of Orthopaedic Surgeons, 2002, pp 271-275. (Originally published by Mosby-Year Book, 1992)

20. Ham SF, Eisma WJ, Schraffordt Koops H, Oldhoff J: The Tikhoff-Linberg procedure in the treatment of sarcomas of the shoulder girdle. *J Surg Oncol* 1993;53:71-77.

Chapter 22

Prosthetic Training

Diane J. Atkins, OTR

Introduction

The amputation of an upper limb involves the loss of a hand and therefore is especially difficult for the patient. The hand functions in prehensile activities, as a sensory organ, and as a means of communication. Any loss will interfere with the individual's productivity and feeling of completeness and will alter his or her interactions with the environment.[1]

Each person with an upper limb amputation is unique, and no two amputations are identical. Because people are so dependent on their arms and hands, the person with an upper limb amputation—particularly a person who has lost both arms—is initially devastated and unprepared to perform even a simple task. Therefore, rehabilitation of these patients can be among the most challenging and rewarding clinical opportunities for a practitioner.

Independence in all functional activities is the goal of almost every person with an upper limb amputation, and this goal is entirely possible except in very short bilateral transhumeral amputations and in bilateral amputations at the shoulder. Every person with an upper limb amputation should be given the opportunity to use a prosthesis, recognizing that it is ultimately that person's choice as to whether the prosthesis will become a part of his or her daily life.

Successful outcomes in rehabilitation for the unilateral and bilateral upper limb amputee are believed to depend on multiple factors. These include early posttraumatic intervention, an experienced team approach, patient-directed prosthetic training, patient education, and patient monitoring and follow-up.

This chapter stresses the importance of adhering to good preprosthetic and prosthetic training principles. Listening to and acknowledging the patient's psychological and functional needs is critically important in achieving the goals of acceptance of the prosthesis and successful function.

Preprosthetic Therapy

The preprosthetic therapy phase begins when the sutures are removed and the wound has healed, generally about 2 to 3 weeks after surgery. This program is managed and monitored primarily by occupational therapy personnel.

The goals of the preprosthetic program are to (1) promote residual limb shrinkage and shaping, (2) promote residual limb desensitization, (3) maintain normal joint range of motion, (4) increase muscle strength, (5) maximize self-reliance in the performance of tasks required for daily living, (6) determine the electrical potential provided by various muscles (in the event that myoelectric prosthetic components are prescribed), (7) inform and guide the patient regarding prosthetic components and options, and (8) explore the patient's goals regarding the future.[2]

Healing of the residual limb usually will be essentially complete by the 21st postoperative day, allowing for a vigorous program of prosthetic preparation.[3] Malone and associates[4] have suggested that the first month after upper limb amputation is the golden period for prosthesis fitting; ie, prosthesis fitting should be initiated during this time to maximize the level of acceptance and use of the prosthesis.

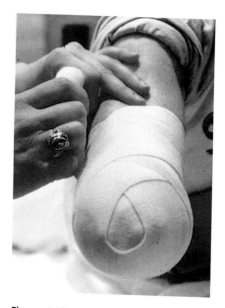

Figure 1 Figure-of-8 wrapping.

Residual Limb Shrinkage and Shaping

Shrinking and shaping of the residual limb is perhaps the most critical aspect of the preprosthetic program. If this is not done properly, significant circulation and wound healing problems can occur.

Compression aids such as elastic bandages, tubular bandages, or shrinker socks are applied to the residual limb to effect shrinking and shaping. A figure-of-8 wrapping method is used to apply more pressure distally than proximally (Figure 1). Elastic bandages should never be applied in a circumferential manner, which can severely compromise circulation.

The wrap should be reapplied at least every 3 to 4 hours, or more frequently if it slips or bunches. The elastic bandage should be worn all day and night except when bathing. An elastic bandage should never be worn more than 48 hours before being replaced with a clean bandage. Elastic bandages should be washed with mild soap and lukewarm water and thoroughly rinsed with clean water.

A preparatory prosthesis might also be applied early in the shaping process. However, a compression bandage is generally preferred because it affords better monitoring of skin healing and points of pressure.

Residual Limb Desensitization

The residual limb is often hypersensitive following surgery and requires desensitization. This can be carried out with gentle massage and tapping techniques. Desensitization can also be accomplished by vibration, constant touch pressure, or the application of various textures to the sensitive areas of the limb.

The amputee should be encouraged to perform these techniques independently, for two reasons. First, only the amputee is aware of his or her tolerance. Second, the amputee can become more in touch with his or her body by practicing desensitization regularly.

When complete healing has occurred, aggressive massage should be performed to prevent adhesions from occurring and to provide additional sensory input. The therapist should explain that this massage will improve the amputee's tolerance to the pressure that will be placed on the residual limb by the prosthetic socket.

Maintenance of Joint Range of Motion

The maintenance of joint range of motion is an essential goal of an effective treatment program. Maintaining scapular, glenohumeral, elbow, and forearm motion is crucial to aid in prosthetic control motions and to maximize the functional potential of the prosthesis.

Pronation and supination of the forearm are critical when using a transradial prosthesis; therefore, significant attention needs to be paid to retaining the motion that still exists between the radius and ulna. Unfortunately, forearm range of motion in the transradial amputee is often neglected and, therefore, this range of motion is lost in as little as 2 to 3 weeks.

Muscle Strengthening

A therapy program to increase upper limb muscle strength can be instituted in conjunction with the range-of-motion program. Active resistance can be applied by the therapist, or progressive resistive exercise with cuff weights attached to the limb can be used. A home program should be provided that contains exercises for general strengthening as well as the specific movements that the amputee will perform when using a prosthesis.

Maximizing Independence

It is critically important to maximize functional independence early in the therapy program. Patterns of dependency can easily occur if the patient is not directed to be independent and self-reliant. Instruction in change of dominance may be necessary. Instruction in one-handed activities is indicated with the unilateral amputee.

The bilateral upper limb amputee presents a unique challenge. These patients are totally dependent following bilateral arm loss, and it is important to express reassurance, support, and realistic optimism to them during this time. Independence can be enhanced by a simple device such as a universal cuff used with an adapted utensil, toothbrush, pen, or pencil.

Myoelectric Site Testing

Electric upper limb components powered by myoelectric control sites are being prescribed with increasing frequency. In such cases, the electric potential generated by various muscles should be determined. A myotester is used for this purpose.

Ideally, the therapist and prosthetist should work together to identify the best myoelectric sites and to discuss the issues of prosthetic design. Reliance on a prosthetist with extensive experience in the fabrication of upper limb prostheses is critically important to guarantee a successful outcome.

The therapist is encouraged to communicate openly with the prosthetist on a frequent basis, not only initially but also when concerns regarding fit or operation arise.[5]

Determining the Appropriate Type of Prosthesis

The individual who has sustained upper limb loss generally has very little knowledge of upper limb prostheses. These persons desperately want and need this information, and one goal of the preprosthetic program is to educate the patient regarding prostheses.

The unique differences between body-powered and electric components should be comprehensively described, and examples of each should be shown and demonstrated if possible. The question of which upper limb prosthetic device is most appropriate for a given patient—an all body-powered, all electric, or a hybrid (combination of body-powered and electric)—is a challenging one. An objective overview of the advantages and disadvantages of body-powered and electric components should be clearly explained.

Advantages of the hook-type, body-powered prosthesis include lighter weight, better durability, increased sensory feedback, less expense, and greater ease in seeing the manipulated object. Advantages of an electric prosthesis include better appearance, moderate or no harnessing, less body movement to operate, greater ability to reach overhead and to grasp larger objects, and better grip strength.[6]

The decision to prescribe an all-electric prosthesis should be made by an experienced amputee rehabilitation team. The amputee should be actively involved with the discussion of prosthetic options and should be given an objective and comprehensive overview of the advantages and disadvantages of the primary elbow, forearm, wrist, hand, and hook components.

It has been my experience that starting simple and providing more complex devices once the basics have been mastered results in significant success for the user of an upper limb prosthesis. Once it has been demonstrated to the rehabilitation team that the amputee actually wears and uses the prosthesis and that there are documented ways in which the amputee's function could be enhanced by an electric elbow, forearm, or hand, then a prescription for this more expensive component can be justified. Third-party payers can more easily justify the required expenditure if this philosophy is followed. Unfortunately, policies that unrealistically limit costs or restrict the patient to one prosthesis per lifetime are becoming increasingly common among managed care insurers, making such staging of care impossible and impeding successful rehabilitation.

A back-up prosthesis is highly recommended for the upper limb amputee and is especially justified if the amputee has demonstrated that the prosthesis is essential to his or her independence. Routine maintenance and repairs are necessary with any prosthesis, and a back-up prosthesis will be used often.

Because of the complexity of managing the fitting and training of proximal bilateral upper limb amputees, referral to a specialized rehabilitation center is strongly suggested. These individuals require many hours of professional attention to solve the many fitting and training challenges posed by such amputations. An experienced physician, prosthetist, and therapist are critically important if success is to be achieved by these individuals.

A careful inventory of the amputee's lifestyle, support system, educational background, and future goals should be taken and discussed. The individual with an amputation should be an integral part of the decision-making process regarding the prosthesis prescription. Involving the patient in decisions that affect his or her own health care helps to restore a sense of control.

Patient Expectations and Assessment

During the period of time from casting until final fitting of the prosthesis, the amputee may eagerly anticipate that the prosthesis will replace, in appearance and function, the amputated limb. Unfortunately, the finished prosthesis is often a disappointment for the amputee. It is perceived as artificial looking, heavy, uncomfortable, and awkward to operate. If the amputee is appropriately oriented to the realities of how the prosthesis looks and operates, he or she will be better prepared to accept its limitations when it is delivered. Therefore, before initiating a program of upper limb prosthetic training, the therapist must orient the amputee as to what the prosthesis realistically can and cannot do. An amputee who has an unrealis-

tic expectation about the usefulness of the prosthesis as a replacement for the lost body part may be dissatisfied with the ultimate functioning of the prosthesis and may reject it altogether. On the other hand, if the expectations of the amputee are more realistic at the beginning of training, then the ultimate acceptance will be based on the ability of the prosthesis to improve the amputee's performance. It is imperative, then, that the therapist be honest and positive about the function of the prosthesis. If the amputee believes in and understands the functional potential of the prosthesis, success is more likely.

During the therapist's first encounter with the amputee, many issues need to be discussed and documented if they have not already been dealt with. These issues include the etiology and onset of the amputation, the age of the patient, dominance, other medical problems, the patient's level of independence, the range of motion of all joints of the residual limb, the muscle strength of the remaining musculature, the shape and skin integrity of the residual limb, the status of the opposite limb, the presence of any phantom pain or residual limb pain, previous rehabilitation experience, revisions, and viable muscle sites for myoelectric control. In addition, the therapist should assess the patient's knowledge regarding prostheses, background education and vocational goals, goals and expectations regarding the prosthesis, and home environment and family support.

Although this list of issues may appear unreasonably long and too lengthy to document, a complete assessment is very important. Not only will it make a significant difference in the therapist's relationship with the patient, but the subsequent success of therapy will be greatly enhanced if this information is gathered before therapy begins.

At the first visit to the occupational therapist, the amputee probably will be carrying the prosthesis in a bag. The therapist should be sensitive to the amputee's feeling of awkward-

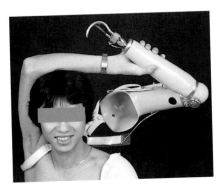

Figure 2 Donning the prosthesis using the "coat" method.

Early Training

During the first couple of visits, several goals should be addressed. These include familiarizing the patient with prosthetic component terminology, training the patient to independently don and doff the prosthesis, orienting the patient to a wearing schedule, and reviewing the care of the residual limb and prosthesis.

Prosthetic Component Terminology
Body-Powered Prosthesis

Considering that the prosthesis has now become the amputee's "arm," it is important that the amputee learn the terminology to identify the major components of the prosthesis. Learning the names of the basic components such as the figure-of-8 harness, cable, elbow unit or elbow hinge, wrist unit, terminal device, and hook or hand will suffice at this time.

Myoelectric Prosthesis

Considering that this prosthesis is now a vital part of the amputee's body, it is particularly important to know the function and names of the major parts, such as the electrodes, battery, glove, and electric hand. The initial visit is an appropriate time to

TABLE 1 Sample Prosthesis Wearing Schedule			
	Morning (AM)	Afternoon (PM)	Evening (PM)
Day 1	9:00-9:30	1:00-1:30	6:00-6:30
Day 2	9:00-10:00	1:00-2:00	6:00-7:00
Day 3	9:00-10:30	1:00-2:30	6:00-7:30
Day 4	9:00-11:00	1:00-3:00	6:00-8:00
Day 5	9:00-11:30	1:00-3:30	6:00-8:30
Day 6	9:00-12:00	1:00-4:00	6:00-9:00
Day 7	All day if no skin problems have occurred		

introduce the battery-charging procedure and the proper use of the battery packs. Instruction manuals are often provided by the manufacturer and should be shared at this time as well.

Donning and Doffing the Prosthesis
Body-Powered Prosthesis

Independence in donning and doffing the prosthesis should be established early by using the "pullover sweater" method. The amputee raises his or her arms overhead as in putting on a pullover shirt or sweater. As an alternative, the "coat" method may also be used. The residual limb is put in the socket first, and the opposite side follows (Figure 2). Bilateral amputees most often use the pullover sweater method.

Myoelectric Prosthesis

The prosthesis should be donned and doffed with the electronics in the off position to avoid unintended movements. A residual limb "pull sock" or "sleeve" may be required for donning the prosthesis to bring the prosthesis in close contact with the limb, particularly for amputees with very short residual limbs. For storage, the prosthesis should be in the off position, and the batteries should be removed. The hand should be fully opened to keep the thumb web space stretched.

Wearing Schedule

The wearing schedule is extremely important to review during this first visit. Initial wearing periods should be no longer than 15 to 30 minutes three times daily, with frequent examination

of the skin for excess pressure or evidence of poor socket fit. This is particularly important if insensate areas and adherent scar tissue are present. If redness persists for more than 20 minutes after the prosthesis has been removed, the patient should return to the prosthetist for socket modifications. If no skin problems are present, wearing periods can be increased in 30-minute increments three times a day. By the end of 1 week, the upper limb amputee should be wearing the prosthesis all day. See Table 1 for an example of a wearing schedule.

Care of the Residual Limb and Prosthesis

Following amputation, the skin of the residual limb is subject to irritation and often to further injury and infection. Appropriate care of the skin is therefore a vital part of rehabilitation. Skin care is covered in detail in chapter 55.

The amputee should be encouraged to inspect the skin of the residual limb daily. If skin disorders develop, the physician should be called promptly. A minor disorder can become disabling if it is neglected or treated incorrectly. Adjustment of the prosthesis is usually necessary, and therefore the prosthetist is generally involved at this time as well.

The residual limb should be washed daily, preferably in the evening, with mild soap and lukewarm water and then rinsed thoroughly with clean water. Soap left to dry on the skin can cause irritation. After rinsing, the skin should be dried thoroughly using patting motions.

The initial visit is an appropriate time to ness and reluctance to put on the prosthesis with others watching. A quiet, nondistracting room with a mirror, plus an atmosphere of acceptance and understanding, is helpful.

Brisk rubbing should be avoided because it can irritate the skin. Lotions, creams, and moisturizers should not be applied to the limb unless specific orders are given by the physician or therapist. Strong disinfectants, such as iodine, should never be used on the skin of the residual limb.

The socket of the prosthesis also should be cleaned often, particularly if the amputee perspires heavily. In warm weather, the socket may require cleaning at least once or twice daily. The socket should be washed with warm water and mild soap. The inside should be thoroughly wiped with a cloth dampened in clean, warm water. The interior of the socket can be allowed to air dry overnight or can be dried thoroughly with a towel if it will be used again immediately.

If residual limb socks are worn, several changes may be necessary during warm weather because of perspiration. Washing the sock as soon as it is taken off, before the perspiration dries on it, will prolong the life of the sock. The sock should be washed in mild soap and warm water and then thoroughly rinsed. The sock should be allowed to dry slowly to avoid shrinkage.

The prosthesis may be cleaned with soap and water, using a soft, damp cloth. Rubbing alcohol can be used to clean the inside of the socket if an odor develops. Some cosmetic gloves that are used with myoelectric prostheses stain easily, so special attention should be paid to avoiding ink, newsprint, mustard, grease, and dirt. A glove-cleansing cream can be obtained from the prosthetist that will remove general soil but not stains. A myoelectric prosthesis should never be immersed in water because it will seriously damage the internal electronic components.

Instruction in Body-Control Motions for a Body-Powered Prosthesis

A body-powered prosthesis is controlled by various muscle groups. Several motions need to be practiced before the prosthesis is actually applied and the upper limb amputee practices controlling the prosthesis. These motions are scapular abduction; chest expansion; shoulder depression, extension, and abduction; humeral flexion; elbow flexion and extension; and forearm pronation and supination.

Scapular Abduction

Spreading the shoulder blades either alone or in combination with humeral flexion will provide tension on the figure-of-8 harness to open the terminal device.

Chest Expansion

This motion should be practiced by deeply inhaling, expanding the chest as much as possible, and then relaxing slowly. Chest expansion is used in a variety of ways for the amputee with a transhumeral amputation, shoulder disarticulation, or scapulothoracic amputation. Some prosthetic designs harness this motion with a cross-chest strap. In some instances of extensive axillary scarring, the cross-chest strap may be used in lieu of the figure-of-8 harness.

Shoulder Depression, Extension, and Abduction

This combined movement is used to operate the body-powered, internal-locking elbow in the prosthesis for the transhumeral amputee. To teach this motion, the therapist should cup one hand under the residual limb and instruct the amputee to press down into the palm. This simulates the motion required to lock and unlock the elbow.

Humeral Flexion

The amputee is instructed to raise the residual limb forward to shoulder level and to push the residual limb forward, sliding the shoulder blades apart as far as possible. This motion applies pressure on the cable and allows the terminal device to open. Scapular abduction and humeral flexion are the basic motions to review with the transradial and more distal amputee.

Elbow Flexion and Extension

A critical goal of therapy in patients with amputations distal to the elbow is to maintain full elbow range of motion. This range will enable the amputee to reach many areas of the body without undue strain or special modifications in the prosthetic design.

Forearm Pronation and Supination

In amputations that retain more than 50% of the forearm, some degree of forearm pronation and supination is maintained. It is very important to maintain as much of this motion as possible. This will enable the amputee to position the terminal device without prepositioning the wrist unit.

Training With the Prosthesis Applied
Introduction to Controlling the Prosthesis
Manual Control of a Body-Powered Prosthesis

After the prosthesis is applied, manual controls should be reviewed. One control should be taught at a time and then combined with others.

Terminal device positioning In the unilateral amputee, the terminal device is positioned in the wrist unit by passive rotation with the opposite hand. In the bilateral amputee, the terminal device must be pressed against a stationary object or held between the amputee's knees. Bilateral cable-controlled wrist rotators may also be prescribed.

Elbow joint Rotation at the elbow turntable is manually adjusted or controlled by leaning the prosthesis against an object.

Shoulder joint The friction shoulder joint is manually adjusted with the opposite hand or by applying pressure against an object such as the arm of a chair. A locking shoulder joint is an option as well.

Wrist unit If the prosthesis has a wrist flexion unit, this can be manually controlled by applying pressure on the button or, for the bilateral am-

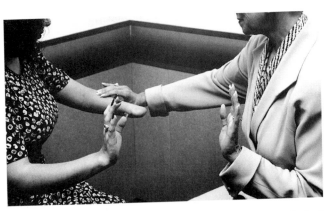

Figure 3 The therapist instructs the patient to imitate the desired muscle contraction in muscle site control training.

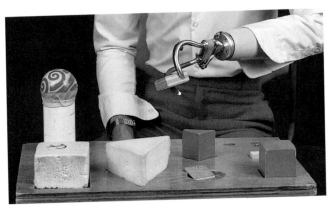

Figure 4 A form board is used in prosthetic training to practice prepositioning the terminal device.

putee, applying pressure against a stationary object.

Body Control Motions for a Body-Powered Prosthesis

The body-control motions described earlier should also be reviewed after the prosthesis has been applied and before functional training. It is essential that the harness be adjusted properly before initiating these exercises. Several ideas are important to remember at this point: (1) In all high proximal levels of upper limb loss, body-powered elbow flexion and extension are greatly enhanced by a forearm lift assist that responds to scapular abduction or chest expansion. Elbow extension is accomplished by gravity if the elbow unit is unlocked. (2) Elbow lock and unlock is one of the most difficult tasks to learn in the operation of a prosthesis. The patient should be taught "down, back, and out" as a reminder to repeat the shoulder depression, extension, and abduction pattern. This pattern not only locks but also unlocks the elbow in an audible two-click cycle. This task should be practiced in a quiet, distraction-free room where it is possible to hear the clicks without difficulty. The motions may need to be exaggerated at first but soon will be barely observable. (3) Before beginning to operate the terminal device, the amputee should practice locking and unlocking the elbow in several positions. (4) In prostheses for shoulder disarticulations and scapulothoracic amputations, the mechanism to lock and unlock the elbow is sometimes a nudge control button attached to the thoracic shell. By depressing this button with the chin, the amputee is able to position and lock the elbow as desired. (5) The therapist should emphasize that the elbow must first be locked in the proper position before the amputee can operate the terminal device. As described previously, biscapular abduction and humeral flexion (as a combined or separate motion) cause the terminal device to open, and relaxing allows it to close.

Myoelectric Prosthesis

Locating appropriate muscle sites superficially is the most important aspect of the successful operation of a myoelectric prosthesis. The muscle groups selected should approximate normal movements as much as possible. The following muscle groups are generally used during muscle site selection:

Transradial and more distal amputations: wrist extensors and flexors are used to open and close the terminal device.

Transhumeral amputations: the biceps is used for elbow flexion and the triceps for elbow extension. The biceps and triceps can also be used for terminal device opening and closing.

Shoulder disarticulations and scapulothoracic amputations: the deltoid, trapezius, latissimus dorsi, or pectoralis muscles can be used for myoelectric control.

It is important to note that the more proximal the level of amputation, the more difficult it becomes for the prosthetist to fit the individual and for the therapist to train that individual.

To help the patient understand the desired muscle contraction, the therapist instructs the amputee to make the desired movement on both sides. For example, the therapist should ask the transradial amputee to raise the sound hand at the wrist (wrist extension) and imagine making that motion with the phantom hand on the affected side (Figure 3). Often a therapist can palpate the wrist flexors and extensors on the residual limb during this exercise. The amputee should be instructed to contract and relax each muscle group separately and on command. Electromyography (EMG), in which the magnitude of the electrical signals from the muscles is measured, is particularly useful for this step. Once the maximum response is found, its location should be marked on the skin. This process is often done with a prosthetist to select the most appropriate muscle site.

When measuring surface potentials with an EMG tester, all the electrodes must have good contact with the skin and must be aligned along the general direction of the muscle fibers. Moistening the skin slightly with water may improve the EMG signal by lowering the skin resistance. EMG testing is begun with the most distal portion of the remnant muscles.

The EMG tester can be used to train the muscles using both visual and auditory feedback. The goals at this point are to increase muscle strength and to isolate muscle contractions. As confidence and accuracy improve, the visual or auditory feedback should be removed. This task teaches the patient to internalize the feeling of each control movement. One advantage of creating this internalized awareness of proper muscle control is that control and strengthening practice can be continued between treatment sessions without the feedback equipment.

The amputee must receive adequate training and practice in initiating these muscle contractions before receiving the myoelectric prosthesis. This will help minimize the anxiety and frustration the individual often experiences while learning to use a myoelectric prosthesis. The amputee's success and effectiveness in using the prosthesis is closely related to the quality of the preprosthetic training. The therapist also needs to recognize muscle fatigue, which frequently occurs during this process, allowing time for muscles to relax during the treatment session.

Controls Practice
Body-Powered Prosthesis
A form board is frequently used to practice prepositioning as well as tension control of the terminal device (Figure 4). Prepositioning involves using both manual and active controls to place the prosthesis in the optimal position for a specific activity. The therapist should be alert for any compensatory body motions the patient might make when approaching an object. Often the amputee will reposition the entire body rather than reposition the elbow and wrist units. A mirror can assist the amputee in seeing the position of the body. It is helpful to instruct the amputee to consider how the arm would have been positioned to approach the object. It is often necessary to remind the amputee to maintain an upright posture and to avoid extraneous body movements.

The five motions basic to hand manipulation are reach, grasp, move, position, and release. A form board can be used to train the amputee to approach, grasp, and release objects differing in shape, weight, firmness, and size. Prehension control can be practiced with a sponge or paper cup. The amputee is instructed to maintain constant tension of the terminal device control cable so as not to overly squeeze the object being held. Approach to an object should be such that the stationary finger makes initial contact with the object and the movable finger moves to grasp it. Flat objects can be moved to the edge of a surface such as a table and then grasped with the terminal device in a horizontal position. Grasp is generally controlled by rubber bands on the terminal device, which can be added as tolerated. Springs may be used as an alternative.

Controls training for the bilateral upper limb amputee may require an extended period of time to perfect. Learning to control the motion of two prostheses separately is a complex motor process. Passing an object such as a ruler back and forth from one terminal device to the other may help in reinforcing this pattern.

Myoelectric Prosthesis
Simple approach, grasp, and release activities are often practiced with a form board on which objects of various shapes, sizes, and firmness are displayed. The amputee should first visualize how the object should be approached and grasped, and then preposition the myoelectric hand. For example, in approaching a glass or cup, the hand should face in, toward the midline, to grasp the glass as a normal hand would. The fingers of the hand should not be positioned downward, because a normal hand does not approach a glass in this position.

As with a body-powered prosthesis, often the patient uses compensatory body motions rather than adjusting or prepositioning the hand first. This action is important to avoid because it appears awkward and often becomes a habit. The transhumeral amputee who uses a body-powered or electric elbow also should make certain the angle of elbow flexion is appropriate. A mirror can help the amputee see the way the body is positioned and visualize how the sound arm would have approached a particular object or activity. The therapist should remind the amputee to maintain an upright posture and avoid extraneous body movements.

Another important aspect of myoelectric training is controlling the gripping force of the terminal device. The amputee learns this by visually observing the degree of muscle contraction that produces a specific result in the myoelectric hand. Styrofoam packing peanuts work well for developing this skill. The amputee must learn how to pick up the peanut without crushing it. Good grasp control through training with materials such as Styrofoam, cotton balls, or sponges helps develop the control needed to handle paper cups, eggs, potato chips, and sandwiches and even to hold another person's hand. Release is accomplished by visualizing a wrist extension contraction, or envisioning the phantom hand up or open. This response should become quite automatic if good preprosthetic training of the muscles has occurred.

Eventually the performance of specific movements will take less cognitive effort, and the movements become automatic. Functional use training can then be introduced into the therapy program.

Functional Use Training
Functional use training is the most difficult and prolonged stage of the prosthetic training process. The success or failure of the amputee's acceptance and use of the prosthesis depends on (1) the motivation of the patient, (2) the comprehensiveness and quality of the tasks and activities practiced, and (3) of critical impor-

TABLE 2 Roles of Body-Powered Hand and Opposite Hand in Bilateral Activities of Daily Living

Activity	Body-Powered Hand	Opposite Hand
Cutting food	Holds fork	Holds knife to cut
Using scissors	Holds material to be cut	Uses scissors
Dressing activities	Holds fabric such as waistband	Tucks in shirt, fastens snap or button (button hook may be used)
Opening jar or bottle	Grasps middle of container with maximum grasp	Unscrews lid or cap
Washing dishes	Manipulates washcloth or sponge (avoiding submerging device)	Holds dish
Drying dishes	Manipulates towel	Holds dish
Using tools	Holds nail or bolt in hook fingers	Uses hammer or wrench
Driving	Assists opposite arm	Turns steering wheel

tance, the experience and enthusiasm of the occupational therapist. The training experience is most effective if the same therapist remains with the amputee throughout the entire process.

It is extremely important to emphasize to the unilateral amputee that the prosthesis will usually play a nondominant role, supplementing the function of the opposite hand. The prosthetic terminal device is most useful for gross prehension activities and to hold and stabilize objects while the opposite hand performs fine motor prehension activities. The prosthesis should be expected to assume no more than 30% of the total function of the task in bilateral upper limb activities, with the opposite arm and hand always dominant.

The amputee who has lost an arm or hand will quickly develop techniques to accomplish tasks unilaterally, and these habits will be difficult to break. It is therefore essential to fit the unilateral amputee within 1 to 2 months of the amputation whenever possible. These individuals definitely show a greater propensity for wearing and successfully using their prostheses. This applies to all amputees, whether fitted with body-powered or electric components. Bilateral skills will be encouraged, self-image is often enhanced, and functional independence is frequently restored.

Training should address activities of daily living that are useful and purposeful. Activities such as cutting food, using scissors, getting dressed, opening a jar or bottle, washing dishes, hammering a nail and using other tools, and driving a car should be practiced so that the amputee will automatically use the prosthesis when encountering the same activity in daily life.

The therapist should review a list of bilateral activities of daily living with the amputee to determine which tasks are the most important for that individual. These are the activities to focus on, stressing throughout the activity that the prosthesis is used to assist the opposite hand. The bilateral activities listed in Tables 2 and 3 are good examples to review and practice. Table 2 describes how activities would be accomplished using a body-powered prosthesis. Table 3 lists similar activities as they would be performed using a myoelectric hand. Several activities are also shown in Figure 5.

With practice, these activities and many others improve and ultimately become automatic. It is extremely important to reinforce and emphasize the fact that activities involving water, including bathing and grooming activities, must be done without a myoelectric hand because of the damaging effects of water on the electric motor and battery. The therapist should also advise myoelectric hand users against subjecting the myoelectric component to excessive vibration, sand, dirt, or the extremes of heat and cold. These too can seriously impair the electronic components.

TABLE 3 Roles of Myoelectric Hand and Opposite Hand in Bilateral Activities of Daily Living

Activity	Myoelectric Hand	Opposite Hand
Opening a jar	Holds the jar	Turns the lid
Tying shoelaces	Holds one shoelace to stabilize	Performs the tying
Using knife and fork	Holds fork to stabilize	Holds knife to cut
Holding a tray	Picks up and releases item	Holds tray
Opening a tube of toothpaste	Holds the tube	Turns the cap
Stirring substance in a bowl	Holds bowl with a strong grip	Holds mixing spoon/fork
Cutting fruit or vegetables	Holds the fruit or vegetable firmly	Holds the knife to cut
Using scissors to cut paper	Holds the paper to be cut	Uses scissors normally
Zipping a jacket from the bottom up	Holds the anchor tab	Manipulates the pull tab at the base and pulls upward
Buckling a belt	Holds buckle end of belt to stabilize it	Manipulates the long end of the belt into the buckle
Donning socks	Holds one side of sock	Holds other side of sock and pulls upward

The importance of correct prepositioning cannot be overemphasized. As a rule, most difficulties in prosthetic use are a result of improper positioning.

A valuable and comprehensive guide to the specifics of training the amputee is found in the classic *Manual of Upper Extremity Prosthetics*.[7]

Vocational and Leisure Activities

Discussing vocational needs and expectations with the amputee is very important. Unfortunately, this is an area that is often overlooked or given only brief attention during the rehabilitation process. This discussion should occur later in the training continuum, when the amputee begins to acknowledge and accept the disability. Although not everyone can return to the exact job held prior to the injury, a review of job responsibilities and expectations can be explored with the therapist. It may be possible to break down the tasks of a job into steps that can be practiced and reinforced in therapy. If the therapist can do an on-the-job site evaluation, it would be a valuable addition to the amputee's comprehensive rehabilitation. If changes and adjustments to the work environment are necessary, the therapist could advise in these modifications.

Recreational and leisure activities are also important to discuss at this time. These activities contribute greatly to an individual's physical and psychological well-being.

Home Instructions

At the conclusion of training, home instructions that include a wearing schedule and prostheses care should be reviewed with the patient and the family. A follow-up appointment should also be made at this time, as well as a list of the rehabilitation team members and their telephone numbers, which will enable the patient to contact the appropriate person when problems arise.[8]

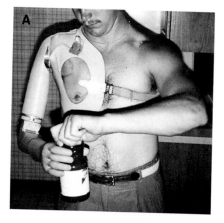
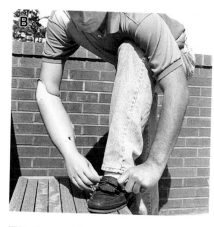
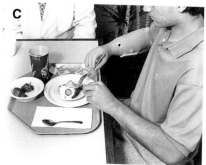
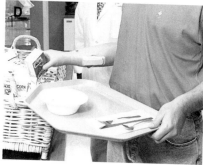

Figure 5 Activities of daily living performed with a myoelectric hand. **A,** To open a jar, the myoelectric hand holds the jar and the sound hand turns the lid. **B,** When tying shoelaces, the myoelectric hand stabilizes and holds, while the opposite hand maneuvers the laces. **C,** The myoelectric hand holds the fork to stabilize the food while the opposite hand holds the knife. **D,** The sound hand is used to hold a tray, and the myoelectric hand can grasp and release items.

Summary

The rehabilitation of a person with upper limb loss can be both challenging and rewarding. Especially in instances of higher level and bilateral amputations, significant training and expertise on the part of the rehabilitation team is essential.

The potential of the person with an amputation is limitless. Amputees have been able to accomplish activities that never would have been expected. The success of a rehabilitation effort does not rest solely on the quality of training to use a prosthesis but is closely intertwined with the quality of the medical management, the quality and fit of the prosthesis, functional training, and conscientious follow-up with the amputee once the rehabilitation phase is complete. Follow-up is critically important and is often overlooked. Perhaps the most important aspect of a successful rehabilitation program, however, is the motivation and the desire of the person with an amputation to become independent. This pivotal ingredient should be cultivated and reinforced by the members of the rehabilitation team. The impact the treatment team makes during this important process will remain with the patient for life.

References

1. Bennett JB, Alexander CB: Amputation levels and surgical techniques, in Atkins DJ, Meier RH III (eds): *Comprehensive Management of the Upper-Limb Amputee.* New York, NY, Springer-Verlag, 1989, pp 1-10.

2. Atkins DJ: Postoperative and preprosthetic therapy programs, in Atkins DJ, Meier RH III (eds): *Comprehensive Management of the Upper-Limb Amputee.* New York, NY, Springer-Verlag, 1989, pp 11-15.

3. Meier RH III: Amputations and prosthetic fitting, in Fisher SV, Helm PA (eds): *Comprehensive Rehabilitation of Burns*. Baltimore, MD, Williams & Wilkins, 1984, pp 267-310.

4. Malone JM, Fleming LL, Robertson J, et al: Immediate, early, and late post-surgical management of upper-limb amputation. *J Rehabil Res Dev* 1984;21:33-41.

5. Atkins DJ: Adult upper-limb prosthetic training, in Atkins DJ, Meier RH III (eds): *Comprehensive Management of the Upper-Limb Amputee*. New York, NY, Springer-Verlag, 1989, pp 39-59.

6. Atkins D: Managing self-care in adults with upper extremity amputations, in Christiansen C (ed): *Ways of Living: Self-Care Strategies for Special Needs*, ed 2. Bethesda, MD, American Occupational Therapy Association, 2000, pp 221-230.

7. Santschi W, Winston M (eds): *Manual of Upper Extremity Prosthetics*, ed 2. Los Angeles, CA, University of California at Los Angeles, 1958.

8. Atkins D: Adult upper limb prosthetic training, in Bowker JH, Michael JW (eds): *Atlas of Limb Prosthetics: Surgical, Prosthetic, and Rehabilitation Principles*, ed 2. Rosemont, IL, American Academy of Orthopaedic Surgeons, 2002, pp 277-291. (Originally published by Mosby-Year Book, 1992.)

Chapter 23

Brachial Plexus Injuries: Surgical and Prosthetic Management

Alexander Y. Shin, MD
Allen T. Bishop, MD
John W. Michael, MEd, CPO

Introduction

Injuries to the brachial plexus can result from a variety of etiologies, including birth injuries, penetrating injuries, falls, and motor vehicle trauma. Closed injuries produce most brachial plexus injuries and are often the result of traction, compression, or a combination of both. Traction injuries occur when the head and neck are violently moved away from the ipsilateral shoulder, often resulting in an injury to the C5-C6 nerve roots, or the upper trunk. Traction to the brachial plexus can result from a violent arm movement. When the arm is abducted over the head with significant force, traction will occur within the lower elements of the brachial plexus (C8-T1 roots or lower trunk). Compression injuries to the brachial plexus can occur between the clavicle and the first rib; these injuries may be secondary to expanding hematomas or malignancies.

Although it is difficult to ascertain the number of brachial plexus injuries that occur annually, the incidence continues to increase with the advent of more extreme sporting activities, more powerful motor sports, and the increasing number of survivors of high-speed motor vehicle accidents (attributed to the use of airbags).[1-9] Most patients with these injuries are males between 15 and 25 years of age.[1,8,10,11] Narakas[12] proposed the "law of seven 70s" to describe the types and mechanisms of injury to the plexus. Based on more than 18 years of experience with more than 1,000 patients with plexus injuries, Narakas estimated that 70% of traumatic brachial plexus injuries are secondary to motor vehicle accidents. Approximately 70% of these motor vehicle accidents involve either motorcycles or bicycles. Of the cycle riders, 70% have multiple injuries. Overall, 70% of patients with brachial plexus injuries have supraclavicular lesions, and of those with supraclavicular lesions, 70% have at least one root avulsed. Of patients who have a root avulsion, at least 70% have avulsions of the lower roots (C7, C8, or T1). Finally, of patients with a lower root avulsion, nearly 70% will experience persistent pain.

Clinical Evaluation

Evaluation of brachial plexus injuries often occurs after acute life-threatening injuries are treated. A thorough physical examination is necessary to determine if the lesion is (1) preganglionic, in which the root is avulsed directly from the spinal cord proximal to the dorsal root ganglion, or (2) postganglionic, in which the root is avulsed or otherwise injured distal to the dorsal root ganglion within the trunk, divisions, cords, or terminal branches. The differences between these lesions have significant prognostic and therapeutic implications. With a preganglionic injury, avulsion of the nerve root has occurred proximal to the spinal root ganglion; there is complete motor and sensory loss in the involved root and denervation of the deep paraspinal muscles of the neck (Figure 1). Several specific clinical findings are pathognomonic for nerve root avulsions associated with brachial plexus injuries: (1) Rhomboid paralysis indicates a C5 nerve root avulsion; (2) serratus anterior paralysis is consistent with avulsion of C5 through C7 nerve roots, and (3) Horner's syndrome (ptosis, miosis, and anhidrosis) is pathognomonic for C8-T1 avulsions (Figure 2). Postganglionic injuries occur distal to the spinal ganglia and have a more favorable prognosis than preganglionic injuries, both in terms of spontaneous recovery and outcomes of surgical reconstruction.

History of Treating Brachial Plexus Injuries

Treatment recommendations for complete root avulsions have varied widely over the past 50 years, and outcomes have ranged from fair to dismal. Just after World War II, the standard approach was surgical reconstruction consisting of shoulder fusion, elbow bone block, and finger tenodesis.[13] In the 1960s, transhumeral amputation combined with shoulder fusion in slight abduction

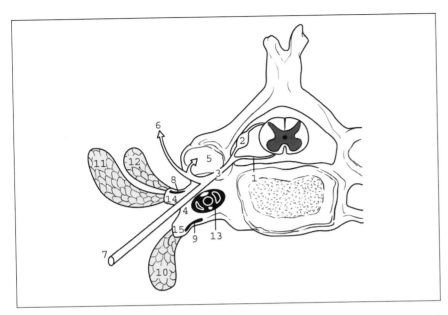

Figure 1 Horizontal cross section of a typical cervical vertebra showing the anatomy of the intervertebral foramen. 1, Anterior spinal root. 2, Posterior spinal root with dorsal root ganglion. 3, Spinal nerve. 4, Transverse process. 5, Articular facet. 6, Posterior branch of spinal nerve. 7, Anterior branch of spinal nerve (plexus root). 8, Posterior transversarius muscle. 9, Anterior transversarius muscle. 10, Anterior scalenus muscle. 11, Middle scalenus muscle. 12, Posterior scalenus muscle. 13, Vertebral pedicle. 14, Posterior tubercle of transverse process. 15, Anterior tubercle of transverse process. Preganglionic injuries occur proximal to 2, the dorsal root ganglion. Injuries distal to this are considered postganglionic. *(Adapted with permission from Herzberg G, Narakas A, Comtet JJ: Surgical approach of the brachial plexus roots, in Alnot JY, Narakas A (eds): Traumatic Brachial Plexus Injuries. Paris, France, Expansion Scientifique, 1996, pp 19-22.)*

and flexion was advocated.[14] The classic article of Yeoman and Seddon[15] noted the tendency for patients to become "one-handed" within 2 years of injury, a clinical outcome deemed unsatisfactory. They reported the lack of good results from the primitive surgical reconstruction of that era; however, outcomes were predominantly good or fair when amputation with shoulder fusion was performed within 24 months of injury. The authors also noted that the loss of glenohumeral motion caused by injury to the suprascapular and axillary nerves limited the effectiveness of body-powered devices and that manual laborers seemed to accept hook prostheses much more readily than did office workers with similar injuries. Although these observations remain valid today, recent advances in brachial plexus reconstruction have produced clinical outcomes superior to those reviewed by Yeoman and Seddon. A better understanding of

the pathophysiology of nerve injury and repair, as well as the recent advances in microsurgical techniques, has allowed reliable restoration of elbow flexion and can provide useful primitive prehension of the hand. Current advances in brachial plexus reconstruction, especially the microvascular reconstructive procedures, as well as the prosthetic/orthotic advances, are the focus of this chapter.

Current Concepts of Surgical Management

The two most important concepts in the surgical management of brachial plexus injuries are (1) the priority of restoring upper arm function, and (2) the implications and timing of surgical reconstruction. The highest priority in restoring the flail extremity is elbow flexion, followed by

shoulder abduction, hand sensibility, wrist extension and finger flexion, and intrinsic function of the hand.

Timing of reconstruction or intervention depends on the mechanism of injury and the type of injury. Immediate exploration and primary repair of the injured portion of the brachial plexus are indicated for sharp, open injuries. If the open injury occurred secondary to impact from a blunt object, the ends of the lacerated nerve should be tagged and addressed 3 to 4 weeks later to excise the zone of nerve injury and place an interposition nerve graft. Patients with gunshot wounds should be observed because most of these injuries are neurapraxic. Early exploration and reconstruction (between 3 and 6 weeks after injury) is indicated in patients with gunshot wounds when there is a high suspicion of root avulsion. Routine exploration (between 3 and 6 months after injury) is typically performed in patients who have partial injuries and partial paralysis in which there is a suspicion of root avulsion. Delayed exploration occurs 6 months after the injury, whereas late exploration occurs after 12 months. Delayed or late surgery often precludes successful direct repair or neurotization because nerve regeneration to the target muscles requires more time than the motor end plate can survive after denervation.

Ideally, electrodiagnostic evaluation should be performed by 3 to 4 weeks after injury, followed by CT myelography to evaluate the status of the cervical roots. The role of MRI in this context continues to evolve; currently, it is considered best for visualizing the dorsal and ventral rootlets but has been less accurate than CT myelography in identifying root avulsion.[16-18] We prefer CT myelography because it appears to be the most sensitive and specific test to identify root avulsion injuries (Figure 3). Consultation with a pain management team and a physical therapist for the hand should be initiated as soon as possible after the injury to address the severe neuritic pain and to prevent joint contractures.[12,15,19-28]

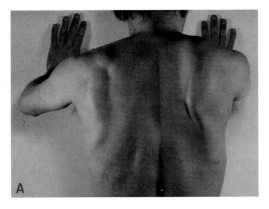
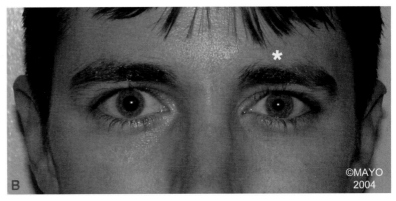

Figure 2 A, Scapular winging is indicative of C5 through C7 root avulsions. **B,** Horner's syndrome (ptosis, miosis, and anhidrosis) is pathognomonic for a C8-T1 avulsion injury. *(Reproduced from the Mayo Foundation, Rochester, MN.)*

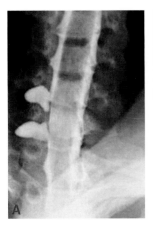
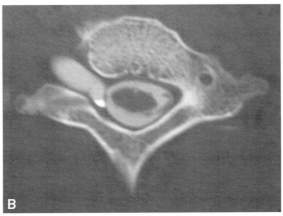

Figure 3 Myelography remains the most sensitive and specific method of detecting root avulsions. **A,** The formation of pseudomeningomyeloceles at C8 and T1 are pathognomonic for root avulsions. **B,** CT myelography further delineates the injury.

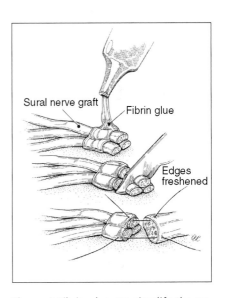

Figure 4 Fibrin glue can simplify the approximation of multiple strands of nerve graft by creating a single large nerve stump when several graft strands are glued together. The graft ends are freshened, and the mass is then coapted to the recipient nerve with several epineurium sutures. *(Reproduced with permission from Hentz VR: Microneural reconstruction of the brachial plexus, in Green DP, Hotchkiss RN (eds): Green's Hand Surgery. Philadelphia, PA, Churchill Livingstone, 1993, pp 1223-1252. Illustration by Elizabeth Roselius,© 1993.)*

Treatment

Surgical treatment of brachial plexus injuries falls into several broad categories, including primary nerve repair, interposition nerve cable grafting, tendon transfers, neurotization, and free-functioning muscle transfers. Tendon transfers should be delayed until evidence shows that further recovery is unlikely. Primary repair is indicated for patients with acute, sharp lacerations. Interposition nerve cable grafting is indicated for those with postganglionic injuries that are less than 6 months old. With neurotization, function is restored by transfer of a functional but less important nerve to a nonfunctioning but more important denervated nerve. Neurotization is indicated for patients with either pre- or postganglionic lesions that have been present for less than 6 months. With a free-functioning muscle transfer, a muscle and its neurovascular pedicle are transplanted to a new location and the motor nerve is neurotized with a functioning motor nerve. Free-functioning muscle transfers are indicated in delayed (3 to 6 months after injury) or late (more than 12 months after injury) presentations.

Nerve Grafts

Sources of donor nerve grafts include the sural nerves, ipsilateral cutaneous nerves, lateral cutaneous nerves of the thigh, saphenous nerve, and the ulnar nerve (if C8 and T1 are avulsed). The size mismatch between the plexus and the individual nerve often requires that multiple strands of bundled nerves be used. These nerve segments may be cabled together with fibrin glue and then sewn in place (Figure 4). In patients with complete avulsions, the ulnar nerve can be harvested as a vascularized nerve graft based on the superior collateral ulnar artery and then effectively used as a free vascularized interposition nerve graft from neurotization sources to the median nerve (Figure 5).

Neurotization

Intercostal nerves can be harvested from the third, fourth, fifth, and sixth ribs and effectively used to provide motor nerves to targeted muscles or sensation to injured sensory nerves.[15,29-36] Each intercostal nerve has a motor and sensory branch and can be easily harvested and neurotized to the target nerves (Figure 6). Each intercostal nerve contains about 1,300 myelinated axons. Thus, two or three intercostal nerves are typically used together. Occasionally, the intercostal nerves require elongation with a nerve graft because the distance to reach the target nerve or muscle is too long. The greatest disadvantage to using a nerve graft is that two lines of coaptation need to be crossed by regenerating nerve fibers. The advantage of using a nerve graft is that the intercostal nerves can be transected more proximally, where the number of motor fibers is greater.

The spinal accessory nerve (cranial nerve XI) can also be used as a donor nerve.[2,7,8,29,32-43] The terminal branch of the spinal accessory nerve can be easily harvested and has about 1,700 myelinated axons. Thus, the spinal accessory nerve is an excellent donor nerve for the suprascapular or axillary nerve to restore shoulder stability or to neurotize a free-functioning muscle transfer (Figure 7).

The ipsilateral phrenic nerve can be used; however, before its use, diaphragmatic and pulmonary function must be assessed.[29,34,35] Hemidiaphragmatic paralysis is an absolute contraindication for phrenic neurotization. Patients with severe chest injury or multiple fractured ribs require careful evaluation of pulmonary function because harvest of the ipsilateral phrenic nerve can further jeopardize pulmonary function. Simultaneous harvesting of intercostal and phrenic nerves restricts pulmonary function in the early postoperative period.[44] Harvest of the phrenic nerve is also contraindicated in young in-

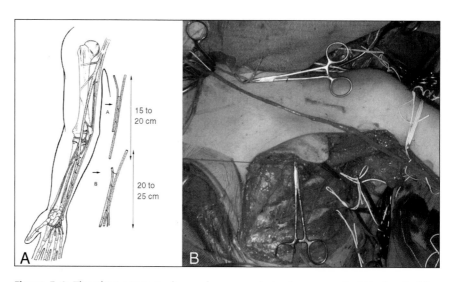

Figure 5 A, The ulnar nerve can be used as a vascularized nerve graft at the level of the arm (vascularized by the ulnar medial inferior pedicle) or at the forearm (vascularized by the ulnar artery). *(Reproduced with permission from Lebreten E, Oberline CH, Alnot JY: The ulnar nerve at the arm and forearm, in Alnot JY, Narakas A (eds):* Traumatic Brachial Plexus Injuries. *Paris, France, Expansion Scientifique, 1996, pp 28-32.)* **B,** A clinical example of a vascularized ulnar nerve graft coapting the contralateral C7 root to the median nerve.

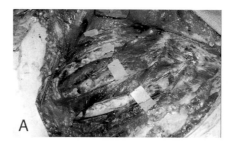

Figure 6 A, Intercostal nerves can be isolated from the inferior portion of the ribs and harvested from the costochondral margin to the midaxillary line. **B,** Each intercostal nerve contains sensory and motor components that can be easily identified with a nerve stimulator and separated for neurotization into muscles and sensory nerves.

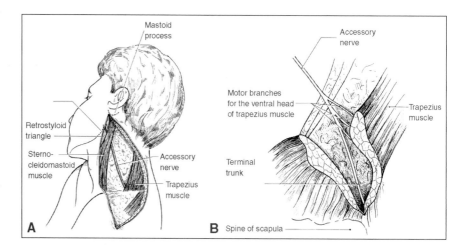

Figure 7 A, The spinal accessory nerve (cranial nerve XI) is a pure motor nerve that can provide about 1,700 myelinated fibers. **B,** The first and second motor branches are typically preserved, and the terminal branch is used for plexus neurotization. *(Reproduced with permission from Alnot JY, Overline CH: Nerves available for neurotization, in Alnot JY, Narakas A (eds):* Traumatic Brachial Plexus Injuries. *Paris, France, Expansion Scientifique, 1996, pp 31-38.)*

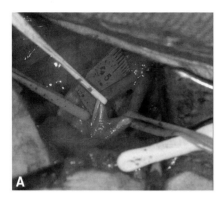 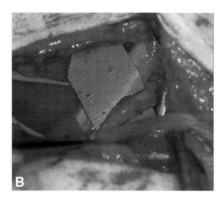

Figure 8 The contralateral C7 root can be harvested with little or no functional deficit in the donor arm. We prefer to use the anterior half of the C7 root (white vessel loop) **(A)** and use a vascularized ulnar nerve graft as the conduit to the median nerve **(B)**.

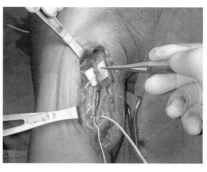

Figure 9 Transferring a portion of an ipsilateral functioning ulnar nerve to the musculocutaneous nerve to provide biceps function. Several fascicles of the ulnar motor nerves are identified and transferred to the musculocutaneous nerve. The ulnar nerve is identified by the vessel loop, and the ulnar nerve to the musculocutaneous nerve is neurotized by these fascicles.

fants and in patients with any diaphragm paralysis. The phrenic nerve is best suited for neurotization of the suprascapular nerve.

Uninjured contralateral C7 root used as donor nerve was first described by Gu and associates[45] in 1992, and by Chuang and associates[46] in 1993. This procedure, however, remains controversial. Based on available reports, transection of the uninjured contralateral C7 root does not result in significant loss of function. By elongating the contralateral C7 root with a vascularized ulnar nerve graft to the ipsilateral median nerve, the contralateral C7 root can be used to neurotize the median nerve or lateral cord. Reduced morbidity has been reported when the anterosuperior portion of C7 is used rather than the entire contralateral C7 root[47] (Figure 8). Donor site morbidity is minimal, initially resulting in paresthesia in the digits affected by the C7 nerve root and mild weakness of pectoralis, triceps, and/or wrist extension.[46-48] The functional loss is typically limited to reduced sensibility in the index finger and some reduced force of the triceps and finger extension. Both the paresthesia and motor weakness diminish during a period of 3 to 6 months.

Oberlin and associates[49,50] described the use of portions of a functioning ipsilateral nerve. In patients with loss of the musculocutaneous nerve, but with preserved ulnar nerve

function (ie, patients with upper trunk injuries or C5-C6 avulsions), several fascicles of the ulnar motor nerves can be transferred to the biceps motor branch of the musculocutaneous nerve at the midhumeral level without significant loss of distal motor or sensory function to the muscles of the hand that are mediated by the ulnar nerve (Figure 9). This transfer is possible because individual ulnar nerve fascicles are mixed at this level, consisting of extrinsic and intrinsic motor fibers as well as sensory fibers. The results are excellent, and donor site morbidity is very low.

Other sources for donor nerves for neurotization include the cervical plexus, the long thoracic nerve, the hypoglossal nerve, and nerve root stumps of postganglionic avulsions at the root-trunk level.

Free-functioning Muscle Transfer

Advances in microsurgical techniques have led to innovations in surgical reconstruction of the upper extremity following brachial plexus injury. Reinnervation of the biceps and shoulder musculature using a combination of nerve grafting and neurotization techniques has resulted in reliable restoration of elbow flexion and shoulder abduction when surgical intervention occurs within 6 to 9 months of injury.[29,30,33,36,46,51-57] In many instances, however, delay in treatment or complete avulsion of the

brachial plexus limits the options for surgical reconstruction.

Free-functioning muscle transfer involves moving a muscle and its motor nerve to a donor site. The number of available extraplexal donor nerves is limited, and the timing of reconstructive procedures is critical. Despite favorable reports of early nerve grafting and transfer techniques, attempts to restore function to long-standing denervated muscle are usually unsuccessful.[30,54,56,57] This lack of success has resulted in free-functioning muscle transfers to be used in conjunction with extraplexal motor nerve transfer to restore function for patients with brachial plexus avulsions or when the time from injury to surgery is longer than 6 months to 1 year.[8,41,58-62] Free-functioning muscle transfers provide reliable elbow flexion when a delay in treatment prevents direct graft or biceps neurotization and proximal muscle strength is insufficient to allow tendon transfers.[8,42,52,58,59,63] With this procedure, circulation in the transferred muscle is restored with microsurgical technique, vessels are anastomosed, and the motor nerve is neurotized with one of the nerves described above. Within several months, the transferred muscle becomes innervated and is reinner-

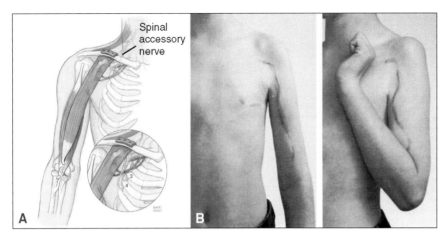

Figure 10 A, If more than 6 months have passed since the time of injury, the fibrotic and denervated biceps is replaced with a free-functioning gracilis muscle that is neurotized by the intercostal nerves. *(Reproduced from the Mayo Foundation, Rochester, MN.)* **B,** This approach can predictably restore elbow function.

vated by the donor nerve. Eventually, the transferred muscle functions independently. A variety of muscles and nerves can be transferred, including the latissimus dorsi with the thoracodorsal nerve, the rectus femoris with the femoral nerve, and the gracilis with the anterior division of the obturator nerve. The gracilis has become one of the most commonly used muscles in brachial plexus reconstruction because of (1) its proximally based muscle neurovascular pedicle, which allows earlier reinnervation, and (2) its length, which can extend into the forearm for hand reanimation. The gracilis can be used to restore biceps function, especially if there is a delay in treatment[39,40] (Figure 10), or as a double-muscle transfer in the novel and revolutionary Doi procedure to restore elbow flexion, wrist extension, and finger flexion in the acute setting.[7,8,64]

Treatment Based on Level of Injury

Pure injuries to the brachial plexus as described below rarely occur. More commonly, injury occurs at more than one level, and patients typically have a combination of pre- and post-

ganglionic injury.[19] Nonetheless, it is instructive to describe the treatment options by pattern of injury.

Preganglionic Injuries

C5-C6

In the C5-C6 preganglionic lesion, there is loss of elbow flexion as well as shoulder abduction. The main goal of treatment is to restore elbow flexion and provide shoulder stability and abduction. Several treatment options can be pursued in injuries less than 6 months old. One option is neurotization of the musculocutaneous motor branch and suprascapular nerve with intercostal nerves (typically two to three nerves) and the terminal branch of the spinal accessory nerve (cranial nerve XI), respectively. Use of the sensory portion of the intercostal nerves with neurotization to lateral cord contribution to the median nerve can provide sensation to the hand. Another option is to perform an Oberlin transfer of motor fascicles of the ulnar nerve to the motor branch of the musculocutaneous nerve and the spinal accessory nerve to the suprascapular nerve. In the late or delayed presentation (more than 12 months), elbow flexion can be restored by a free-functioning single gracilis transfer neurotized by the spi-

nal accessory nerve or intercostal nerves. Shoulder fusion can be pursued later if the shoulder becomes problematic.

C5 through C7

Injuries involving the C5 through C7 nerve roots add radial palsy to the clinical picture presented above. Not only does the sensory loss in the hand increase but all active extension at the wrist, hand, and fingers is lost as well. Neurotization of the posterior cord can be helpful to restore wrist extension; however, restoring elbow flexion and shoulder function remains the priority. If there are not enough donor nerves to neurotize the posterior cord, either a static or spring-assisted wrist, hand, and finger extension can be added to the previous orthosis.[27]

C8-T1

Injuries involving the C8-Tl nerve roots are generally associated with good shoulder and elbow function but loss of finger flexor, extensor, and intrinsic function. Surgical exploration of the plexus at this level is often futile because the nerve roots are often so avulsed that they cannot be repaired. Treatment of injuries at this level remains controversial because restoration of intrinsic function of the hand remains untenable. In these situations, the great distance and time the nerve has to regenerate to reach the intrinsic muscles appears to exceed the survivability of the motor end plates. However, intercostal neurotization to the ulnar nerve has been reported to achieve grade III motor recovery.[31]

Surgical reconstruction by tendon transfers is often especially successful in these patients and can restore significant function. Patients who sustain a concomitant traumatic transradial amputation should be able to operate a body-powered or switch-controlled terminal device. Loss of forearm innervation eliminates myoelectric control sites below the elbow. Patients with C8-Tl type injuries have the best chance of orthotic success because motor loss, not sensory loss, is significant. Although the finger flexors and intrinsics are paralyzed, sensory loss is limited to the ring and small fingers, neither of which are involved in pinch prehension.

Complete Plexus Injury

The complete plexus type injury has the greatest loss of function. Not only is the arm totally flail and anesthetic but chronic pain is also frequently present. Prior to the advances of brachial plexus surgery during the past decade, these patients had the lowest long-term success rate, regardless of treatment. Historically, these patients were relegated to transhumeral amputation plus shoulder fusion and a prosthesis.[11,13,15,19,25,27,28,65] Outcomes for this group have greatly improved, however, with more complex neurotizations, the ability to use extraplexal nerve sources (phrenic, contralateral C7), and free-functioning muscle transfers.[8,29,33,35,46-48,57] In this group of patients, the smallest gains in function make significant improvements in clinical outcome.

In complete avulsion of the plexus (C5 through C8, T1), the main goal of surgery is to restore elbow function, followed by shoulder abduction. Within 6 months of injury, and barring any intraplexal nerve injury, several neurotization plans can be pursued. One basic approach with limited goals of shoulder stability and abduction with elbow flexion is the neurotization of the suprascapular nerve with the spinal accessory nerve and the musculocutaneous motor nerve with intercostal nerves. Adding a hemi-cross C7 neurotization extended by a vascularized ulnar nerve graft to the median nerve provides potential wrist and finger flexion and sensibility in the median nerve distribution. Alternatively, the neurotization of the suprascapular nerve with the phrenic nerve, spinal accessory nerve to the musculocutaneous motor nerve (elongated with a sural nerve graft), and neurotization of the intercostal nerves to the median nerve can be performed.

The use of a double free-functioning gracilis muscle transfer described by Doi and associates[8] has given the hope of prehension to patients with complete plexus lesions. The goals of this two-stage operation are to restore elbow flexion and extension, as well as wrist extension and finger flexion. In the first stage, the plexus is explored and a free-functioning gracilis is harvested and neurotized by the spinal accessory nerve (Figure 11). The gracilis is attached proximally to the clavicle and it is routed distally under the brachioradialis and flexor carpi ulnaris pulley to the radial wrist or finger extensors. The vascular anastomoses are to the thoracoacromial artery and venae comitantes. The suprascapular nerve can be neurotized with the accessory phrenic nerve, if present (as in 25% to 38% of patients). Approximately 2 to 3 months later, the second stage is performed (Figure 12). The second gracilis is harvested and the motor and sensory intercostal nerves from ribs three through six are harvested. The gracilis is attached proximally to the second rib and is routed subcutaneously along the medial side of the arm and attached to the flexor tendons. Then, it is neurotized with two of the motor intercostal nerves. The sensory intercostal nerves are neurotized to the median nerve to provide palmar sensation. The transferred gracilis is vascularized by the thoracodorsal vessels. The remaining two motor intercostal nerves are neurotized to the radial nerve innervating the triceps.

We have slightly modified the double free-functioning muscle transfer originally described by Doi and associates.[7,8,40-42,59,60,64,66] In the first stage, we secure the gracilis muscle to the wrist extensors as opposed to finger extensors; we believe that this helps promote finger flexion through a tenodesis effect. In addition, we have altered the route of the first gracilis muscle transfer to create a more effective pulley at the elbow using the flexor carpi ulnaris muscle. When the brachioradialis muscle is used to cre-

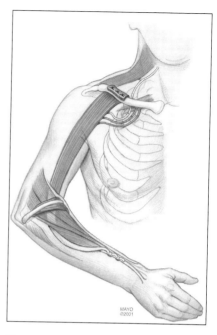

Figure 11 Reanimation of the complete brachial plexopathy. In this two-stage procedure, the first stage involves exploration of the plexus and a free-functioning muscle transfer for elbow flexion and wrist extension. The contralateral gracilis is harvested along with its motor nerve. The proximal end of the gracilis is secured to the lateral clavicle, and the artery and vein are anastomosed to the thoracoacromial vessels. The gracilis is neurotized by the spinal accessory nerve (cranial nerve XI). The distal tendon portion of the gracilis is placed under the brachioradialis and is woven into the radial wrist extensors. *(Reproduced from the Mayo Foundation, Rochester, MN.)*

ate an elbow pulley, bowstringing of the first gracilis muscle transfer at the elbow gradually occurs, limiting strength and motion, resulting in an elbow flexion contracture. We detach the distal portion of the flexor carpi ulnaris and create a pulley at the level of the proximal forearm as described by the late David Khoo, MD (personal communication, 1996) (Figure 13). This technique creates a more effective pulley and should improve muscle excursion and strengthen wrist extension.

When transferred for elbow flexion, the major vascular pedicle should be placed in proximity to the thoracoacromial trunk in the infraclavicular fossa. To do so, the proximal graci-

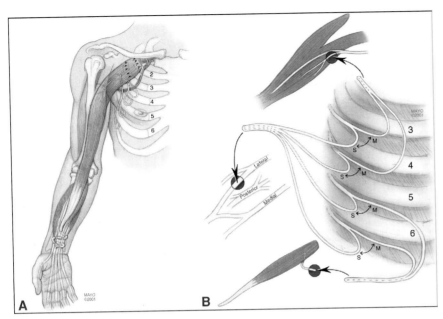

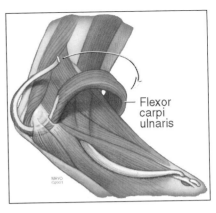

Figure 12 The second stage of the double free-functioning muscle transfer is performed 6 to 8 weeks later and involves harvest of the second ipsilateral gracilis. **A,** The proximal end of the gracilis is secured to the lateral aspect of the second rib, and the vessels are anastomosed to the thoracodorsal vessels. The intercostal nerves from ribs three through six are harvested, and the motor and sensory branches are separated. The motor intercostal nerves from ribs three and four are neurotized into the motor branch for the triceps muscle, and the motor nerves from ribs five and six are neurotized into the free gracilis muscle. **B,** The sensory intercostal nerves are then neurotized into the lateral cord contribution to the median nerve. The gracilis is tunneled under the medial aspect of the arm, and the tendon is woven into the flexor digitorum profundus and flexor pollicis longus tendons. M = motor intercostal nerve, S = sensory intercostal nerve. *(Reproduced from the Mayo Foundation, Rochester, MN.)*

Figure 13 When the brachioradialis muscle is used to create an elbow pulley, bowstringing of the first gracilis muscle transfer at the elbow gradually occurs, thus limiting strength and motion and resulting in an elbow flexion contracture. To create a more effective pulley, the distal portion of the flexor carpi ulnaris is detached and a pulley is created at the level of the proximal forearm. *(Reproduced from the Mayo Foundation, Rochester, MN.)*

lis tendon is passed beneath the clavicle and secured to its superior border. It is tunneled subcutaneously to the antecubital fossa, where it is later secured to the biceps tendon. The obturator nerve branch to the gracilis may be repaired to the spinal accessory nerve or to two intercostal motor nerves, either of which should be harvested if possible to allow direct nerve repair distal to the clavicle.

We recently reported the results of single free-muscle transfers performed at our institution.[67] Of 15 patients who underwent these transfers, 14 had recovered at least M3 strength based on more than 1-year follow-up. Of these 14 patients, all but one had an arc of motion of 90° or greater and could support a 2-kg weight. The transfer of two free-functioning gracilis muscle grafts, combined with nerve transfers for triceps function and hand sensibility, is a demanding

reconstructive effort performed in two separate, lengthy surgical procedures. When performed soon after injury in patients with avulsions of four or five nerve roots, this procedure offers the possibility of hand grasp and release, sensory recovery in the hand, and active elbow flexion and extension.

Using a double free-muscle transfer, Doi and associates[8] were able to restore good to excellent elbow flexion in 96% of their patients. In our experience, eight patients have had at least 1 year of follow-up after the second-stage transfer. Transfer for combined elbow flexion and wrist extension lowered the percentage of patients achieving ≥ M4 elbow flexion strength compared with elbow flexion alone. In our patients, 79% of the free-functioning muscle transfers for elbow flexion alone (single transfer) and 63% of similarly innervated mus-

cles transferred for combined motion (first stage of the Doi procedure) achieved ≥ M4 elbow flexion strength ($P > 0.05$). This result is not surprising in that the muscles must use some of their strength and excursion to extend the wrist or digits and invariably lose some effect because of bowstringing at the elbow.

Grasp function after the double free-muscle procedure relies on recovery of some triceps function to stabilize the elbow during contraction of the gracilis muscle. Thus, this procedure is most successful in patients with adequate muscle strength and absence of significant adhesions. In the series by Doi and associates,[8] 65% of patients achieved more than 30° of total active motion of the fingers with the second muscle transfer. Such function allows only rudimentary grasp in many patients. Grasp function, however, is difficult to achieve with other methods. Previous efforts at restoring prehension in patients with a brachial plexus injury have been unsuccessful because of the long length of nerve that must be repaired and the prolonged time of reinnervation; this combination may exceed the time that the injured motor end plates will survive. Therefore, these results must still be regarded as a significant advance in these otherwise irreparable avulsion injuries. Our experience is nearly identical to that of Doi. Five of eight of our patients recovered at least 30° of total active digit motion. Two of the remaining three patients lost the gracilis muscle because of venous thrombosis soon after surgery. Currently, the only other alternative that offers the possibility of hand function after root avulsion injuries is the contralateral C7 nerve root used in combination with a vascularized ulnar nerve conduit.

Postganglionic Injuries

Postganglionic plexus injuries that have been present for less than 6 months should be treated with interposition cable grafting or selective neurotization if possible. These injuries are often found concomitantly with preganglionic injuries and thus treatment with a combination of neurotization and cable grafting is required. The use of intraoperative somatosensory evoked potentials will allow the surgeon to determine if the proximal portion of the avulsed nerve is in continuity with the spinal cord; in this situation, intraplexal nerve grafting is the treatment of choice. If the proximal portion of the avulsed nerve is not in continuity with the spinal cord, neurotization or free muscle transfers can be performed.

Other Considerations

To successfully use the hand, the shoulder must be stable to allow positioning of the hand and forearm in space. In most patients with brachial plexus injuries, the remaining muscles are insufficient for successful tendon transfer about the shoulder. Tendon transfer of the trapezius and the levator scapulae has been attempted in patients with upper brachial plexus injuries in which rotator cuff, deltoid, and biceps function has been lost.[68] Although the shoulder will no longer subluxate inferiorly, active function in

forward flexion and abduction is not generally possible. Thus, most of these patients would benefit from shoulder fusion. Shoulder fusion works best when scapular control has been preserved through adequate function of the serratus anterior and the trapezius muscles.[69] Occupation is also a factor. Employment as a manual laborer, for example, suggests that shoulder fusion should be considered. Many patients, however, are best served by leaving the shoulder in its flail condition if they do not report pain from chronic traction and their occupation makes a mobile flail shoulder more cosmetically acceptable than a fused shoulder.

Orthotic and Prosthetic Considerations
Prosthetic Approaches

Transhumeral amputation plus shoulder fusion is still a viable approach to complete and untreatable plexus lesions, although many authors have noted that a significant percentage of such patients discard their prostheses over time.[70,71] Leffert's[72] excellent text notes that arthrodesis of the flail or weak shoulder is widely accepted because it is both predictable and uncomplicated. However, fusion increases the leverage on the scapula from the weight of the arm plus prosthesis/orthosis. Leffert suggests that trapezius and serratus anterior strength must be good (or preferably normal) to provide sufficient control; motion will be smoother if the levator scapulae and rhomboids are also functioning.

Rowe[73] has noted that shoulder fusion attitudes originally intended for pediatric poliomyelitis survivors are not optimal for brachial plexus injuries. Rowe recommends shoulder fusion with the humerus in 20° of abduction, 30° of forward flexion, and 40° of internal rotation. Fusion in this attitude permits scapular motion, when combined with motion produced by the prosthetic elbow, to al-

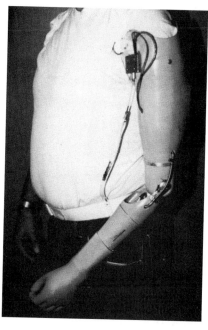

Figure 14 Microswitch control of an externally powered prosthesis is readily feasible because only a few millimeters of motion are required to fully operate either the elbow, the terminal device, or both. In this case, 11 mm of shoulder elevation fully operates both the electric elbow and the electric hand.

low the patient to reach all four major functional areas: face, midline, perineum, and rear trouser pocket.

Numerous harnessing variants have been developed to maximize the limited excursion remaining after brachial plexus injuries.[74] Although the complicated harnessing that is required because of the limited active motion remaining after the injury may make donning or doffing the prosthesis independently more difficult, some patients find body-powered components a good choice. Unlocking the elbow mechanism is often inconsistent because of limited shoulder movement, so a friction elbow or nudge control is frequently used.

With the widespread availability of externally powered components,[75] limited body excursion is now less problematic. Microswitch control requires only a few millimeters of motion and can be used to operate an electric hand,[76] an electric elbow, or both[77] (Figure 14). Myoelectric control may also be feasible because even

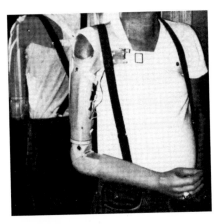

Figure 15 If two reliableEMG sites are available following a brachial plexus injury, proportional myoelectric control may be possible. A multiposition microswitch, controlled in this case by a few millimeters of chest expansion, allows the amputee to direct EMG control to the elbow, wrist, or hand motors. Thus, one pair of EMG signals provides proportional control of three degrees of freedom: flex-extend, pronate-supinate, and open-close.

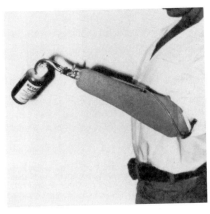

Figure 16 Nerve grafting plus shoulder fusion may result in good elbow control and proprioception. A relatively simple self-suspending transradial prosthesis may be then used to provide grasp even though the skin of the residual limb is insensate. *(Reproduced with permission from Leffert RD:* Brachial Plexus Injuries. *New York, NY, Churchill Livingstone, 1985, p 176.)*

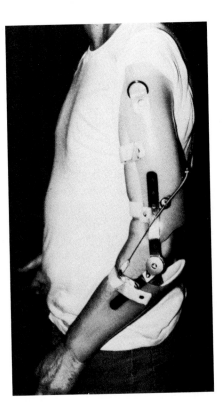

Figure 17 A body-powered elbow orthosis provides active flexion and reduces shoulder subluxation. An optional locking mechanism may be used to stabilize the elbow in several different positions. *(Reproduced with permission from Leffert RD:* Brachial Plexus Injuries. *New York, NY, Churchill Livingstone, 1985, p 153.)*

very weak muscles may generate sufficient signal to operate an externally powered device. It can be argued that myoelectric control for the terminal device is preferable for precise grasp. It may also be possible to use myoelectric control for both elbow and hand function (and perhaps for wrist rotation as well), but control sites will likely be on the chest or back (Figure 15). Advances in available prosthetic components have multiplied the options available for amputees with brachial plexus injuries and have increased the percentage of those who can actuate an active prosthesis. Whether this will result in increased long-term use remains to be documented.

In the presence of lesions that spare some elbow function, transradial amputation is sometimes performed. This may also be necessary because of the original trauma or because of vascular complications.[76] Prosthetic fitting is often complicated by residual weakness at the shoulder or elbow or both. Dralle[78] reported on a patient with good shoulder control and elbow flexors but no triceps function. When the amputee attempted to operate a body-powered hook, the force generated along the control cable forced the elbow into full flexion. It was necessary to use an outside locking joint normally intended for elbow disarticulation to stabilize the arm; difficulty in operating the lock because of the triceps absence was noted. Van Laere and associates[76] reported a case complicated by complete absence of elbow and shoulder function. Following surgical arthrodesis of the shoulder, a switch-operated electric hand and passive friction elbow joints were incorporated into a prosthesis that the patient reportedly used for many daily activities. Leffert[72] has reported success with transradial fittings provided that the amputee can sense elbow position. It is all-important to attempt to preserve the elbow if there is proprioceptive feedback from the joint because the usefulness and degree of acceptance of the prosthesis will be much enhanced by it. Even if the elbow is flail and the skin over the proposed residual limb is insensate, proprioception may be intact and a useful prosthetic fitting may be obtained without residual limb breakdown (Figure 16).

Flail Arm Orthoses

In view of the substantial percentage of amputees with brachial plexus injuries who reject prosthetic devices, it has been argued that orthotic restoration is an equally plausible alternative.[70,79-84] Figure 17 depicts one example of a custom arm orthosis that was successfully used when some useful hand function remained following a partial brachial plexus injury. Wynn Parry[85] has reported on his experience with a series of more than 200 patients and states that 70% continue to use a flail arm orthosis for work or hobby activities after 1 year. Originally developed in London during the early 1960s,[83] the Stanmore flail arm orthosis consists of a series of modules that can be interconnected to provide any degree of control desired (Figure 18). For the

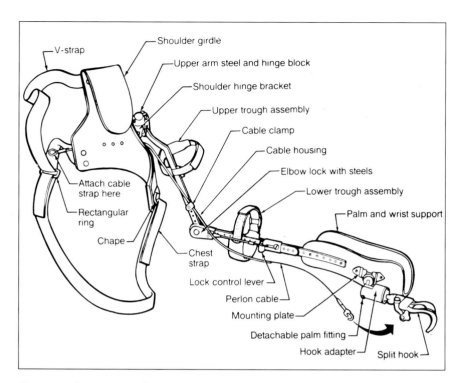

Figure 18 The Stanmore flail arm orthosis uses a series of modules to stabilize the arm following a brachial plexus injury.

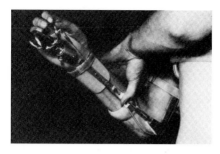

Figure 19 When a body-powered hook is mounted to the Stanmore orthosis, it functions like a prosthesis even though the flail arm remains intact. *(Reproduced with permission from Wynn Parry CB: Brachial plexus injuries. Br J Hosp Med 1984;32:130-139.)*

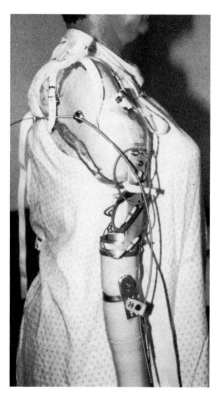

Figure 20 The complex and sometimes anomalous neuromuscular deficits that are commonly associated with brachial plexus injuries often make a prior determination of prosthetic components impossible. In such instances, a diagnostic or evaluation prosthesis allows clinical assessment of patient tolerance for weight, various harness configurations, and component alternatives. Once therapy training has been successfully completed with the evaluation device, the definitive prosthesis design can be determined and provided.

completely flail arm, a body-powered prosthetic hook mounted adjacent to the patient's hand is used to provide grasp (Figure 19). In essence, the patient has a prosthesis over the flail arm.[85] Incomplete lesions may require only the elbow or shoulder control modules.

Rehabilitation

Modern surgical advances have resulted in a much less uniform range of impairment following brachial plexus injuries, and the prosthetist-orthotist is now faced with an unpredictable array of residual functions. Muscle transfers sometimes result in powerful electromyographic (EMG) signals suitable for myoelectric control in unexpected anatomic locations. Nerve transfers further complicate the issue because anomalous neuroanatomy may preclude precise myoelectric control despite a grossly powerful signal. Finally, muscle fatigue is frequently overlooked and virtually impossible to predict. It is frustrating for all involved when the brachial plexus injury survivor can operate a sophisticated device flawlessly in therapy or the clinic but does not use it at home long-term because the small mass of functioning remnant muscle becomes totally fatigued after 1 or 2 hours of effort.

As a result of all these factors, a diagnostic prosthesis[76] is strongly recommended (Figure 20) and an interdisciplinary team approach encouraged for these singularly complicated cases.[77,80,86,87] A thorough physical examination including manual and EMG muscle testing is required to assess rehabilitation potential. Because patients with brachial plexus injuries often have a lengthy recovery period, most will have become accustomed to functioning unilaterally, which can significantly reduce enthusiasm to master an adaptive device. It is therefore imperative that the patient be actively involved in all prescription decisions from the outset; without a motivated and cooperative individual, even heroic prosthetic/orthotic interventions are doomed to failure.

Wynn Parry[87] recommends use of a full-arm orthosis during the recov-

ery period, beginning as soon as the patient has come to terms with the se-

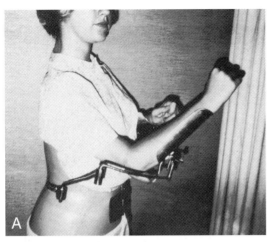
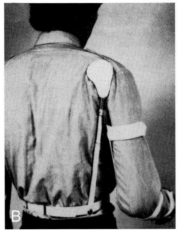
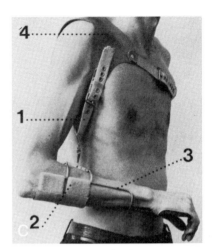

Figure 21 A, A pelvic hemigirdle is sometimes used to unweight the flail arm; a counterbalanced forearm assembly is characteristic of a "gunslinger" orthosis. **B,** For slender individuals, a spring-loaded metal rod attached to a waist belt can help unweight the arm. **C,** Cool[88] has proposed using the weight of the paralyzed forearm, acting across a fulcrum near the radial head, to provide a vertical antisubluxation force to the humerus. (Figure C is reproduced with permission from Cool JC: Biomechanics of orthoses for the subluxed shoulder. *Prosthet Orthot Int* 1989;13:90-96.)

rious and potentially permanent nature of his or her injuries. He also notes that fitting more than a year after injury is much less successful. Robinson[81] has suggested 6 to 8 weeks postinjury as the optimal time for orthotic intervention, ie, "when the patient is beginning to accept the implications of his or her injury and yet has not become too one-handed."

Once surgical reconstruction and spontaneous recovery are complete, amputation and a trial with a prosthesis can be considered. The decision to choose amputation is always difficult; the opportunity to meet another brachial plexus injury amputee who has successfully mastered a prosthesis may be helpful. Psychological and social work consultation may be useful to help the patient discuss the altered body image and employment possibilities that will follow amputation. The presence of chronic pain complicates prosthetic/orthotic intervention. In those cases in which humeral traction worsens the pain, special care must be taken to prevent the weight of the device from displacing the arm downward at the shoulder. This is often a difficult task because conventional prosthetic harnessing supports axial loads via pressure on the ipsilateral trapezius or by encumbering the contralateral shoulder; neither ap-

proach is ideal in the presence of a brachial plexus injury.

One alternative is to unweight the arm with a strut along the axillary midline, attached to a waist belt or to a well-molded pelvic hemigirdle. Cool[88] from the Netherlands has reported a clever approach using the weight of the paralyzed forearm acting across a fulcrum at the radial head level to literally lever the humerus back into the glenoid fossa (Figure 21). Although more than 1,600 patients have been fitted in Europe, this approach has not been widely used in North America.

In general, any device for patients with a brachial plexus injury should be as lightweight as possible to minimize inferior shoulder subluxation. Because external power is often required, a trial with an appropriately weighted test socket can help determine tolerance for the added weight of powered components.

Limb Function Prerequisites

Simpson[89] has summarized the prerequisites for upper limb function as follows:

- Proximal stability
- Placement in space
- Functional grasp

It is useful for both the physician and the prosthetist-orthotist to keep these

principles in mind when evaluating the patient with a brachial plexus injury.

Proximal stability is absolutely essential for successful fitting. The shoulder girdle and elbow flexors must be strong enough to support the arm or arm remnant plus the orthotic/prosthetic device. If body-powered control is anticipated, they must also be able to resist the forces generated during cable actuation. This force typically varies between 2 kg (4.4 lb) and 10 kg (22 lb), depending on the grip strength desired at the terminal device (Figure 22).

When shoulder stability is marginal, a trial with exercises to improve muscular control may be warranted. Functional electric stimulation can also be helpful in strengthening residual musculature. In the absence of intrinsic stability, the prosthetic or orthotic device must stabilize the arm by extending well onto the torso. Many patients find this approach awkward or uncomfortable, although some will tolerate it (Figure 23).

Although Rorabeck[90] has suggested transhumeral amputation without shoulder arthrodesis, an unstable shoulder will always compromise prosthetic function. Surgical stabilization is often the most practical approach to providing proximal sta-

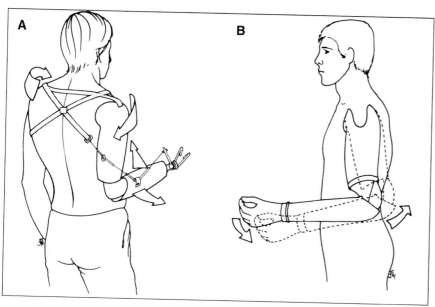

Figure 22 A, A body-powered control applies forces along the control cable that tend to flex the elbow and externally rotate the shoulder. B, The weight of externally powered components applies elbow extension and shoulder extension forces. In either case, proximal stability must be provided via muscle strength, surgical fusion, or prosthetic/orthotic control.

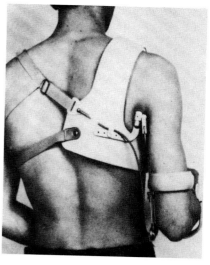

Figure 23 Prosthetic/orthotic shoulder control requires large flanges extending well onto the torso, which many patients find cumbersome or objectionable.

bility despite requiring several weeks of immobilization for the bony fusion to occur. Malone and associates[77] have suggested that postsurgical fitting with a prosthesis immediately following arthrodesis may be useful.

Elbow stability can be provided by a variety of locking mechanisms. Unfortunately, many orthoses require use of the uninvolved hand for unlocking. Wrist stability is readily achieved because orthoses that fix the hand in slight wrist extension are well known and well tolerated. Thumb and finger stabilization is determined individually by following accepted orthotic principles.

Placement in space is closely related to stability and is imperative to provide a useful work envelope and thereby allow the individual to reach above, below, in front of, and behind the body. In cases where residual shoulder musculature can steady the arm but not support its weight when reaching out, the utility of the prosthetic/orthotic device is severely compromised. Orthotic control of the shoulder is cumbersome and requires extensions onto the torso, as noted

previously. Again, surgical stabilization via fusion may be preferable.

Elbow placement is more readily provided by Bowden cable harnessing adapted from transhumeral prosthetic principles or through the use of externally powered components. Because the weight of the arm/orthosis/prosthesis provides a reliable extension moment, a locking mechanism is not always required. A flexion moment generated by biscapular shoulder abduction, for example, can be readily controlled by the patient to precisely counterbalance the extension forces due to gravity. This is particularly effective when weak elbow flexors are present but shoulder stability is good. Springs or elastics can also be used to help counterbalance the weight of the forearm (Figure 24).

Functional grasp is readily restored in a variety of ways. Body-powered hooks of the voluntary-opening type are the traditional approach and are often effective. In addition to being lightweight and durable, they provide a constant, limited pinch force without continued exertion by the patient. Electric hands or hooks are increasingly common and offer powerful

grip forces with minimal exertion. Switch control is used when necessary, but myoelectric control generally offers more precise grip force, provided that suitable muscle sites can be found.

Sophisticated orthoses can also restore grasp to the paralyzed hand by using either mechanical or external power. Most are variations of the "wrist-driven" styles originally developed for individuals with quadriplegia (Figure 25). Other approaches include mounting a prosthetic hook near the palm of the paralyzed hand and the use of adaptive utensil cuffs for various specific activities.

Mastery of any prosthetic/orthotic device is believed to be contingent on its effectiveness in augmenting functional activities. Actively including the patient in the decision-making process, particularly in the choice of specific components and design options, increases the success rate. One key to long-term usage is to identify specific tasks important to the individual that will be facilitated by using the device.

A major limitation of all current prosthetic/orthotic grasp modalities is the absence of sensation, which requires close attention to visual cues by the user. As Simpson[89] has noted, when control of the arm becomes the

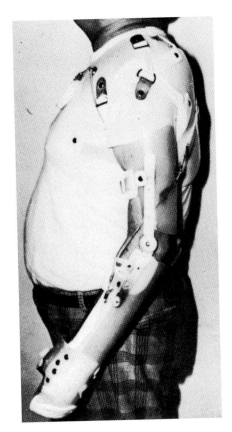

Figure 24 Biscapular shoulder motion may sometimes be harnessed to provide active elbow flexion despite significant paresis. Various mechanical flexion assists can help counterbalance the weight of the forearm and hand. *(Reproduced with permission from Leffert RD:* Brachial Plexus Injuries. *New York, NY, Churchill Livingstone, 1985, p 153.)*

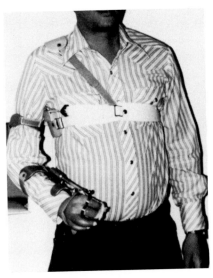

Figure 25 Orthoses originally designed for individuals with quadriplegia may be useful following brachial plexus injuries. This version uses switch control to operate a miniature electric motor that opens and closes the fingers.

main task, the rate of rejection increases significantly. The difficulties involved in using the insensate "blind" hand are well documented. The alternative of teaching the individual with a brachial plexus injury one-handed independence should always be carefully considered and is frequently the most effective solution long term.[91]

Conclusion

Injuries to the brachial plexus can be devastating and often drastically change the lives of the individuals who sustain them. In the past, clinical outcomes were dismal, resulting in little more than trick movement in the flail extremities. Based on the

work of the pioneers of brachial plexus surgery during the past several decades, a better understanding of these injuries and novel approaches to treatment have emerged. These advances have given both patients and surgeons new options that offer hope for improved clinical outcomes.

Despite recent surgical advances, brachial plexus injuries present one of the greatest challenges to the rehabilitation team. Providing grasp is only the first step and is often the easiest to accomplish. Practical restoration of the ability to place the arm in space can be difficult, while provision of external shoulder stability is cumbersome at best. Surgical stabilization by shoulder fusion should always be carefully considered if functional use of the affected limb is desired. Residual neuromuscular deficits make fitting the amputee with a brachial plexus injury a complicated undertaking. The use of a diagnostic prosthesis before determination of the final prescription is highly recommended because of the complexity of interrelated factors.

The longer the time lapse between injury and functional use of the arm, the greater the likelihood of a poor

result. Early provision of a flail arm orthosis may be useful to encourage two-handed activities during the recovery phase. Timely surgical intervention should enhance residual function.

Leffert[72] has emphasized the importance of educating brachial plexus injury survivors who are considering prosthetic fitting about what is realistically possible. Patients often come with totally unrealistic ideas of "bionic arms" depicted in the popular media. Unless they give up such fantasies, they are unlikely to be satisfied with their results. Whenever possible, patients with brachial plexus injuries contemplating amputation should have the opportunity to see and talk with other patients who have already undergone the procedure.

The ideal environment to manage brachial plexus injuries is a multidisciplinary clinic specializing in this most challenging problem. Despite recent advances in both surgical and prosthetic-orthotic technique, many individuals with brachial plexus injuries will find that the functional capabilities of the affected limb remain significantly limited because of the magnitude of the functional loss they have sustained.

References

1. Allieu Y, Cenac P: Is surgical intervention justifiable for total paralysis secondary to multiple avulsion injuries of the brachial plexus? *Hand Clin* 1988;4: 609-618.

2. Allieu Y, Privat JM, Bonnel F: Paralysis in root avulsion of the brachial plexus: Neurotization by the spinal accessory nerve. *Clin Plast Surg* 1984;11:133-136.

3. Azze RJ, Mattar Junior J, Ferreira MC: et al: Extraplexual neurotization of brachial plexus. *Microsurgery* 1994;15: 28-32.

4. Brandt KE, Mackinnon SE: A technique for maximizing biceps recovery in brachial plexus reconstruction. *J Hand Surg [Am]* 1993;18:726-733.

5. Brunelli G: Direct neurotization of severely damaged muscles. *J Hand Surg [Am]* 1982;7:572-579.

6. Brunelli G, Monini L: Direct muscular

neurotization. *J Hand Surg [Am]* 1985; 10:993-997.

7. Doi K, Kuwata N, Muramatsu K, et al: Double muscle transfer for upper extremity reconstruction following complete avulsion of the brachial plexus. *Hand Clin* 1999;15:757-767.

8. Doi K, Muramatsu K, Hattori Y, et al: Restoration of prehension with the double free muscle technique following complete avulsion of the brachial plexus: Indications and long-term results. *J Bone Joint Surg Am* 2000;82:652-666.

9. Frampton VM: Management of brachial plexus lesions. *J Hand Ther* 1988;1:115-120.

10. Allieu Y: Evolution of our indications for neurotization: Our concept of functional restoration of the upper limb after brachial plexus injuries. *Chir Main* 1999;18:165-166.

11. Malone J, Leal J, Underwood J, et al: Brachial plexus injury management through upper extremity amputation with immediate postoperative prostheses. *Arch Phys Med Rehabil* 1982;63:89-91.

12. Narakas A: The treatment of brachial plexus injuries. *Int Orthop* 1985;9:29-36.

13. Hendry HAM: The treatment of residual paralysis after brachial plexus lesions. *J Bone Joint Surg Br* 1949;31:42.

14. Fletcher I: Traction lesions of the brachial plexus. *Hand* 1969;1:129-136.

15. Yeoman PM, Seddon HJ: Brachial plexus injuries: Treatment of the flail arm. *J Bone Joint Surg Br* 1961;43:493-500.

16. Carvalho GA, Nikkhah G, Matthies C, et al: Diagnosis of root avulsions in traumatic brachial plexus injuries: Value of computerized tomography myelography and magnetic resonance imaging. *J Neurosurg* 1997;86:69-76.

17. Doi K, Otsuka K, Okamoto Y, et al: Cervical nerve root avulsion in brachial plexus injuries: Magnetic resonance imaging classification and comparison with myelography and computerized tomography myelography. *J Neurosurg* 2002;96:277-284.

18. Nakamura T, Yabe Y, Horiuchi Y, et al: Magnetic resonance myelography in brachial plexus injury. *J Bone Joint Surg Br* 1997;79:764-769.

19. Leffert R: Rehabilitation of the patient with a brachial plexus injury. *Neurol Clin* 1987;5:559-568.

20. Meredith J, Taft G, Kaplan P: Diagnosis and treatment of the hemiplegic patient with brachial plexus injury. *Am J Occup Ther* 1981;35:656-660.

21. Millesi H: Brachial plexus injuries: Management and results. *Clin Plast Surg* 1984;11:115-120.

22. Millesi H: Trauma involving the brachial plexus, in Omer G, Spionner M (eds): *Management of Peripheral Nerve Problems.* Philadelphia, PA, WB Saunders, 1980, pp 565-567.

23. Robinson C: Brachial plexus lesions: Part I. Management. *Br J Occup Ther* 1986;49:147-150.

24. Robinson C: Brachial plexus lesions: Part 2. Functional splintage. *Br J Occup Ther* 1986;49:331-334.

25. Rorabeck C: The management of flail upper extremity in brachial plexus injuries. *J Trauma* 1980;20:491-493.

26. Wynn P: Brachial plexus injuries. *Br J Hosp Med* 1984;32:130-139.

27. Wynn P: Rehabilitation of patients following traction lesions of the brachial plexus. *Clin Plast Surg* 1984;11:173-179.

28. Wynn PCB: The management of injuries of the brachial plexus. *Proc R Soc Med* 1974;67:488-490.

29. Chuang DC: Neurotization procedures for brachial plexus injuries. *Hand Clin* 1995;11:633-645.

30. Chuang DC, Yeh MC, Wei FC: Intercostal nerve transfer of the musculocutaneous nerve in avulsed brachial plexus injuries: Evaluation of 66 patients. *J Hand Surg [Am]* 1992;17:822-828.

31. Dolenc VV: Intercostal neurotization of the peripheral nerves in avulsion plexus injuries. *Clin Plast Surg* 1984;11:143-147.

32. Hattori Y, Doi K, Fuchigami Y, et al: Experimental study on donor nerves for brachial plexus injury: Comparison between the spinal accessory nerve and the intercostal nerve. *Plast Reconstr Surg* 1997;100:900-906.

33. Merrell GA, Barrie KA, Katz DL, et al: Results of nerve transfer techniques for restoration of shoulder and elbow function in the context of a meta-analysis of the English literature. *J Hand Surg [Am]* 2001;26:303-314.

34. Nagano A, Yamamoto S, Mikami Y: Intercostal nerve transfer to restore upper extremity functions after brachial plexus injury. *Ann Acad Med Singapore* 1995;24:42-45.

35. Songcharoen P: Brachial plexus injury in Thailand: A report of 520 cases. *Microsurgery* 1995;16:35-39.

36. Waikakul S, Wongtragul S, Vanadurongwan V: Restoration of elbow flexion in brachial plexus avulsion injury: Comparing spinal accessory nerve transfer with intercostal nerve transfer. *J Hand Surg [Am]* 1999;24:571-577.

37. Allieu Y, Cenac P: Neurotization via the spinal accessory nerve in complete paralysis due to multiple avulsion injuries of the brachial plexus. *Clin Orthop* 1988;237:67-74.

38. Allieu Y, Chammas M, Picot MC: Paralysis of the brachial plexus caused by supraclavicular injuries in the adult: Long-term comparative results of nerve grafts and transfers. *Rev Chir Orthop Reparatrice Appar Mot* 1997;83:51-59.

39. Chung DC, Carver N, Wei FC: Results of functioning free muscle transplantation for elbow flexion. *J Hand Surg* 1996;21:1071-1077.

40. Doi K, Sakai K, Ihara K, et al: Reinnervated free muscle transplantation for extremity reconstruction. *Plast Reconstr Surg* 1993;91:872-883.

41. Doi K, Sakai K, Kuwata N, et al: Double free-muscle transfer to restore prehension following complete brachial plexus avulsion. *J Hand Surg [Am]* 1995;20:408-414.

42. Doi K, Sakai K, Kuwata N, et al: Reconstruction of finger and elbow function after complete avulsion of the brachial plexus. *J Hand Surg [Am]* 1991;16:796-803.

43. Samardzic M, Grujicic D, Antunovic V, et al: Reinnervation of avulsed brachial plexus using the spinal accessory nerve. *Surg Neurol* 1990;33:7-11.

44. Gu YD, Ma MK: Use of the phrenic nerve for brachial plexus reconstruction. *Clin Orthop* 1996;323:119-121.

45. Gu YD, Zhang GM, Chen DS, et al: Seventh cervical nerve root transfer from the contralateral healthy side for treatment of brachial plexus root avulsion. *J Hand Surg [Br]* 1992;17:518-521.

46. Chuang DC, Wei FC, Noordhoff MS: Cross-chest C7 nerve grafting followed by free muscle transplantations for the treatment of total avulsed brachial plexus injuries: A preliminary report. *Plast Reconstr Surg* 1993;92: 717-727.

47. Songcharoen P, Wongtrakul S, Mahaisavariya B, et al: Hemi-contralateral C7 transfer to median nerve in the treatment of root avulsion brachial plexus injury. *J Hand Surg [Am]* 2001; 26:1058-1064.

48. Gu YD, Chen DS, Zhang GM, et al: Long-term functional results of contralateral C7 transfer. *J Reconstr Microsurg* 1998;14:57-59.

49. Oberlin C, Alnot JY, Comtet JJ: Vascularized nerve trunk grafts: Technic and results of 27 cases. *Ann Chir Main* 1989;8:316-323.

50. Oberlin C, Beal D, Leechavengvongs S, et al: Nerve transfer to biceps muscle using a part of ulnar nerve for C5-C6 avulsion of the brachial plexus: Anatomical study and report of four cases. *J Hand Surg [Am]* 1994;19:232-237.

51. Chuang DC, Lee GW, Hashen F, et al: Restoration of shoulder abduction by nerve transfer in avulsion brachial plexus injury: Evaluation of 99 patients with various nerve transfers. *Plast Reconstr Surg* 1995;96:122-128.

52. Krakauer JD, Wood MB: Intercostal nerve transfer brachial plexopathy. *J Hand Surg [Am]* 1994;19:829-835.

53. Leechavengvongs S, Witoon CK, Uerpairojkit C, et al: Nerve transfer to biceps muscle using a part of the ulnar nerve in brachial plexus injury (upper arm type): A report of 32 cases. *J Hand Surg [Am]* 1998;23:711-716.

54. Mikami Y, Nagano A, Ochiai N, et al: Results of nerve grafting for injuries of the axillary and suprascapular nerves. *J Bone Joint Surg Br* 1997;79:527-531.

55. Narakas A, Hentz VR: Neurotization in brachial plexus injuries: Indication and results. *Clin Orthop* 1988;237: 43-56.

56. Ruch DS, Friedman AH, Nunley JA: The restoration of elbow flexion with intercostal nerve transfers. *Clin Orthop* 1995;314:95-103.

57. Songcharoen P, Mahaisavariya B, Chotigavanich C: Spinal accessory neurotization for restoration of elbow flexion in avulsion injuries of the brachial plexus. *J Hand Surg [Am]* 1996; 21:387-390.

58. Akasaka Y, Hara T, Takahashi M: Free muscle transplantation combined with intercostal nerve crossing for reconstruction of elbow flexion and wrist extension in brachial plexus injuries. *Microsurgery* 1991;12:345-351.

59. Doi K, Sakai K, Fuchigami Y, et al: Reconstruction of irreparable brachial plexus injuries with reinnervated free-muscle transfer: Case report. *J Neurosurg* 1996;85:174-177.

60. Doi K, Shigetomi M, Kaneko K, et al: Significance of elbow extension in reconstruction of prehension with reinnervated free-muscle transfer following complete brachial plexus avulsion. *Plast Reconstr Surg* 1997;100: 364-372.

61. Manktelow RT: Functioning muscle transplantation, in Manktelow RT (ed): *Microvascular Reconstruction: Anatomy, Applications and Surgical Techniques.* New York, NY, Springer-Verlag, 1986, pp 151-164.

62. Manktelow RT, Zuker RM, McKee NH: Functioning free muscle transplantation. *J Hand Surg [Am]* 1984; 9:32-39.

63. Berger A, Flory PJ, Schaller E: Muscle transfers in brachial plexus lesions. *J Reconstr Microsurg* 1990;6:113-116.

64. Doi K: New reconstructive procedure for brachial plexus injury. *Clin Plast Surg* 1997;24:75-85.

65. Shurr D, Blair W: A rationale for treatment of complete brachial plexus palsy. *Orthot Prosthet* 1984;38:55-59.

66. Doi K, Hattori Y, Kuwata N, et al: Free muscle transfer can restore hand function after injuries of the lower brachial plexus. *J Bone Joint Surg Br* 1998;80: 117-120.

67. Bishop AT, Barrie KA, Steinmann SP: Gracilis free muscle transfer for restoration of function following complete brachial plexus avulsion. Presented at the 56th Annual Meeting of the American Society for Surgery of the Hand, October 4-6, 2001, Baltimore, MD.

68. Saha A: Surgery of the paralyzed and flail shoulder. *Acta Orthop Scand* 1967; 97:5-90.

69. Leffert R, Seddon H: Infraclavicular brachial plexus injuries. *J Bone Joint Surg Br* 1965;47:9-22.

70. Perry J, Hsu J, Barber L, Hoffer MM: Orthoses in patients with brachial plexus injuries. *Arch Phys Med Rehabil* 1974;55:134-137.

71. Ransford AO, Hughes SPF: Complete brachial plexus lesions. *J Bone Joint Surg Br* 1977;59:417-420.

72. Leffert RD: *Brachial Plexus Injuries.* New York, NY, Churchill Livingstone, 1985.

73. Rowe CR: Re-evaluation of the position of the arm in arthrodesis of the shoulder in the adult. *J Bone Joint Surg Am* 1974;56:913.

74. Schottstaedt ER, Robinson GB: Functional bracing of the arm. *J Bone Joint Surg Am* 1955;38:477-499.

75. Michael JW: Upper limb powered components and controls: Current concepts. *Clin Prosthet Orthot* 1986; 10:66-77.

76. Van Laere M, Duyvejonck R, Leus P, et al: A prosthetic appliance for a patient with a brachial plexus injury and forearm amputation: A case report. *Am J Occup Ther* 1977;31:309-312.

77. Malone JM, Leal JM, Underwood J, et al: Brachial plexus injury management through upper extremity amputation with immediate postoperative prostheses. *Arch Phys Med Rehabil* 1982;63: 89-91.

78. Dralle AJ: Prosthetic management of a below-elbow amputation with brachial plexus injury. *Orthot Prosthet* 1977;31:39-40.

79. Chu DS, Lehneis HR, Wilson R: Functional arm orthosis for complete brachial plexus lesion. *Arch Phys Med Rehabil* 1987;68:594.

80. Frampton VM: Management of brachial plexus lesions. *J Hand Ther* 1988; 1:115-120.

81. Robinson C: Brachial plexus lesions: Part 1. Management. *Br J Occup Ther* 1986;49:147-150.

82. Robinson C: Brachial plexus lesions: Part 2. Functional splintage. *Br J Occup Ther* 1986;49:331-334.

83. Wardlow M: A modular orthosis for brachial plexus lesions. *Inter Clin Info Bull* 1979;17:9-12.

84. Wynn Parry CB: The management of injuries to the brachial plexus. *Proc R Soc Med* 1974;67:488-490.

85. Wynn Parry CB: Brachial plexus injuries. *Br J Hosp Med* 1984;32:130-139.

86. Shurr DG, Blair WF: A rationale for treatment of complete brachial plexus palsy. *Orthot Prosthet* 1984;38:55-59.

87. Wynn Parry CB: Rehabilitation of patients following traction lesions of the brachial plexus. *Clin Plast Surg* 1984; 11:173-179.

88. Cool JC: Biomechanics of orthoses for the subluxed shoulder. *Prosthet Orthot Int* 1989;13:90-96.

89. Simpson DC: The hand/arm system, in Murdoch G (ed): *Prosthetic and Orthotic Practice*. London, England, E Arnold, 1968.

90. Rorabeck CH: The management of the flail upper extremity in brachial plexus injuries. *J Trauma* 1980;20:491-493.

91. Frampton VM: Management of brachial plexus lesions. *Physiotherapy* 1984;70:388-392.

Chapter 24

Aesthetic Prostheses

Thomas Passero, CP
Kim Doolan

Introduction

The importance of prosthetic appearance and function cannot be overemphasized and is well documented.[1-10] Often, an amputee more readily accepts and uses a prosthesis if it mimics the appearance of the lost digit or limb. Aesthetic prostheses are more frequently indicated for upper rather than lower limb amputees, probably because of the increased visibility of the upper limbs during most activities.

Misconceptions regarding the role of aesthetics in the selection of a prosthesis are common. An aesthetic or cosmetic restoration is sometimes considered to be a last resort that is offered only if the patient rejects mechanical devices. A comprehensive treatment plan, however, considers all available prostheses appropriate for the type and level of amputation, including aesthetic prostheses. A thorough examination, combined with careful assessment of the amputee's goals and desires, enables the health care team to prioritize restoration of normal appearance among the criteria for prosthetic design.

The prescription for a prosthesis is based on the anatomic state of the residual limb, including the level of amputation, length, shape, and range of motion. The intended functional outcomes or uses of the prosthetic device(s) are also key considerations. The prescription process should identify the prosthetic components

and design that are most likely to successfully meet the needs of the patient.

The prosthesis should reproduce a realistic appearance with regard to both texture and color. Although a variety of materials have been used for aesthetic restorations, silicone is generally preferred because of its versatility, durability, and compatibility with human tissue.[5,11-13] Ideally, prostheses should be custom made to intimately fit the contours of the residual digit or limb.

History

In the 1950s, the French physician Jean Pillet emphasized the profound impact of the loss of even a single digit on the amputee's body image, self-esteem, and psychological status.[8] He established clinics around the world and pioneered the use of silicone prostheses that were sculpted and painted to match the individual patient. Twenty years later, Horst Buckner, a German prosthetist, developed a new method to cover mechanical prosthetic components, such as body-powered and electric hands, with lifelike silicone skins. Today, many fabrication techniques use multiple grades of silicone, and aesthetic prostheses are produced at both large and small facilities.

Function

The functional capabilities of aesthetic prostheses are surprisingly complex and vary with the level of amputation. Upper limb applications include manipulative activities such as prehension, pushing, and pulling, as well as balance, support, stabilization, proprioception, and communication.[1,4,6,8,14,15] Most patients with an upper limb prosthesis use the entire surface of the prosthesis and not just the terminal device. Common examples include stabilizing a book on the forearm, sandwiching a grocery bag between the hip and prosthesis, and pushing up from a chair by placing weight against the prosthetic elbow.

Although active prehension with a prosthetic hook or hand is critical for bilateral upper limb amputees, it is less important for many unilateral arm amputees. Several studies have confirmed that active grasp and release does not occur continuously, even for excellent prosthetic users. "If active manipulation of a terminal device is seen as the determinant for good prosthetic use, then the number of 'good' users found would be less than 25%."[1] Several international trials have reported that 58% to 76% of the amputees studied wear their prosthesis for at least 8 hours each day.[1,4] The inevitable conclusion is that a person wearing a prosthesis finds a use for it, including activities that do not involve active grasp and release.[4]

The potential functions of an aesthetic prosthesis depend on the complexity of involvement (ie, unilateral or bilateral amputation) and the use of passive, mechanical, or electric components. A single aesthetic prosthesis used on an index finger, for example, actively functions in prehensile activities such as writing and grasping small objects, or during activities requiring striking, such as use of a keyboard.[8] A partial hand prosthesis for a hand without a thumb and forefinger provides functional opposition to the remaining fingers. For the unilateral total hand amputee, an aesthetic hand prosthesis provides opposition to the sound hand while performing bimanual activities. In addition, a prosthetic hand can be used to communicate, balance, stabilize, and push or pull objects without active grasping.

Aesthetic prostheses for lower limb amputees have some limitations because they can interfere with the multidirectional forces and motions generated during ambulation.[16,17] This will be discussed in a subsequent section.

Psychological Considerations

A prosthetic limb with a realistic appearance provides subtle psychosocial advantages, similar to the nonfunctional advantages provided by the painted pupil, iris, and sclera of a prosthetic eye. An aesthetic prosthesis partially restores both the active and passive functional capabilities that were lost with amputation, including normal appearance.

Whether small parts or entire lengths of limbs are removed, it is impossible to predict an individual's reaction to determine what prosthetic designs will best meet his or her needs. A patient may do better if initially provided with a prosthesis that mimics the appearance of the lost limb. This is especially true of upper limb amputees who cannot conceal their changed body as easily as lower limb amputees. A prosthesis with a natural appearance allows patients to blend in and not be singled out as different, even when using their prosthesis in public. Once the amputee has accepted the change in body image, wearing more obvious terminal devices, such as hooks or electrically powered grippers, may be more acceptable. Unfortunately, some amputees who were provided with metal tool-like devices shortly after the amputation later report having felt so self-conscious that once rehabilitation was completed, their prosthesis was placed in a closet and never worn again. Pillet and Mackin[8] expressed the importance of personal appearance to the patient as follows: "Often the disfigurement is more pronounced in the mind of the amputee than others. However, the man who finds himself unable to take his hand from his pocket, even though it is very 'functional,' may be as handicapped as if it were lost."

Early Fitting and Rehabilitation

The importance of fitting a prosthesis as soon after amputation as possible is well established. Malone and associates[18] wrote that the first month after amputation should be considered the "golden period" during which fitting of an upper limb prosthesis would lead to the best long-term outcome. Amputees who have delayed fittings do not seem to master the use of their prosthesis as thoroughly or use it as spontaneously as do amputees who have been fitted shortly after surgery.

Therapy

Expert training in the effective use of prostheses to replace the hand or entire arm is important to ensure that the patient receives the full potential benefit of the prosthesis. Fraser[1] argues for expanding the role of the prosthesis to include more than just grasping actions. "If the role of the prosthesis in supporting, stabilizing, pushing, pulling, holding, and facilitating balance in everyday life situations is accepted as more useful than that of manipulation of small objects in the clinic situation; this could...influence training" as well as the design of componentry and composition of surface and subsurface materials. Thus, training must not be limited to controlling prehension, particularly for patients with a unilateral arm amputation. Hubbard and associates[2] argue that most unilateral amputees use their prosthesis as gross motor assists, not for fine motor activities.

The therapist best serves the amputee by using protocols that not only teach control of prosthetic components (terminal devices, wrists, elbows, shoulders) but also how to most efficiently complete activities of daily living and occupational tasks. These activities include using the exterior of the artificial limb to stabilize, lift, move, and compress external objects. These latter functions are readily accomplished with aesthetic prostheses.

Patient Compliance With Prosthetic Use

In their classic study, Millstein and associates[6] wrote, "For any prosthesis to be accepted and used by the amputee, it must be comfortable, functional, and have a pleasing appearance." Other characteristics described as priorities include light weight, durability, ease of cleaning, longevity of operation (up to 12 hours), and suitability for driving. Amputees also frequently request that the prosthesis be as unnoticeable as possible and not get in the way. Consideration of these factors when choosing the type of prosthesis and related components increases the chances that the patient will wear the prosthesis.

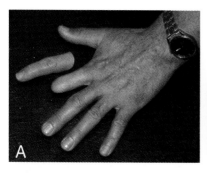 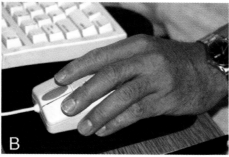

Figure 1 **A,** Index figure prosthesis. **B,** Index figure prosthesis in use.

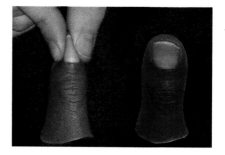

Figure 2 Silicone fingernail.

Initial Assessment

The initial patient assessment is the same regardless of the type of prosthesis under consideration. Once the assessment has been completed and it is determined that an aesthetic prosthesis is indicated, then the residual limb must be prepared for the prosthetic fitting. The wound should be completely healed, and the volume of the residual limb should be reasonably stable. Wrapping the digit or limb with a compressive material will accelerate volume reduction. The limb volume must be stable if suction is to be used as the sole means of suspension. If significant atrophy of the residual limb occurs, the subsequent loss of the vacuum seal will result in displacement of the device and, in some instances, the prosthesis will fall off the arm or digit. Even for prostheses not suspended by suction, unwanted movement within a loose-fitting socket can affect function and/or cause skin irritation and breakdown.

Considerations for Prostheses for Upper Limb Amputees

Malone and associates[18] observed that there is no standard prosthetic prescription for upper limb amputees. In part, this is because no upper limb prosthesis, however elegant, can restore more than a small portion of the complex functions that have been lost. An optimal level of functional rehabilitation is often achieved by

providing prosthetic devices that are optimized for different specific activities and situations. Different upper limb prostheses are increasingly being used for different activities. Some transradial amputees, for example, will use a myoelectric prosthesis with an electronic gripper at work when powerful prehension is of the utmost importance. A more basic body-powered prosthesis with a cable-operated hook may be used in the workshop because of its rugged nature, and an aesthetic prosthesis might be used for social occasions.

Finger Prostheses

Finger and partial finger amputations are among the most common types of partial hand loss.[5] The National Limb Loss Information Center indicates that 88% of the 26,000 upper limb amputations in 1996 involved the loss of fingers.

The benefits of silicone restoration of digital amputations are well documented and include a range of functional and psychological improvements, in addition to a much more normal appearance[7-9,19,20] (Figure 1).

The length of the remaining finger or fingers is a primary consideration in the selection of the method of suspension (suction or mechanical), length of the prosthesis (whether the proximal edge of the prosthesis terminates at the proximal interphalangeal or metacarpophalangeal joint), shape of the restoration, and use of either a hard acrylic or soft silicone fingernail.

Although suction is the primary means of retention of most digital prostheses, the use of osseointegration

has advantages,[21] including increased pinch force and the transfer of deep pressure sensation. The risks of osseointegration are the same as those for other similar surgical procedures. This procedure is especially useful when the length of the residual digit is insufficient for retention of a conventional prosthesis. Other means of retaining prostheses on short residual limbs include medical adhesives, incorporation of vacuum chambers in the distal portion of the prosthesis,[22] or use of adjacent finger(s) and rings to anchor the prosthesis to the hand in a manner similar to that used for a dental crown and bridge.

Suction is the primary means of suspension for most finger prostheses. Therefore, the residual finger must have an appropriate shape (ideally, cylindrical or bulbous) and be of sufficient length, usually at least 1 to 1.5 cm.[5,8] Suspension by suction is usually unreliable with shorter residual digits that have a conical shape. In such situations, the previously mentioned alternate methods could be used. If the involved hand has multiple short residual fingers, it may be necessary to cover the entire hand with an aesthetic glove to create a device that is firm enough to withstand the force required to grasp and hold objects.

If the residual digit has sufficient length, a half finger prosthesis is preferred by most patients. A half finger prosthesis terminates at the proximal interphalangeal joint and has a feathered proximal edge to minimize the transition between the silicone and the natural tissue and to avoid limit-

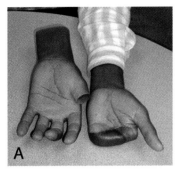
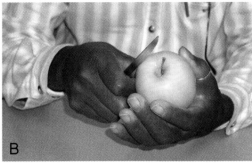

Figure 3 A partial hand device **(A)** can be used to perform tasks of daily living **(B)**.

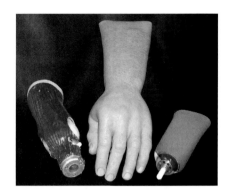

Figure 5 Roll-on suction liners with mechanical locking mechanisms allow the patient to interchange multiple terminal devices, including an aesthetic hand prosthesis with internal armature.

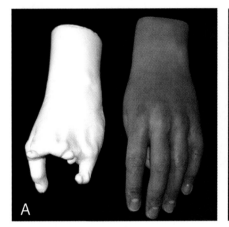
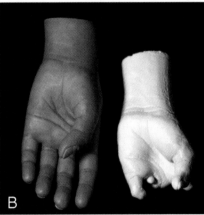

Figure 4 A, Dorsal view of hand and mold for prosthesis. **B,** Palmar view of hand and mold.

ing joint range of motion. When the length of the remaining digit is insufficient to secure a half finger restoration, a full finger prosthesis terminating at the metacarpophalangeal joint is recommended. A full finger prosthesis may also be used even with a more distal amputation when anticipated activities will generate sufficient forces to displace a half finger restoration. Because the termination of a full finger prosthesis occurs at the base of the proximal phalanx, a ring can be used both to enhance the attachment and to minimize the transition line.

A half finger prosthesis is generally indicated for patients who have a partial nail and nail bed after a distal tip amputation or for those with an amputation at the base of the nail. An acrylic nail is probably not feasible for these patients because the mounting mechanism protrudes into the prosthesis. In this situation, a silicone nail can be used (Figure 2). Unlike acrylic

nails, silicone nails should not be painted. In addition, the silicone cannot be extended beyond the length of the fingertip.

Thumb Prostheses

Thumb prostheses present unique challenges because of the desired mobility and stability of the prosthesis.[5] A full-length prosthesis is generally indicated to maintain adequate stability, given the presence of soft tissue in the web space between thumb and index finger and the extreme range of motion and significant force generated during prehension. For maximum stability, a glove-type partial hand prosthesis may be preferable.

Internal Armatures

In partial or full hand prostheses, a semirigid internal armature may be added to provide additional stability. Functionally, the armature adds a skeletal or structural component to

the flexible silicone skin of the prosthesis. The armature is often made of braided stainless steel, but other materials can be used as long as they are sufficiently durable to be repeatedly reshaped by the amputee. Armatures allow the amputee to flex or extend the fingers of the prosthesis, effectively positioning them for specific tasks.

Partial Hand Prostheses

A partial hand prosthesis should be considered for either acquired or congenital deficiencies in which there is total loss of one or more digits at or proximal to the metacarpophalangeal joint (Figure 3). When functional digits remain, the design must be carefully optimized to minimize interference with their movements. Proximal termination of the prosthesis is usually planned so that a watch or bracelet can be worn to minimize evidence of the transition between silicone and natural skin.

An example of such a restoration is shown in Figure 4. The mold depicts a congenital unilateral limb deficiency. Design options included exposing the thumb and little finger, which are able to oppose and grasp, or completely containing them inside of the prosthesis. In this case, a full restoration that provided the most normal appearance was selected based on the patient's vocational requirements.

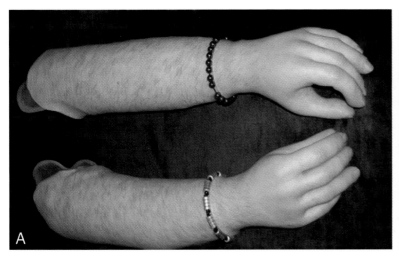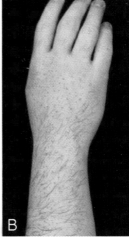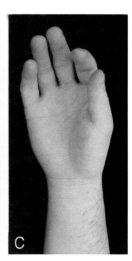

Figure 6 Myoelectric (**A**) and passive (**B** and **C**) transradial devices.

The use of an armature with a partial hand prosthesis is helpful in providing firm resistance to the intact fingers, thumb, or opposing hand during opposition or bimanual activities. In patients who have retained most of their metacarpals, however, it may be impossible to provide an armature because there is insufficient space within the prosthesis to anchor it firmly.

Full Hand Prostheses

Patients with amputations through the wrist require a full hand prosthesis. The major challenge in making a full hand prosthesis is to identify the most effective socket design to stabilize the restoration without encumbering the patient.[8] During the last decade, roll-on suction liners with mechanical locking mechanisms have been increasingly popular for upper limb prostheses. This type of suspension allows the patient to interchange multiple terminal devices, including an aesthetic hand prosthesis with internal armature (Figure 5).

Transradial Prostheses

For a patient with a unilateral arm amputation, a passive aesthetic prosthesis provides good function, is lightweight, and offers the most natural appearance. The sound hand is used for activities requiring dexterity. The passive prosthetic hand is used to assist the sound hand during various activities.

An aesthetic restoration is still possible when a mechanical or electric hand is provided, but compromises in the dimensions and shape of the wrist, palm, and fingers are needed because of the configuration of the internal mechanisms. These hands can be covered with a custom-made silicone skin for enhanced cosmesis as well as active prehension by the terminal device (Figure 6). Silicone coverings resist staining better than the vinyl covers that are typically provided with these hands.

Prostheses for Amputations at Transhumeral and Higher Levels

For passive transhumeral prostheses, the silicone skin can be made in one piece, encompassing the entire prosthesis up to the axilla. This use of silicone provides the most realistic appearance, although the silicone will inevitably distort unnaturally at the elbow or shoulder during flexion. A concealed, internal mechanical elbow joint is manipulated with the opposite hand, prepositioned, and locked for specific activities (Figure 7).

Silicone coverings most often terminate at the elbow to minimize interference with movement of the body-powered or electrically actuated

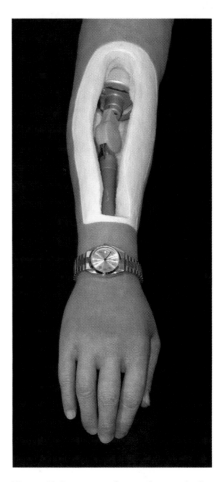

Figure 7 Cutaway of transhumeral device showing embedded passively operated elbow.

elbow. A continuous cover to the axilla creates marked resistance to elbow flexion, which drains the batteries of an electric prosthesis or forces the pa-

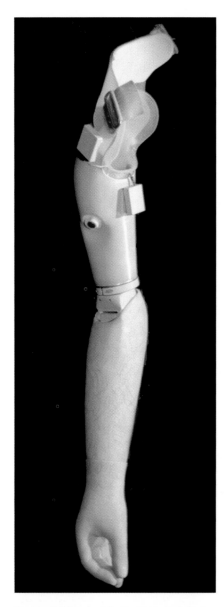

Figure 8 Myoelectrically operated device with custom silicone cover.

tient to generate excessive forces to operate a body-powered device (Figure 8).

Bilateral Upper Limb Prostheses

The rehabilitation process for a bilateral upper limb amputee is more complicated than for patients with a unilateral limb loss. A bilateral transhumeral amputee has only a 25% to 50% likelihood of achieving total independence (DJ Atkins, unpublished data, 1999, Reno, NV). Referring these amputees to a specialized

and experienced rehabilitation team of physicians, prosthetists, occupational therapists, and psychotherapists will help to optimize clinical outcome.

Pillet and Mackin[8] have observed that physical impairment is so great for the bilateral amputee that it overshadows the aesthetic concern, but such a concern is in fact not diminished in these patients. Most bilateral upper limb amputees initially focus on prostheses that restore active grasp and release. Interest in obtaining an aesthetic prosthesis, however, often increases over time, particularly for patients living in cultures that place a high value on physical appearance.

Patients with Congenital Deficiencies

Parents have great expectations for their children and learning that their newborn has a congenital limb deficiency can cause them to despair about their child's future. Fitting an infant with a natural-looking prosthesis to make his or her appearance more like that of other children can help the process of parental acceptance.[2,3,8,10] Early prosthetic fitting encourages the child to use the prosthesis to meet age-appropriate functional milestones.[3]

The types of prosthesis fitted may vary as the child matures. Most infants begin with passive terminal devices, although some are initially fitted with myoelectrically controlled or body-powered prostheses. Preschool children are often unconcerned with the appearance of the prosthesis, but this can change when the child reaches adolescence. Adults with a congenital limb deficiency may request an aesthetic prosthesis to facilitate social interactions in work situations, particularly if their occupation involves frequent interactions with the general public.

Considerations for Lower Limb Prostheses

Aesthetic restorations for lower limb amputations are routinely provided, although not as frequently as for upper limb amputees. A lower limb prosthesis can often be easily concealed under clothing and footwear. The material currently used for aesthetic restorations of lower limbs is not as durable as those used for upper limb prostheses. Custom aesthetic restorations are currently most commonly used for patients with toe or partial foot amputations. The aesthetic restorations are more frequently requested by female than male amputees. Many lower limb amputees have expressed a desire for a more lifelike artificial limb. Efforts to develop new lower limb prostheses to better withstand the forces of ambulation are ongoing.

Toe, Partial Foot, and Foot Prostheses

As the extent of the amputation progresses from distal to more proximal levels of the foot, aesthetic prostheses require internal and/or supplemental structural components to control unwanted foot movement, protect compromised tissue, and distribute the transmission of forces generated during walking. These devices may be called orthoses or prostheses because they typically contain elements of both types of devices[16] (Figure 9). These structural appliances can then be covered with a custom silicone skin to provide an aesthetic external appearance.

Syme, Transtibial, and Transfemoral Prostheses

If the entire foot is lost, the functional characteristics of silicone prostheses are limited to the psychosocial benefits associated with having a more normal appearance. In these patients, conventional prosthetic components are provided. After the prosthesis is fitted and the dynamic alignment

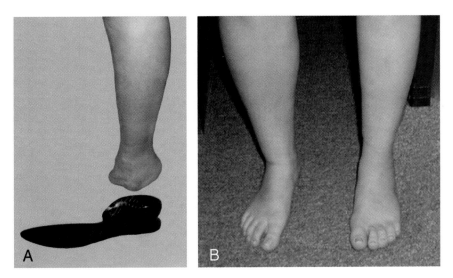

Figure 9 A, Partial foot over custom fiber sole. **B,** Patient wearing the finished foot. *(Courtesy of Jack Uellendahl, CPO.)*

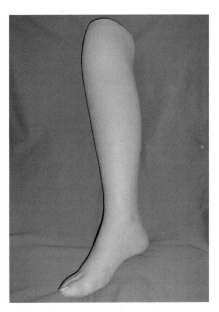

Figure 10 Transtibial prosthesis. *(Courtesy of Liberating Technologies Inc, Hollister, MA.)*

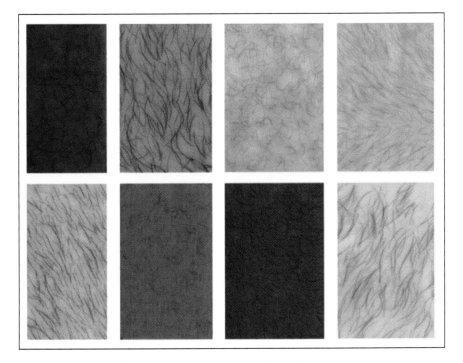

Figure 11 Samples of hair that can be used in prosthesis development.

Nails

Fingernails and toenails can be made from either a hard acrylic material or a softer, flexible silicone. The most realistic appearance is achieved with acrylic, which can be formed to match any nail shape, length, and color. Acrylic nails can also be painted by the user with commercially available nail polish. Silicone nails are soft and flexible, cannot be extended beyond the tip of the finger, and should not be painted with nail polish. Acrylic nails are commonly used for finger prostheses when the residual finger length is not an issue and in most partial and full hand restorations; they are less commonly used in prostheses for lower limb restorations.

Hair

Even if the color, shape, and texture of the silicone skin are perfectly matched, prostheses for patients with moderate to dense body hair are not acceptable without an attempt to reproduce their hair pattern. This is accomplished by painting the illusion of hair into the silicone, or by applying synthetic or human hair into or onto

process is completed, silicone coverings are fitted over the prosthesis. For transtibial coverings, the silicone terminates at the proximal edges of the prosthetic socket (Figure 10). The considerations relevant to elbow coverings also apply to transfemoral coverings as a continuous cover distorts during knee flexion and inhibits knee motion. Therefore, transfemoral cov-

erings generally terminate at the knee. The colors of the foot, leg, hair, and nails are incorporated into the prosthesis so that the appearance in open-toed footwear is natural. Increased forces and wear associated with walking, coupled with the high cost of silicone manufacturing, limit the applications for this type of restoration for lower limb amputees.

the skin in a pattern similar to that of the patient (Figure 11).

Color Changes

Human skin is dynamic, exhibiting cyclical color changes that may be subtle or dramatic. These changes can be internal and physiologic, such as the changes caused by surface capillary dilation. Color changes may also be external and environmental, such as suntanning. Unlike human skin, silicone is static. When the silicone of a prosthesis is pigmented, the color is carefully matched to the colors of the amputee's skin at the time it is painted. Once applied, the color cannot easily be changed. If the patient's skin darkens significantly, the prosthesis also needs to be darkened to maintain an acceptable match.

To solve this problem, the patient can obtain two devices that represent the extremes of lightness and darkness typical of their skin color changes. Another option is to obtain a prosthesis that accepts a surface pigment, which is applied to deepen or darken the color. Normal exposure to ultraviolet light causes this surface pigment to fade to the original lighter shade.

Conclusion

The role of aesthetics in prosthetic restoration should not be overlooked, especially when treating individuals with upper limb deficiencies and partial foot amputations. The concept that prostheses mimicking normal appearance are somehow nonfunctional is obsolete. Aesthetic prostheses should be provided whenever appropriate to address the intertwined functional and psychosocial deficits experienced by individuals with limb loss.

References

1. Fraser CM: An evaluation of the use made of cosmetic and functional prostheses by unilateral upper limb amputees. *Prosthet Orthot Int* 1998;22:216-224.

2. Hubbard S, Bush G, Naumann S: Myoelectric prostheses for the limb-deficient child. *PMR Clinics North Am* 1991;2:847-866.

3. Hubbard SA, Kurtz I, Heim W, et al: Powered prosthetic intervention in upper extremity deficiency, in Herring JA, Birch JG (eds): *The Child With a Limb Deficiency*. Rosemont, IL, American Academy of Orthopaedic Surgeons, 1998, pp 417-431.

4. Kyberd PJ, Davey JJ, Dougall Morrison J: A survey of upper-limb prosthesis users in Oxfordshire. *JPO* 1998;10: 85-91.

5. Michael JW, Buckner H: Options for finger prostheses. *JPO* 1994;6:10-19.

6. Millstein SG, Heger H, Hunter GA: Prosthetic use in adult upper limb amputees: A comparison of the body powered and electrically powered prostheses. *Prosthet Orthot Int* 1986;10: 27-34.

7. O'Farrell DA, Montella BJ, Bahor JL, et al: Long-term follow-up of 50 Duke silicone prosthetic fingers. *J Hand Surg* 1996;21:696-700.

8. Pillet J, Mackin EJ: Aesthetic restoration, in Bowker JH, Michael JW (eds): *Atlas of Limb Prosthetics*, ed 2. St. Louis, MO, Mosby-Year Book, 1992, pp 227-235.

9. Pilley MJ, Quinton DN: Digital prostheses for single finger amputations. *J Hand Surg* 1999;24:539-541.

10. Uellendahl J, Heelan J: Prosthetic management of the upper limb deficient child. *Phys Med Rehabil* 2000;14: 221-235.

11. Burkhart A, Weitz J: Oncological applications for silicone gel sheets in soft tissue contractures. *Am J Occup Ther* 1990;45:460-462.

12. Ohmori S: Effectiveness of silastic sheet coverage in the treatment of scar keloid. *Plast Surg* 1988;12:95-99.

13. Quinn KJ: Silicone gel in scar treatment. *Burns* 1987;13:533-540.

14. Atkins D: Adult upper limb prosthetic training, in Bowker JH, Michael JW (eds): *Atlas of Limb Prosthetics*, ed 2. St. Louis, MO, Mosby-Year Book, 1992, pp 277-291.

15. Bennett JB, Alexander CB: Amputation levels and surgical techniques, in Atkins DJ, Meier RH (eds): *Comprehensive Management of the Upper Limb Amputee*. New York, NY, Springer-Verlag, 1990, pp 1-10.

16. Condie DN, Stills M: Prosthetic and orthotic management, in Bowker JH, Michael JW (eds): *Atlas of Limb Prosthetics*, ed 2. St. Louis, MO, Mosby-Year Book, 1992, pp 403-412.

17. Inman V, Ralston HJ, Todd F: Prosthetics, in Rose J, Gamble JG (eds): *Human Walking*, ed 2. Baltimore, MD, Williams & Wilkins, 1994, pp 165-199.

18. Malone JM, Fleming LL, Roberson J, et al: Immediate, early and late postsurgical management of upper limb amputation. *J Rehabil Res Dev* 1984;21: 33-40.

19. Allison A, Mackinnon SE: Evaluation of digital prostheses. *J Hand Surg [Am]* 1992;17:923-926.

20. Beasley RW, de Beze GM: Prosthetic replacements for the thumb. *Hand Clin* 1992;8:63-69.

21. Manurangsee P, Isariyawut C, Chatuthong V, et al: Osseointegrated finger prostheses: An alternative method for finger reconstruction. *J Hand Surg [Am]* 2000;25:86-92.

22. Herring HW, Romerdale EH: Prosthetic finger retention: A new approach. *O&P* 1983;37:28-30.

Chapter 25

Bilateral Upper Limb Prostheses

Jack E. Uellendahl, CPO

Introduction

Bilateral upper limb amputation is a profound loss. Performing basic and routine tasks such as eating and self care becomes difficult or impossible without assistance. Prostheses and other assistive devices can enable users to regain some of their lost ability to manipulate objects and successfully complete a wide variety of tasks. Replacing the many exquisite features of the physiologic hand, however, is currently impossible. The completion of even simple manual tasks requires an amazing amount of complex manipulation. These words, for example, were typed using 10 fingers working in concert. Each finger performs independent and sometimes coordinated simultaneous functions, relying on sensation and precise positioning to accurately produce the intended result. These abilities are taken for granted until they are lost.

The goal of prosthetic rehabilitation for the bilateral upper limb amputee is to enable the individual to achieve functional independence and to participate successfully in vocational as well as recreational pursuits. Although bilateral prosthetic arm replacement offers only a small amount of the functions lost, users can perform many activities that would otherwise be impossible. Subtle details of socket fit, control system configuration, and suspension can sometimes mean the difference between long-term success and failure. Unlike the person with a unilateral arm amputation, the person with bilateral upper limb amputations cannot compensate for the inadequacies of a prosthesis with the use of an intact physiologic arm.[1] Therefore, it is paramount that every detail of prosthetic design be optimized. Given the current inability to duplicate the diverse and complex functions of the human arm, prosthetic systems should be viewed as tools, with each component being best suited for certain uses. Success relies on the selection of the most appropriate components for the desired tasks, matching those components with optimal control sources and interfacing them with the human body in a comfortable and functional manner. Of equal importance is the user's dedication and motivation to succeed in the face of adversity.

Patient Evaluation

Given the complexity of bilateral upper limb loss and the fluid nature of the early rehabilitation period, thorough evaluation of the new bilateral upper limb amputee should occur over a period of time. Most often, patients who sustain bilateral upper limb amputations have experienced a traumatic injury, so there are medical issues in addition to limb loss. Ideally, a team of experienced professionals should be working in concert to address the many issues facing the new amputee. The treating or consulting professionals may include an orthopaedic surgeon, physiatrist, prosthetist, occupational therapist, physical therapist, psychologist, nurse, and a social worker. An invaluable adjunct to the care and treatment provided by these professionals is patient access to peer support whenever available.

Patient factors that affect prosthetic component and control scheme selection include cognitive level, mechanical aptitude, family life, occupation, hobbies, and self-image. Residual limb length, and strength and range of motion of the joints of the upper limbs, including scapulothoracic motion, should be carefully evaluated as these will have direct implications regarding the method of prosthetic fitting. The general strength and flexibility of the lower limbs should be assessed as well. With more proximal amputations, foot use should be encouraged, with training dedicated to exploring and developing the manipulative capabilities of the feet (Figure 1). At the conclusion of the initial evaluation process, a defined plan for the selection of the prosthetic components and control scheme should be in place. However, the team needs to be flexible throughout the rehabilitation process. The configuration of the prosthesis will almost inevitably evolve in response to the changing needs and abilities of the user. Such changes can be ex-

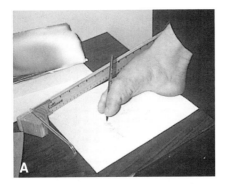 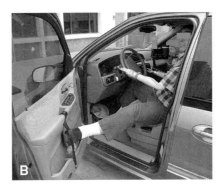

Figure 1 A, Persons with congenital bilateral upper limb deficiency often develop remarkable dexterity and manipulative foot function. **B,** Adults with acquired bilateral upper limb loss usually do not develop this kind of foot function but may find foot use an efficient alternative to prosthetic function for tasks away from the body. *(Reproduced with permission from Fenstermacher Photo Release.)*

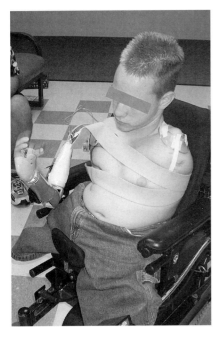

Figure 2 This teenage boy with congenital quadrimembral limb deficiency demonstrates the use of his prototype prosthesis. The control scheme provides dedicated variable-speed control of the hand, wrist, and elbow using two-site myoelectric control of the hand, a linear transducer for elbow operation controlled by scapular abduction, and a pair of FSRs positioned near his mobile right acromion for wrist rotation. *(Reproduced with permission from Gentry Photo Release.)*

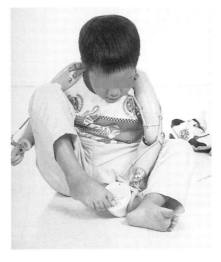

Figure 3 A young boy with acquired bilateral very short transhumeral amputations demonstrates the superior manipulative function provided by his sensate feet, as he stabilizes the object with his prosthesis.

jects that differ in size, shape, and texture. Information about the characteristics of an object would be relayed to the user through a sensory feedback system. Proprioception regarding the speed of prosthetic movement, the force exerted, and the position of the prosthetic device would be inherent. The hand would be lightweight and durable. Currently available state-of-the-art prosthetic prehensors are far from this ideal. Available technology can be optimized, however, by considering the needs of each individual and then comparing the attributes of each prosthetic component and control scheme to the ideal.

Although this chapter focuses primarily on the management of adult amputees, many of the concepts presented have application for the management of children. Pediatric patients, however, cannot be treated simply as small adults because of their small size and sometimes immature cognitive ability. With a small body size comes decreased physical ability to generate useful force and excursion and a lower tolerance for weight and prosthesis complexity. Congenital bilateral limb deficiency is very rare, and the issues regarding prosthetic fitting for children with this deficiency can be quite different from those of adult bilateral upper limb amputees (Figure 2). On the positive side, children with congenital limb deficiency are often much more adaptable than adults and will do remarkable things with their residual limbs and their feet[2] (Figure 3). The section on pediatric issues provides more detail about this unique cohort of patients.

Staging of Care

A prosthesis should be fit as soon as possible, preferably within the first 30 to 90 days, for all patients with either unilateral or bilateral acquired arm amputation. The first 30 days after amputation have been referred to by Malone and associates[3] as the golden period of fitting for upper limb pros-

consider the advantages and disadvantages of various components and control options for a specific individual. To give structure to this thought process, it is useful to understand the attributes of the "ideal" prosthesis and then compare these attributes to existing technologies. The ideal prosthesis would fully restore the appearance and function of the limbs lost. Considering prosthetic prehensors, this would mean that the ideal prehensor would be a hand. Control of the hand would be subconscious and natural. The hand would be capable of manipulating a wide variety of ob-

pected and are considered part of the normal recovery process from such a massive functional loss.

Throughout the evaluation process, the prosthetist should carefully

thetic devices, based on clinical evidence that optimal acceptance and practical use of a prosthesis are most likely to occur during this period. Early postoperative fitting has multiple advantages, including decreased edema and pain, accelerated wound healing, improved patient rehabilitation, decreased length of hospital stay, increased prosthetic use, maintenance of some continuous type of proprioception input through the residual limb, and improved psychological adaptation to amputation. In patients who have injuries or other complicating factors that make fitting within the golden period impractical or impossible, prosthetic use may be delayed. In many patients, one side may be ready to fit before the other, and it is advisable to do so. Indeed, initially providing a prosthesis on only one side is often desirable. For most patients with bilateral upper limb amputations, it is beneficial to begin prosthetic training using a simplified component configuration and control scheme as this is easier for the patient to master initially. Especially for patients with higher level amputations, "gadget overload" is a practical concern, as each limb may have multiple dynamically positioned components. In these situations, it is generally advisable to introduce new components sequentially to allow the user to become accustomed to each new device before increasing the overall complexity of the artificial limbs.

Given the dynamic nature of prosthetic rehabilitation of the bilateral upper limb amputee, it is useful to develop short- and long-term goals. As the amputee's skills develop, and as his or her medical condition stabilizes, and priorities change in response to the realities of the challenges of daily life, so too, the prosthetic devices and use pattern will change. The process of rehabilitation can be expected to take 6 months to 1 year or more, depending on the level of limb loss, the extent of other complicating factors, and how quickly the amputee adapts. An invaluable tool during this period of change is

the prototype prosthesis, as will be discussed later in this chapter. The prototype prosthesis allows the amputee and the team to evaluate various prosthetic systems before deciding on a definitive prescription. Short-term goals will generally focus on mastering basic daily functional use of the prostheses for tasks such as donning, eating, and toileting. Long-term goals may include dressing, vocational skills, and avocational pursuits. During this period of experimentation, the amputee should spend most of his or her time at home, periodically returning to the rehabilitation facility for prosthetic modifications and additional training. In this way, the user will be better able to determine which prosthetic systems work best in a real-life situation and to identify specific problems that need attention during the next visit with the team.

Complete independence is expected to be achieved in all patients except those who have lost both limbs above the elbow or who have other limiting factors. Strongly motivated bilateral transhumeral amputees can sometimes attain complete independence in accomplishing their daily regimen, but realizing this goal can take an extended period of time.

Socket Design

Socket designs for bilateral amputees do not differ substantially from those for unilateral amputees, except that it is even more crucial to permit as much range of motion as practical. Because of the absence of both hands, however, it is important to consider ease of donning and flexibility in positioning of the prostheses. Positioning flexibility includes range of motion of the intact physiologic joints with the prostheses donned, and, in some patients, the ability to reposition the prosthesis at the limb-socket interface in a manner that increases functionality (Figure 4). Although the socket may not always be completely self-suspending, the interface should fit snugly and work with the suspen-

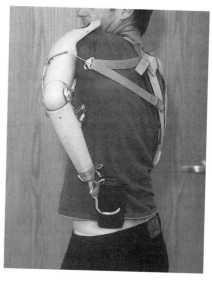

Figure 4 The functional envelope can sometimes be expanded by repositioning the prosthesis on the limb to produce more useful function. This man demonstrates retrieving his wallet from his back pocket, requiring hook operation behind his back.

sion system so that the prosthesis feels firmly connected to the user under conditions of dynamic use. This intimate fit will not only provide optimal control of the positioning of the prosthesis but will also minimize the sensation of weight. The socket is the foundation of the prosthetic system, and any shortcomings in socket design will adversely affect the success of the prosthesis. This is true for both body-powered and electronic control systems. There should be minimal lost motion, so that as the residual limb begins to move, the prosthesis responds immediately.

Transradial amputees using body-powered control will most often benefit from flexible hinges as these components allow them to retain active use of physiologic forearm rotation. In patients with significant remaining forearm rotation, it is critical that the socket shape capture the maximum amount of available motion. Supracondylar socket designs do not allow physiologic forearm rotation, so this important disadvantage must be considered carefully. Self-suspending sockets such as those typically used for myoelectric control, and to a

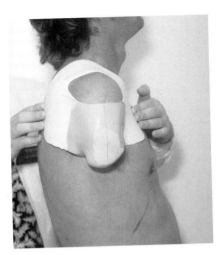

Figure 5 The half-and-half socket provides an integral shoulder saddle offering good suspension and comfort. Use of a passive prosthesis on one side is sometimes indicated when no functional prosthesis is desired. Here the passive prosthesis provides a firm anchor point for the harness of the contralateral prosthesis and provides a more normal appearance for this amputee with a very short right transhumeral amputation and a left interscapulothoracic amputation.

lesser extent, for body-position control, are generally best donned by pushing the residual limb into the socket because of the obvious difficulty of pulling in with a stockinette. The Northwestern University self-suspending socket[4] offers particular advantages for bilateral transradial fittings in which supracondylar suspension is desired because it tends to offer good range of motion at the elbow and is easily donned by pushing in. The Northwestern socket can also be modified with a cutout over the olecranon, which reduces heat buildup and improves cosmesis, especially when the elbow is extended.[5] On rare occasions when pulling in is deemed necessary, a nylon donning bag is an effective tool and can be used independently by some patients.

Sockets for the transhumeral prosthesis should also provide a close coupling of the residual limb and the prosthesis to maximize prosthetic function. Ideally, the socket design should cause little or no restriction of motion at the next proximal joint. Therefore, open shoulder designs[6] are

preferred because they allow relatively free range of motion at the shoulder joint, especially when sufficient limb length remains. Another option for socket design is the half-and-half socket described by Sauter. This socket uses a flexible silicone proximal section that is fitted over the shoulder region and is fabricated as an integral part of the socket. The deltoid area is cut out laterally to improve flexibility and air circulation within the socket. The socket is rigid distally from the axilla level[7] (Figure 5). This design works particularly well with a completely myoelectric prosthesis, in which case the only function of the harness is to hold the silicone piece in place on the shoulder. Another option similar to the half-and-half socket is the flexible shoulder suspension system in which a strip of Lycra-backed neoprene or similar material replaces the silicone saddle and is attached to the wings of the standard open shoulder socket.[1] Closed shoulder designs are best used for short residual limbs when there is insufficient leverage to use the full range of physiologic shoulder motion. The closed shoulder socket offers good stabilization of the prosthesis on the user and a convenient and secure anchor point for the harness lateral suspension strap.

The design of a shoulder disarticulation interface requires sufficient surface area to effectively stabilize the prosthesis on the amputee. Because of the length of the prosthesis lever arm and the weight of the components, there is a strong tendency for rotation at the prosthesis-user interface, especially as the terminal device is moved away from the body. Therefore, the socket perimeter should extend sufficiently onto the torso to resist these forces. The use of a frame-type socket will allow the requisite stabilization, facilitate heat dissipation, and minimize weight. If body-powered control is used, the frame should capture as much body motion as possible, particularly biscapular abduction. Any loss of motion will limit prosthetic function. If the components are con-

trolled myoelectrically, it may be advantageous to allow the shoulder to move independently of the frame to prevent movement of the electrodes on the skin, resulting in loss of control. Shoulder motion can often be used to activate various electronic inputs. In this configuration, the weight of the prosthesis anchors the frame to the user, whereas the shoulder is free to move independently. Several shoulder disarticulation frame variations are in use today. When designing a frame for an individual, the prosthetist should consider control sources, harness attachments, and mounting of the mechanical shoulder joint mechanism, in addition to the above-mentioned design objectives. These design requirements will dictate the optimal frame geometry for each prosthesis.

Harnessing

Conventional harnessing serves the dual role of suspension and control of the body-powered prosthesis. In designing a harness system for the bilateral upper limb amputee, it may be useful to consider suspension and control separately. When electrically powered components are used, or when the socket design provides suspension, the harness requirements are altered. Cognizance of these factors can result in simpler, less restrictive harness designs and ultimately a prosthesis that is more comfortable to wear. In situations in which right and left prostheses are harnessed together, each prosthesis serves as the anchor point for the other. This design has advantages but can sometimes lead to inadvertent activation of the opposite limb (sometimes referred to as cross-control) in fully body-powered systems. One solution would be to provide a fully body-powered prosthesis on one side and a fully electronic prosthesis on the other. In this situation, the difference in control methods makes it much easier for the amputee to control the arms independently.

In some patients with bilateral upper limb amputations, a socket may be

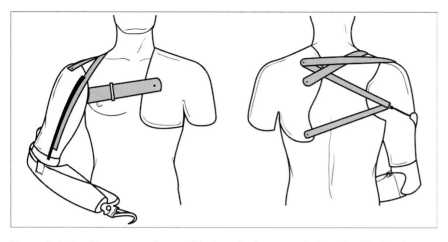

Figure 6 A shoulder cap can be provided on the interscapulothoracic side for the person with interscapulothoracic/transhumeral amputations.

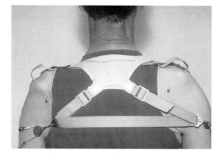

Figure 7 A leather pad can be provided to replace the cross point of the webbing harness, thereby spreading the load over a larger area and helping to position the control attachment straps lower on the back for greater excursion.

fitted for the sole purpose of providing a secure anchor for the contralateral prosthesis. One example is the interscapulothoracic/transhumeral bilateral design in which a frame-type socket or shoulder cap provides a firm anchor for suspension and control of the transhumeral prosthesis and can be shaped to provide shoulder symmetry under clothing (Figure 6). The bilateral transradial amputee using body-powered control is generally fitted with a standard figure-of-8 harness, typically incorporating a ring at the cross point for free movement of the straps, along with flexible hinges and a triceps pad. Compared with the unilateral figure-of-8 harness, the bilateral version eliminates the axilla loop, which is a frequent area of discomfort. Thus, the bilateral harness is well tolerated by almost all patients and is also easy to don and doff independently. Bilateral myoelectrically controlled prostheses at the transradial level typically require no harness.

Similarly, the bilateral transhumeral amputee wearing body-powered systems is usually fitted with a figure-of-8 harness. If cable excursion is limited, it is advisable to use a harness design without a ring to limit any loss of motion that occurs when the harness straps rotate on the ring. Either a standard sewn cross point or a leather pad may be beneficial in such situations. The leather pad has the additional advantage of routing the control attachment straps more inferiorly on the scapulae, thereby increasing the available excursion (Figure 7). Another useful modification is the cross-back strap, which also keeps the control attachment straps low on the scapulae. A double-ring harness offers another option to accomplish this result (Figure 8). Harness configurations for bilateral fittings in patients with differing amputation levels require careful planning and customization to provide optimal stabilization, suspension, and control. Figure 9 shows examples of successful harness designs for patients with asymmetric limb loss.

Components
Terminal Devices

The new bilateral upper limb amputee is likely to prefer to be fitted with prosthetic hands, an intuitive choice given the societal expectation that available technology can replace the function and appearance of the physiologic hand. The rehabilitation team must gently educate the patient and family so both come to realize that the current state of the art is not this versatile. Most body-powered hands are mechanically inefficient, offer little grip force, and have proved to be of very limited functional use.

Compared with body-powered hands, electrically powered prehensors offer a much tighter grip that can be

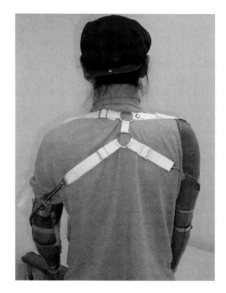

Figure 8 The double-ring harness increases available excursion by positioning the control attachment straps lower on the scapulae, as seen in this transhumeral/transradial example.

maintained without significant exertion, but their control systems offer little direct proprioceptive feedback.[8] If having an anthropomorphic appearance is critical to the patient, then at least one electrically powered hand is generally warranted.

Cable-driven grippers, such as the split hook, offer direct proprioception via the cable and harness system. Component movement and forces are sensed by the controlling body part when the harness compresses the underlying skin,[8] as will be discussed in detail later in this chapter.

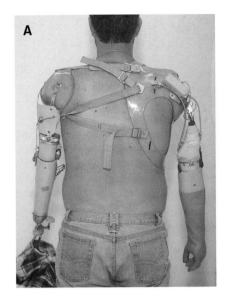 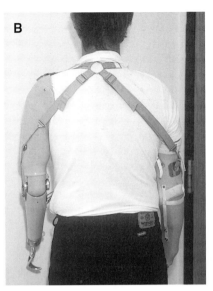 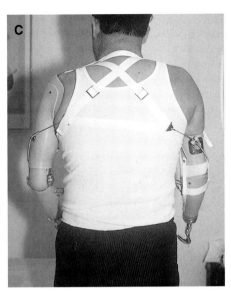

Figure 9 A, An example of a harness for shoulder disarticulation/transhumeral combination in which the transhumeral prosthesis is entirely body powered and the hybrid shoulder disarticulation prosthesis uses myoelectric control of the terminal device and body-powered control of the elbow. A single anterior chest strap allows independent donning and doffing. **B,** A simple figure-of-8 ring harness can be used for the transhumeral/transradial amputee if sufficient excursion is available. **C,** In situations in which excursion is limited, a sewn cross-point and a cross-back strap are usually advisable to maximize excursion.

Bilateral electronic hands and grippers have been most successful in patients with transradial or wrist disarticulations. An electrically powered device provides prehension forces three to six times the force possible with the typical voluntary-opening split hook, making the grip more secure for bilateral users.[1] As electronic hands and the means of controlling them gradually improve, their utility for the bilateral amputee should be continually reevaluated. At present, few persons with bilateral amputations choose hand-like prehension devices for long-term use, despite the strong preference expressed for such devices at the initial fitting. Anthropomorphic devices are bulky and obstruct the view of the object being grasped. In my experience, most users prefer body-powered split hooks for dominant side function. The slender fingers of the split hook allow relatively good visual access to the work area and the objects being handled. As the person with bilateral acquired amputations gradually comes to terms with the magnitude of loss and his or her altered self-image, practical considerations such as ease of use for fine grasping tasks often outweigh the un-natural appearance of the body-powered hook.

For bilateral fittings, it is generally advisable to use two different types of prehensors to provide greater grasp versatility. One common strategy is to provide a hook with canted fingers on the dominant side and a lyre-shaped hook on the opposite side. The canted hook allows good visual feedback of objects being manipulated, and the lyre-shaped hook provides better stability for gripping large cylindrical objects. Another clinically successful terminal device combination is a canted hook on the dominant side and an electrically powered prehensor on the other side. This combination provides the fine manipulation capabilities of a split hook with the superior gripping forces of an electronic prehensor. In my experience, this combination has been particularly well accepted by the transhumeral/shoulder disarticulation amputee.

Voluntary-opening hooks are used primarily for bilateral amputees because these components maintain grip without requiring the amputee to generate constant cable tension. Another reason that these hooks are commonly used is that they are avail-able in a wide variety of shapes, sizes, and specific prehension patterns. Voluntary-closing hooks are less commonly used by bilateral amputees even though body-powered voluntary-closing hooks offer both excellent feedback regarding prehension forces and good grip strength. Requisite continuous cable tension or the need for a locking mechanism to maintain grasp, as well as the limited number of design configurations for voluntary-closing hooks, appears to restrict the use of voluntary-closing hooks.

Task-specific terminal devices should always be considered for the bilateral amputee. These devices are generally used with quick-disconnect wrist components to facilitate interchange between a utilitarian hook and specific-use devices such as work tools and kitchen utensils. One innovative approach uses a hands-free tool exchanger that permits automatic release and exchange of one task-specific device for another.

Wrists

Wrist flexion is particularly helpful for body-centered activities, such as feeding, dressing, oral and facial hygiene, and toileting. Therefore, wrist

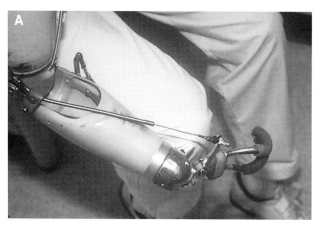

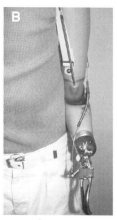

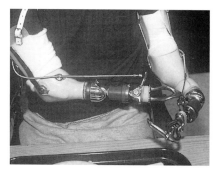

Figure 11 Midforearm flexion facilitates hook placement for midline activities when elbow range of motion is limited.

Figure 10 The four-function forearm setup allows body-powered control of wrist flexion and rotation. **A,** The wrist flexion lock is actuated by pulling against the knee; the unlocked wrist is flexed by pulling on the control cable and extended by an elastic tension band. **B,** Wrist rotation is unlocked by depressing a lock lever against the torso; cable tension causes the unlocked wrist to supinate the terminal device; pronation is provided by an internally mounted coil spring.

flexion should be provided on the dominant side, if not bilaterally. Wrist rotation is essential for effective orientation of the prehension device. If a cable-actuated prehensor is used, the range of wrist rotation will be limited because the control cable crosses the joint. The combination of an electronic rotator and an electronic prehension device does not limit wrist rotation because no control cable is needed to activate the prehensor.[1] Continuous wrist rotation can be useful for certain activities such as turning a water spigot.

Locking wrist components are usually more useful than friction designs. Bilateral amputees must apply high forces through their prostheses to accomplish various tasks. When friction devices are used, the friction must be very strong for it to be stable during these tasks, which then makes it difficult to reposition the device.

Positive-locking components make the prosthesis a rigid extension of the body that can maintain position under high loads and yet be repositioned with ease when unlocked. One noteworthy body-powered system is the four-function forearm setup originally described by Robinson and Caywood (Figure 10). This system has been used successfully by short transradial, transhumeral, and shoulder

disarticulation amputees.

In my experience, the preferred system for transhumeral amputation and shoulder disarticulation patients is the body-powered system based on this four-function forearm setup;[9] this system uses a common control cable to position four different body-powered prosthetic components: (1) split hook, (2) wrist flexion unit, (3) wrist rotation unit, and (4) elbow. The simplicity of the control method is a mixed blessing. An advantage of this method is that the same physiologic control motion is used to position each of the four components, thus conserving available control sources. The control arrangement, however, is sequential in that only one device can be positioned at a time. Therefore, it is not possible to produce coordinated movements involving two or more components. The straightforward method of control and the inherent proprioceptive feedback appear to outweigh these disadvantages for most users.[1]

Midforearm flexion offers a nonanthropomorphic solution to limited range of motion and has been particularly useful for the short or very short transradial amputee. By placing the flexion device more proximal in the prosthesis, a greater arc of motion is achieved at the terminal de-

vice, which improves the ease of midline tasks. A greater amount of cable excursion is required in the flexed position, depending on the cable system configuration (Figure 11).

Elbows

Selection of the most appropriate elbow should include careful evaluation of weight, control options, and compatibility with the other desired components. Body-powered elbows are lighter and faster than electrically powered units, but they provide very little live lift. Electrically powered elbows have greater lifting capacity but are heavier and lack the proprioceptive feedback inherent in the cable control of body-powered elbows.[1]

A spring lift assist or automatic forearm balance should be considered for all body-powered elbow fittings. These devices allow the prosthetist to optimize and balance the force/excursion requirements with the abilities and needs of a particular user.

In bilateral amputees who require two elbows, it is sometimes beneficial to provide one body-powered type and one electrically powered type. The two elbows complement each other as the electrically powered side offers greater live lift capacity and the body-powered elbow makes precise positioning easier.[1]

Rigid elbow hinges are rarely appropriate for bilateral transradial amputees because these hinges prohibit active pronation and supination. One exception is the step-up hinge that requires twice the force for motion but

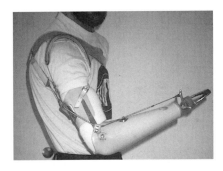

Figure 12 A fair-lead cable can be used to assist elbow flexion so long as sufficient extension force can be generated to stabilize the elbow during hook operation.

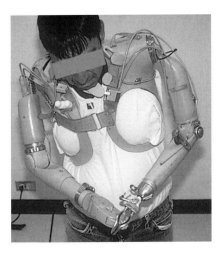

Figure 13 Locking humeral rotation makes it simple to move the terminal device transversely yet provides a rigid limb to resist high forces when locked. This bilateral shoulder disarticulation amputee demonstrates the ability to bring his terminal devices into contact with each other, allowing bimanual manipulation. *(Reproduced with permission from Fenstermacher Photo Release.)*

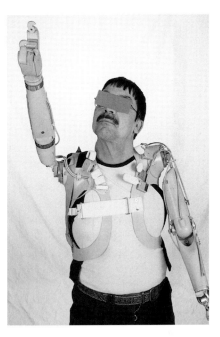

Figure 14 A locking shoulder joint allows this bilateral shoulder disarticulation amputee to operate the terminal device overhead. This terminal device is controlled by a linear transducer using shoulder elevation, providing reliable variable-speed control. *(Reproduced with permission from Fenstermacher Photo Release.)*

moves the forearm 2° for every 1° of residual limb flexion. The disadvantages of the step-up hinge include poor forearm cosmesis when the elbow is flexed, the extent of which is dependent on the length of the residual limb. The disadvantages of this specialized elbow joint are sometimes outweighed by the increased range of motion afforded. A fair-lead cable housing also can be used with these hinges to supplement elbow flexion force as long as the user has sufficient elbow extension force to stabilize the forearm during operation of the terminal device. This same cabling method using standard single-pivot hinges can be advantageous for the user who has weak elbow flexor strength on presentation, as long as an adequate range of passive flexion range is available and there is enough extension force to resist further flexion during operation of the terminal device (Figure 12).

Humeral Rotation

All internal locking elbow systems routinely used in North America, whether body-powered or electrically powered, include a mechanism simulating passive humeral rotation that is stabilized by friction. Locking humeral rotation may be beneficial for bilateral fittings and for selected unilateral arm amputees, offering the same relative advantages as a locking wrist unit. Rimjet Corporation (Sarasota, FL) offers a locking humeral ro-

tator designed to interface with the ubiquitous Hosmer Dorrance E-400 mechanical elbow (Hosmer Dorrance, Campbell, CA), although it is possible to adapt this rotator for other elbows, including electronic ones.[1,10] The lock is operated by a control cable that can be actuated through a harness strap that is parallel with the elbow lock control strap or by a chin-actuated nudge control (Figure 13).

Shoulder Joints

The bilateral amputee who requires a prosthetic shoulder joint will benefit from a device that locks in position for the same reasons as those described for locking wrist and humeral components. The LTI-Collier joint (Liberating Technologies Inc, Holliston, MA) provides a positive locking feature for flexion-extension as well as friction for abduction control. This joint locks at 10° intervals. The lock can be operated either by a cable nudge control or with an electronic actuator. The rigidity of the locked shoulder joint allows the person to use the prosthesis more effectively as an extension of the body.[1] For bilateral amputees, the ability to

operate the terminal device overhead is invaluable, as it increases the scope of practical work that can be accomplished with the artificial arm (Figure 14).

Prosthesis Control

The two basic categories of currently available prosthetic controls are body position control and myoelectric control. Body position control refers to voluntary movement of anatomic structures and the excursion and/or forces produced by those motions (Table 1). Cable-operated components are the most common examples of this type of control, but body motions are also useful to operate electronic inputs such as switches, servos, and pressure transducers (Figure 15). Myoelectric control uses the electrical by-product of voluntary muscle contractions, as discussed in chapter 12. Unlike many cable control systems, myoelectric control is generally independent of proximal joint position,

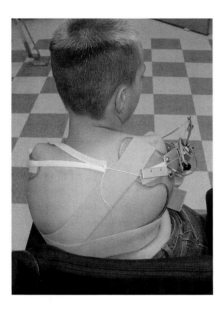

Figure 15 A linear transducer activated by contralateral scapular abduction provides variable-speed control of the prosthetic elbow for this boy with bilateral shoulder-level limb deficiencies. *(Reproduced with permission from Gentry Photo Release.)*

TABLE 1 Body Position Control Sources

Primary Work Sources Producing Good Force and Excursion

Glenohumeral flexion

Scapular/biscapular abduction

Control sources for mechanical locks and electronic inputs

Glenohumeral extension/abduction/shoulder depression

Shoulder elevation

Chest expansion

Abdominal expansion

Chin nudge

Glenohumeral adduction

Other (any movable body part)

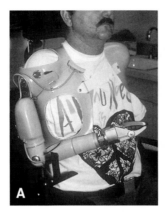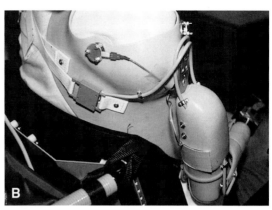

Figure 16 This patient has quadrimembral amputations plus paraplegia. He uses a single multifunctional prosthesis to achieve partial independence in self-feeding and manipulation of simple objects. **A,** The wrist rotator, positioned at midforearm, is controlled by a rocker switch using his chin. The wheelchair-mounted bracket assists with internal and external rotation of the humeral turntable. Wrist flexion is achieved using a conventional flexion wrist. **B,** An electronic elbow is operated with a pair of FSRs mounted anteriorly and posteriorly within the socket, and the terminal device is controlled using scapular abduction and a harness pull switch. Coordinated elbow flexion and wrist rotation are possible and are useful for self-feeding.

which can make the prosthesis easier to use.

When developing a prescription for the upper limb amputee, it is critical to understand the relationship between available control sources and the types of components these sources can most effectively control. Component selection should be based on a careful analysis of which devices

and control options will facilitate the intended function of the user.

For the bilateral amputee, the reliability of the control system is of paramount importance. A control source is reliable only when each and every control command results in the desired component function. In addition, a component should never operate inadvertently. Whenever a control command fails to produce the desired result, the overall utility of the prosthesis is severely compromised. Therefore, control systems that are overly complicated or that rely on a marginal control source are rarely successful for long-term use. Training for prosthetic use is often essential in maximizing the reliability of prosthesis control. However, if training fails to produce consistently reliable control function, then an alternative control method is indicated.

In the context of operation of multiple components, control options are described as either dedicated or sequential. Sequential control means that two or more components are controlled from a common source, making simultaneous control impossible. Dedicated control assigns separate control sources to each prosthetic component. Although it is a more complex approach, dedicated control

allows immediate use of each component and, sometimes, results in simultaneous control of two components for the production of coordinated movements.[1,8] The use of a body-powered elbow and myoelectric hand, for example, allows the amputee to reach out and open the terminal device in one fluid motion, similar to the function of the natural arm.

For bilateral fittings, dedicated control is always preferable. For amputations at higher levels, achieving dedicated control poses a significant challenge because of the increased number of potential prosthetic joints and the limited number of available control sources. It may be necessary to combine sequential and dedicated controls to provide all of the desired functions. In these complex situations, component functions should be prioritized, and those that are frequently needed or are interrelated should be assigned separate control sources (Figure 16).

Body-Powered Control

Cable actuation of body-powered prostheses provides users with a wealth of proprioceptive feedback through the physiologic joints harnessed to the prosthetic components.[11] Users of these devices can

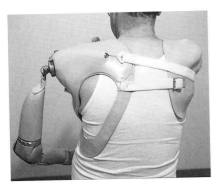

Figure 17 Biscapular abduction using a linear transducer provides elbow control for this patient with a bilateral humeral neck amputation. In this patient, only one side is fitted with a prosthesis. The contralateral side provides a suspension anchor point and a valuable control source for body motion control.

readily perceive the position and speed of movement of the prosthetic components.[1] Body-powered cable-operated devices offer many of the desirable characteristics of the control theory proposed by Childress,[12] based on the work of Simpson,[13] which states: "The most natural and most subconscious control of a prosthesis can be achieved through use of the body's own joints as control inputs in which joint position corresponds (always in a one-to-one relationship) to prosthesis position, joint velocity corresponds to prosthesis velocity, and joint force corresponds to prosthesis force."

This type of control is referred to as extended physiological proprioception (EPP). Although implementation of EPP control is possible with electronic components,[11,14-16] it requires fast, high-performance components to produce optimal results. Presently, EPP control is not commercially available, and available elbow components do not offer the required performance.

Given the inherent feedback provided by the cable and harness system, body-powered elbow control is more useful than any currently available electric control when adequate force and excursion exist. Childress[12] and Doubler and Childress[14] conducted tracking studies to provide evidence

that this type of control is superior to on-off and proportional velocity control. Body-powered control of an elbow is very graceful, the rate of motion is nearly normal, and positioning of the prehensor in space is very accurate. Body-powered control of a prosthetic elbow can become subconscious, as illustrated when the bilateral transhumeral amputee gestures with his limbs, gracefully flexing and extending his mechanical elbows as he speaks.

Cable efficiency is critically important to the success of many body-powered fittings, particularly for patients with high-level amputations. Careful attention should be devoted to producing the straightest line of pull and to using materials that offer the least amount of frictional loss, such as a Spectra cable in a Teflon-lined housing.[17]

Myoelectric Control

The most physiologically natural method of controlling an electronic hand is through myoelectric control. Myoelectric control looks very natural because the muscle activity is inside the socket and is invisible, in contrast to control methods that require body motions of more proximal body segments.[8] The most physiologically natural and inconspicuous control is achieved by the transradial amputee by using myoelectric signals from the forearm flexors to close the hand and signals from the extensors to open it. When the transradial socket is self-suspending, the harness can be eliminated. This results in a greater range of function than with a cable-driven terminal device because the position of the prosthesis and operation of the terminal device are not restricted by harness straps.

More proximal muscles can also be used effectively for grasp and release control. Flexor-extensor patterns are associated with grasp and release. Although persons with higher level amputations cannot use the actual muscle groups directly responsible for hand function, they can use remnant muscle patterns that are normally as-

sociated with grasp and release. The transhumeral amputee could therefore use the biceps to close the hand and the triceps to open the hand because of a flexion pattern closely associated with grasping and an extensor pattern associated with releasing.[8] Childress[12] described this as the myoprehension principle, suggesting that myoelectric control is more intuitive for the amputee. As noted, a major disadvantage of all myoelectric systems is the lack of direct feedback from the control system regarding the position, velocity, and force of the component. Thus, users of a myoelectrically controlled system must rely primarily on visual feedback as they manipulate their environment using the prosthesis.[8]

Switch Control

Switches are the most simple and basic input devices for activation of electronic components. A variety of switches has been used for prosthesis control, including pull, push, rocker, and toggle designs. Most switches provide only single-speed control and, therefore, are not optimally suited for terminal device operation or elbow or wrist rotation. Switches are best used for lock activation and mode selection when using a sequential control scheme. Simple switches are also used to turn power on and off, which is especially useful in situations in which the standard power switch for a particular component is inconveniently located or inaccessible to the bilateral amputee.

Servo Control

Servo control may be thought of as a more sophisticated type of switch control in which the speed of the prosthetic component is variable and is controlled by small body motions, usually through a harness system (Figure 17). Servo controllers can use either position or force as the input signal. A position servo has a transducer at the harness that measures excursion. This excursion information is then electronically processed and actuates the electronic component, similar to the operation of a body-powered system but requiring far less effort. A force-activated servo is quite similar to a position-controlled servo, except that no excursion is required with a force-activated servo. A transducer measures the force applied and drives the electronic component so that the speed of movement is proportional to that applied force.[8]

Force Sensing Resistor Control

Force Sensing Resistors (FSRs) are very thin input devices that can be placed either inside the socket, where the residual limb may press against them, or outside of the prosthesis, so some other body part might act on them (Figure 18). FSRs are typically used to provide proportional control in response to the pressure exerted.

Regardless of the type of control arrangement used, it should impose the minimum amount of mental loading on the user. In other words, the control of the prosthesis should not be so complicated as to make it the primary object of the user's attention.[1] Faced with the complexity of high-level bilateral fittings, sometimes one seemingly small change in the control strategy can cause a chain reaction of control source interaction and render the prosthesis impractical for daily tasks.[1] Although hybrid (electric- and body-powered) components and hybrid input devices may provide the most desirable results, these systems can be technically demanding, requiring a high degree of creativity and specialized knowledge on the part of the prosthetist. In my experience, the benefits realized by the users of hybridized systems far outweigh the technical difficulties in producing these systems. The key to optimal prosthesis design for the bilateral upper limb amputee is careful attention to details.

Prototype Prostheses

Because of the large variety of components and controls available to the

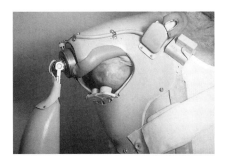

Figure 18 For this bilateral humeral neck amputee, a mobile residual humerus provides excellent control of the electronic terminal device using a pair of FSRs.

upper limb amputee, it is often advisable to set up a clinical trial of the proposed design using a prototype prosthesis. For the patient with a high-level arm amputation, this trial period can be critical to the long-term outcome of prosthetic rehabilitation as there is so little available evidence to make conclusive recommendations for components. Critical to the success of this approach is the availability of all component options and the technical ability to mix and match components from different manufacturers. The foundation of the prototype prosthesis is a well-fitted interface for evaluation. A prototype prosthesis may be used for periods of time ranging from a few hours for very straightforward fittings to several months for difficult situations in which several prosthetic options must be evaluated. Through the use of a prototype prosthesis, the amputee, the family, and other concerned parties can evaluate and validate the efficacy of any particular prosthetic component/control configuration through first-hand experience before completion of the definitive prosthesis[8] (Figure 19).

Fitting Considerations by Level
Partial Hand

In patients with one or both limbs amputated at the partial hand level, the main prosthetic considerations are to provide effective prehension and to

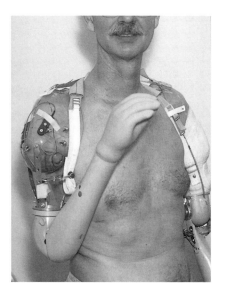

Figure 19 Prototype prostheses are an invaluable tool in the development of an optimal prosthesis. The well-fitted socket serves as the foundation for the prototype arm, and modular construction allows trials with various prosthetic component and control options. The bilateral transhumeral amputee shown ultimately decided that body-powered control bilaterally best served his needs.

limit the sensate area that is covered or encumbered by the device. Opposition posts (Figure 20), handi-hooks (Figure 21), and even myoelectric prostheses can be fitted at the partial hand level. Opposition posts are particularly useful whenever one or more movable digits remain. These devices are simple, lightweight, and generally cover the least amount of area. A handi-hook provides the ability to grasp and release in patients who lack one or more movable digits; when these devices are fitted loosely, users can "sneak" out of the socket, leaving it attached by the control system while they manipulate objects using their sensate residual hand. Wrist motion should be unrestricted by the prosthesis as much as possible. Myoelectric hands offer strong grip forces but also cover all of the sensate skin of the hand, so this drawback must be considered.

Transradial

Body-powered hooks and myoelectric systems have been proved effective for

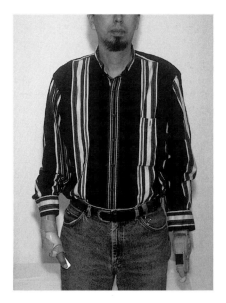

Figure 20 An opposition post can provide a simple and robust device to enhance the function of a partial hand amputation with one or more movable digits remaining. This man with transradial/partial hand amputations finds his partial hand side most useful for fine motor tasks primarily because of the wealth of information provided by his sensate thumb.

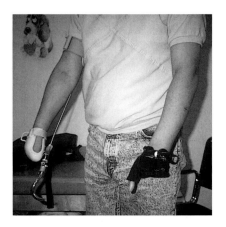

Figure 21 For the partial hand amputee with no movable digits remaining, the handi-hook prosthesis can offer a functional grasp. This design permits free motion at the wrist, improving the utility of the device.

the bilateral transradial amputee. Body-powered hooks are robust, lightweight, and offer the best fine manipulation capabilities. Myoelectric hands offer good cosmesis and a powerful grip force with acceptable manipulative function. Myoelectric systems for transradial amputees do

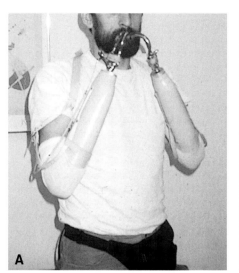

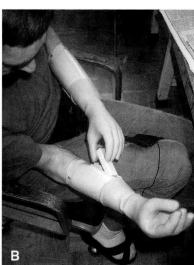

Figure 22 This bilateral wrist disarticulation amputee is shown wearing both his body-powered and his myoelectric prostheses. **A,** Both systems allow full elbow range of motion and retain forearm rotation by design. **B,** Electric-powered hands provide greater grip force and a more natural appearance than the voluntary-opening split hooks. This amputee finds both sets of prostheses valuable and can match the most appropriate design with a particular activity.

not require a harness, thereby increasing the scope of work of the terminal device. Some users find both types of prostheses useful and routinely switch between them depending on the type of activities pursued (Figure 22). As discussed for the partial hand amputee, sensation is of critical concern for the transradial amputee. Exposed skin can be desirable, especially for patients with longer transradial amputations or wrist disarticulations. For the blind bilateral transradial amputee, sensation is required for function. In these patients, surgical interventions such as a Krukenberg procedure or a toe transfer to the forearm such as the Vilkki procedure (Figure 23) should be seriously considered to produce a limb with manipulative capabilities.[18]

Transhumeral

Body-powered systems seem to offer the best long-term results for the bilateral transhumeral amputee. However, electronic terminal devices and elbows provide greater forces and, in some patients, can complement the function of a body-powered prosthesis worn on the dominant side. The ability to easily and securely position the terminal device in space becomes

more difficult as physiologic joints are lost. As noted, positive-locking wrists and locking humeral rotators should be considered for this patient population. Because of the loss of glenohumeral rotation in the transhumeral prosthesis, it may be beneficial for the surgeon to perform an angulation osteotomy to enhance the amputee's ability to actively position the prosthesis in space[19] (Figure 24).

Independent donning of both transhumeral prostheses is a primary goal for this population. This goal is almost always achieved when body position control is used but may be quite difficult when myoelectric control is used, because a very snug socket is required to ensure consistent skin-to-electrode contact. In my experience, nearly all bilateral upper limb amputees ultimately prefer a body-powered prosthesis incorporating a four-function forearm setup on the transhumeral side compared with myoelectric or hybrid control options that they have tried. Despite this experience, electronic control of one or more components may be advantageous for some patients, particularly when the requisite force and/or ex-

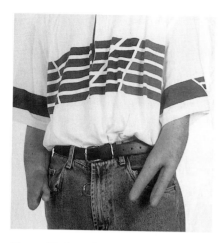

Figure 23 Sensation is critical for blind bilateral transradial amputees, and thus active prostheses have little to offer. For this patient, a Krukenberg procedure performed on the left side and a Vilkki procedure on the right provide a variety of gripping options.

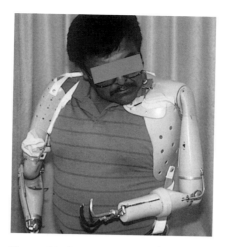

Figure 24 This transhumeral/shoulder disarticulation amputee benefits from an angulation osteotomy on his right arm that facilitates physiologic humeral rotation, which improves rotational stability and provides added positioning control of the prosthesis.

cursion for body-powered control are unavailable.

Suspension/control options, such as silicone suction sockets with integral myoelectric contacts and novel electronic control input options currently under development, may offer functional advantages for bilateral upper limb amputees. The development of methods to easily don the prostheses independently will be critical in order for such technology to be practical for bilateral transhumeral amputees.

Shoulder Disarticulation

When fitting the bilateral shoulder disarticulation amputee, it is generally advisable to start with as simple a prosthetic system as possible. Often, only the dominant side is fit initially. The complexity of control methods should be minimized, starting perhaps with only an activated terminal device and elbow. As the patient becomes acquainted with the use of the prosthesis, wrist function can be added, followed by addition of humeral rotation and a locking shoulder joint. The nondominant prosthesis can be fitted once the user has gained confidence in the use of the prosthesis on the dominant side. Complexity on the nondominant side can be staged

in a similar manner as used for the dominant prosthesis. In my practice, the dominant prosthesis of the bilateral pair is configured with mechanical, cable-actuated components similar to the four-function setup, and the nondominant side incorporates either all electric or hybrid components to provide complimentary functions.[1] The electronic prosthesis should use dedicated variable-speed control of the prehensor, wrist, and elbow whenever possible.

Case Studies

Case Study 1

A 28-year-old man who lived with his wife and their 3-year-old child sustained bilateral transradial amputations as a result of an electrical injury. His limbs were amputated at the midforearm level bilaterally, and he had no other injuries that would limit prosthetic rehabilitation. Sixty days after the accident, his limbs were well healed. At this time, prosthetic options were presented. Follow-up discussions focused on the advantages and disadvantages of myoelectric hands and cable-operated hooks. The initial prosthetic prescription called for body-powered preparatory pros-

theses. Once the residual limbs stabilized in size, myoelectrically controlled prostheses also were provided. Compression was provided by elasticized stockinettes whenever the prostheses were not worn to reduce swelling and prevent rebound edema. The initial terminal devices were both voluntary-opening devices, with a canted Hosmer 5X hook (Hosmer Dorrance) on the dominant right side and a lyre-shaped Dorrance 555 (Hosmer Dorrance) on the left. Two hook tension bands were provided on each hook initially to reduce the amount of force required for operation. More hook tension is provided, in half-band increments, as quickly as the amputee can tolerate the added pressure in the sockets and on the harness straps. Six to eight tension bands are expected to be used on each terminal device to provide a reasonable amount of pinch force. Wrist flexion units are mounted on constant friction wrists bilaterally. The prostheses are suspended using flexible hinges, triceps pads, and a Northwestern University ring harness. The amputee quickly learned to use the prostheses for daily self-care activities and was able to don and doff the arms independently after the first week of training. Under the care of a local occupational therapist, the patient returned home for continued practice and for discovery of the functional challenges he would face.

Upon the patient's return to the rehabilitation facility 3 months later, he demonstrated basic competency in feeding, oral/facial hygiene, dressing, and toileting. He and his family were very eager for new prostheses with myoelectric hands. He was particularly interested in the better appearance of such hands but also stated that the increased grip strength would be of great value. Myoelectric prostheses were provided, including Northwestern University self-suspending sockets, microprocessor-based two-site proportional myoelectric control, electronic wrist rotators with a quick-disconnect feature, and interchangeable electronic hands and

Otto Bock greifers (Otto Bock, Duderstadt, Germany). The amputee was pleased with the appearance and found certain activities, such as pulling up his socks, easier to perform with the greater pinch force. He also found manipulation of small objects to be more difficult than with the cable-operated hooks. He realized that although neither type of device is ideal, both have advantages. After 3 years, the patient still used both body-powered and myoelectric prostheses on a routine basis and could perform all necessary self care with both sets of prostheses. He used the body-powered prostheses exclusively on his job as an inspector for the power company (where he was employed at the time of his injury) because of problems with occasional inadvertent opening or closing of the electronic hands when near sources of high-powered electronic interference, but he generally preferred the myoelectric prostheses for use when not in his work environment.

Case Study 2

A 48-year-old man who lived on a 300-acre farm with his wife and two grown sons, where they grow floral greenery, lost both arms as a result of an accident involving the power take-off on his tractor. His dominant right arm was amputated at the midtranshumeral level, and he had a left shoulder disarticulation. Thirty days after the injury, he was seen at a rehabilitation facility for prosthetic fitting and training. The transhumeral limb was well healed, but his left side still had some open wounds and was quite sensitive to touch.

This patient had a very pragmatic attitude toward prostheses. From the first consultation, he expressed an interest in wearing the most functional prostheses so that he could continue to be productive on the farm. He had known other amputees who were farmers in his community and readily accepted the utilitarian appearance of a hook-type prehensor. Initially, he was fitted with a body-powered prosthesis on the right side and only a frame-style cap on the left side, designed to avoid the unhealed areas. The cap serves as a secure anchor point for the suspension and control of the right transhumeral prosthesis. A Hosmer 5XA hook (Hosmer Dorrance) is used, along with a wrist flexion unit and a constant friction wrist. The lever for the flexion lock is extended by attaching an 18-mm metal washer so the amputee can actuate it without assistance by pulling it against his knee, hip, or other object. An internal locking elbow with a lift assist is fitted with an adjustable elbow flexion attachment fixture to optimize the amount of force and excursion required to operate the prosthesis. The prosthetic sockets are worn over a T-shirt that has been tailored to fit snugly over the residual limbs, acting as a one-piece cotton torso sock. A Spectra control cable inside a Teflon-lined housing was used to reduce friction as much as possible. The plan was to complete training and practice with this relatively simple component configuration and then to add dynamic wrist rotation and flexion using a four-function forearm setup within approximately 1 month.

Upon the amputee's return to the rehabilitation facility 1 month after his initial fitting, he was progressing nicely using his single prototype prosthesis. He could feed himself some foods after assisted setup, he could dress himself partially, and he was nearly independent in toileting with a bidet, requiring assistance in redressing. The new wrist setup was installed, and the left shoulder disarticulation was fitted with an electrically powered prosthesis using a temporary socket as a foundation. By using a fully electrically powered prosthesis on the left side, separation of control can be readily achieved, and all biscapular abduction and glenohumeral motions can be devoted to the operation of the dominant side prosthesis.

This control system was designed to provide variable-speed dedicated control of elbow, prehension, and wrist rotation. Initially, a linear transducer was used to produce variable-speed control of the Boston electronic elbow operated by shoulder elevation harnessed using a "lift-through" socket design. Constant-speed control of a greifer is provided by a simple rocker switch activated by chin nudge control. During the next 4 months, incremental changes were made to the prosthetic design to gradually meet the original design objectives. At the end of this time, variable-speed control of the prehensor and wrist rotator was achieved using FSRs paired in a rocker configuration and activated by nudge control. A third FSR was used to cycle the lock for the LTI-Collier (Liberating Technologies, Inc) shoulder joint in an alternating fashion (ie, one push locks, one push unlocks) also activated by the chin. The locking shoulder joint permits terminal device activation above shoulder level, a function not possible on the right transhumeral side because of the limited bony lever arm. When the terminal device is overhead, the chin nudge control prevents visual tracking of objects being grasped. To alleviate this problem, control of the terminal device was changed to shoulder elevation using the linear transducer, and the elbow was controlled proportionally using a pair of FSRs in a chin-activated rocker fashion. Although the patient used his right body-powered transhumeral prosthesis for most daily tasks, he found the increased gripping and lifting capabilities of the electronic prosthesis invaluable. One year after the final fitting, the patient could independently don and doff both prostheses; prepare certain simple meals, although his wife assisted with most of the setup; toilet himself in his own home, using a bidet and strategically mounted hooks to assist in pulling up his pants; and complete daily oral/facial hygiene using an electric razor and toothbrush mounted on a flexible gooseneck.

Summary

Successful rehabilitation of the bilateral upper limb amputee is best achieved with the collaboration of an experienced team. Bilateral upper limb amputees, particularly those with amputation at a high level, benefit greatly from prosthetic fitting and require other assistive technologies, including automobile modification, communication devices, self-care devices, and nonprosthetic manipulators.[20] All of these modalities augment the function of the user who is faced with the tremendous functional loss of amputation of both arms. Each new bilateral upper limb amputee must be approached as an individual whose particular needs, goals, and desires should be the focus of the team. The fitting methods and philosophies discussed here should only serve as examples of successful prosthetic rehabilitation. Variations are required based on the unique presentation of the individual, taking into account his or her expressed preferences for particular prosthetic options.

Experience has shown that careful attention to socket fitting, provision of a control system that is reliable and simple to use, and minimizing the weight of the prosthetic device are critical for successful rehabilitation. Prostheses that are successful in the long term offer the bilateral amputee comfort, aesthetics, proprioceptive feedback, donning independence, control reliability, variable-speed control, and positive locking joints.[1]

Clinical fittings are based on available components and control strategies suitable for their operation. As new components and control schemes emerge, they should be evaluated with an open mind, and their potential utility for bilateral upper limb amputees should be considered carefully. Fitting the bilateral upper limb amputee is an art as much as a science, and potential solutions should not be limited to previous options. Despite the many limitations of state-of-the-art arm prostheses, bilateral amputees often make good use of these tools, as they strive for functional independence and meet the challenges of daily life.

References

1. Uellendahl JE, Heckathorne CW: Creative prosthetic solutions for the person with bilateral upper extremity amputations, in Atkins D, Meier R (eds): *Functional Restoration of Adults and Children With Upper Extremity Amputation.* New York, NY, Demos Medical Publishing, 2004, pp 225-237.

2. Uellendahl JE, Heelan JR: Prosthetic management of the upper limb deficient child, Alexander M, Molnar G (eds): *Physical Medicine and Rehabilitation: State of the Art Reviews.* Philadelphia, PA, Hanley & Belfus, 2000, vol 14, no 2, p 232.

3. Malone JM, Fleming LL, Roberson J, et al: Immediate, early, and late postsurgical management of upper-limb amputation. *J Rehabil Res Dev* 1984;21:33-41.

4. Billock JN: The Northwestern University supracondylar suspension technique for below-elbow amputations. *Orthot Prosthet* 1972;26:16-23.

5. Sauter WF, Naumann S, Milner M: A three-quarter type below-elbow socket for myoelectric prostheses. *Prosthet Orthot Int* 1986;10:79-82.

6. McLaurin CA, Sauter WF, Dolan CM, Hartmann GR: Fabrication procedures for the open shoulder above-elbow socket. *Artif Limbs* 1969;13:46-54.

7. Bush G: *Powered Upper Extremity Prosthetics Programme: Above Elbow Fittings.* Hugh MacMillan Rehabilitation Centre, Rehabilitation Engineering Department Annual Report, 1990, pp 35-37.

8. Uellendahl JE: Upper extremity myoelectric prosthetics. *Phys Med Rehabil Clin N Am* 2000;11:639-652.

9. Uellendahl J, Heckathorne C: Prosthetic component control schemes for bilateral above-elbow prostheses, in *Proceedings of the Myoelectric Control Symposium.* University of New Brunswick, 1993, pp 3-5.

10. Ivko JJ Sr: Independence through humeral rotation in the conventional transhumeral prosthetic design. *J Prosthet Orthot* 1999;11:20-22.

11. Heckathorne CW: Manipulation in unstructured environments: Extended physiological proprioception, position control, and arm prostheses, in *Proceedings of the International Conference on Rehabilitation Robotics,* 1990, pp 25-40.

12. Childress DS: Upper-limb prosthetics: Control of limb prostheses, in Bowker JH, Michael JW (eds): *Atlas of Limb Prosthetics: Surgical, Prosthetic, and Rehabilitation Principles,* ed 2. Rosemont, IL, American Academy of Orthopaedic Surgeons, 2002, pp 175-198. (Originally published by Mosby-Year Book, 1992.)

13. Simpson DC: The choice of control system for the multi-movement prosthesis: Extended physiological proprioception (E.P.P.), in Herberts P, Kadefors R, Magnusson R, Petersen I (eds): *The Control of Upper-Extremity Prostheses and Orthoses.* Springfield, IL, Charles C Thomas Publishers, 1974, pp 146-150.

14. Doubler JA, Childress DS: Design and evaluation of a prosthesis control system based on the concept of extended physiological proprioception. *J Rehabil Res Dev* 1984;21:19-31.

15. Heckathorne C, Childress D, Grahn E, Strysik J, Uellendahl J: E.P.P. control of an electric hand by exteriorized forearm tendons, in *Proceedings of the Eighth World Congress of the International Society for Prosthetics and Orthotics.* 1995, p 101.

16. Heckathorne CW, Uellendahl J, Childress DS: Application of a force-actuated position servo controller for electric elbows, in *Proceedings of the Seventh World Congress of the International Society for Prosthetics and Orthotics.* 1992, p 315.

17. Carlson LE, Veatch BD, Frey DD: Efficiency of prosthetic cable and housing. *J Prosthet Orthot* 1995;7:96-99.

18. Vilkki SK: Free toe transfer to the forearm stump following wrist amputation: A current alternative to the Krukenberg operation. *Handchir Mikrochir Plast Chir* 1985;17:92-97.

19. Marquardt E, Neff G: The angulation osteotomy of above-elbow stumps. *Clin Orthop* 1974;104:232-238.

20. Weir RF: Robotics and manipulators, in Olson DA, DeRuyter F (eds): *Clinician's Guide to Assistive Technology.* St. Louis, MO, Mosby, 2002, pp 281-293.

Chapter 26

Prosthetic Adaptations in Competitive Sports and Recreation

Robert Radocy, MS

Introduction

A continuing challenge in prosthetics is providing technology that allows the amputee to compete and excel in sports and recreation while using an upper limb prosthetic device. Creative solutions currently exist, and new designs are continually evolving.[1-3] See the lists of resources and product manufacturers provided at the end of this chapter for further information.

In the 1990s, research and development on activity-specific prostheses intensified at the urging of amputees who were interested in participating competitively in sports and recreational activities. Many prosthesis users experience great satisfaction and self-assurance when they can successfully return to a favorite sport or recreation. This chapter focuses on multiple approaches to achieving performance using specialized prosthetic accessories, custom prostheses, and modified sports and recreational equipment.

General Considerations
Patient Assessment

A thorough assessment of the patient's physical capabilities (muscle hypertrophy, strength, range of motion, etc), as well as personal sports and recreational goals is critical and provides a baseline from which to develop a prosthetic rehabilitation plan.

Social and cultural assessments related to family and peer support are important, and understanding the patient's motivation, cooperation, and communication capabilities enhances the therapeutic process.

The patient must understand that successful prosthetic and physical rehabilitation is a prerequisite for optimal performance. A state-of-the-art prosthesis will not provide optimal performance to a user who is not physically capable of taking advantage of its features. Conversely, optimal performance will not be achieved with a prosthesis that does not provide a level of technical sophistication that matches or challenges the user's physical capabilities.

Function

Function, performance, and limb morphology are interrelated. Bimanual performance becomes increasingly difficult to achieve with higher levels of limb loss or bilateral involvement. High-level transhumeral absence forces unilateral dominance and performance, and function and performance options decrease with higher levels of limb absence. Because unilateral transradial absence is the most common upper limb absence, most prosthetic solutions are designed for this level.

Sports and recreational activities are highly function-specific. Duplicating the biomechanics required in a particular activity is the primary challenge. Adequate prehension is sometimes a consideration but not always. Gross motor movement is most likely required. Because pain limits performance, secure and comfortable suspension is paramount.

Insurance and Funding

Few private insurance policies cover avocational prostheses, even though such care is routinely provided by the Shriners and Scottish Rite hospitals and the United States Department of Veterans Affairs. Consumer demand and the influence of proactive national organizations such as the Amputee Coalition of America (ACA) may lead to progress in obtaining insurance coverage. Workers' compensation insurance related to limb loss is more progressive and usually includes prostheses for sports and recreation.

Safety

Safety must be viewed from two perspectives. First, a prosthesis must allow the user to perform activities safely. Second, it must be safe to use around others, protecting them from injury as well. In competitive physical contact sports, padding the definitive prosthesis with 5-mm-thick neoprene with nylon laminated to both sides (divers' wet suit material) provides an excellent cushion. The neoprene can be sized to be slightly smaller than the diameter of the prosthesis and de-

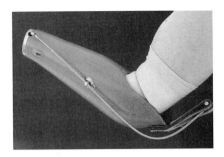

Figure 1 Self-suspending prosthesis design with broad brim and cross-bar strap. *(Courtesy of TRS Inc, Boulder, CO.)*

signed to slip over the device, providing a snug, nonslip cover. Neoprene sleeves also add buoyancy in the water; a 5-mm-thick cover will float a conventional transradial prosthesis.

For high school sports or intercollegiate athletic programs, specific waivers may be required to allow the athlete to compete while wearing a prosthesis. Local or regional athletic authorities can provide written waivers for high school sports such as basketball, where the use of a conventional prosthesis is generally prohibited. Rule books for high school sports can be obtained from the National Federation of State High School Associations (see list of resources). Recreational, intramural, and community programs usually do not have such rigid regulations.

Prosthesis Design Considerations
Socket Designs and Options

A supracondylar or self-suspending prosthesis is very useful in providing adequate suspension without inhibiting range of motion. A wide brim around the socket transfers distal prosthetic loads to the humerus and creates additional leverage-enhancing cable excursion during elbow flexion, when a cross-bar assembly is properly applied (Figure 1).

A self-suspending socket designed with a partial liner (padding) over the elbow condyles and olecranon pro-

vides a prosthesis that the user can tolerate under the severe loads that are generated during sports and recreational activities. Roll-on liners made of silicone or equivalent materials provide an excellent interface between the limb and the prosthesis and can significantly enhance performance. Prostheses to be used in water sports usually require some type of roll-on liner or external suspension sleeve because of the inherent lubricity of water. The high levels of surface friction or traction created by roll-on liners serve to increase suspension.

Liners differ in design and elasticity. Some types of shorter limbs benefit more from custom-made liners; other limbs generate adequate suspension with standardized molded liners. Liner thickness and stretch characteristics are factors that affect suspension and performance. Some liners have both longitudinal and circumferential elasticity, whereas others have limited or no longitudinal stretch. Users with short residual limbs will prefer liners with little or no longitudinal stretch. Longitudinal stretch can result in limb migration and loss of suspension, especially in activities where direct distal pulling is involved or where forearm or elbow flexion and extension under resistance is required (exercises such as triceps press-downs or latissimus pull-downs). Thicker liners can provide some additional comfort around bony prominences but do add to the overall bulk of the prosthesis. If a thin liner is used, a partial liner of padding is suggested, as described earlier.

Harnesses

Many sports prostheses do not require a harness. Harnesses can limit or restrict the range of motion required for a particular activity, such as the motion needed to carry through a golf swing. In activities that require active controlled prehension, a cable and harness can be used. Controlled prehension also can be achieved by an externally powered prosthesis. A modified, adjustable excursion, such as a Northwestern

figure-of-9 harness, provides excellent terminal device operation without the cumbersomeness and discomfort sometimes associated with a traditional figure-of-8 harness system. Specialized axilla padding options improve comfort. Polypropylene strap materials and traditional Dacron webbing provide options in harness design, construction, strength, color, and comfort.

Power Options

Most custom sports prostheses are designed around conventional body-powered technology, which has proved to be durable and reliable. Shock, vibration, and exposure to high-moisture or water environments typically have required the use of body-powered systems. However, externally powered prostheses have been used in sports and recreational activities, and their lack of cable and harness suspension may improve the user's performance. As advances occur in the technology of externally powered prostheses, including improved resistance to water and the ability of the components to withstand shock and vibration, the use of externally powered limbs in these situations will no doubt expand.

Materials

A custom sports prosthesis should fit well, be comfortable, support weight, and handle a variety of loads. A wide variety of high-strength materials and resins lend themselves to high-performance prostheses. Use of Kevlar and carbon-reinforced fabrics, ultra-high molecular weight polyethylenes, and compatible resins results in strong, lightweight prostheses that provide safe, reliable bimanual performance. Stainless steel or titanium reinforcement is sometimes used in the construction of prostheses, prehensors, and sports accessories. Other materials include structural nylons, aircraft-grade aluminum, and a variety of modern, resilient elastomers such as polyurethane.

Alignment

Alignment is an important factor when designing and constructing a prosthesis. Alignment is always a factor in a lower limb system but may not be as closely monitored in the fabrication of upper limb prostheses. Proper alignment is crucial to performance. Because many sports and recreational activities demand a wide range of upper limb motion, such as gross motor arm activity, an excessively preflexed prosthesis can limit performance. A prosthesis with a neutral or preextended alignment (socket to arm centerline) may be a better alternative. Additionally, the wrist mounting angle must be considered. Slight changes in wrist angle can cause the load on the residual limb to shift, sometimes causing discomfort or creating instability.

Archery and weight lifting are two activities in which alignment is especially important. In archery, a significant distal load occurs on the arm holding the bow. If the alignments of the socket to arm centerline and the wrist to arm centerline are not accurate, balancing this load on the residual limb becomes very difficult and the load feels unstable. The shorter the residual limb, the greater the role alignment plays in the design. The bow must load the prosthesis, residual limb, upper arm, and shoulder properly for stability and shooting accuracy. Improper alignment can result in three undesirable situations: (1) the user may not be able to draw the bow; (2) the user may draw the bow but once it is drawn, may be incapable of supporting it comfortably; or (3) the user may draw and support the bow but not be able to shoot the arrow accurately because of the forces and torque induced into the system. Similar problems can arise in weight lifting. For example, bench pressing requires a strong stable prosthetic platform. Improper alignment may create intolerable or unstable load conditions that compromise safety. Alignment that facilitates the specific tasks desired must be carefully fac-tored into the prosthetic design. Experimentation with loads and forces before the final lamination process can help avoid the need and expense of refabrication.

Cosmesis

In most sports and recreational activities, function rather than cosmesis is the goal. However, in activities such as dance, aerobics, and floor exercise, where cosmesis may be a concern, efforts should be made to create a prosthesis that is lifelike in contour, texture, and color. Muscle definition can be sculpted into the prosthetic foam before lamination to enhance cosmesis. A flat exterior finish rather than a glossy finish might be preferred. Soft cosmetic covers might be an option but are not always practical because of their limited durability.

Biomechanical Considerations

To achieve maximum performance with a prosthesis in a particular sport or recreational activity, the biomechanical aspects and demands of the activity need to be understood and duplicated as much as possible. Duplicating the biomechanics provides for the control and transfer of energy and motion from the body and torso through the anatomic and prosthetic limbs, resulting in or facilitating some predetermined action.

In some instances, the prosthetic limb can be used to generate energy (ie, prehension via a cable or external power source). However, its primary use is to transfer energy or, in some instances, store energy and then transfer it. Prosthetic components or accessories that provide or allow for various degrees of freedom enable the efficient transfer of energy and power. Biomechanics in the upper limb primarily provide for the following motions: (1) basic prehension (opposed thumb grasp and cylindrical grasp), (2) wrist flexion and extension, (3) forearm pronation and supination, (4) elbow flexion (forearm flexion and extension), and (5) humeral flexion, extension, abduction, and adduction.

These motions rarely occur in isolation but in progressive and coordinated harmony to create a limb action. An example is the "wrist break" that occurs in normal limbs when a baseball bat or similar object is swung through completely. A baseball bat swing that culminates in a wrist break and follow-through is a complicated interaction of not only humeral, forearm, and wrist biomechanics, but also biomechanics that involve the torso, hips, and lower limbs.

Traditional prosthetic limb technology provides for only certain degrees of freedom and therefore, only certain motions. Specialized prosthetic components and accessories can fill this gap.

Activities

Sports and recreational activities can be grouped according to their biomechanical demands, and parallel solutions can apply to activities that have similar biomechanical requirements. Certain activities are unique, however, and specific accessories or solutions have been devised to enhance performance in these areas.

Ball Sports, Aerobics, Dance, Tumbling, Skating

This large and varied group of activities, including soccer, volleyball, basketball, and similar sports, shares some biomechanics. These activities usually involve the need for bimanual control (two-handed opposition and manipulation), energy storage, stability, balance, and safety. Traditional prehension (opposed thumb and forefinger grasp) are not necessarily important. Historically, cosmetic hands were used to try to meet these needs; however, they were not designed to provide the strength, durability, and function that more modern accessories can provide.

Anthropomorphic terminal devices that enhance bimanual control

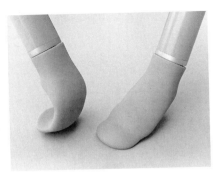

Figure 2 Super Sport Hands. *(Courtesy of TRS Inc, Boulder, CO.)*

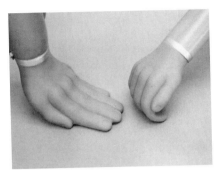

Figure 3 Free Flex Hands. *(Courtesy of TRS Inc, Boulder, CO.)*

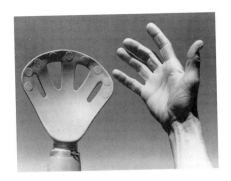

Figure 4 Rebound Basketball Hand. *(Courtesy of TRS Inc, Boulder, CO.)*

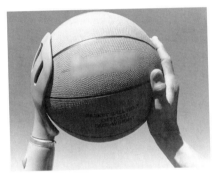

Figure 5 Rebound Basketball Hand. *(Courtesy of TRS Inc, Boulder, CO.)*

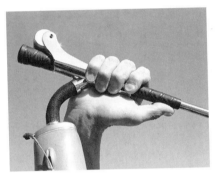

Figure 6 Amputee Golf Grip. *(Courtesy of TRS Inc, Boulder, CO.)*

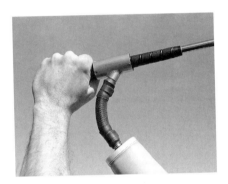

Figure 7 Golf Pro, right hand model. *(Courtesy of TRS Inc, Boulder, CO.)*

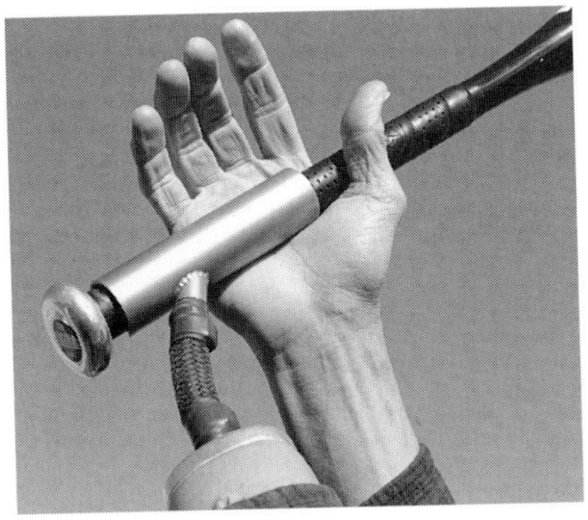

Figure 8 Grand Slam baseball bat accessory. *(Courtesy of TRS Inc, Boulder, CO.)*

and function are available and have been designed to be flexible, safe, and store energy (Figures 2 and 3). When external force is applied to these devices, they produce an action similar to wrist and hand flexion and extension. The Rebound Basketball Hand (TRS Inc, Boulder, CO) (Figures 4 and 5) takes the concept to a higher level of complexity by attempting to duplicate certain hand and finger me-

chanics used in controlling a basketball.

Externally powered hands might have some application in some of these activities, but their configuration does not allow for accurate bimanual ball control. They also do not provide the energy storage needed for duplicating dynamic wrist and hand action.

Baseball, Softball, Golf, Bowling

These activities involve a complex combination of biomechanical elements. Prehension is important but secondary to the development and smooth transfer of kinetic energy into the projectile involved. Duplicating the degrees of freedom that occur in the forearm and wrist allows for the transfer of energy into the ball. A variety of studies have been conducted on how to duplicate the biomechanics involved. Simple mechanical joints such as ball-and-socket joints and universal-type joints have been tested

and found to be reliable, but they have certain limits to their range of motion. Another alternative that has proved effective is the flexible coupling. A flexible coupling was possibly first used by prosthetist J. Caywood (Robin-Aids) in developing a golf device.

A high-strength flexible couple can provide a smooth, efficient, and controlled transfer of energy. The Amputee Golf Grip, Golf Pro devices, and Grand Slam baseball and softball bat accessories (TRS Inc) (Figures 6 through 8) use the flexible coupling design. The Amputee Golf Grip and the Grand Slam devices require the grasp of the opposite hand to help engage the devices. The Golf Pro differs in that it slides up the shaft of the golf club and "jam fits" onto the grip.

A variety of other individual, custom solutions have evolved to suit specific needs and preferences in golf. In some designs, the golf clubs are equipped with "snap on" connectors to fit directly into the end of the pros-

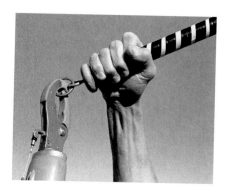

Figure 9 Power Swing Ring. *(Courtesy of TRS Inc, Boulder, CO.)*

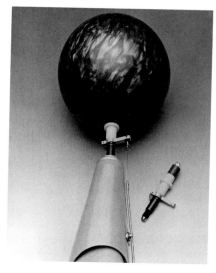

Figure 10 Bowling Ball Adaptor. *(Courtesy of Hosmer Dorrance Corp, Campbell, CA.)*

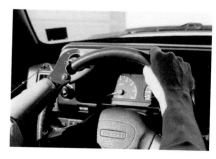

Figure 11 Grip prehensor for the steering wheel. *(Courtesy of TRS Inc, Boulder, CO.)*

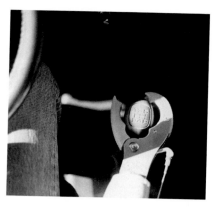

Figure 12 Grip prehensor for a stick shift. *(Courtesy of TRS Inc. Boulder, CO.)*

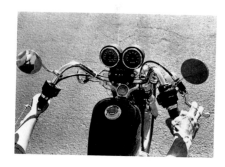

Figure 13 Grip prehensor for a motorcycle. *(Courtesy of TRS Inc, Boulder, CO.)*

thesis with no flexible joint. Other designs attempt to "lock in" the angle of club swing and limit the degrees of freedom involved. This is accomplished by using a single-axis hinge-type joint mounted at the appropriate angle.

Wooden bats can be easily modified. The Power Swing Ring (TRS Inc) uses a simple swivel mechanism that is attached to the bottom of the bat (Figure 9).

In all cases, hand dominance needs to be considered, as well as the side of the hand absence. Significant variances in the design of prosthetic accessories are dictated by these differences. A device designed to allow an amputee with a left hand absence to swing "right handed" in either golf or baseball usually will not work for an amputee with a right hand absence with a similar swing. An array of accessories has evolved to accommodate these differences.

Bowling biomechanics parallel many of the motions of golf and baseball. Instead of swinging an object to hit a projectile, however, bowling requires a pendulum action of the arm and a hand release to deliver the ball. Because bowling is essentially a unilateral activity, a person missing a hand has the option of relearning to bowl with the nondominant hand. This may be preferred over trying to use a prosthetic accessory.

The Bowling Ball Adapter (Hosmer Dorrance Corp, Campbell, CA) (Figure 10) can be used by those who wish to use their prosthesis for ball control. The device uses an expandable plug controlled by cable excursion to release the bowling ball. The ball requires minor customization to receive the plug adapter.

Steering, Driving, Riding

Activities that involve vehicle riding and control have similar biomechanical demands. These activities require spontaneous grasp and release capability. Bimanual control and adequate prehension usually are needed to manipulate throttles, clutches, and brake and shift levers simultaneously or in a synchronous manner. Appropriate hand grasp configuration (opposed thumb and forefinger) is needed to conform to the rounded or cylindrical controls.

Spontaneous release is important to free the rider from the vehicle controls in the event of a spill or crash. Modern voluntary-closing prehensors (Figures 11 through 13) work well in these applications. Most vehicle controls require arm and elbow extension and flexion. These biomechanical motions control voluntary-closing-type devices. Gross motor activity in general helps to maintain prehension without the need for additional cable excursion control. Release is automatic when cable tension is relaxed.

Externally powered terminal devices and hands function well in controlling most vehicles, with the exception of watercraft, which is usually prohibited because of the likelihood of prosthesis immersion in water. The prehension of approximately 25 kg (of force) produced by myoelectric and similar devices is adequate for controlling vehicles in most situations. Quick release of the controls is possible, although not as instantaneous as release by the human hand.

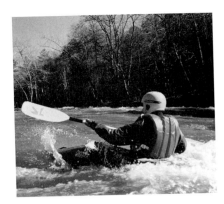

Figure 14 Grip 3 prehensor for kayaking. *(Courtesy of TRS Inc, Boulder, CO.)*

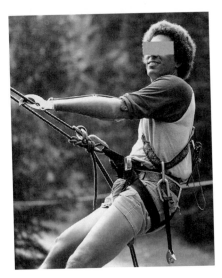

Figure 16 Grip prehensor for mountaineering. *(Courtesy of TRS Inc, Boulder, CO.)*

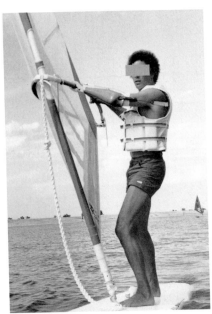

Figure 15 Grip 3 prehensor for windsurfing. *(Courtesy of TRS Inc, Boulder, CO.)*

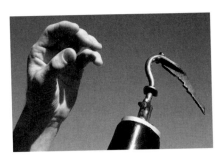

Figure 17 Custom mountaineering accessory. *(Courtesy of TRS Inc, Boulder, CO.)*

Split hooks and other voluntary-opening types of cable-activated prosthetic devices usually are not adequate because of the gripping configuration and inability to maintain grasp under cable load. Typically they "pry off" controls. Some swivel ring adapters exist to enable split hooks to better control automobile steering wheels.

Locking onto vehicle handlebars, steering wheels, and other controls is unsafe and should be avoided. Mountain bicycles, off-road motorcycles, snowmobiles, all-terrain vehicles, and personal watercraft require control and extra strength under most riding situations. Maintaining grasp and control while pulling or pushing on the handlebars or steering wheel is

necessary. Selecting a prosthetic accessory that provides all the necessary requirements is important to ensure safe, reliable control.

Special "dual-action" bicycle brake levers (TRS Inc) allow both front and rear brakes to be actuated with one hand. Hydraulic systems on motorcycles and other vehicles can be modified to operate both the front and rear brakes simultaneously or synchronously. Specialty custom shops and vehicle dealerships usually can help modify vehicles for safe control.

Water Sports, Mountaineering, Hockey

These activities, including canoeing, kayaking, windsurfing, water skiing, and fishing, require strength, prehen-

sion, and quick grasp and release capability. They differ from the last series of activities in that they usually require a separate piece of equipment that is controlled bimanually. Gross motor upper limb activity is typical. Pulling and pushing, including the mechanics of humeral flexion, extension, abduction, and adduction and elbow flexion and extension, are involved. Body-powered voluntary closing prehensors such as the Grip 3 (TRS Inc) (Figures 14 and 15) have proved to function well, providing the necessary prehension and rapid grip and release capability. Voluntary-opening devices are not recommended because of their lower grip force. Wet suits can inhibit the action of a cable and harness system; however, wearing the harness outside the wet suit can usually eliminate the problem. Externally powered arm electronics may be compromised in water sports activities.

Mountaineering requires gripping strength and reaching, grasping, and rope handling capabilities. Voluntary-closing prehensors (Figure 16) have performed satisfactorily for many mountaineering and climbing tasks, but a plethora of specialized equipment exists in this sport. Specialized training is required to ensure safety. Individual custom aids (Figure 17) have been developed by some enthusiasts to more successfully participate in this type of activity.

Locking a prosthetic device onto a kayak or canoe paddle, windsurfer boom, or ski rope handle can have fatal consequences. Loss of control in rough conditions can cause the participant to be thrown into and under the water with no easy way to release the prosthetic grasp. In water skiing, the speeds can be great enough to cause severe injury because of the impact or dragging that ensues if release is not accomplished.

Fishing, except fly fishing and surf casting, does not typically involve dynamic upper limb motion. A prosthesis serves to either power the reel or control the rod. Direct attachment of

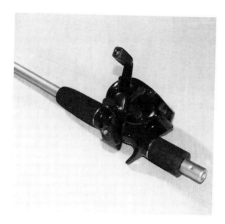

Figure 18 Prosthetic fishing accessory. *(Courtesy of Texas Assistive Devices, Brazoria, TX.)*

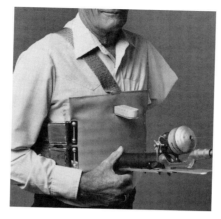

Figure 19 Chest harness fishing platform. *(Courtesy of The Free Handerson Co, Valier, MT.)*

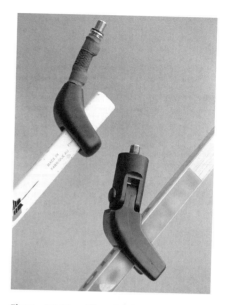

Figure 20 Slap Shot hockey accessories. *(Courtesy of TRS Inc, Boulder, CO.)*

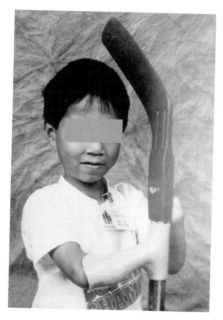

Figure 21 Custom Canadian hockey accessory. *(Courtesy of War Amps of Canada, Scarborough, Ontario, Canada.)*

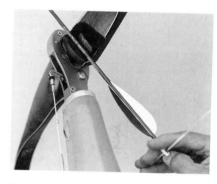

Figure 22 Grip prehensor for a bow and arrow. *(Courtesy of TRS Inc, Boulder, CO.)*

the pole into the prosthesis is possible with an accessory made for that purpose (Figure 18). Another alternative is a flexible rubber snow ski and fishing accessory from Hosmer Dorrance, which provides a passive grip.

Handling the reel with a prosthesis and the rod in the anatomic hand is preferred by some fishers. An externally powered terminal device, myoelectric hand, or a voluntary closing prehensor will provide enough prehension for control of the reel. Modifying or padding the reel handle can facilitate grasping it with a prosthesis, thereby improving control. Other alternatives include custom prosthetic reel adapters, electrically powered fishing reels (available from Access to Recreation; see Resources), and chest harness–supported fishing rod holders and apparatus that provide improved function for the high-level unilateral amputee or persons with hemiplegia (Figure 19).

A hockey stick can be controlled with a prosthesis by holding the stick either at the top end or down on the shaft. In both cases, wrist and forearm biomechanics need to be duplicated for efficient control and performance in puck handling. A simple swivel and ring or ball-and-socket joint may suffice as a top-end control mechanism. More sophisticated hockey accessories are commercially available from TRS Inc that provide both the degrees of freedom needed and the type of hockey stick attachment that accommodates either style of stick handling (Figure 20).

Numerous custom adaptations have been developed for individual amputees, especially for young athletes. Prosthetists in Canada, in particular, have focused on prosthetic adapters for hockey to meet their patients' needs (Figure 21).

Archery, Weight Lifting

A variety of prosthetic approaches have been taken to facilitate these activities. Devices for shooting a bow are designed to accommodate either holding the bow or drawing the bowstring. Some designs involve mechanisms for connecting the bow directly to the end of the prosthesis. Other designs use a modified voluntary closing prehensor (Figures 22 and 23) to hold the bow. The modifications temporarily lock the prehensor onto the bow handle. Externally powered hands can create the required gripping configuration and prehensive strength to handle a bow. Slightly modifying the bow's handle will improve control whether a prehensor or a myoelectric hand is used. A simple cushioned gripping surface formed around the bow's handle allows for

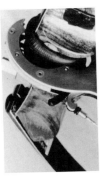
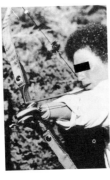
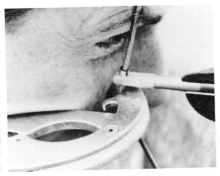

Figure 23 Grip prehensors for archery. *(Courtesy of TRS Inc, Boulder, CO.)*

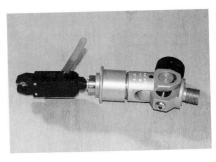

Figure 24 Archery accessory. *(Courtesy of Texas Assistive Devices, Brazoria, TX.)*

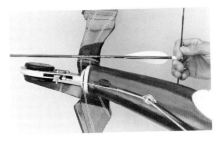

Figure 25 Custom archery equipment. *(Courtesy of TRS Inc, Boulder, CO.)*

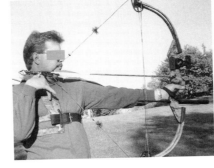

Figure 26 Custom archery equipment. *(Courtesy of Wright Bow Brace, Ltd.)*

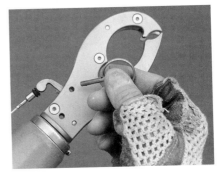

Figure 27 Grip prehensor with locking pin accessory. *(Courtesy of TRS Inc, Boulder, CO.)*

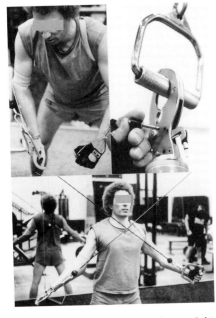

Figure 28 Grip prehensors for weight training. *(Courtesy of TRS Inc, Boulder, CO.)*

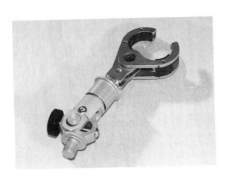

Figure 29 N-Abler weight lifting accessory. *(Courtesy of Texas Assistive Devices, Brazoria, TX.)*

ease of centering and balancing the bow in the prosthesis. Centering the hand or prehensor provides for a smooth draw and release of the arrow. No torque is induced into the bow because of "too tight" grasp or imbalance in holding.

Archers missing a hand can now draw the bowstring using modified commercially available release aids used by archers. The release aid connects via an adapter directly into the end of the prosthesis, hooks onto the bowstring, and can be activated by triggering a lever (Figure 24). Custom designs have evolved as well to suit the individual archer's needs and preferences (Figures 25 and 26).

Weight lifting typically involves heavy loads and a wide range of motion; therefore, a high-performance prosthesis is needed to handle these loads and accommodate the biomechanics involved. Voluntary-closing prehensors modified with a locking pin (Figures 27 and 28) have proved to satisfy most of these demands. Split hooks and other voluntary-opening–type devices usually are not appropriate. Externally powered devices also can provide access but are more limited in application because of their prehension range, durability, and electronic controls.

Custom weight lifting devices have been developed as well. A simple barbell- and dumbbell-holding accessory has been designed to fit into the N-Abler prosthetic adapter from Texas Assistive Devices (Figure 29). TRS designed the Black Iron Master (Figure 30), a custom alternative accessory for extreme conditions and professional-level performance and competition.

Designs that can be used with a variety of equipment types, such as barbells and dumbbells and Universal

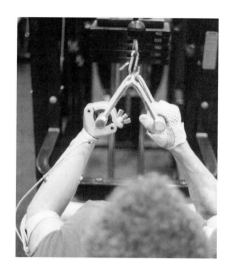

Figure 30 Black Iron Master. *(Courtesy of TRS Inc, Boulder, CO.)*

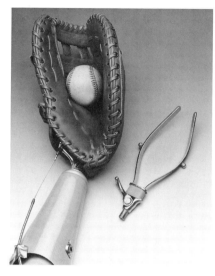

Figure 31 Baseball Glove Attachment. *(Courtesy of Hosmer Dorrance Corp, Campbell, CA.)*

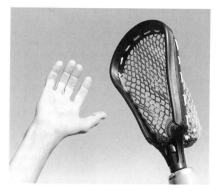

Figure 32 Hi Fly Fielder. *(Courtesy of TRS Inc, Boulder, CO.)*

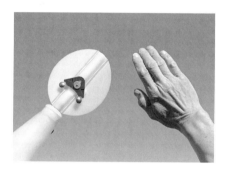

Figure 33 Freestyle Swimming accessory. *(Courtesy of TRS Inc, Boulder, CO.)*

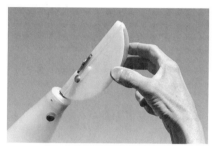

Figure 34 Freestyle Swimming accessory. *(Courtesy of TRS Inc, Boulder, CO.)*

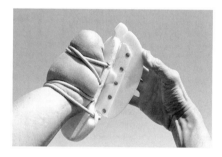

Figure 35 Swim Fin. *(Courtesy of TRS Inc, Boulder, CO.)*

and Nautilus equipment, provide the prosthetic user with greater flexibility in training a broader range of muscle groups. Designs such as a self-suspending socket with a partial padded liner, carbon fiber reinforcement, and a roll-on liner provide for added comfort, performance, and safety.

Swimming, Fielding/Catching

Grouping swimming with fielding and catching may at first seem odd, but the biomechanics of controlled pronation and supination are common to these activities. In swimming, a natural pronation and supination occurs in "feathering" the hand during power and retrieval arm strokes and motions. In baseball and softball catching, the forearm must be pronated or supinated to cover body

zones above and below the waist while fielding balls. Powered or controlled pronation and supination (wrist rotation) are not readily available with a prosthesis. Externally powered systems do provide some terminal device rotation, but the action is slower than would be required for competently fielding a ball in most situations.

The Baseball Glove Attachment by Hosmer Dorrance (Figure 31) provides one alternative. The cable-operated, voluntary-opening device with extended hook fingers is designed to fit into a first baseman's glove. The player with a longer forearm can pronate naturally and use this device. The midlevel to short transhumeral user cannot pronate and supinate naturally. The terminal device and glove must be manually

rotated and reoriented to field in all body zones. In many fielding situations, this is not practical or possible.

An alternative is the Hi Fly Fielder system (Figure 32) by TRS. This system replaces the glove entirely with a ball catching accessory that is styled after a lacrosse stick head. A large custom mesh pocket provides for bi-directional catching. The user can catch forehanded or backhanded, and pronation and supination are not required for fielding.

Similarly, pronation and supination in swimming can be avoided. In a flexible paddle system, such as the Freestyle Swimming accessory from TRS (Figures 33 and 34), the paddle flares open to create the resistance required in the power stroke, and during stroke recovery the flaps fold back, allowing water to push past the paddle. This concept was first envisioned by Canadian prosthetist Robert Gabourie as overlapping fins between fixed fingers. TRS simplified the design into the "butterfly wing"

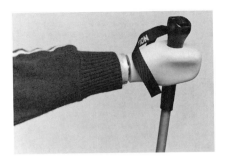

Figure 36 Ski Hand/Fishing Hand. *(Courtesy of Hosmer Dorrance Corp, Campbell, CA.)*

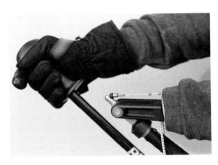

Figure 37 Ski 2. *(Courtesy of TRS Inc, Boulder, CO.)*

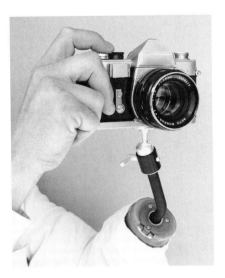

Figure 38 Amp-U-Pod camera accessory. *(Courtesy of TRS Inc, Boulder, CO.)*

paddle concept for ease in manufacturing and to allow for easy modification to match different hand displacements.

A swimmer with a long residual limb can use a simple rigid paddle attached to the forearm to create the resistance necessary in the power stroke, yet "feather" the paddle, reducing resistance during recovery. Curved paddles and flat paddle designs have been tried; however, depending on the stroke employed, the curved paddle has the tendency to submarine and cause a loss of stroke volume. Another design, the Swim Fin (Figure 35), allows for a flexible paddle design without a prosthesis for persons with shorter limbs. This system is convenient and less costly than a custom swimming prosthesis.

Using a roll-on silicone or similar liner in any swimming prosthesis can help suspension. Additionally, a prosthesis that places the flexible swimming paddle closer to the end of the residual limb will provide the user with better control.

Other Specialized Activities
Firearms Handling (Rifle and Pistol Shooting)

Certain firearms, such as pistols, can be safely handled with a voluntary-closing prehensor or an externally powered prosthesis. Because safety is the primary objective and concern, the prehensor or hand is used for gripping and/or stabilizing the pistol, not for triggering. Rifles and shotguns typically require modification for safe handling and control. The forearm of

the gun must be held or stabilized by the prosthesis in some manner. A pistol grip or swivel ring can be added to the forearm and grasped by a hook, prehensor, or hand. A military strap is useful for adding stability for aiming and firing. Triggering is possible, but the lack of tactile sensitivity in all terminal devices makes triggering with a prosthesis a safety concern and a questionable practice.

In all cases, modifications to firearms should not be performed by the prosthetic manufacturing facility unless personnel are certified in the gunsmith trade. A certified gunsmith, qualified and knowledgeable in firearms, should be contracted to modify guns for use with a prosthesis.

Snow Skiing (Alpine and Nordic)

Snow skiing involves upper limb activity for balance and ski pole control. The biomechanics involved include humeral flexion, extension, abduction, and adduction. Elbow flexion and wrist flexion and extension can also be involved. A prosthetic device needs to be able to adapt to a ski pole. The ability to easily disconnect from the ski pole is useful when ski lifts must be boarded. Alpine skiing uses poles primarily for balance, while Nordic skiing usually requires poles for propulsion.

Two manufactured ski devices are currently available. The Ski Hand/Fishing Hand (Hosmer Dorrance) (Figure 36) is available in several sizes. It is a simple prosthetic device that allows the ski pole to fit into a hole in the flexible rubber hand. The pole op-

erates like a pendulum and can be snapped forward using a forceful humeral flexion. The elasticity of the Ski Hand causes the pole to rebound to its original configuration. The Ski 2 (Figure 37) is a prosthetic device for holding a ski pole that can be cable operated much like a voluntary-closing prehensor. Humeral flexion tightens the cable, causing the pole to pivot forward for a pole plant. An elastic bias returns the pole to its retracted position. Both devices require the removal of the standard ski pole grip. The Ski 2 allows for easy pole installation and removal, unlike the Ski Hand, which requires the pole to be force fit into the hand.

Cameras and Photography, Musical Instrument Adapters, Pool and Billiards

The primary prosthetic objectives for these activities include positive attachment of accessories, stable mounting, and angular adjustment. The Amp-U-Pod (TRS Inc) (Figure 38) is a simple accessory that adapts to any camera equipped with a tripod receiver mount. The device is a lockable ball-and-socket adapter on which the camera is mounted directly to the end of the prosthesis. The Amp-U-Pod facilitates focusing, meter adjustments, and film changing, while providing a stable mounting platform for filming.

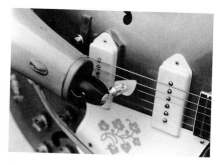

Figure 39 Guitar adaptor accessory. *(Courtesy of TRS Inc, Boulder, CO.)*

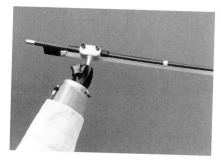

Figure 40 Violin adaptor accessory. *(Courtesy of TRS Inc, Boulder, CO.)*

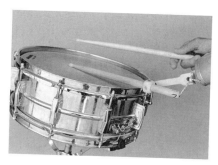

Figure 41 Drum Stick Adaptor. *(Courtesy of TRS Inc, Boulder, CO.)*

Musical instrument accessories are specific to the instrument involved, but a lockable ball-and-socket mount can provide an adjustable platform on which to attach musical instrument holders. Guitar picks and violin bows (Figures 39 and 40) can be more easily controlled with a prosthesis using these types of adapters.

Playing the drums requires a more complex adapter. The Drum Stick Adapter (TRS Inc) (Figure 41) is a commercially available alternative. This accessory holds the stick under elastic tension while allowing it to pivot. The user can duplicate a variety of drumming techniques.

Pool and billiards require prosthetic stability, as well as flexibility in guiding the pool cue. The Hustler (TRS Inc) (Figure 42) is a commercially available option that provides a stable and versatile mount for positioning and controlling the cue.

Summary

As consumer demand has developed for specialized sports prostheses, emphasis has been placed on the goal of achieving competitive bimanual per-

formance. Careful assessment of the patient's capabilities, requirements, and desires is necessary to ensure a more successful outcome, and assessment of the biomechanical demands of the activity provides insight into possible prosthetic solutions. Successfully duplicating those biomechanical motions required by the activity enhances performance using a prosthesis. Safety is also an integral concern and needs to be factored into the prosthetic equation.

A variety of commercially available and custom accessories have been developed for persons missing one or both hands. Prosthetic aids and accessories or modifications to sports and recreational equipment open the doors to successful, competitive, two-handed performance in activities ranging from archery to windsurfing.

Provision of a well-designed prosthesis with specialized terminal devices will enable the upper limb amputee to participate in a broad range of normal recreational and sporting activities. In many cases, performance is currently limited not by the available prosthetic technology but by the physical capabilities of the participants.

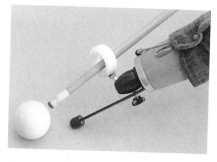

Figure 42 Hustler pool/billiards accessory. *(Courtesy of TRS Inc, Boulder, CO.)*

References

1. Radocy B: Upper-extremity prosthetics: Considerations and designs for sports and recreation. *Clin Prosthet Orthot* 1987;11:131-153.

2. Radocy B: Upper-limb prosthetic adaptations for sports and recreation, in Bowker JH, Michael JW (eds): *Atlas of Limb Prosthetics: Surgical, Prosthetic, and Rehabilitation Principles*, ed 2. Rosemont, IL, American Academy of Orthopaedic Surgeons, 2002, pp 325-344. (Originally published by Mosby-Year Book, 1992.)

3. Radocy B, Beiswenger W: A high performance, variable suspension, transradial prosthesis. *J Prosthet Orthot* 1995;7:65-67.

Manufacturer Contact Information

Fillauer, Inc
2710 Amnicola Hwy.
Chattanooga, TN 37406
(800) 251-6398
www.fillauer.com

Hosmer Dorrance Corp
561 Division St.
Campbell, CA 95008
800-827-0070
hosmer@hosmer.com

Texas Assistive Devices, LLC
9483 County Road 628
Brazoria, TX 77422
(979) 798-1185
www.n-abler.org

TRS, Inc
3090 Sterling Circle, Studio A
Boulder, CO 80301-2338
(303) 444-4720
Fax (303) 444-5372
800-279-1865
www.oandp.com/trs

T/Wright Archery
PO Box 1541
Lethbridge, Alberta, Canada, T1J 4K3

Resources

Access to Recreation Inc
Equipment for the Physically Challenged (catalog)
www.accesstr.com

Active Living (magazine) *Healthy Lifestyles for Today's Amputees*
PO Box 2660
Niagra Falls, NY 14302
tel: (800) 725-7136
fax: (905) 957-6017
activeliv@aol.com
www.activelivingmagazine.com

America's Athletes With Disabilities
www.americasathletes.org

Amputee Coalition of America (ACA)
www.amputee-coalition.org

Amputee Golfer (magazine)
www.nagagolf.org/Magazine

Assistive driving resources. *In Motion* 1998;8.

Association of Driver Educators for the Disabled (ADED)
www.driver-ed.org

CHAMP, The War Amps Child Amputee Program
CHAMP Newsletter
www.waramps.ca

Department of Veterans Affairs Prosthetic and Sensory Aids Service
Mailing Code 113
Washington, DC 20420
(202) 273-8515
Fax (202) 273-9110

Disabled Sports/USA (DS/USA)
www.dsusa.org

Handicapped Scuba Association (HSA) International
www.hsascuba.com

Keeping Fit (booklet)
Abilities Unlimited
www.oandp.com/abilities

Little League Challenger Division (A special division for children with disabilities)
www.littleleague.org

National Amputee Golf Association (NAGA)
info@nagagolf.org

National Federation of State High School Associations Rule Books
www.nfhs.org

National Mobility Equipment Dealers Association (NMEDA)
www.nmeda.org

National Sports Center for the Disabled
www.nscd.org

Orthotic & Prosthetic Assistance Fund, Inc
opaf@opfund.org

Palaestra (magazine of adapted physical education)
www.palaestra.com

Physically Challenged Bowhunters of America, Inc (PCBA)
www.pcba-inc.org

Sports Anyone? (booklet)
American Orthotic and Prosthetic Association (AOPA)
info@aopanet.org

United Foundation for Disabled Archers (UFFDA)
bowtwang@runestone.net

Chapter 27

Future Developments: Hand Transplantation

Christopher H. Allan, MD

Introduction

Limb transplantation has been technically feasible for many years. The surgical techniques allowing for microvascular anastomoses and coaptation of nerves were developed in the 1960s. These techniques have been refined greatly, such that replantation of amputated hands and digits is now commonplace. The obstacle to widespread use of limb transplantation is the potential for morbidity and mortality due to the long-term immunosuppression presently required to prevent rejection of the allograft, although new drugs and techniques of drug delivery are under study and may reduce this barrier. There are significant ethical concerns over subjecting patients to these risks to treat a non–life-threatening condition. Despite these concerns, at the time of this writing, at least 18 hand transplants have been performed worldwide since 1998. This cohort of patients represents an ongoing experimental group, lessons from which will guide the future of composite tissue allograft transplantation. In some modified form, this procedure will likely change forever our treatment options for the patient with limb loss.

While prostheses remain the gold standard for replacing lost limbs, the goal of replacing the limb with a new living one has become a reality, albeit a highly controversial one. Successful midforearm-level upper limb transplants have now been performed in several centers worldwide, with thus far a 100% survival rate of the allografted limbs in the present era. An earlier transplant in 1964 failed, and the first patient in the modern era of hand transplantation (1998 to the present) requested elective removal of his transplant. One other transplanted hand has since been removed as well.

History

The first hand transplant was reported in 1964 in Ecuador and survived for 2 weeks before rejection occurred, despite a regimen of immunosuppressive medications consistent with knowledge at that time. Substantial scientific progress in immunosuppression has since been made.[1,2] The next attempt at hand transplantation took place in 1998 in Lyons, France, and involved a 48-year-old man who had lost his right forearm and hand to a circular saw injury in 1984, at which time he underwent replantation.[3] The original replanted limb was electively amputated for lack of function in 1989. Nine years later, transplantation of a midforearm-level allograft upper limb from a 41-year-old brain-dead male donor was successful, resulting in a viable graft. After several episodes of rejection, the patient eventually opted to discontinue immunosuppressive therapy and requested that the allografted hand be removed. Several months after the French transplant, in January 1999, a team in Louisville, Kentucky, performed the first hand transplant in the United States. Strategies for patient selection and evaluation, surgical procedure, immunosuppressive regimen, and postoperative rehabilitation were similar for the two groups.

Hand transplants have since been performed in China, Italy, Austria, and several other countries.[2] At least 18 such procedures have now been undertaken, six for bilateral hand loss, and return of function is being closely monitored.[4] Because the risks of long-term immunosuppression are believed to be so great, it is difficult to make the case for single limb allograft transplant; some surgeons believe that the procedure should be reserved for patients with loss of both hands. A survey of the audience at the 2001 meeting of the American Society for Surgery of the Hand revealed that more than 90% of surgeons in attendance would consider the procedure for themselves in the event of bilateral hand loss, whereas fewer than 5% would wish to undergo hand transplantation for loss of a single hand.

Patient Selection and Preoperative Testing

The selection criteria used by the Louisville group[2,5] included patient age

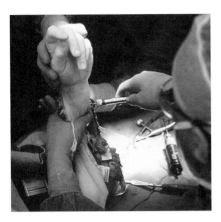

Figure 1 Stabilizing donor hand and forearm to recipient forearm bones. (© Copyright Jewish Hospital; Kleinert, Kutz and Associates Hand Care Center; and University of Louisville, Louisville, KY. Photo by John Lair.)

between 18 and 65 years, overall good health, amputation at the wrist level, and human immunovirus–negative and hepatitis B–negative status. Preoperative workup included HLA typing, cytomegalovirus and Epstein-Barr serology, electromyography (EMG) and angiography of the involved limb, and limb and chest radiographs. Other teams[6] have included MRI of the involved limb. Psychiatric and psychological evaluation and testing are required as well. An advocate not associated with the transplant team is selected by the patient, and a team of health care professionals in the patient's home area is established for close follow-up after surgery. Informed consent is obtained in writing and is filmed.

In each of the first two hand transplants (Lyons, France; Louisville, Kentucky, United States) the donor and recipient had mismatches at all six HLA alleles. Donors were adult males matched with recipients for bone size and skin tone.[2]

Surgical Procedure

The surgical procedures followed by both groups have been described in detail and are quite similar.[3,5] The donor limb is removed through or near the elbow joint, perfused with University of Wisconsin transplant solution via the brachial artery, and cooled. Excess skin is removed, and arteries (radial, ulnar, and anterior interosseous), veins (cephalic and basilic), nerves (median, ulnar, and radial sensory), and tendons (dorsal and palmar forearm muscles or tendons) are then identified and tagged for later suture. Dorsal and palmar incisions are made on the recipient limb under tourniquet control, and the corresponding structures are identified.

The radius and ulna are cut transversely on both donor and recipient limbs and stabilized with compression plates and screws (Figure 1). With the Louisville patient, a pronation contracture required release of the pronator teres. With the Lyons patient, autogenous bone grafting was necessary. Following skeletal stabilization, vascular anastomoses (arteries first) are performed with No. 8-0 or 9-0 suture. The French team reported 12.5 hours of ischemic time from donor death to arterial anastomosis; the Louisville team reported "cold ischemic time" of 310 minutes. Next, the nerves are reapproximated, followed by muscle and tendon units. Tendon ends are woven through muscle when length allows, approximated end to end, or joined using a Pulvertaft weave technique.[6] Tendon grafts (taken from the patient's feet) and transfers were used with the first Louisville transplant because of the patient's shortened and atrophic forearm musculature. Tendon transfers comprised brachioradialis to flexor carpi radialis, extensor carpi ulnaris to extensor pollicis longus, and extensor carpi radialis brevis to extensor digitorum communis. Other tendons were repaired directly, with the middle, ring, and little finger profundus tendons conjoined. Autogenous skin grafting was used at the time of wound closure in each of the first two transplant patients. The operated limb was then splinted and postoperative monitoring begun in a similar fashion to that followed after replantation (anticoagulation, antibiotics, frequent vascular checks). The principal difference was the immuno-suppressive therapy regimen, which is not used when using a patient's own limb.

Immunosuppression

The required immunosuppressive therapy and its associated toxicity (nephrotoxicity, myeloproliferative and lymphoid tumors) are the main obstacles to widespread use of limb transplantation.[7] Transplanted organs, including hands, are recognized as foreign by host T cells. T and B cell lines clonally expand and in their activated form invade the graft and destroy it.[1] Various steps in this process are targeted by several immunosuppressive medicines. One risk with all of these medicines is that the host's ability to recognize and attack other threats to the host, such as infectious organisms or neoplastic cells, is impaired. For this reason, immunosuppression carries a risk of infection or malignancy, both of which can threaten quality of life and can result in patient death.

Hand allografts comprise many different tissue types with different antigenicities, which can also complicate therapy. Any successful regimen must prevent rejection of all these tissue types.

Animal studies have shown that single-agent protocols (ie, one drug designed to reduce toxicity) work only if used in high doses for the rest of the patient's life, and risks of respiratory and other complications are correspondingly high. Therapy with multiple agents can be as successful with lower doses and lower toxicities.

In work with a swine model, Lee and associates[8] reported that complete major histocompatibility complex matching can decrease requirements for immunosuppression, allowing long-term graft survival after only 12 days of cyclosporin-A.

Presently, hand transplant patients are treated with both an induction phase, characterized by higher doses of medications, and a maintenance phase of immunosuppression. Combined therapies are used to minimize toxicity of any one agent and to effectively block T cell activation at various steps. Corticosteroids are paired with cyclosporin-A or FK-506 (tacrolimus), which prevent T cell clonal expansion against the transplant but risk renal toxicity, hypertension, dyslipidemia, and diabetes mellitus. They can also be paired with antiproliferative agents (azathioprine or mycophenolate mofetil), which risk bone marrow suppression or gastrointestinal symptoms and cytomegalovirus infection. Corticosteroids inhibit cytokine production by T cells and macrophages but can cause hypertension, dyslipidemia, and glucose intolerance.

In addition to these risks, cost is another factor complicating the use of immunotherapy. Immunosuppression accounts for approximately 80% of the present cost of hand transplantation. For these reasons, there is great interest in reducing or eliminating the need for these costly toxic drugs in transplantation. The goal of immunosuppression—host tolerance of the grafted part—can theoretically be attained in other ways than with immunosuppression. The pathway that seems most promising is hematopoietic chimerism.

Chimerism is the coexistence of two genetically different populations of cells in the same animal.[1] This requires depletion of the host's immune system via anti–T cell cytotoxic drugs or irradiation (during which time the host is at risk for infection), followed by grafting of donor bone marrow into the recipient. The mechanism of host tolerance to donor graft thus induced is not clear but may involve deletion of thymus T cells targeting the donor.[9] Various strategies are being investigated. One laboratory recently reported delayed rejection in a rat hindlimb transplant model when chimeric donor limb allografts were created through removal of donor bone marrow and replacement with recipient bone marrow.[10] Some authors report that chimerism need not be lifelong to induce lasting tolerance.[11]

The risk of graft versus host disease (GVHD) is present when establishing chimerism. The donor T cells used to establish mixed chimerism are immunocompetent and can identify and respond to foreign tissue. In GVHD, donor T cells can react to recipient tissues as foreign; this is particularly a risk when the recipient's own immune system is suppressed, as is often done to protect a transplanted organ. Results of the graft cells reacting against host tissues can include skin rash, peeling or blistering skin, inflammation of the stomach and intestines with resulting nausea and cramping, and liver involvement with resultant jaundice. In studies in a rat hindlimb model, GVHD did not develop until levels of donor T cell chimerism exceeded 50%.[7] In most protocols, the level of chimerism achieved has ranged from 2% to 10%, suggesting low risk of GVHD.[1]

These strategies are not clinically applicable yet, but they hold promise for reducing requirements for the immunosuppressive protocols presently in use. Given the present risks associated with these protocols, the future of hand transplantation may well rest on the success or failure of efforts in this area.[12]

Functional Results

The work done by the Louisville group when preparing to embark on their program of hand transplantation suggested that the expected functional outcome might parallel that seen after hand replantation. Not surprisingly, sensibility and intrinsic hand muscle function (which rely on nerve regeneration) recover less well than extrinsic muscle function (which relies on tendon repairs or grafts), both after replantation and after transplant. Thus, restoration of grip, for example, exceeds that of fine manipulation. Still, overall results of replantation exceed those of amputation and prosthesis use. Early results suggest that the same is true after hand transplantation.[13,14]

The Louisville group reported that a Tinel's sign developed in the first patient's fingertips after 6 months.

Monofilament testing reported at 14 months showed "diminished or loss of protective sensibility." The first hand transplant at Lyons showed sensibility intact to deep pressure only. No data were reported for the first two Chinese transplants. The Louisville patients could distinguish hot and cold in the palm of the transplanted hand by 20 weeks. EMG at 6 months demonstrated potentials in the radial and ulnar nerves only. EMG at 12 months showed the ulnar lumbricals were innervated, as was the adductor pollicis, although this muscle demonstrated only 3/5 motor power on clinical examination. By 11 months, the patient could use his transplanted hand to help tie shoes and pick up small objects.[2]

In September 2003, hand surgeon and transplantation researcher W.P. Andrew Lee, MD, reported observations made during his recent visit to six hand transplant centers worldwide.[4] He noted that most patients were hospitalized for several months after transplantation surgery and underwent daily hand therapy for 6 to 12 months. All but one of the 11 patients he met and examined had had rejection episodes, and many had major complications (eg, skin necrosis, osteomyelitis) requiring periods of prolonged hospitalization. All patients continued to receive systemic immunosuppressive medications. His examinations of these 11 patients showed that most had recovered protective sensation, but only about half could localize sensation to a specific digit. Only two showed any evidence of reinnervation of the intrinsic muscles of the transplanted hand. Like other reports, his findings suggest that the functional outcome after hand transplantation is similar to that seen after hand replantation, but that it comes at a much higher cost in terms of hand therapy and pharmacotherapy.

Future Possibilities

The growing field of tissue engineering has as its goal the combining of a scaffold, multipotent cells, and appropriate cytokines to "build" living tissues.[15] Use of host mesenchymal stem cells or other cell types leads to a construct comprising these cells and their offspring, inhabiting a scaffold of extracellular matrix components produced by these autogenous cells to replace the original scaffold. In this way, replacement body parts might be constructed that are host-derived and not seen as foreign by host immune defenses.

Hands are quite complex, with multiple tissue types and functions, and represent an extreme test of tissue engineering principles. Creating a scaffold to mimic any one of the components of a hand may seem straightforward, but combining tissue-engineered tendons moving tissue-engineered bones and joints fed by tissue-engineered vessels and given sensibility by tissue-engineered nerves is a daunting task. One strategy used in vascular grafts recognizes that the perfect scaffold may be the part itself. Cadaver arteries have been decellularized, removing donor material and leaving the organized collagen scaffold behind. This scaffold is then "seeded" with autogenous cells, which populate the graft in culture and lead to a living replacement part compatible with the recipient. In canine studies such tissue-engineered grafts have survived and been shown to be functional for as long as 6 months.[16]

Manipulating the many tissues in a hand in a similar manner may not be feasible; for example, decellularization of skin (the most immunogenic of the tissues in a hand transplant) has thus far been limited to the dermis.

Lee and associates[10] addressed the bone marrow component of the allograft, generally an early target of host immune response. Slowing, but not preventing, rejection was shown in a rat vascularized limb tissue transplantation model wherein allergenic bone marrow was replaced with host marrow, leading to a chimeric allograft.

Summary

Hand transplantation may be viewed as what some surgeons call "a procedure in search of an indication," if only because of the toxicity of present immunosuppressive regimens. The technical aspects of the procedure combine knowledge already developed in prior transplantation and extremity surgical disciplines. Function of the allograft, while poor regarding sensibility, is clearly better than a prosthesis. With more than 1 million persons in the United States alone living with an amputation, the demand for limb transplantation would likely be great if the procedure and its associated medical treatment were made safe and widely available.[17] Work on inducing tolerance will help solve this problem if chronic immunosuppression is rendered unnecessary. Finally, regenerative healing and tissue engineering may contribute to this area as well. Hand transplantation is an exciting development holding great promise. It is fascinating to speculate on the form this chapter will take in the next edition of this text.

References

1. Siemionow M, Ozer K: Advances in composite tissue allograft transplantation as related to the hand and upper extremity. *J Hand Surg [Am]* 2002;27: 565-580.

2. Cendales LC, Breidenbach WC III: Hand transplantation. *Hand Clin* 2001;17:499-510.

3. Dubernard JM, Owen E, Herzberg G, et al: Human hand allograft: Report on first 6 months. *Lancet* 1999;353: 1315-1320.

4. Amadio PC: What's new in hand surgery. *J Bone Joint Surg Am* 2004;86:442-448.

5. Jones JW, Gruber SA, Barker JH, Breidenbach WC: Successful hand transplantation: One-year follow-up. Louisville Hand Transplant Team. *N Engl J Med* 2000;343:468-473.

6. Lanzetta M, Dubernard JM, Owen ER, et al: Surgical planning of human hand transplantation. *Transplant Proc* 2001;33:683.

7. Kann BR, Hewitt CW: Composite tissue (hand) allotransplantation: Are we ready? *Plast Reconstr Surg* 2001;107: 1060-1065.

8. Lee WP, Rubin JP, Bourget JL, et al: Tolerance to limb tissue allografts between swine matched for major histocompatibility complex antigens. *Plast Reconstr Surg* 2001;107:1482-1492.

9. Manilay JO, Pearson DA, Sergio JJ, Swenson KG, Sykes M: Intrathymic deletion of alloreactive T cells in mixed bone marrow chimeras prepared with a nonmyeloablative conditioning regimen. *Transplantation* 1998; 66:96-102.

10. Lee WP, Butler PE, Randolph MA, Yaremchuk MJ: Donor modification leads to prolonged survival of limb allografts. *Plast Reconstr Surg* 2001;108: 1235-1241.

11. Bourget JL, Mathes DW, Nielsen GP, et al: Tolerance to musculoskeletal allografts with transient lymphocyte chimerism in miniature swine. *Transplantation* 2001;71:851-856.

12. Brenner MJ, Tung TH, Jensen JN, Mackinnon SE: The spectrum of complications of immunosuppression: Is the time right for hand transplantation? *J Bone Joint Surg Am* 2002;84: 1861-1870.

13. Graham B, Adkins P, Tsai TM, Firrell J, Breidenbach WC: Major replantation versus revision amputation and prosthetic fitting in the upper extremity: A late functional outcomes study. *J Hand Surg [Am]* 1998;23:783-791.

14. Breidenbach WC III, Tobin GR II, Gorantla VS, Gonzalez RN, Granger DK: A position statement in support of hand transplantation. *J Hand Surg [Am]* 2002;27:760-770.

15. Musgrave DS, Fu FH, Huard J: Gene therapy and tissue engineering in orthopaedic surgery. *J Am Acad Orthop Surg* 2002;10:6-15.

16. Wilson GJ, Courtman DW, Klement P, Lee JM, Yeger J: Acellular matrix: A biomaterials approach for coronary artery bypass and heart valve replacement. *Ann Thorac Surg* 1995;60(suppl 2):S353-S358.

17. Dillingham TR, Pezzin LE, Mackenzie EJ: Limb amputation and limb deficiency: Epidemiology and recent trends in the United States. *South Med J* 2002;95:875-883.

Chapter 28

New Developments in Upper Limb Prosthetics

Hans Dietl, PhD

Introduction

The field of upper limb prosthetics has held great interest for generations of prosthetists, scientists, and engineers who have worked to make their progressive concepts and dreams a reality. However, only concepts that fulfill three criteria have prevailed, specifically (1) successful integration into the movement scheme of the patient, (2) reliability, and (3) manageability by the prosthetist (D Atkins, Houston, TX, unpublished data, 1995). Many technical and scientific institutions presently support work in this area. This chapter presents a general overview of current approaches to research and development.

Prosthetic Hands

The field of hand prosthetics constantly struggles with the challenge of fulfilling two basically incompatible requirements: providing the best possible cosmetic replacement for a lost limb and achieving maximal functionality. As a result, research in the field focuses on the development of prosthetic hands that strive to imitate the natural hand as closely as possible and the development of prehensors that are optimized to suit a given function.

Externally Powered Prosthetic Hands
Kinematics

The classic construction of most prosthetic hands is based on forceps kinematics, in which the thumb and finger face each other. This type of hand has only one degree of freedom. The advantage of this type of hand is its robust construction; its disadvantages are its unnatural motion and functional limitations in grasp geometry. Nevertheless, some of the newest developments continue to incorporate this kinematics concept. Examples include the new Motion Control Hand[1] (Motion Control, Salt Lake City, UT) (Figure 1) and the hand concept of Nishihara and associates (K Nishihara et al, Glasgow, Scotland, unpublished data presented at the International Society of Prosthetists and Orthotists [ISPO] World Congress, 2001).

Control Options

Although the kinematics of currently available hand systems may not have changed much, significant progress has been made in control options to help the amputee operate these devices with greater ease and precision. Multiple control options are now available, allowing better customization of the prosthetic system to the demands of the individual user and numerous adjustments for fine-tuning of the controls. Using a computer, the prosthetist can modify various parameters of every component integrated into the prosthesis (H Dietl, PhD, Glasgow, Scotland, unpublished data presented at the ISPO World Congress, 2001).

State-of-the-art hands now have integrated sensors that reduce the user's need to concentrate on controlling the grasping action.[2] For example, on-board sensors for hand control can signal when to adjust grasping force (both magnitude and direction), opening width, and speed of movement.[3] Different types of sensors are used. For example, force measurement is usually based on strain gauge sensors

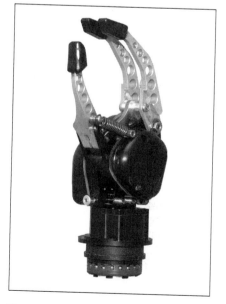

Figure 1 Motion Control Hand (Motion Control, Salt Lake City, UT).

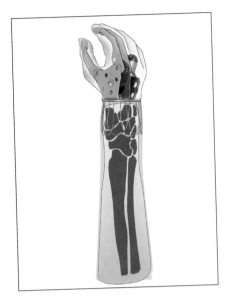

Figure 2 Transcarpal hand (Otto Bock HealthCare, Vienna, Austria).

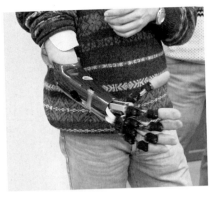

Figure 3 Mechanical structure of the Karlsruhe hand.

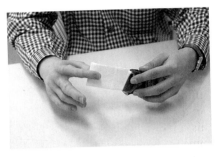

Figure 4 Pincer-grasp mechanism of the Karlsruhe hand.

or force-sensitive resistors.[4,5] For touch and slip detection, Kyberd and Chapell[6] use a combined optical-acoustical sensor. Trials with piezo-electric sensors,[4] as well as sensors based on the magnetic Hall effect, have also been conducted.[7] These sensors can serve as the signal sources for feedback systems. Electrical stimulation has proved to be most promising for force feedback.[8] However, work remains to eliminate the interference between the electromyographic (EMG) signals and the feedback stimulation pulse. Some groups have experimented with temperature feedback.[9] Better functionality for the patient could result in a secondary benefit. A group of German psychologists reported that increasing prosthetic function correlates with a reduction in phantom pain.[10-12] These authors theorize that a functional prosthesis that includes a feedback mechanism should significantly reduce phantom pain.

The improved quality of hand controls combined with increased battery capacities allows faster hand movements. Patient trials with the recently launched SensorHand Speed (Otto Bock HealthCare, Vienna Austria) indicate that the increased speed results

in a more frequent use of the hand functions.

One alternative to the widely used pincer-type grasping style is the Electrohand 2000 for Children[13] (Otto Bock HealthCare). In this hand, a polycentric mechanism coordinates the movement of the fingers and thumb, improving grasping geometry and resulting in more lifelike finger movement. Typical desktop activities are easier to perform and require less compensatory arm movement. The limited durability and elasticity of contemporary materials used for cosmetic covers, such as polyvinyl chloride and silicone, have discouraged more widespread use of this concept. However, because this concept has proved to be beneficial to the patient, it is likely to be incorporated into the next generation of prosthetic hands, replacing the classic pincer-grasp kinematics.

There is significant interest in developing powered components for amputation levels distal to the wrist. Some research designs for long residual limbs have an electromechanical drive in the fingers.[14] Currently, one commercially available electromechanical hand allows fitting to mid-metacarpal amputation levels while offering reasonable cosmesis[15] (Figure 2).

The Anthropomorphic Hand

Another alternative to the classic pincer-grasp geometry is the anthropomorphic hand, which attempts to

imitate the grasp kinematics of a sound hand as closely as possible. The advantage of this principle is that the fingers curl around objects better, so less grip force is required. Unlike the pincer grasp, which has only one degree of freedom, the anthropomorphic hand has additional degrees of freedom, making various grasping patterns possible, including a power grasp and lateral or key pinch.

The Karlsruhe Project

One innovative new concept is being explored at the Research Center in Karlsruhe, Germany[16] (S Schulz, CH Pylatiuk, Glasgow, Scotland, unpublished data presented at the ISPO World Congress, 2001). Hydraulic actuators flex and extend the finger joints and the wrist joint. Each finger has three joints, which correspond to the metacarpophalangeal joint, the proximal interphalangeal joint, and the distal interphalangeal joint (Figure 3). The base joint of the thumb allows movement in three planes, resulting in several grasp patterns. The wrist also allows rotation in all planes.

The actuators are flexible tubular structures that bridge the joints; joint flexion is caused by inflation and distention of the flexible chambers. Pressure and fluid flow are generated by a hydraulic micropump positioned in the metacarpal area of the hand, together with the electric power source and the microvalves. This mechanism allows various grasp patterns (Figure 4) and therefore represents the closest approximation of the natural hand to date. Because most of the elements are made of lightweight plastics, the total weight of the mechanism is approximately the same as that of a conventional lightweight prosthesis. Although this design still lacks a sufficient number of control inputs for the various degrees of freedom, this disadvantage is partially overcome by a hierarchical control system that produces predefined movement patterns. The maximum force at the fingertips achieved so far is 12 N. Although the adaptability of the flexible fingers combined with the soft silicone glove that covers the hand reduces the grip force required, some important activities of daily living cannot be performed with this hand at this time. If this new concept proves to be feasible for performing activities of daily living, then it will become essential to find new principles for controlling the multiple degrees of freedom it offers.

Another ongoing anthropomorphic hand project is Kyberd's Southampton Hand[17,18] (Oxford Orthopaedic Engineering Centre, Oxford, England). The drive for this hand is conventionally operated, using direct-current motors and cables for actuation. This project focuses on intelligent control using integrated sen- sors.[19]

All anthropomorphic hand projects attempt to create a functional hand prosthesis with improved cosmesis. However, no project has been commercially successful to date because the materials currently available cannot withstand the strain imposed by these kinds of hand mechanisms.

Drive Mechanisms

Most commercial hand designs still use conventional direct-current motors to power the hand. However, two research groups are exploring the use of ultrasonic motors[20] (K Nishihara et al, Glasgow, Scotland, unpublished data presented at the ISPO World Congress, 2001). The benefits of ultrasonic motors are high motor torque, which allows a reduction in the weight and size of the transmission, and reduced noise. Also, these motors cannot

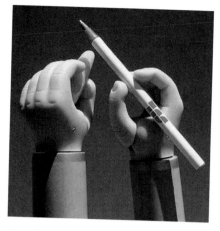

Figure 5 Lite Touch hand (TRS Inc, Boulder, CO).

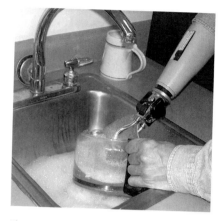

Figure 6 Electronic terminal device (Motion Control, Salt Lake City, UT).

be back-driven, so items grasped remain secure in the fingers. The major shortcomings of ultrasonic motors are poor efficiency and the need for high voltage, both of which result in more rapid drain of the batteries.

Power systems using hydraulic actuators are used by the Karlsruhe group and by Instituto Nazionale Assicurazione contro gli Infortuni sul Lavoro (INAIL) in Rome, Italy. INAIL uses this system for a powered elbow. A hydraulic micropump is the actuation force for both the hand drive and the elbow drive.

Body-Powered Prosthetic Hands

Unfortunately, only limited progress has been made in improving body-powered prosthetic hands. The main shortcoming of these devices is their poor efficiency, caused in large part by the resistance of the protective glove that covers the mechanism. Most of the energy that the user puts into the device is lost as friction. Herder[21] reported some innovative concepts to address this concern by the use of "rolling links." The efficiency problem has been overcome with the design of the Lite Touch Hand (TRS Inc, Boulder, CO), a compromise between cosmetic design and hook functionality (Figure 5). The findings of Weiss and associates,[11] with respect to the role of biofeedback-controlled prosthetics in the reduction of phantom pain, has

the potential to stimulate new interest in the traditional technique of muscle cineplasties. This could create a renewed demand for body-powered prosthetic hands optimized for cineplasty control, as occurred in the years following World War II when cineplasties were more commonly performed.[22]

Externally Powered Hooks

Several styles of externally powered hooks have established their usefulness. The fundamental requirement in these types of prostheses is robustness, which eliminates complex anthropomorphic features. In the future, sensors will be integrated into powered hook terminal devices, as has already been done in some electric hands. Waterproof electric hooks have recently been developed and will expand the range of electrical terminal devices for performing activities of daily living (Figure 6).

Mechanical Hooks

Mechanical hooks are the most commonly used of all terminal devices. A wide variety of styles is available, but only a few are used frequently. Many innovative designs for voluntary-closing devices are available for both pediatric patients and adults. Also, for the first time in decades, new designs for voluntary-opening devices are being released commercially, including an energy-optimized two-load hook that produces nearly constant grip

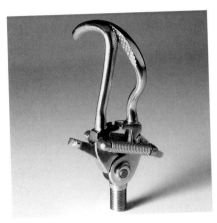

Figure 7 Two-load hook (Otto Bock HealthCare, Vienna, Austria).

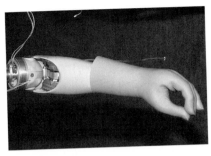

Figure 8 Electronic elbow prototype, forearm assembly (Otto Bock HealthCare, Vienna, Austria).

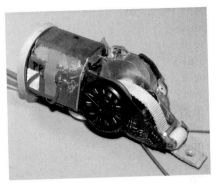

Figure 9 Electronic elbow prototype, drive unit (Otto Bock HealthCare, Vienna, Austria).

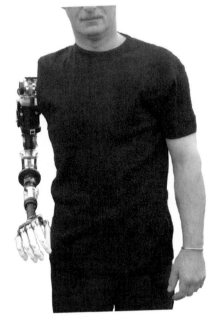

Figure 10 Edinburgh Modular Arm (Bioengineering Centre, Edinburgh, Scotland).

force over a wide range of opening widths (Figure 7).

Elbows
Body-Powered and Hybrid Elbows

Many new components that can be operated by a variety of harness-based control options are now available, as are programmable electronic controls. Innovative solutions such as the Automatic Forearm Balance[13] (AFB) and electronic locks permit more dynamic control of body-powered elbows with reduced effort by the patient.

Electrically Powered Elbows

Innovations in electrically powered elbows include programmable controls, improved adjustability, and increased battery capacity. Patient compliance will significantly improve if these control schemes can be better integrated into the body movement of the patient so that the prosthetic arm movements are less robot-like. One approach is to create devices in which at least two degrees of freedom are controlled simultaneously. Typically, the prehensor is controlled by myosignals, whereas the elbow is controlled by some additional input, such as a force sensor, that is integrated into a harness. The logical next step is the application of extended physiological proprioception (EPP), a concept advocated by Doubler and Childress[23] in 1984. However, to implement EPP would require an elbow drive with greater speed and force than is currently available. With the response time available in today's elbows, the patient would complain that the artificial arm is delaying the movement.

Elbow designs are now being explored to facilitate the implementation of EPP. One example is an experimental elbow based on the ErgoArm family of prosthetic elbows (Otto Bock Healthcare) (Figure 8). In this design, the elbow axis has an electric locking mechanism. Elbow flexion and extension are achieved by a complex drive consisting of a brushless direct-current motor, a gear train that allows continuous gear reduction, and an electronic servomechanism that adjusts the gear reduction ratio (Figure 9). For energy efficiency, the drive is supported by an AFB mechanism that counterbalances the weight of the forearm, wrist, and terminal device, thus reducing the demand on the elbow motor. The servomechanism disengages the gear train automatically for an energy-efficient free arm swing. Position and force sensors provide inputs for the control of this device. A myoelectric arm using this system can go from extension to full elbow flexion in 0.5 seconds when nothing is being held in the terminal device and actively lift 6 kg of weight in approximately 6 seconds.

Complete Electronic Arm Systems

Some research centers are developing complete electronic arm systems. In addition to having a powered prehensor, wrist, and elbow joint, the shoulder joint is also powered in these designs. In the prototype developed by Gow and associates,[24] the movement of the shoulder joint is reduced to one degree of freedom in the sagittal plane, the prehensor is an anthropomorphic hand, and the electromechanical actuators are modular, which allows different assemblies to be combined (Figure 10). Although the system is designed as a complete arm, the individual components can also be used for lower level amputations. For example, each finger contains a direct-current motor and a gear train and can therefore be used for finger replacement as well as for metacarpal amputation levels. A prosthetic hand for metacarpal amputation levels is currently in clinical testing (JR Ronald et al, Glasgow, Scotland, unpublished data presented at the ISPO World Congress, 2001) (Figure 11).

Based on the findings of British research teams, the European Community funded the Totally Modular Prosthetic Arm with High Workability (TOMPAW) project, which focused on the modularity aspects, optimized functionality, cosmesis, and optimization for use with osseointegrated patients. Bergomed AB (Vadstena, Sweden) is finishing the concept for a commercially available product system (Figure 12).

Schärer[25] uses standard components for the elbow and the prehensor but has designed a shoulder joint that allows spherical motion by means of three actuators. Control signals originate from three EMG electrodes using a control scheme based on the concept of a neural network.

Signal Acquisition for Prosthesis Control

Myoelectric Signals

New electrodes are being developed that will be much less sensitive to electromagnetic interference and increase the performance reliability of electronic prostheses. For example, some commercially available electrodes improve common mode rejection, which significantly reduces such problems as interference by cellular telephones (PH Kampas, Glasgow, Scotland, unpublished data presented at the ISPO World Congress, 2001).

Body Movement

It has been common practice for centuries to use a harness to capture the user's body movement to both control and power a prosthesis. Recently, many new electronic controls that can be operated by small body movements have become commercially available. For example, a microprocessor-controlled linear transducer incorporated into a lightweight harness can be used to supplement myoelectric inputs or to replace a missing myoelectric input.

Contact Forces

Contact forces generated by the residual limb have long been used to control prosthetic functions. One common application of this control option uses microswitches, as in the case of the initial fittings of the Edinburgh Modular Arm (Bioengineering Centre, Edinburgh, Scotland). The typical "on-off" microswitch provides single-speed (digital) control of the prosthesis, analogous to the power window button in an automobile.

By using Force Sensing Resistors, variable-speed (proportional) control can be achieved because the resistance is proportional to the contact pressure. Proportional control is analogous to the accelerator pedal in an automobile, where increased pressure translates into increased speed.

To avoid damage to this kind of sensor, good protection against moisture is necessary. Researchers at Rutgers University have designed a pneumatic sensor consisting of a pad made of closed-cell foam and a connected electronic pressure sensor that they claim can reliably detect movement of a single tendon in the residual limb. This would allow the independent control of each finger of an anthropomorphic hand. Prototypes of such sensors have been successfully applied to test fittings in which an anthropomorphic hand with an RC-servo drive (servo drive used in radio-controlled model cars) for each finger is used.[26]

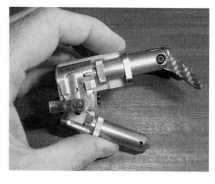

Figure 11 ProDigit hand derived from Edinburgh Modular Arm project (Bioengineering Centre, Edinburgh, Scotland).

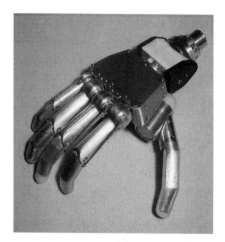

Figure 12 Anthropometric hand (Bergomed AB, Vadstena, Sweden).

Implantable Sensors

Little progress has been made in developing implantable devices to control an artificial limb. Current research has been focused on two primary approaches: (1) implantable myoelectrodes, which would lead to a better differentiation of muscle groups, and (2) direct neural coupling, which would add neural feedback.

The potential patient group for implantable electronic devices is rather small; therefore, definitive answers have been difficult to obtain. Researchers are attempting to apply the knowledge acquired from the field of functional electrical stimulation to the field of prosthetic limbs[27] (B Andrews et al, Glasgow, Scotland, unpublished data presented at the ISPO World Congress, 2001).

Controls

Most widely used controls are still based on proportional relationships between the EMG signal amplitudes, from the contraction of the involved muscle groups, and the intended action of the prosthetic component—such as speed of movement, magnitude of grip force, or position.[1] Closed-loop controls like the Southampton Adaptive Manipulation Scheme (SAMS) (Oxford Orthopaedic Engineering Centre) principle[17] or the Otto Bock Dynamic Mode Control (DMC) principle (R Kaitan, unpublished data presented at Weltkongress Orthopädie und Reha-Technik, 1994) feed back information internally, resulting in more precise and reliable user control.

The SUVA grasp stabilization system (Schweizerische Unfall Versicherungs Anstalt—Swiss Insurance Agency, Lucerne, Switzerland) is an additional control loop that activates once an object has been grasped.[3] A sensor measures the force vector between the hand and the grasped object and monitors changes in this vector. If the change indicates a potential risk of dropping the item, the grip force is increased to a level that stabilizes the grasp. This mechanism allows the user to pay less attention to the prosthetic device.

Another approach uses the combined EMG signals from electrodes or electrode arrays that are applied to the residual limb. These multiple signals are processed by a neural network that generates the output for the simultaneous control of all degrees of freedom of a prosthetic arm. Laboratory results have been promising,[28-30] especially from projects that combine neural networks with fuzzy logic.[31] However, these control systems are not yet sufficiently reliable to integrate this type of control in prostheses for activities of daily living.

Prosthesis Adjustment

Sophisticated controls require precise monitoring of the fitting and training procedures. Many software-based tools are now commercially available for this purpose. Animated Prosthetics (Greensboro, NC) offers a system that allows wireless programming and adjustment of the prosthesis by a personal digital assistant. This type of system is very convenient for the patient and makes the adjustment process easier because the patient is not physically tethered to the computer. Otto Bock offers an adjustment system for different levels of complexity. In most cases, only a few adjustments are required, making the software simple to use. When necessary, an expert system can be invoked that is much more complex but provides numerous adjustments to refine the control algorithms for more difficult fittings (H Dietl, PhD, Glasgow, Scotland, unpublished data presented at the ISPO World Congress, 2001).

Sockets and Suspension

The small population of upper limb amputees and the complexity of the components that must be integrated into their prostheses make research into this area very challenging. No specific tools are available for computer-aided socket design of upper limb prostheses. Most upper limb sockets use materials and design concepts that have proved successful for the larger population of lower limb amputees.[32-34] However, considerable work is being done to improve liner technology for myoelectric prostheses. Daly[35] inserts metal contacts into roll-on silicone socket liners and connects them to the preamplifiers of a myoelectric system. Motion Control now offers contacts and cables that are specifically designed for use with such elastomeric liners. Gröpel integrates the cables and skin contacts in custom-made liners directly. How-

ever, donning and doffing a prosthesis that incorporates the EMG sensors is complicated for the user.

Another disadvantage of methods that modify existing commercial liners is the increased risk of electromagnetic interference from the cable connections between the preamplifiers and the skin contact elements. For example, Müller and associates[36] extended the surface of standard Otto Bock electrodes and equipped the liner with stainless-steel rivets for conducting EMG signals. Problems occurred in clinical use as a result of electromagnetic disturbances created by the movement between the electrode surface and the rivet surface. A solution to these problems will be an important advance because patient comfort can be improved significantly by use of today's elastomer liner technologies.

Conclusion

Progress in arm prostheses remains evolutionary rather than revolutionary. Regretfully, it may take years before a new concept becomes a commercially available component that can make its way into daily clinical practice. The limited budgets for research and development in this field, compared with that for other technologically driven industries, and the demanding reliability requirements for prosthetic limbs make research in this area singularly challenging.

References

1. Sears HH, Shaperman J: Proportional myoelectric hand control: An evaluation. *Am J Phys Med Rehabil* 1991;70: 20-28.

2. Chappell PH, Kyberd PJ: Prehensile control of a hand prosthesis by a microcontroller. *J Biomed Eng* 1991;13: 363-369.

3. Puchhammer G: Der taktile Rutschsensor: Integration miniaturisierter Sensorik in einer Myo-Hand. *Orthopädie-Tehnik* 1999;7:564-569.

4. Tura A, Lambert C, Davalli A, Sacchetti R: Experimental development of

a sensory control system for an upper limb myoelectric prosthesis with cosmetic covering. *J Rehabil Res Dev* 1998; 35:14-26.

5. Okuno R, Yoshida M, Akazawa K: Development of biometric prosthetic hand controlled by electromyogram. *IEEE* 1996;9:103-108.

6. Kyberd PJ, Chappell PH: Characterization of an optical and acoustic touch and slip sensor for autonomous manipulation. *Meas Sci Technol* 1992;3: 969-975.

7. Kyberd PJ, Chappell PH: A force sensor for automatic manipulation based on the Hall effect. *Meas Sci Technol* 1993;4:281-287.

8. Wang G, Zhang X, Zhang J, Gruver WA: Gripping force sensory feedback for a myoelectrically controlled forearm prosthesis. *IEEE* 1995;1:501-504.

9. Davalli A: Biofeedback for upper limb myoelectric prosthetics, in *AAATE 99, 5th European Conference for the Advancement of Assistive Technology*. Amsterdam, The Netherlands, IOS Press.

10. Flor H, Elbert T, Knecht S, et al: Phantom-limb pain as a perceptual correlate of cortical reorganization following arm amputation. *Nature* 1995;375:482-484.

11. Weiss TH, Miltner WHR, Adler T, et al: Decrease in phantom limb pain associated with prosthesis-induced increased use of an amputation stump in humans. *Neurosci Lett* 1999;272: 131-134.

12. Weiss TH, Miltner WHR: Die Bedeutung der sensomotorischen Funktionalität von Prothesen für die Entwicklung von Phantomschmerz und kortikaler Plastizität. *Orthopädie-Technik* 2003;1:11-15.

13. Dietl H: Tendenzen in der Entwicklung von Prothesen für die obere Extremität. *Orthopädie-Technik* 1997;2: 126-132.

14. Weir RF, Grahn EC, Duff SD: A new externally powered, myoelectrically controlled prosthesis for persons with partial-hand amputations at the metacarpals. *J Prost Orthot* 2001;14: 26-31.

15. Dietl H, Gröpel W: Versorgung nach Teilhandamputationen mit myoelektrischen Komponenten. *Orthopädie-Technik* 2001;1:21-23.

16. Schulz S, Pylatiuk CH, Bretthauer G: A New ultralight anthropomorphic hand. *Proceedings of the International Conference on Robotics and Automation.* New Jersey, IEEE, 2001, pp 2437-2441.

17. Kyberd PJ, Chappell PH: The Southampton Hand: An intelligent myoelectric prosthesis. *J Rehabil Res Dev* 1994;31:326-334.

18. Kyberd PJ, Evans M, te Winkel ST: An intelligent anthropomorphic hand with automatic grasp. *Robotica* 1998; 16:531-536.

19. Kyberd PJ, Mustapha N, Carnegie F, Chappell PH: A clinical experience with hierarchically controlled myoelectric hand prosthesis with vibrotactile feedback. *Prosthet Orthot Int* 1993;17:56-64.

20. Rodriguez H, Pons JL, Ceres R: Precise speed control of a travelling wave ultrasonic motor for prosthetic hands. *Proceedings of the IFAC Conference on Mechatronic Systems.* Darmstadt, Germany, 2000, pp 401-406.

21. Herder JL: *Energy-Free Systems: Theory, Conception and Design of Statically Balanced Spring Mechanisms.* Delft, The Netherlands, Delft University of Technology, 2001. Dissertation.

22. Weir RF: A century of the Sauerbruch-Lebsche-Vanghetti muscle cineplasty: The US experience. *Proceedings of the 9th World Congress of the International Society for Prosthetics and Orthotics.* Amsterdam, The Netherlands, 1998, pp 198-199.

23. Doubler JA, Childress DS: An analysis of extended physiological proprioception as a prosthesis control technique. *J Rehabil Res Dev* 1984;21:5-18.

24. Gow DJ, Douglas W, Geggie C, Monteith E, Stewart D: The development of the Edinburgh Modular Arm system. *Proc Instn Mech Engrs* 2001;215(part H):291-298.

25. Schärer C: *Mikroprozessorsteuerung für eine Armprothese mit trainierbarer Befehlserkennung.* Zürich, Switzerland, Swiss Federal Institute of Technology, 1993. Dissertation.

26. Craelius W, Abboudi RL, Newby NA: Control of a multi-fingered prosthetic hand. *Proceedings of ICORR'99.* Stanford, CA, Stanford University, 1999, pp 255-259.

27. Herberts P, Kadefors R, Kaiser E, et al: Implantation of micro-circuits for myoelectric controls of prostheses. *J Bone Joint Surg Br* 1997;50:780-791.

28. Englehart K, Hudgins B, Parker PA: A wavelet-based continuous classification scheme for multifunction myoelectric control. *IEEE* 2001;48:302-311.

29. Huang HP, Chen CY: Development of a myoelectric discrimination system for a multi-degree prosthetic hand. *IEEE Robotics and Automation Society Proceedings.* 1999, pp 2392-2397.

30. Yeh EC, Chung WP, Chan RC, Tseng CC: Development of neural network controller for below-elbow prosthesis using single-chip microcontroller. *Biomed Eng* 1993;5:24-30.

31. Chan FHY, Yang YS, Lam FK, Zhang YT, Parker PA: Fuzzy EMG classification for prosthesis control. *IEEE Trans Rehabil Eng* 2000;8:305-311.

32. Daly W: Upper extremity socket design options. *Phys Med Rehabil Clin N Am* 2000;11:627-638.

33. Uellendahl JE, Heelam JR: Prosthetic management of the upper limb deficient child. *Phys Med Rehabil* 2000;14: 221-235.

34. Uellendahl JE: Upper extremity myoelectric prosthetics. *Phys Med Rehabil Clin N Am* 2000;11:639-652.

35. Daly W: Clinical application of roll-on sleeves for myoelectrically controlled transradial and transhumeral prostheses. *J Prosth Orthot* 2000;12:88-91.

36. Müller N, Lehmann A, Vietz W, Zapfe J: Silikonliner für myoelektrische Unterarmprothesen. *Orthopädie-Technik* 2000;10:876-879.

Section III

The Lower Limb

Chapter 29

Normal Gait

Jacquelin Perry, MD

Introduction

Walking relies on each limb repeating a sequence of integrated joint motions under muscle control to simultaneously advance the body along the desired line of progression and to maintain weight-bearing stability.[1] Superimposed on these two basic functions are actions that absorb the impact of limb loading and minimize energy cost. These functions are accomplished by the interplay of free joint mobility and muscle action; the latter is selective in both timing and intensity.[2]

Walking is also an interplay of opposing forces. Muscles generate the active force needed to initiate, accelerate, and decelerate the rate of displacement of the limb. The masses of the limb segments, influenced by gravity and inertia, present opposing forces, the most prominent of which is the ground-reaction force during stance phase (Figure 1). Because individual muscle force cannot be measured directly, a system has been devised by which muscle force values can be deduced from the measurable factors of limb dimensions, body weight, joint motion, and ground-reaction forces.[3] The resulting calculated values identify the external mechanical moments of gait. Then, by applying the principle that a force in one direction generates an equal and opposite force in the resisting object, the external moments are translated into internal moments to identify muscle action based on the mechanics of the limb.[1,4,5] Joint power is calculated using the product of moment and joint velocity to differentiate the intervals of muscle energy generation or absorption.[6]

Divisions of the Gait Cycle

Each sequence of lower limb action, from initial floor contact by one foot to the next instant of initial floor contact by the same foot, is called a gait cycle, or stride. The instant of floor contact by the foot is designated the beginning of the gait cycle because it is a consistent, conspicuous event that is readily visualized or measured. Some call this onset event "heel strike," but because either the heel or forefoot may touch the floor first, I prefer the term initial contact (IC).[2] A step, which is one half of a gait cycle (gc), consists of the events that occur from IC by one limb to IC by the opposite limb, ie, right IC to left IC or vice versa.

To facilitate differentiation of the numerous events occurring within a gait cycle, two basic systems for subdividing the cycle have been devised. The floor contact pattern was the first approach. Later attempts to better explain the interplay of the asynchronous joint motions resulted in the second approach, which groups the

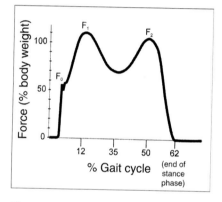

Figure 1 Vertical ground-reaction force during the stance phase of one gait cycle. F_0 = Impact peak force. F_1 = Loading response peak force. F_2 = Preswing push-off peak force. *(Reproduced with permission from Powers CM, Heino JG, Rao S, Perry J: The influence of patellofemoral pain on lower limb loading during gait. Clin Biomech 1999;14:722-728.)*

events into functional patterns of the limb and identifies the phases of gait.

Floor Contact Pattern

The simplest subdivision of the gait cycle divides the cycle into two periods: the period of floor contact (stance phase) and the period of mid-air limb advancement (swing phase), which is initiated by "toe-off." The gait cycle is divided into 100 percentage points, with 0% representing the moment when the foot first contacts the ground and 100% representing the next IC. The timing of events within the gait cycle is indicated by

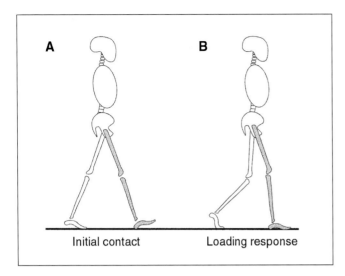

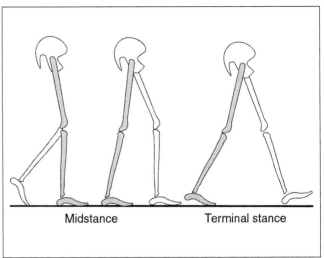

Figure 2 Weight acceptance gait phases showing limb posture and critical events (reference limb shaded). **A,** Initial contact (contact by heel). **B,** Loading response (shock-absorbing knee flexion). *(Adapted with permission from Perry J: Phases of gait, in Perry J (ed): Gait Analysis: Normal and Pathological Function. Thorofare, NJ, SLACK, 1992, pp 12-14.)*

Figure 3 SLS gait phases showing limb posture and critical events (reference limb shaded): midstance (left, foot flat, ankle neutral; and right, foot flat, ankle dorsiflexed, center of body mass over toe) and terminal stance (heel rise, ankle dorsiflexed, center of body mass beyond toe). *(Adapted with permission from Perry J: Phases of gait, in Perry J (ed): Gait Analysis: Normal and Pathological Function. Thorofare, NJ, SLACK, 1992, pp 12-14.)*

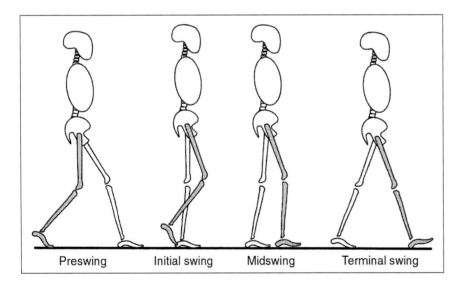

Figure 4 Swing limb advancement showing limb posture and critical events (reference limb shaded): preswing (forefoot contact, ankle plantar flexed, knee flexed), initial swing (peak knee flexion, swing foot opposite stance limb), midswing (foot clear, tibia vertical, peak hip flexion), and terminal swing (hip flexed, knee extended, ankle dorsiflexed). *(Adapted with permission from Perry J: Phases of gait, in Perry J (ed): Gait Analysis: Normal and Pathological Function. Thorofare, NJ, SLACK, 1992, pp 12-14.)*

giving the percentage at which they occur; eg, for an event that occurs one third of the way through the gait cycle, the indication would be 33% gc.

At the average normal velocity of approximately 80 m/min, stance phase occupies 62% of the gait cycle and swing phase involves 38%. Walking at slower speeds lengthens stance time and shortens swing time proportionally. Conversely, the faster the walking speed, the shorter the stance phase.

The stance phase can be further subdivided into periods of double- and single-limb support.[7] Each step begins with initial double-limb stance, during which period weight is transferred from the trailing to the leading foot. The average duration of double-limb stance is 12% of the gait cycle. When one foot lifts for swing, the function of the other limb changes to single-limb support (SLS). The average duration of SLS is 38% gc. At the end of stance, both limbs are again in contact with the ground as weight is transferred from the now-trailing foot to the lead foot. This interval is called terminal stance and represents 12% gc.

Phases of Gait

The second system of subdividing the gait cycle is based on phases of gait. Researchers who observed the complex interaction of hip, knee, and ankle motion identified a total of eight limb patterns that displayed a unique functional significance. These are the phases of gait. The functions of these eight gait phases combine to accomplish three tasks:[2] weight acceptance, SLS, and swing limb advancement (Figures 2 through 4). Each of these tasks meets several objectives required for normal gait. This information is summarized in Table 1.

TABLE 1 Tasks and Phases of Gait

Task	Phases of Gait	Objectives
Task A: Weight acceptance (Figure 2)	• Initial contact (initiates the heel rocker for progression and impact reduction)	Limb stabilization to support the fall of body weight
	• Loading response (knee flexion for shock absorption)	Shock absorption Preservation of progression
Task B: Single-limb support (Figure 3)	• Midstance (forward roll of limb over the supporting foot)	Progression
	• Terminal stance (advancement of the body beyond the supporting foot)	Weight-bearing stability
Task C: Swing limb advancement (Figure 4)	• Preswing (transition from stance to swing)	Foot clearance of the floor
	• Initial swing (floor clearance as limb advances)	Forward swing of the limb
	• Midswing (final thigh advancement)	
	• Terminal swing (final reach for step length, preparation for stance)	Preparation of the limb for stance

Each individual joint performs a sequence of motions, which reflects the actions needed to accomplish the objectives of gait. The dominant pattern of motion is in the sagittal plane, although motion does occur in other planes, including minor rotation needed for one limb to pass the other and to help maintain lateral balance. Each motion is associated with a dedicated pattern of muscle control. The function of each joint is best appreciated by relating the motion pattern of the joint to the three basic tasks of walking.

Function of the Ankle Joint

The ankle passes through four arcs of motion during each gait cycle (Figure 5), which are alternating periods of plantar flexion and dorsiflexion. The primary objective of the motion pattern of the ankle is progression. The foot also contributes to progression by its sequence of floor contact: heel only (0% to 12% gc), foot flat (12% to 31% gc), forefoot (31% to 62% gc), and swing (62% to 100% gc).[2]

Weight Acceptance
Motion

The dominant motion is a brief, but critical, arc of plantar flexion followed by dorsiflexion. Initial contact is made by the heel with the ankle at neutral. Loading the heel initiates rapid ankle plantar flexion (6° by 5% gc). This drops the forefoot toward the floor, but forefoot contact is delayed by the onset of ankle dorsiflexion. At this point the rounded surface of the heel functions as a supporting rocker over which the foot and tibia roll forward until the forefoot contacts the floor (12% gc). At the end of the loading response, the ankle is at neutral and the tibia is vertical.

Two functions are accomplished: (1) The impact of abrupt floor contact is partially absorbed by the initial foot drop, and (2) progression is preserved by the stimulation of rapid tibial advancement (180°/s) to overcome the static posture favored by the nearly vertical alignment of the limb.

Muscle Control

The pretibial muscles control the posture of the foot throughout weight acceptance. Already active in swing to support the foot, the anterior muscles abruptly increase their intensity as body weight is dropped onto the heel. The anterior tibialis is dominant at 35% of its maximum manual muscle test electromyography (MMT/EMG$_{max}$), whereas the extensor digitorum longus and extensor hallucis average 20% of MMT/EMG$_{max}$. Pretibial muscle action ceases when the forefoot contacts the floor (12% gc).

Kinetics

A small and brief internal dorsiflexor moment follows initial heel contact during the first 4% of the gait cycle. This indicates activity of the pretibial muscle group to control the falling foot. The power identifies that the muscle action is eccentric and that it is most intense at the onset of the motion (0.3 W/kg·m by 3% gc).[6] Progression of the body weight vector over the heel then advances the vector anterior to the ankle joint axis and initiates a plantar flexion moment. Joint power, however, indicates a low level of generative muscle action. This is consistent with concentric pretibial muscle activity moving the ankle toward dorsiflexion. The late onset of electromyographic (EMG) activity in the soleus at this time identifies an interval of antagonistic cocontraction, which supports the contradiction between the moment and joint power data.

Single-Limb Support
Motion

From a neutral position at the onset of SLS, the ankle progressively dorsiflexes, attaining 10° of dorsiflexion by the end of the task. During this arc of motion the mode of foot support changes. Midstance is an interval of foot flat support. Combined heel and forefoot floor contact provides stability as dorsiflexion of the ankle (7° at 31% gc) advances the center of pres-

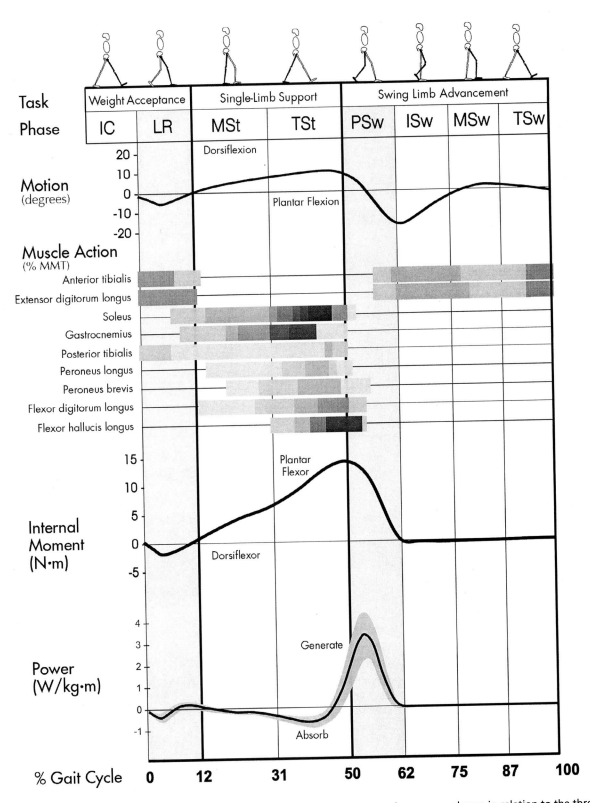

Figure 5 Normal ankle reference data for motion, muscle action, internal moment, and power are shown in relation to the three tasks and eight phases of motion. IC = Initial contact, LR = Loading response, MSt = Midstance, TSt = Terminal stance, PSw = Preswing, ISw = Initial swing, MSw = Midswing, TSw = Terminal swing. Column shading indicates phases within that task. *(Adapted with permission from The Pathokinesiology Service & The Physical Therapy Department (eds): Observational Gait Analysis. Downey, CA, Los Amigos Research & Education Institute, 2001, pp 11-21.)*

sure to the forefoot. During terminal stance, as the rounded metatarsal heads act as a forefoot rocker, the heel rises and the ankle reaches 11° of dorsiflexion at 45% gc. The combination of foot and ankle action advances the center of body mass beyond the foot.

Muscle Control

The soleus and gastrocnemius muscles control the rate of ankle dorsiflexion. Both muscles become active in loading response, and the intensity of the action continues to increase until the ankle approaches maximum dorsiflexion near the end of terminal stance (soleus: 88% of MMT at 43% gc; gastrocnemius: 79% of MMT at 40% gc). Muscle activity then rapidly decreases, terminating by the end of single stance (50% gc).[8] The perimalleolar muscles (so named because they wrap closely around the malleoli) also are commonly identified as ankle plantar flexors, but with limited leverage and small mass, they are incapable of controlling weight-bearing tibial rotation.

Kinetics

The small plantar flexor moment present at the onset of SLS continually increases in intensity throughout SLS to reach a peak of 14 N·m by the time the other foot contacts the floor (50% gc). This moment indicates progressively stronger action of the dominant plantar flexor muscle group. Calculation of joint power indicates this muscle action to be energy absorbing and eccentric.

Swing Limb Advancement

The third arc of ankle motion (preswing, terminal double support) and fourth arc of ankle motion (swing) both contribute to limb advancement. These two motion patterns have very different mechanics, so they will be reviewed separately.

Preswing: Motion

The preswing phase is a period of abrupt unloading of the trailing limb by rapid transfer of body weight to the other limb. Relief from full body weight frees the joints to respond to their trailing alignment. The response at the ankle is rapid plantar flexion to 18° below neutral. While this motion is occurring, the tibia and foot are rolling forward over the point of floor contact. At the same time, the point of support advances beyond the transverse axis of the forefoot, thereby removing the force that has been stabilizing the foot on the floor. The mobile metatarsophalangeal (MTP) joint becomes the preswing area of support. This could be classified as a fourth rocker; its function is to facilitate preparation of the limb for swing.

Preswing: Muscle Control

The source of the energy for this large and rapid arc of ankle plantar flexion has been long debated. Neither the soleus nor the gastrocnemius muscle exhibits evidence of EMG activity during preswing. The long toe flexors are still active, but they are too small to produce a force capable of moving the limb. Rather than neural control, the force moving the ankle into plantar flexion is a by-product of the rapid curtailment of the strong dorsiflexion moment that developed during terminal stance. This releases the final accumulation of soleus muscle energy (without EMG stimulation) as motion rather than static restraint. Physiologically, this represents a rapid change in the mode of muscle contraction, from eccentric to concentric. In clinical terms, this is called "rebound." The rapid transfer of body weight also frees the limb to respond to the final soleus output.

Preswing: Kinetics

Two force patterns are generated at the ankle during preswing. These are curtailment of the internal plantar flexion moment and the generation of high mechanical power.

Floor contact by the lead foot signifies the onset of preswing and that unloading of the trailing limb already is in progress. Forward alignment of the center of body mass, having exceeded the limits of stability, has initiated the fall of body weight onto the leading limb. The early rate of weight transfer is indicated by the impact experienced by the loading heel. A typical ground-reaction force sample shows 60% of body weight received within 20 ms.[9] Unloading of the preswing limb occurs at the same rate. This rapid change in load initiates a sequence of three significant events. The external dorsiflexion moment at the ankle is terminated, and this releases the residual gastrocnemius-soleus muscle energy. With the significantly unloaded limb presenting only a minor antagonistic moment, the residual gastrocnemius-soleus energy, now in a concentric mode, initiates ankle plantar flexion (without EMG stimulation), and the pattern of preswing limb motion begins.

The simultaneous occurrence of a high internal moment at the onset of preswing and the rapid rate of ankle plantar flexion combine to generate a prominent spike of mechanical power. Although the spike is brief because of quick dissipation of the plantar flexion moment, the timing identifies it as the "push-off force," which initiates forward advancement of the limb.

Swing: Motion

With the onset of toe-off, the ankle begins its final arc of dorsiflexion during initial swing. Neutral alignment is reached by the middle of midswing (80% gc) and is maintained through terminal swing.

Swing: Muscle Control

Ankle dorsiflexion is provided by the anterior tibialis and long toe extensor muscles, the activity of which begins just before toe-off and quickly attains a moderate intensity (30% of MMT). In midswing, once the foot is appropriately positioned, the activity of these muscles often temporarily diminishes or even ceases; however, the intensity increases quickly during terminal swing.

Swing: Kinetics

During the three phases of swing, the relatively small mass of the foot (average, 0.45 kg) is insufficient to produce a detectable moment. A brief period of power absorption during initial swing reflects a minor concentric response to lift the foot.

Function of the Foot Joints

Only two joints of the foot have sufficiently large arcs of motion to be isolated during gait. These are the subtalar joint and the MTP joints.

Subtalar Joint
Motion

An early, brief arc of calcaneal eversion (5° at 5% gc) occurs in response to initial contact by the heel and is followed by a slow yield of an additional few degrees through early midstance.[10] Then, the subtalar joint gradually reverses toward neutral by early terminal stance. Analysis of the motion of the calcaneus shows a persistent eversion of approximately 2°. During swing, the forefoot registers slight inversion.

Muscle Control

Eversion following heel contact stimulates a prompt response by the muscles that control inversion. The anterior tibialis, already active during swing, immediately increases its intensity, but it ceases when its dorsiflexion action terminates. The posterior tibialis also responds promptly, and its activity persists throughout the stance phase. In addition, its intensity increases with heel rise. Lateral restraint of potential subtalar inversion is provided by the peroneus longus and peroneus brevis muscles. Subtalar control during swing phase is provided by the dorsiflexor muscles. The anterior tibialis inverts the forefoot, and the extensor digitorum longus and peroneus tertius muscles provide eversion. The result is balanced dorsiflexion.

Metatarsophalangeal Joints
Motion

Heel rise during terminal stance phase is accompanied by dorsiflexion at the MTP joints. The limb is in a trailing position, and the forefoot (metatarsal heads) provides support. The forward roll of body weight over the forefoot both lifts the hindfoot and diminishes the area of the forefoot providing support. The toes are included in the supporting area. During terminal stance phase, the MTP joints dorsiflex 20°; this extension may reach 55° during preswing.

Muscle Control

Resistance to the dorsiflexion moment imposed by heel rise is provided by the toe flexor muscles (flexor hallucis longus and flexor digitorum longus) and the intrinsic muscles. Stabilization of the toes enlarges the area of forefoot support. The intrinsic muscles augment the toe control provided by the long muscles.

Function of the Knee

The knee performs four arcs of motion during a gait cycle. A sequence of flexion followed by extension occurs during both the stance and swing phases (Figure 6).

Weight Acceptance (Arc 1)
Motion

In response to the heel rocker rotating the tibia forward, the knee rapidly flexes from a relatively stable position of 5° flexion at initial contact to 18° at the end of the loading response (12% gc). This motion is the major source of shock absorption to lessen the stress of rapid limb loading, but the final position does not allow weight bearing without dynamic control.

Muscle Control

Throughout weight acceptance, the hamstrings and quadriceps act synergistically, exchanging dominance as needed. At initial contact, protective flexion is emphasized, with the EMG intensity of the medial hamstrings (semimembranosus and semitendinosus) being relatively greater than that of the quadriceps. The flexor muscle action then subsides, and the activity of the quadriceps increases notably in intensity, to 30% of MMT, to stabilize the flexed knee for the transfer of body weight.

Kinetics

At the onset of stance, an immediate but brief flexor moment occurs (peak: 4 N·m at 3% gc). Power is generated that, when related to the accompanying EMG activity, indicates initial dominance of knee flexor musculature to prevent knee hyperextension; however, this period is characterized by cocontraction of the quadriceps and hamstrings. By 5% of the gait cycle, the knee moment develops an extensor orientation. Power absorption during the end of weight acceptance indicates that the extensor muscles are providing an eccentric force to stabilize the passively flexing knee.

Single-Limb Support (Arc 2)
Motion

At the onset of SLS, the knee progressively reduces its flexion throughout midstance and early terminal stance. Maximum extension (3° of flexion) is reached at 36% gc and maintained for a short time, until 42% gc, when the knee reverses its motion, toward flexion.

Muscle Control

Continuation of the prior quadriceps action at a lesser intensity actively extends the knee. By 20% gc, however, the EMG for all four of the vasti muscles ceases. Further knee extension is a passive reaction to remote forces that advance the body over the supporting foot.

Kinetics

Although the extensor moment, which peaked earlier, rapidly declines to zero by the middle of midstance, the accompanying generative power indicates that a brief interval of concentric extensor muscle action occurs

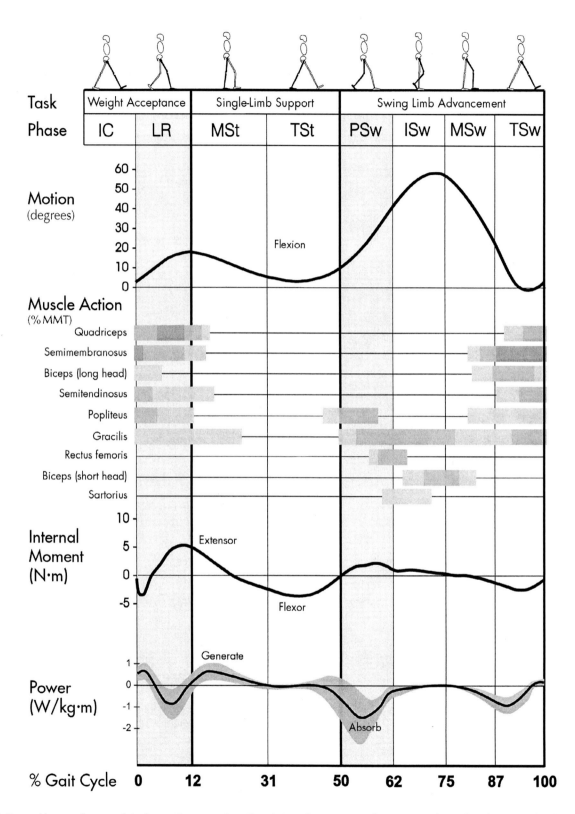

Figure 6 Normal knee reference data for motion, muscle action, internal moment, and power are shown in relation to the three tasks and eight phases of motion. IC = Initial contact, LR = Loading response, MSt = Midstance, TSt = Terminal stance, PSw = Preswing, ISw = Initial swing, MSw = Midswing, TSw = Terminal swing. Column shading indicates phases within that task. *(Adapted with permission from The Pathokinesiology Service & The Physical Therapy Department (eds):* Observational Gait Analysis. *Downey, CA, Los Amigos Research & Education Institute, 2001, pp 11-21.)*

at this time. These data correlate with the segment velocity pattern, which shows that the transfer of energy from the decelerating tibia to the femur facilitates knee extension.[11] Continuing anterior displacement of the body weight vector introduces a moderate flexion moment, which peaks at 3 N·m during terminal stance. The lack of significant power and EMG activity at this time indicates that this is a passive event.

Swing Limb Advancement (Arcs 3 and 4)
Motion

The knee moves through two large arcs of motion of similar duration. The first is flexion, to elevate the foot for floor clearance, followed by extension, to complete step length in preparation for stance.

Knee flexion is essential for the swinging limb to clear the floor.[12] Three gait phases are involved: terminal stance, preswing, and initial swing. In terminal stance, knee flexion is initiated by the center of pressure moving beyond the stable area of the forefoot. The pushing action of the ankle during preswing rapidly increases knee flexion to 40° by toe-off (62% gc), which represents two thirds of the arc needed for toe clearance. Finally, an additional 20° is gained during initial swing by a combination of active knee and hip flexion. Peak flexion is 60° by 70% gc.

After reaching maximum flexion during initial swing, the knee quickly reverses the direction of motion, toward extension, through midswing and into late terminal swing. After reaching zero extension, the knee flexes 2° to 3°.

Muscle Control

Direct muscle control of this large arc of knee flexion is subtle, with the source being low-intensity activity (13% to 17% of MMT) of several small muscles. The popliteus is consistently active during the last 5% of terminal stance and during early preswing, but otherwise its timing varies.

Fiber alignment implies that the popliteus may contribute internal tibial rotation to unlock the extended knee. Three muscles contribute during initial swing: the short head of the biceps femoris, the sartorius, and the gracilis.

Muscle control of the extending knee involves a synergistic sequence. First, a reduction of the flexor influence by the gracilis and short head of the biceps femoris occurs. By the middle of midswing, activation of the long hamstrings (semimembranosus, long head of the biceps femoris, and semitendinosus) introduces a two-joint whip effect, which aids inhibition of the forward swing of the thigh at the hip while also avoiding hyperextension at the knee. At the onset of terminal swing, the quadriceps muscles introduce knee extension.

Kinetics

A small extensor moment is created during preswing despite the relatively large arc of knee flexion (40°). Also, measurements of the associated power show a prominent peak of energy absorption (1.5 W/kg·m) despite the absence of significant EMG activity in the knee flexors. These apparently inconsistent facts suggest that the rapid knee motion contributes to the power peak.

Both moment and power are minimal during initial swing and midswing. During terminal swing, a modest flexor moment and accompanying peak of energy absorption occur. This indicates that flexor activity is dominant in the extensor and flexor muscle cocontraction that EMG studies show occur at this time.

Function of the Hip

The hip has just two arcs of motion during the gait cycle, one of flexion and one of extension (Figure 7). In addition, two intervals of static posturing supplement this movement. Defining hip motion is difficult because not only the movement of the thigh but also that of the pelvis, which may alter its alignment during

gait, must be considered.[13] Further, the sagittal axis between the pelvic landmarks used in the laboratory for gait analysis (the anterior and posterior superior iliac spines) tilts downward 10° anteriorly from the vertical, resulting in a measured hip angle between the thigh and pelvis that is 10° greater than the angle of the thigh relative to the reference axis of the laboratory. During normal gait, the pelvis tilts a mere 5°, but during pathologic gait, pelvic deviations can be significant. Laboratory gait analysis is oriented to calculating hip motion, while the observing eye follows the thigh. The hip is the focus of the discussion presented here.

Weight Acceptance (Posture 1)
Motion

At IC the hip is flexed 30°, and this posture is maintained until the end of the loading response. Abrupt loading of the limb initiates a contralateral pelvic drop in the coronal plane, which reaches 4° by the end of the loading response. This is noted at the hip as adduction. The forward pelvic rotation of 10° is equivalent to the external rotation of the hip.

Muscle Control

Maximum involvement of hip musculature occurs during the task of weight acceptance. The two primary hip extensors, the adductor magnus and the lower gluteus maximus, are activated in late terminal swing and quickly increase in intensity, peaking at IC (adductor magnus, 40% of MMT; lower gluteus maximus, 25% of MMT). This intensity has diminished by the middle of the task, and the action ceases by the end of the loading response. The hamstring muscles, which begin their action during midswing, continue during the loading response at a slightly reduced intensity (semimembranosus, 23% of MMT; long head of the biceps femoris, 10% of MMT).

Lateral support of the hip by the abductor muscles also is most intense

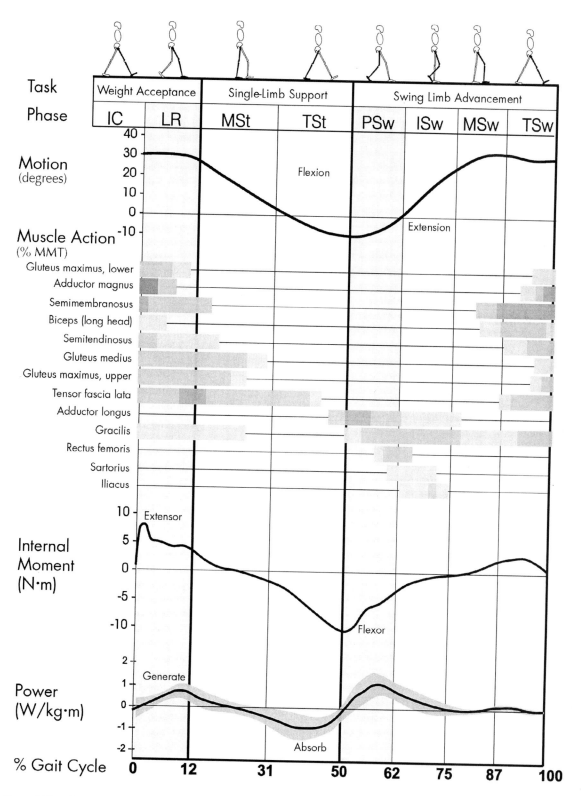

Figure 7 Normal hip reference data for motion, muscle action, internal moment, and power are shown in relation to the three tasks and eight phases of motion. IC = Initial contact, LR = Loading response, MSt = Midstance, TSt = Terminal stance, PSw = Preswing, ISw = Initial swing, MSw = Midswing, TSw = Terminal swing. Column shading indicates phases within that task. *(Adapted with permission from The Pathokinesiology Service & The Physical Therapy Department (eds): Observational Gait Analysis. Downey, CA, Los Amigos Research & Education Institute, 2001, pp 11-21.)*

during weight acceptance.[14] The mean intensities are moderate, with the gluteus medius averaging 28% of MMT, the upper gluteus maximus averaging 23% of MMT, and the tensor fascia lata averaging 18% of MMT.

Kinetics

The immediate peak extensor moment (7 N·m at 3% gc) is consistent with the moderately strong EMG activity of the hip extensors, particularly that of the adductor magnus muscle. Continuation of a slightly reduced extensor moment occurs, which is consistent with the interpretation that extensor muscles are supporting the flexed hip. The increasing arc of generative power, which peaks at the end of the phase, indicates that the extensor muscles are contracting concentrically to initiate active hip extension.

Single-Limb Support (Arc 1)
Motion

As the contralateral limb prepares to lift the foot (at 10% gc), the hip begins to extend, an action that continues throughout midstance and terminal stance. Maximum hyperextension (−15°) is reached at the end of terminal stance.

Muscle Control

Contraction of the primary hip extensor muscles has ceased activity, but the activity of the medial hamstring group (the semimembranosus and semitendinosus) persists into single stance. The abductor muscles continue their activity through most of midstance and terminal stance. The semiposterior orientation of these muscles to the hip indicates that they would contribute some extensor control. The tensor fascia lata, which has an anterior alignment, remains active into early terminal stance, providing a dynamic limit to extension.

Kinetics

At the onset of single stance, the magnitude of the extensor moment and power generation rapidly decline. Both the development of a flexor mo-

ment during terminal stance and the power calculation showing muscle absorptive action are not consistent with the minimal flexor EMG.

Swing Limb Advancement (Arc 2, Posture 2)
Motion

With the onset of preswing, the hip begins to flex. This action continues through initial swing and early midswing. Maximum flexion of 35° is attained at the end of midswing (86% gc). Then, during terminal swing, the hip assumes a final posture at 30° of flexion.

Muscle Control

As the flexing hip moves through its arc, a transfer of control from one set of muscles to another occurs. During preswing, flexion is provided by two muscles that combine adduction and flexion: the adductor longus (contracting at its highest intensity, 30% of MMT) and the gracilis, which contracts at a low intensity (18% of MMT). The combination of flexion and adduction accompanies the shift of body weight toward the contralateral limb. During initial swing, shortly after toe-off, the iliacus and sartorius become active at a low intensity (18% of MMT) and continue through the phase. Also, the gracilis increases its intensity (to 28% of MMT) during early initial swing. During terminal swing, the extensor function of the hamstrings actively terminates hip flexion. The semimembranosus (33% of MMT at 88% gc) is more active than the long head of the biceps femoris and the semitendinosus (20% of MMT at 98% gc).

Kinetics

With contralateral foot contact signifying the onset of preswing, the magnitude of the flexion moment of the hip declines rapidly. Power calculations show, however, that the muscle action becomes concentric to advance the thigh. During terminal swing, extensor moment is small and concentric power is minimal, which is con-

sistent with the small reduction in hip flexion recorded during this period.

Function of the Pelvis

The pelvis follows the swing limb as it moves forward. Conversely, the pelvis appears to rotate backward relative to the stance limb. At IC, the weight-accepting limb and that side of the pelvis are at the maximum forward rotation (5°) relative to the center of the body. Forward swing of the contralateral limb rotates the pelvis to a transverse neutral alignment in midstance. By the end of terminal stance, the weight-bearing side of the pelvis is relatively posterior (5°). The pelvis also has a 5° anterior tilt. The abrupt transfer of body weight causes a contralateral pelvic drop in the coronal plane, which is recorded as 4° elevation of the pelvis on the stance limb.

Function of the Total Limb
Weight Acceptance

Weight acceptance is the most challenging task of walking (Figure 8). At weight acceptance, approximately 60% of body weight is almost instantaneously dropped onto the forward limb. The nearly erect alignment of the limb, with the thigh only 20° from vertical, favors stability over progression.

Initial Contact (0% gc)

As the heel contacts the floor, the hip is flexed 20°, the knee is extended (5° of flexion), and the ankle is dorsiflexed to neutral. The heel rocker is set.

Loading Response (0% to 12% gc)

The mechanics of the heel rocker facilitate two functions: preservation of progression and shock absorption. Loading the heel initiates ankle plantar flexion, with a peak foot drop velocity of 300°/s, softening the impact of initial floor contact (Figure 1).

Prompt pretibial muscle response limits the arc to 6° at 5% gc and preserves the heel rocker by initiating ankle dorsiflexion.

Heel contact also initiates subtalar eversion as another shock-absorbing response. The combined action of the inverting muscles (anterior tibialis and posterior tibialis) limits subtalar eversion to 5°. This muscle action continues until the forefoot contacts the floor.

The foot and tibia continue rolling forward on the heel rocker until forefoot contact occurs (at 12% gc), when a stable, foot flat posture is attained. The energy of the foot rolling forward on the heel is transmitted to the tibia by the contracting pretibial muscles, propelling the tibia forward at a peak velocity of 180°/s. This rapid tibial advancement initiates knee flexion and interrupts the shock of rapid limb loading. A prompt increase in quadriceps activity preserves weight-bearing stability by limiting knee flexion to 18°. The early interval of rapid foot drop also shortens the duration of the heel rocker, which reduces the period of peak quadriceps response. Simultaneous response by the primary hip extensors stabilizes the flexed hip and, by controlling the femur, also contributes to knee stability. Synergistic action by the hamstrings both provides circumferential control of the knee and augments the hip extensors.

Kinetics

Floor impact initiates an immediate peak moment (3% gc) at both the hip and knee, but the direction of the reactions differ. At the hip, the moment of 8 N·m represents the peak response of the primary hip extensor muscles. Continuing support is provided by a smaller extensor moment (5 N·m).

At the knee the immediate peak moment is a flexor moment, which implies action by the hamstrings to oppose potential knee hyperextension. The moment then reverses, to an extensor moment, in response to the rapid tibial advancement initiated by

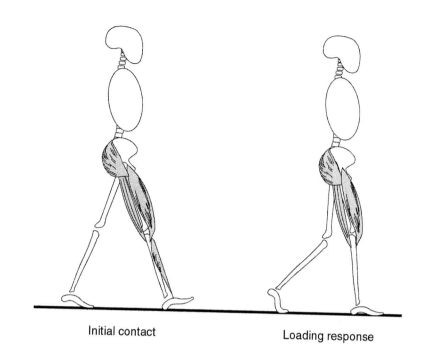

Figure 8 Total limb function during weight acceptance. Limb posture and critical muscles for the involved phases are shown. *(Adapted with permission from Perry J: Total limb function, in Perry J (ed):* Gait Analysis: Normal and Pathological Function. *Thorofare, NJ, SLACK, 1992, pp 151-158.)*

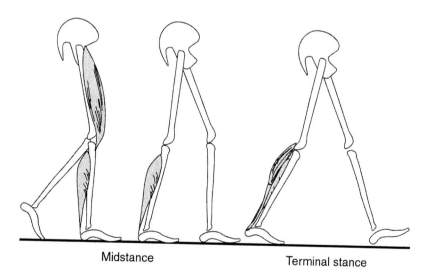

Figure 9 Total limb function during SLS. Limb posture and critical muscles for the involved phases are shown. *(Adapted with permission from Perry J: Total limb function, in Perry J (ed):* Gait Analysis: Normal and Pathological Function. *Thorofare, NJ, SLACK, 1992, pp 151-158.)*

the heel rocker. A dorsiflexion moment at the ankle controls the foot.

By the end of weight acceptance, the limb attains a posture of dynamic stability. The foot is flat and the ankle is neutral, but there are residual flexor moments at the hip and knee, which still require active muscle control.

Single-Limb Support

SLS is shown in Figure 9. During this prolonged period of progression, energy is conserved as direct muscle control is replaced with passive control to maintain knee and hip stability during the last half of the task.

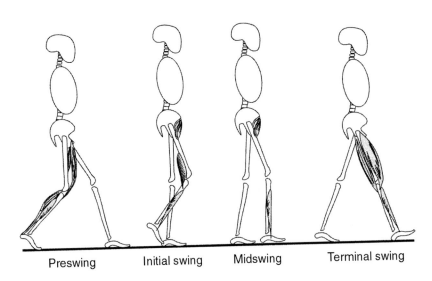

Preswing   Initial swing   Midswing   Terminal swing

Figure 10 Total limb function during swing limb advancement. Limb posture and critical muscles for the involved phases are shown. *(Adapted with permission from Perry J: Total limb function, in Perry J (ed):* Gait Analysis: Normal and Pathological Function. *Thorofare, NJ, SLACK, 1992, pp 151-158.)*

Midstance (12% to 31% gc)

At the onset of SLS, the supporting area is limited to the dimensions of the weight-bearing foot. As the ankle advances to 5° of dorsiflexion, the body weight vector reaches the forefoot (metatarsal heads). Graduated soleus and gastrocnemius action slows the rate of tibial progression to 48°/s, and the progressional velocity of the femur is increased to 140°/s by the quadriceps, which act concentrically at this point. When neutral knee extension is reached (by 23% gc), the quadriceps muscle relaxes. The hip uses this accelerated advancement of the femur over a slowed tibia as a remote source of extensor control.

Terminal Stance (31% to 50% gc)

Continuing progression of the body weight vector over the anterior forefoot significantly increases the intensity of the EMG activity of the soleus and gastrocnemius muscles. The accompanying heel rise contributes significantly to the plantar flexor moment. Advancement of the thigh over the relatively stable tibia passively extends the knee and hip until the end of terminal stance. The tensor fascia lata may be active to restrain hip extension. Then, as the foot becomes unstable, flexion of the limb slowly begins.

Kinetics

Throughout SLS, the plantar flexor moment at the ankle is accompanied by significant EMG activity of the soleus and gastrocnemius. The increasing intensity of the eccentric action is demonstrated by the power pattern, which shows progressively greater energy absorption. The plantar flexor moment at the ankle is the source of remote knee and hip control.

Swing Limb Advancement

Figure 10 illustrates swing limb advancement. Two modes of limb mechanics are involved in this task: forward swing of the foot for step length and preparation of the limb for stance.

Preswing (50% to 62% gc)

This final phase of stance is a period of double support during which preswing is simultaneous with contralateral weight acceptance. Rapid forward transfer of body weight favors the mechanics of preswing. Unloading of the limb releases the energy stored by the soleus and gastrocnemius muscles during their prior eccentric activity in terminal stance. The resulting rapid ankle plantar flexion initiates 40° of knee flexion and energizes the limb to swing forward.

Several factors contribute to preswing limb advancement. The posture of the limb at the end of terminal stance is critical: it is in trailing alignment, with only the forefoot contacting the floor, while the ankle is maximally dorsiflexed and the hip is at the end of its extensor range. Both tensed muscle groups are active. The knee has been unlocked as the support area of the foot rolls forward beyond the center of the metatarsal heads during late terminal stance and is free to respond. Also, EMG activity in the popliteus is a constant finding.

The rapid transfer of body weight to the contralateral limb at the onset of preswing releases the stored energy in the hip and ankle musculature. A rapid sequence of motion follows. Most prominent is the arc of ankle plantar flexion. Passive tension stored in the previously active gastrocnemius and soleus muscles is released rapidly by the fall of body weight onto the contralateral limb. Because there is no EMG activity, the release of stored energy is assumed to be the push-off force that advances the tibia and flexes the knee.

Hip flexor control also contributes to the initiation of knee flexion. The stored flexor energy is released, and the adductor longus and gracilis muscles, while acting to limit the rate of medial fall, also initiate advancement of the thigh from its trailing position.

Initial Swing (62% to 75% gc)

Two critical motions are completed during initial swing: knee flexion and hip flexion. Maximum knee flexion (60° by 72% gc) lifts the toe for floor clearance. This amount of knee flexion is required because the trailing posture of the lower leg places the foot into a toe-down position. The contributing muscles are the short head of the biceps femoris, the sartorius, and the gracilis, all of which contract at low intensities.

Active hip flexion advances the thigh. This is accomplished by the continued activity of the preswing muscles with the addition of the iliacus and the sartorius. At an individual's optimum gait velocity, the plantar flexion thrust (push-off) of the ankle relieves the hip flexor muscles of their function, conserving energy. The timing between peak knee flexion and thigh advancement is critical for clearance of the floor by the toe because the ankle still lacks full dorsiflexion (−7°).

Midswing (75% to 87% gc)

With the swing foot ahead of the supporting limb, the knee begins extending for greater step length. The resulting vertical tibia necessitates continuing ankle dorsiflexion for foot clearance of the floor. Near the end of midswing, rapid onset of hamstring muscle action inhibits further advancement of the thigh and also avoids excessive forward swing of the tibia from inertia. By the end of midswing, the hip and knee are both flexed 30° and the ankle is dorsiflexed to neutral.

Terminal Swing (87% to 100% gc)

Knee extension is the final swing motion. This action both completes step length and positions the limb for stance. Prompt activation of the quadriceps at the beginning of the phase extends the knee, and continuing action of the hamstrings prevents hyperextension. At the end of terminal swing, the limb is positioned for optimum initial contact.

Kinetics

Control of the limb during preswing includes a significant power peak at each joint. At both the ankle and hip, motion-inducing moments include a significant arc of generative energy (30° ankle plantar flexion and 10° hip flexion). In contrast, the dominant force pattern that contributes to the 35° arc of flexion of the knee is an extensor moment with absorptive power. Thus the hip and ankle motion is due to active muscle contraction, whereas knee function is passive.

Summary

The normal pattern of limb motion and muscle control accomplishes the basic objectives of walking, progression with weight-bearing stability, through an optimum interplay of the forces generated by positional demand and muscle control. Normal function also minimizes the energy cost of walking, allowing the customary adult walking speed of approximately 80 m/min.[15] Because physical fitness is reflected in a person's self-selected walking speed, inability to walk at a normal speed is an early sign of physical impairment. Therefore, knowledge of the normal motion pattern of walking is a valuable tool for the health professional to use when examining a patient.

Focusing on just the basic determinants of walking speed, stride length, and cadence can be very informative. Stride length depends on both dynamic stability and the mechanics of progression. Dynamic stability is the result of selective timing and intensity of the controlling muscles, and progression is gained from the effectiveness of the four foot rockers: heel, ankle, forefoot, and MTP joint. Cadence, or the rate of stepping, depends on the ease of initiating swing and of accepting the transfer of body weight at the onset of stance. Accomplishing these basic determinants of walking speed relies on the mechanics defined by the eight phases of gait.

References

1. Inman VT, Ralston HJ, Todd F, Lieberman JC (eds): *Human Walking*. Baltimore, MD, Williams and Wilkins, 1981.

2. Perry J (ed): *Gait Analysis: Normal and Pathological Function*. Thorofare, NJ, SLACK, 1992.

3. Bressler B, Frankel JP: The forces and movements in the leg during level walking. *Trans ASME* 1950;72:27-36.

4. Cappozzo A, Figura F, Marchetti M: The interplay of muscular and external forces in human ambulation. *J Biomech* 1976;9:35-43.

5. Meglan D, Todd F: Kinetics of human locomotion, in Rose J, Gamble JG (eds): *Human Walking*, ed 2. Baltimore, MD, Williams & Wilkins, 1994, pp 73-99.

6. Winter DA: Energy generation and absorption at the ankle and knee during fast, natural, and slow cadences. *Clin Orthop* 1983;175:147-154.

7. Eberhardt HD, Inman VT, Bresler B: The principal elements in human locomotion, in Klopsteg PE, Wilson PD (eds): *Human Limbs and Their Substitutes*. New York, NY, Hafner Publishing, 1968, pp 437-471.

8. Sutherland DH, Cooper L, Daniel D: The role of the ankle plantar flexors in normal walking. *J Bone Joint Surg Am* 1980;62:354-363.

9. Powers CM, Heino JG, Rao SS, Perry J: The influence of patellofemoral pain on lower limb loading during gait. *Clin Biomech* 1999;14:722-728.

10. Powers CM, Reischl S, Rao SS, Perry J: Abstract: Quantification of foot pronation using 3D motion analysis. *J Sports Phys Ther* 1997;25:67.

11. Rao SS, Boyd LA, Mulroy SJ, Bontrager EL, Gronley JK, Perry J: Segment velocities in normal and transtibial amputees: Prosthetic design implications. *IEEE Trans Rehabil Eng* 1998;6:219-226.

12. Brinkmann JR, Perry J: Rate and range of knee motion during ambulation in healthy and arthritic subjects. *Phys Ther* 1985;65:1055-1060.

13. Perry J: Scientific basis of rehabilitation. *Instr Course Lect* 1985;34: 385-388.

14. Lyons K, Perry J, Gronley JK, Barnes L, Antonelli D: Timing and relative intensity of hip extensor and abductor muscle action during level and stair ambulation: An EMG study. *Phys Ther* 1983;63:1597-1605.

15. Waters RL, Mulroy SJ: The energy expenditure of normal and pathologic gait. *Gait Posture* 1999;9:207-231.

Chapter 30

Amputee Gait

Jacquelin Perry, MD

Introduction

The walking ability of a person with a lower limb amputation is determined by both the mechanical quality of the prosthesis[1] and the physiologic quality of the residual limb.[2] The primary determinants of residual limb quality are passive joint mobility and muscle strength. Knee flexion contractures greater than 10° were found to be the most significant obstacle to recovering the ability to walk.[3] The disuse that accompanies illness or injury is an insidious cause of muscle weakness. In addition, the most common indications for lower limb amputation in the United States—diabetes mellitus and peripheral vascular disease—impose physiologic limitations on muscle strengthening. A direct correlation has been found between muscle weakness and walking speed in persons with transtibial amputations.[4] Thus, the initial rehabilitation program to prevent contracture formation and muscle weakening from disuse is a critical determinant of the future ability of individuals with a lower limb amputation to walk on a prosthesis.

Advances in prosthetic design have significantly increased the amputee's options. The basic qualities of the prosthetic feet currently available fall into three categories: anatomic, biomechanical, and dynamic. The first approach combines anatomic reproduction with an articulated, single-axis ankle joint. This design continues to be preferred in the United Kingdom for its mobility.[5] However, greater weight, limited durability, and arcs of uncontrolled motion in an insensate artificial foot have been persistent adverse qualities. The second type of foot, developed to circumvent the limitations of a mechanical joint, is a unitary biomechanical solid ankle–cushion heel (SACH) foot that was developed by the University of California, Berkeley (UCB) Prosthetic Project. In this foot, stability, mobility, and durability are effectively integrated by the creative combination of a solid ankle, cushion heel, dense foam forefoot, and rocker contour.[6] The SACH foot became the standard for function, economy, and durability, but limitation of progression has remained a drawback. In the third type of foot, developed to improve progression without sacrificing stance stability, the basic design of the biomechanical foot has been enhanced by the introduction of "dynamic-response" materials. Two basic designs have evolved: those with a short spring inside the foot area, such as the Seattle Foot (Model & Instrument Works, Inc, Seattle, WA), and those with a longer spring that extends from the toes up into the shank, such as the Flex-Foot Modular III (Ossur, Reykjavik, Iceland). Several variations of each are available. Function at the hip and knee is also being addressed with newer materials and mechanical designs. The functional effects of these advances have been documented by gait analysis, which includes kinematics, dynamic electromyography (EMG), kinetics, and stride analysis. These measurements also serve as clinical standards for individual patient management.

Transtibial Amputee Gait

The many prosthetic feet currently available for the individual with a transtibial amputation differ in heel, ankle, and forefoot mobility because of variations in design and material. Although these variations introduce functional differences, the prosthetic feet have an underlying similarity, that of providing the fundamental functions required for walking. For each stage of the gait cycle, the fundamental functions are presented first, followed by a review of the unique characteristics of the different prosthetic designs that have been identified by comparative studies.

The numerous comparisons of the different prosthetic feet have addressed selected designs and functions. Here, as in most gait research projects, examples of the four basic structural classes are discussed. Hence, the data cited will mostly relate to the single-axis (Otto Bock, Minneapolis, MN), SACH (Kingsley

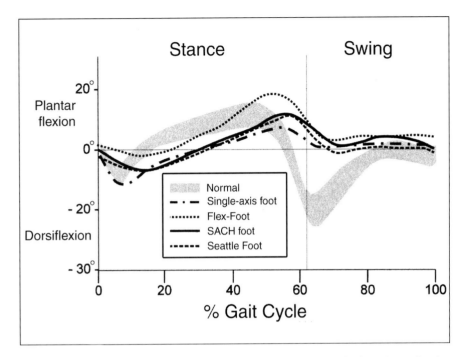

Figure 1 Ankle motion of four different prosthetic feet during self-selected speed gait in persons with a unilateral transtibial amputation, compared with normal.[7,11]

Manufacturing Co, Costa Mesa, CA), foot spring only (Seattle Foot, Model & Instrument Works; Seattle Systems, Poulsbo, WA), and the shank-foot spring (Flex-Foot) (Flex-Foot, Aliso Viejo, CA; Ossur) designs.

Weight Acceptance
Ankle/Foot

Initial heel contact at the onset of stance imparts significant energy to both the foot and the tibia. The hindfoot of all prosthetic feet includes some means of lessening the impact of abrupt heel loading. These response mechanisms, however, differ significantly from normal and also vary with the design of the prosthesis.

Prostheses with a single-axis ankle joint initiate a short period of plantar flexion at the same rate as a normal ankle. With only a terminal bumper for motion control, however, the magnitude of the free foot drop exceeds normal joint motion by 50%.[7,8] The common response to this hypermobility is to choose a harder bumper. As a result, both the arc of plantar flexion and the duration of recovery to neutral are exaggerated.[5,9,10]

The composite prosthetic feet simulate ankle plantar flexion by compression of an elastomeric heel cushion (SACH foot; Seattle Lite foot, Seattle Systems) or posterior spring blade (Flex-Foot). The rate of loading response in plantar flexion in these feet is approximately half of normal[8,11] (Figure 1). With a Flex-Foot, the result is a shorter than normal arc of motion, whereas the slower response of the SACH and Seattle Lite heels yields a prolonged arc of motion.

The shock-absorbing capability of prosthetic cushion heels has been quantified by the reduction of the peak acceleration at heel strike. Gait measurements were made for five subjects walking with six types of prosthetic feet. Each series of measurements was repeated with the subjects wearing two styles of shoes, sports and leather. Among the prosthetic feet, no significant difference in shock-absorbing capability was found. The sports shoes registered notably greater shock absorption than did the leather shoes in 80% of the comparisons. Only with the two stiffest feet was no difference between

shoe styles demonstrated. The random pattern of the prosthetic foot data suggested functional similarity among the prosthetic feet, in contrast to the strong differences between shoe styles. Further definition was prevented by wide variations among individual trials and a loss of data.

The second response to initial heel contact is the transfer of the energy of the foot into a heel rocker to rotate the foot and tibia forward.[12] All of the prosthetic designs have a similar loading response. The tibial shank rotates forward at about half of the normal rate. As a result, heel-only support is significantly prolonged, averaging 21% of the gait cycle (gc) (normal, 12% gc) before attaining foot-flat floor contact.[8] This slow rate of foot drop extends the heel-only mode of limb support into the period of single stance.[13] Even a delay in contralateral toe-off (16% gc versus 12% gc) does not resolve the problem.[8] Throughout this delay in attaining foot-flat weight bearing, instability is prolonged as the dorsiflexion moment remains in effect.

There are notable differences in the duration of heel-only support among prosthetic foot types. The most prolonged occurs with the SACH foot (27% gc)[5] and the shortest with the single-axis ankle (17% gc). In between are the Seattle Lite foot (21% gc) and Flex-Foot (19% gc). The finding that a highly mobile articulated ankle and a relatively stiff composite prosthetic foot (SACH foot, Seattle Foot, and Flex-Foot) cause a functionally significant delay in forefoot contact suggests that some mechanism other than ankle mobility is involved. Knee control may be the related factor.

Knee

Motion The peak knee flexion that follows initial heel contact during prosthetic gait differs significantly from normal function both in magnitude and timing (Figure 2). Advancement of the tibia over the prosthetic heel occurs at a rate approximately half of normal. The resulting arc of knee flexion is far less than normal (range, 6° to 10° versus 18°).[11,14,15] In addition, peak flexion is delayed until 19% or 20% gc, which is significantly later than normal (12% gc). All of the prosthetic foot designs present the same pattern of knee flexion.

Muscle Control Throughout weight acceptance, the quadriceps muscle group contracts vigorously to control the rate of knee flexion for weight-bearing stability. Whereas the arc of knee flexion is approximately half that of the normal range,[11,16] the intensity of the quadriceps EMG is equal to or greater than normal, and the duration of quadriceps activity is markedly prolonged. Peak quadriceps EMG intensity during prosthetic gait is 40% of maximum manual muscle test (MMT) versus the normal 29%[15] (Figure 3). In addition, both of the major hamstrings (biceps femoris[14] and semimembranosus[15]) register significantly higher than normal EMG during weight acceptance and have prolonged activity through most of stance (Figure 4). This pattern of action implies a deliberate effort to restrict the knee flexion of the residual tibia to an arc significantly shorter than normal. Also, the increased knee flexion that accompanies the hamstring muscle response to provide greater support to the flexed posture of the hip necessitates additional quadriceps control.

The reason for reduced flexion in individuals with a transtibial amputation is not clear, but it can be related to the anatomy of the extensor system of the knee. The normal knee flexes 20° in response to rapid weight transfer at the onset of stance. An analysis of the quadriceps demand with a mechanical model showed that knee flexion of both 5° and 15° required 20% of maximum strength.[17] The equalizing factor during the first 10° to 15° of knee flexion was the increase in quadriceps leverage as the femur rocked posteriorly on the tibia and the simultaneous change in articular contact areas[18,19] (Figure 5, *A*). The length of the patellar tendon lever arm is maximal at 15° of flexion because of the enlarged sagittal contour of the distal femur.[17] Be-

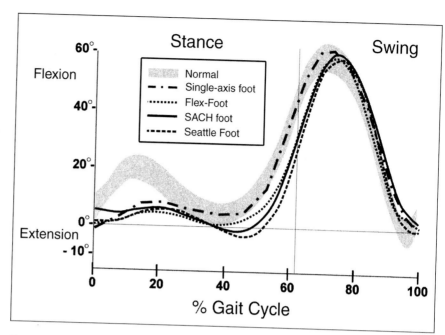

Figure 2 Knee motion of four different prosthetic feet during free-speed gait in persons with a unilateral transtibial amputation, compared with normal.[7,11]

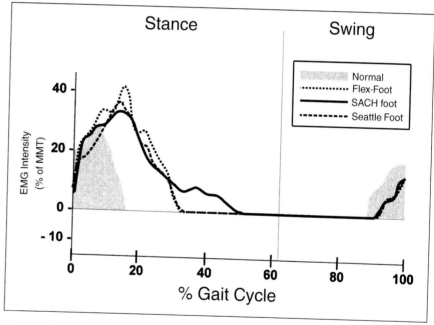

Figure 3 EMG activity of the vastus lateralis, representing quadriceps muscle action, during free-speed gait in persons with transtibial amputations using three different prosthetic feet.[15]

yond this position, further flexion is gained by the combined roll and slide of the femur on the posterior surface of the tibia (Figure 5, *B*). Although this decreases the leverage of the patella, the quadriceps force is significantly increased by greater sarcomere length. The mechanical model also showed

that weight bearing on a knee flexed 30° required a significantly greater quadriceps torque (up to 50%). In the transtibial amputee, a greater quadriceps force would increase distal tibial pressure against the socket, and this may be what the transtibial amputee is avoiding.

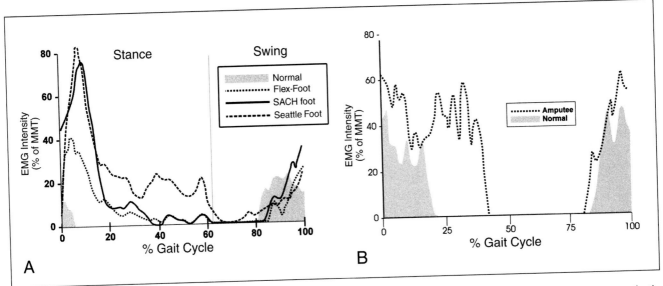

Figure 4 Hamstrings muscle action during free-speed gait in persons with transtibial amputations using three different prosthetic feet.[15] **A,** Biceps femoris, long head. **B,** Semimembranosus.

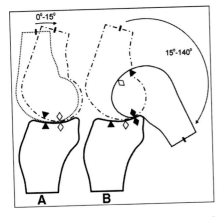

Figure 5 Joint surface contact pattern of the femur and tibia during knee flexion.[18] **A,** Flexion from 0° to 15°: equal posterior displacement on both joint surfaces (rocker effect). **B,** Flexion from 15° to 140°: The femoral surface continually changes, but tibial contact remains relatively constant (roll and glide).

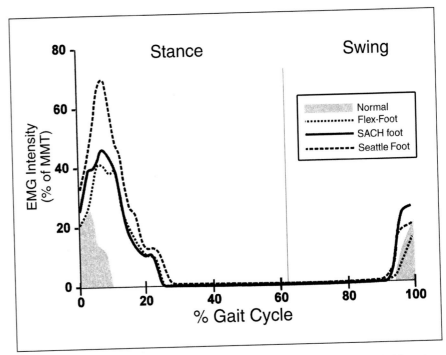

Figure 6 EMG activity of the lower portion of the gluteus maximus muscle (a hip extensor) while walking at a self-selected speed. The intensity is greater than normal with all three types of prosthetic feet. Prolonged activity ceases shortly after the end of heel-only support (average, 22% gc). *(Adapted with permission from Kapandji IA (ed): Physiology of the Joints. London, England, E&S Livingstone, 1970, p 89.)*

Studies of the gait mechanics of a person with a Syme ankle disarticulation tend to confirm that tibial stability within the prosthesis is important (J Perry, MD, unpublished data, 1989). Both transtibial amputees and those who have undergone the Syme procedure use similar types of prostheses, but the Syme procedure preserves sufficient tibial length for weight bearing on the end of the residual limb. Also, the increased contact provided by the length of the tibia and the broad distal surface of the Syme procedure would be expected to notably enhance stability of the prosthesis. Gait analysis of an individual with a Syme ankle disarticulation showed a peak knee flexion of 14° during limb loading, a position very close to normal.

One difficulty in comparing quadriceps strength in a limb with a transtibial amputation with that of an in-

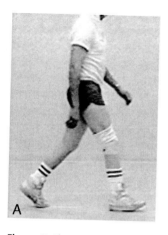
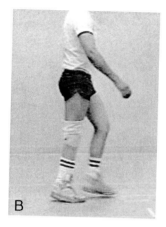
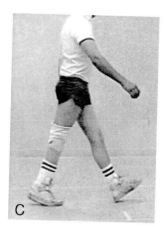
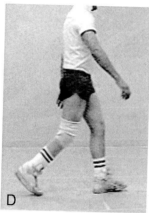

Figure 7 Floor contact pattern in a person with a transtibial amputation using a SACH foot. **A,** End of weight acceptance: Forefoot contact still lacking. **B,** Early single-limb support: The premature heel rise is obvious. **C,** Terminal stance: Step length is gained by increased heel rise, which, combined with an extended knee, elevates the body mass. **D,** Preswing: Rapid drop of body weight onto the forward limb initiates a visibly vigorous quadriceps response.

tact limb is the effect of the resistance applied against the proximal tibia. Theoretically, muscle moment is the same at both ends of the distal bone, but the internal mobility of the knee presents a unique situation. Resistance against the upper tibia opposes the anterior drawer that normally accompanies quadriceps activity when the knee is flexed less than 30°. This reduces the patellar lever, with resulting weakness of knee extension.[20] In the patient with borderline quadriceps strength, a snug fit of the prosthesis against the tibia could be an aggravating factor.

Hip

The motion pattern of the hip in the gait of individuals with a transtibial amputation is similar to normal except for an average 10° increase in flexion.[11,14,21] Dynamic EMG shows a significant increase above normal in the intensity and duration of the hip extensor function of the gluteus maximus (Figure 6). The accompanying vigorous action of the biceps femoris and semimembranosus, which, incidentally, increases quadriceps demand, confirms that the primary role of these muscles is hip control.[11,15]

Analysis of hip kinetics during walking demonstrates an increase in the internal extension moment in loading,[14] which correlates with the greater EMG reported. The corresponding posture would be a slight forward lean to lessen the extensor moment at the knee and, thereby, also reduce the need for quadriceps power to stabilize the knee.

Single-Limb Support
Ankle

Having attained weight-bearing stability, the limb and body mass advance over the single supporting foot. All prosthetic feet accomplish some tibial progression, although the mechanics differ. The SACH foot, limited by a solid keel, allows little foot-flat stability. Instead, the prolonged heel-only contact during the loading response is almost immediately exchanged for premature heel rise as the shank advances beyond vertical[5] (Figure 7). The final heel rise is twice the normal elevation. In contrast, the flexible shank of the Flex-Foot allows a prolonged period of foot-flat stability as the shank advances (Figure 8). The Flex-Foot also provides significantly greater ankle dorsiflexion (20°) in terminal stance than the other prosthetic foot designs (13°).[5,11,16] The cited arcs imply more mobility than that of the normal ankle (10° dorsiflexion), yet the prosthetic stride length is shorter than normal. This inconsistency stresses the difficulty of defining the ankle axis of a prosthesis. When total tibial advancement is assessed, however, progression is only 67% of nor-

mal with the Flex-Foot and 33% with the SACH foot.[22]

The arcs of dorsiflexion identified during walking are compatible with instrumented stiffness tests. Nine individual designs fall into two very different categories.[23] The stiffer ones, with a deformation value of 0.076 to 0.061 N/m, are designs using intrinsic foot flexibility (SACH and Seattle Lite feet), whereas the flexible shaft design of the less stiff prosthetic feet (Flex-Foot; and College Park Foot, College Park Industries, Fraser, MI) presented half as much resistance to deformation (0.038 to 0.028 N/m).

Knee

Motion From its limited flexion at the end of the loading response, the knee slowly extends. Maximum extension to neutral is attained near the end of terminal stance (45% gc), then the knee begins to flex. Consistent with its greater arc of ankle dorsiflexion, the Flex-Foot tends to initiate knee flexion slightly sooner.

Muscle Control Continuing quadriceps activity at a diminishing intensity provides active knee extension. Generally, this muscle relaxes as midstance ends (30% gc), but it may continue until 40% gc. Prolonged quadriceps activity is particularly likely with a SACH foot.

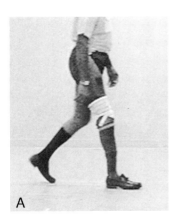
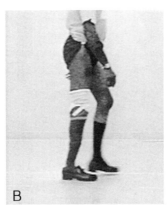
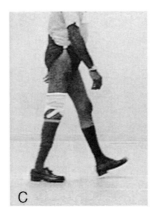
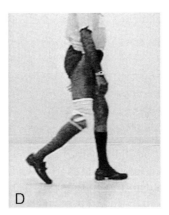

Figure 8 Floor contact pattern in a person with a transtibial amputation using a Flex-Foot. **A,** End of weight acceptance: The onset of forefoot contact initiates stable flat-foot support. **B,** Early single-limb support: Prosthetic "ankle" dorsiflexion continues foot-flat support while the tibia advances. **C,** Terminal stance: The combination of continuing foot-flat support and excessive prosthetic "ankle" dorsiflexion allows a longer step without elevation of the body. **D,** Preswing: Unloading body weight from the trailing limb allows the prosthetic ankle to rebound to neutral.

Hip

Motion As the body rolls forward over the supporting foot, the limb falls into a trailing position as the hip joint extends. The hip of the prosthetic limb uses less hyperextension (10°) than does the opposite limb (20°),[21] which is consistent with the reduced arc of tibial progression at the foot.

Muscle Control The duration of hip extensor muscle action differs with prosthetic foot mobility. Only the gluteus maximus consistently ceases activity shortly after the heel-only support ends (about 21% gc) (Figure 6). The biceps femoris EMG has a similar early drop in intensity, but lower levels of muscle action persist until the end of stance (Figure 4, A). The consistency of the gluteus maximus EMG compared with the variability of the biceps femoris reaction implies that the knee is more directly influenced by prosthetic foot mechanics than is the hip. The differences in the response of the biceps femoris reflect the mode of tibial progression provided by the various prosthetic designs. The premature heel rise of the SACH foot over a rigid but favorably contoured keel initiates an early forefoot rocker, which facilitates advancement of the tibia, and shank flexibility provides a similar advantage to the Flex-Foot. Con-

versely, prostheses dependent on intrafoot flexibility for tibial progression have a material-imposed delay. These interpretations have yet to be statistically supported by the published data because of the small number of subjects tested in the comparison studies. Statistical power analysis indicates that 25 subjects would be needed to document a difference in stride length,[11] yet the detailed comparisons of the gait of different prosthetic designs have included only 5 or 10 subjects.[5,11,14-16,21,22,24-26]

Preswing Limb Advancement

Ankle

The onset of double-limb support signifies the beginning of body weight transfer from the prosthetic foot to the intact limb. Each limb is significantly affected.

Rapid unloading of the trailing limb releases the energy stored in the dorsiflexed prosthetic foot. The reaction, a fast arc of "ankle" plantar flexion for "push-off," is merely a reversal of the prior dorsiflexion motion. None of the prosthetic feet moves beyond the zero position[11] (Figure 1).

The Flex-Foot, by attaining the greatest dorsiflexion in terminal stance (23° versus 12°), has the fastest rate of plantar flexion (71% of normal),[8] but the motion ends at 5° of

dorsiflexion. The push-off rate for the single-axis and Seattle Lite feet averages 61% of normal, and these feet have a smaller arc of motion.

Opposite Limb Demand

The second effect of weight transfer is the load imposed on the opposite limb.[11,24,27,28] Most prosthetic foot designs significantly increase the loading force transferred to the opposite limb, averaging 130% of body weight compared with the normal 111%. In contrast, the opposite limb's vertical force in persons using a Flex-Foot (110% of body weight) does not exceed a normal response.[16,29,30] The functional difference between these prosthetic feet resides in the ability to move forward over the prosthetic limb, which is identified by the arc of terminal stance dorsiflexion. The increased rate of weight transfer is also evidenced by the rapid onset and magnitude of the vastus lateralis EMG. Although the magnitude of heel rise has not been measured, the very premature heel rise of the SACH foot is a well-recognized consequence of its restricted tibial advancement. The substitution of heel rise for limited dorsiflexion would elevate the body as the foot rolls forward on the forefoot rocker, thereby creating a greater drop onto the opposite limb. These limb-loading mechanics have been related to an increased incidence

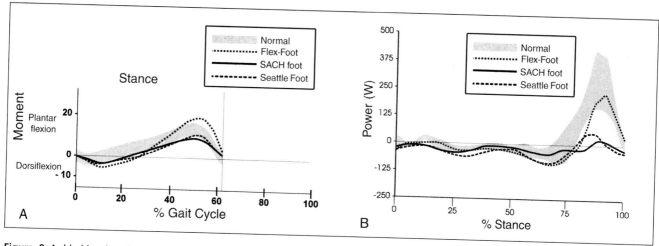

Figure 9 Ankle kinetics of three different prosthetic feet generated during the stance phase of free-speed gait in persons with a unilateral transtibial amputation, compared with normal. **A,** Ankle moment. **B,** Ankle power. *(Adapted with permission from Gitter A, Czerniecki JM, DeGroot DM: Biomechanical analysis of the influence of prosthetic feet on below-knee amputee walking. Am J Phys Med Rehabil 1991;70:142-148.)*

of knee osteoarthritis in elderly persons with a long experience of walking with a transtibial amputation.[31] Another demand on the opposite leg is a longer stance time of 66% gc versus 63% gc for the prosthetic limb.

Kinetics

Moments define the balance of the limb's antagonistic forces (muscle action) in the designated plane derived from the postures and motions used during walking. Power identifies the influence of speed on the moments, with the outcome defined as acceleration (generative) or deceleration (absorptive).[32]

The dominant intervals of the prosthetic gait are weight acceptance, terminal stance, and preswing. Each joint has a dominant force pattern in one of these intervals.

Weight Acceptance

At the ankle, the response to the impact of initial heel contact is a small internal dorsiflexion moment that reaches its peak magnitude of 4 N·m by 10% gc and then persists for another 8% to 14% of gc before forefoot contact occurs.[13,14] The duration of the dorsiflexion moment does not vary significantly among the prosthetic foot designs (Figure 9, A). No notable power is generated at the ankle during weight acceptance.

Loading the knee generates a markedly reduced extensor moment. The normal peak moment is 0.70 N·m; for the transtibial amputee, the peak moment is less than 10% of this value[15] (Figure 10). This reduction in moment is consistent with the limited arc of flexion that occurs during loading response and has been interpreted as an energy-saving situation.

The less flexible prosthetic feet (the SACH and Seattle feet) experience a slight reversal of the knee moment toward flexion, and the usual power peaks are absent. Although the Flex-Foot has a slight extensor moment, it also lacks any significant peaks of power at the knee.[14]

The realignment of the knee moments of the SACH and Seattle prosthetic feet (and, to a lesser extent, the Flex-Foot moments) toward flexion implies increased hamstring flexor muscle action (Figure 10, A). The corresponding sharp increase in hip extensor power (Figure 11, A) suggests a forward trunk lean as a means of reducing the knee moment. The logical stimuli for this postural adaptation are the challenge to balance over the limited area of support provided by the heel and a need to reduce the knee extensor demand. Power generation is minor during weight acceptance (Figure 10, B).

The hip shows a reverse pattern as both the magnitude of the moment and the power increase (Figure 11, A). The timing of their peaks differs, however. The peak extensor moment is delayed, occurring at 10% gc versus the normal 3% gc. Hip power increases immediately following heel strike (Figure 11, B). Peak power averages 16 W for prosthetic feet compared with the normal 6 W. Hence, the kinetic data indicate a significant increase in extensor muscle activity at the hip and a decrease in extensor muscle activity at the knee.

Terminal Stance

Throughout the period of single-limb support, a progressively greater plantar flexor moment develops as the body weight vector advances over and beyond the foot. The responses of prosthetic feet differ significantly (Figure 9, A). By the end of terminal stance, the peak plantar flexor moment of the Flex-Foot is twice as great as that of the SACH and Seattle feet, which is closely related to the amount of dorsiflexion permitted by each foot design.[11]

During this action, power is absorbed at an increasing rate (Figure 9, B). Power storage with the SACH foot is minimal, but it is notably increased in both the Flex-Foot and the Seattle

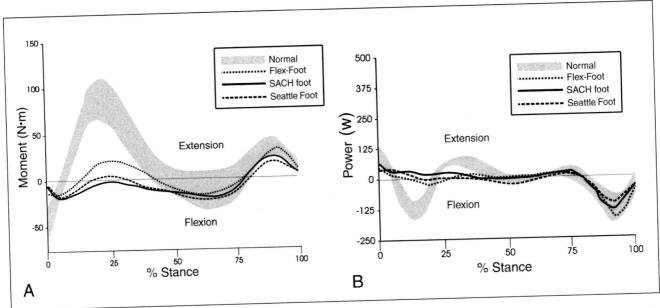

Figure 10 Knee kinetics of three different prosthetic feet generated during the stance phase of free-speed gait in persons with a unilateral transtibial amputation, compared with normal. **A,** Knee moment. **B,** Knee power. *(Adapted with permission from Gitter A, Czerniecki JM, DeGroot DM: Biomechanical analysis of the influence of prosthetic feet on below-knee amputee walking. Am J Phys Med Rehabil 1991;70:142-148.)*

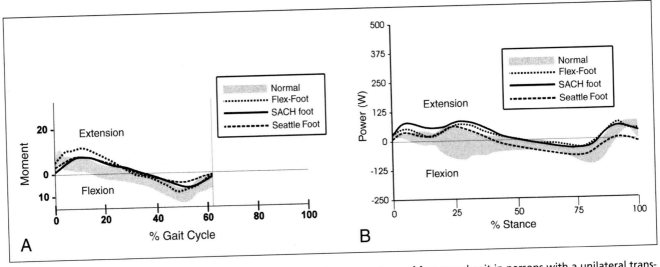

Figure 11 Hip kinetics of three prosthetic feet generated during the stance phase of free-speed gait in persons with a unilateral transtibial amputation, compared with normal. **A,** Hip moment.[11] **B,** Hip power. *(Adapted with permission from Gitter A, Czerniecki JM, DeGroot DM: Biomechanical analysis of the influence of prosthetic feet on below-knee amputee walking. Am J Phys Med Rehabil 1991; 70:142-148.)*

Foot. These differences are reflected in their preswing response.

Preswing

The relatively fast rate of unloading the limb by weight transfer transforms the plantar flexor force into a spike of generative power, commonly identified as the push-off force of the foot (Figure 9, *B*). With little energy absorption capability, the SACH foot generates minimal power. Conversely, the more flexible Flex-Foot creates a power spike five times as great, and the concentric power of the Seattle Foot lies midway between the two, although all are significantly less than normal.

The knee has a moderate extensor moment during preswing, with notable absorptive power (Figure 10). This is an interval of rapid, vital, passive flexion in response to the push-off action of the ankle, which seldom needs restraint. The calculated power reflects the interaction of high-speed motion and low force.

The hip has a relatively normal power pattern during the later phase of stance. In preswing there is a small burst of generative power consistent with the hip flexor action assisting in preparation for swing (Figure 11, *B*).

Energy

The reductions in the knee extensor moment and power peaks are interpreted as energy-saving mechanics provided by the newer, dynamic-response prosthetic feet. Yet, the kinetics of the various prosthetic designs differ little from that of the SACH foot. Direct determinations of the energy costs of prosthetic gait by measurement of oxygen use show a significant increase over normal with all prosthetic foot designs.[33] Individuals with transtibial amputations accommodate this increase in two ways. Those who are limited physiologically by dysvascular disease keep the rate of oxygen use within 10% of normal by limiting walking speed (60 m/min, compared with 86 m/min).[2] In contrast, physically fit amputees (typically, those with a traumatic amputation) accept a higher energy rate (47% greater than normal) in order to walk at a nearly normal speed (83 m/min). For both groups, the energy expenditure per meter traveled is costly (45% greater than normal).[33] None of the prosthetic foot designs shows any significant difference in the energy requirement of walking.

These higher energy values relate closely to the EMG evidence of greater hip and knee muscle activity during weight acceptance and the continuation of this activity through much of stance. The stimulus appears to be the prolonged tibial instability imposed by heel-only support. This support pattern, in turn, is related to two significant situations, the short arc of loading-response knee flexion and the fixed orthogonal relationship between forefoot and shank. To attain a stable foot-flat posture, the prosthetic shank must be vertical, as the apparent "plantar flexion" is merely a marker of displacement from heel compression, not a drop of the forefoot on the shank. With the knee held in relative extension, the whole body must advance with the tibia until it

becomes vertical. This imposes an increased demand on the quadriceps.

The higher intensity of the hip extensor EMG, unlike the merely prolonged quadriceps EMG, implies voluntary protection of the transected tibia. Increased hip extensor muscle action is a well-recognized protective gait for a weak quadriceps. A slight forward trunk lean reduces the external flexor moment at the knee, thereby decreasing the pull of the quadriceps. In the amputee with a transected tibia, anterior displacement of the distal tibia would be similarly reduced.

To date, efforts to reduce the energy cost of prosthetic gait have focused on improving push-off. Yet, the major muscle group normally responsible for this action, the gastrocnemius-soleus complex, is lost with the transtibial amputation, which leaves the hip flexors as the source of swing-phase limb advancement. Although the hip flexor muscles are activated with each step, overuse symptoms are rarely noted, as the flexion arc is only 30°. The peak intensity of normal function is 20%, a state that allows full muscle oxygenation.[34] The gait mechanics identified in this chapter strongly indicate that efforts to reduce the energy cost of walking for amputees should be redirected to the functions involved in weight acceptance.

Conclusions

For persons with transtibial amputations, the biomechanical demands of weight acceptance necessitate heightened muscular control by both the prosthetic and sound limbs and are thus likely responsible for much of the elevated energy cost of transtibial amputee gait.

Muscular exertion on the prosthetic side during weight acceptance results from insufficient knee flexion and persistent ankle dorsiflexion, which perpetuate the postural instability created by the heel rocker moment. The various cushion heel designs allow the forefoot to sink toward the floor but do not alter its alignment relative to the tibia,

whereas the instability introduced by the unrestricted mobility of the single-axis foot (twice the rate of a normal ankle) further augments the need for muscular effort. A design that represents a functional compromise between these two extremes is needed.

Muscular exertion of the sound limb during weight acceptance results from the excessive ground-reaction force created by prosthetic foot designs, which maximize tibial advancement by heel rise as a substitute for inadequate ankle dorsiflexion.

Transfemoral Amputee Gait

Amputations through the femur not only deprive patients of the limb segments that contain and control the knee and foot, but also weaken the musculature controlling the hip. Surgical division of the tendons and muscles allows the residual muscle fibers to retract because the viscoelastic sarcomeres have lost their tether,[35] and undue shortening of the sarcomeres entails the loss of muscle force.[36]

An additional threat to optimal function is the hip's natural resting posture. Experimental distension of the hip by sterile plasma injection has identified that intra-articular pressure (indicative of capsular tension) is lowest when the hip is in 30° of flexion, 15° of external rotation, and abduction. Hence, this is the posture the injured hip spontaneously assumes. Consequently, early rehabilitation must include both vigorous contracture prevention and extensor muscle strengthening.

Motion
Ankle/Foot

All prosthetic foot designs initiate stance with the heel. Active inhibition of knee flexion by the transfemoral amputee has two effects: (1) heel-only support is continued until the limb is erect, and (2) the locked knee extends the influence of the heel rocker to the

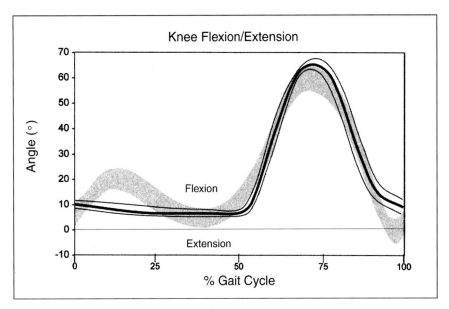

Figure 12 The motion pattern of the prosthetic knee during stance phase in persons with a unilateral transfemoral amputation. The data are mean (bold line) and standard deviation (thin lines) for 25 subjects. Normative data (shaded region) are provided for comparison. The width changes shape as it represents the standard deviation for the respective groups. *(Adapted with permission from Boonstra AM, Schrama JM, Eisma WH, Hof AL, Fidler V: Gait analysis of transfemoral amputee patients using prostheses with two different knee joints.* Arch Phys Med Rehabil *1996;77:515-520.)*

femur, thereby accelerating the progression of the whole limb over the supporting heel.

The magnitude of knee flexion on the prosthetic limb is indicative of the quality of swing-phase knee control.[37] For example, during slow gait, a hydraulic dampening system is prone to retard flexion excessively, as is indicated by a reduction in the maximum knee flexion. Conversely, during fast walking, a constant-friction mechanical knee allows excessive knee flexion because of inadequate restraint.

Premature midstance plantar flexion by the sound limb assists toe clearance of the prosthetic limb by lifting the body. Vaulting is the clinical term for this event. Excessive plantar flexion during preswing denotes an extra push-off effort to facilitate progression of the prosthetic limb during weight acceptance.

Knee

Most prosthetic knees obligate persons with transfemoral amputation to avoid flexion during stance so that the knee does not collapse (Figure 12). As

the end of terminal swing approaches, the knee is fully extended (0°). Loading of the limb may initiate 5° of flexion, but generally the joint is maintained at 0° throughout stance. Then, just before toe-off, knee flexion begins in order to meet the floor clearance requirements of swing. Knee flexion is rapid, with approximately 65° of flexion attained by midswing. Once peak flexion is reached, the knee rapidly extends in preparation for the next period of stance.

Recently, prosthetic knees that permit 5° to 12° of stable knee flexion during loading response have become available. Gait studies have shown that although such "stance flexion" occurs, the magnitude of knee flexion is less than normal and occurs later in the gait cycle. Peak knee flexion in midswing occurs too late to assist in toe clearance. In fact, the normal limb has a critical arc of knee flexion of 40° in preswing to supplement the final 20° attained in initial swing as hip flexion advances the limb.

A pneumatic swing-control knee joint reduces the rate and magnitude

of knee flexion. The 5° reduction (compared with the knee flexion allowed by a four-bar mechanical knee joint) shortens the duration of swing. Despite this aid, the swing phase of a prosthetic knee is still slower than that of the sound limb.[38]

Microprocessor-controlled hydraulic knees, such as the Intelligent Knee (Chas. A. Blatchford & Sons, Ltd, Basingstoke, Hampshire, England) and the C-Leg (Otto Bock HealthCare, Inc, Minneapolis, MN) have recently become available. They use on-board computers to monitor limb motion and to readjust resistance to flexion and extension up to 50 times per second.[39] Preliminary gait analysis has demonstrated a significant reduction in energy cost.

Published reports, which have been limited primarily to subjective disciplines, suggest improved walking ease. In one study, 12 amputees using the Intelligent Knee noted the ability to vary their speed and a reduction in energy demand, which enabled them to walk farther.[40] One user reported that the C-Leg eliminated the need to pull the hip extensors back to stabilize the knee.[41] Measured energy cost for one user demonstrated a 10% reduction in demand when walking with the C-leg compared with a customary prosthesis.[42]

The control mechanisms that enable the C-Leg to reduce the energy cost of walking have not been reported, but by comparing the hip and knee motion patterns of one amputee fitted with a C-Leg to the typical gait of persons walking with a customary transfemoral prosthesis and the mean normal gait pattern, the general approach can be deduced. The most impressive contribution of the C-Leg microprocessor knee joint was replication of the normal pattern of swing-phase knee flexion. Although the onset of knee flexion was slightly delayed, the abrupt initiation of a fast arc in mid preswing (55% gc) provided the range needed for ground clearance. At normal toe-off (62% gc), the knee was flexed 35°. Toe lift, aided by the slightly dorsiflexed pros-

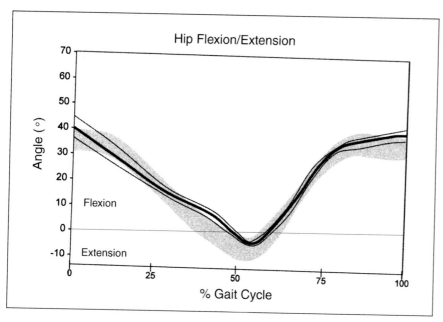

Figure 13 The motion pattern of the hip in persons with transfemoral amputations. (Data [unpublished] courtesy of Ayyapa.)

thetic foot (5°), would be adequate. Continuation of this fast rate of knee motion also attained 58° of flexion by 73% gc. Both magnitude and timing met the tight requirements for ground clearance by a swinging limb. During midswing, the knee's motion reversed into extension, and continuing movement at a rapid rate (similar to that of the flexion arc) provided timely extension for stance. By mid terminal swing, the knee had extended to 5° of flexion.

The motion pattern during stance implied either less concern by the amputee for replicating the normal pattern of knee motion or a more demanding situation. The gross motion pattern appeared to be similar to normal, but the initial flexion wave provided by the C-Leg was smaller and its peak delayed (10° of flexion at 20% gc) compared with normal (20° of flexion at 12% gc). The transfemoral prosthesis customarily has no loading response flexion; hence, the C-Leg represented a compromise: a partial, rather than full, shock-absorbing wave. This implied a limited ability to reproduce the normal rate and magnitude of the knee's response to limb loading.

The motion pattern of initiating thigh retraction immediately after initial contact, rather than preserving the normal loading response flexion, supported this interpretation. As the hip actively extended from 35° of flexion at initial contact, the femur would simultaneously become more vertical. This, in turn, would move the body weight vector closer to the knee, and the combined effects would reduce the added effort required to stabilize the knee. The duration of loading response, however, also could be prolonged (20% gc versus 12% gc), as decreased knee flexion required the whole limb to roll forward until the vertical shank permitted foot-flat support. On the other hand, the C-Leg can provide the knee flexion needed for reciprocal limb support during stair descent. The difference may be the result of the control required to allow an arc of flexion while also stabilizing the knee against a rapid increase in body load compared with allowing a previously stabilized limb to yield into an arc of flexion.

There were indications that the end of stance required hip control adaptation. The prolonged dorsiflexion of the prosthetic foot for step length would inadvertently flex the pros-

thetic knee. Prolongation of hip extension into the middle of preswing provided the necessary compensation to stabilize the limb until body weight was transferred to the other limb. This allowed the knee to be readied to respond to the subsequent rapid initiation of flexion required for swing.

Thus, the basic phasing of stance stability and swing progression was determined by active hip control. The C-Leg, by superimposing timely magnitudes of force within the knee, reduces the energy demand of walking and provides a more normal gait pattern for persons walking with a transfemoral prosthesis.

Hip

The pattern of hip motion recorded for persons with transfemoral amputations represents displacement of the prosthesis as the femur is obscured by the socket. A significant difference from normal gait is the abruptness of the postural change (Figure 13). At initial contact, the hip is flexed approximately 37°.[43] As the limb is loaded, the hip immediately begins to extend, reaching 5° of hyperextension by the end of single stance (50% gc). Then, during the next 25% of the gait cycle, the hip flexes to 35° at a rate of motion twice that used for hip extension. This is followed by a slow advancement to the final flexed position.

Significant motion of the residual limb within the prosthetic socket has been identified by ultrasound.[44] In the sagittal plane, initial contact is followed by a rapid 7° arc of extension. This position is maintained until the end of terminal stance (Figure 14, A). Then, in preswing, the residual limb rapidly reverses to a peak of 7° of flexion by toe-off. This flexed position is maintained until neutral alignment is regained in terminal swing. In the coronal (frontal) plane, a similar pattern of rapid abduction and subsequent release occurs, but swing involves only a minor interval of adduction (Figure 14, B). For most individuals with transfemoral amputations, the range of hip motion by the

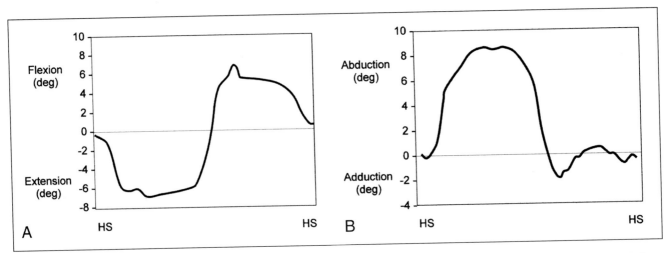

Figure 14 Motion of the residual femur within the socket recorded by ultrasound during level walking by a person with a transfemoral amputation. **A**, Flexion/extension. **B**, Abduction/adduction. HS = heel strike. *(Adapted with permission from Convery P, Murray KD: Ultrasound study of the motion of the residual femur within a trans-femoral socket during gait. Prosthet Orthot Int 2000;24:226-232.)*

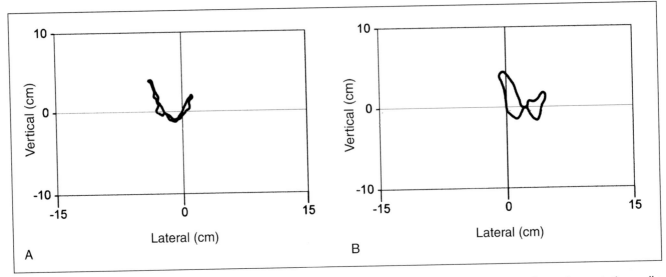

Figure 15 Transverse planar motion of the pelvis generated during one gait cycle as a person with a transfemoral amputation walks on a level surface. **A**, Good walker. **B**, Poor walker. *(Adapted with permission from Tazawa E: Analysis of torso movement of transfemoral amputees during level walking. Prosthet Orthot Int 1997;21:129-140.)*

prosthetic limb is about 80% of that used by the opposite limb. Femoral displacement is augmented with measurable arcs of pelvic and trunk motion.

Pelvis

A combination of sagittal and coronal plane tilting presents as figure-of-8 patterns of motion. The magnitude of the three-dimensional motion varies with the quality of the walker (Figure 15). Anterior rotation and tilt accompany the swinging limb. As the trunk remains erect, compensatory lumbar extension (lordosis) occurs. Pelvic mobility is greater in these amputees than the 4° average of persons with intact limbs.[45]

Trunk

Throughout each stride the trunk also experiences three-dimensional motion (measured at shoulder level). Planar analysis shows the trunk follows a figure-of-8 pattern of lateral and vertical motion.[46] Good walkers use a tight, symmetric motion pattern, which remains within a 7-cm area (Figure 16, *A*). Less able walkers display asymmetric displacement patterns, which may cover twice the area (Figure 16, *B*). The upper trunk also follows a sequence of reciprocal forward rotation in the horizontal plane. The shoulder generally is higher on the side without the prosthetic limb, although good walkers keep their shoulders level. Arm swing was found to be a balancing factor. Poorer walkers use greater arcs of pelvic motion.

Muscle Control

Jaegers and associates[47] used surface EMG to identify the action of the su-

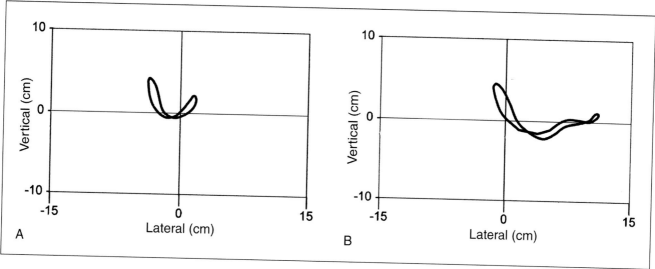

Figure 16 One cycle of trunk motion recorded at shoulder level as a person with a transfemoral amputation walks on a level surface. **A,** Good walker. **B,** Poor walker. *(Adapted with permission from Tazawa E: Analysis of torso movement of trans-femoral amputees during level walking. Prosthet Orthot Int 1997;21:129-140.)*

perficial muscles controlling the hip. The authors defined phasing as the interval of peak intensity excluding the lowest 12%, which was assumed to include cross talk from adjacent musculature. This approach probably was adequate for isolating the signals of the three large rectangular muscles (erector spinae, gluteus maximus, and gluteus medius). All of the other muscles, however, are narrow rectangles in intimate contact with their neighbors, and only the peak EMG could be accepted because of the ease of signal travel among contiguous muscle tissue. This limitation applied to the hamstrings (biceps femoris and semitendinosus), the adductors (magnus and longus), and the hip flexors (sartorius and rectus femoris). Also, the depth of the primary hip flexor, the iliacus, made it unavailable. Despite these limitations, significant information was gained.

The peak signal intensity from similar anatomic areas showed a notable increase in EMG intensity for all the muscles of the subjects with transfemoral amputations, compared with the signals of able-bodied control subjects (Figure 17). Peak action of the residual limb muscles ranged between 50% and 75% of maximum, whereas in the normal control subject the action did not exceed 25% of

maximum. The signals with a likely cross talk origin were excluded. The prolonged action of the gluteus maximus (Figure 17, *A*) and gluteus medius (Figure 17, *C*) indicated the need for vigorous support of the hip throughout single stance as well as limb loading. The change in the dominant intensity of the transfemoral hamstrings to loading response (Figure 17, *B*), rather than in the terminal swing to decelerate the swinging limb, was further evidence of the need for strong extensor muscle action at the time the limb is accepting body weight.

Several functional qualities are displayed by the EMG pattern of the hip flexor muscles (Figure 17, *D*). Peak activity of the adductor longus musculature in preswing is consistent with the normal function of limiting abduction as body weight is transferred to the other limb. The intense sartorius EMG activity implies that the sartorius is the primary synergist of the iliacus (which could not be sampled with surface electrodes). The phasing of the sartorius preswing through initial swing and a single high peak is consistent with the long fibers' unique capability to rapidly move the limb through a large arc of hip flexion, whereas the limited strength of rapidly shortening muscle

fibers is indicated by the magnitude of the muscles' EMG activity. The prolongation of the rectus femoris through swing indicates the better endurance of shorter fibers.

The EMG patterns for the transfemoral hip extensor, abductor, and flexor muscles are consistent with the pattern of sustained residual limb displacement within the socket recorded with ultrasound.[44]

The relative effectiveness of the hip muscles following amputation varied significantly with the level of limb removal, the extent of intramuscular fatty degeneration,[48] and whether or not muscle length was preserved by tenodesis at the time of the amputation. For example, loss of the distal third of the adductor magnus results in a 70% reduction of the muscle's moment arm.[35] The other adductor muscles and the accessory hip flexors have a similar fate. Disruption of the iliotibial band impairs the gluteus maximus.[48] Gottschalk and Stills[35] recommend tenodesis of the adductor magnus and tenodesis of the hamstring muscles, which has been found to preserve normal tissue quality. On three-dimensional MRI reconstructions of the hip and thigh muscles, significant atrophy has been identified in experienced walkers with a unilateral transfemoral amputation of traumatic

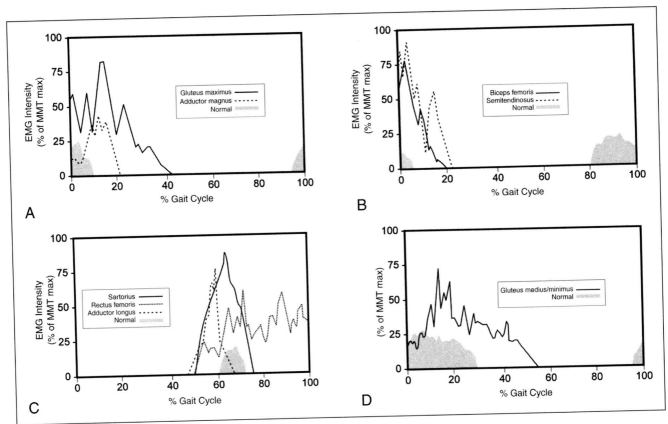

Figure 17 Muscular control of the hip during free-speed gait of individuals with a transfemoral amputation as measured by EMG. **A**, Hip extensor muscles. **B**, Hamstring muscles. **C**, Hip abductor muscles. **D**, Hip flexor muscles. *(Adapted with permission from Jaegers SM, Arendzen JH, de Jongh HJ: An electromyographic study of the hip muscles of transfemoral amputees in walking.* Clin Orthop *1996; 328:119-128.)*

origin. The average atrophy of the primary hip extensors (gluteus maximus and adductor magnus) was 38%, whereas 60% atrophy characterized the long muscles such as the hamstrings, sartorius, and rectus femoris. Even the noninvaded muscles (iliopsoas and gluteus medius) displayed a 22% loss. Hence, a transfemoral amputation significantly impairs muscle control of the residual thigh. This further explains why so few persons with amputations of dysvascular origin recover an effective gait.

Other Limb Demand

The gait of persons with transfemoral amputation depends on several compensatory functions by the sound limb to overcome the performance limitations of prostheses.[49-51] Each of these functions requires the sound limb to exert greater effort than limb normal gait. All phases of stance are involved.

The ground-reaction force of the stance limb during weight acceptance is higher than normal with most prosthetic feet.[51] In meeting this added demand, the sound limb uses increased ankle and knee motion,[49] generates greater knee and hip extensor moments, and creates higher power at the hip.[50] The cause of this increased demand is the limited dorsiflexion of the prosthetic foot.[52] For example, the Seattle Lite foot, which depends on intrinsic flexibility, has minimal dorsiflexion. This means that most of the tibial advancement is gained by premature heel rise. In contrast, the Springlite foot (Otto Bock HealthCare) gains significant dorsiflexion through its flexible shank. As a result of these different prosthetic foot mechanics, the ground-reaction force during weight acceptance (F1) generated by the Seattle Lite foot with its foot spring is significantly greater

than normal. In contrast, the loading force is not increased with the Springlite foot, which has a longer shank-foot spring.[52] This difference is attributable to the fact that the heel rise elevates the body center when dorsiflexion is limited, which does not occur with a flexible shank. Hence, the free drop of the higher body mass is the stimulus for the greater loading force on the opposite side.

Midstance is normally a period of progressive dorsiflexion. The sound limb interrupts this action with increased activation of its ankle plantar flexor muscles to compensate for the delay in prosthetic knee flexion needed for toe clearance in swing.[37,49] Recent data from studies of microprocessor-controlled hydraulic prosthetic knees have demonstrated a reduction in the tendency of the ankle plantar flexor to vault, along with a

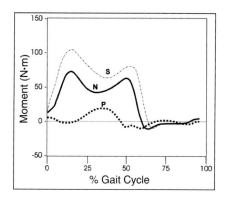

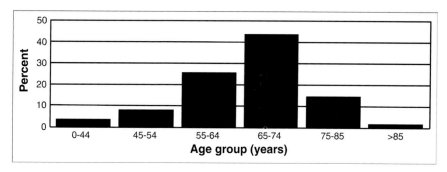

Figure 19 Distribution of amputations in veterans discharged in 1992 by age group.

Figure 18 Support moment of the limbs in persons with transfemoral amputations, compared with normal gait. The support moment is calculated as the moving sum of the limb's hip extensor, knee extensor, and ankle plantar flexor moments during the gait cycle. S = sound limb, N = normal gait, P = prosthetic limb. *(Adapted with permission from Seroussi RE, Gitter A, Czerniecki JM, Weaver K: Mechanical work adaptations of above-knee amputee ambulation. Arch Phys Med Rehabil 1996;77:1209-1214.)*

more normal range of knee flexion in preswing.

At the end of stance, the push-off power generated by the sound limb significantly exceeds that of normal gait. These increases in net ankle joint moment and power indicate a significant increase in work by the plantar flexor muscles of the sound limb.[49]

The total support moment of the limb is the sum of the ankle, knee, and hip moments. For the group of eight subjects studied, the average total support moment for the sound limb was 25% greater than that exerted in able-bodied gait[50] (Figure 18). This is an underestimation of the measured increase in physiologic cost (45% per meter walked) for persons with transfemoral amputations.[53] In contrast, the total support moment pattern is minimal for the prosthetic limb. These findings of greater moment patterns for the sound limb present a strong argument for strengthening the hip extensors of both limbs and the ankle plantar flexors of the sound limb.

Conclusion

Walking with a transfemoral prosthesis is an arduous task that requires

significant functional contributions by the intact limb and trunk during each stride. The residual limb function is hampered by loss of musculature, lack of direct connection between the human thigh and prosthetic knee, and persistent limitations in the prosthetic foot. The sound limb augments transfemoral prosthetic gait by providing increased moments and powers generated at the ankle, knee, and hip.

Progress in prosthetic foot design has been directed toward increasing flexibility while preserving stability. In conflict is the increased rigidity, which may result from efforts to ensure durability. A broad array of designs is available to persons with an amputation, but the advantages of each model continue to be offset by some disadvantages. None has significantly lessened energy cost, nor increased walking speed or symmetry. Dominance of one design over the others has yet to be demonstrated for persons dependent on a transfemoral prosthesis, though the trend favors flexibility.

Outcome

With the advances in limb salvage for the management of trauma and tumors, the limbs of most young adults are preserved today; however, amputation remains a common means of preserving the life and ambulatory ability of persons impaired by peripheral vascular disease and diabetes mellitus. The current etiology of more than 80% of amputations is dysvascular disease, with an equal di-

vision between peripheral vascular disease and diabetes in the United States.[54-57] Less than 10% result from trauma.

The age of most amputees now lies between 55 and 75 years, and the number reaching age 85 is increasing.[54-59] Among the 5,180 veterans discharged with an amputation in 1992, the highest incidence of amputations (44%) occurred in those age 65 to 74 years. The incidence was significantly lower for both the younger and older age groups (Figure 19). A similar relationship between age and amputation frequency was reported by the Nova Scotia Rehabilitation Centre.[57] Of their 132 patients, 68% were age 60 to 79 years; there were markedly fewer amputations in the younger and older patient groups.

Improved medical and surgical procedures also have permitted preservation of the knee in more patients. As a result, the most frequent amputation level today is transtibial (63%), and only 30% are transfemoral. The exception to this pattern is seen in local programs emphasizing partial foot amputations. In the survey of amputations among veterans, 44% were within the foot, with a corresponding reduction in transtibial procedures.[55]

The effects of a recent amputation superimposed on the complications of aging and coexisting pathologies have challenged the rehabilitation programs that were designed for young adults. The best approach to providing elderly patients with a prosthesis remains a challenge because prosthesis use has a high failure rate among frail, older amputees. The

TABLE 1 Stride Characteristics of Unilateral Lower Limb Amputation Gait in Males

Amputation	No. of patients	Age (y)	Velocity (m/min)	Stride Length (m)	Cadence (steps/min)
Traumatic					
Transtibial[16,25,56]	26	30	76	1.4	97
Transfemoral[10,37,38,54,60,61]	110	35	54	1.3	85
Dysvascular					
Syme procedure[56]	14	57	54	1.1	98
Transtibial[4,9,10,16,24,26,56]	99	57	61	1.2	88
Transfemoral[56]	13	60	36	1.0	72
Normal[4]	46	77	86	1.5	115

effectiveness of medical management and rehabilitation have been assessed from three primary aspects: survival, walking ability, and function.

Survival is significantly influenced by comorbidity.[55] Among the 5,180 veterans who underwent amputation in 1992, the calculated 6-year survival rate for those who had a forefoot amputation was 50%, whereas cardiovascular disease reduced this prediction to 30%, and renal disease to 20%. Diabetes did not show an adverse influence on survival rate.

Walking ability is defined by the person's stride characteristics. Gait velocity is the basic measure,[60-62] as persons spontaneously choose a walking speed that is the optimum balance between progression and energy cost.[63] A good correlation with disability has been identified.[60,61] Also, the amputee's stride characteristics define the walking ability associated with the different classes of amputation.[53,62] Of the two basic components of velocity, stride length and cadence, stride length delineates the effectiveness of the limb mechanics that contribute to progression. Cadence is less significant because it has a voluntary quality, which allows some modification of walking speed.

The stride characteristics of amputees are modified primarily by the extent of limb loss and the etiology of the amputation. Subdividing lower limb amputation according to the major etiologies of trauma and dysvascular disease differentiates patients

with normal physiologic health from those in whom it is compromised (energy and strength limitations). The multiple classes of limb loss remain clinically pertinent, but only unilateral transtibial amputations, transfemoral amputations, and the Syme ankle disarticulation are performed with adequate frequency to permit group comparisons. To provide a perspective on the significance of amputee disability, the stride characteristics of the male subjects with a lower limb amputation cited in the literature have been tabulated (Table 1). Too few of the reports included data on female amputees to permit assessment of this group. There is a significant difference in the peak age range between traumatic (30 to 35 years) and dysvascular (65 to 75 years) amputees. Few persons with transfemoral amputations of dysvascular origin regain an ability to walk, and those who do have the slowest velocity (36 m/min). This is barely half of the walking speed used for a normal stroll.[64] Trauma causes a similar, but less severe, functional difference between transtibial and transfemoral amputees (76 m/min versus 54 m/min). Only persons with transtibial amputations of traumatic origin have a walking speed within the ranges used by able-bodied persons. This attests to their physiologic health, which tolerates excessive energy expenditure.

Step counting with a microprocessor system that stores the number of

footswitch contacts over many days expands gait analysis to include the measurement of endurance.[57] Among 48 subjects with unilateral amputations equally divided between the transtibial and transfemoral levels, a significant difference in walking endurance developed after the first 100 days. From a common step pattern of 900 steps per day, the transtibial amputees progressively increased their walking to 2,000 steps per day by 300 days, while the transfemoral amputees made no further gains. The progress of a small group of bilateral transtibial amputees was similar to that of the transfemoral amputees. Transtibial amputees older than age 65 years also showed the same limitation as the transfemoral amputees.

Function

The simplest assessment of an amputee's ability to use a prosthesis is a mere "yes" or "no." Positive responses were as high as 94% in Australia,[54] but 16% of amputees in Finland and Nova Scotia said "no."[56,64] A more discriminating criterion is the length of time the prosthesis is worn per day. Use per day varied from 7 hours[54] to 12 hours,[53] and the overall proportion of the walking day was 60% to 66%. This incidence increased to 79% for individuals with a transtibial amputation, but was only 40% for those with transfemoral amputations. Wearing the prosthetic limb part of the day (4 hours) was less frequent (12% to 25%). Age was found to be significant for the transfemoral amputees when ambulatory independence was considered. Among individuals in their seventh decade of life, 44% walked without assistance, but the percentage dropped to 10% for those in their eighth decade of life. None of the five persons older than 80 years was independent.[56] For transtibial amputees, only reaching the age of 80 years made a difference in ambulatory independence.

Lifestyle evaluations almost always assess the discharge residence, which is home for 90% of individuals with lower limb amputation in countries that provide home adaptations.[54,65] An interesting assessment of independence at home was the measure of the number of steps needed per day.[65] Personal care required an average of 315 steps and food preparation an average of 727 steps, for a total of 1,042 steps per day. The average daily distance walked was 560 m. The social activities of persons with an amputation are limited by their inability to drive (25%) and inability to use public transportation (9%). Most of their activities are sedentary hobbies. Return to work is no longer an absolute criterion of rehabilitation success because many individuals with an amputation are of retirement age (65 years and older).

Many individuals with lower limb amputation, whose average age is 65 years, use a walking aid for both indoor and outdoor ambulation. The incidence of persons with a transtibial amputation who walk without any aids is estimated between 15%[59] and 22%,[65] compared with only 11% for those with transfemoral prostheses. Seventy-one percent of transtibial amputees and 52% of transfemoral amputees use one cane for independent walking. Dependence on two canes or a frame walker indicates a severe limitation in walking ability, with gait velocities of 35 m/min or less. New research is needed to address the unique needs of a growing population of elderly, physiologically limited persons with lower limb amputation.

References

1. Klute GK, Kallfelz CF, Czerniecki JM: Mechanical properties of prosthetic limbs: Adapting to the patient. *J Rehabil Res Dev* 2001;38:299-307.

2. Waters RL, Perry J, Antonelli D, Hislop H: Energy cost of walking of amputees: The influence of level of amputation. *J Bone Joint Surg Am* 1976;58: 42-46.

3. Munin MC, Espejo-De Guzman MC, Boninger ML, Fitzgerald SG, Penrod LE, Singh J: Predictive factors for successful early prosthetic ambulation among lower-limb amputees. *J Rehabil Res Dev* 2001;38:379-384.

4. Powers CM, Boyd LA, Fontaine CA, Perry J: The influence of lower-extremity muscle force on gait characteristics in individuals with below-knee amputations secondary to vascular disease. *Phys Ther* 1996;76: 369-385.

5. Goh JC, Solomonidis SE, Spence WD, Paul JP: Biomechanical evaluation of SACH and uniaxial feet. *Prosthet Orthot Int* 1984;8:147-154.

6. Murphy EF: Lower-extremity components, in *Orthopaedic Appliances Atlas: Artificial Limbs*. Chicago, IL, American Academy of Orthopaedic Surgeons, 1960, vol 2, pp 129-261.

7. Perry J, Boyd LA, Rao SS, Mulroy SJ: Prosthetic weight acceptance mechanics in transtibial amputees wearing the Single Axis, Seattle Lite, and Flex foot. *IEEE Trans Rehabil Eng* 1997;5: 283-289.

8. Rao SS, Boyd LA, Mulroy SJ, Bontrager EL, Gronley JK, Perry J: Segment velocities in normal and transtibial amputees: Prosthetic design implications. *IEEE Trans Rehabil Eng* 1998;6:219-225.

9. Sterling HM, Perry J, Gronley JK, Torburn L: Rehab R&D Progress Report. 1986; 19-20.

10. Skinner HB, Abrahamson MA, Hung RK, Wilson LA, Effeney DJ: Static load response of the heels of SACH feet. *Orthopedics* 1985;8:225-228.

11. Torburn L, Perry J, Ayyappa E, Shanfield SL: Below-knee amputee gait with dynamic elastic response prosthetic feet: A pilot study. *J Rehabil Res Dev* 1990;27:369-384.

12. Van Jaarsveld HWL, Grootenboer HJ, De Vries J: Accelerations due to impact at heel strike using below-knee prosthesis. *Prosthet Orthot Int* 1990;14: 63-66.

13. Winter DA, Sienko SE: Biomechanics of below-knee amputee gait. *J Biomech* 1988;21:361-367.

14. Gitter A, Czerniecki JM, DeGroot DM: Biomechanical analysis of the influence of prosthetic feet on below-knee amputee walking. *Am J Phys Med Rehabil* 1991;70:142-148.

15. Powers CM: Rao S, Perry J: Knee kinetics in trans-tibial amputee gait. *Gait Posture* 1998;8:1-7.

16. Barth DG, Schumacher L, Sienko-Thomas S: Gait analysis and energy cost of below-knee amputees wearing six different prosthetic feet. *J Prosthet Orthot* 1992;4:63-75.

17. Perry J, Antonelli D, Ford W: Analysis of knee-joint forces during flexed-knee stance. *J Bone Joint Surg Am* 1975; 57:961-967.

18. Kapandji IA (ed): *The Physiology of Joints: Annotated Diagrams of the Mechanics of the Human Joints*. London, England. E&S Livingstone, 1970, pp 88-89.

19. Lindahl O, Movin A: The mechanics of extension of the knee-joint. *Acta Orthop Scand* 1967;38:226-234.

20. Otis JC, Gould JD: The effect of external load on torque production by knee extensors. *J Bone Joint Surg Am* 1986; 68:65-70.

21. Barr AE, Siegel KL, Danoff JV, et al: Biomechanical comparison of the energy-storing capabilities of SACH and Carbon Copy II prosthetic feet during the stance phase of gait in a person with below-knee amputation. *Phys Ther* 1992;72:344-354.

22. Wagner J, Sienko S, Supan T, Barth D: Motion analysis of SACH vs Flex-Foot™ in moderately active below-knee amputees. *Clin Prosthet Orthot* 1987;11:55-62.

23. Geil MD: Energy loss and stiffness properties of dynamic elastic response prosthetic feet. *J Prosthet Orthot* 2001; 13:70-73.

24. Culham EG, Peat M, Newell E: Analysis of gait following below-knee amputation: A comparison of the SACH and single axis foot. *Physiother Can* 1984;36:237-242.

25. Lehmann JF, Price R, Boswell-Bessette S, Dralle A, Quested K: Comprehensive analysis of dynamic elastic response feet: Seattle Ankle/Lite Foot versus SACH foot. *Arch Phys Med Rehabil* 1993;74:853-861.

26. Doane NE, Holt LE: A comparison of the SACH and single axis foot in the gait of unilateral below-knee amputees. *Prosthet Orthot Int* 1983;7:33-36.

27. Snyder RD, Powers CM, Fontaine C, Perry J: The effect of five prosthetic feet on the gait and loading of the sound limb in dysvascular below-knee amputees. *J Rehabil Res Dev* 1995;32: 309-315.

28. Hurley GR, McKenney R, Robinson M, Zadravec M, Pierrynowski MR:

The role of the contralateral limb in below-knee amputee gait. *Prosthet Orthot Int* 1990;14:33-42.

29. Perry J, Shanfield S: Efficiency of dynamic elastic response prosthetic feet. *J Rehabil Res Dev* 1993;30:137-143.

30. Powers CM, Torburn L, Perry J, Ayyappa E: Influence of prosthetic foot design on sound limb loading in adults with unilateral below-knee amputations. *Arch Phys Med Rehabil* 1994; 75:825-829.

31. Lemaire ED, Fisher FR: Osteoarthritis and elderly amputee gait. *Arch Phys Med Rehabil* 1994;75:1094-1099.

32. Inman VT, Ralston HJ, Todd F (eds): *Human Walking.* Baltimore, MD, Williams & Wilkins, 1992, pp 85-88.

33. Torburn L, Powers CM, Guiterrez R, Perry J: Energy expenditure during ambulation in dysvascular and traumatic below-knee amputees: A comparison of five prosthetic feet. *J Rehabil Res Dev* 1995;32:111-119.

34. Edwards RH, Hill DK, McDonnell M: Myothermal and intramuscular pressure measurements during isometric contractions of the human quadriceps muscle. *J Physiol* 1972;224:58-59.

35. Gottschalk FA, Stills M: The biomechanics of trans-femoral amputation. *Prosthet Orthot Int* 1994;18:12-17.

36. Wang K, McCarter R, Wright J, Beverly J, Ramirez-Mitchell R: Viscoelasticity of the sarcomere matrix of skeletal muscles: The titin-myosin composite filament is a dual-stage molecular spring. *Biophys J* 1993;64:1161-1177.

37. Murray MP, Mollinger LA, Sepic SB, Gardner GM, Linder MT: Gait patterns in above-knee amputee patients: Hydraulic swing control vs constant-friction knee components. *Arch Phys Med Rehabil* 1983;64:339-345.

38. Boonstra AM, Schrama JM, Eisma WH, Hof AL, Fidler V: Gait analysis of transfemoral amputee patients using prostheses with two different knee joints. *Arch Phys Med Rehabil* 1996;77: 515-520.

39. Conley P: A Healthy Harmony. Physical Therapy Products, May/June 2003, 18-20.

40. Datta D, Howitt J: Conventional versus microchip controlled pneumatic swing phase control for trans-femoral amputees: User's verdict. *Prosthet Orthot Int* 1998;22:129-135.

41. Taylor MB, Clark E, Offord EA, Baxter C: A comparison of energy expenditure by a high level trans-femoral amputee using the Intelligent Prosthesis and conventionally damped prosthetic limbs. *Prosthet Orthot Int* 1996;20: 116-121.

42. Wilson M: Computerized prosthetics. *PT Magazine* 2001;(Dec): 35-38.

43. Boonstra AM, Schrama J, Fidler V, Eisma WH: The gait of unilateral transfemoral amputees. *Scand J Rehabil Med* 1994;26:217-223.

44. Convery P, Murray KD: Ultrasound study of the motion of the residual femur within a trans-femoral socket during gait. *Prosthet Orthot Int* 2000; 24:226-232.

45. Perry J (ed): *Gait Analysis: Normal and Pathological Function.* Thorofare, NJ, SLACK Inc, 1992.

46. Tazawa E: Analysis of torso movement of trans-femoral amputees during level walking. *Prosthet Orthot Int* 1997; 21:129-140.

47. Jaegers SM, Arendzen JH, de Jongh HJ: An electromyographic study of the hip muscles of transfemoral amputees in walking. *Clin Orthop* 1996;328: 119-128.

48. Jaegers SM, Arendzen JH, de Jongh HJ: Changes in hip muscles after above-knee amputation. *Clin Orthop* 1995;319:276-284.

49. Nolan L, Lees A: The functional demands on the intact limb during walking for active trans-femoral and trans-tibial amputees. *Prosthet Orthot Int* 2000;24:117-125.

50. Seroussi RE, Gitter A, Czerniecki JM, Weaver K: Mechanical work adaptations of above-knee amputee ambulation. *Arch Phys Med Rehabil* 1996;77: 1209-1214.

51. van der Linden ML, Solomonidis SE, Spence WD, Lin N, Paul JP: A methodology for studying the effects of various types of prosthetic feet in the biomechanics of trans-femoral amputee gait. *J Biomech* 1999;32:877-889.

52. Jones L, Hall M, Schuld W: Ability or disability? A study of the functional outcome of 65 consecutive lower limb amputees treated at the Royal South Sydney Hospital in 1988 1989. *Disabil Rehabil* 1993;15:184-188.

53. Waters RL, Hislop HJ, Perry J, Antonelli D: Energetics: Application to the study and management of locomotor disabilities: Energy cost of normal and pathologic gait. *Orthop Clin North Am* 1978;9:351-356.

54. Mayfield JA, Reiber GE, Maynard C, Czerniecki JM, Caps MT, Sangeorzan BJ: Survival following lower-limb amputation in a veteran population. *J Rehabil Res Dev* 2001;38:341-345.

55. Anderson AD, Cummings V, Levine SL, Kraus A: The use of lower extremity prosthetic limbs by elderly patients. *Arch Phys Med Rehabil* 1967;48: 533-538.

56. Holden JM, Fernie GR: Extent of artificial limb use following rehabilitation. *J Orthop Res* 1987;5:562-568.

57. Sapp L, Little CE: Functional outcomes in a lower limb amputee population. *Prosthet Orthot Int* 1995;19: 92-96.

58. Baker PA, Hewison SR: Gait recovery pattern of unilateral lower limb amputees during rehabilitation. *Prosthet Orthot Int* 1990;14:80-84.

59. Andriacchi TP, Ogle JA, Galante JO: Walking speed as a basis for normal and abnormal gait measurements. *J Biomech* 1977;10:261-268.

60. Crowinshield RD, Brand RA, Johnston RC: The effects of walking velocity and age on hip kinematics and kinetics. *Clin Orthop* 1978;132:140-144.

61. Skinner HB, Effeney DJ: Gait analysis in amputees. *Am J Phys Med* 1985;64: 82-89.

62. Rose J, Ralston HJ, Gamble JG: Energetics of walking, in Rose J, Gamble JG (eds): *Human Walking,* ed 2. Baltimore, MD, Williams & Wilkins, 1994, pp 45-72.

63. Murray MP, Mollinger LA, Gardner GM, Sepic SB: Kinematic and EMG patterns during slow, free, and fast walking. *J Orthop Res* 1984;2:272-280.

64. Pohjolainen FT, Alaranta H, Karkkainen M: Prosthetic use and functional and social outcome following major lower limb amputation. *Prosthet Orthot Int* 1990;14:75-79.

65. Holden JM, Fernie GR: Minimal walking levels for amputees living at home. *Physiother Can* 1983;35:317-320.

Chapter 31

Visual Analysis of Prosthetic Gait

Susan L. Kapp, CPO

Introduction

Clinicians frequently use visual gait analysis when evaluating the results of fitting with a prosthesis. Visual inspection, also referred to as observational gait analysis, or OGA, is conducted while the patient is walking. The clinic team verifies that the prosthesis is functioning well overall and that the patient has mastered prosthetic gait skills. The prosthetist looks for socket problems, suspension shortcomings, alignment or component adjustment mistakes, and errors in component prescription. A therapist who specializes in amputee management looks for subtle gait and postural errors that can result in asymmetric, more energy-consuming ambulation. A physician who specializes in amputee rehabilitation can readily detect changes in the patient's physical condition and spot important clues about more subtle problems such as errors in the thickness of the prosthetic socks being worn.

OGA is based on visual assessment of motion to identify kinematic asymmetries in all three planes. Effective OGA requires a thorough knowledge of the biomechanics of gait and the functional features of each component of the prosthesis. The overall goal of OGA is to verify that the amputee's gait is smooth, symmetric, and confident. Any deviations from this goal require further investigation and are acceptable only if the cause has been identified and cannot be rectified.

Clinicians worldwide use OGA because it is the least costly method for gait analysis, no specialized equipment is required, no measuring devices encumber the amputee, and it is not very time consuming. However, a number of studies have shown that it is not as accurate or repeatable as computerized gait analysis (CGA).[1,2] OGA is sufficient to make qualitative judgments about various aspects of gait, but only CGA can provide quantifiable results. Another significant shortcoming of OGA is that it is very difficult to assess motion that crosses multiple planes. Finally, only visible characteristics, such as kinematic variables, can be assessed with OGA. To measure forces or to calculate torques generated, CGA is required.

Prosthetists receive specialized training and practice in OGA, with an emphasis on optimizing prosthetic alignment and component adjustments based on OGA plus amputee feedback regarding forces, which cannot be observed. Despite its inherent subjectivity, evidence is emerging that experienced prosthetists tend to reach similar end points in dynamic alignment based on OGA. Geil[3] compared the results of five alignments done by five prosthetists using visual analysis. He concluded that the consistency among practitioners with varying levels of experience suggests that automated alignment is probably feasible but may not be necessary. Blumen-

tritt[4] has suggested that, for transtibial prostheses, the load line on the prosthetic side should be 10 mm to 30 mm ahead of the knee. He used a static laser line to identify the knee position that best corresponded to biomechanical rules of alignment and found that experienced prosthetists tended to obtain this result when performing dynamic alignment trials using OGA.

Static Alignment

Prior to initial OGA, the prosthetist verifies that socket weight bearing and suspension are adequate and that gross alignment and component adjustments are correct. During the static phase of alignment, the length of the prosthesis is evaluated by palpating the iliac crests while weight is applied to both limbs evenly. During static standing, the prosthetic socket should be slightly flexed such that the patient can stand comfortably without excessive lumbar lordosis. Weight should be borne evenly along the sole of the shoe, and the pylon should not have an excessive medial or lateral lean. The prosthetic foot should match the heel height of the shoe. This relationship is confirmed when the top of the prosthetic foot is parallel to the floor. The external rotation of the prosthetic foot should closely match that of the sound side. In a transfemoral prosthesis, the knee center generally should fall 6 mm behind a line connecting the trochanter and the ankle. This measurement will vary somewhat, with knees offering more inherent stability when placed on or slightly anterior to this reference line.

Dynamic Alignment

Once the gross alignment, length, and adjustments have been verified, then dynamic alignment trials can begin by having the patient ambulate within parallel bars. If the socket of the prosthesis is securely attached to the alignment components and the patient is able to ambulate safely after gait has been optimized within the parallel bars, dynamic alignment may continue with free walking. The patient is viewed in both the sagittal and coronal (frontal) planes as he or she walks. Each phase of gait is evaluated for optimum alignment, and any deviation is noted and corrected. By analyzing each phase of gait, the observer can systematically identify elements that are less than optimal. Once the alignment is fine tuned, the patient will ambulate with the most energy-efficient gait. For new amputees, recovery from the debilitating effects of surgery and gait training may take several months, so repeated dynamic alignment trials will be necessary. For experienced amputees, dynamic alignment can proceed more quickly. For active individuals, dynamic alignment may include observational gait analysis on a treadmill or jogging track.

Clinicians must first evaluate overall movement of the body as a whole and then focus in on each body seg-ment in each plane to identify specific problems. Areas to observe include the foot/ground relationship during stance, symmetry of steps, prosthetic and nonprosthetic knee motion, and pelvic motion (Trendelenburg). Finally, patient feedback is sought regarding limb comfort, perceived hip and knee forces, and overall effort required to walk.

Rancho Los Amigos National Rehabilitation Center has developed a format to record observational gait analysis results (Figure 1). The specific sequence of decision-making is less important than approaching OGA in a systematic and comprehensive manner.

The first step is to observe gross gait. Most gait deviations are best visualized from the side, usually with the prosthesis closest to the observer. Experienced clinicians tend to stand at right angles to the line of progression near the middle of the walkway, to see sagittal plane motion in isolation. Then, with the clinician standing behind the patient, coronal plane problems can be observed as the patient moves away from and toward the observer. Finally, transverse plane problems are noted.

The second step includes observation of kinematics at each body segment. Slow motion analysis of digital video is very helpful in isolating phases of gait and clarifying deviations but has not been shown to result in more accurate OGA. Attempts to measure angles between limb segments based on video images alone have never been validated. Once gait deviations are detected, their cause can be inferred, and the alignment or adjustment of the prosthetic components is modified to reduce their magnitude.

The study guides shown on pages 388 through 394 summarize commonly observed transtibial and transfemoral gait deviations and typical prosthetic and patient causes. The study guides also indicate in which plane the deviation is best viewed. They are intended to be a summary of the most commonly encountered clinical problems but not an exhaustive listing of all possible deviations or causes. For most problems, OGA can identify the deviation, but further investigation is required to determine the causes and therefore the remedy. Intermittent deviations are often due to inconsistencies in the patient's gait and indicate the need for more gait training, more time to adapt to a new prosthesis, or both.

References

1. Rietman JS, Postema K, Geertzen JHB: Gait analysis in prosthetics: Opinions, ideas and conclusions. *Prosthet Orthot Int* 2002;26:50-57.

2. Krebs DE, Edelstein JE, Fishman S: Reliability of observational kinematic gait analysis. *Phys Ther* 1985;65: 1027-1033.

3. Geil MD: Variability among practitioners in dynamic observational alignment of a transfemoral prosthesis. *J Prosthet Orthot* 2002;14:159-164.

4. Blumentritt S: A new biomechanical method for determination of static prosthetic alignment. *Prosthet Orthot Int* 1997;21:107-113.

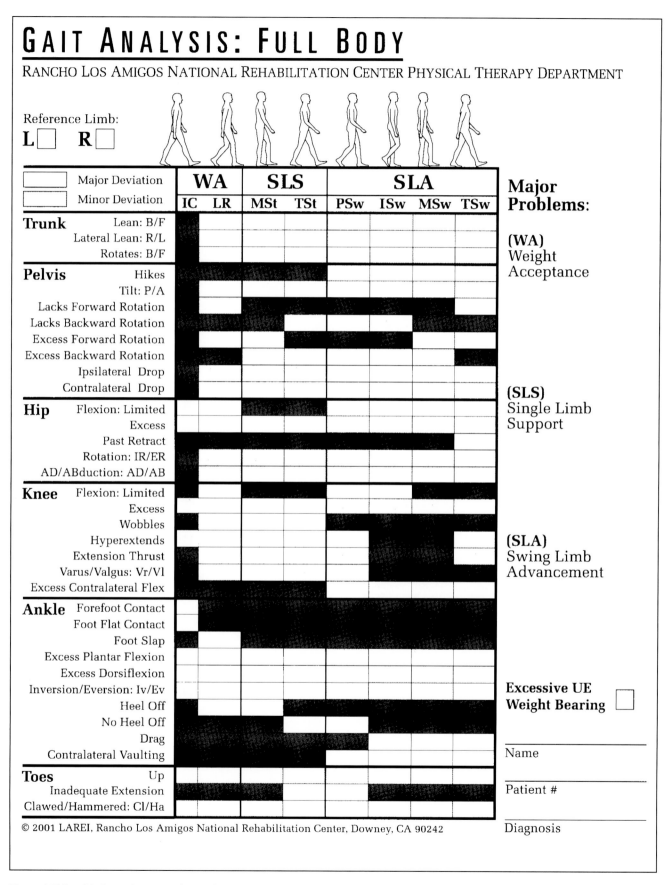

GAIT ANALYSIS: FULL BODY
RANCHO LOS AMIGOS NATIONAL REHABILITATION CENTER PHYSICAL THERAPY DEPARTMENT

Reference Limb:
L ☐   R ☐

☐ Major Deviation
☐ Minor Deviation

		WA		SLS		SLA			
		IC	LR	MSt	TSt	PSw	ISw	MSw	TSw
Trunk	Lean: B/F								
	Lateral Lean: R/L								
	Rotates: B/F								
Pelvis	Hikes								
	Tilt: P/A								
	Lacks Forward Rotation								
	Lacks Backward Rotation								
	Excess Forward Rotation								
	Excess Backward Rotation								
	Ipsilateral Drop								
	Contralateral Drop								
Hip	Flexion: Limited								
	Excess								
	Past Retract								
	Rotation: IR/ER								
	AD/ABduction: AD/AB								
Knee	Flexion: Limited								
	Excess								
	Wobbles								
	Hyperextends								
	Extension Thrust								
	Varus/Valgus: Vr/Vl								
	Excess Contralateral Flex								
Ankle	Forefoot Contact								
	Foot Flat Contact								
	Foot Slap								
	Excess Plantar Flexion								
	Excess Dorsiflexion								
	Inversion/Eversion: Iv/Ev								
	Heel Off								
	No Heel Off								
	Drag								
	Contralateral Vaulting								
Toes	Up								
	Inadequate Extension								
	Clawed/Hammered: Cl/Ha								

Major Problems:

(WA)
Weight
Acceptance

(SLS)
Single Limb
Support

(SLA)
Swing Limb
Advancement

**Excessive UE
Weight Bearing** ☐

_____
Name

_____
Patient #

_____
Diagnosis

© 2001 LAREI, Rancho Los Amigos National Rehabilitation Center, Downey, CA 90242

Figure 1 This table is used to record OGA in a systematic and comprehensive manner. *(Reproduced with permission from the Pathokinesiology Service and the Physical Therapy Department (eds): Observational Gait Analysis. Downey, CA, Rancho Los Amigos Research and Education Institute, 2001, p 72.)*

Transtibial Gait Deviations
(study guide)

Initial Contact (Heel Strike)	Deviation	Possible Causes
Best viewed from the side 	Knee fully extended	• Faulty suspension, does not maintain knee in 5° to 10° of flexion • Insufficient preflexion of the socket • Foot too anterior
	Knee excessively flexed (greater than 10°)	• Faulty suspension (maintains knee in greater than 10° of flexion) • Possible flexion contracture
Goals • Knee maintained in 5° to 10° of flexion • Stride length equal to that of sound side	Unequal stride length	• Faulty suspension (may limit range of motion of knee) • Poor gait pattern

Loading Response (Heel Strike to Foot Flat)	Deviation	Possible Causes
Best viewed from the side 	Knee flexion is not smooth or controlled, may look "jerky"	Weak quadriceps
	Knee flexion is abrupt and uncontrolled	• Foot too posterior • Socket too flexed (foot is excessively dorsiflexed) • Heel on shoe too high • Plantar flexion bumper or heel wedge in foot too firm • Shoe does not allow heel cushion to compress sufficiently
Goals • Smooth knee flexion to approximately 20° • Approximately 3/8-in heel compression • No piston action	Knee remains extended and patient "rides" the heel through to midstance	• Foot too anterior • Insufficient socket flexion (foot plantar flexed) • SACH heel too soft (if greater than 3/8 inch) • Heel on shoe too low • Excessive use of knee extensors (poor gait pattern)
	Piston action, patient may be dropping too deeply into the socket (best viewed in the coronal plane as patient walks away from observer)	• Suspension too loose • Not enough prosthetic socks • Faulty socket modifications (not enough support under medial tibial flare or patellar tendon)

Midstance	Deviation	Possible Causes
Best viewed from the front	Pylon leans medially	• Too much adduction in the socket • Foot may be outset
	Pylon leans laterally	• Not enough adduction in the socket • Foot may be inset
	½-in varus moment not apparent (for some patients this may be desirable to reduce torque)	• Foot relatively outset
	Varus moment excessive (greater than ½ inch is never desirable)	• Foot too inset • Medial-lateral socket dimension too wide
	Less than 2 inches between feet at midstance	• Foot inset (narrow base gait)
	Greater than 4 inches between feet at midstance	• Foot too outset
Goals • Pylon vertical • Socket displaced laterally by about ½ inch (duplicates varum moment at midstance) • 2 to 4 inches between medial side of the feet (as the swing foot passes the stance foot) • No excessive lateral trunk bending	Lateral trunk bending at midstance to the prosthetic side	• Prosthesis too short • Residual limb pain (patient leans laterally to reduce torque) • Prosthesis too long • Foot too outset

Terminal Stance (Heel-Off)	Deviation	Possible Causes
Best viewed from the side	Heel-off occurs early and abruptly. The patient appears to "drop off" the foot at the end of stance phase.	• Toe lever arm too short due to excessive posterior position of the foot • Foot may be excessively dorsiflexed (socket is in too much flexion)
	Heel-off is delayed. The patient's knee may tend to hyperextend. The patient may describe a feeling of "walking uphill."	• Toe lever arm is too long due to excessive anterior placement of the foot • The foot may be plantar flexed (insufficient socket flexion)
Goals • Heel-off should occur smoothly and effortlessly prior to initial contact on the sound side • Immediately after heel-off, the knee should begin to flex in preparation for toe-off		

Presswing (Toe-Off) Best viewed from the side	Deviation	Possible Causes
	"Drop off" (patient appears to fall too quickly to the sound side)	• Foot too posterior • Foot too dorsiflexed (excessive socket flexion)
	Socket drops away from the residual limb (evident when the anterior socket gaps or the posterior proximal socket brim drops distally in relation to the popliteal region)	• Suspension too loose (for supracondylar sockets) or indentation located too high above the femoral condyles (for patellar tendon–bearing supracondylar-suprapatellar sockets) • Patient may not be wearing enough prosthetic socks

Goals
- Smooth transfer of body weight to the sound side
- Socket remains adequately suspended as swing phase is initiated

Swing Best viewed from the side	Deviation	Possible Causes
	Foot "whips" medially or laterally during initial swing	• Cuff suspension tabs not aligned evenly • Prosthetic socket rotated medially or laterally with respect to the line of progression
	Prosthetic foot touches the floor during midswing	• Prosthesis too long • Suspension too loose • Knee flexion may be limited by the socket or suspension system • Muscle weakness or lack of gait training

Goals
- During initial swing (viewed from the posterior), the heel of the foot should accelerate smoothly with no tendency to "whip" medially or laterally.
- During midswing, the prosthetic foot should swing through without touching the floor. The patient should not have to exert extra effort to ensure foot clearance.

Transfemoral Gait Deviations
(study guide)

Initial Contact (Heel Strike)	Deviation	Possible Causes
Best viewed from the side **Goals** • Smooth controlled plantar flexion • Knee extension stability • Equal step length	Knee instability	• Knee set too far anterior • Excessive resistance to plantar flexion (plantar flexion bumper or heel cushion too firm) • Increased shoe heel height causing an anterior leaning pylon • Initial socket flexion insufficient to give hip extensors a biomechanical advantage • Patient may have weak hip extensors
	Unequal step length (short prosthetic side step)	• Painful socket causes patient to quickly transfer weight to sound side • Insufficient knee friction or extension aid can cause excessive heel rise resulting in uneven timing • Unstable knee • Patient insecurity, lack of balance, or muscle weakness
	Foot slap (rapid toe descent)	• Plantar flexion bumper or heel cushion in foot too soft • Patient forces heel compression to ensure knee stability

Loading Response (Heel Strike to Foot Flat)	**Deviation**	**Possible Causes**
Best viewed from the side **Goals** • Foot remains on the line of progression during plantar flexion	External foot rotation	• Plantar flexion bumper or heel cushion in foot too firm • Excessive toe-out • Socket rotation from loose fit • Socket rotation as a result of tight medial/posterior wall angle • Patient has poor muscle control

Midstance	**Deviation**	**Possible Causes**
Best viewed from the side **Goals** • Vertical pylon • Narrow-based gait, 2 to 4 inches between medial side of the feet (as the swing foot passes the stance foot) • No excessive lateral trunk bending	Abducted gait (prosthesis held away from midline throughout the gait cycle)	• Pubic ramus pressure • Pain at the distal lateral femur • Lateral wall not shaped to provide adequate femur support • Prosthesis too long • Excessive socket abduction built into the prosthesis • Pelvic band position too far from ilium • Patient has weak or contracted abductors • Patient insecurity, lack of balance, or habit
	Lateral trunk bending	• Prosthesis too short • Excessive foot outset • Insufficient socket adduction • Wide medial-lateral socket dimension • Lateral wall not shaped to provide adequate femur support • Pubic ramus pressure • Pain at the distal lateral femur • Patient has weak or contracted hip abductors • Patient has short residual limb
	Toe rotation does not match sound side	• Improper foot rotation

Terminal Stance (Heel-Off)	Deviation	Possible Causes
Best viewed from the side	Pelvic rise (hill climbing)	• Toe lever too long
	Drop off (excessive pelvic drop with forward progression)	• Toe lever too short
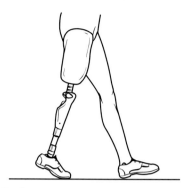	Excessive lumbar lordosis	• Insufficient initial socket flexion • Improperly shaped posterior wall causing painful ischial weight bearing • Patient has hip flexion contracture • Patient has weak hip extensors or weak abdominal muscles • Patient has short residual limb decreasing the functional lever arm

Goals
• Center of gravity follows smooth arc without perceptible rise and fall of head
• Normal step length on sound side without excessive lumbar lordosis

Preswing (Toe-Off)	Deviation	Possible Causes
Whips best viewed from the back; other deviations best viewed from the side	Medial whip (abrupt medially directed motion of the heel with external rotation of the knee) Back view	• Knee axis in excessive external rotation • Socket donned with too much external rotation • Socket contours do not adequately accommodate contracting muscles • Silesian belt worn too tightly • Patient has weak limb musculature
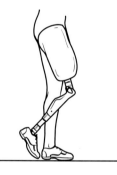	Lateral whip (abrupt laterally directed motion of the heel with internal rotation of the knee) Back view	• Knee axis in excessive internal rotation • Socket donned with too much internal rotation • Socket contours do not adequately accommodate contracting muscles • Patient has weak limb musculature
	Socket drops away from the residual limb Side view	• Inadequate suspension
	Inadequate or delayed knee flexion Side view	• Excessive mechanical resistance to knee flexion • Prosthesis aligned with too much stability
	Uneven heel rise Sagittal view	• Incorrect resistance to knee flexion • Incorrectly adjusted extension bias • Patient may forcibly flex hip or give too little or no hip flexion

Goals
• Hip, knee, and foot swing through on the line of progression
• Smooth hip and knee flexion with "quadriceps-like" control
• Heel rise equal to sound side
• Socket remains secure on the residual limb

Initial and Midswing	**Deviation**	**Possible Causes**
Circumduction best viewed from the back; vaulting best viewed from the side **Goals** • Center of gravity reaches the summit on its smooth, rhythmic path over the prosthetic foot	Circumduction (flexion, abduction, and external rotation followed by adduction; prosthesis swings on a laterally curved line) Back view	• Excessive mechanical resistance to knee flexion • Prosthesis aligned with too much stability • Extension bias too strong • Prosthesis too long • Medial brim pressures • Inadequate suspension • Patient lacks confidence or has inadequate hip flexion
	Vaulting (rising on the toe of the sound side to clear the prosthetic foot) Side view	• Prosthesis too long • Excessive mechanical resistance to knee flexion • Prosthesis aligned with too much stability • Extension bias too strong • Inadequate suspension • Patient habit

Terminal Swing	**Deviation**	**Possible Causes**
Best viewed from the side **Goals** • Smooth and noiseless deceleration to full extension • Equal step length	Excessive terminal impact	• Insufficient knee friction • Extension bias too strong • Worn or absent extension bumper • Patient strongly and deliberately extends hip to ensure knee extension at initial contact
	Unequal step length (long prosthetic side step)	• Insufficient initial socket flexion to accommodate a hip flexion contracture

Chapter 32

Energy Expenditure of Walking in Individuals With Lower Limb Amputations

Robert L. Waters, MD
Sara J. Mulroy, PhD, PT

Introduction

Measurement of physiologic energy expenditure has proved to be a reliable method of quantitatively assessing the penalties imposed by pathologic gait. This chapter outlines the basic principles of exercise physiology relevant to human locomotion and details the impact of lower limb amputation on the energy expenditure of walking. The chapter also compares the effects of various levels of amputation and patients' capacity to tolerate the increased energy requirements and examines the effectiveness of rehabilitation interventions.

Energy Sources and Measurement

After several minutes of exercise at a constant submaximal workload, the rate of oxygen (O_2) consumption reaches a level sufficient to meet the energy demands of the tissues. The cardiac output, heart rate, respiratory rate, and other parameters of physiologic workload also plateau, and a steady-state condition is achieved. The rate of O_2 consumption at this time reflects the energy expended during the activity.

Aerobic Versus Anaerobic Metabolism

During continuous exercise, both aerobic and anaerobic metabolic processes may occur, depending on the exercise workload. During mild or moderate exercise, the O_2 supply to the cell and the capacity of aerobic energy–producing mechanisms are usually sufficient to satisfy adenosine triphosphate (ATP) requirements, and exercise can be sustained for a prolonged time without the individual reaching an easily definable point of exhaustion.[1] During more strenuous exercise, both anaerobic and aerobic oxidation processes occur. From a practical standpoint, the anaerobic pathway provides muscle with an immediate supply of additional energy for sudden and short-term strenuous activity. Anaerobic oxidation is limited, however, by the individual's tolerance for acidosis resulting from the accumulation of lactate. The point of onset of anaerobic metabolism is heralded by a rise in the serum lactate level, a drop in pH, and a rise in the ratio of expired carbon dioxide (CO_2) to inspired O_2.[2]

Measurements Used in Metabolic Studies

Table 1 lists terms and units used in metabolic studies.

TABLE 1 Terms and Units Commonly Used in Metabolic Studies

Basal metabolic rate (BMR) The minimum level of energy required to sustain the body's vital functions in the waking state.

Calorie A gram-calorie is the amount of heat energy required to raise 1 g of water 1°C. A kilogram-calorie is the amount of heat energy required to raise 1 g of water 1,000°C. Because of the equivalence between caloric expenditure and O_2 consumption during aerobic activities (5 g-calories = 1 mL O_2 consumed), the terms energy expenditure and O_2 consumption can be used interchangeably in this context.

O_2 cost The amount of energy required to perform a task. During level walking, the O_2 cost is the amount of O_2 consumed per kilogram of body weight per unit distance traveled (mL/kg·m), or rate of O_2 consumption divided by walking speed. Also called physiologic work.

O_2 pulse The rate of O_2 consumption divided by the heart rate. Indicates the exercise efficiency of the active muscle.

Rate of O_2 consumption Equal to the milliliters of O_2 consumed per kilogram body weight per minute (mL/kg·min). Also called power requirement.

Respiratory Exchange Ratio (RER) The ratio of CO_2 production to O_2 consumption under exercise conditions. An RER greater than 0.90 is indicative of anaerobic activity, and an RER greater than 1.00 is indicative of severe exertion.

V_{O_2max} The highest rate of O_2 consumption attained during exercise of large muscle groups at sea level. The higher the O_2 uptake, the greater the aerobic energy output. V_{O_2max} is an indicator of physical fitness. Also called maximal aerobic capacity.

Units of Energy

The energy units used in metabolic studies are the gram-calorie (cal) and the kilogram-calorie (Kcal). Because the direct measurement of heat production in subjects while they exercise is impractical, caloric consumption is calculated indirectly based on the volume of O_2 consumption and CO_2 production.

Units of Power and Work

The terms power and work describe energy expenditure. The power requirement of an activity is the same as the rate of O_2 consumption, which is defined as milliliters of O_2 consumed per kilogram of body weight per minute (mL/kg·min). Physiologic work is the amount of energy required to perform a task.

Physiologic work (O_2 cost) during level walking is defined as the amount of O_2 consumed per kilogram of body weight per unit distance traveled (mL/kg·m) and is determined by dividing the rate of O_2 consumption by the speed of walking. By comparing the energy cost of pathologic gait with the corresponding value for normal gait, it is possible to determine the gait efficiency.

The rate of O_2 consumption relates to the level of physical effort; the O_2 cost is a measurement of the total energy required to perform the task of walking. Oxygen cost will be higher either when O_2 consumption is higher at a normal walking speed or when the walking speed is lower at a normal rate of O_2 consumption. In the latter case, the patient will not experience physical stress or fatigue, and the high energy cost is not clinically significant.

Respiratory Exchange Ratio

The respiratory exchange ratio (RER) is the ratio of CO_2 production to O_2 consumption under exercise conditions.[2] Sustained strenuous exercise resulting in an RER greater than 0.90 is indicative of anaerobic activity.[1] A ratio greater than 1.00 is indicative of severe exertion.

Maximal Aerobic Capacity

The maximal aerobic capacity ($V_{O_{2max}}$) is the highest O_2 uptake an individual can attain during physical work while breathing air at sea level.[1] It is the single best indicator of physical fitness.[3] Generally an individual will reach $V_{O_{2max}}$ within 2 to 3 minutes of exhausting work.

Age influences the $V_{O_{2max}}$. Up to approximately age 20 years, the $V_{O_{2max}}$ increases. Thereafter, the $V_{O_{2max}}$ declines, primarily because of a decrease in both maximum heart rate and stroke volume, and also because individuals usually exercise less as they age.

Because body size and composition affect the amount of O_2 consumed, $V_{O_{2max}}$ is divided by body weight to enable comparisons between subjects. Differences in body composition and hemoglobin level account for a higher $V_{O_{2max}}$ in men than in women. Although the $V_{O_{2max}}$ per kilogram of fat-free body mass is not significantly different between men and women, the absolute $V_{O_{2max}}$ is 15% to 20% higher in men because men generally have lower body fat and higher hemoglobin levels than do women.[1,2] Similarly, the $V_{O_{2max}}$, when normalized by body weight, is 10% to 15% higher in children age 6 to 12 years than in a 20-year-old adult.[4]

The $V_{O_{2max}}$ also depends on the type of exercise performed. The O_2 demand is directly related to the muscle mass involved; therefore, the $V_{O_{2max}}$ during upper limb exercise is lower than during lower limb exercise. For any given workload, however, heart rate and intra-arterial blood pressure are higher in upper limb exercise than in lower limb exercise.[5] The reduction in available muscle mass that occurs with lower limb amputation reduces the individual's $V_{O_{2max}}$, with greater decrements at higher amputation levels.[6]

Heart Rate

Increased heart rate, or tachycardia, is the symptom most closely associated with strenuous exercise. In the ab-sence of cardiac disease, a linear relation exists between the rate of O_2 consumption and heart rate. At a given rate of O_2 consumption, higher heart rates are associated with lower limb exercise than with upper limb exercise.[1] The ratio of O_2 uptake to heart rate is called the O_2 pulse, an indicator of cardiovascular exercise efficiency. A higher O_2 pulse value indicates greater exercise efficiency. Deconditioning, which can be caused by inactivity or disease that impairs the delivery of O_2 to the cells, decreases the O_2 pulse value.

Training

A physical conditioning program can increase aerobic capacity by increasing several factors: cardiac output, the capacity of the cells to extract O_2 from the blood, the hemoglobin level, and muscle mass (hypertrophy). All of these changes lead to increased fat utilization as the primary source of energy.[2] As a result, less lactate is formed during exercise, and endurance is increased. Other effects of aerobic training include a decrease in the resting and submaximal heart rates; lowered blood pressure; and an increase in stroke volume and, therefore, cardiac output.

Aerobic fitness level as a result of training, muscle fiber type, capillary density, and changes in the oxidative capabilities of the muscles determines the percentage of the $V_{O_{2max}}$ that can be sustained during endurance exercise without triggering anaerobic metabolism.[2,7] The contribution of anaerobic metabolic pathways normally begins when the O_2 uptake reaches between 55% and 65% of the $V_{O_{2max}}$ in healthy, untrained subjects, but in highly trained athletes, it may not begin until O_2 uptake exceeds 80% of the $V_{O_{2max}}$.[8-11] Experienced endurance athletes tend to compete at exercise levels just above the point of onset of blood lactate accumulation.[12,13]

A sedentary lifestyle has the opposite effect of physical conditioning on $V_{O_{2max}}$.[14,15] Not only does atrophy of peripheral musculoskeletal structures occur, but there is a decline in stroke volume and cardiac output and an increase in resting and exercising heart rate as a result of inactivity. Bed rest for 3 weeks has been shown to result in a 27% decrease in the Vo_{2max} by decreasing cardiac output and stroke volume and affecting other factors.[15] In addition, any disease process of the respiratory, cardiovascular, muscular, or metabolic system that restricts the supply of O_2 to the cells will also decrease the Vo_{2max}.

A special problem confronting many older patients with vascular amputations is limited exercise ability. Physical work capacity, Vo_{2max}, and O_2 pulse are reduced not only by aging but also by commonly associated diseases such as arteriosclerotic disease of the heart and peripheral vascular system. Diabetes, which is common in vascular amputees, increases the frequency of these disorders.

Resting and Standing Metabolism

The basal metabolic rate (BMR) is the minimum rate of energy use required to sustain the body's vital functions in the waking state.[2] The BMR is proportional to the surface area of the body as well as to the percentage of lean body mass, and this in part accounts for a 5% to 10% difference in BMR between women and men. The BMR decreases approximately 2% for every 10 years of age, through adulthood.[2] This reduction in BMR with age coincides with the progressive change in body composition that results in a lower proportion of lean muscle mass and a higher percentage of fat and bone.

The BMR is approximately the same as the resting metabolic rate when a person is recumbent.[16] In the sitting position, O_2 uptake is slightly increased.[17] Quiet standing further elevates the rate of O_2 consumption by approximately 22%, to an average of 3.5 mL/kg·min for men and 3.3 mL/kg·min for women.[18] These results are in agreement with the elec-

tromyographic studies that demonstrated that minimal muscular activity is required for normal standing.[19,20] In the normal individual, postural reflexes balance alignment of the center of gravity close to the center of rotation of the hip, knee, and ankle joints so that the muscle forces required for standing are minimal. This is another example of energy conservation in human lower limb design.

Normal Walking
Range of Customary Walking Speeds

Most adults prefer to walk at speeds from 1.0 to 1.67 m/s (60 to 100 m/min).[21-23] In a study of adult pedestrians age 20 to 60 years who were unaware they were observed, the mean walking speed for men, 1.37 m/s (82 m/min), was significantly higher than that for women, 1.23 m/s (74 m/min).[21] Similar values were obtained in energy expenditure studies performed on an outdoor, circular track when subjects were instructed to select their natural customary walking speed (CWS).[23] Patients in this study were also tested at their customary slow and fast speeds. The customary slow, normal, and fast walking speeds in adults age 20 to 59 years ranged from approximately 0.62 to 1.65 m/s (37 to 99 m/min).[23]

At speeds greater than 100 m/min, the individual chooses whether to walk or to run. Thorstensson and Roberthson[24] found the transition point between walking and running in men occurred at an average of 1.88 m/s (113 m/min), with a tendency for longer-legged men to make the transition at a higher speed. Running becomes more efficient than walking at speeds greater than approximately 2.22 m/s (133 m/min).[22]

In children the CWS is slower than in adults, averaging 1.17 m/s (70 m/min) for children age 6 to 12 years and 1.22 m/s (73 m/min) for teenagers.[23,25] Stride length in children is shorter than in adults

(1.165 m versus 1.42 m) because of their smaller stature, whereas cadence is faster (120 steps/min versus 112 steps/min) to compensate for the shorter stride.

Walking at a Controlled Speed Versus a Self-Selected Speed

Although it is convenient to measure energy expenditure at a controlled walking speed on a treadmill, this approach has several disadvantages. First, the CWS varies greatly in different patient populations depending on the extent of disability. Also, patients with gait disabilities may have difficulty adjusting to walking on a treadmill. For these reasons, most investigators prefer to conduct testing on a track, allowing patients to select their own CWS.

Energy Expenditure at the CWS

At the CWS, the rate of O_2 consumption for adults age 20 to 59 years and those age 60 to 80 years does not differ significantly, averaging 12.1 and 12.0 mL/kg·min, respectively[23] (Table 2). The rate of O_2 consumption is higher in teenagers and children, averaging 12.9 and 15.3 mL/kg·min, respectively. Expressed as a percentage of the Vo_{2max}, the rate of O_2 consumption at the CWS requires approximately 28% of the Vo_{2max} of an untrained normal subject age 6 to 12 years, 32% of the Vo_{2max} of an adult age 20 to 59 years, and nearly 48% of the Vo_{2max} of an adult age 60 to 80 years.[4,25-27] The RER is less than 0.85 for normal subjects of all ages at their CWS, indicating anaerobic metabolism is not required.[23]

In a study of sedentary and active adults, the older subjects (age 66 to 86 years) had a lower rate of O_2 consumption at their CWS than did the younger subjects (age 18 to 28 years) for the sedentary groups only, whereas the O_2 consumption values for the active groups were similar across age. This may have been the result of a purposeful effort to keep ex-

TABLE 2 Energy Expenditure at CWS and FWS at Various Ages in Able-Bodied Persons*

Age (years)	Velocity (m/min)		Rate of O_2 Consumption (mL/kg·min)		% Vo_{2max}	O_2 Cost (mL/kg·m)		Heart Rate (beats/min)		RER	
	CWS	FWS	CWS	FWS	CWS	CWS	FWS	CWS	FWS	CWS	FWS
6 to 12	70	88	15.3	19.6	28	0.22	0.22	114	127	0.84	0.87
13 to 19	73	99	12.9	19.1	N/A	0.18	0.20	97	117	0.76	0.82
20 to 59	80	106	12.1	18.4	32	0.15	0.19	99	124	0.81	0.92
60 to 80	74	90	12.0	15.4	48	0.16	0.17	103	119	0.84	0.92

*Waters and associates[23,25,26]
N/A = not available

ertion within the aerobic range.[23,28] The fact that CWS walking requires less than 50% of the Vo_{2max} in normal subjects in all age groups and does not require anaerobic activity accounts for the perception that walking requires little effort in healthy individuals. It is significant that as they age, individuals demonstrate progressively smaller aerobic reserves (the Vo_{2max} declines); this makes it more difficult to compensate for the physiologic penalties imposed by gait disorders that commonly accompany aging. This decline in Vo_{2max} has been attributed to reduced muscle strength in older persons, which requires the recruitment of a greater proportion of available motor units with a higher percentage of fast-twitch fibers for a given walking speed.[28]

Energy Expenditure at the Customary Fast Walking Speed

When children, teenagers, and adults age 20 to 59 years are asked to walk at a customary (self-selected) fast walking speed (FWS), the average rate of O_2 uptake is approximately the same, averaging 19.6, 19.1, and 18.4 mL/kg·min, respectively[23,25,26] (Table 2). The value for adults age 60 to 80 years is significantly lower, however (15.4 mL/kg·min), and there is a corresponding decline in the average FSW. The decrease in the rate of energy expenditure in older subjects is similar in magnitude to the decline observed in other parameters of physiologic performance such as muscle strength. The decline in the CWS and FWS is associated with a decrease in the Vo_{2max} that is independent of age.[29]

The average RERs for children, teenagers, adults age 20 to 59, and adults age 60 to 80 at their self-selected FWS were 0.87, 0.82, 0.92, and 0.92, respectively.[23] These findings indicate that able-bodied adults customarily set their FWS just above the threshold where anaerobic metabolism is triggered. Interestingly, long distance runners also select an exercise rate slightly above the anaerobic threshold.[2]

Relationship Between Rate of O_2 Consumption and Walking Speed

In normal walking, the rate of O_2 consumption depends on walking speed.[22,30-36] The plot of this energy/speed relation is approximately linear within the customary range of walking speeds, below 1.67 m/s (100 m/min)[23,37] (Figure 1). Above that point, O_2 consumption increases faster than does speed. Within this customary range of walking speeds, higher-order regressions do not improve data fit in comparison to a linear.[23]

Children walk less efficiently than do adults. Their BMR is higher and their cadence is faster to compensate for a shorter stride length, resulting in a higher rate and cost of O_2 consumption than in adults. A child's lower body weight, however, results in a higher aerobic reserve per kilogram of body weight than in adults.

The plots of the energy/speed relation for all age groups are relatively flat. This indicates that normal gait is quite efficient throughout the customary range of walking speeds (Figure 1).

Ralston[32] demonstrated that if the relationship between rate of O_2 consumption and speed is determined by a second-order equation, the equation relating O_2 cost to speed yields a curve that is concave upward with a minimum value at 1.33 m/s (80 m/min). This is approximately the average speed of unobserved adult pedestrians, 1.30 m/s (78 m/min).[21] This close relationship between the most economical walking speed and the normal self-selected walking speed has been confirmed by numerous investigators.[28,38,39]

Range of Average Walking Distances

Functional ambulation involves traversing a certain distance to perform a specific activity. Average walking distances for various activities of daily living were measured in a variety of areas in Los Angeles, California.[40] The authors found that in an urban environment and with an automobile available, and given a normal walking speed of 1.33 m/s (80 m/min), most activities of daily living require less than 5 minutes of walking. As a person's walking speed declines with age or pathology, however, the same activities can require 10 to 15 minutes of walking, which may be difficult for many individuals to sustain without a rest.

Loading

Studies in which weights were placed on the body in various locations found that the increase in the rate of O_2 consumption depended on the location of the loads.[18,41-43] Loads that were placed peripherally had a much greater effect than did loads placed over the trunk. Placement of a 20-kg load on the trunk of a male subject did not result in a measurable increase in the rate of O_2 consumption.[18] On the other hand, a 2-kg load placed on each foot increased the rate of O_2 consumption by 30%. This finding is predictable because during walking, forward foot acceleration is much greater than trunk acceleration and, therefore, greater effort is required to move the same amount of weight. These findings indicate the importance of minimizing weight, especially distally, when designing lower limb orthoses or prostheses.

Despite the increased rate of O_2 consumption while walking with added loads, studies show that self-selected speeds declined only minimally.[42,43] One exception was an experiment in which subjects held weights in their hands and pumped them while walking for 20 minutes.[44] The rate of O_2 consumption with pumping was closer to that seen with fast walking, even with no added weight. To maintain a normal walking speed with the increased weight would have shifted the energy demand to levels that were not sustainable.

The increased load of body weight carried by obese persons has also been shown to increase the rate of O_2 consumption when walking speed is held constant.[45,46] The self-selected walking speed in a group of severely obese women was found to average 1.18 m/s (71 m/min),[47] compared

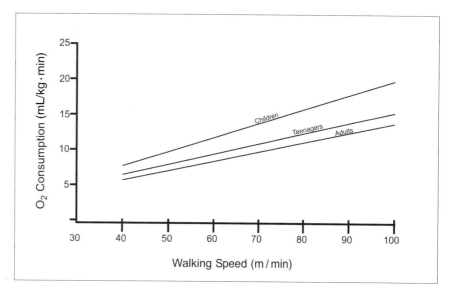

Figure 1 Relationship between the rate of O_2 consumption and speed of walking for children, teenagers, and adults without disability.

with the 80 m/min walking speed observed in women in the study cited earlier.[21] Even at this reduced speed, the rate of O_2 consumption was much higher: 56% of the V_{O_2max} compared with 36% in a group of normal-weight control subjects. This rate of exertion is greater than that demanded by fast walking in normal adults. Conversely, Foster and associates[46] found that weight loss reduces the rate of O_2 consumption during walking. A group of obese individuals displayed a greater than expected reduction in O_2 consumption following a weight loss program. The average weight loss was 21 kg, or 20% of body weight, while the reduction in energy rate was 31%.

Walking and the Unilateral Lower Limb Amputee

Despite the considerable body of literature on the energy expenditure of walking in persons with lower limb amputations,[6,48-60] a direct comparison of the results of the different studies is difficult, for several reasons. First, the studies do not consistently distinguish young amputees, whose amputations are usually traumatic, from older amputees, whose amputa-

tions are usually vascular, although gait performance differs significantly between the two groups. Second, often no distinction is made between amputees who use upper limb assistive devices and those who do not. Third, the adequacy of prosthetic fit and duration of experience are not often specified, despite the common clinical observation that patients with inadequately fitted prostheses, or those who have worn a prosthesis for only a short time, walk less efficiently than do more experienced patients with well-fitted prostheses.

Prosthesis Versus Crutches

Lower limb amputation with or without prosthetic replacement imposes energy penalties for ambulation. If the patient chooses walking without a prosthesis, increased energy is required for upper limb weight bearing on crutches. If the patient chooses a prosthesis, increased energy is required to use the remaining proximal muscles to substitute for lost muscle function distal to the amputation.

Crutch walking without a prosthesis may be a primary or secondary means of transportation for unilateral amputees when necessary if a prosthesis is unavailable or inadequate. A study of unilateral amputees compared walking with a prosthesis with

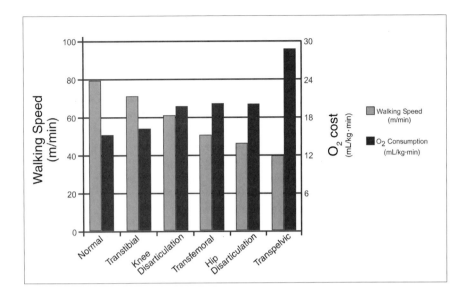

Figure 2 Comparison of O_2 consumption and CWS with a prosthesis in individuals with unilateral traumatic amputations at different levels.

walking without a prosthesis using instead a unilateral non–weight-bearing crutch-assisted (swing-through) gait.[6] The study revealed that all the amputees, with the single exception of persons with vascular transfemoral amputations, had a lower rate of energy expenditure, heart rate, and O_2 cost when using a prosthesis. This difference was insignificant in the vascular transfemoral group, which probably relates to the fact that even with a prosthesis, most of these patients relied on crutches for some support, increasing the energy demand and heart rate. Traugh and associates[61] also compared energy expenditure with and without a prosthesis in middle-aged and elderly patients with transfemoral amputations and reported the same findings.

A study of a group of young patients (mean age, 32 years) with recent lower limb fractures confirmed the extreme cardiovascular demand of crutch walking using a unilateral non–weight-bearing gait.[62] After 5 min of crutch walking, the rate of O_2 consumption increased 32%, the heart rate increased 53% (to 153 beats/min), and the RER was 1.05, indicating significant anaerobic metabolism. After 10 minutes of ambulation, each parameter worsened further, approaching peak values for maximal upper limb exercise. This severe demand accounts for the common clinical finding that patients who require a non–weight-bearing crutch-assisted gait have a restricted sphere of ambulatory activities. Because the maximal aerobic capacity normally declines with age, older patients have more difficulty meeting the strenuous demands of crutch ambulation than do younger patients. If pulmonary, cardiac, or other disease processes further restrict O_2 delivery, the patient will have even greater difficulty meeting the energy demand.

It may be concluded that a well-fitted prosthesis that results in a satisfactory gait not requiring crutches significantly reduces the physiologic energy demand. Because crutch walking requires more exertion than walking with a prosthesis, patients with transtibial or transfemoral amputations should not be required to attempt to crutch walk without a prosthesis before the initiation of prosthetic prescription and training.

Prosthetic Ambulation
Level of Amputation

Several investigators have used linear or second-order equations to describe the energy/speed relation, or the metabolic cost of walking at various speeds, in persons with transtibial amputations.[48-51] The rate of O_2 consumption in transtibial amputees is 20% higher than in normal subjects at various walking speeds.[50] Studies of persons with transfemoral amputations indicate that values for the energy/speed relation are greater in persons with transfemoral amputations than for persons with transtibial amputations.[48,52]

Two studies in which patients were tested at CWS under similar conditions illustrate the importance of the level of amputation. In the first study,[6] energy expenditure was measured in subjects with unilateral transtibial amputations, knee disarticulations, and transfemoral amputations following amputation secondary to trauma or vascular disease. Patients had worn their prostheses at least 6 months and did not use upper limb assistive aids (with the exception of some transfemoral amputees in the vascular group). In the second study,[53] healthy individuals with hip disarticulations and transpelvic amputions were tested at their CWS using a similar methodology. These subjects with surgical amputations met the following criteria: they were young, healthy at the time of testing, had not received radiation or chemotherapy for at least 6 months before testing, had no evidence of tumor recurrence, had worn their prosthesis for at least 6 months, and did not use crutches. The O_2 cost increased at each higher amputation level, from the transtibial to the transpelvic level (Figure 2). Patients with higher level amputations had a less efficient gait and higher O_2 cost than those with lower level amputations.

The average rate of O_2 consumption at CWS did not depend on amputation level and was approximately the same as the value for able-bodied subjects (Table 3). The CWS, however, did depend on the level of amputation, decreasing with each higher amputation level in both the traumatic and surgical amputation

TABLE 3 Energy Expenditure in Unilateral Amputees Walking With a Prosthesis

	Velocity (m/min)	Rate of O_2 Consumption (mL/kg·min)	% Vo_{2max}	O_2 Cost (mL/kg·m)	Heart Rate (beats/min)	RER
Traumatic Amputees*						
Transtibial	71	12.4	35	0.16	106	0.83
Knee disarticulation	61	13.4		0.20	109	
Transfemoral	52	10.3	37	0.20	111	0.90
Surgical Amputees†						
Hip disarticulation	47	11.1		0.24	99	
Transpelvic	40	11.5		0.29	97	
Vascular Amputees*						
Syme ankle disarticulation	54	9.2	43	0.17	108	0.85
Transtibial	45	9.4	42	0.20	105	0.82
Transfemoral	36	10.8	63	0.28	126	0.96

*Waters and associates[6]
†Nowroozi and associates[53]

groups. Interestingly, a study of patients with vascular amputations showed that individuals with Syme ankle disarticulations had a faster CWS than those with transtibial amputations.[54]

These findings indicate that subjects with amputations adapt to the inefficient gait (higher O_2 cost) caused by progressively higher level amputations by selecting a slower CWS at which the mean rate of O_2 consumption does not significantly exceed the normal rate (Figure 1). Clearly, as more joints and muscles of the leg are lost at higher level amputations, the greater the loss of normal locomotor mechanisms and, therefore, the greater the energy cost and the disability.[55]

Other studies of lower limb amputees walking at CWS also have shown higher than normal energy cost per meter, but whether the increased cost resulted from the slower walking speed or the higher rate of O_2 consumption depended on the level of amputation and the physical fitness of the subjects.[49,56-60] Several studies demonstrated that the rate of O_2 con-

sumption in amputees at their CWS, which was slower than normal, was approximately the same as for normal subjects.[49,56,57,60]

In contrast, other investigators have found that some individuals, especially young persons with traumatic transtibial amputations, are able to tolerate the increased rate of O_2 consumption required to maintain a walking speed that is close to normal. In a study that included subjects with only nonvascular transtibial amputations, but with a wide range in age (22 to 75 years), walking speed was found to be 10% lower and rate of O_2 consumption was 20% higher than in the younger (nonamputee) control subjects.[58] Baseline O_2 consumption during quiet standing was found to be a strong predictor of the rate of O_2 consumption during walking. Subjects with higher quiet standing O_2 consumption had higher rates of O_2 consumption during walking, indicating that a higher fitness level allowed the subjects to accept the higher O_2 demand created by the amputation and maintain a more normal walking speed. Age also correlated negatively

with energy rate, but factoring in age did not improve the prediction beyond the effects of baseline Vo_{2max}.

Torburn and associates[59] confirmed the significance of physical fitness in maintaining a CWS despite an increased rate of O_2 consumption. Subjects with traumatic transtibial amputations had a normal CWS of 1.37 m/s (82 m/min) with an elevated rate of O_2 consumption of 17.7 mL/kg·min. Their heart rate was only slightly increased (113 beats/min), and the RER was 0.86, indicating that anaerobic metabolism was not required. Physical fitness is also critical to maximizing the walking ability of persons with transfemoral amputations. Gitter and associates[63] studied a group of young, physically fit individuals with unilateral traumatic transfemoral amputations. They were found to walk at a CWS of 1.2 m/s (72 m/min) with a rate of O_2 consumption of 13.7 mL/kg·min, considerably faster than reported in other studies of transfemoral amputees that included older, less physically fit subjects. Other studies have shown that aerobic conditioning exercises both increase walking speed (by 8%) and decrease rate of O_2 consumption (by 6% to 10%) in subjects with transtibial and transfemoral amputations.[64,65] Achieving and maintaining both cardiovascular fitness and muscle strength, therefore, are critical to the economy of walking and the long-term functional status of individuals with lower limb amputations.

Traumatic Versus Vascular Amputees

The data in Table 2, which describe the energy expenditure in able-bodied persons, also can be used to compare energy expenditure in younger persons with traumatic amputations to that of older individuals with vascular amputations at the transtibial level. As shown in Table 3, the CWS and rate of O_2 consumption have been found to be significantly higher in subjects with traumatic transtibial

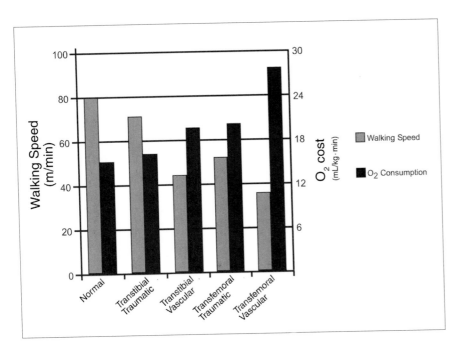

Figure 3 Comparison of O_2 consumption and CWS in individuals with traumatic versus vascular amputations at different levels.

amputations than in those with vascular transtibial amputations. This finding has been confirmed consistently in other studies.[58-60,66,67] It is probable that the higher exercise capacity of a younger person with a traumatic amputation allows a higher CWS than in an older person with a vascular amputation. The higher O_2 cost seen in individuals with vascular amputations than in those with traumatic amputations at the same level reflects the increased disability associated with age, deconditioning, and disease (Figure 3). The fact that the CWS, rate of O_2 consumption, and energy cost in persons with traumatic transtibial amputations were very similar to those in patients with ankle joint fusion relates to the fact that both groups have a similar biomechanical penalty (loss of ankle joint mobility) without the concomitant effects of advanced age or disease.[68]

Increased activity of the hip and knee musculature can compensate for the restriction of ankle joint mobility and the additional loss of power from the ankle plantar flexor muscles in individuals with transtibial amputations.[69-71] This demand is met with relative ease in the young, physically fit individual, but it represents a much greater challenge for the older patient with a vascular amputation, in whom aerobic capacity and muscle strength are likely to be reduced. Czerniecki and Gitter[71] studied a group of young, fit men with unilateral transtibial amputations who were fitted with prostheses. They found that the hip extensor muscles of the residual limb during stance phase and the hip flexor muscles of the residual limb during swing phase as well as the hip and knee muscles on the contralateral limb demonstrated increased mechanical work during running compared with the same muscles in able-bodied control subjects. Powers and associates[70] studied a group of individuals with vascular transtibial amputations and found that hip extensor strength on the amputated side was the strongest predictor of both CWS and FWS. These results further emphasize the importance of muscle strength to optimizing gait after an amputation.

When walking speed is controlled during treadmill ambulation, the difference in performance between individuals with traumatic amputations and those with vascular amputations is reflected in the rate of O_2 consumption. Huang and associates[67] studied treadmill ambulation at several speed and grade combinations. They documented an average increase in rate of O_2 consumption of 123% and 164%, respectively, in individuals with traumatic and vascular transtibial amputations, compared with an able-bodied control group. Oxygen pulse, reflecting exercise efficiency level, was lower than normal in the vascular amputees but not in the traumatic amputees. The RER was 0.90 for the vascular group, indicating anaerobic metabolism was required, whereas the RERs for the other two groups were in the aerobic range (0.83 and 0.81 for the traumatic and able-bodied groups, respectively). This study demonstrated the mechanical penalty of transtibial amputation, as seen in the traumatic group, and the additional impact of age and disease in those with vascular amputations.

Most older patients who have transfemoral amputations from vascular disease are not successful long-term prosthetic ambulators. Only a small percentage of these patients are functional ambulators.[6,72] Most who are able to walk have a very slow gait velocity and, if crutch assistance is required, an elevated heart rate.[6,60] In contrast, persons with traumatic transfemoral amputations have an adequate gait.[6,63,73,74] It may be concluded that every effort must be made to protect dysvascular limbs early, so that transfemoral amputation does not become necessary. If amputation is required, every effort should be made to amputate below the knee.

Residual Limb Length

Gonzalez and associates[56] evaluated patients with transtibial amputations with residual limbs ranging from 14 to 19 cm in length. All patients wore a patellar tendon–bearing prosthesis except for one, who had a conventional hard socket with a thigh corset. No significant differences were noted in walking speed or energy expenditure between patients with short and long residual limbs. Gailey and associates[58] found a weak negative correlation ($r = -0.32$) between residual limb length and rate of O_2 consumption at CWS in a group of 39 subjects with transtibial amputations. An evaluation of 27 vascular and traumatic amputees with residual limb lengths ranging from 9 to 24 cm revealed no significant differences in walking velocity, rate of O_2 consumption, or O_2 cost related to residual limb length.[75] Of particular clinical importance is the finding that a residual limb as short as 9 cm will result in performance superior to that reported for individuals with amputations at the knee disarticulation and transfemoral levels.

Among subjects with transfemoral amputations, James[76] found that residual limb length had little effect on torque about the hip, except for adduction. He attributed the effect on adduction to the fact that the adductor muscles insert onto the entire length of the femur and are therefore most affected by differences in residual limb length. Studies are lacking that relate speed and energy expended to residual limb length in persons with transfemoral amputations.

Prosthesis Type

Recent improvements in prosthetic design have resulted in a greatly expanded choice of prostheses for persons with both transtibial and transfemoral amputations. For example, prostheses with the dynamic elastic response foot (DERF) have been developed for the transtibial amputee. The intent of this design is to store and return mechanical energy during the stance phase of walking, thereby partially replacing the function of the triceps surae and reducing the metabolic energy requirement. Energy cost studies comparing the DERF with the conventional solid ankle–cushion heel (SACH) foot have been equivocal, with modest improvements in walking speed and energy cost seen in younger subjects with traumatic amputations.[59,66,69,77,78] Huang and associates[67] tested treadmill ambulation at several velocities and grades in transtibial amputees who wore three different types of prosthetic feet: a multiple-axis foot, a single-axis foot (sagittal only), and a SACH foot. They found the prosthetic foot type had no impact on the rate of energy consumption, but they did find elevated energy consumption in the transtibial amputees compared with able-bodied control subjects. This finding indicates that the lack of active muscle at the ankle has a greater impact on the energy cost than the presence or absence of ankle joint mobility. Other studies have shown that the addition of weight (0.4 to 1.5 kg) to the prosthesis does not increase the energy cost of walking for subjects with transtibial amputations as long as the added mass is not concentrated at the distal end of the prosthesis.[58,79,80]

In an attempt to improve the gait of the individual with a transfemoral amputation, a new socket, the Contoured Adducted Trochanteric-Controlled Alignment Method (CAT-CAM) socket, was designed to hold the femur in adduction and improve the grip on the pelvis. This socket has been demonstrated to improve walking speed by 10%, O_2 cost by 21%, and rate of O_2 consumption by 20% over that required with the traditional quadrilateral-shaped socket.[81,82]

Another modification to prostheses for transfemoral amputees is the addition of a microprocessor-controlled knee extension damper. This device detects the swinging speed of the prosthetic shank and adjusts the rate of knee extension of the pneumatic knee joint to match the subject's walking speed. Studies have demonstrated that this "intelligent" knee prosthesis provides a more mechanically efficient gait over a greater range of speeds. Energy cost was reduced between 5% and 10%, particularly at walking speeds faster than CWS.[83,84]

Children With Lower Limb Amputations

Herbert and associates[85] compared the energy consumption of children with and without transtibial amputations. They found that children with an amputation walked at a speed similar to that of their able-bodied counterparts, but at a higher level of energy consumption. The level of energy expenditure was well below the anaerobic threshold in both groups. This indicates that maintaining a normal walking speed did not require a strenuous effort on the part of the children with transtibial amputations.

Bilateral Amputees

Few energy expenditure studies have been performed on subjects with bilateral lower limb amputations.[8,49,75,86] The data, as summarized in Table 4, must be interpreted cautiously because relatively few subjects have been studied. This limited information indicates that the bilateral lower limb amputee expends greater effort than does the unilateral amputee (Figure 4). As with unilateral amputees, level of amputation affects performance: vascular patients with Syme disarticulations walked faster and had a lower O_2 cost than did vascular patients with transtibial amputations, and persons with traumatic transtibial amputations performed more efficiently than did persons with transfemoral amputations.

The distinction between traumatic and vascular amputations has an even greater functional significance in bilateral amputees, as is shown in Table 4. Persons with traumatic transtibial amputations walked faster and at a lower energy cost than did their counterparts with vascular transtibial amputations. Subjects with traumatic amputations were able to tolerate a higher rate of O_2 consumption at a similar heart rate. Subjects with traumatic transfemoral amputations had both higher rates of O_2 consumption and reduced velocity. No subjects with bilateral vascular amputations at the transfemoral level were able to ambulate long enough to complete the testing protocol. This is not surprising given that individuals with unilateral vascular transfemoral amputations

TABLE 4 Energy Expenditure in Bilateral Amputees Walking With Prostheses*

	Velocity (m/min)	Rate of O$_2$ Consumption (mL/kg·min)	O$_2$ Cost (mL/kg·m)	Heart Rate (beats/min)
Traumatic Amputees†				
Transtibial	67	13.6	0.20	112
Transfemoral	54	17.6	0.33	104
Vascular Amputees†				
Syme ankle disarticulation	62	12.8	0.21	99
Transtibial	40	11.6	0.31	113
Amputees wearing Stubby Prostheses‡	46	9.9	0.22	86

*Both amputations at same level
†Waters and associates[75]
‡Wainapel and associates[87]

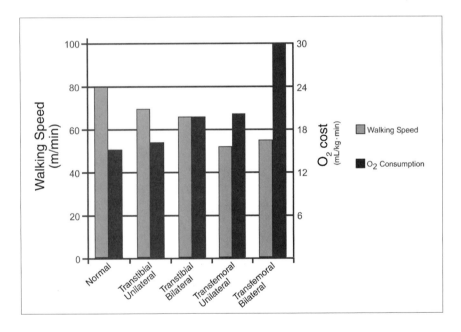

Figure 4 Comparison of O$_2$ consumption and CWS in individuals with unilateral versus bilateral traumatic amputations at different levels.

use 63% of their maximal capacity with an RER of 0.96, indicating significant anaerobic metabolism, to achieve even a reduced velocity. Amputation of the second limb imposes too large a penalty on this compromised population to permit functional ambulation.

Hoffman and associates[88] confirmed the high energy demands of walking with bilateral transfemoral amputations. They recorded energy consumption in five young subjects with traumatic transfemoral amputations at both self-selected and imposed walking speeds. Two of the subjects walked without any assistive devices; the other three used a unilateral single-point cane. The self-selected speed of 0.82 m/s (49 m/min) corresponded with the most efficient velocity (lowest O$_2$ cost). The rate of O$_2$ consumption was 49% greater than that in an age- and weight-matched control group (15.5 compared with 10.5 mL/kg·min). At the slowest imposed speed of walking (0.3 m/s, or 18 m/min), the rate of O$_2$ consumption of the subjects with amputations was 11.1 mL/kg·min, approximately the same as that of the able-bodied subjects at CWS. The level of physical fitness of the individuals with bilateral amputations allowed them to tolerate the higher rate of energy consumption to maintain the moderately reduced self-selected velocity.

Gonzalez and associates[56] pointed out that considering approximately 24% to 35% of patients with amputations from diabetes mellitus lose the remaining leg within 3 years, it is important to preserve the knee joint even if the residual limb is short. This is because a unilateral transtibial amputee who undergoes another transtibial amputation would still expend 24% less energy than a patient with a unilateral transfemoral amputation. Patients with bilateral vascular amputations rarely achieve a functional ambulation status if one amputation is at the transfemoral level.

Use of Stubby Prostheses

Wainapel and associates[87] measured energy expenditure in a 21-year-old patient with bilateral knee disarticulations who walked on stubby prostheses ("stubbies") while using a walker. The patient walked faster with the stubbies and the walker, though at a slightly greater rate of O$_2$ consumption, than with conventional prostheses and crutches. Similarly, Crouse and associates[86] studied a subject with bilateral transfemoral amputations and found that O$_2$ consumption was 23% lower when the subject used stubbies than with long-leg prostheses. Walking on stubbies is cosmetically unacceptable for most patients (except for gait training or limited walking in the home), but the data from these case studies illustrate that it can result in a functional gait.

Summary

Measurement of physiologic energy expenditure provides a method to determine the energy penalty of gait disability and a patient's functional performance ability. The O_2 cost relates directly to the extent of the patient's gait disability. The rate of O_2 consumption indicates the physiologic effort of walking at the selected speed.

The use of upper limb assistive devices (cane, crutches, or walker) for weight bearing requires significant upper limb effort. This results in an elevated rate of energy expenditure and heart rate. Patients not requiring upper limb weight bearing on assistive devices typically adapt to the disability by reducing their walking speed so that the rate of O_2 consumption does not significantly exceed normal limits. Exceptions include patients who have increased cardiovascular fitness and muscle strength, which allows them to tolerate higher rates of energy consumption to maintain a more normal walking speed. The penalty lower limb amputation imposes on the energy cost of walking increases with each higher level of amputation.

Muscle strengthening exercise programs can improve the patient's ability to compensate for gait disabilities. Aerobic conditioning exercise increases cardiovascular capacity, which reduces the relative effort of submaximal workloads. Both types of physical fitness can improve the long-term functional capacity of patients with impaired walking ability. Maintenance of ideal body weight also is recommended for individuals with lower limb amputation to minimize the impact of the disability on walking and other weight-bearing functions.

Acknowledgments

The authors wish to thank the staff of the Pathokinesiology Laboratory at Rancho Los Amigos National Rehabilitation Center, Downey, CA; Jacquelin Perry, MD, Medical Consultant at Rancho Los Amigos; and the students in the Department of Physical Therapy, University of Southern California, who assisted in patient testing.

References

1. Astrand PO, Rodahl K (eds): *Textbook of Work Physiology*. New York, NY, McGraw-Hill, 1977, pp 447-480.

2. McArdle WD, Katch FI, Katch VL (eds): *Exercise Physiology: Energy, Nutrition, and Human Performance*, ed 2. Philadelphia, PA, Lea & Febiger, 1986.

3. Waters RL, Hislop HJ, Perry J, Antonelli D: Energetics: Application to the study and management of locomotor disabilities. Energy cost of normal and pathologic gait. *Orthop Clin North Am* 1978;9:351-356.

4. Astrand PO: Physical performance as a function of age. *JAMA* 1968;205:729-733.

5. Astrand PO, Saltin B: Maximal oxygen uptake and heart rate in various types of muscular activity. *J Appl Physiol* 1961;16:977-981.

6. Waters RL, Perry J, Antonelli D, Hislop H: Energy cost of walking of amputees: The influence of level of amputation. *J Bone Joint Surg Am* 1976;58:42-46.

7. Holloszy JO, Coyle EF: Adaptations of skeletal muscle to endurance exercise and their metabolic consequences. *J Appl Physiol* 1984;56:831-838.

8. Davis JA: Anaerobic threshold: Review of the concept and directions for future research. *Med Sci Sports Exerc* 1985;17:6-21.

9. Mickelson TC, Hagerman FC: Anaerobic threshold measurements of elite oarsmen. *Med Sci Sports Exerc* 1982;14:440-444.

10. Rhodes EC, McKenzie DC: Predicting marathon time from anaerobic threshold measurements. *Phys Sportsmed* 1984;12:95-98.

11. Wasserman K, Whipp BJ, Koyal SN, Beaver WL: Anaerobic threshold and respiratory gas exchange during exercise. *J Appl Physiol* 1973;35:236-243.

12. Coyle EF, Martin WH, Ehsani AA, et al: Blood lactate threshold in some well-trained ischemic heart disease patients. *J Appl Physiol* 1983;54:18-23.

13. LaFontaine TP, Londeree BR, Spath WK: The maximal steady state versus selected running events. *Med Sci Sports Exerc* 1981;13:190-193.

14. Bassey EJ, Bennett T, Birmingham AT, Fentem PH, Fitton D, Goldsmith R: Changes in the cardiorespiratory response to exercise following bed-rest in hospital patients. *J Physiol* 1971;15:79-81.

15. Saltin B, Blomqvist G, Mitchell JH, Johnson RL Jr, Wildenthal K, Chapman CB: Response to submaximal and maximal exercise after bedrest and training. *Circulation* 1968;3(suppl 5):1-78.

16. Durnin JV, Passmore R (eds): *Energy, Work and Leisure.* London, England, Heinemann Educational Books, 1967.

17. Passmore R, Durnin JV: Human energy expenditure. *Physiol Rev* 1955;35:801-840.

18. Inman VT, Ralston HJ, Todd F (eds): *Human Walking.* Baltimore, MD, Williams & Wilkins, 1981.

19. Joseph J (ed): *Man's Posture: Electromyographic Studies.* Springfield, IL, Charles C. Thomas, 1960.

20. Perry J (ed): *Gait Analysis: Normal and Pathological Function.* Thorofare, NJ, Slack Inc, 1992.

21. Finley FR, Cody KA: Locomotive characteristics of urban pedestrians. *Arch Phys Med Rehabil* 1970;51:423-426.

22. Falls HB, Humphrey LD: Energy cost of running and walking in young women. *Med Sci Sports* 1976;8:9-13.

23. Waters RL, Lunsford BR, Perry J, Byrd R: Energy-speed relationship of walking: Standard tables. *J Orthop Res* 1988;6:215-222.

24. Thorstensson A, Roberthson H: Adaptations to changing speed in human locomotion: Speed of transition between walking and running. *Acta Physiol Scand* 1987;131:211-214.

25. Waters RL, Hislop HJ, Thomas L, Campbell J: Energy cost of walking in normal children and teenagers. *Dev Med Child Neurol* 1983;25:184-188.

26. Waters RL, Hislop HJ, Perry J, Thomas L, Campbell J: Comparative cost of walking in young and old adults. *J Orthop Res* 1983;1:73-76.

27. Astrand I, Astrand PO, Hallback I, Kilbom A: Reduction in maximal oxygen uptake with age. *J Appl Physiol* 1973;35:649-654.

28. Martin PE, Rothstein DE, Larish DD: Effects of age and physical activity status on the speed-aerobic demand relationship of walking. *J Appl Physiol* 1992;73:200-206.

29. Cunningham DA, Rechnitzer PA, Pearce ME, Donner AP: Determinants of self-selected walking pace across

ages 19 to 66. *J Gerontol* 1982;37: 560-564.

30. Bobbert AC: Energy expenditure in level and grade walking. *J Appl Physiol* 1960;15:1015-1021.

31. Booyens J, Keatinge WR: The expenditure of energy by men and women walking. *J Physiol* 1957;138:165-171.

32. Ralston HJ: Energy-speed relation and optimal speed during level walking. *Int Z Angew Physiol* 1958;17:277-283.

33. Corcoran PJ, Brengelmann GL: Oxygen uptake in normal and handicapped subjects, in relation to the speed of walking beside a velocity-controlled cart. *Arch Phys Med Rehabil* 1970;51:78-87.

34. Cotes JE, Meade F: The energy expenditure and mechanical energy demand in walking. *Ergonomics* 1960;3:97-119.

35. Dill DB: Oxygen used in horizontal and grade walking and running on the treadmill. *J Appl Physiol* 1957;20:19-22.

36. Erickson L, Simonson E, Taylor HL, Alexander H, Keys A: The energy cost of horizontal and grade walking on the motor-driven treadmill. *Am J Physiol* 1946;145:391-401.

37. Bunc V, Dlouha R: Energy cost of treadmill walking. *J Sports Med Phys Fitness* 1997;37:103-109.

38. Gleim GW, Stachenfeld NS, Nicholas JA: The influence of flexibility on the economy of walking and jogging. *J Orthop Res* 1990;8:814-823.

39. Farley CT, McMahon TA: Energetics of walking and running: Insights from simulated reduced-gravity experiments. *J Appl Physiol* 1992;73: 2709-2712.

40. Lerner-Frankiel MB, Vargas S, Brown M, Krusell L, Schoneberger W: Functional community ambulation: What are your criteria? *Clin Manag Phys Ther* 1986;6:12-15.

41. Duggan A, Haisman MF: Prediction of the metabolic cost of walking with and without loads. *Ergonomics* 1992;35: 417-426.

42. Skinner HB, Barrack RL: Ankle weighting effect on gait in able-bodied adults. *Arch Phys Med Rehabil* 1990;71: 112-115.

43. Barnett SL, Bagley AM, Skinner HB: Ankle weight effect on gait: Orthotic implications. *Orthopedics* 1993;16: 1127-1131.

44. Morrow SK, Bishop PA, Ketter CA: Energy costs of self-paced walking with handheld weights. *Res Q Exerc Sport* 1992;63:435-437.

45. Maffeis C, Schutz Y, Schena F, Zaffanello M, Pinelli L: Energy expenditure during walking and running in obese and nonobese prepubertal children. *J Pediatr* 1993;123:193-199.

46. Foster GD, Wadden TA, Kendrick ZV, Letizia KA, Lander DP, Conill AM: The energy cost of walking before and after significant weight loss. *Med Sci Sports Exerc* 1995;27:888-894.

47. Mattsson E, Larsson UE, Rossner S: Is walking for exercise too exhausting for obese women? *Int J Obes Relat Metab Disord* 1997;21:380-386.

48. Ganguli S, Datta SR, Chatterjee BB, Roy BN: Metabolic cost of walking at different speeds with patellar tendon-bearing prosthesis. *J Appl Physiol* 1974; 36:440-443.

49. Huang CT, Jackson JR, Moore NB, et al: Amputation: Energy cost of ambulation. *Arch Phys Med Rehabil* 1979;60: 18-24.

50. Molen NH: Energy-speed relation of below-knee amputees walking on a motor-driven treadmill. *Int Z Angew Physiol* 1973;31:173-185.

51. Pagliarulo MA, Waters R, Hislop HJ: Energy cost of walking of below-knee amputees having no vascular disease. *Phys Ther* 1979;59:538-543.

52. James U: Oxygen uptake and heart rate during prosthetic walking in healthy male unilateral above-knee amputees. *Scand J Rehabil Med* 1973;5: 71-80.

53. Nowroozi F, Salvanelli ML, Gerber LH: Energy expenditure in hip disarticulation and hemipelvectomy amputees. *Arch Phys Med Rehabil* 1983;64: 300-303.

54. Waters RL, Lundsford BR: Energy cost of paraplegic locomotion. *J Bone Joint Surg Am* 1985;67:1245-1250.

55. Eberhart HD, Elftman H, Inman VT: The locomotor mechanism of the amputee, in Klopsteg PE, Wilson PD (eds): *Human Limbs and Their Substitutes.* New York, NY, Hafner, 1968, pp 472-480.

56. Gonzalez EG, Corcoran PJ, Reyes RL: Energy expenditure in below-knee amputees: Correlation with stump

length. *Arch Phys Med Rehabil* 1974;55: 111-119.

57. James U, Nordgren B: Physical work capacity measured by bicycle ergometry (one leg) and prosthetic treadmill walking in healthy active unilateral above-knee amputees. *Scand J Rehabil Med* 1973;5:81-87.

58. Gailey RS, Wenger MA, Raya M, et al: Energy expenditure of trans-tibial amputees during ambulation at self-selected pace. *Prosthet Orthot Int* 1994; 18:84-91.

59. Torburn L, Powers CM, Guiterrez R, Perry J: Energy expenditure during ambulation in dysvascular and traumatic below-knee amputees: A comparison of five prosthetic feet. *J Rehabil Res Dev* 1995;32:111-119.

60. Pinzur MS, Gold J, Schwartz D, Gross N: Energy demands for walking in dysvascular amputees as related to the level of amputation. *Orthopedics* 1992; 15:1033-1037.

61. Traugh GH, Corcoran PJ, Reyes RL: Energy expenditure of ambulation in patients with above-knee amputations. *Arch Phys Med Rehabil* 1975;56: 67-71.

62. Waters RL, Campbell J, Perry J: Energy cost of three-point crutch ambulation in fracture patients. *J Orthop Trauma* 1987;1:170-173.

63. Gitter A, Czerniecki J, Weaver K: A reassessment of center-of-mass dynamics as a determinate of the metabolic inefficiency of above-knee amputee ambulation. *Am J Phys Med Rehabil* 1995;74:332-338.

64. Pitetti KH, Snell PG, Stray-Gundersen J, Gottschalk FA: Aerobic training exercises for individuals who had amputation of the lower limb. *J Bone Joint Surg Am* 1987;69:914-921.

65. Lane JM, Kroll MA, Rossbach PG: New advances and concepts in amputee management after treatment for bone and soft-tissue sarcomas. *Clin Orthop* 1990;256:22-28.

66. Casillas JM, Dulieu V, Cohen M, Marcer I, Didier JP: Bioenergetic comparison of a new energy-storing foot and SACH foot in traumatic below-knee vascular amputations. *Arch Phys Med Rehabil* 1995;76:39-44.

67. Huang GF, Chou YL, Su FC: Gait analysis and energy consumption of below-knee amputees wearing three

different prosthetic feet. *Gait Posture* 2000;12:162-16.

68. Waters RL, Barnes G, Husserl T, Silver L, Liss R: Comparable energy expenditure after arthrodesis of the hip and ankle. *J Bone Joint Surg Am* 1988;70: 1032-1037.

69. Torburn L, Perry J, Ayyappa E, Shanfield SL: Below-knee amputee gait with dynamic elastic response prosthetic feet: A pilot study. *J Rehabil Res Dev* 1990;27:369-384.

70. Powers CM, Boyd LA, Fontaine CA, Perry J: The influence of lower-extremity muscle force on gait characteristics in individuals with below-knee amputations secondary to vascular disease. *Phys Ther* 1996;76: 369-385.

71. Czerniecki JM, Gitter A: Insights into amputee running: A muscle work analysis. *Am J Phys Med Rehabil* 1992; 71:209-218.

72. Steinberg FU, Garcia WJ, Roettger RF, Shelton DJ: Rehabilitation of the geriatric amputee. *J Am Geriatr Soc* 1974; 22:62-66.

73. James U, Oberg K: Prosthetic gait pattern in unilateral above-knee amputees. *Scand J Rehabil Med* 1973;5:35-50.

74. Jaegers SM, Vos LD, Rispens P, Hof AL: The relationship between comfortable and most metabolically efficient walking speed in persons with unilateral above-knee amputation. *Arch Phys Med Rehabil* 1993;74:521-525.

75. Waters RL, Perry J, Chambers R: Energy expenditure of amputee gait, in Moore WS, Malone JM (eds): *Lower Extremity Amputation*. Philadelphia, PA, WB Saunders, 1989, pp 250-260.

76. James U: Maximal isometric muscle strength in healthy active male unilateral above-knee amputees: With special regard to the hip joint. *Scand J Rehabil Med* 1973;5:55-66.

77. Colborne GR, Naumann S, Longmuir PE, Berbrayer D: Analysis of mechanical and metabolic factors in the gait of congenital below knee amputees: A comparison of the SACH and Seattle feet. *Am J Phys Med Rehabil* 1992;71: 272-278.

78. Lehmann JF, Price R, Boswell-Bessette S, Dralle A, Questad K: Comprehensive analysis of dynamic elastic response feet: Seattle Ankle/Lite Foot versus SACH foot. *Arch Phys Med Rehabil* 1993;74:853-861.

79. Gailey RS, Nash MS, Atchley TA, et al: The effects of prosthesis mass on metabolic cost of ambulation in non-vascular trans-tibial amputees. *Prosthet Orthot Int* 1997;21:9-16.

80. Lehmann JF, Price R, Okumura R, Questad K, de Lateur BJ, Negretot A: Mass and mass distribution of below-knee prostheses: Effect on gait efficacy and self-selected walking speed. *Arch Phys Med Rehabil* 1998;79:162-168.

81. Flandry F, Beskin J, Chambers RB, Perry J, Waters RL, Chavez R: The effect of the CAT-CAM above-knee prosthesis on functional rehabilitation. *Clin Orthop* 1989;239:249-262.

82. Gailey RS, Lawrence D, Burditt C, Spyropoulos P, Newell C, Nash MS: The CAT-CAM socket and quadrilateral socket: A comparison of energy cost during ambulation. *Prosthet Orthot Int* 1993;17:95-100.

83. Taylor MB, Clark E, Offord EA, Baxter C: A comparison of energy expenditure by a high level trans-femoral amputee using the Intelligent Prosthesis and conventionally damped prosthetic limbs. *Prosthet Orthot Int* 1996;20: 116-121.

84. Buckley JG, Spence WD, Solomonidis SE: Energy cost of walking: Comparison of "Intelligent Prosthesis" with conventional mechanism. *Arch Phys Med Rehabil* 1997;78:330-333.

85. Herbert LM, Engsberg JR, Tedford KG, Grimston SK: A comparison of oxygen consumption during walking between children with and without below-knee amputations. *Phys Ther* 1994;74: 943-950.

86. Crouse SF, Lessard CS, Rhodes J, Lowe RC: Oxygen consumption and cardiac response of short-leg and long-leg prosthetic ambulation in a patient with bilateral above-knee amputation: Comparisons with able-bodied men. *Arch Phys Med Rehabil* 1990;71: 313-317.

87. Wainapel SF, March H, Steve L: Stubby prostheses: An alternative to conventional prosthetic devices. *Arch Phys Med Rehabil* 1985;66:264-266.

88. Hoffman MD, Sheldahl LM, Buley KJ, Sandford PR: Physiological comparison of walking among bilateral above-knee amputee and able-bodied subjects, and a model to account for the differences in metabolic cost. *Arch Phys Med Rehabil* 1997;78:385-392.

Chapter 33

Prosthetic Suspensions and Components

John W. Michael, MEd, CPO

Introduction

The variety of commercially available components and suspension options for lower limb prostheses has grown steadily in recent years, offering today's clinician a multitude of high-quality alternatives. The challenge is to keep abreast of these new developments in prosthetic rehabilitation to make the most appropriate choice for each individual amputee.

Fortunately, these commercial products, numbering in the hundreds, can be organized conceptually into a handful of logical groupings, based primarily on their biomechanical performance or engineering design.[1] Once these functional groups have been identified, key indications and limitations can readily be determined, and inappropriate choices can be quickly ruled out.[2] In consultation with the prosthetist, the rehabilitation team must then select a specific solution from the appropriate alternatives for each individual.

This chapter provides an overview of the key characteristics of the functional groupings of prosthetic suspensions and components. Specific applications illustrating these general principles are discussed in later chapters.

Suspension

Gravity, momentum, and other forces inherent in ambulation cause the prosthesis to displace on the residual limb, particularly during the swing phase of gait. Each millimeter of displacement creates a greater pseudarthrosis at the socket interface, compromising the amputee's comfort and control of the prosthesis. Weight bearing usually reverses the displacement to some extent, as the residual limb is pushed back into the socket during stance phase.

This chronic reciprocating movement of the residual limb within the socket is often referred to as pistoning, and it must be minimized for successful use of the prosthesis. Pistoning has many undesirable effects, including the generation of shear stresses on the skin and functional elongation of the prosthesis during swing phase.[3]

Over the centuries, many different methods to suspend the artificial limb from the body have been developed in an effort to keep pistoning to an absolute minimum. Suspensions can be classified into one of four functional classes. The most effective in reducing pistoning are atmospheric pressure suspensions, followed by anatomic suspensions, strap suspensions, and, finally, hinge suspensions.

Atmospheric Pressure Suspensions

Available evidence clearly indicates that atmospheric pressure suspensions, or "suction" suspensions, provide the most secure external attachment to the residual limb.[4] Consequently, they are the preferred mode of suspension whenever feasible. Until skeletal attachment becomes a viable option, these suspensions should be considered for every amputee.

Suction Sockets

The Germans are credited with the first widespread application of the concept of creating a relative vacuum inside the socket to achieve suspension.[5] This technique was unknown in the United States until after World War II, but once it became part of the curriculum in the prosthetic training programs, the method was widely accepted and applied. For nearly 50 years, the suction socket was the suspension design of choice for transfemoral amputees.

In the original implementation, the skin of the thigh remnant serves as a gasket to seal the brim of the socket against air infiltration. To be effective, the skin must be pliable and free of artifacts such as deep scar channels that might compromise the seal. The prosthetist must carefully reduce the circumference of the socket during the fitting trials, avoiding constriction of the blood flow yet ensuring that the skin never loses contact with the socket, even during vigorous activities. Volume reduction tables were developed, based on clinical ex-

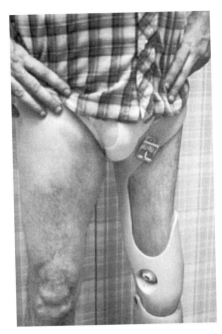

Figure 1 Patient wearing a suction socket. The flexible inner socket shown here is fabricated from a clear thermoplastic material and contained within a rigid weight-bearing frame. *(Courtesy of CPO Services, Inc.)*

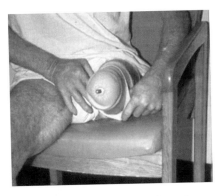

Figure 2 The ICEROSS is invaginated over the residual limb and adheres to the skin by a combination of friction and atmospheric pressure. It is usually tethered to the distal end of the socket, thus suspending the prosthesis. *(Courtesy of CPO Services, Inc.)*

perience with hundreds of successful fittings, to provide an initial guideline for rectification of the positive model of the patient's residual limb to create a suction socket.

A valve installed in the distal aspect of the socket is temporarily removed for donning, allowing air to be expelled as the residual limb is drawn into the socket. Once the soft tissues have displaced all of the air, the valve is reattached. The socket is then held onto the residual limb by normal atmospheric pressure, much as a suction cup is anchored onto a glass window (Figure 1). To remove the prosthesis, the amputee opens the valve; when the outside air has equalized the pressure inside the socket, it can be slipped off easily.

Long-term experience has demonstrated that this is an excellent method for suspension provided that the residual limb volume is relatively constant and the patient can don the socket correctly each time. Originally, the soft tissues were pulled into the socket with the aid of a thin tube of fabric called a pull sock; however,

many alternatives are now available, including elastic bandages. Use of an absorbable lotion to lubricate the proximal thigh tissues now often supplements or supplants the pull-in technique.

The suction socket must fit precisely so that all of the air is expelled and the skin is in full contact with the socket walls at all times. When there is a small void in the socket, the vacuum becomes concentrated in this local area and skin damage quickly results. Over time, the high stresses in such voids lead to capillary breakages, serous fluid drainage, thickening and furrowing of the skin, and in severe cases, to malignancy.[6] Consequently, the provision of total contact is now considered routine in almost every case.

There are three practical limitations to the use of a suction socket—inability to maintain the vacuum seal, inability to don or doff the socket consistently, and inability of the skin to tolerate direct contact with the hard socket walls.

Additional problems can be created by clinical conditions such as various skin defects, volume fluctuations due to intermittent edema or similar complications, and upper limb involvement that compromises hand function and makes donning difficult. Amputees with relatively bony residual limbs, such as transtibial levels, have

not done well with traditional suction sockets because of difficulties maintaining the skin-socket seal over the long term.

Internal Roll-On Locking Liners

Researchers have developed alternative methods that use atmospheric pressure for suspension in an effort to overcome these limitations. One of the most notable is the roll-on liner originally developed by Ossur Kristinsson of Iceland.

In the 1980s, prosthetist and transtibial amputee Ossur Kristinsson[7] reported success fitting many levels of lower limb amputation with a custom-fabricated pliable liner made from silicone rubber. He inverted the thin, elastomeric liner and rolled it onto the residual limb much as a condom is applied. This created an interface between the residual limb and prosthesis. Because the silicone adheres to the skin, the liner provided protection against shear forces. Limb socks were applied over the silicone liner to accommodate volume fluctuations. A sturdy cord was then attached to the distal tip of the liner and used to draw the liner-limb combination into the socket. Once the cord was anchored in a cleat, the amputee was essentially tethered to the socket via the silicone liner.

Kristinsson called this socket the Icelandic Roll-On Suction Socket (ICEROSS), and clinical experience worldwide gradually verified that this suspension method is broadly applicable.[8] Amputees appreciate being able to don and doff the prosthesis from a seated position (Figure 2), particularly if they have bilateral limb loss or have difficulty balancing on one leg. Clinicians appreciate the ability to provide the security of suction suspension while still allowing the use of limb socks to manage volume changes.

In the decades that followed, automatic lock assemblies were developed that engage a pin protruding from the end of the liner; these "shuttle locks" are now preferred by many clinicians.[9] Gradually, the application of these silicone suction sockets, or "3S" suspensions, expanded from the original transtibial application to include transfemoral and upper limb amputees as well.[10] Prefabricated liners are now available in a variety of shapes and configurations, making it easier and less costly to provide such suspension.

In the past decade, interest in thicker roll-on suction sockets has grown. These thicker sockets may provide additional cushioning and pressure dissipation, along with the shear protection and secure suspension offered by the original Icelandic design.

Some amputees find the distal tethering uncomfortable, which has led to the development of other methods to anchor the roll-on liner to the socket. For example, some liners are suspended by a vacuum created within the socket. In this application, the liner is rolled onto the skin to create a suction seal between the residual limb and the inner surface of the liner. When the amputee pushes the liner-covered residual limb into the socket with the aid of a small amount of lubricant, air is expelled through a one-way valve. This creates a second vacuum that anchors the outer surface of the liner to the inner wall of the socket. A knee sleeve is usually provided to create a seal between the socket walls and thigh tissues.

This vacuum also can be augmented by the use of a suction pump that is self-energizing during ambulation. Many amputees who use this augmented suction suspension report that once the vacuum reaches a certain level, they have a sensation of enhanced proprioception and improved control over the prosthesis as if all pseudarthrosis has been eliminated. The vacuum pump also draws perspiration away from the skin, which amputees find more comfortable. Preliminary studies also suggest that augmented suction suspension can reduce daily residual limb volume changes, although the reasons for this have not yet been established.[11]

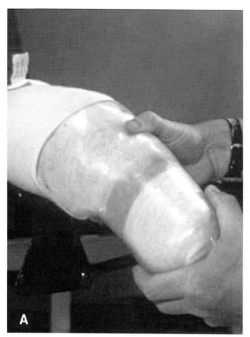
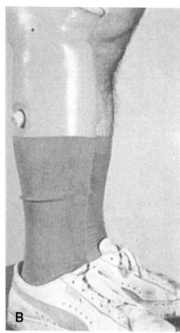

Figure 3 Hypobaric sock. **A,** A silicone rubber band impregnated into the textile hypobaric sock seals against the skin and the inner socket wall. **B,** A one-way valve expels the air in the socket during weight bearing, and the resulting vacuum suspends the prosthesis. *(Courtesy of Sid Fishman, PhD.)*

Hypobaric Socks

A third common method of providing atmospheric pressure suspension involves the use of textile limb socks in which a silicone band is impregnated to create a gasket that creates a seal between the skin and inner socket walls (Figure 3). One advantage is that the textile material can wick perspiration away from the skin. Because the silicone band does not always provide a complete seal, these socks are always used in combination with a one-way valve that automatically expels any air infiltration each time the amputee steps onto the prosthesis.

Elastomeric Knee Sleeves

One of the simplest methods of providing a suction seal for transtibial amputees employs an elastic rubber sleeve that extends onto the thigh. To create an effective vacuum seal, approximately 2 cm of rubber must seal against the socket; an equal amount must extend onto the thigh, above the level of the limb socks. Although suspension is most secure when used with an expulsion valve, many pa-

tients find that the elastomeric sleeve alone is sufficient.

The biggest disadvantage to suspension sleeves is that they are readily damaged by contact with environmental surfaces during normal use and must therefore be replaced at regular intervals. Sleeves also tend to restrict full knee flexion and retain perspiration and may irritate the skin. Still, because of their simplicity, sleeve suspensions remain popular with many amputees and clinicians.

Only air-impervious sleeves provide atmospheric pressure suspension.[12] Sleeves made from various textile materials or perforated rubbers provide purely mechanical suspension and function more like strap suspensions, which are discussed later in this chapter.

Many clinicians recommend the use of sleeves as supplemental suspension, to augment the primary suspension for special activities such as playing sports or walking in snow, mud, or sand. Sleeves are also commonly used for pediatric patients, where simplicity is of primary importance (Figure 4).

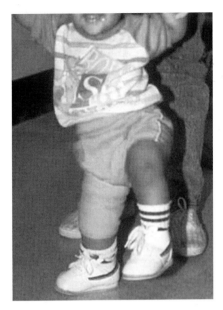

Figure 4 Child wearing a rubber knee sleeve, which is one of the simplest methods of creating a vacuum seal to suspend the socket. *(Courtesy of CPO Services, Inc.)*

Anatomic Suspensions

When the use of suspension alternatives based on atmospheric pressure is not feasible, generally the next best choice is attachment of the prosthesis by taking advantage of anatomic contours. Although the localized forces inherent in anatomic suspension create higher pressures than the suction variants, most patients tolerate this well after an initial period of weaning into the prosthesis.

Fenestrations

In the case of many congenital malformations as well as hindfoot amputations, the irregular contours of the residual limb provide an excellent method of stabilizing the socket.[13] Creation of a fenestration is often necessary to permit the irregular shape to slide into the socket comfortably. Sometimes the socket is split into approximately equal halves. If possible, the fenestration should be small and covered with a "door" to secure the limb in place. The posterior-opening Syme design shown in Figure 5 illustrates this concept. Sometimes the door is omitted, and a strap or elastic

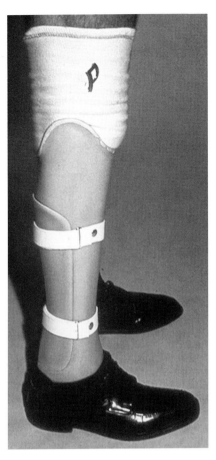

Figure 5 Posterior-opening Syme prosthesis. A fenestration in the socket allows the bulbous end of the Syme disarticulation to pass by the narrower region above the ankle. When the "door" that covers the opening is in place, it suspends the prosthesis over the supramalleolar region. *(Reproduced with permission from Otto Bock HealthCare.)*

sleeve over the socket provides the suspension.

Hidden Panels

Socket strength is significantly reduced when it is necessary to cut an opening, even with careful reinforcement. Consequently, various alternatives to fenestrations have been developed.

Firm but resilient foam can be molded over the positive model of the residual limb to fill the undercut areas. The exterior surface of the foam is then sculpted by hand to blend into the overall shape of the limb, and a one-piece rigid socket is molded over the entire assembly. The result is a small filler of foam that bridges the

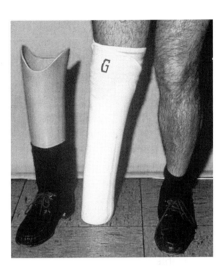

Figure 6 Prosthesis using a hidden foam panel for suspension. The panel in this example has been incorporated into a thin insert fabricated from polyethylene foam. *(Reproduced with permission from Otto Bock HealthCare.)*

gap between the socket and the limb contours. Because the foam is resilient, it can be shimmed slightly to create a mild compression force for a snug fit.

To don the prosthesis, the amputee applies the proper thickness of limb sock and places the hidden panel filler carefully in place. The panel is then held in position by pulling a thin nylon stocking over the limb sock and filler, unless it has been incorporated into a thin polyethylene foam liner (Figure 6). Once the prosthesis has been donned, the friction and compression forces stabilize the panel and suspend the socket.

Expandable Inner Wall

When the irregularities of the residual limb are not too pronounced, it is sometimes possible to create a double-wall socket with localized areas of flexibility.[14] The inner socket is laminated with rigid plastic except in the immediate area of the undercuts, which is saturated with a flexible resin. Molten wax is then poured to fill the region that contains the flexible resin. The wax is allowed to cool and solidify and is then hand-sculpted to blend into the overall limb contours similar to the hidden panel method noted above. A rigid outer socket is then laminated over the inner socket wax model so that it chemically bonds to all exposed plastic. A small hole is drilled through the outer socket in the region of the wax, which is then melted by applying local heat until it liquefies and drains out. This creates a hollow area between the flexible inner section and the rigid outer wall. To apply this prosthesis, the amputee must force the residual limb to expand the flexible area until the irregular areas have slipped past and the socket is fully donned. When the flexible area returns to its normal contours, the prosthesis is suspended.

This very difficult fitting technique is rarely used except for selected pediatric patients. The relatively fleshy limb remnants of children tolerate the forces required to don and doff this type of prosthesis more readily than do adult residual limbs.

Supracondylar Wedges

One of the most common forms of anatomic suspension involves the use of a wedge of firm material that fits into the area above the medial femoral condyle, just proximal to the adductor tubercle. For most amputees, a localized wedge in this region can provide excellent suspension plus some measure of rotational control. This method is widely used in both transtibial and knee disarticulation prostheses.

In a hard-socket design, the wedge is often removed for donning. After the residual limb is in place, the wedge is slipped into the socket and suspends the prosthesis. A transtibial socket can also be fabricated so that the proximal medial wall is removed for donning and then clipped into place for ambulation.

In a soft-socket design, a molded cushioning liner is donned first and then the residual limb in its liner is inserted into the hard outer socket. The supracondylar wedge usually is molded into the liner when it is fabricated (Figure 7). Because the wedge is always held precisely in place by the liner itself, this simplifies donning

and doffing and makes this suspension particularly suitable for people with visual impairments or hand involvements.

In addition to providing suspension for transtibial prostheses, the supracondylar wedge also adds a measure of additional mediolateral control. This is particularly advantageous for a relatively short transtibial amputation, and is often combined with a suprapatellar configuration that helps limit socket hyperextension.[15] Supracondylar suspension is also frequently combined with other suspensions, such as external suspension sleeves, to supplement the primary suspension and/or to add mediolateral stability.

Strap Suspensions

Hundreds of methods of strapping on a prosthesis have been described in the literature.[16] Strap suspensions are easy for the amputee to adjust and therefore readily accommodate volume fluctuations. This is an advantage when medical treatments such as dialysis result in an unstable residual limb volume, or during the period when postoperative edema is rapidly resolving. Unfortunately, even with the addition of a waist belt, strap suspensions inevitably allow significant pistoning and may be less comfortable than atmospheric pressure methods or anatomic suspensions.

Suprapatellar Cuff

The suprapatellar cuff, also known as the patellar tendon–bearing (PTB) strap, is one of the most common types of strap suspension. It is designed to fit snugly against the suprapatellar tendon during swing phase, suspending the prosthesis over the proximal edge of the patella, and to gradually relax when the knee is flexed beyond 60° so that sitting is comfortable. The strap that encircles the thigh is primarily intended to hold the cuff in place during sitting and should never be fastened so tight that it affects the vascular supply. For added security, many patients use a cloth waist belt in combination with a

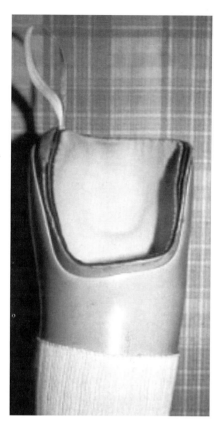

Figure 7 Supracondylar wedge suspension. Here, the supracondylar wedge is incorporated into the soft liner, simplifying donning and doffing. *(Courtesy of CPO Services, Inc.)*

cuff strap (Figure 8). An elastic billet is used to connect the thigh cuff to the waist belt.

Fork Strap and Waist Belt

A webbing or leather strap that looks like an inverted Y can be attached to a waist belt to provide another option for suspension. Because the fork strap is typically used only in combination with metal side joints and a leather thigh lacer, this suspension is quite rare.

Silesian Belt

A custom-made fabric or leather strap that encircles the pelvis and suspends a transfemoral prosthesis is often referred to as a Silesian belt or Silesian bandage, named after the region of Silesia, located in what is now Germany, where this concept was first developed (Figure 9). Numerous variations are described in the literature.

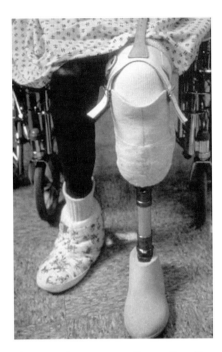

Figure 8 The suprapatellar cuff, often used along with a waist belt as shown here, is easily adjusted to accommodate volume changes in the residual limb. *(Courtesy of CPO Services, Inc.)*

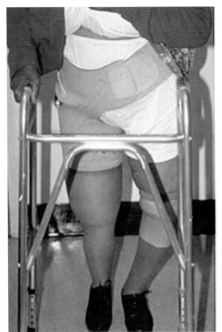

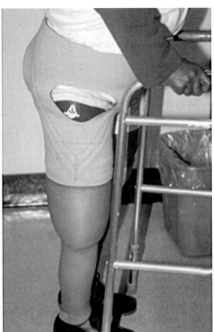

Figure 10 Elastic suspension belt. *(Courtesy of CPO Services, Inc.)*

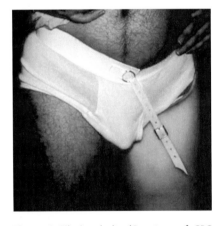

Figure 9 Silesian belt. *(Courtesy of CPO Services, Inc.)*

In addition to suspending the prosthesis, Silesian belts and related variants also provide a measure of rotational stability.[17] This can be advantageous when the residual limb has poor tone and the amputee is unable to control rotation with voluntary muscle contractions. The standard Silesian belt does not provide significant mediolateral stability.

In the past decade, prefabricated suspensors resembling modified biking shorts have become increasingly popular. These elastic suspension belts are often made from wetsuit material with selective reinforcement. They fasten about the waist with a simple Velcro closure. Because they are not attached permanently to the prosthesis, as is the case with most Silesian belts, the patient can remove elastic suspension belts for laundering (Figure 10).

Hinge Suspensions

Prior to World War II, nearly all lower limb prostheses in the United States were suspended by metal hinges that attached to a leather pelvic belt or thigh lacer. Because of the bulk, weight, and discomfort associated with such bracing, these suspensions have become increasingly rare.

They persist primarily because they offer far more mediolateral stability than other alternatives. This is sometimes a critical consideration, particularly for extremely short residual limbs. They are also commonly prescribed for satisfied previous wearers. Unfortunately, even optimally fitting hinge suspensions allow pistoning during swing phase.

Thigh Lacer With Side Joints

Prior to the development of the PTB socket design in the 1950s, it was considered impossible for the transtibial residual limb to bear all of the body's weight long term. The use of metal hinges at the knee, in combination with a tightly laced leather thigh corset, was ubiquitous. A significant percentage of weight-bearing forces were transferred to the thigh musculature, thus relieving pressure on the residual limb.

This remains one of the primary indications today for the use of "joints and lacer" suspension—to partially unload a fragile residual limb.[18] The bracing effect of the metal hinges also stabilizes the knee in the coronal (frontal) plane and provides a positive hyperextension stop (Figure 11). This is sometimes helpful when knee laxity is a major concern.

Hip Joint and Pelvic Belt

In a prosthesis suspended by a hip joint and pelvic belt, the metal hinge controls coronal plane motion while

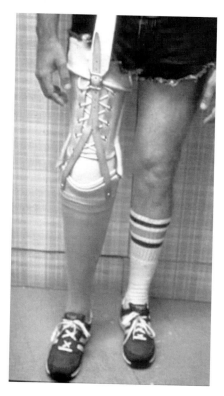

Figure 11 Thigh lacer with side joints. *(Courtesy of CPO Services, Inc.)*

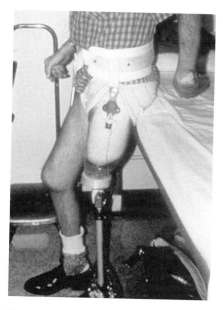

Figure 12 Hip joint and pelvic belt suspension. *(Courtesy of CPO Services, Inc.)*

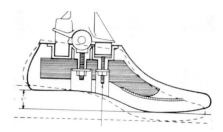

Figure 13 Single-axis foot. Once the plantar surface of this foot is in contact with the floor, the GRF instantly moves forward and passes through the articulation until midstance, when the anterior stop prevents further dorsiflexion motion at the ankle. *(Reproduced with permission from DAW Industries.)*

permitting free flexion and extension (Figure 12). It also provides some degree of rotational control if the abdomen is not too fleshy. Because amputees object to the bulk and restricted movement inherent in such a suspension, a trial with alternatives is generally recommended. In patients who walk with a Trendelenburg lurch because of the limited femoral leverage offered by a very high amputation level, however, gait is sometimes improved when a hip joint is provided.[19]

Suspension Summary

Tables 1 and 2 summarize the key characteristics of transtibial and transfemoral suspension alternatives. Suction alternatives are preferred because they minimize pistoning and enhance control of the prosthesis, but they are not always feasible. Cumbersome hinge suspensions are rarely necessary but do have limited indications. Local experience and patient preference also influence the selection of specific suspensions.

Ankle-Foot Mechanisms

Prosthetic ankle-foot devices can be classified into five conceptual groups based on their biomechanical performance.[20] Although many recent developments attempt to combine the performance of two or more functional groups and are therefore considered hybrid designs, the original five classifications have proved to be clinically useful in characterizing components that are currently available.

Each functional group of components shares common indications and limitations. This makes it easy to identify good candidates, rule out poor candidates, and generate a functionally appropriate prescription recommendation.[21] The prosthetist must then choose a specific commercial ankle-foot assembly from the appropriate functional group based on clinical experience. This process should provide the highest reliability and performance for each individual amputee's needs, with the lowest cost and weight penalties.

Single-Axis Ankle-Foot

Prior to 1950, the articulated foot with a single-axis ankle was the only widely available option for lower limb

prostheses. Because of its long history as a prosthesis, this is also one of the most thoroughly studied devices.

Although it may seem intuitively attractive to have a foot that moves in the sagittal plane through a range similar to that of the biologic ankle, this is not always the most clinically effective approach. Providing the variable restraint offered by functioning muscles in a simple mechanical fashion has proved to be quite difficult.

Numerous scientific studies have concluded that the primary biomechanical distinction of the single-axis foot, compared with alternatives, is that it reaches foot flat most quickly.[22] As soon as the prosthetic foot is in full contact with the ground, the net ground-reaction force (GRF) vector instantly moves forward to fall through the ankle joint (Figure 13). This rapid anterior movement of the GRF also generates an extension moment at the knee, which increases passive knee stability. This gives rise to the primary indication for the use of a single-axis foot—to increase knee stability.

Unfortunately, the ankle mechanism itself adds significant mass to the terminal end of the prosthesis and requires ongoing service. Because amputees generally prefer the lightest and most maintenance-free foot option, the single-axis design is now generally reserved for cases in which knee stability is a major concern. It is rarely applied to transtibial prostheses, when the amputee presumably

TABLE 1 Overview of Transtibial Suspension

Generic Class	Examples	Primary Indication	Major Advantages	Chief Limitations
Atmospheric pressure	Roll-on locking liners; hypobaric socks; augmented vacuum systems; elastomeric knee sleeves	Whenever clinically feasible	Minimizes pistoning; best proprioception; greatest range of motion	Precise fit, consistent donning necessary; works best with stable residual limb volume
Anatomic	Supracondylar wedge, with or without suprapatellar extension	To increase knee stability, for short residual limb or ligamentous laxity	Easy to don and doff, even with limited hand function or vision; supracondylar wedge adds mediolateral stability; suprapatellar extension limits knee hyperextension	Restricts full knee flexion; suspension pressure is localized
Straps	Cuff; cuff + waist belt; fork strap + waist belt	Residual limb volume changes anticipated	Amputee-adjustable; good auxiliary suspension	Some pistoning; waist belt may be uncomfortable; tight cuff may impair circulation
Hinges	Thigh corset (joints and lacer)	Damaged knee or residual limb	Maximum mediolateral and anterior-posterior stability; partial unloading of residual limb	Heavy, bulky, awkward to don; allows significant pistoning

can voluntarily control the knee, because the abrupt increase in the knee extension moment that this mechanism generates might prove harmful to the ligaments over time.

Solid Ankle–Cushion Heel Foot

In the 1950s, research at the University of California culminated in the development of what is now termed the solid ankle–cushion heel (SACH) foot. Compared with the single-axis design, the SACH foot represented a lighter, more durable, lower cost, and maintenance-free alternative. It quickly became very popular worldwide and has proven to be a very versatile, albeit basic, foot design.

In a typical SACH configuration (Figure 14), the posterior third of the foot consists of an open-cell foam rubber that readily compresses under load in early stance. As the heel compresses, the foot is lowered toward the ground, effectively simulating plantar flexion motion. As momentum carries the body forward, the heel gradually rebounds and the GRF moves anteriorly. By late stance, when the heel comes off the ground, the GRF is located at the tip of the rigid wooden

TABLE 2 Overview of Transfemoral Suspension

Generic Class	Examples	Primary Indication	Major Advantages	Chief Limitations
Atmospheric pressure	Suction socket with valve; roll-on locking liner; hypobaric sock; augmented vacuum systems	Whenever clinically feasible	Minimizes pistoning; best proprioception; greatest range of motion	Precise fit, consistent donning necessary; works best with stable residual limb volume
Anatomic	Supracondylar wedge for knee disarticulation	Knee disarticulation or congenital malformations	Good suspension; rotational control	Suspension pressure is localized
Straps	Silesian belt variants; prefabricated elastic suspension belts	Residual limb volume changes anticipated	Amputee-adjustable; good auxiliary suspension; controls rotation	Some pistoning; belt may be uncomfortable; donning properly takes skill
Hinges	Pelvic joint and belt	Short residual limb or weak hip abductors	Maximum mediolateral support; partial rotational control	Heavy, bulky, awkward to don; allows significant pistoning; can be uncomfortable when sitting

inner keel. The flexible toe segment flexes and permits rollover to occur.

Despite its mechanical simplicity, the SACH foot results in very smooth motion clinically. Although it has been displaced by more dynamic foot designs in recent decades,[23] the SACH foot remains the lightest, simplest, and lowest cost option available. It is popular for infants and toddlers and is often used in preparatory limbs and for patients whose physical condition precludes ambulating more than a few steps at a time.

Multiaxial Ankle-Foot

Multiaxial feet contain a mechanism that offers a limited range of coronal plane inversion and eversion as well as sagittal plane plantar flexion and dorsiflexion. Because the weight and maintenance frequency are similar to that of single-axis designs and the cost is only slightly higher, many clinicians prefer to offer multiaxial feet when an articulated ankle is desired.

Prior to the 1970s, multiaxial feet were not particularly durable; however, subsequent improvements have substantially increased their reliability. Although the rubber elements that limit the extremes of motion must be replaced as they wear out, the added

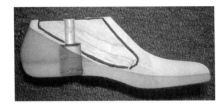

Figure 14 The SACH foot has no mechanism that requires servicing. (*Courtesy of CPO Services, Inc.*)

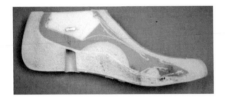

Figure 16 Cross section of a flexible-keel foot. (*Courtesy of CPO Services, Inc.*)

mobility outweighs the disadvantage of periodic servicing for many patients.

The classic indication for use of a multiaxial foot is to accommodate uneven surfaces encountered in the amputee's vocational or avocational activities. This device essentially functions like a universal joint so that the foot is in uniform contact with the ground even if the surface is not level (Figure 15). The compliance of this device is also believed to contribute to socket comfort by absorbing some of the impact of walking.[24] Most, but not all, feet of this type also provide transverse plane motion.

These components are commonly prescribed for use by surveyors, golfers, hikers, and others who routinely negotiate irregular terrain. However, many community ambulators prefer the added ankle mobility offered by multiaxial devices because they are helpful in crossing sidewalks, parking lots, lawns, and other common irregular surfaces.

Flexible-Keel Foot

For centuries, conventional wisdom held that a prosthetic foot must have a rigid forefoot to provide sufficient stability for amputee ambulation. In the early 1980s, an innovative design developed by an American prosthetist

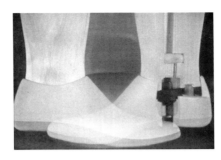

Figure 15 Multiaxial feet. (*Reproduced with permission from Otto Bock Health-Care*)

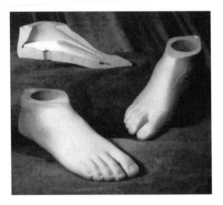

Figure 17 Dynamic-response feet. (*Reproduced with permission from Seattle Systems, Inc.*)

shattered this illusion.[25] As the cross-section in Figure 16 illustrates, this foot is composed almost entirely of resilient polyurethane rubber except for a small rigid section where it bolts onto the prosthesis.

The keel in this example is made from solid rubber and extends beyond the metatarsal region into the toe area of the foot. As a result, the forefoot is very flexible and can accommodate irregularities by bending into pronation or supination. The flexible keel also facilitates rollover, and amputees find this makes walking easier.

The plantar surface of this design is reinforced with high-strength webbing straps analogous to the plantar fascia of the biologic foot. As the amputee shifts weight onto the forefoot, the plantar straps tighten and gradually stiffen the toe to allow pushoff. This is similar to the well-known windlass effect in the normal foot.

Flexible-keel feet are well accepted by many amputees, and they are sometimes used in preparatory limbs because of the smooth rollover provided. They are also increasingly popular in pediatric prostheses, particularly for smaller, lighter preschool-age children. They are not recommended for activities that require a fast push-off, such as sprinting, because it takes a few moments for the flexible keel to stiffen enough to aid propulsion.[26]

Dynamic-Response Foot

Dynamic-response feet are characterized by a spring-like keel that deflects under load, stores potential energy, and releases it in the latter part of stance phase[27] (Figure 17). Since their development in the mid 1980s, dynamic-response feet have grown steadily in clinical acceptance to the point that they are now one of the most commonly prescribed components.

This design was originally developed to address amputee complaints that the solid keel of the SACH and single-axis feet were too stiff to permit comfortable ambulation at more than a moderate pace, precluding jogging or similar recreational activities. Initially, this innovation was embraced by highly active amputees who were delighted to be able to participate in a wider range of recreational and sport activities.

With increasing clinical experience, however, it became clear that most amputees preferred a dynamic-response foot, even for routine walking.[28] Dynamic-response feet are now considered broadly applicable to encourage the amputee to achieve a higher activity level. Perhaps the only contraindication for such feet would be if the amputee is unable or unwilling to load the forefoot, in which case, the forefoot spring would be nonfunctional.

Studies have demonstrated that dynamic-response feet vary in their ability to store and release energy and that those made from carbon fiber composites are generally more efficient than designs using lower cost

TABLE 3 Overview of Prosthetic Feet and Ankles

Generic Class	Basic Function	Primary Indication	Major Advantages	Chief Limitations
Single-axis	Simplicity	Limited ambulation or maximum durability required	Inexpensive and durable	Rigid forefoot; not energy-efficient
SACH	Rapid foot flat	To enhance knee stability	Biomechanical stability in early stance	Abrupt dorsiflexion stop increases knee hyperextension moment; increased weight, maintenance, initial cost
Multiaxial	Hindfoot inversion/eversion; internal/external rotation	To accommodate uneven surfaces	Reduces stresses on skin and prosthesis	Increased weight, maintenance, initial cost
Flexible-keel	Smooth, easy rollover	To make ambulation easier	Comfortable and reliable	Limited pushoff; increased cost
Dynamic-response	Dynamic pushoff	To increase activity level	Subjective sense of dynamic responsiveness	Increased cost

plastics.[29] In the configuration that has been shown to be the most dynamic (Figure 18), the spring extends from the toe region proximal to the ankle; the longer a given spring, the greater is its capacity to store kinetic energy.[30]

However, not all patients prefer the foot with the greatest measured energy return. In addition, even the most effective dynamic-response foot design still falls far short of providing the propulsion of a normal limb.[31] Although many investigators have shown that dynamic-response feet are the most energy-efficient option for sports and recreational activities, few studies have demonstrated any energy advantage at normal walking speeds on level surfaces.[32]

Hybrid Designs

Manufacturers have recently produced several designs that combine a multiaxial ankle with a dynamic-response foot, in an effort to offer the advantages of both concepts. Growing clinical acceptance suggests that this hybridization has been effective.[33] Multiaxial ankles combined with flexible-keel feet are also available, but these are less common.

Ankle-Foot Components Summary

Table 3 summarizes the characteristics of ankle-foot components. They are prescribed based primarily on the amputee's activity level and functional aspirations. The prosthetist chooses the specific commercial product from

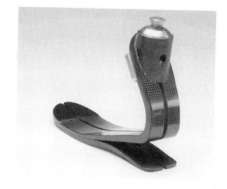

Figure 18 Spring element from a dynamic-response foot. In this design, the spring extends from the toe region to the calf region. *(Reproduced with permission from Freedom Innovations, Inc.)*

within the appropriate functional classification that is believed to offer the

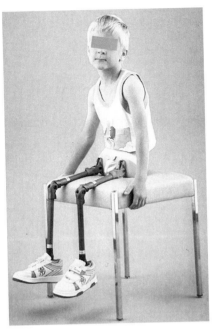

Figure 19 Child wearing prostheses with single-axis knees. *(Reproduced with permission from Otto Bock HealthCare.)*

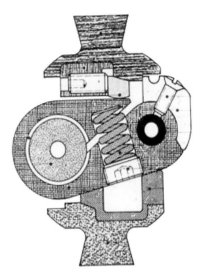

Figure 20 Most stance-control knees use a friction-brake mechanism for added stance stability. In the cross section depicted here, weight bearing compresses the spring and causes the knee to clamp against the cylindrical brake bushing. Unweighting the prosthesis allows the spring to open the clamping mechanism so that the lower leg can swing freely. *(Reproduced with permission from Otto Bock HealthCare.)*

greatest value, function, and durability without adding excessive weight.

Prosthetic Knee Mechanisms

Prosthetic knees can be grouped into five functional classes based on their biomechanical performance.[34] This initial classification suggests primary indications and specific limitations and provides a convenient guideline for prescription. Once the appropriate functional class has been determined, the prosthetist must then choose the specific product that he or she believes will offer the greatest durability and functional performance with the lowest cost and weight penalty.

Single-Axis Knee

Until World War II, the only prosthetic knee that was widely available in the United States was a basic hinge design that allowed the lower leg to bend freely during the swing phase of gait (Figure 19). Because of its mechanical simplicity, the single-axis knee remains the least expensive and most maintenance-free option. It is still widely used in children's prostheses, where rugged simplicity is a primary consideration. It is also sometimes recommended for amputees who live in remote areas and cannot arrange regular prosthetic follow-up.

Unfortunately, the basic single-axis knee has two major biomechanical deficiencies. First, the knee has no inherent stability, and therefore must be carefully controlled by the amputee with every step to prevent collapse of the prosthesis.[35] Because the typical new amputee today is an elderly individual with concomitant medical problems, such perfect control of every step is often an unrealistic expectation.

Equally important, with a free-swinging knee, the lower leg is essentially a pendulum with a rate of swing limited by its length. As a consequence, the amputee is forced to walk at a constant, slow speed. Attempts to accelerate result in excessive knee flexion in early swing, which slows the cadence even further. Even with the addition of a friction adjustment or a spring extension aid, the cadence is still severely restricted.[36]

Because of these dual biomechanical shortcomings, basic single-axis knees are increasingly rare. Amputees with sufficient strength and reflexes to safely control such a device are also able to vary their walking speed; therefore, it is rarely an optimal choice for adults. Pediatric application is more common, in part because the shorter lower leg swings at a faster rate than the longer pendulum of the adult prosthesis.

Stance-Control Knee

The stance-control knee is the most commonly prescribed prosthetic knee design worldwide.[37] These mechanisms typically have a weight-activated friction brake. As the amputee applies weight to the prosthesis in early stance, the brake is engaged and the resulting friction holds the knee securely (Figure 20). Stance-control knees are sometimes used in preparatory prostheses because their simplicity and safety help new amputees learn to walk on a prosthesis.[38]

To flex the knee, the amputee must shift weight onto the opposite leg. Once the prosthesis is fully unloaded, the brake mechanism is released so the lower leg can then swing freely. Most patients have no trouble learning to walk in this fashion, even though it results in an abnormal gait pattern.

The requirement to shift weight off the prosthesis prematurely to allow knee flexion presents few problems at slow cadences. However, if the amputee tries to walk at a more normal speed, the lack of knee flexion under partial weight bearing during late stance phase significantly disrupts the gait pattern. For this reason, stance-control knees are most appropriate for limited ambulators who are capable of walking only at a slow pace because of cardiopulmonary restrictions or similar comorbidities.

The use of bilateral friction-brake knees may present a risk to the amputee in the event of a fall, because it will be impossible to voluntarily bend the knees and control the direction of collapse. Accordingly, for bilateral amputees, the stance-control knee is best used on only one side, if at all.

Polycentric Knee

Polycentric knees can be identified by the multiple articulations they contain, with four axis points being the most common configuration. Because the four axes are connected by four linkage bars, this type of polycentric knee is also called a four-bar knee. Five-, six-, and seven-bar designs are also now commercially available.[39]

Polycentric designs offer several biomechanical advantages and are increasingly popular as a result. A key distinction is that the functional center of rotation is generally located outside the knee joint itself. In a four-bar type of polycentric knee, the instantaneous center of rotation (ICOR) can be determined geometrically by drawing straight lines through the posterior and anterior axes (Figure 21). The point where these lines intersect is the ICOR—the point in space where this knee effectively articulates.[40]

In a typical design, the ICOR is located posteriorly and proximally to the mechanical knee axes. The posterior position makes this knee inherently stable because the GRF is located far anteriorly, thus generating a strong extension moment. As the amputee starts to flex the knee, the ICOR changes; typically, it moves more anteriorly and distally with each additional degree of knee flexion.

Once the knee has been flexed a few degrees, the ICOR falls in front of the GRF and a flexion moment is created. This combination of a posterior ICOR at extension and a much more anterior ICOR after a few degrees of knee flexion makes the typical polycentric knee very stable in early stance and yet relatively easy to flex in late stance, even under partial weight bearing. The proximal location of the ICOR also gives the amputee a leverage advantage over an articulation at the anatomic knee center, making it

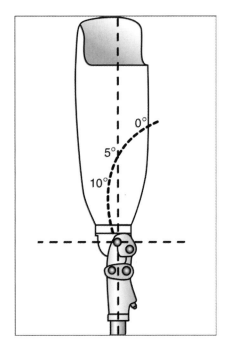

Figure 21 Polycentric knees have an initial ICOR that typically falls proximal and posterior to the mechanical axes. As the knee is flexed, the ICOR usually moves in an anterior and distal direction, as shown here, along a characteristic arc called the centrode. (*Reproduced with permission from James Breakey, PhD, CP.*)

easier to voluntarily control the prosthesis.[41]

Polycentric knees offer yet another biomechanical advantage—additional toe clearance at midswing. The actual ground clearance can increase as much as 3 cm for some knee designs,[42] thus significantly reducing the risk of tripping on environmental obstacles.

Because of these biomechanical advantages, polycentric knees are widely prescribed. Many clinicians advocate their use over friction-brake stance-control components when added stability is desired. Polycentric knees also work very well bilaterally, providing stability without preventing voluntary knee flexion under partial weight bearing.

In addition to polycentric designs that offer enhanced stability, a second group of polycentric knees is designed to minimize the protrusion beyond the socket in flexion.[43] As shown in Figure 22, the linkage in these knees

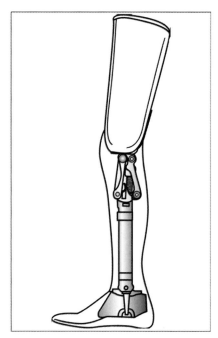

Figure 22 One special class of polycentric knees is designed to minimize the protrusion beyond the end of the socket in flexion. They are intended for use with knee disarticulation and similar very long residual limbs. (*Reproduced with permission from Otto Bock HealthCare.*)

pulls the lower leg back under the socket at 90° of flexion; this design is ideal for knee disarticulations and similarly very long residual limbs.[44]

In recent years, complex polycentric knees featuring five-, six-, or seven-bar linkages have become available. Most offer more stance-phase functions than four-bar designs, such as a geometric lock that automatically engages and disengages during ambulation. Some provide a limited range of controlled knee flexion during the loading response phase of gait, simulating this shock-absorbing motion of the biologic knee (Figure 23). Gait studies have confirmed that these stance-flexion knees result in a more biomechanically normal gait pattern.[45]

Manual Lock Knee

Manual lock knees provide maximum stability by locking the knee in full extension throughout the gait cycle. Because swing-phase knee flexion is eliminated, the prosthesis is functionally too long; therefore, the amputee

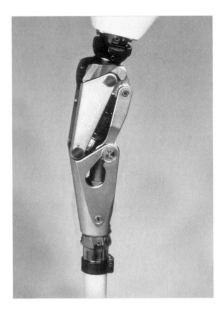

Figure 23 Polycentric knee with more complex linkage to provide controlled knee flexion in early stance phase. *(Reproduced with permission from Otto Bock HealthCare.)*

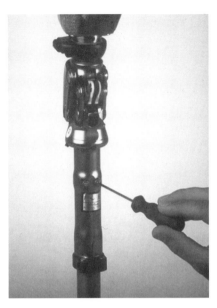

Figure 24 This hybrid knee combines the stability of a polycentric knee with the cadence response of a pneumatic fluid-control cylinder. The individual adjustment valve allows the prosthetist to independently set the amount of knee flexion and knee extension resistance. *(Reproduced with permission from Otto Bock HealthCare.)*

must hip-hike, vault, circumduct, or abduct the prosthesis to clear the floor. These necessary compensations not only result in an abnormal gait but are also believed to increase the energy cost of ambulation. It is customary to shorten a prosthesis with a manual lock knee approximately 1 cm to facilitate toe clearance; however, this means that the amputee will seem to step into a hole with each gait cycle.

Because of the abnormal gait compensations required, the manual lock knee can be considered the knee of last resort and should not be used if a polycentric or other design will suffice. If it must be used temporarily, because of patient weakness or similar considerations, the manual lock knee should be replaced with a more functional mechanism as soon as feasible, before the gait faults become habitual.

It appears that a locked knee does not provide a more energy-efficient gait than a free-swinging knee,[46] but it may permit feeble elderly patients to walk more rapidly[47] and therefore be preferred for this population.[48] Locked knees should rarely be used bilaterally because they prevent the

amputee from bending the knee in the event of a fall.

Locked knees are routinely provided for toddlers and small children until they have developed sufficient balance to walk with a free-swinging knee.[49] Recent studies have challenged the assumption that this practice is justified, however, because even very young children fitted with a polycentric or similar free-swinging knee learn to master its use and appear to develop a more mature gait pattern earlier than those who transition from a locked knee prosthesis.[49]

Fluid-Controlled Knee

The term fluid-controlled knee refers to a prosthetic knee that incorporates a pneumatic or hydraulic unit to control knee motion.[50] Research has shown that fluid-controlled knees provide a smoother, more normal swing-phase movement and automatically compensate for moderate changes in the amputee's cadence.[51] They are therefore indicated whenever the amputee is capable of walking at variable speeds.

Because pneumatic knees use air as the control medium, their function is not affected by ambient temperature; they may be preferable in bitterly cold climates where the thickening of hydraulic fluid could be a concern. The primary limitation to pneumatic knees is that they may not provide sufficient resistance for very vigorous activities because gases such as air are compressible.[52] In clinical experience, however, they are well accepted by the amputee and provide good swing-phase control for many people.

Hydraulic knees, in contrast, use an incompressible liquid to control knee motion. For this reason, they can provide as much swing-phase resistance as necessary,[53] and some are designed to provide hydraulic stance stability as well. Because only a small volume of liquid is required for swing-phase control, some hydraulic knees are considerably smaller and lighter than pneumatic models.

Fluid-controlled knees are more complicated and therefore more costly than simpler mechanical devices, and they require periodic servicing to replace worn seals. However, many amputees consider the increase in function well worth the additional cost and maintenance.

Hybrid Knees

In an effort to offer the amputee a more versatile knee component, designers have created knees that combine the features of one or more of the generic functional groups discussed above. One of the most clinically popular combinations uses a polycentric knee with its biomechanical advantages and adds a hydraulic or pneumatic fluid-controlled unit to provide variable cadence swing-phase control[54] (Figure 24).

Another hybrid knee with hydraulic control (Figure 25) provides hydraulic swing-phase control for variable cadence; hydraulic stance control, in the form of yielding resistance to knee flexion during the first half of stance phase; and an optional manual lock, for added safety during activities such as climbing ladders.[55] Compo-

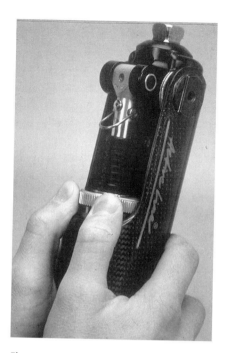

Figure 25 This hybrid knee has a hydraulic knee control cylinder that offers independently adjustable swing resistance as well as a yielding stance-flexion resistance for added stability. *(Reproduced with permission from Otto Bock HealthCare)*

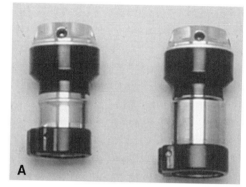
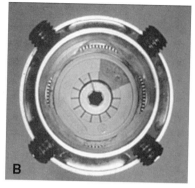

Figure 26 Torque absorber. **A,** Side view. **B,** The device shown can be adjusted, as shown in the transverse view, to increase or decrease the resistance to motion. *(Reproduced with permission from Otto Bock HealthCare.)*

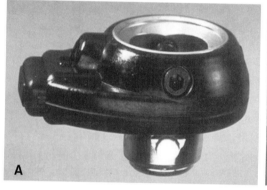
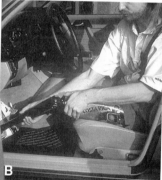

Figure 27 Positional rotator. **A,** Side view. **B,** Amputee uses the device to enter a vehicle. *(Reproduced with permission from Otto Bock HealthCare.)*

nents that provide stance security as well as variable cadence swing-phase resistances are often called "stance and swing" units.

Microprocessor Control

The recent addition of microprocessor control to automatically adjust the resistance of fluid-controlled knees while the amputee is walking has proved its clinical value.[56] Scientific studies suggest that microprocessor control makes the gait kinematics more normal[57] and may result in a more energy-efficient gait.[58] Amputee acceptance of this technology has been very encouraging.[59]

The use of microprocessor control in lower limb components is expected to increase steadily in future years, enabling the amputee to engage in a greater range of normal activities of daily living. In addition to providing the ability to adjust the stance stability and swing-phase control of the prosthesis while the person is walking, microprocessor control can provide specialized resistances that facilitate work

tasks such as standing during surgery or hairdressing, and recreational activities such as a bent-knee stance for golfing or skiing.

Knee Components Summary

Table 4 summarizes the characteristics of the functional classes of prosthetic knees, allowing the clinic team to quickly rule out biomechanically inappropriate alternatives and to focus on those components most suitable for the individual. In many instances, hybrid designs that combine the characteristics of two or more functional classes are preferred. Microprocessor control makes the knee component self-adjusting, and although presently limited to fluid-controlled mechanisms, may be applied to other functional classes in the future.

Other Functional Components

No discussion of lower limb prosthetic components would be complete without mentioning several items that provide additional functional capabilities in the prosthesis. These devices are typically located in the shin or thigh region of the prosthesis.

Torque Absorber

The torque absorber (Figure 26) is a small component that permits controlled transverse rotation[60] and thereby absorbs many of the stresses that would normally be transmitted from the floor to the prosthetic components and ultimately to the amputee's skin.[61] The torque absorber may be used in lieu of a multiaxial ankle, or to supplement the movement provided by a multiaxial foot. For bilateral amputees, torque absorbers are

TABLE 4 Overview of Prosthetic Knees

Generic Class	Basic Function	Primary Indication	Major Advantages	Chief Limitations
Single axis (Constant friction)	Simplicity	Single-speed walking only if hip control is good or better or when maximum durability is required	Inexpensive and durable	Fixed cadence and low stability
Stance-control	Increased weight-bearing stability	General debility; poor hip control	Improved knee stability	Delayed swing phase; must unload fully to flex or sit
Polycentric	Positive stability and ease of flexion for swing phase; special design available that provides sitting cosmesis for long residual limbs	To enhance knee stability; special design available for knee disarticulation	Stable without disrupting swing phase; special design provides cosmesis for long residual limbs	Increased weight, maintenance, initial cost
Manual lock	Knee of last resort	Ultimate knee stability	Eliminates knee flexion	Abnormal gait; awkward sitting
Fluid-controlled	Permits cadence change; micro-processor control offers most normal gait pattern	Able to vary walking speed	Variable cadence; more natural gait; hydraulic stance control adds stability	Increased initial cost; may involve increased weight or maintenance

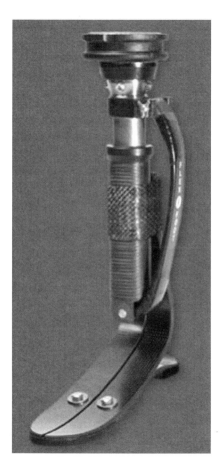

Figure 28 Dynamic-response foot with an integrated vertical shock absorber. Separate vertical shock-absorbing mechanisms are also available, including units that also provide torque absorption in the transverse plane. *(Reproduced with permission from OSSUR.)*

sometimes used in pairs in each prosthesis, to provide twice as much rotary motion and thereby facilitate a reciprocal gait.

Positional Rotator

The positional rotator is a locking turntable, generally located just proximal to the prosthetic knee, that allows the amputee to passively rotate the lower leg (Figure 27). This capability facilitates sitting, dressing, entering a vehicle, and similar everyday activities. As a general guideline, a positional rotator should be considered whenever there is sufficient space between the knee and the socket for this component.

Shock-Absorbing Pylon

In recent years, telescoping spring-loaded pylons have become available. These components are intended to partially replace the biomechanical shock absorption that is lost when the leg is amputated.[62]

Although scientific data are limited,[63] clinical acceptance of these components suggests that the amputee perceives an increase in comfort while using a shock-absorbing pylon, particularly for activities such as descending stairs or stepping down from a curb or vehicle. These components (Figure 28) are routinely recommended for active amputees who engage in recreational or competitive sport, because of the higher impacts involved in such activities,[64] yet they have also been well accepted by general community ambulators.

Conclusion

It is rarely possible to prescribe prosthetic components and suspensions solely on the basis of scientific evidence because of the dearth of available objective data. It is always possible, however, to recommend specific devices based on a logical rationale. One of the most widely accepted approaches is to match the biomechanical performance of the prosthetic components to the individual amputee's functional goals and physical abilities.

To facilitate this approach, lower limb components and suspensions can be grouped conceptually into specific classes based on their performance characteristics. This allows inappropriate choices to be quickly identified and ruled out. The clinic team can then focus on selecting the optimal specific design for each individual amputee, based on the best currently available scientific evidence and local clinical experience.

References

1. Staros A, Rubin G: Prescription considerations in modern above-knee prosthetics. *Phys Med Rehabil Clin N Am* 1991;2:311-324.

2. Michael JW: Prosthetic knee mechanisms. *Phys Med Rehabil: State of the Art Rev* 1994;8:147-164.

3. Meier RH, Meeks ED, Herman RM: Stump-socket fit of below-knee prostheses: Comparison of three methods of measurement. *Arch Phys Med Rehabil* 1973;54:553-558.

4. Grevsten S, Eriksson U: Stump-socket contact and skeletal displacement in a suction patellar-tendon bearing prosthesis. *J Bone Joint Surg Am* 1974;56: 1692-1696.

5. Canty TJ: Suction socket for above knee prosthesis. *United States Naval Med Bull* 1949;49:216-233.

6. Levy SW: Skin problems of the leg amputee. *Prosthet Orthot Int* 1980;4: 37-44.

7. Kristinsson O: The ICEROSS concept: A discussion of a philosophy. *Prosthet Orthot Int* 1993;17:49-55.

8. Fillauer CE, Pritham CH, Fillauer KD: Evolution and development of the Silicone Suction Socket (3S) for below-knee prostheses. *J Prosthet Orthot* 1989;1:92-103.

9. Heim M, Wershavski M, Zwas ST, et al: Silicone suspension of external prostheses: A new era in artificial limb usage. *J Bone Joint Surg Br* 1997;79: 638-640.

10. Jain AS, Stewart CPU: The use of the shuttle lock system for problem transfemoral suspension. *Prosthet Orthot Int* 1999;23:256-257.

11. Goswami J, Lynn R, Street G, et al: Walking in a vacuum-assisted socket shifts the stump fluid balance. *Prosthet Orthot Int* 2003;23:107-113.

12. Chino N, Pearson JR, Cockrell JL, et al: Negative pressures during swing phase in below-knee prostheses with rubber sleeve suspension. *Arch Phys Med Rehabil* 1975;56:22-26.

13. Doyle W, Goldstone J, Kramer D: The Syme prosthesis revisited. *J Prosthet Orthot* 1993;5:95-99.

14. Meyer LC, Bailey HI, Friddle D: An improved prosthesis for fitting the ankle-disarticulation amputee. *ICIB* 1970;9:11-15.

15. Breakey JW: Criteria for use of supracondylar and supracondylar-suprapatellar suspension for below-knee prostheses. *Orthot Prosthet* 1973; 27:14-18.

16. Pritham CH: Suspension of the below-knee prosthesis: An overview. *Orthot Prosthet* 1979;33:1-19.

17. Kapp SL: Transfemoral socket design and suspension options. *Phys Med Rehabil Clin N Am* 2000;11:569-583.

18. Shem KL, Breakey JW, Werner PC: Pressures at the residual limb-socket interface in transtibial amputees with thigh lacer-side joints. *J Prosthet Orthot* 1998;10:51-55.

19. Swanson VM: The anatomical above-knee suspension belt. *J Prosthet Orthot* 1992;4:119-125.

20. Michael JW: Overview of prosthetic feet. *Instr Course Lect* 1990;39:367-372.

21. Czerniecki JM, Gitter A: Prosthetic feet: A scientific and clinical review of current components. *Phys Med Rehabil* 1994;8:109-128.

22. Doane NE, Holt LE: A comparison of the SACH and single axis foot in the gait of unilateral below-knee amputees. *Prosthet Orthot Int* 1983;7:33-36.

23. Lehmann JF, Price R, Boswell-Bessette S, et al: Comprehensive analysis of dynamic elastic response feet: Seattle Ankle/Lite foot versus SACH foot. *Arch Phys Med Rehabil* 1993;74: 853-861.

24. Van Leeuwen JL, Speth LAWM, Daanen HAM: Shock absorption of below-knee prostheses: A comparison between the SACH and the multiflex foot. *J Biomech* 1990;23:441-446.

25. Campbell JW, Childs CW: The S.A.F.E. foot. *Orthot Prosthet* 1980;34:3-16.

26. Michael J: Energy storing feet: A clinical comparison. *Clin Prosthet Orthot* 1987;11:154-168.

27. Wing DC, Hittenberger DA: Energy-storing prosthetic feet. *Arch Phys Med Rehabil* 1989;70:330-335.

28. Murray DD, Hartvikson WJ, Anton H, et al: With a spring in one's step. *Clin Prosthet Orthot* 1988;12:128-135.

29. Gitter A, Czerniecki JM, Degroot DM: Biomechanical analysis of the influence of prosthetic feet on below-knee amputee walking. *Am J Phys Med Rehabil* 1991;70:142-148.

30. Alaranta H, Kinnunen A, Karkkainen M, et al: Practical benefits of Flex-Foot in below-knee amputees. *J Prosthet Orthot* 1991;3:179-181.

31. Czerniecki JM, Gitter A: Insights into amputee running: A muscle work analysis. *Am J Phys Med Rehabil* 1992; 71:209-218.

32. Torburn L, Powers CM, Guiterrez R, et al: Energy expenditure during ambulation in dysvascular and traumatic below-knee amputees: A comparison of 5 prosthetic feet. *J Rehabil Res Dev* 1995;32:111-119.

33. Crandall RC, Anderson TF, Backus B, et al: Clinical evaluation of an articulated, dynamic-response prosthetic foot in teenage transtibial and Syme-level amputees. *J Prosthet Orthot* 1999; 11:92-97.

34. Michael JW: Modern prosthetic knee mechanisms. *Clin Orthop* 1999;361: 39-47.

35. Radcliffe CW: Functional considerations in the fitting of above-knee prostheses. *Artif Limbs* 1955;2:35-60.

36. Murphy EF: The swing phase of walking with above-knee prostheses. *Bull Prosthet Res* 1964;10:5-39.

37. Fishman S, Berger N, Watkins D: A survey of prosthetics practice: 1973-74. *Orthot Prosthet* 1975;29:15-20.

38. Romo HD: Prosthetic knees. *Phys Med Rehabil Clin N Am* 2000;11:595-607.

39. Breakey JW, Marquette SH: Beyond the four-bar knee. *J Prosthet Orthot* 1998;10:77-80.

40. Radcliffe CW: Four-bar linkage prosthetic knee mechanisms: Kinematics, alignment and prescription criteria. *Prosthet Orthot Int* 1994;18:159-173.

41. Greene MP: Four bar linkage knee analysis. *Orthot Prosthet* 1984;37: 15-24.

42. Gard SA, Childress DS, Vellendahl JE: The influence of four-bar linkage knees on prosthetic swing-phase floor clearance. *J Prosthet Orthot* 1996;8: 34-40.

43. Gardner HF, Peizer E: Some physiological and prosthetic considerations in the selection of amputation sites about the knee. *Bull Prosthet Res* 1969; 10:26-33.

44. Oberg K: Knee mechanisms for through-knee prostheses. *Prosthet Orthot Int* 1983;7:107-112.

45. Gard SA, Childress DS: What determines the vertical displacement of the body during normal walking? *J Prosthet Orthot* 2001;13:64-67.

46. Traugh GH, Corcoran PJ, Reyes RL: Energy expenditure of ambulation in patients with above-knee amputations. *Arch Phys Med Rehabil* 1975;56: 67-71.

47. Isakov E, Susak Z, Becker E: Energy expenditure and cardiac response in above-knee amputees while using prostheses with open and locked knee mechanisms. *Scand J Rehabil Med* 1985;12:108-111.

48. Devlin M, Sinclair LB, Colman D, et al: Patient preference and gait efficiency in a geriatric population with transfemoral amputation using a free-swinging versus a locked prosthetic knee joint. *Arch Phys Med Rehabil* 2002;83:246-249.

49. Wilk B, Karol L, Halliday S, et al: Transition to an articulating knee prosthesis in pediatric amputees. *J Prosthet Orthot* 1999;11:69-74.

50. Staros A, Murphy EF: Properties of fluid flow applied to above-knee prostheses. *Bull Prosthet Res* 1964;10:40-65.

51. Staros A: The principles of swing-phase control: The advantages of fluid mechanisms. *Prostheses Braces Tech Aids* 1964;13:11-16.

52. Radcliffe CW, Lamoreux L: UCBL Pneumatic Swing-Control Unit for above-knee prostheses: Design, adjustment and installation. *Bull Prosthet Res* 1968;10:73-89.

53. Sekikawa S, Sugano S, Yamamoto S: Relationship between the mechanical properties of knee joints of above-knee prostheses and amputee gait. *Gait Posture* 1995;3:268-269.

54. Zarrugh MY, Radcliffe CW: Simulation of swing phase in above-knee prostheses. *J Biomech* 1976;9:283-292.

55. Hinterbuchner C, Sakuma J, Levy D: Hydraulic swing and stance phase control for above-knee amputees. *Arch Phys Med Rehabil* 1975;56:179-182.

56. Kocher L: Das kniegelensystem C-LEG-klinische versorgungsstatistik (the C-LEG knee system: Evaluation of clinical results). *Med Orthop Tech* 2001;121:129-134.

57. Kirker S, Keymer S, Talbot J, et al: An assessment of the intelligent knee prosthesis. *Clin Rehabil* 1996;10: 267-273.

58. Taylor MB, Clark E, Offord EA: A comparison of energy expenditure by a high level trans-femoral amputee using the Intelligent Prosthesis and conventionally damped prosthetic limbs. *Prosthet Orthot Int* 1996;20: 116-121.

59. Datta D, Howitt J: Conventional versus microchip controlled pneumatic swing phase control for trans-femoral amputees: User's verdict. *Prosthet Orthot Int* 1998;22: 129-135.

60. Racette W, Breakey JW: Clinical experience and functional considerations of axial rotators for the amputee. *Orthot Prosthet* 1977;31:29-33.

61. Levens AS, Inman VT, Blosser JA: Transverse rotation of the segments of the lower extremity in locomotion. *J Bone Joint Surg Am* 1948;30:859-872.

62. Miller LA, Childress DE: Analysis of a vertical compliance prosthetic foot. *J Rehabil Res Dev* 1997;34:52-57.

63. Hsu MJ, Nielsen DH, Yack HJ, et al: Physiological measurement of walking and running in people with transtibial amputations with 3 different prostheses. *J Orthop Sports Phys Ther* 1999;29: 526-533.

64. Hsu MJ, Nielsen DH, Yack J, et al: Physiological comparisons of physically active persons with transtibial amputation using static and dynamic prostheses versus persons with non-pathological gait during multiple-speed walking. *J Prosthet Orthot* 2000;12:60-67.

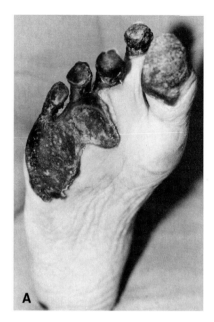
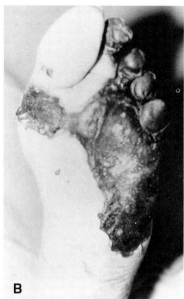
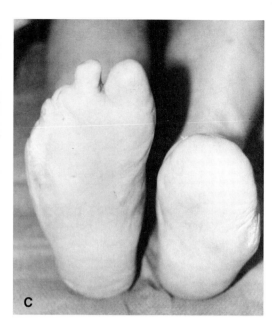

Figure 7 Plantar views of feet of a 60-year-old man with lupus erythematosus and bilateral dry gangrene. Right foot **(A)** and left foot **(B)** show good perfusion proximal to lines of demarcation. **C,** Eleven months after radical débridement of the right foot and Lisfranc disarticulation of the left foot. *(Reproduced with permission from Bowker JH, San Giovanni TP: Amputations and disarticulations, in Myerson MS (ed): Foot and Ankle Disorders. Philadelphia, PA, WB Saunders, 2000.)*

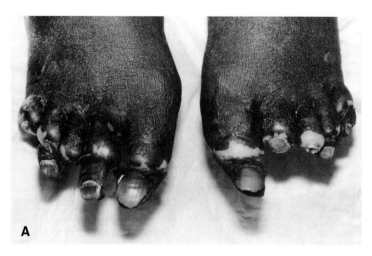
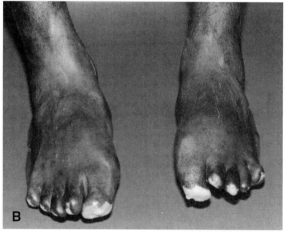

Figure 8 A, Feet of a 41-year-old man with acquired immunodeficiency syndrome who awoke from septic coma with partial necrosis of all toes. Treatment consisted of keeping the toes dry and protected from trauma. **B,** Twenty months later, completed autoamputations are evident. *(Reproduced with permission from Bowker JH, San Giovanni TP: Amputations and disarticulations, in Myerson MS (ed): Foot and Ankle Disorders. Philadelphia, PA, WB Saunders, 2000.)*

and viable tissue, a regimen of minor débridement, oral antibiotics, and local application of drying agents such as povidone-iodine may avert the conversion of dry to wet gangrene. As each toe sloughs its necrotic portion, usually through a joint, the wound will have largely or completely closed (Figure 8). This approach is especially appropriate when the patient is not a candidate for limb bypass surgery be-cause of health status yet has not de-veloped critical limb ischemia requir-ing a major amputation (Figure 9). Most important, areas of dry gan-grene must never be treated with soaks, whirlpool baths, wet dressings, or débriding agents. Moistening the junction of viable and gangrenous tis-sue encourages bacterial and fungal growth, converting an easily managed condition to an emergent one.

Infection

Wet (infective) gangrene may spread along fascial planes and tendon sheaths with alarming rapidity, abet-ted by several factors. Continued weight bearing, commonly seen in di-abetic patients lacking protective sen-sation, causes the dispersal of pus ac-cumulating under pressure. As definitive treatment is delayed be-cause of lack of protective sensation

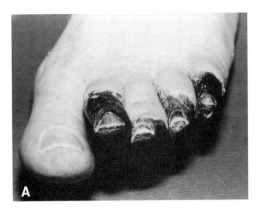
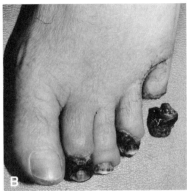
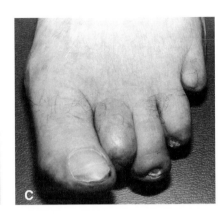

Figure 9 A, Left foot of 77-year-old man with diabetes mellitus and a 30-year history of smoking. Note partial dry gangrene of the lateral four toes. Vascular reconstruction was not feasible because of his cardiac status. **B,** Three months later, apparent gangrene had receded in all toes, and the fifth toe had sloughed through the proximal interphalangeal joint. **C,** Six months later, there was considerable tissue salvage by allowing completion of autoamputation without surgical interference. (*A and C are reproduced with permission from Bowker JH: Transtibial amputation, in Murdoch G, Wilson AB Jr (eds):* Amputation Surgery: Surgical Practice and Patient Management. *Oxford, England, Butterworth–Heinemann, 1996, pp 43-58.) (B is reproduced with permission from Bowker JH, San Giovanni TP: Amputations and disarticulations, in Myerson MS (ed):* Foot and Ankle Disorders. *Philadelphia, PA, WB Saunders, 2000.)*

and attendant denial, single-species infections soon become polymicrobial. The wound can be probed with a sterile cotton-tipped applicator. If bone is contacted, a presumptive diagnosis of osteomyelitis can be made, even without the use of expensive bone scans.[13] Confirmation is obtained by coned-down radiographs. Aerobic and anaerobic cultures should be taken at this time, allowing presumptive selection of antibiotics pending the results of cultures and antibiotic sensitivity tests. Because most diabetic foot infections are polymicrobial, broad-spectrum antibiotics should be administered intravenously. The length of foot that can be salvaged is often profoundly affected by the behavioral and temporal factors already noted, so surgical débridement must be undertaken promptly to avert further tissue loss. If a definitive débridement must be delayed more than a few hours, the abscess should be drained in the emergency department to control further spread of infection. This can be performed with or without ankle block anesthesia, depending on the severity of sensory loss from diabetic neuropathy. Decompressive incisions must respect all normal weight-bearing skin surfaces such as the heel pad, lateral sole, and the surface di-

rectly plantar to the metatarsal heads. Incisions should be longitudinally oriented to avoid as many vascular and neural structures as possible. By unnecessarily extending an incision into the heel pad or proximal to the ankle joint, a more proximal ablation, such as a Syme ankle disarticulation, may be severely compromised.

The interdependence of serum glucose levels and infection control relates to the negative effect of chronic hyperglycemia on leukocyte function and on tissue resistance to infection. Serum glucose control should be initiated promptly, although this may be difficult in the face of infection, reinforcing the need for assistance from an internist as well as early formal débridement of all necrotic and infected tissue, including bone, in the operating suite. However, it may be unsafe to strive for tight serum glucose control until the patient is metabolically stable postoperatively.

General Surgical Technique (All Levels)

If the criteria for level selection are met and the standards for wound healing are correctly factored in, no amputation level in the foot need be

excluded on the basis of etiology. Longitudinal rather than transverse amputation should be the goal whenever functionally feasible. Narrowing the foot rather than shortening it greatly simplifies postoperative shoe fitting. Conversely, the surgeon should also consider the possibility that a failed forefoot or midfoot amputation performed because of infection may eliminate the opportunity for a Syme ankle disarticulation. Therefore, the surgeon must be reasonably sure that the initial level selection is logical.

In cases of foot infection, a careful and thorough débridement is the first step. Although the preoperative examination, radiographs, and vascular assessment provide valuable guidance, at the beginning of débridement the surgeon cannot be certain of the full proximal extent of an infective process or the viability of remaining tissues. The patient and family should be told that the procedure is, therefore, somewhat exploratory in nature and that based on further information obtained during the operation, the surgeon will be as conservative as possible in removal of tissue.

Both plantar and dorsal incisions may be required to fully drain all abscess pockets. All of the central plantar spaces described by Grodinsky[14] can be opened by the extensile plantar incision described by Loeffler and Ballard.[15] This incision begins posterior to the medial malleolus and ends distally between the first and second metatarsal heads. From there it may be extended as deeply into the first web space as necessary. Depending on the extent of the infection, all or part of this incision may be used. Distal infections may track across the entire distal foot pad, requiring a transverse incision at the base of the toes. Two parallel incisions may be required to obtain full exposure of a dorsal infection, but they should be as widely separated as possible. Even then, the intervening skin bridge may necrose because of septic thrombosis of its small skin vessels. After removal of obviously necrotic tissue, the dorsal and plantar surfaces of the foot should be firmly stroked proximally to distally along tissue planes to discover and empty remaining pockets of pus. These pockets are then probed to their proximal end, opened widely, and débrided. If a severe midfoot infection is present but the heel pad is spared, an open Syme ankle disarticulation is indicated. Extension of infection along tendon sheaths proximal to the ankle joint or into the heel pad or ankle joint generally precludes anything but an open true ankle disarticulation and a delayed transtibial amputation. Even when the extent of involvement is initially uncertain, preliminary exploration with aggressive débridement rarely adds much time to the overall procedure. All poorly vascularized tissues, such as tendons, joint capsules, volar plates, and articular cartilage, should be treated as foreign bodies and removed as part of a thorough débridement. If this is not done, the wound may remain open for months until these structures sequestrate. All well-vascularized tissue should be saved for secondary reconstruction regardless of configuration to assist in preserving foot length for maximum function. The guillotine approach, in contrast, will preclude creative use of

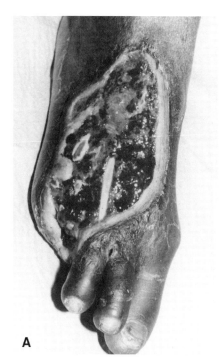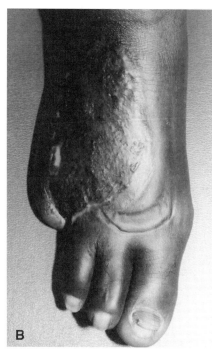

Figure 10 A, Right foot of 52-year-old woman with diabetes mellitus following disarticulation of the fourth and fifth toes and necrotic dorsal skin for wet gangrene. The wound is ready for split-thickness skin grafting on a bed of granulation tissue. **B,** Three months after grafting. The graft has now tolerated shoe wear for many years. *(Reproduced with permission from Bowker JH: Partial foot amputations and disarticulations. Foot Ankle Clin North Am 1997;2:153.)*

otherwise salvageable tissues in preservation of forefoot length.

Redébridement of a wound may be necessary for several reasons. First, it is often difficult to be certain that all infected and necrotic tissue has been removed primarily. Second, some areas of skin that initially appeared viable may have become frankly necrotic. Finally, the infection may have persisted despite the débridement and antibiotic use. Therefore, manually stripping the infected areas from proximal to distal every 24 to 48 hours to locate pockets of infection that may have escaped initial detection is a sound practice. Limited secondary débridements can be done at bedside or, if more extensive or the patient requires ankle block anesthesia, in the operating room.

When primary wound closure can be accomplished safely, other factors should be considered. To absorb the shear and direct (normal) forces generated during gait, the soft-tissue envelope must be mobile. The envelope is ideally formed of plantar skin, subcutaneous tissue, and investing fascia. Although muscle tissue is an integral part of the soft-tissue envelope in more proximal amputations, it is not available at all these levels. Adherence of skin directly to bone must be minimized to prevent ulceration from shear forces during walking. This is best accomplished by avoiding coverage with split-thickness skin grafts on the distal, lateral, and plantar surfaces of the residual foot whenever possible.[16] Conversely, split-thickness skin grafts placed dorsally, even on granulated bony surfaces, can last indefinitely with reasonable care (Figure 10). To prevent further damage to skin with compromised vascularity, such skin should never be handled with forceps during surgery. Proper contouring of all bone ends will prevent damage to the soft-tissue envelope from within wherever it is compressed between bone and the prosthesis, orthosis, or shoe. To prevent equinus contracture of the ankle

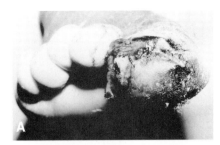

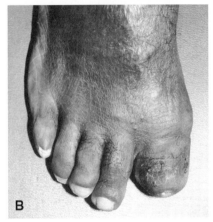

Figure 11 A, Right foot of a 49-year-old man with diabetes mellitus who has wet gangrene of the great toe and adequate perfusion proximally. **B,** After interphalangeal disarticulation following conservative débridement and primary closure over Kritter flow-through irrigation system. *(Reproduced with permission from Bowker JH: Surgical techniques for conserving tissue and function in lower-limb amputation for trauma, infection, and vascular disease.* Instr Course Lect *1990; 39:355-360.)*

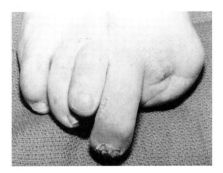

Figure 12 Right foot of a 46-year-old man with diabetes mellitus who has osteomyelitis of the distal phalanx of the second toe with mallet deformity of the distal interphalangeal joint. Disarticulation of the distal phalanx was curative. Previous MTP disarticulation of the great toe left the insensate second toe exposed to trauma. *(Reproduced with permission from Bowker JH: Minor and major lower limb amputations in diabetes mellitus, in Bowker JH, Pfeifer MA (eds):* Levin and O'Neal's The Diabetic Foot, *ed 6. St. Louis, MO, Mosby, 2001.)*

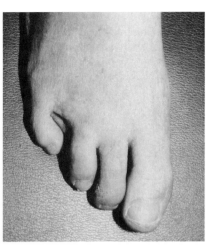

Figure 13 Medial shift of right fifth toe closed the gap from earlier disarticulation of the fourth toe, restoring a smooth distal contour to the forefoot. No further ulcerations occurred during an 8.5-year follow-up period. *(Reproduced with permission from Bowker JH: Role of lower limb amputation in diabetes mellitus, in Levin ME, O'Neal LW, Bowker JH (eds): The Diabetic Foot, ed 5. St. Louis, MO, Mosby-Year Book, 1993, pp 433-455.)*

joint in foot ablations proximal to the MTP joints, postoperative casting in slight dorsiflexion for 3 to 4 weeks is recommended. By weakening the plantar flexors relative to the dorsiflexors, immobilization results in a residual foot with better muscle balance.

Toe Disarticulations
Method

Even when osteomyelitis is present in the distal phalanx of the great toe, sufficient skin can often be salvaged to permit an interphalangeal disarticulation. The remaining proximal phalanx will aid with balance and result in a much better gait than results after disarticulation at the MTP joint. This

is due to preservation of the flexor hallucis brevis complex, including the sesamoids and hence the windlass mechanism (Figure 11). To achieve closure of the wound without tension, trimming the condylar prominences and shortening the proximal phalanx by removing the articular cartilage are often necessary. When a more radical resection of the proximal phalanx is required, Wagner[17] recommends leaving just its base, to keep both the sesamoids and the plantar fat pad beneath the metatarsal head. The joint capsule is left intact, helping to limit proximal spread of infection.

The first MTP joint is the next site of election if the entire proximal phalanx is involved. After division of the flexor hallucis brevis insertions on the proximal phalanx, the sesamoid bones will displace proximally, exposing the prominent crista on the plantar surface of the metatarsal head. The sesamoids may also become troublesome bony prominences just proximal to the metatarsal head. For this reason the sesamoids, with their fibrocartilaginous plate, should be excised and the crista removed with a rongeur. Following removal of the articu-

lar cartilage, the head should be smoothed carefully with a file.

Osteomyelitis of the distal phalanx of a lesser toe often occurs following ulceration of a mallet toe associated with loss of protective sensation. This is most commonly noted in the second toe in patients with a long second metatarsal bone, especially following disarticulation of the great toe, but may occur in any lesser toe (Figure 12). Removal of the infected distal phalanx both shortens and straightens the toe, reducing the risk of future ulceration.

If the third or fourth toe alone is disarticulated, the adjacent toes will tend to close the gap and restore a good contour to the distal forefoot (Figure 13). Amputation of the fifth toe alone may leave a wide fifth metatarsal head prominent laterally. In this case, the lateral condyle of the metatarsal head should be trimmed sagittally. Leaving a lesser toe isolated by removing toes on either side will increase the susceptibility of the isolated toe to deformity and injury (Figure 14).

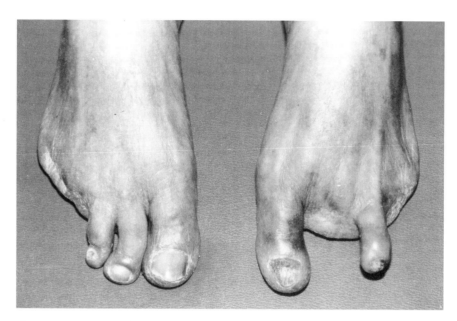

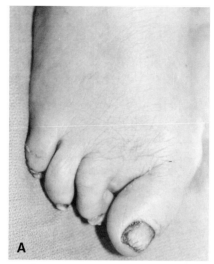

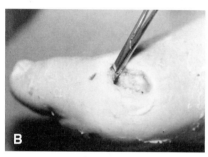

Figure 14 A striking difference is evident in the distal forefoot contours of the pictured insensate right and left feet. On the right foot, the remaining lesser toes are protected by the great toe. On the left foot, the fourth toe is constantly exposed to minor trauma and should have been removed with the other lesser toes, leaving the great toe to contribute to forward propulsion and easy shoe fitting. *(Reproduced with permission from Bowker JH: Minor and major lower limb amputations in diabetes mellitus, in Bowker JH, Pfeifer MA (eds):* Levin and O'Neal's The Diabetic Foot, *ed 6. St. Louis, MO, Mosby, 2001.)*

Figure 15 Result of right second toe disarticulation in an 87-year-old man with diabetes mellitus. **A,** Hallux valgus deformity secondary to loss of lateral support of second toe. **B,** Ulcer over bunion penetrating MTP joint. *(Reproduced with permission from Bowker JH, San Giovanni TP: Amputations and disarticulations, in Myerson MS (ed):* Foot and Ankle Disorders. *Philadelphia, PA, WB Saunders, 2000.)*

Disarticulation of the second toe at the MTP joint may create a special problem because it removes lateral support from the great toe that is required to prevent a hallux valgus (bunion) deformity. This iatrogenic bony prominence may lead to a pressure ulcer in an insensate foot (Figure 15). The probability of this occurrence can usually be reduced by removing the second metatarsal through its proximal metaphysis along with the toe. Following this ray amputation, the first and third metatarsals will normally approximate each other, narrowing the foot and resulting in a good cosmesis and function (Figure 16).

Occasionally, dry gangrene will occur in all five toes without significant change in perfusion proximally. In this case, disarticulation of all five toes can be accomplished with primary coverage of the metatarsal heads, provided the dorsal and plantar incisions are both made as far distally as possible in the web spaces. Removal of the artic-

ular cartilage and volar plates will increase the amount of skin available for closure (Figure 17).

Special Considerations

Walking function will be most affected by disarticulation of the great toe at the metacarpophalangeal joint because the role of the first ray in the final transfer of weight during late stance phase is lost. This effect was studied by Mann and associates[18] in 10 patients with an average age of 23 years who had undergone pollicization of the great toe. They found a shift in the end point of progression of the moving center of plantar pressure during stance from the second metatarsal head to the third. This occurred despite a dropping of the first metatarsal head following loss of the great toe and its stabilizing windlass mechanism. In this group, reported symptoms after an average of 3 years were minimal except for difficulty in movements requiring flexion of the

great toe during active sports. Whether significant problems will occur with aging is not known, but to prevent this, the authors suggested that the base of the proximal phalanx be left to preserve the windlass mechanism or that the insertion of the plantar aponeurosis and intrinsic muscles be sutured into the distal metatarsal to stabilize it.[18] These measures may not be possible in cases of infection or severe trauma. Loss of lesser toes, in contrast, appears to cause little clinical difficulty. Walking impairment following great toe disarticulation is minimized by provision of a shoe with a stiff sole, molded soft insert, and filler.

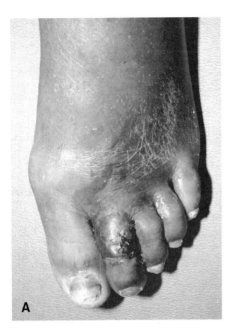 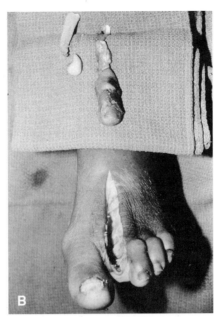 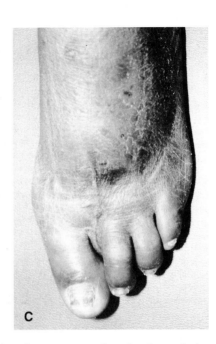

Figure 16 Left foot of a woman with diabetes mellitus who has osteomyelitis of the second ray from a penetrating ulcer beneath the prominent metatarsal head. **A,** Dorsal view demonstrates swelling centered over the second ray. **B,** Intraoperative view shows dissolution of the metatarsal neck and resected tissue. **C,** Postoperative view shows forefoot narrowing with no significant hallux valgus because of lateral support provided by the third toe.

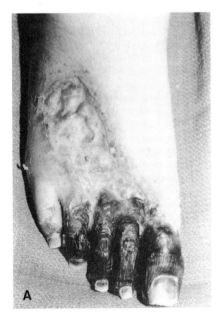 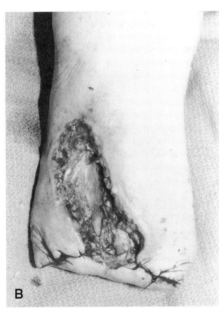 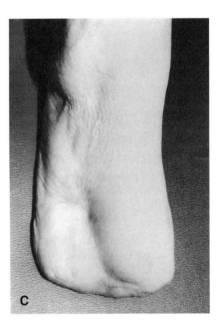

Figure 17 A, Right foot of a 63-year-old woman with lupus erythematosus and dry gangrene caused by microemboli. **B,** Intraoperative view showing partial closure after disarticulation of all five toes and débridement of necrotic dorsal skin. Because of arteritis, postoperative hyperbaric oxygen treatments were given. The dorsal defect healed by wound contraction. **C,** Seven years later, patient has excellent gait in a rocker-soled shoe with custom inlay. (**A** and **C** are reproduced with permission from Bowker JH: Partial foot amputations and disarticulations. *Foot Ankle Clin North Am* 1997;2:153.) (**B** is reproduced with permission from Bowker JH, San Giovanni TP: Amputations and disarticulations, in Myerson MS (ed): *Foot and Ankle Disorders.* Philadelphia, PA, WB Saunders, 2000.)

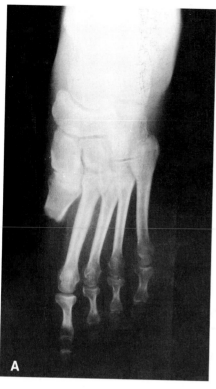
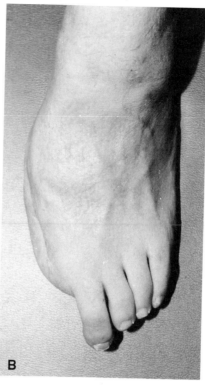

Figure 18 A, Radiograph of a left foot after radical first ray amputation for diabetic infection. Insufficient metatarsal shaft remains for effective orthotic support of the medial column. **B,** Planovalgus position of the foot secondary to loss of medial column support is evident. (*Reproduced with permission from Bowker JH: Medical and surgical considerations in the care of patients with insensate dysvascular feet.* J Prosthet Orthot *1992; 4:23-30.*)

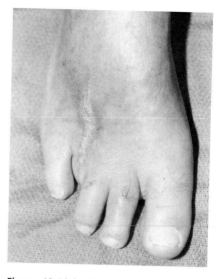

Figure 19 Right foot of a man with diabetes mellitus who underwent fourth ray amputation for osteomyelitis that healed by secondary intention. Narrowing of the forefoot and excellent distal forefoot contour are evident. (*Reproduced with permission from Bowker JH, San Giovanni TP: Amputations and disarticulations, in Myerson MS (ed):* Foot and Ankle Disorders. *Philadelphia, PA, WB Saunders, 2000.*)

Ray Amputations
Methods

In ray amputation, a toe and part or all of the metatarsal are removed. With the first or medial ray, as much metatarsal shaft length should be left as possible to allow for effective elevation of the medial arch with a custom-molded insert (Figure 18). The insert should be fitted into a shoe with a rigid rocker bottom. Preservation of first metatarsal length is often simple because the usual cause of infection is a penetrating ulcer under the first metatarsal head. In addition to the great toe, only a portion of the head may need to be removed to eradicate the infection, leaving all uninfected portions of the head and shaft. The extent of osteomyelitis in a metatarsal can generally be determined visually. Curettage of the marrow cavity is recommended. The bone should be beveled on the plantar as-

pect to avoid an area of increased pressure during latter stance phase.

A single amputation of ray 2, 3, or 4 affects only the width of the forefoot. Resection should be performed through the proximal metaphysis where the involved ray intersects with the adjacent metatarsals, leaving the tarsometatarsal joints intact (Figure 19). The fifth metatarsal should be transected obliquely with an inferolateral-facing facet. The uninvolved half to three quarters of the shaft is left to enhance the weight-bearing area and to retain the insertion of the peroneus brevis tendon (Figure 20).

In cases of massive forefoot infection, multiple lateral ray resections may be required. In this situation, the lateral metatarsals can be divided obliquely, with each affected metatarsal being cut somewhat longer with progression toward the first ray (Figure 21). If all but the first ray are involved, the first ray can be left complete (Fig-

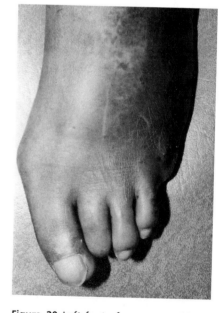

Figure 20 Left foot of a woman with diabetes mellitus who underwent fifth ray amputation. The proximal half of the shaft was left to maintain the weight-bearing area and retain the insertion of the peroneus brevis tendon. (*Reproduced with permission from Bowker JH: Minor and major lower limb amputations in diabetes mellitus, in Bowker JH, Pfeifer MA (eds):* Levin and O'Neal's The Diabetic Foot, *ed 6. St. Louis, MO, Mosby, 2001.*)

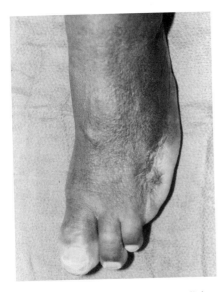

Figure 21 Left foot of a man with diabetes mellitus who underwent fourth and fifth ray amputations. He walks well in an in-depth shoe with custom-molded inlay and lateral filler. *(Reproduced with permission from Bowker JH, San Giovanni TP: Amputations and disarticulations, in Myerson MS (ed):* Foot and Ankle Disorders. *Philadelphia, PA, WB Saunders, 2000.)*

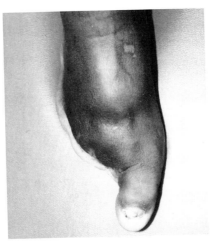

Figure 22 Right foot of a 62-year-old man with diabetes mellitus 3 years after the lateral four rays were excised obliquely for a severe foot abscess. The first ray is intact. Walking function with a customized shoe is excellent with preservation of the medial arch and rollover in terminal stance. *(Reproduced with permission from Bowker JH, San Giovanni TP: Amputations and disarticulations, in Myerson MS (ed):* Foot and Ankle Disorders. *Philadelphia, PA, WB Saunders, 2000.)*

ure 22). This strategy will retain both rollover function and full foot length in the shoe and, with proper pedorthic fitting, is preferable to a transmetatarsal amputation.[17,19,20] Removal of two or more medial rays is a poor choice, both functionally and cosmetically, as is removal of two or more central rays (Figure 23). In any ray amputation, the inciting ulcer is easily excised with a No. 11 blade through the full thickness of the tissues plantar to the bone. If the resulting wound is clean and small enough, it can be closed primarily with a single deeply spaced skin suture. Otherwise, it can be left open to contract and heal secondarily.

Special Considerations

Major reduction of first metatarsal length is devastating because an intact medial column is essential to proper foot balance during both stance and forward progression. The effectiveness of orthotic restoration of the medial arch will depend on the length of first metatarsal shaft preserved. Single lesser ray amputations can provide an excellent result both functionally and cosmetically. Because only the width of the forefoot is reduced, rollover function and overall foot balance during terminal stance appear to remain essentially normal. Proper pedorthic fitting can compensate for removal of several lateral rays when done conservatively. Barefoot walking is impaired in all but the single lesser ray amputations.

When a penetrating ulcer destroys the first MTP joint, leaving the great toe viable, rather than a first ray amputation, the joint alone can be removed through a medial longitudinal incision. The inciting ulcer should be excised as described above. All avascular tissues, including the sesamoid complex, remaining articular cartilage, joint capsule, flexor tendons, and infected cancellous bone, should be removed. The extensor hallucis longus tendon can usually be retained (Figures 24 and 25). If the wound appears clean at the conclusion of the procedure, it can be closed loosely over a Kritter flow-through irrigation

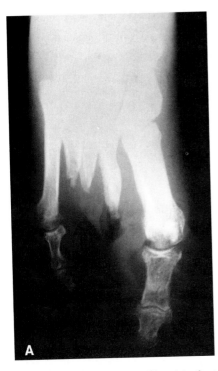

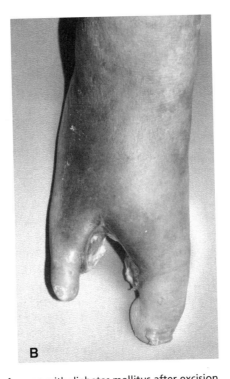

Figure 23 A, Radiograph of the right foot of a man with diabetes mellitus after excision of the three central rays for an abscess. *(Reproduced with permission from Bowker JH: Minor and major lower limb amputations in diabetes mellitus, in Bowker JH, Pfeifer MA (eds):* Levin and O'Neal's The Diabetic Foot, *ed 6. St. Louis, MO, Mosby, 2001.)* B, The cosmetic and functional result is poor. Transmetatarsal amputation was required to correct chronic plantar ulceration. Initial oblique excision of all lateral rays might have prevented this outcome.

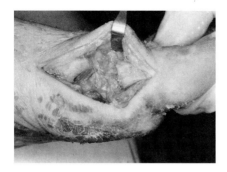

Figure 24 Intraoperative medial view of the left forefoot of a man with diabetes mellitus after excision of a chronically infected first MTP joint demonstrates the plantar bevel of the distal metatarsal metaphysis. Joint infection followed penetration from an ulcer plantar to the sesamoids. *(Reproduced with permission from Bowker JH: Partial foot amputations and disarticulations. Foot Ankle Clin North Am 1997;2:153.)*

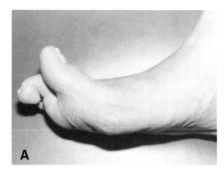 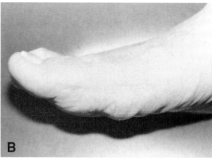

Figure 25 Right foot of a man with diabetes mellitus 14 months after excision of the first MTP joint for septic arthritis. **A,** In active dorsiflexion, the extensor hallucis longus was intact. **B,** When active plantar flexion is attempted, absence of extension contracture is evident. *(Reproduced with permission from Bowker JH, San Giovanni TP: Amputations and disarticulations, in Myerson MS (ed): Foot and Ankle Disorders. Philadelphia, PA, WB Saunders, 2000.)*

system,[21] which is described later. Temporary stabilization with Kirschner wires may be useful in some cases.

Transmetatarsal Amputation
Method

Transmetatarsal amputation should be considered when two or more medial rays or more than one central ray must be amputated. For maximum function, it is important to save as much metatarsal shaft length as can be covered with good plantar skin distally, avoiding the use of skin graft distally and plantarly (Figure 26). Residual dorsal defects are easily managed with split-thickness skin grafts, with good assurance they will not break down later with proper footwear. To assist in obtaining maximum forefoot length and to ensure distal coverage of the metatarsal shafts with durable skin, plantar and dorsal transverse skin incisions are made at the base of the toes. At closure, the flaps are trimmed to fit without redundancy or tension. To help preserve length, the metatarsal cuts should begin medially, within the cancellous bone of the dis-

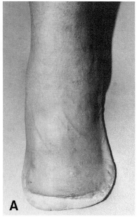 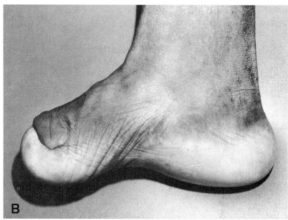

Figure 26 Dorsal **(A)** and lateral **(B)** views of an ideal transmetatarsal amputation. Note the position of the distal plantar flap, the overall length of the residual forefoot, the maintenance of the medial arch, and the absence of equinus deformity. *(Reproduced with permission from Bowker JH: Minor and major lower limb amputations in diabetes mellitus, in Bowker JH, Pfeifer MA (eds): Levin and O'Neal's The Diabetic Foot, ed 6. St. Louis, MO, Mosby, 2001.)*

tal first metatarsal if possible. The 15° transverse angle that parallels the metacarpophalangeal joints and normal toe break of the shoe should be reproduced. Plantar beveling of the metatarsal shafts will reduce distal plantar pressures during gait. If a large plantar forefoot ulcer is present, it can be excised in a longitudinal elliptical manner and the wound closed in a "T" fashion (Figure 27). A Kritter flow-through irrigation system is useful in removing detritus. If the patient has active or passive ankle dorsiflexion above a neutral position, postoperative casting following transmetatarsal

amputation should prevent equinus deformity. If no passive dorsiflexion is present, a percutaneous fractional lengthening is indicated to reduce distal pressures over the metatarsal shafts followed by provision of an appropriately padded ankle-foot orthosis (AFO). If drop foot is present secondary to nerve trauma, transfer of a posterior muscle-tendon unit may also be performed for its tenodesis effect. A well-padded rigid dressing should be applied before discharge with the foot in a plantigrade or slightly dorsiflexed position to protect the wound and prevent equinus contracture. The cast

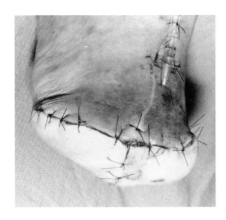

Figure 27 Intraoperative view of a right transmetatarsal amputation in a 62-year-old man with diabetes mellitus. Infection was initiated by a large penetrating ulcer beneath the second metatarsal head. Wide elliptical excision of the ulcer required a T-shaped closure. The Kritter flow-through irrigation system with widely spaced sutures allows egress of irrigation fluid. *(Reproduced with permission from Bowker JH, San Giovanni TP: Amputations and disarticulations, in Myerson MS (ed):* Foot and Ankle Disorders. *Philadelphia, PA, WB Saunders, 2000.)*

is changed weekly until the wound is sound, when a shoe with filler and stiff rocker sole and any indicated AFO previously fabricated can be fitted.

Special Considerations

Published healing rates for transmetatarsal amputations have varied widely. Geroulakos and May[22] noted healing in 68% of a group of 34 diabetic and nondiabetic patients with dry gangrene, but no follow-up regarding function was offered. Hobson and associates[23] reported a 50% healing rate in 30 amputees selected for gangrene, rest pain, or infection; likewise, the authors presented no functional data. Both groups of patients were chosen for this level of amputation on clinical grounds alone, including extent of gangrene and skin appearance. Durham and associates[24] reported that 53% of 43 open transmetatarsal amputations healed by wound contraction or split-thickness skin grafting in a mean time of 7.1 ± 5.6 months, with 21 of 23 patients (91%)

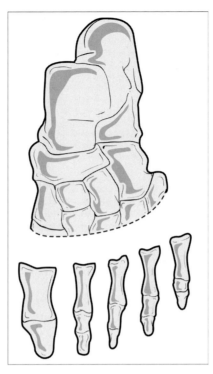

Figure 28 "Hidden amputation" of Baumgartner, used in lieu of transmetatarsal amputation. Diagram shows the position of the toes, which have retracted to the level of proximal bony resection after about 6 months. *(Reproduced with permission from Baumgartner R: Forefoot and hindfoot amputations, in* Surgical Techniques in Orthopaedics and Traumatology. *Paris, France, Elsevier SAS, 2001, p 3.)*

becoming independent walkers. Unfortunately, the authors provided no long-term data regarding durability of the scarred or grafted wounds.[24] Pinzur and associates[25] reported 81% healing in 58 patients with both short transmetatarsal amputations and Lisfranc disarticulations. Again, functional follow-up data were not provided. The work of McKittrick and associates,[26] published in 1949, demonstrates what a high level of clinical acumen can achieve. Prior to the availability of any laboratory determinations of tissue perfusion, the authors obtained healing in 196 of 215 diabetic patients (91%). Criteria for healing included gangrene limited to the toes, controlled infection, absence of dependent rubor, and a venous filling time of less than 25 seconds. They noted that palpable pedal pulses were

unnecessary and that the incision should not traverse infected areas. They also reported a satisfactory outcome in walking function in 78% of patients.

Following transmetatarsal amputation, the shoe sole should be fitted with a steel shank or carbon fiber stiffener with a rocker to avoid distal ulcers from a flexible sole wrapping around the end of the residual foot. A distal filler will also be needed to maintain the shape of the toebox. Some patients may elect a custommade short shoe, but because of the shortened forefoot lever arm this will result in an unequal drop-off gait. Another option for a short transmetatarsal amputation is an AFO with an anterior shell to provide improved stability and balance. A variety of inframalleolar prostheses for this level have been successfully fitted.

For selected lesions involving several metatarsals in which the toes are intact, in lieu of a transmetatarsal amputation, Baumgartner[20] has described a "hidden amputation." In this procedure, the distal two thirds of each metatarsal is resected through cancellous bone. After about 6 months, with soft-tissue contraction, the toes retract to the level of proximal bony resection (Figure 28).

Tarsometatarsal (Lisfranc) Disarticulation
Method

Disarticulation at the tarsometatarsal joints, described by Lisfranc[27] in 1815, is most useful in cases of trauma and selected cases of foot tumor. It can also be used in cases of infection, if patients are selected carefully so as not to risk failure of a Syme ankle disarticulation. With a significant loss of forefoot lever length, the massive triceps surae can easily overpower the relatively weaker dorsiflexors, leading to equinus contracture. To help maintain a balanced residual foot, the insertions of the peroneus brevis, peroneus longus, and anterior tibial tendons must be preserved. Careful dissection will spare the proximal insertions of the peroneus longus and anterior tibial tendons on the medial cuneiform. As reinforcement, the distal insertions of these tendons can be carefully dissected off the first metatarsal base and sutured to the proximal slips. The "keystone" base of the second metatarsal should be left in place to help preserve the proximal transverse arch. The first, third, and fourth metatarsals can be disarticulated, while a portion of the base of the fifth metatarsal is left to preserve the insertion of the peroneus brevis tendon. Equinus contracture can be avoided by performing a primarily percutaneous fractional heel cord lengthening followed by application of a rigid dressing with the foot in a plantigrade or slightly dorsiflexed position.[4] Another method that has been successful in lieu of heel cord lengthening is cast immobilization of the residual foot in dorsiflexion for 3 to 4 weeks to weaken the triceps surae relative to the ankle dorsiflexors (Figure 29).

In the Bona-Jaeger procedure, the line of resection is between the navicular and cuneiforms medially, then through the cancellous bone of the cuboid laterally in line with the medial disarticulations. Careful dissection will preserve the plantar arteries, which lie adjacent to the second and third cuneiform bones. Although the procedure preserves some foot length, dorsiflexion power is diminished. Baumgartner[20] recommends fusion of the midtarsal (Chopart) joints to prevent their secondary dislocation, but only if normal sensation and perfusion are present. Tarsometatarsal (Lisfranc) disarticulation is preferred over the Bona-Jaeger procedure because of preservation of the ankle dorsiflexion insertions.

Special Considerations

Tarsometatarsal disarticulations represent a major loss of forefoot length with a corresponding decrease in barefoot walking function. To restore

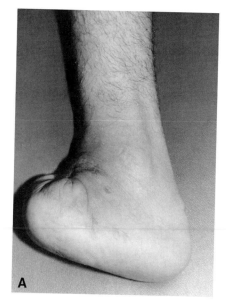 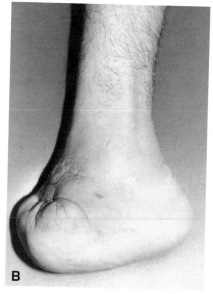

Figure 29 Lateral views of the right foot of a young man with traumatic Lisfranc disarticulation demonstrate the range of ankle motion achieved by preservation of the midfoot insertions of the extrinsic muscles and postoperative casting in dorsiflexion. **A,** Maximum active dorsiflexion. **B,** Maximum active plantar flexion. *(Reproduced with permission from Bowker JH, San Giovanni TP: Amputations and disarticulations, in Myerson MS (ed):* Foot and Ankle Disorders. *Philadelphia, PA, WB Saunders, 2000.)*

fairly normal late-stance-phase gait, a customized close-fitting fixed-ankle prosthesis or orthosis is typically prescribed. This is then placed into a shoe with a rigid rocker bottom.

Midtarsal (Chopart) Disarticulation
Method

The Chopart disarticulation is through the talonavicular and calcaneocuboid joints. Like the Lisfranc disarticulation, it is most useful in trauma and selected cases of foot tumor. It is rarely applicable to diabetic foot infections because of the proximity of the infection to the heel pad. At the time of disarticulation, all ankle dorsiflexors are divided. Without restoration of dorsiflexor function and weakening of the plantar flexors, severe equinus deformity from myostatic contracture of the unopposed triceps surae is inevitable, with weight bearing becoming painful as it shifts from the heel pad to the distal talus and calcaneus. Active dorsiflexion can be restored to this extremely short re-

sidual foot by attachment of the anterior tibial tendon to the talus, either through a drill hole in the talar head or with sutures or staples to a groove in the head.[28] To further restore a relative balance between dorsiflexors and plantar flexors, I have found removal of 2 to 3 cm of the Achilles tendon to be more effective than lengthening it. This is accomplished through a separate longitudinal incision, leaving the sheath of the tendon in place to allow rapid reconstitution at its new length. A rigid dressing should be applied with the hindfoot in slight dorsiflexion for about 6 weeks to prevent equinus contracture of the hindfoot as well as allow secure healing of the anterior tibial tendon to the talus. Removal of the sharp anteroinferior corner of the calcaneus is also recommended to provide comfortable stance and gait.

Marquardt[29] believes that anterior tibial tendon transfer to the talus alone is inadequate because the transferred muscle elevates only the talus while the continued plantar flexion force on the calcaneus by the triceps surae produces separation and insta-

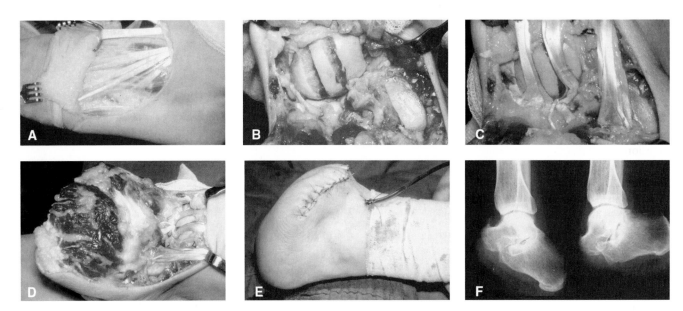

Figure 30 Marquardt tenomyoplastic modification of the midtarsal (Chopart) disarticulation with triple dorsiflexor tenodesis. **A,** Lateral intraoperative view of the left foot (toes to left). The anterior tibial tendon is retracted medially, and the extensor hallucis longus tendon is retracted distally. Note the extensor digitorum longus tendons and the length of the plantar flap. **B,** Anterior view shows two longitudinal grooves in the talus (to left) and one in the calcaneus (right). The grooves will receive the anterior tibial, extensor hallucis longus, and extensor digitorum longus tendons. **C,** The tendons are in place, sutured to the plantar capsular and fascial structures. **D,** Full-thickness plantar flap (to left) includes short flexor muscle bellies for distal padding. **E,** Completed procedure with drain just before casting. Note the plantigrade position of the heel pad. **F,** Lateral radiograph after Marquardt modification demonstrates range of active dorsiflexion and plantar flexion. (Courtesy of Professor G Neff.)

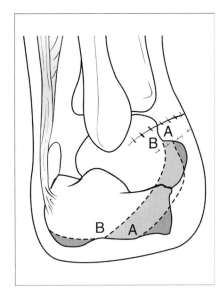

Figure 31 Diagram showing amount of bone removed from the talus and calcaneus to provide a smoother, more comfortable end-bearing surface in the event of an equinus deformity. The amount of bone resected in the zone demarcated by lines A-A and B-B depends on the quality and quantity of soft tissue available for closure. *(Reproduced with permission from Baumgartner R: Forefoot and hindfoot amputations, in Surgical Techniques in Orthopaedics and Traumatology, Paris, France, Elsevier SAS, 2001, p 4.)*

bility of the subtalar joint over time. He has developed a tenomyoplastic operation that elevates both bones. The anterior tibial and extensor hallucis longus tendons are placed in separate grooves in the talar head, and the common extensors are placed in another groove in the anterior calcaneus. With the hindfoot held in dorsiflexion, the tendons are sutured to the plantar capsular and fascial structures (Figure 30). The hindfoot is casted in dorsiflexion until the tenodeses are sound.

Baumgartner[20] recommends postoperative external fixation of Chopart disarticulations to limit equinus deformity. Nonetheless, he anticipates what he considers inevitable equinus contracture by reshaping the distal talus and calcaneus to allow less painful anterior weight bearing in equinus (Figure 31). The heel pad, of course, is not plantigrade. If weight bearing becomes painful because of severe equinus, Baumgartner[20] recommends lengthening of the Achilles tendon followed by wedge resection and ar-

throdesis of the subtalar joint with transfer of the anterior tibial tendon to the lateral border of the residual foot. The heel pad again becomes plantigrade, and the vertical clearance for a prosthetic foot is increased by 1 to 2 cm (Figure 32).

Some cases of equinus contracture following Chopart disarticulation can be treated without reattaching the dorsiflexors. Active dorsiflexion with restoration of heel pad weight bearing is obtained by partial Achilles tendon excision and cast immobilization for 3 to 4 weeks with restoration of comfortable prosthetic gait. This simple salvage procedure, recommended by Burgess,[30] avoids revision to a Syme ankle disarticulation or higher level (Figure 33).

Because a prosthesis for this level eliminates both ankle and subtalar motion without necessarily preventing deformity, several authors have recommended arthrodesis of both the subtalar and ankle joints following Chopart disarticulation.[31,32] They cite advantages of absolute prevention of equinus deformity by ankle fusion and prevention of progressive talocalcaneal instability by subtalar fusion.

Special Considerations

Although Chopart disarticulation does allow direct end bearing, it has no inherent rollover function. With preservation of full limb length and a stable heel pad, the amputee can walk without a prosthesis for short distances. This is in contrast to the Syme procedure, after which a prosthesis is essential to both heel pad stability and limb-length equality. Nonetheless, the prosthesis is essential for functional walking. A close-fitting rigid ankle prosthesis or orthosis and a shoe with a rigid rocker sole are generally required to permit good late-stance-phase gait.

Immediate Postoperative Management

Primary closure is usually indicated for ablation as a result of ischemia. In cases of trauma, however, discovery of foreign material or removal of vascularly compromised tissue may be incomplete at the conclusion of the first procedure. Secondary closure at 7 to 10 days, following any necessary redébridement, greatly reduces the chances of infection and subsequent wound dehiscence.

In some cases of low-grade foot infection, if the wound had little or no initial purulence and is visually clean following débridement (no compromised tissue or residual pus), a primary loose closure can be done. If the wound has sufficient volume, it can be closed over a Kritter flow-through irrigation system.[21] A 14-gauge polyethylene venous catheter is passed into the depths of the wound from an adjacent site by means of its integral needle. The needle is discarded and the catheter is sutured to the skin and connected to a bag of normal saline. The fluid exits the wound between widely spaced simple skin sutures at the rate of 1 L per day for 3 days (Fig-

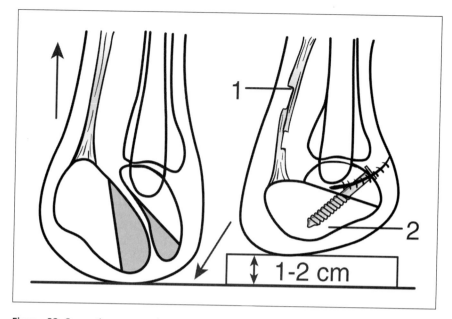

Figure 32 Corrective surgery for severe painful equinus in a Chopart residual foot. The drawing on the left illustrates the deformity and amount of bone to be removed for wedge resection of the subtalar joint. Drawing on the right shows (1) Achilles tendon lengthening with restoration of the plantigrade hindfoot and (2) completed subtalar arthrodesis with internal fixation. *(Reproduced with permission from Baumgartner R: Forefoot and hindfoot amputations, in* Surgical Techniques in Orthopaedics and Traumatology, *Paris, France, Elsevier SAS, 2001, p 4.)*

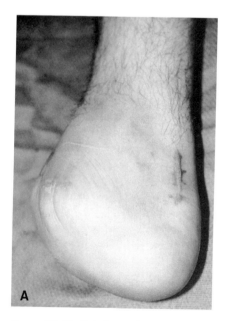
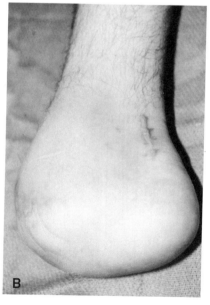

Figure 33 Medial views of the right foot of a 17-year-old man with a traumatic Chopart disarticulation. He presented with distal anterior pain while walking in a prosthesis secondary to severe equinus deformity. These photographs were taken 3 weeks after excision of 2 cm of Achilles tendon and casting in dorsiflexion to restore the plantigrade position of the hindfoot. Note the medial incision. **A,** Maximum active dorsiflexion. **B,** Maximum active plantar flexion. *(Reproduced with permission from Bowker JH, San Giovanni TP: Amputations and disarticulations, in Myerson MS (ed):* Foot and Ankle Disorders. *Philadelphia, PA, WB Saunders, 2000.)*

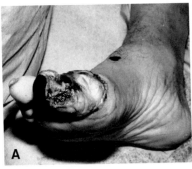
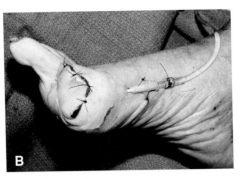

Figure 34 A, Wet gangrene of the right great toe in a man with diabetes mellitus. The phalanges were infected, but some lateral skin was salvageable. Forefoot perfusion was adequate. B, Closure of the MTP disarticulation with a lateral toe flap. Note the widely spaced sutures, which allow egress of irrigation fluid, and the catheter sutured to the skin.

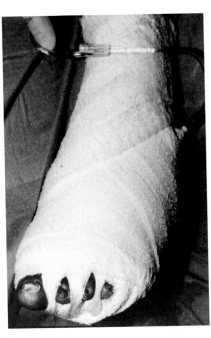

Figure 35 Kritter flow-through irrigation system installed in a left second ray amputation wound at conclusion of surgery. Note the bulky bandage used to absorb irrigation fluid; the outer of the three rolls is replaced every few hours.

ure 34). The fluid, containing residual wound detritus, is collected in an absorbent dressing (Figure 35). The outer layers of the dressing are changed every 4 to 5 hours.[33] After removal of the system on the third day, the edges of the wound are gently compressed by the surgeon. If any signs of purulence are present, the sutures are removed and wound packing commenced. If patients have been carefully selected, however, purulence should be uncommon. The chief advantage is primary healing, usually within 3 weeks. The need for secondary closure or healing by secondary intention over several months, often augmented by skin grafting, is avoided.

The management of open amputations or disarticulations resulting from trauma or infection is quite straightforward. Moderately wet saline gauze dressings, gently packed into all recesses of the wound, are appropriate in most cases. The advantages of this method are low cost and ease of execution. Requiring only clean technique, it is easily taught to the patient and family members before discharge. The dressing is changed every 8 hours, which is sufficient time for the gauze to adhere to the wound surface and débride detritus with each change. If the wound is producing excessive fluid, the gauze may be used dry until this ceases. Conversely, if the wound is too dry, or if a vital tendon or joint capsule is ex-

posed, a wet-to-wet method is useful. Four hours after each dressing change, the dressing is rewetted exteriorly with saline to prevent critical tissues from drying. Repeated exposure of the wound surface to povidone-iodine or hydrogen peroxide can be cytotoxic to granulation tissue and is not recommended.[34,35] If Pseudomonas colonization occurs, as evidenced by a greenish tinge to the dressing, a 0.25% solution of acetic acid can be used for a few days to suppress it. Use must be limited because its bactericidal activity is exceeded by its fibroblast toxicity.[36] Maceration of the wound by soaks or whirlpool treatments is not indicated.

Every 24 to 48 hours, the surgeon should manually strip the wound from proximal to distal to locate previously undetected pockets of infection, which may require débridement. Pre- and postoperative nutritional support must include sufficient caloric intake to compensate for a poor initial serum albumin level, as well as the catabolic effects of infection and bed rest. Multivitamins as well as additional iron, zinc, and vitamin C provide essential elements for collagen formation in wound healing.[37,38] Oral hyperalimentation in patients with diabetes mellitus will require appropriate adjustments of hypoglycemic medication to prevent iatrogenic hyperglycemia. Before discharging the patient to outpatient status, the surgeon should observe for-

mation of granulation tissue throughout the depths of the wound. The diabetologist consulted to assist with preoperative control of serum glucose levels should provide the patient with a management program that will continue to assist in wound healing after discharge by decreasing tissue glycation.

The most important aspect of postoperative management in these cases is patient compliance with the program. This includes avoidance of weight bearing until the wound is sound enough for suture removal, adequate nutrition, avoidance of vasoconstrictors such as nicotine and caffeine, and tight control of serum glucose levels in patients with diabetes mellitus. Walking should be limited to the absolute minimum, and the foot should be kept elevated whenever the patient is not walking to reduce the negative effect of edema on wound healing. During the first few weeks, the wound should be evaluated weekly. In the case of closed wounds, the partial weight-bearing cast can be removed at 3 weeks postoperatively, and ankle and subtalar motion resumed. In the case of open ablations, it is often possible to allow protected weight bearing, using heel-bearing weight-relief shoes.

Summary

Amputations and disarticulations within the foot offer important advantages over more proximal levels, including direct weight bearing with proprioceptive feedback along normal neural pathways. The degree to which full walking function can be restored prosthetically or orthotically is relative to the loss of forefoot lever length and associated muscles. Retention of even the hindfoot, however, provides for much greater independence and energy conservation than higher levels such as transtibial or transfemoral amputations. This is especially important for elderly patients. In addition, amputation levels within the foot result in the least alteration of body image, often requiring only shoe modifications or a limited orthosis or prosthesis.

With convergent advances in wound healing, tissue oxygenation, and antibiotic therapy, as well as improvements in vascular and amputation surgery techniques, today's surgeons have the opportunity to consider the foot rather than the tibia or femur as the site of election for amputations as a result of a variety of traumatic, ischemic, or infectious conditions.

References

1. Bowker JH: Partial foot amputations and disarticulations. *Foot Ankle Clin North Am* 1997;2:153.

2. Millstein SG, McCowan SA, Hunter GA: Traumatic partial foot amputations in adults: A long-term review. *J Bone Joint Surg Br* 1988;70:251-254.

3. McCollum PT, Walker MA: The choice between limb salvage and amputation: Major limb amputation for end-stage peripheral vascular disease. Level selection and alternative options, in Bowker JH, Michael JW (eds): *Atlas of Limb Prosthetics: Surgical, Prosthetic and Rehabilitation Principles*, ed 2. Rosemont, IL, American Academy of Orthopaedic Surgeons, 2002, pp 25-38. (Originally published by Mosby-Year Book in 1992.)

4. Livingston R, Jacobs RI, Karmody A: Plantar abscess in the diabetic patient. *Foot Ankle* 1985;5:205-213.

5. Cianci P, Hunt TK: Adjunctive hyperbaric oxygen therapy in treatment of diabetic foot wounds, in Bowker JH, Pfeifer MA (eds): *Levin and O'Neal's The Diabetic Foot*, ed 6. St. Louis, MO, Mosby-Year Book, 2001, p 416.

6. Pecoraro RE: The nonhealing diabetic ulcer: A major cause for limb loss. *Prog Clin Biol Res* 1991;365:27-43.

7. Matos LA, Nunez AA: Enhancement of healing in selected problem wounds, in Kindwall EP (ed): *Hyperbaric Medicine Practice*. Flagstaff, AZ, Best Publishing, 1994, p 589.

8. McCollum PT, Spence VA, Walker WF, et al: Oxygen-induced changes in the skin as measured by transcutaneous oximetry. *Br J Surg* 1986;73:882-885.

9. Sheffield PJ: Tissue oxygen measurements, in Davis JC, Hunt TK (eds): *Problem Wounds: The Role of Oxygen*. New York, NY, Elsevier, 1988, p 17.

10. Harward TRS, Volay R, Golbranson F, et al: Oxygen inhalation: Induced transcutaneous PO_2 changes as a predictor of amputation level. *J Vasc Surg* 1985;21:220-227.

11. Wattel F, Mathieu D, Coget JM, et al: Hyperbaric oxygen in chronic vascular wound management. *Angiology* 1990;41:59-65.

12. Karanfilian RG, Lynch TG, Zirul VT, et al: The value of laser-Doppler velicometry and transcutaneous oxygen tension determination in predicting healing of ischemic forefoot ulcerations and amputations in diabetics. *J Vasc Surg* 1986;5:51-5161.

13. Grayson MI, Gibbons GW, Balogh K, et al: Probing to bone in infected pedal ulcers: A clinical sign of underlying osteomyelitis in diabetic patients. *JAMA* 1995;273:721-723.

14. Grodinsky M: A study of fascial spaces of the feet. *Surg Gynecol Obstet* 1929;49:737-751.

15. Loeffler RD Jr, Ballard A: Plantar fascial spaces of the foot and a proposed surgical approach. *Foot Ankle* 1980;1:11-15.

16. Harris WR, Silverstein EA: Partial amputations of the foot: A follow-up study. *Can J Surg* 1964;7:6-11.

17. Wagner FW Jr: Partial-foot amputations: Surgical procedures, in Bowker JH, Michael JW (eds): *Atlas of Limb Prosthetics: Surgical, Prosthetic and Rehabilitation Principles*, ed 2. Rosemont, IL, American Academy of Orthopaedic Surgeons, 2002, pp 389-401. (Originally published by Mosby-Year Book in 1992.)

18. Mann RA, Poppen NK, O'Kinski M: Amputation of the great toe: A clinical and biochemical study. *Clin Orthop* 1988;226:192-205.

19. Bowker JH, San Giovanni TP: Amputations and disarticulations, in Myerson MS (ed): *Foot and Ankle Disorders*. Philadelphia, PA, WB Saunders, 2000, pp 466-503.

20. Baumgartner R: Forefoot and hindfoot amputations. Editions Scientifique et Médicales Elsevier SAS (Paris) *Surgical Techniques in Orthopaedics and Traumatology*. 55-700-C-10, 2001, pp 1-6.

21. Kritter AE: A technique for salvage of the infected diabetic foot. *Orthop Clin North Am* 1973;4:21-30.

22. Geroulakos G, May ARL: Transmetatarsal amputation in patients with peripheral vascular disease. *Eur J Vas Surg* 1991;5:655-658.

23. Hobson MI, Stonebridge PA, Clason AE: Place of transmetatarsal amputations: A 5-year experience and review of the literature. *J R Coll Surg Edinb* 1990;35:113-115.

24. Durham JR, McCoy DM, Sawchuck AP, et al: Open transmetatarsal amputation in the treatment of severe foot infection. *Am J Surg* 1989;158:127-130.

25. Pinzur MS, Kaminsky M, Sage R, et al: Amputations at the middle level of the foot. *J Bone Joint Surg Am* 1986;68:1061-1064.

26. McKittrick LS, McKittrick JB, Risley TS: Transmetatarsal amputation for infection or gangrene in patients with diabetes mellitus. *Ann Surg* 1949;130:826-935.

27. Lisfranc J: Nouvelle méthode opératoire pour l'amputation du pied dans son articulation tarsométatarsienne:

Méthode précédée des nombreuses modifications qu'a subies celle de Chopart. Paris, France, Gabon, 1815.

28. Letts M, Pyper A: The modified Chopart's amputation. *Clin Orthop* 1990;256:44-49.

29. Marquardt E: Die Chopart-Exartikulation mit Tenomyoplastik. *Z Orthop* 1973;111:584-586.

30. Burgess EM: Prevention and correction of fixed equinus deformity in mid-foot amputations. *Bull Prosthet Res* 1966;10:45.

31. Menager D, Chiesa G, Ha Van G, LeFèvre B, Camilleri A: Conuite à tenir devant une amputation de Chopart traumatique. *Méd Chir Pied* 1988;4:35.

32. Persson BM, Söderberg B: Pantalar fusion for correction of painful equinus after traumatic Chopart's amputation: A report of 2 cases. *Acta Orthop Scand* 1996;67:300-302.

33. Bowker JH: The choice between limb salvage and amputation: Infection, in Bowker JH, Michael JW (eds): *Atlas of Limb Prosthetics: Surgical, Prosthetic and Rehabilitation Principles*, ed 2. Rosemont, IL, American Academy of Orthopaedic Surgeons, 2002, pp 39-43. (Originally published by Mosby-Year Book in 1992.)

34. Rodeheaver G, Bellamy W, Kody M, et al: Bacterial activity and toxicity of iodine-containing solutions in wounds. *Arch Surg* 1982;117:181-186.

35. Oberg MS, Lindsey D: Editorial: Do not put hydrogen peroxide or povidone iodine into wounds! *Am J Dis Child* 1987;141:27-29.

36. Lineaweaver W, Howard R, Soucy D, et al: Topical antimicrobial toxicity. *Arch Surg* 1985;120:267-270.

37. Sieggreen MY: Healing of physical wounds. *Nurs Clin North Am* 1987;22:439-447.

38. Stotts NA, Washington DF: Nutrition: A critical component of wound healing. *AACN Clin Crit Care Nurs* 1990;1:585-594.

Chapter 35

Amputations and Disarticulations Within the Foot: Prosthetic Management

David N. Condie, CEng
Roy Bowers, SRProsOrth

Introduction

The successful prosthetic management of partial foot amputations demands a clear understanding of the functions of the normal foot and the biomechanical consequences of each amputation variant. Depending on the extent of the amputation, the functional problems range from simple to severe. The range of currently available prosthetic solutions may also be considered as a continuum ranging from very simple toe fillers to the more complex designs favored by some patients with Chopart amputations. Armed with this knowledge, the clinician can then make appropriate decisions regarding the materials and prosthetic designs to be used for each individual.

Biomechanics
Normal Foot Function

The normal foot is an extremely complex structure, the detailed function of which is still only partially understood. This discussion will be restricted to a brief consideration of the load-bearing structure and the function of the foot joints during normal walking. Further information on these and the other ankle-foot mechanisms may be obtained by consulting the relevant literature.[1-4]

The foot is the means whereby the ground-reaction forces generated during physical activities are transmitted to the body structure. During

normal level walking, these loads are directed initially onto the heel, the specially adapted fatty tissues of which are ideally suited to the absorption of the high forces generated at impact and during the subsequent loading of the limb. Once the foot is flat and until the heel leaves the ground as push-off is initiated, the supporting forces are shared between the heel and the forefoot, with only a small contribution from the lateral aspect of the midfoot. This method of load transmission is commonly attributed to the arch structure of the foot, even though it is now clearly understood that its effectiveness is a function of a number of neuromuscular mechanisms. Once the heel leaves the ground, the increased ground force associated with push-off is transmitted through the area defined by the metatarsal heads and the pads of the toes. As body weight is transferred to the contralateral limb, this load reduces and localizes on the plantar surface of the hallux.

The functions of the joints of the foot have been the subject of endless investigation. The ability of the foot to alter its shape and alignment is of considerable importance in adapting to variations in the slope of the walking surface. A more subtle but equally important role, however, concerns the absorption of the longitudinal rotations of the lower limbs that occur with each stride (Figure 1).

Internal rotation of the tibia commences during the swing phase and continues after heel contact until the foot is flat on the ground. During this phase, the foot pronates about the subtalar joint axis, thereby maintaining the normal toe-out position of the foot. Elevation of the lateral margin of the foot, which is a consequence of hindfoot pronation, is counteracted by supination of the forefoot, thus ensuring that ground contact is achieved across the entire forefoot. After the foot is flat on the ground, the tibia rotates externally and the foot supinates about the subtalar joint axis to absorb this motion, thus preventing slippage occurring between the foot and the ground. The associated elevation of the medial margin of the foot is counteracted by pronation of the forefoot, enabling the maintenance of full forefoot loading. After the heel leaves the ground, the foot pronates, transferring the area of support medially onto the first metatarsal head and then the hallux as the foot loses contact with the ground.

During the initial loading phase, the midtarsal joint acts in concert with the subtalar joint. Thereafter, as the subtalar joint supinates, the midtarsal joint locks and stiffens the long arch of the foot to prepare it for the increased dorsiflexion moment that it is subjected to after the heel leaves the ground.

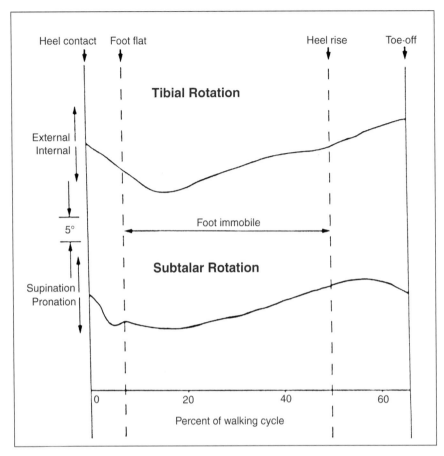

Figure 1 Longitudinal rotations of the leg and associated subtalar joint motions during walking.

Functional Loss After Amputation

The loss of normal foot function after amputation is progressively more severe the more proximal the site of amputation. The extent of the loss may be summarized as relating to three primary aspects of foot function: load-bearing capacity, stability, and dynamic function.

Any partial foot amputation reduces the forefoot load-bearing area, and any amputation proximal to the metatarsal heads totally eliminates this load-bearing site. Ironically, the magnitude of the forefoot ground-reaction force has been shown to increase following partial foot amputation because of the reduced forefoot lever arm when the patient attempts to walk in a normal manner.[5-8]

Similarly, any amputation proximal to the metatarsal heads removes the contribution that these structures make to the normal mediolateral stability of the foot. The natural shape of the longitudinal arch of the foot results in a residual foot with an apparently supinated forefoot, which if left untreated will inevitably result in compensatory pronation of the hindfoot.

As the level of amputation moves proximally, the active flexion of the first metatarsophalangeal joint at final push-off is eliminated, followed by loss of the supinatory/pronatory capability of the forefoot. Fortunately, if the amputation surgery has been performed according to the best current practice, both ankle and subtalar joint function most likely will be preserved, although midtarsal joint function will

be lost following tarsometatarsal and transtarsal amputation.[9-13]

Prosthetic Assessment and Designs

Devices used in the management of partial foot amputations are frequently referred to as both prostheses and orthoses; sometimes the term "prosthosis" is used. Many of these designs incorporate principles used in foot orthoses or ankle-foot orthoses (AFOs), as well as those used in lower limb prostheses. Shoe modifications are also commonly provided to enhance function for these levels of loss; therefore, a knowledge of pedorthic principles is important.

As with all levels of amputation, assessment of a number of factors must precede prescription. The amputee's control of the remaining joints of the foot and ankle must be assessed. The presence of muscle imbalance and joint instability or deformity, either fixed or correctable, should be noted. The tissue coverage at the amputation site and the sensitivity and any adherence of the scar should be assessed. Vascularity, sensation, and the presence of neuropathy must be noted, and the foot should be checked for callosities or other skin lesions. The ability to comfortably bear weight through the residual foot and the amputee's balance should be checked. The patient's aspirations with regard to activity level and the cosmetic appearance of the prosthesis are of major importance and will help influence the prescription process, because higher levels of function are often at the expense of cosmesis.

The methods of compensation for each of the more commonly encountered amputation levels will be discussed in detail, but one important biomechanical issue should be mentioned here. When the surgery is confined to the toes, prosthetic forefoot loading, which is most significant after heel-off, may simply be transferred directly onto the metatarsal heads and any remaining toes. When the surgery involves removal of the metatarsal heads, however, this force is anteriorly offset from the residual plantar tissues. This action results in an external moment that will, unless resisted, cause the prosthesis to rotate (in the direction of dorsiflexion) relative to the residual foot (Figure 2). The management of this particular requirement is one of the most critical issues to be considered in the selection, manufacture, and fit of prostheses for these more proximal levels of amputation.

Amputation of the Toes

The functional loss associated with the amputation of one or more toes is primarily a reduction in the forefoot load-bearing area, resulting in increased pressure on the metatarsal heads, which are also more exposed by the removal of the toes. These symptoms will be most pronounced if the hallux is removed, when foot function also will be compromised by the loss of active flexion of the first metatarsophalangeal joint, which normally occurs at the end of push-off. For normal walking, the loss of the toes is not a major functional problem, but loss of the great toe makes running and participation in competitive sports more difficult because of the loss of active push-off.

Cosmetic issues need to be addressed. Most prostheses for toe amputations consist of a toe filler to reinstate normal foot shape and prevent deformation of the shoe, which also may be a cause of discomfort. Some patients elect to pack the shoe with soft foam or cloth. Alternatively, the prosthesis may consist of a modified insole (inlay), with a built-up foam section acting as a replacement for the lost digits (Figure 3). If required, this foam section may be formed in a manner that resists any tendency of the remaining toes to deviate in the transverse plane. In contrast, when the hallux has been removed, the prosthesis is best custom fabricated to a plaster model of the foot. Modifications at the amputation site re-

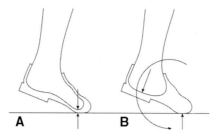

Figure 2 A, Amputation of the toes: ground-reaction force transferred directly onto metatarsal heads. **B,** Amputation proximal to the metatarsal heads: ground-reaction force results in a dorsiflexion moment.

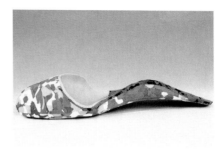

Figure 3 Modified insole (inlay) with filler for amputation of the toes.

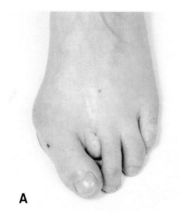

Figure 4 A, Foot with amputation of one of the central toes. **B,** Toe spacer improves the alignment of the remaining toes.

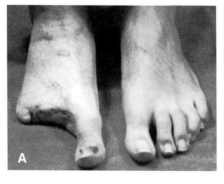

Figure 5 A, Amputation of the second through fifth toes. **B,** Silicone prosthesis in place.

distribute pressure away from this area and onto the medial longitudinal and transverse metatarsal arches, resulting in improvements in comfort and gait.

The provision of a toe spacer may be beneficial in patients where one of the central toes has been removed (Figure 4). For these designs, a plaster

model of the foot is not generally required for fabrication of the prosthesis.

Silicone replacement of the toes offers optimum cosmesis (Figure 5), but this highly specialized technique may be unavailable at some prosthetic facilities, and specialist manufacturers may need to be consulted. The psy-

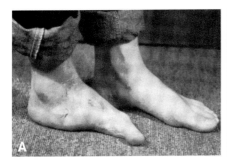
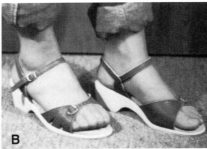

Figure 6 A, Ray amputation of the right foot. **B,** Silicone prosthesis in place.

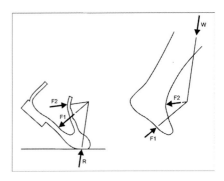

Figure 7 Forces occurring between the residual foot and the socket of a trans-metatarsal amputation prosthesis at push-off. F1 = force at plantar surface of the residual foot; F2 = force at dorsal surface of the residual foot; R = ground-reaction force; W = body weight.

chological benefits of a foot that appears normal when wearing open shoes or sandals can be very significant and should not be underestimated.

Any tendency of the shoe to deform may be resisted by reinforcing the sole with a steel plate or a footplate composed of a carbon composite material; however, this material should not be too rigid, or normal foot "third rocker" will be inhibited.[11] When further pressure reduction is required at the amputation site, a rocker sole with its apex behind the metatarsal heads may be added to the shoe.

Ray Amputations

The functional consequences of amputation of one or more rays of the foot depend on the position and extent of the tissues removed. In every instance, there will be a reduction in the forefoot load-bearing area, resulting in increased pressure on the remaining forefoot plantar tissues, which may be a problem for insensate patients or patients with diabetes mellitus. If the amputation includes either the first or fifth rays, either singly or with adjacent rays, there is an associated loss of mediolateral foot stability affecting the patient's balance. Additionally, supination and pronation of the forefoot will be virtually eliminated.

The stability of the prosthesis on the residual foot requires intimacy of fit. It therefore typically takes the form of an insole that is custom-molded to a plaster model of the residual foot, consisting of a soft,

pressure-sensitive material next to the skin, reinforced with a firmer, more durable base layer, which will improve both its function and longevity. The prosthesis is built up to reinstate normal foot shape, thus restoring mediolateral stability and indirectly facilitating subtalar joint function. Silicone prostheses combine these functions with excellent cosmetic restoration (Figure 6).

If necessary, mediolateral stability may be further enhanced by wedging the prosthesis itself, or by the addition of either a wedge or flare to the shoe. The use of a prosthesis will prevent deformation of the shoe and may remove the need for split size or custom-made footwear.

Transmetatarsal Amputation

The functional loss that occurs when the amputation procedure involves the removal of the metatarsal heads is substantially greater than in toe amputations. In these amputations, the entire normal forefoot load-bearing capacity is eliminated. In addition, forefoot mediolateral stability will be impaired, which may result in pronation of the hindfoot. Finally, forefoot supination and pronation are largely eliminated.

The removal of the metatarsal heads means that it is no longer practical to transfer the forefoot ground-reaction force (R) directly onto the plantar surface of the residual foot; therefore, the rotational stability of the patient/prosthesis interface will require special attention. Attempts should be made to use the remaining

surface of the longitudinal arch of the foot both as a load-bearing area (F1) and to restore mediolateral stability. However, for this mechanism to be effective, it will be necessary for the prosthetic socket to generate a posteriorly directed force (F2) on the dorsum of the residual foot (Figure 7). This same force generates a moment that resists the tendency of the prosthesis to rotate (in the direction of dorsiflexion) relative to the residual foot when weight is applied to the prosthetic forefoot.

Some designs of prostheses for this level are similar to the molded insole type used for toe amputations, functioning as forefoot fillers maintained in correct relation to the residual foot by the patient's shoe. Better results can be achieved by custom fabrication to a plaster model, which has been carefully shaped so as to transfer the forefoot ground-reaction force behind the cut bone ends. If correctable, the arches of the foot should be reinstated, and this is best done during casting. If the arches are not correctable, the prosthesis must accommodate and support them to prevent further deformation.

A preferred option is to construct a prosthesis with a molded or laminated socket, built up to replace the lost forefoot, including a soft liner or anterior pad if required.[14] This prosthesis resembles a modified Univer-

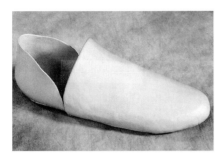

Figure 8 Transmetatarsal prosthesis with hinged laminated socket to facilitate donning.

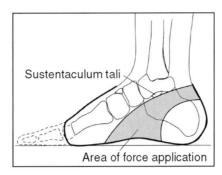

Figure 9 Loading the sustentaculum tali to resist pronation of the hindfoot.

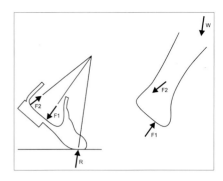

Figure 10 Tarsometatarsal and transtarsal amputation prostheses/perimalleolar designs. Forces occurring between the residual foot and the socket at push-off. F1 = force at plantar surface of residual foot; F2 = force at calcaneus; R = ground-reaction force; W = body weight.

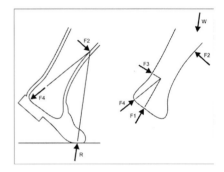

Figure 11 Tarsometatarsal and transtarsal amputation prostheses/high-profile designs. Forces occurring between the residual foot and the socket at push-off. F1 = force at plantar surface of residual foot; F2 = anterior force at socket brim; F3 = posterior force at heel level; F4 = oblique force created by combination of F1 and F3; R = ground-reaction force; W = body weight.

sity of California Biomechanics Laboratory (UCBL) foot orthosis, covering the dorsum of the foot. The plastic socket may be hinged to facilitate donning (Figure 8). The tendency of the foot to pronate can be addressed either by medially wedging the prosthesis to support the forefoot or by applying a pronation-resisting force to the area of the sustentaculum tali in the socket[15] (Figure 9).

The addition of a rocker sole to the shoe, with its apex proximal to the amputation site, can further relieve the cut bone ends. This also has the effect of reducing the moment that tends to cause rotation of the prosthesis relative to the residual foot at end-stance.

Tarsometatarsal and Transtarsal Amputations

Inevitably, the functional loss and the associated demands for successful prosthetic management are greatest when the surgery entails complete removal of all the metatarsals (tarsometatarsal or Lisfranc's amputation) or amputation through the midtarsal joint (transtarsal or Chopart's amputation). All of the functional limitations described for transmetatarsal amputation will be present. In addition, the shape of the residual foot and the much-reduced surface area available make the task of interfacing a prosthesis to it even more challenging.

As mentioned earlier, use of appropriate surgical procedures, even with these most proximal partial foot

amputations, can result in retention of a useful degree of ankle and even subtalar joint function. Conversely, when this is not the case, the unresisted action of the intact calf muscles will inevitably produce a deformed equinovarus position of the residual foot over time.

The designs of prostheses that have been produced for these amputation levels are categorized as perimalleolar and high-profile designs. Perimalleolar designs include inframalleolar designs, where the proximal trimline is below the malleoli, and supramalleolar designs, where the proximal trimline encloses the malleoli. The choice of which category and which variant within that category to employ will depend on a number of factors that will be discussed later. First, however, it is important to fully understand the biomechanical basis on which each category functions.

In perimalleolar designs, it is appropriate to attempt to use the residual plantar surface of the hindfoot (F1) to replace the support normally provided by the absent forefoot between heel-off and toe-off. As with transmetatarsal amputations, achieving this goal requires the prosthetic socket to generate a posteriorly directed force on the dorsum of the residual foot. Unfortunately, because of its more restricted area of application and its much shorter lever arm, this force is not capable of successfully resisting the dorsiflexing moment created by the prosthetic forefoot ground-reaction force (R) if the patient attempts to walk normally. As a

result, the socket will tend to rotate relative to the residual foot.

An alternative biomechanical solution to this problem, which was described as early as 1955, is to shape the socket so that it grasps the calcaneus firmly mediolaterally.[16] As the socket attempts to "dorsiflex," this action is resisted by downward forces (F2) generated on both sides of the calcaneus (Figure 10).

High-profile designs of prostheses for these amputation levels solve this problem in an entirely different and generally more satisfactory manner. In these designs, the forefoot dorsiflexion moment is resisted by a force

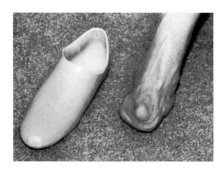

Figure 12 Slipper-type elastomer prosthesis (STEP).

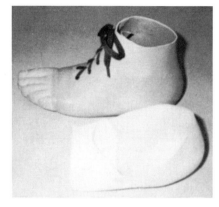

Figure 13 Imler prosthesis.

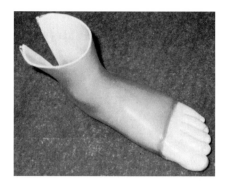

Figure 14 Lange silicone prosthesis.

couple created by socket interface forces located anteriorly at the socket brim (F2) and posteriorly at heel level (F3). This latter force combines with the plantar support force (F1) to create a single, oblique force (F4). Obviously, the higher the trimline and hence the wider the separation between F2 and F3, the lower will be their magnitude and consequently the pressure on the residual foot at their sites of application (Figure 11).

One final biomechanical consideration must be mentioned before discussing prescription criteria and related design issues. Irrespective of which category of device is supplied, if the user attempts to simulate normal push-off, requiring the generation of a significant forefoot ground-reaction force, the construction of the device must be stiff enough to withstand the resulting dorsiflexion moment without deforming.

In most respects, the similarities between tarsometatarsal and transtarsal amputations mean that they can be considered together. In both cases, if control of the talocrural or subtalar joints is impaired and results in deformity, this must be addressed whenever possible by realigning these joints during the casting procedure and with further modification of the positive cast. If mobile, the heel pad must be stabilized in the correct position to avoid medial deviation.

A number of prosthetic designs are available for these amputation levels, and prescription will depend on sev-

eral factors, including the functional and cosmetic aspirations of the amputee, the presence of joint instability or deformity, the ability to tolerate full body weight, and the sensitivity of the amputation site.

Perimalleolar Designs

Many popular modern designs of prostheses for these amputation levels terminate around the level of the ankle joint. Inframalleolar designs of prostheses are unobtrusive and combine reasonable function and good comfort with very satisfactory cosmesis. They permit the amputee to make use of the talocrural and subtalar joints, but it should be noted that this is appropriate only in patients in whom there is no requirement for significant joint realignment, restriction of motion, or augmentation of function[17] (Figure 12). If necessary, minor realignment of the subtalar joint can be achieved by appropriate wedging of the prosthesis or by wedging or flaring the shoe.

In all perimalleolar designs, resistance to the end-stance dorsiflexion moment is achieved by the intimacy of the socket fit over the anterior/dorsal aspect of the residual foot and, importantly, by the firm grip on either side of the calcaneus. Skillful modification of a plaster model of the foot is an important factor in achieving success. The use of soft interface padding, or silicone or polyurethane liners, which have excellent pressure and shear management properties,

also may be beneficial. Naturally, for slipper designs to be successful, the amputee must be able to tolerate full plantar surface weight bearing.

The major shortcomings of perimalleolar designs are related to suspension problems, discomfort at the anterior aspect of the residual foot at end-stance, and inability to generate adequate push-off, all of which limit the activity level of the user. Some of these shortcomings may be overcome by providing a prosthesis in the form of a bootie that encloses more of the residual foot, with a corresponding reduction in contact pressure. The stability of the prosthesis on the residual foot also is improved, as is suspension. A number of designs with varying degrees of flexibility have been used successfully and combine reasonable levels of function and cosmesis (Figures 13 and 14). Some of these prostheses are fitted with zip or Velcro closures to facilitate donning.[18,19]

Originally introduced for their excellent cosmetic appearance, silicone prostheses (Figure 15) have proved particularly successful for amputees with adherent or fragile scar tissue. In addition, they permit successful restoration of balance and a more normal gait when appropriately reinforced to achieve the degree of rigidity required to match the amputee's functional needs.[20] As a general rule, greater rigidity is indicated for the more active user. A lost wax method is used to create a negative impression of the required foot shape, and pure reinforced silicone is used to form the socket and the foot simultaneously. Pigment is added to the silicone to closely match the basic tissue color of the individual, with more detailed color matching done at the time of fitting. These sockets may be flexible enough to allow the residual foot to be pushed into the prosthesis after lubrication with skin lotion.

The anticipated activity level of the user is perhaps the most important factor to be considered when deciding on a suitable prescription for the tarsometatarsal or transtarsal amputee. There is no scientific evidence that perimalleolar designs allow the more active user to generate the forefoot ground-reaction force necessary to achieve normal push-off. In contrast, a recently published Swedish study clearly demonstrates the ability of users of a modern high-profile design to successfully generate and transmit these forces to their residual foot.[21]

High-Profile Designs

The absence of push-off at the end of stance phase seriously compromises the quality of gait. This situation is analogous to the problem faced by nonamputees with inadequate plantar flexor strength, who are often successfully treated with a rigid AFO. Prostheses based on a rigid AFO design (Figure 16), albeit with an appropriate sole plate and forefoot filler, prevent dorsiflexion by blocking the ankle at an appropriate angle.[22,23] An important socket interface force required to resist dorsiflexion is located anteriorly at the socket brim. Therefore, a prosthesis constructed with an anterior shell and a posterior opening is more appropriate than the posterior shell AFO-type designs (Figure 17). Naturally, this anterior shell approach will require the plaster model to be modified to protect the tibial crest and the amputation site. Some modern designs incorporate a full-length energy-storing footplate of carbon composite material, built up with a foam material to create the desired foot shape.[21]

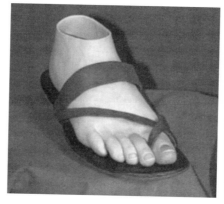
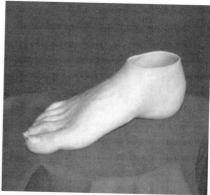

Figure 15 Silicone prosthesis by M. Alaric, Paris. *(Reproduced with permission from Soderberg B, Wykman A, Schaarschuch R, Persson BM: Silicone prosthesis, in Partial Foot Amputations: Guidelines to Prosthetic and Surgical Management. Helsingborg, Sweden, AB Boktryck, 2001, pp 80-85.)*

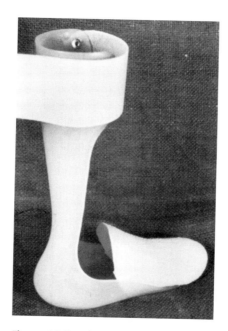

Figure 16 Prosthesis based on a modified AFO. *(Reproduced with permission from Stills ML: Partial foot prostheses/orthoses. Clin Prosthet Orthot 1988;12:14-18.)*

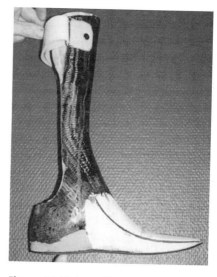

Figure 17 High-profile design prosthesis with anterior tibial shell and footplate of carbon fiber. *(Reproduced with permission from Soderberg B, Wykman A, Schaarschuch R, Persson BM: The chopart amputation, in Partial Foot Amputations: Guidelines to Prosthetic and Surgical Techniques. Helsingborg, Sweden, AB Boktryck, 2001, pp 51-59.)*

The angle at which the ankle is aligned is important. An anterior tibial tilt of 5° to 10° is desirable if a smooth rollover in late stance is to be achieved.[24] It is the anterior tilt angle of the tibia relative to the floor that is important, rather than the true angle of the talocrural joint, because the heel height of the footwear always must be considered (Figure 18, *A*). This alignment should avoid the need

for a rocker sole on the footwear, which otherwise might be required, and might still be required if the desired angle of dorsiflexion cannot be achieved. If necessary, a wedge build-up under the heel may be incorporated to accommodate any equinus deformity (Figure 18, *B*). If the wedge is made from a compressible material, plantar flexion will be simulated in a manner similar to the solid

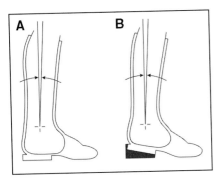

Figure 18 Preferred anterior tilt angle of 5° to 10°. **A,** Normally achieved by ankle dorsiflexion. **B,** A heel wedge is required in the presence of an equinus deformity.

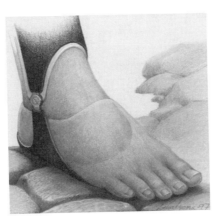

Figure 19 Prosthesis based on a jointed high-profile design permits plantar flexion while blocking dorsiflexion at an appropriate angle. *(Reproduced with permission from Soderberg B, Wykman A, Schaarschuch R, Persson BM: Evaluation of different prosthetic solutions for Lisfranc amputees, in* Partial Foot Amputations: Guidelines to Prosthetic and Surgical Management. *Helsingborg, Sweden, AB Boktryck, 2001, pp 76-79.)*

ankle–cushion heel (SACH) prosthetic foot. However, when an accommodation for equinus is necessary, the length of the prosthesis will be increased, requiring a compensatory lift on the contralateral side.

Excessive toe-in of this style of prosthesis can lead to the development of a varus moment at the knee. Therefore, it is important to ensure that the forefoot section of the prosthesis is formed so that its rotational alignment matches the sound side. It also has been suggested that making the soleplate stiffer on the lateral side will help resist this varus knee moment.[21]

The use of a rigid high-profile design will sacrifice all movement about the remaining joints of the foot and ankle; however, because these movements are often reduced or absent, this may not represent a serious loss. In any case, the loss of these movements may be worthwhile to achieve improvements in comfort and gait. SACH modification to the heel of the footwear will improve shock attenuation in early stance and simulate plantar flexion, but careful selection of footwear with a compressible heel, eg, a sports shoe, may make this modification unnecessary. A more sophisticated approach is to incorporate an ankle joint in the prosthesis that permits plantar flexion but blocks dorsiflexion at the appropriate angle, thus permitting more normal ankle joint motion (Figure 19).

In some cases, the combination of a very small plantar surface area of the residual foot and the presence of a fixed equinovarus deformity makes distal weight bearing impractical. In these situations, a prosthesis employing proximal weight-bearing techniques similar to those seen in transtibial prostheses is indicated.[23,25] In general, patients who perform at higher activity levels will derive benefit from the provision of prostheses with higher trimlines.

Summary

A comfortable socket, a balanced foot, and an optimal gait pattern are the clinical objectives for all users of partial foot prostheses. The choice of the particular design to be used will depend on a number of factors and requires a careful assessment of the user and a full appreciation of the individual's aspirations. New materials and fabrication techniques have permitted the development of both cosmetically and functionally improved designs that may make partial foot amputation a practical alternative to higher amputation where the pathology permits.

References

1. Condie DN: Biomechanics, in Helal B, Rowley DI, Crachiollo A, Myerson MS (eds): *Surgery of Disorders of the Foot and Ankle.* London, England, Martin Dunitz, 1996, pp 37-46.

2. Wright DG, Desai ME, Henderson BS: Action of the subtalar and ankle-joint complex during the stance phase of walking. *J Bone Joint Surg Am* 1964;46:361-382.

3. Elftman H: The transverse tarsal joint and its control. *Clin Orthop* 1960;16:41-45.

4. Levens AS, Inman VT, Blosser JA: Transverse rotations of the segments of the lower limb in locomotion. *J Bone Joint Surg Am* 1948;30:859-872.

5. Chrzan JS, Giurini JM, Hurchik JM: A biomechanical model for the transmetatarsal amputation. *J Am Podiatr Med Assoc* 1993;83:82-86.

6. Kavanagh PR, Ulbrecht JS, Wu G, et al: The diabetic foot with partial amputation: A biomechanical study. *J Biomech* 1994;27:606.

7. Boyd LA, Rao SS, Burnfield JM, et al: Forefoot rocker mechanics in individuals with partial foot amputation. *Gait Posture* 1999;9:144.

8. Kelly VE, Mueller MJ, Sinacore DR: Timing of peak plantar pressure during the stance phase of walking: A study of patients with diabetes mellitus and transmetatarsal amputation. *J Am Podiatr Med Assoc* 2000;90:18-23.

9. Parziale JR, Hahn KK: Functional considerations in partial foot amputation. *Orthop Rev* 1988;17:262-266.

10. Letts M, Pyper A: The modified Chopart amputation. *Clin Orthop* 1990;256:44-49.

11. Wagner FW: Partial foot amputations: Surgical procedures, in Bowker JH, Michael JW (eds): *Atlas of Limb Prosthetics.* Rosemont, IL, American Academy of Orthopaedic Surgeons, 2002, pp 389-402. (Originally published by Mosby-Year Book, 1992.)

12. Moore JW: Prostheses orthoses and shoes for partial foot amputees. *Clin Podiatr Med Surg* 1997;14:775-784.

13. Perry J: *Gait Analysis: Normal and Pathological Function.* Thorofare, NJ, Slack, 1992.

14. Collins SN: A partial foot prosthesis for the transmetatarsal level. *Clin Prosthet Orthot* 1988;12:19-23.

15. Colson JM, Berglund G: An effective design for controlling the unstable subtalar joint. *Orthot Prosthet* 1979;33: 39-49.

16. MacDonald A: Chopart amputation: The advantages of a modified prosthesis. *J Bone Joint Surg Br* 1955;37: 468-470.

17. Childs C, Staats T: The slipper type partial foot prosthesis, in *Advanced Below-knee Prosthetic Seminar*. Los Angeles, CA, UCLA Prosthetics and Orthotic Education Program, Fabrication Manual, 1983.

18. Imler CD: Imler Partial Foot Prosthesis: IPFP— The Chicago boot. *Orthot Prosthet* 1985;39:53-56.

19. Lange LR: The Lange silicone partial foot prosthesis. *J Prosthet Orthot* 1991; 4:56-61.

20. Kulkarni J, Curran B, Ebdon-Parry M, Harrison D: Total contact silicone partial foot prostheses for partial foot amputations. *Foot* 1995;5:32-35.

21. Soderberg B, Wykman A, Schaarschuch R, Persson BM: *Partial Foot Amputation*. Helsingborg, Sweden, Swedish Orthopaedic Association Publications, 2001.

22. Stills ML: Partial foot prostheses/orthoses. *Clin Prosthet Orthot* 1988; 12:14-18.

23. Rubin G, Cohen E: Indications for variants of the partial foot prosthesis. *Orthop Rev* 1985;14:49-56.

24. Glancy J, Lindseth RE: The polypropylene solid-ankle orthosis. *Orthot Prosthet* 1972;26:14-26.

25. Cohen-Sobel E, Caselli MA, Rizzuto J: Prosthetic management of a Chopart variant. *J Am Podiatr Med Assoc* 1994;84:505-510.

Chapter 36

Ankle Disarticulation and Variants: Surgical Management

John H. Bowker, MD

Introduction

In 1843, James Syme, then Professor of Surgery at the University of Edinburgh, described his innovative operation, now known as the Syme ankle disarticulation, as "disarticulation through the ankle joint with preservation of the heel flap to permit weight-bearing on the end of the stump.[1] Because the procedure preserves weight bearing on the heel pad along normal proprioceptive pathways, gait with a Syme ankle disarticulation is more energy efficient than with a transtibial amputation and requires minimal prosthetic gait training, chiefly the equalization of stride length and time in stance phase. From the patient's viewpoint, a Syme ankle disarticulation is a less destructive procedure than a transtibial amputation.[2] The heel pad is remarkably activity tolerant, even if insensate, as in many patients with diabetes mellitus, provided the heel pad is held directly under the tibia by an intimately fitted socket. Careful prosthetic follow-up is essential to maintain this position because calf atrophy inevitably occurs. The main limitation of the procedure is cosmetic; it results in distal bulkiness of the malleoli and heel pad that is reflected to a variable degree in the prosthetic socket, depending on the surgical technique selected. Despite this disadvantage, the benefit to the patient of being able to comfortably engage in a wide range of activities suggests that much more frequent use of this procedure is indicated.

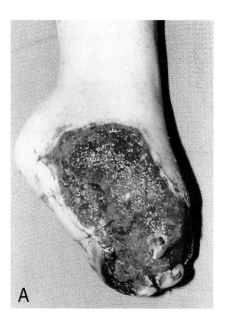 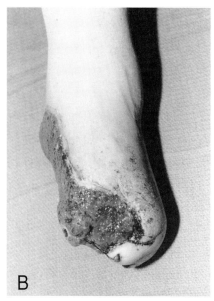 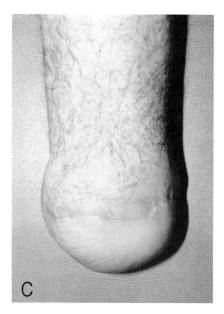

Figure 1 A 32-year-old man sustained work-related trauma to his left foot. **A,** Medial view of the foot showing loss of skin proximal to the site of a standard Syme incision. **B,** Anterior view showing sufficient lateral skin to compensate for lack of medial skin. **C,** Anterior view 3 years after Syme procedure. The individual works, stands, and walks up to 16 to 18 hours daily without difficulty. *(Reproduced with permission from Bowker JH, San Giovanni TP: Amputations and disarticulations, in Myerson MS (ed): Foot and Ankle Disorders. Philadelphia, PA, WB Saunders, 2000.)*

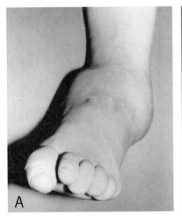
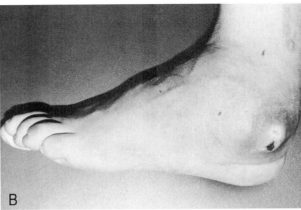
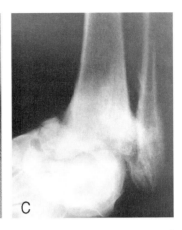

Figure 2 A 32-year-old woman with type 1 diabetes mellitus was seen 1 year after sustaining a nondisplaced bimalleolar fracture of the left ankle that was treated in a cast for 6 weeks. Loss of protective sensation to the level of the tibial tubercle was undetected by the surgeon. **A,** Anterior view of the foot showing medial displacement. **B,** Use of an ankle-foot orthosis to attempt control of this irreducible and increasing deformity caused a pressure ulcer over the lateral malleolus. **C,** AP radiograph shows dissolution of the ankle joint, talus, and subtalar joint with varus deformity. *(Reproduced with permission from Bowker JH, San Giovanni TP: Amputations and disarticulations, in Myerson MS (ed): Foot and Ankle Disorders. Philadelphia, PA, WB Saunders, 2000.)*

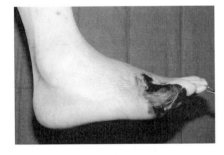

Figure 3 Right foot of a 66-year-old man with diabetes mellitus with dry gangrene of the distal forefoot. The posterior tibial artery was patent, making the patient a good candidate for a Syme ankle disarticulation.

Patient Selection

Ankle disarticulation with preservation of the heel pad is suitable for treating several conditions. One example is severe forefoot trauma that spares the heel pad but leaves insufficient soft tissue to close a midtarsal (Chopart) disarticulation (Figure 1). The procedure is also a reasonable choice in selected cases of severe diabetic neuroarthropathy of the hindfoot and/or ankle joint (Figure 2). It offers a more rapid return to weight-bearing status than does ankle/subtalar arthrodesis because it requires no fusion or fibrous ankylosis of the involved bones. It can also be considered in dry gangrene of the

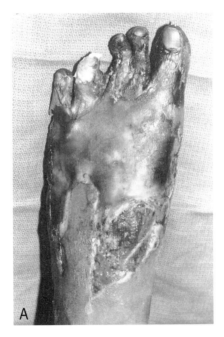
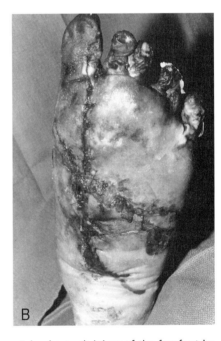

Figure 4 The left foot of a 41-year-old man sustained a crush injury of the forefoot by forklift truck. The hindfoot was spared, permitting ankle disarticulation. **A,** Dorsal view. **B,** Plantar view. *(Reproduced with permission from Bowker JH, San Giovanni TP: Amputations and disarticulations, in Myerson MS (ed): Foot and Ankle Disorders. Philadelphia, PA, WB Saunders, 2000.)*

forefoot due to occlusion of the distal arterial arch of the foot from peripheral vascular disease (Figure 3) or with severe crush injuries if the posterior tibial artery is patent (Figure 4). With wet gangrene of the forefoot, common in patients with diabetes mellitus, Syme ankle disarticulation is useful, but care must be taken to do a

staged procedure if infection is too close to the heel pad to risk primary closure (Figure 5). A much less common condition for which the Syme procedure is sometimes appropriate is congenital arteriovenous fistulae of the foot resulting in marked overgrowth. With this condition, repeated hemorrhage from minor trauma may occur despite embolization procedures. In carefully selected patients, the heel pad can be salvaged (Figure 6). Another unusual condition is severe varus deformity associated with progressive hemiatrophy. Children with unilateral or bilateral total longitudinal deficiency of the fibula, partial longitudinal deficiency of the tibia, or partial longitudinal deficiency of the femur may also benefit from Syme ankle disarticulation with care taken to preserve the distal tibial and fibular physes[3,4] (Figure 7).

Indications

The main indication for a Syme ankle disarticulation is a foot with the requisite blood flow to the heel pad through the posterior tibial artery in which a more distal functional level cannot be salvaged. A secondary indication is a midfoot infection that is too close to the heel pad to risk a Lisfranc (disarticulation between the tarsus and metatarsus) or Chopart disarticulation. In such cases, the Syme wound is left open initially to allow local control of the infection before secondary closure. The Syme procedure is also a good choice for patients with expectation of a high level of walking activity. It is also particularly advantageous for obese individuals because the end–weight-bearing provided by a Syme procedure is better tolerated than the peripheral weight-bearing that results from a transtibial amputation.

Contraindications

Absolute contraindications to a Syme ankle disarticulation include inadequate circulation to the heel pad via the posterior tibial artery, infection within the heel pad, and severe traumatic damage to the skin or fatty compartments of the heel pad. Significant tibial deformity may prevent placement of the heel pad in good weight-bearing alignment, resulting in displacement of the heel pad.[2] In addition, some patients may object to the appearance of the residual limb

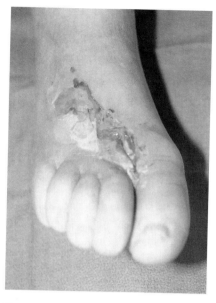

Figure 5 Extensive wet gangrene of the forefoot in a patient with diabetes mellitus precluded even Chopart disarticulation. The heel pad and posterior tibial artery were intact, allowing a Syme procedure.

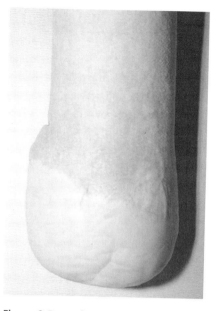

Figure 6 Foot of a young woman several years after a Syme ankle disarticulation performed for congenital arteriovenous fistulae of the foot. No new fistulae developed, but residual distended veins are seen extending to the incision line on the right.

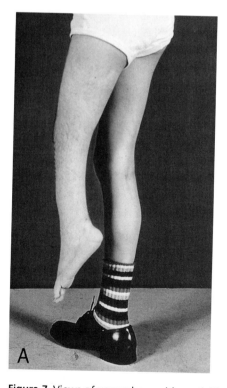

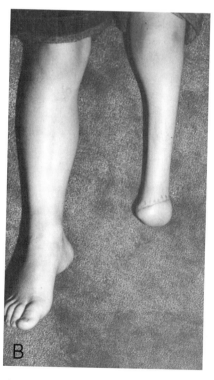

Figure 7 Views of young boys with partial longitudinal deficiency of the left femur and total longitudinal deficiency of the left fibula. **A,** Preoperative view of one boy showing limb-length discrepancy and equinus deformity. **B,** Postoperative view of another boy following Syme ankle disarticulation showing the residual limb ready for prosthetic fitting. *(Reproduced with permission from Bowker JH, San Giovanni TP: Amputations and disarticulations, in Myerson MS (ed): Foot and Ankle Disorders. Philadelphia, PA, WB Saunders, 2000.)*

and the prosthesis; this must be anticipated and resolved before surgery. Some surgeons have been reluctant to recommend this procedure for young female patients, but Baumgartner[5] and others believe that with appropriate preoperative counseling and modern prosthetic techniques, the Syme procedure can be confidently recommended for this group. Because the patient's cooperation is essential to both the short-term and long-term success of this procedure, the surgeon should be aware that failure is likely in a patient with a history of reckless noncompliance with medical advice or overt psychosis. In addition, patients with end-stage renal disease who require dialysis are unlikely to heal because of poor retention of serum proteins.[6-8]

Relative contraindications include problems that may be controllable, at least to some extent, by the treatment team. Unless these conditions show some improvement preoperatively, they must be considered absolute contraindications. They include lymphangitis ascending to the leg, low serum albumin due to malnutrition or nephropathy, and congestive heart failure.

Preoperative Considerations
Adequate Blood Flow

In preparation for a Syme ankle disarticulation, the surgeon must be certain that there is adequate perfusion of the heel pad, which occurs largely through the posterior tibial artery (Figure 8). If a bounding posterior tibial pulse can be felt, no further investigation is needed. If a pulse cannot be felt, a portable Doppler device may be used. This is, however, of limited use in patients with diabetes mellitus because artificially high values may be obtained from incompressible, heavily calcified arteries. In this case, or if edema is present, real-time flow may be observed directly by means of duplex ultrasound angiography.

The absolute necessity of adequate posterior tibial blood flow to the heel pad cannot be overemphasized. During the 1960s, Sarmiento[9] performed a series of Syme ankle disarticulations in a group of 38 patients with forefoot gangrene without regard to the presence of palpable pedal pulses; 19 (50%) failed. The author also performed the procedure on a second group of 15 patients who were required to have a palpable posterior tibial pulse. Of these, 12 healed, for a failure rate of 20%. Francis and associates[10] reported that 19 of 22 patients (86%) with a palpable posterior tibial pulse healed primarily. Laughlin and Chambers[11] evaluated the predictive value of Doppler waveform configuration in 52 patients with diabetes mellitus before surgery. Of 29 patients, 26 (90%) with either a triphasic waveform or a normal pulse healed, compared with only 13 of 23 patients (57%) with a monophasic waveform.

If a patient with diabetes mellitus presents with severe forefoot ischemia or ischemic ulceration and has no discernible posterior tibial pulse, consultation with a vascular surgeon may be indicated. Patients with diabetes typically have occlusion of the posterior tibial and peroneal arteries in the calf with retained patency of the vessels in the foot. Angioplasty or bypass procedures may improve distal flow sufficiently to allow healing distal to the transtibial level. Weaver and associates[12] reported on 35 patients ranging in age from 40 to 77 years, of whom 31 (89%) had diabetes mellitus. A vascular procedure was performed in 22 patients with the most compromised blood flow immediately before a Syme ankle disarticulation. Primary healing occurred in 19 (86%), compared with 77% in those in whom vascular intervention was deemed unnecessary. In another series of 13 patients who had vascular intervention an average of 3 months before a Syme procedure, 12 (92%) healed.[11]

Wound Healing Potential

Wound healing potential must also be assessed, including the patient's nutri-

tional status, as reflected in the serum albumin level. Levels less than 3.0 g/dL can be indicative of starvation, significant renal disease, acute stress, or a combination of these factors. Patients who are immunosuppressed as indicated by a total lymphocyte count less than 1,500/mm³ may also have decreased wound healing potential. Dickhaut and associates[13] retrospectively reviewed Syme healing rates in 23 patients with diabetes who had adequate blood flow and in whom serum albumin levels and total lymphocyte counts had been obtained on admission. Healing occurred in only 43% of those with a serum albumin level less than 3.5 g/dL and a total lymphocyte count less than 1,500/mm³, in contrast with 86% of those with higher values. Pinzur and associates[8] concluded from a similar study that a minimum serum albumin level of 3.0 g/dL was sufficient. The dietary needs of the patient with low serum albumin levels can usually be met by oral hyperalimentation. For patients with diabetes mellitus, caloric increase must be matched with appropriate increases in medication to prevent iatrogenic hyperglycemia.

Diffuse tissue glycation resulting from chronic hyperglycemia may have a negative effect on wound healing as well. The presence of chronic hyperglycemia can be inferred from repeated glycohemoglobin levels in excess of 7%. Several studies have shown poor healing in hyperglycemic rats, with wounds exhibiting decreased leukocytosis and impaired neovascularization as well as decreased nitric acid synthesis, granulation tissue mass, collagen content, and wound strength.[14-17] Perioperative control of very high serum glucose levels is therefore important, although this may be difficult to achieve if infection persists despite the use of antibiotics, indicating the need for prompt surgical management. Tight control of serum glucose levels should be delayed until the patient has recovered from the stress of

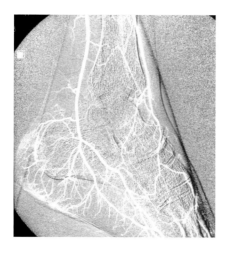

Figure 8 Lateral view of a posterior tibial arteriogram showing its major contribution to heel pad circulation. *(Courtesy of Professor G. Neff.)*

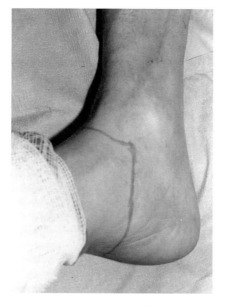

Figure 9 Syme procedure. Medial view of a right foot showing the transverse incision line across the ankle joint, continuing as a stirrup incision anterior to the heel pad. The necrotic toes have been wrapped to exclude them from the surgical field. *(Reproduced with permission from Bowker JH, San Giovanni TP: Amputations and disarticulations, in Myerson MS (ed): Foot and Ankle Disorders. Philadelphia, PA, WB Saunders, 2000.)*

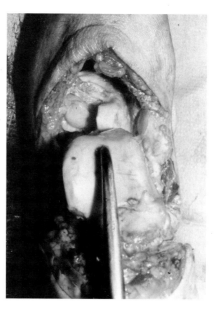

Figure 10 Syme procedure. A bone hook has been placed in the talar dome to provide anteroplantar traction on the foot. Note the flexor hallucis longus tendon just posterior to the talus, clearly demarcating the safe area lateral to the medial neurovascular structures. *(Reproduced with permission from Bowker JH, San Giovanni TP: Amputations and disarticulations, in Myerson MS (ed): Foot and Ankle Disorders. Philadelphia, PA, WB Saunders, 2000.)*

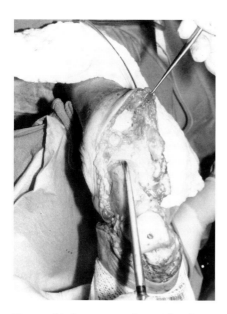

Figure 11 Syme procedure. The bone hook has been transferred to the calcaneal tuberosity to put tension on the Achilles tendon to facilitate its separation from the calcaneus. *(Reproduced with permission from Bowker JH, San Giovanni TP: Amputations and disarticulations, in Myerson MS (ed): Foot and Ankle Disorders. Philadelphia, PA, WB Saunders, 2000.)*

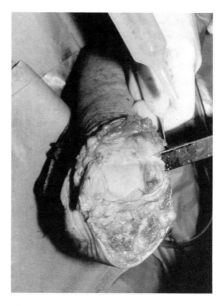

Figure 12 Syme procedure. Shortening and narrowing of the malleoli is accomplished easily with a sharp osteotome. *(Reproduced with permission from Bowker JH, San Giovanni TP: Amputations and disarticulations, in Myerson MS (ed): Foot and Ankle Disorders. Philadelphia, PA, WB Saunders, 2000.)*

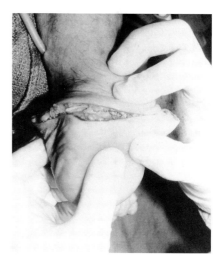

Figure 13 Syme procedure. Prior to closure, flap lengths are carefully checked. If the fit is too loose, skin is removed from the proximal flap. If too tight, the tibia will need to be appropriately shortened, which is accomplished most accurately with a broad saw. *(Reproduced with permission from Bowker JH, San Giovanni TP: Amputations and disarticulations, in Myerson MS (ed): Foot and Ankle Disorders. Philadelphia, PA, WB Saunders, 2000.)*

surgery, to avoid life-threatening iatrogenic hypoglycemia.

Infection Control

A major preoperative management goal for any forefoot or midfoot infection is prevention of the proximal spread of infective material along tissue planes. The first measure required is prohibition of all further weight bearing; the second is prompt initial drainage of any abscess in the emergency department if an operating suite is not available soon after medical clearance. Decompressive incisions must respect the heel pad if a Syme ankle disarticulation is to remain feasible. Deep wound cultures, both aerobic and anaerobic, should be obtained and broad-spectrum antibiotics begun because most diabetic foot infections are polymicrobial. The antibiotics administered initially, pending culture and sensitivities confirmation, should be effective against *Staphylococcus* and *Streptococcus* as well as common gram-negative bacilli and anaerobes.[18-20]

Surgical Technique

A Syme ankle disarticulation, although not a technically difficult procedure, must be done with meticulous attention to preservation of the posterior tibial neurovascular structures and the vertically oriented fat-filled chambers of the heel pad, which provide shock absorption on heel contact. These points are well illustrated and discussed in the classic articles by Syme[1] and Harris.[21]

With the patient in the supine position and a thigh tourniquet in place, an anterior transverse incision is made at the level of the ankle joint, ending medially and laterally at points 1 cm distal and 1 cm anterior to the midline of each malleolus. These two points are connected by a stirrup incision, placed just anterior to the heel pad (Figure 9). If the tourniquet is inflated, the incisions may be taken directly to bone; otherwise, the neurovascular structures should be dealt with as the wound is deepened. Care must be taken to find and shorten all anterior

sensory nerves to avoid their entrapment in the incisional scar. These include the branches of the superficial peroneal nerve and the deep peroneal nerve, which must be separated from its accompanying vessels and shortened.

Following incision of the anterior ankle capsule, the foot can be plantar flexed with the aid of a large bone hook inserted into the talar dome (Figure 10). Alternatively, as suggested by Öznur,[22] a Steinmann pin can be placed transversely in the posterior talus and attached to a traction bow or Ilizarov half ring with traction on the talus applied through a cord attached to weights or the surgeon's foot. Care must be taken to pass the pin from medial to lateral to avoid damage to the posterior tibial artery. Traction will assist in locating the tendon of the flexor hallucis longus, an important landmark that lies directly posterior to the talar body and just medial to the neurovascular bundle. With the collateral ligaments under tension, they can be safely divided at the talar body with the neurovascular bundle protected by gentle retraction. The soft tissues are gently stripped from the superior, medial, and lateral surfaces of the calcaneus with care to avoid penetration of the cortex, especially in osteoporotic bone. Bruising of the posterior tibial vessels is to be avoided because it may lead to thrombosis with loss of heel pad perfusion.

The bone hook is then transferred to the posterior aspect of the calcaneal tuberosity to expose and put tension on the Achilles tendon (Figure 11). The tendon is gently separated from the calcaneus, taking care to avoid buttonholing the thin posterior heel skin. The foot is then further plantar flexed and the heel pad is freed subperiosteally from the plantar calcaneal surface. The calcaneal origin of the plantar fascia is divided transversely to complete the disarticulation. The inside of the heel pad should be palpated carefully to reveal any flakes of cortical bone left from stripping of the calcaneus. These should be meticulously removed to

avoid growth of painful bony masses.

Provision of a durable and comfortable weight-bearing surface is the next concern. Harris[21] recommended removing a 1-cm slice of the distal tibia, effectively removing the malleoli. This is best done with a wide-blade saw to ensure that the distal tibial surface is parallel to the floor during weight bearing. Sarmiento[9] advised removing 1.2 cm of the distal tibia and narrowing the malleoli to fit a more cosmetic prosthesis with an expandable liner. Wagner[6] also modified the traditional technique used in patients with diabetes mellitus by shortening and narrowing the malleoli but leaving the cartilage of the plafond intact (Figure 12). He also recommended that the procedure be done in two stages in cases of forefoot infection to reduce the theoretic chance of recurrent infection. Other authors[5,7,23] have reported that both stages can be safely combined provided that infection is not adjacent to the heel pad. Prior to closure, the fit of the heel pad should be checked (Figure 13). If too loose, excess skin can be removed from the proximal skin edge. If too snug, 0.5 to 1.0 cm should be removed from the tibia and fibula. If infection is close to the heel pad, the skin incision should be made more distal and the wound left open for 7 to 10 days to see if débridement and antibiotics have controlled the infection. Secondary closure without wound tension will require that the tibia be shortened as described by Harris[21] to accommodate interval shrinkage of the heel pad flap and to remove the exposed plafond cartilage.

Elmslie[24] attempted to improve the cosmetic appearance of the residual limb following a Syme procedure by using an incision that radically reduced the surface area of the heel pad and by transecting the tibia and fibula 2.5 cm proximal to the ankle joint. These two modifications greatly diminished the weight-bearing surface of both the heel pad and the distal tibia, leading to painful prosthetic gait (Figure 14).

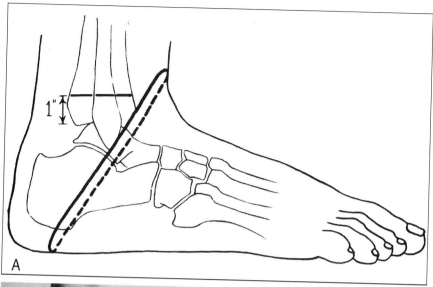

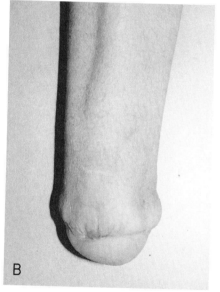
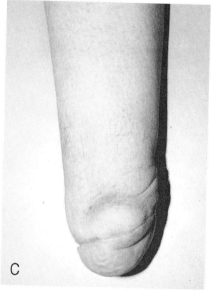

Figure 14 Elmslie's modification of the Syme procedure. **A,** Diagram shows placement of the incision, which removes a major portion of the heel pad, and location of transection of the tibia and fibula, proximal to the ankle joint 1 in (2.5 cm). (Reproduced with permission from *Carson's Modern Surgical Surgery*. London, England, 1924.) **B,** Anterior and **C,** lateral views of a right limb that underwent an Elmslie-type procedure 6 years earlier for trauma. Walking in a prosthesis was painful because of the small weight-bearing surface of the truncated heel pad.

drain tube can be run between layers of cast padding and out the top of the cast, allowing its removal without disturbing the cast after 24 to 48 hours. When a Syme ankle disarticulation has been done for infection, it may be more appropriate to use a continuous closed irrigation stem to minimize recurrence of infection. Just before closure, a double-lumen catheter, such as a Shirley drain or Foley catheter, is modified and inserted through a lateral stab wound[6] (Figure 15). A Foley catheter is prepared by dividing it obliquely proximal to the balloon. The smaller tube is attached to a bag of saline solution and the larger one to a sterile urine collection bag. One liter of saline solution is passed through the wound every 8 hours until the outflow is clear, usually by 2 to 3 days postoperatively. Every 4 hours, the wound is flushed by occluding the larger egress tube for 5 minutes, then releasing it. A cast is applied immediately upon removal of the catheter, carefully molding the heel pad to a central and slightly forward position under the tibia. The cast is reapplied in the same manner at weekly intervals for 4 to 5 weeks, when a walking heel is added (Figure 16). This temporary prosthesis is changed whenever it becomes loose, but at least every 2 weeks, until limb volume has stabilized. At that time, measurements for a prosthesis are taken, and a new walking cast is worn until the prosthesis is ready.

Occasionally, major anterior or medial skin defects proximal to the ankle joint can be closed with salvaged sole skin extending distally from the heel pad. Careful trimming and rotational placement of the flap are essential. The initial bulkiness of the sole flap will resolve with progressive weight bearing in temporary prostheses (Figures 17 and 18).

Expected Functional Outcome

Both the Syme ankle disarticulation and transtibial amputation retain the

The heel pad flap can be accurately and securely centered under the tibia by suturing the plantar fascia to the anterior tibial cortex through drill holes. Alternatively, Smith and associates[25] recommend tenodesing the Achilles tendon through drill holes in the posterior tibial cortex to neutralize the pull of the triceps surae on the heel pad, thus preventing its posterior displacement. Other methods include taping or transfixing the heel pad to the tibia by a threaded or smooth pin, but these do not offer the security of direct suture of the plantar fascia or Achilles tendon to the tibia, when these latter techniques are combined with casting.

Prior to closure and cast application, consideration should be given to draining the large dead space created by removal of the talus and calcaneus to prevent hematoma formation. In trauma cases, a nonsutured suction

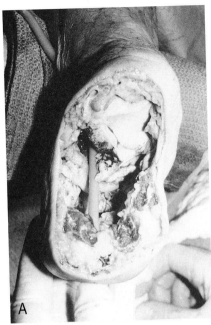
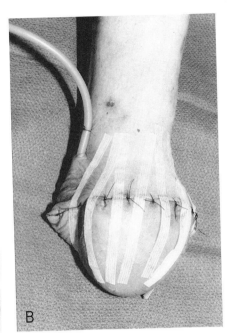

Figure 15 Syme procedure. **A,** Note placement of the catheter posterolateral to the fibula. Also note the oblique division of the catheter, which opens both lumens. **B,** Note the wide spacing of the sutures and the supplemental use of adhesive paper strips. The modified Foley catheter provides continuous irrigation with normal saline solution. Note that "dog ears" have not been trimmed to avoid narrowing of the heel flap pedicle. *(Figure 2,B reproduced with permission from Bowker JH, San Giovanni TP: Amputations and disarticulations, in Myerson MS (ed): Foot and Ankle Disorders. Philadelphia, PA, WB Saunders, 2000.)*

knee joint. A distinct advantage of the Syme, however, is preservation of end–weight-bearing along normal proprioceptive pathways through the heel pad (Figure 19). Gait studies demonstrate that patients with Syme disarticulations have increased cadence and velocity and consume less oxygen per meter traveled than do persons with more proximal level amputations or disarticulations.[26]

Minimal prosthetic gait training is required following a Syme procedure, chiefly the equalization of stride length and time spent in stance phase. Even an insensate heel pad is remarkably activity tolerant, as noted by Srinivasan,[27] who reported that pressure sores of the heel pad developed in only 3 of 20 persons (15%) with Hansen's disease (leprosy) at an average of 5 years after Syme ankle disarticulation, despite loss of protective sensation.

Careful maintenance of the heel pad in a central weight-bearing position beneath the tibia is essential. In the absence of careful initial prosthetic alignment of the heel pad and ongoing adjustments/refitting as necessary as normal atrophy occurs, the heel pad may migrate posteriorly or in the coronal plane, even within the prosthesis, leading to painful weight-bearing and/or ulceration (Figure 20). In a review of the literature, Smith and associates[25] found that heel pad migration ranged from 7.5% to 45%, but in their series of 10 patients in whom Syme disarticulation was augmented by Achilles tenodesis to the posterior tibia, all heel pads remained stable at an average of 18.5 months.

One of the advantages of the Syme procedure is that it allows weight bearing directly on the heel pad without a prosthesis, at least for short distances. Gaine and McCreath[2] studied 46 patients who had undergone Syme disarticulations, at an average follow-up of 22 years after surgery. They found that 32 patients (70%) could bear weight directly on the heel pad without a prosthesis in their home. Another ten

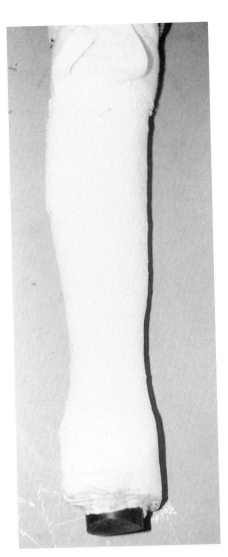

Figure 16 Syme procedure. A temporary weight-bearing prosthesis is applied after 4 to 5 weeks of non–weight-bearing casts, changed weekly. The temporary prosthesis is changed every 10 to 14 days until the leg volume has stabilized, when the definitive prosthesis is fitted. It is important that the heel pad be continuously held in weight-bearing line by casting until fitting is accomplished. *(Reproduced with permission from Bowker JH, San Giovanni TP: Amputations and disarticulations, in Myerson MS (ed): Foot and Ankle Disorders. Philadelphia, PA, WB Saunders, 2000.)*

of this group were considered to have "poor" residual limbs due to uncontrollable heel pad mobility or tibial cuts that were too proximal or not parallel to the floor when the patient was in the standing position. Nine of these ten were unable to bear weight without a prosthesis because of pain. The

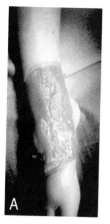 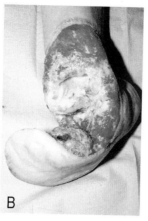 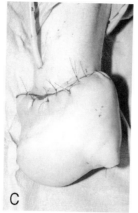 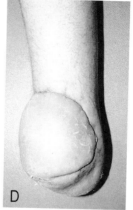 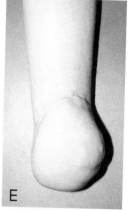

Figure 17 A 29-year-old woman with type 1 diabetes mellitus sustained extensive loss of skin over the anterior foot, ankle, and leg following a spider bite. Note the intact heel pad. **A,** Preoperative view. **B,** Same lower limb about 10 days after open ankle disarticulation with salvage of the heel pad and contiguous sole skin flap. **C,** Wound closure with sole flap used to cover anterior defect. Note the extreme bulkiness of the flap. **D,** Same limb 7 weeks later, after the patient had walked in two temporary prostheses. Note the good incorporation of the sole flap and reduction in bulkiness. **E,** Same limb 9 months after closure. The patient had been successfully fitted with a Syme prosthesis.

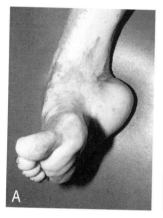 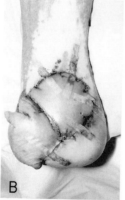 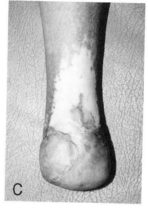

Figure 18 A 63-year-old woman with hemiatrophy of the right foot was treated with a Syme ankle disarticulation. **A,** Note the fixed varus deformity of the foot and extensive scarring of the medial ankle and leg. **B,** Medial view 2 days postoperatively. At the time of surgery, a portion of skin from the sole of the foot was used as a flap to cover the defect created by repositioning of the heel pad. Note the edema and duskiness of the sole flap. **C,** Medial view 8.5 months later. The flap was well incorporated and the woman was a successful ambulator in a prosthesis.

80% at both 3 and 5 years. In another series, Birch and associates[29] evaluated 10 young adults (age 18 to 26 years) who had undergone Syme ankle disarticulation between the ages of 2 and 12 years for fibular deficiencies. The surgical criteria were equinovalgus ankle, 5 cm or more of tibial shortening, and absence of at least two lateral rays. All 10 wore a prosthesis without difficulty and all were reported to have normal psychological adjustment to their impairment. Nine of the 10 participated in recreational sports, two in high school football.

Variants of Ankle Disarticulation

The Syme ankle disarticulation, because it involves removal of the talus and calcaneus, provides enough vertical clearance to fit a variety of dynamic-response prosthetic feet. In some patients, however, the heel pad remains unstable unless constrained by the socket, making it impossible to walk prosthesis-free without the risk of displacing the heel pad.

To allow the hindfoot amputee to walk securely without the need for an expensive prosthesis, Pirogoff[30] advocated a calcaneotibial arthrodesis to maintain heel pad stability and mini-

authors then compared 25 of these patients with 25 transtibial amputees in regard to level of activity and general function. The groups were found to be quite similar, although those who had undergone disarticulation in childhood had fewer problems with function and the residual limb. Two patients had a Syme ankle disarticulation in one leg and a transtibial amputation in the other leg; they preferred the Syme ankle disarticulation because its more natural proprioceptive feedback allowed easier limb placement while walking or stairclimbing.[2,28]

Laughlin and Chambers[11] assessed functional level in a series of 20 patients who had undergone Syme disarticulations 27 months postoperatively. Eighteen (90%) were community ambulators, 11 (55%) could walk 3 or more blocks, and 16 (80%) could climb stairs. All 18 community ambulators wore a prosthesis the entire day.[11] Weaver and associates[12] reported successful prosthetic fitting of 28 of 29 patients (97%) with Syme disarticulations who achieved primary healing. They noted cumulative ambulatory rates of 92% at 1 year and

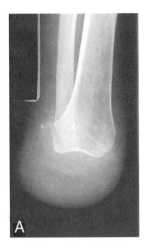
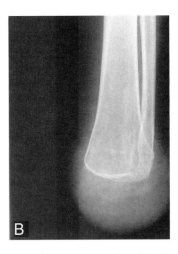
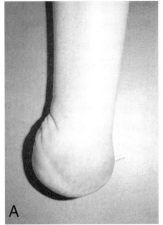
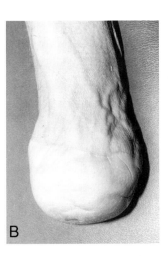

Figure 19 Mature Syme ankle disarticulation. **A,** Lateral and **B,** AP radiographs. Note the thickness of the fatty heel pad, which provides excellent weight-bearing characteristics when contained within a prosthesis socket. Also note the well-centralized position of the heel pad in both views. *(Figure 19 B is reproduced from Bowker JH: Minor and major lower limb amputations in persons with diabetes mellitus, in Bowker JH, Pfeifer MA (eds): Levin and O'Neal's The Diabetic Foot, ed 6. St. Louis, MO, Mosby, 2001.)*

Figure 20 A woman who underwent a Syme disarticulation of the left limb sustained a fixed posteromedial displacement of the heel pad 1 year after the initial surgery while walking in a prosthesis that no longer fit intimately because of tissue atrophy. **A,** Preoperative appearance of the limb. **B,** Appearance of the residual limb 7 years after surgical release and realignment of the heel pad beneath the tibia. The woman was actively wearing the prosthesis 14 to 16 hours daily. *(Figure 20 B is reproduced from Bowker JH: Minor and major lower limb amputations in persons with diabetes mellitus, in Bowker JH, Pfeifer MA (eds): Levin and O'Neal's The Diabetic Foot, ed 6. St. Louis, MO, Mosby, 2001.)*

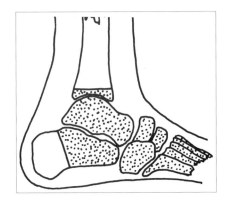

Figure 21 Diagram showing the original Pirogoff calcaneotibial arthrodesis. Stippled areas of bone are excised. *(Courtesy of Professor G. Neff.)*

mize limb-length discrepancy while walking barefoot or in a simple boot. This procedure has been widely used in Europe over many decades for injuries sustained during war. The original procedure is as follows: After midtarsal disarticulation, the talus is removed. The calcaneus is then sectioned in the frontal (vertical) plane and its anterior portion is discarded. The distal tibia is divided transversely through the cancellous metaphysis and the calcaneus is then rotated forward 90° to contact the denuded inferior tibia[30] (Figure 21). The two bones are then securely fixed.

A disadvantage of the original Pirogoff method compared with the Syme procedure is that the thinner skin over the posterior aspect of the calcaneus becomes weight bearing, rather than the plantigrade fleshy heel pad. To correct this shortcoming, several modifications have been proposed. In the Lefort-Neff variation (G Neff, MD, personal communication, 2003), the superior calcaneus is sectioned in the transverse (horizontal) plane. The calcaneus is shifted proximally and anteriorly, thus keeping the heel pad plantigrade. The malleoli are trimmed to improve cosmesis, but the calcaneal tuberosity is retained to assist in suspension of the prosthesis (Figure 22). To provide a more cosmetic prosthetic fitting, Camilleri and associates[31] recommend shifting the calcaneus anteriorly, directly beneath the tibia, after excising the superior one third of the bone. This eliminates posterior protrusion of the tuberosity. The anterior projection of the calcaneus and the malleoli are trimmed to match the width of the tibial metaphysis (Figure 23). With these methods, firm fixation is essential to encourage

bony union. Baumgartner[5] recommends an external fixator for 6 to 8 weeks, and Camilleri and associates[31] place screws across the denuded surfaces. Transection of the Achilles tendon is advised to reduce the posterior displacement force on the calcaneus.[5]

The Pirogoff procedure as modified is well suited to selected cases of trauma. Livingston and associates[32] also advocate it for cases of diabetic foot infection. Baumgartner,[5] however, does not recommend it in patients with neuropathy because of the typically prolonged time for bony union to occur in these cases. The Boyd[33] calcaneotibial arthrodesis is similar to the modified Pirogoff procedure. Following midtarsal disarticulation, the calcaneus is divided transversely just distal to the peroneal tubercle. Cancellous bone is exposed on the superior calcaneus, distal tibia, and malleoli. The calcaneus is shifted anteriorly and superiorly and fixed securely to the tibia (Figure 24). This procedure is also subject to malunion or nonunion if the bones are not well fixed (Figures 25 and 26).

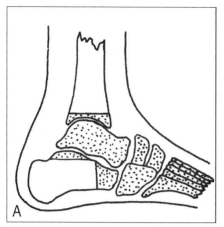
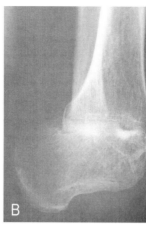
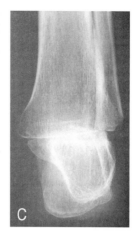
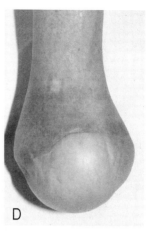

Figure 22 The Lefort-Neff modification of the Pirogoff procedure. **A,** Diagram of the Lefort-Neff modification. Note that the heel pad will remain plantigrade as the calcaneus is shifted anteriorly and superiorly to contact the osteotomized tibia. Stippled areas of bone are excised. **B,** Lateral and **C,** AP radiographs of a lower limb that underwent the Lefort-Neff modification of the Pirogoff procedure. Note the prominence of the calcaneal tuberosity, which assists in suspension of the prosthesis. **D,** Anterior view. Note the plantigrade heel pad. *(Courtesy of Professor G. Neff.)*

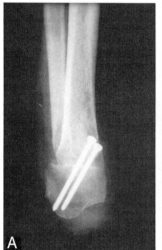
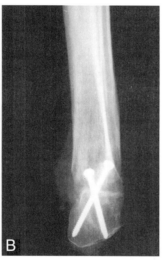
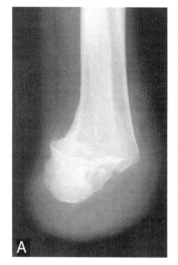
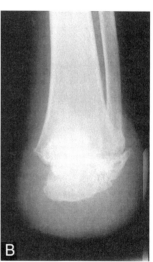

Figure 23 Radiographs of a lower limb that underwent the Camilleri modification of the Pirogoff procedure. **A,** Lateral view. Note the anterior translation of the calcaneal tuberosity to a position directly beneath the tibia. Also note that the anterior portion of the calcaneus has been excised. **B,** AP view. Note the centralized position of the calcaneus and its fixation with crossed screws. *(Courtesy of Dr. D Ménager.)*

Figure 24 Radiographs of a lower limb that underwent a Boyd amputation. **A,** Lateral and **B,** AP radiographs. Note the posterior prominence of the calcaneal tuberosity, which assists in suspension of the prosthesis.

As noted above, the original impetus for development of the Pirogoff procedure and its variants was provision of a stable heel pad with less limb-length discrepancy to allow a comfortable gait without a prosthesis. It is ironic that the length advantage of these procedures has made it difficult, until recently, to fit a foot that has undergone ankle disarticulation because of insufficient vertical clearance from the ground. With the de-velopment of low-profile Syme feet and carbon fiber technology, however, it is now possible to fit a dynamic-response foot even within the 3- to 4-cm space distal to the residual limb following a Pirogoff procedure.[32]

Summary

Ankle disarticulation and its variants should be considered in lieu of a trans-tibial amputation whenever foot trauma or infection has left the hind-foot unaffected. By preserving heel pad weight bearing along normal proprioceptive pathways, these procedures at the ankle provide a more energy-efficient gait than does trans-tibial amputation and also require minimal prosthetic gait training. The heel pad is remarkably activity toler-ant, even if insensate, provided that it is held firmly in place under the tibia by an intimately fitted prosthetic

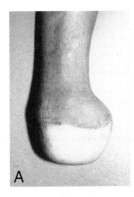
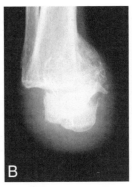
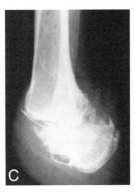
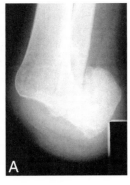
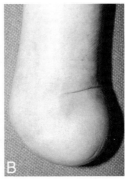

Figure 25 Right lower limb of a 57-year-old woman who underwent a Boyd amputation. **A,** Note the poor cosmesis due to a medial shift of the calcaneus. **B,** AP radiograph showing malunion. **C,** Lateral radiograph showing both excessive posterior displacement of the calcaneus and inadequate fixation with wire loops. *(Reproduced with permission from Bowker JH, San Giovanni TP: Amputations and disarticulations, in Myerson MS (ed): Foot and Ankle Disorders. Philadelphia, PA, WB Saunders, 2000.)*

Figure 26 Lower limb of patient who underwent a Boyd amputation. **A,** Lateral radiograph showing posterior displacement of the calcaneal fragment subsequent to inadequate fixation to the inferior tibia. The patient was unable to bear weight on the limb because of pain. **B,** Corresponding lateral photograph of the same limb. Note the prominence of the distal anterior tibia and the posterior prominence of the calcaneal fragment with proximal creasing of the skin. The residual limb was successfully converted to a Syme ankle disarticulation by excision of the calcaneal fragment.

socket. Careful prosthetic follow-up is essential to maintain this position, as calf atrophy inevitably develops. Although achieving a cosmetically acceptable distal socket contour is more difficult than with a transtibial prosthesis, the fact that ankle disarticulation and its variants allow the amputee to engage comfortably in a wide range of activities should lead to much more frequent use of these procedures.

References

1. Syme J: On amputation at the ankle joint. *Lond Edinb Mon J Med Sci* 1843; 26:93-96.

2. Gaine WJ, McCreath SW: Syme's amputation revisited. *J Bone Joint Surg Br* 1996;78:461-467.

3. Mazet R Jr: Syme's amputation: A follow-up study of fifty-one adults and thirty-two children. *J Bone Joint Surg Am* 1968;50:1549-1563.

4. Kruger LM: Lower limb deficiencies: Surgical management, in Bowker JH, Michael JW (eds): *Atlas of Limb Prosthetics: Surgical, Prosthetic, and Rehabilitation Principles*, ed 2. Rosemont, IL, American Academy of Orthopaedic Surgeons, 2002, p 795. (Originally published by Mosby-Year Book in 1992.)

5. Baumgartner R: *Forefoot and Hindfoot Amputations*. Paris, France, Editions Scientifiques et Mèdicales Elsevier, SAS, 2001, pp 4-5.

6. Wagner FW Jr: The Syme ankle disarticulation: Surgical procedures, in Bowker JH, Michael JW (eds): *Atlas of Limb Prosthetics: Surgical, Prosthetic, and Rehabilitation Principles*, ed 2. Rosemont, IL, American Academy of Orthopaedic Surgeons, 2002, p 413. (Originally published by Mosby-Year Book in 1992.)

7. Bowker JH, Bui VT, Redman S, et al: Syme amputation in diabetic dysvascular patients. *Orthop Trans* 1988;12: 767.

8. Pinzur MS, Morrison C, Sage R, Stuck R, Osterman H, Vrbos L: Syme's two-stage amputation in insulin-requiring diabetics with gangrene of the forefoot. *Foot Ankle* 1991;11:394-396.

9. Sarmiento A: A modified surgical-prosthetic approach to the Syme's amputation. A follow-up report. *Clin Orthop* 1972; 85:11-15.

10. Francis H, Robert JR, Clagett P, Gottschalk F, Fisher DF: The Syme amputation: Success in elderly diabetic patients with palpable ankle pulses. *J Vasc Surg* 1990;12:237-240.

11. Laughlin RT, Chambers RB: Syme amputation in patients with severe diabetes mellitus. *Foot Ankle* 1993;14:65-70.

12. Weaver FA, Modrall JG, Baek S, et al: Syme amputation: Results in patients with severe forefoot ischemia. *Cardiovasc Surg* 1996;4:81-86.

13. Dickhaut SC, DeLee JC, Page CP: Nutritional status: Importance in predicting wound healing after amputation. *J Bone Joint Surg Am* 1984;66:71-75.

14. Fahey TJ III, Sadaty A, Jones WG II, Barber A, Smoller B, Shires GT: Diabetes impairs the late inflammatory response to wound healing. *J Surg Res* 1991;50:308.

15. Schaffer MR, Tantry U, Efron PA, Ahrendt GM, Thornton FJ, Barbul A: Diabetes-impaired healing and reduced wound nitric oxide synthesis: A possible pathophysiologic correlation. *Surgery* 1997;121:513- 519.

16. Yue DK, McLennan S, Marsh M, et al: Effects of experimental diabetes, uremia and malnutrition on wound healing. *Diabetes* 1987;36:295-299.

17. Yue DK, Swanson B, McLennan S, et al: Abnormalities of granulation tissue and collagen formation in experimental diabetes, uraemia and malnutrition. *Diabet Med* 1986;3:221-225.

18. Grayson ML: Diabetic foot infections: Antimicrobial therapy. *Infect Dis Clin North Am* 1995;9:143-161.

19. Lipsky BA: Evidence-based antibiotic therapy of diabetic foot infections.

FEMS *Immunol Med Microbiol* 1999;
267-276.

20. Lipsky BA, Berendt AR: Principles and practice of antibiotic therapy of diabetic foot infections. *Diabetes Metab Res Rev* 2000;16(suppl 1):S42-S46.

21. Harris RI: Syme's amputation: The technical details essential for success. *J Bone Joint Surg Br* 1956;38:614-632.

22. Öznur A: Syme ankle disarticulation: A simplified technique. *Foot Ankle Int* 2001;22:484-485.

23. Pinzur MS, Smith D, Osterman H: Syme ankle disarticulation in peripheral vascular disease and diabetic infection: The one-stage versus two-stage procedure. *Foot Ankle Int* 1995; 16:124-127.

24. Elmslie RC: Section on amputations, in *Carson's Modern Operative Surgery.*

London, England, Cassel & Company, 1924, p 132.

25. Smith DG, Sangeorzan BG, Hansen ST, Burgess EM: Achilles tendon tenodesis to prevent heel pad migration in the Syme's amputation. *Foot Ankle* 1994;15:14-17.

26. Waters RL, Perry J, Antonelli D, Hislop H: Energy costs of walking of amputees: The influence of level of amputation. *J Bone Joint Surg Am* 1976;58: 42-46.

27. Srinivasan H: Syme's amputation in insensitive feet: A review of twenty cases. *J Bone Joint Surg Am* 1973;55: 558-562.

28. Murdoch G: Syme's amputation. *J R Coll Surg Edinb* 1976;21:15-30.

29. Birch JG, Walsh SJ, Small JM, et al: Syme amputation for the treatment of fibular deficiency: An evaluation of

long-term physical and psychological functional status. *J Bone Joint Surg Am* 1999;81:1511-1518.

30. Pirogoff NI: Osteoplastic elongation of the bones of the leg in amputation of the foot. *Voyerno Med J* 1854;68:83.

31. Camilleri A, Anract P, Missenard G, Lariviére JY, Ménager D: Amputations et désarticulations des membres: Membre inférieur, in Encyclopédie Médico-Chirurgicale: Paris, France, Editions Scientifiques et Médicales Elsevier, SAS, 2000, pp 6-8.

32. Livingston R, Jacobs RL, Karmody A: Plantar abscess in the diabetic patient. *Foot Ankle* 1985;5:205-213.

33. Boyd HB: Amputations of the foot with calcaneotibial arthrodesis. *J Bone Joint Surg* 1939;21:997-1000.

Chapter 37

Ankle Disarticulation and Variants: Prosthetic Management

Gary M. Berke, MS, CP

Introduction

Nearly a century ago, Marks' *Manual of Artificial Limbs* noted that "amputations through the ankle articulations with or without the malleoli, flaps formed of heel tissues, provide stumps that can be fitted with artificial limbs in advantageous ways."[1] As surgical techniques and technologically advanced components continue to evolve, the potential functional ability of the lower limb amputee is enhanced and the Syme ankle disarticulation may become more prevalent. Ankle disarticulation is arguably the most functional level of amputation because the length of the residual limb leaves a significant lever arm to distribute forces and control a prosthetic device.[2] In addition, unlike the more distal amputation levels, the complete replacement of the foot equalizes limb length and facilitates near-normal gait, activity level, and energy consumption in healthy individuals. Advantages and disadvantages of ankle disarticulation with regard to prosthesis use are summarized in Table 1.

This chapter discusses the value of ankle disarticulation and provides the historical basis for the design and construction of prostheses for this patient population. Methods of evaluation, staging of care, design considerations, design alternatives, and components for an appropriate ankle disarticulation prosthesis are reviewed. A discussion of the biome-chanics of gait and alignment and its relationship to the strength and function of a prosthesis follows. A clear understanding of the mechanics, biomechanics, and function involved in prosthesis wear in this population is critical to improving the effectiveness of ankle disarticulation prostheses. Finally, two case studies are described.

Evaluation and Staging of Care

As with any amputation, evaluation of the patient with an ankle disarticulation is critical. The residual limb should be free from open wounds, and care should be taken to assess areas of thin skin, especially around the anterior distal scar line. Strength and range of motion of the remaining joints of the affected limb as well as the contralateral limb should be evaluated. The activity level before amputation and the ambulation goals of the patient should be noted. These factors will have a significant effect on the type of prosthesis prescribed. Evaluation must include an assessment of the patient's ability to comfortably bear weight on the distal end of the residual limb, as well as the presence (or absence) of the medial and distal malleoli. The position of the distal heel pad—medial, lateral, or centralized—should also be noted. Stability of the pad will determine

TABLE 1 Prosthetic Advantages and Disadvantages of a Syme Ankle Disarticulation

Advantages	Disadvantages	Contraindications for Prosthetic Fitting
Full weight-bearing potential on the distal end of the residual limb	Bulbous nature of distal end complicates cosmetic prosthesis	Poor heel pad integrity
Natural gait pattern	Healing is sometimes difficult	Open wound or unhealed surgical site
Self-suspending prosthesis; allows walking without a prosthesis for short distances, if necessary	Limited room distally hinders foot selection and significantly complicates the alignment procedure	Medialized or unstable heel pad
Minimal disturbance to growth potential in children	Some designs have poor structural integrity[3]	Pain independent of prosthesis or ambulation
Early fitting		

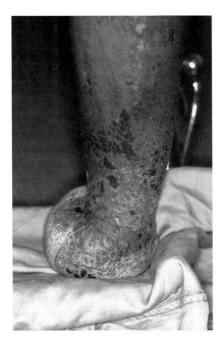

Figure 1 Severe medial shift of the heel pad following ambulation without a prosthesis.

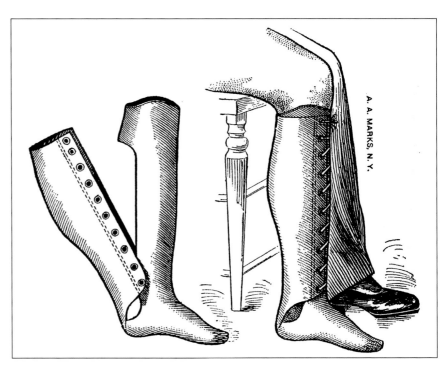

Figure 2 Historical ankle disarticulation prosthesis. *(Reproduced from Marks GE (ed): Manual of Artificial Limbs: An Exhaustive Exposition of Prosthesis. New York, NY, AA Marks, 1907, p 37.)*

whether the patient should ambulate without a prosthesis. A hypermobile pad may shift to the side during ambulation without a prosthesis, making later prosthetic fitting extremely difficult (Figure 1). Knee joint instability must be noted and addressed either by alignment or by extending the prosthesis above the knee with supracondylar support or a thigh lacer.

One of the advantages of ankle disarticulation is that the patient can be fitted immediately after the amputation with a partial weight-bearing cast applied by the surgeon or prosthetist. A standard cast with good padding and a walking post on the distal end will allow early limited weight bearing and controlled ambulation with an assistive device. The first prosthesis may be fitted soon after suture removal, assuming adequate healing has occurred. The patient may begin full weight bearing upon fitting of the first prosthesis and usually will begin ambulating without an assistive device within the first few weeks. Physical therapy for gait training is not usually required unless significant gait anomalies or other medical complications are present.

Design Considerations

For comfortable transmission of the forces for ambulation and to provide ease of donning and doffing, the prosthesis must have the following features[4]: (1) The prosthesis must provide comfortable support of the limb on the distal end, the proximal portion of the socket brim, or both. (2) Firm support must be provided against the anteroproximal surface of the leg to absorb the significant pressures present at the time of push-off. Careful fitting against the wedge-like medial and lateral surface of the tibia or application of a patellar tendon force can satisfy this requirement. (3) Similar support must be provided against the posterior surface of the leg to absorb pressures that occur at the time of heel contact. (4) Within the socket, there must be provision for the shifting of the center of pressure against the distal end of the residual limb during gait. Prevention of the relative motion between the stump and the socket in an anteroposterior

direction is critical to comfort and continued skin protection. The horizontal component of the force against the posterior distal regions of the residual limb must be accommodated during push-off, as well as anterior distal pressure during heel strike. (5) Adequate stabilization must be provided against the torques about the long axis of the leg. Three-point stabilization against the medial and lateral flares at the anterior/proximal margin of the tibia and a flattening of the posterior/proximal contour can be highly effective in providing the necessary torque resistance. If insufficient stabilization is provided, torques acting on the distal end of the residual limb will result in skin abrasion. (6) Finally, the prosthesis must provide adequate relief for the bulbous distal end to allow for ease in donning as well as suspension.

The design of the ankle disarticulation prosthesis is unique (Figure 2). Ankle disarticulation results in an end-bearing residual limb; consequently, the prosthesis may be designed with less proximal pressure

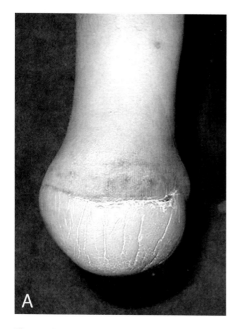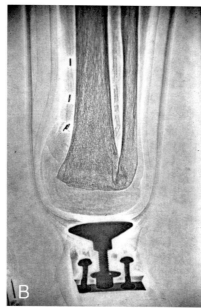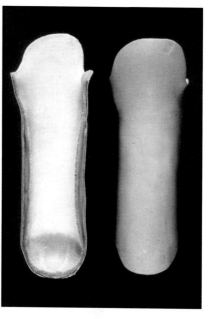

Figure 3 A, Anterior view of a conventional Syme ankle disarticulation. **B,** Xeroradiograph of a Syme ankle disarticulation residual limb within a prosthetic device. The distal malleoli have been removed, and the self-suspending prosthesis is fitted with a soft interface.

Figure 4 Cross section of an expandable silicone bladder ankle disarticulation prosthesis, fabricated using the "lost wax" method. The tubular shape of the outside wall allows the limb to pass through the narrower portion of the expandable liner.

than is required for transtibial prostheses. The distal circumference, being larger than the ankle circumference, is both an advantage and disadvantage to the user. The advantage is that this bulbous end may be used to suspend the prosthesis. Application of carefully contoured pressure proximal to the malleoli can comfortably and effectively keep the prosthesis in close contact with the residual limb during swing phase. The disadvantage is that the large distal segment is often cosmetically unappealing because of its location and size. Some authors recommend removing the medial and lateral aspects of the malleoli to reduce the bulk of the residual limb; however, care must be taken to not affect the suspension benefit. Despite the bulbous nature of the limb, contact throughout the residual limb must be preserved to spread the pressures of ambulation over the entire residual limb (Figure 3).

Design Alternatives

Radcliffe[4] observed that the highest stresses in a prosthetic socket will occur where the transverse cross section

is the smallest. During normal ambulation, the socket will undergo three types of stress—compression stresses from direct thrust load, bending stresses resulting from a tendency for the structure to bow posteriorly, and bending stresses from the tendency to bow laterally.[4] At heel strike, moderate compressive loads occur on the posterior side of the prosthesis, and tensile loads occur on the anterior side. During the terminal stance phase of the gait cycle, significant compressive loads occur on the anterior surface of the socket and substantial tensile loads occur on the posterior aspect. When the structure of the socket is breached, as with a window or hole to permit donning, the rigidity and durability of the structure is significantly compromised. Several socket variations have been developed to address this concern.

The "stovepipe" prosthesis can be fabricated in a variety of ways. One method incorporates a removable liner (usually high-density closed cell foam) that maintains the shape of the limb on the inside and is tubular in shape on the outside. The rigid outer

socket is tubular in shape (oval or nearly round in cross section) and therefore very strong, with the overall circumference being determined by the circumference of the bulbous distal end and liner.

The liner usually must be split on one or two sides to allow the bulbous distal end to pass through the narrower circumference of the ankle region of the liner. Permutations of this basic design are limited only by materials and creativity. Silicone bladders, elastic liners,[5] and double-wall sockets fabricated by the "lost wax" method all can provide suspension and ease in donning and doffing but are difficult to adjust. These are the strongest and most durable type of ankle disarticulation sockets because there is a uniform cross-sectional area without any breach of the rigid external structure (Figure 4).

The Canadian ankle disarticulation prosthesis, first described in 1954 by the Veterans Administration in Canada, is a bivalved socket with a posterior door that extends to the proximal brim of the socket, allowing easy insertion of the limb into the device. The door is buckled or strapped in place for ambulation. Such posterior opening designs are structurally weak, with high stress concentrations where the abbreviated anterior panel meets the hemispherical base. With an end-bearing residual limb, the tensile forces on the anterior panel are actually increased, compared with the same posterior opening device without end bearing.[4] Reinforcing the device with materials resistant to tensile stress at the critical junctures is therefore essential.

In 1959, the Veterans Administration Prosthetics Center in New York described the medial-opening Syme prosthesis.[6] The opening on the medial side resembles a small door and terminates well below the proximal trimline of the socket. The opening is usually medial because of the prominence of the medial malleolus and the natural curvature of the residual limb.[7] The opening must be large enough to accommodate the distal residual limb, but not so large as to compromise structural integrity. In a prosthesis with a medial window, the anterior edges of the medial opening are under significant compressive stresses during the late stance phase of gait. (Because the posterior edges are under only moderate compression at early stance phase and are usually not involved in structural failure, they are not discussed in this chapter.) To increase the resistance to local compressive stress, the wall thickness of the socket must be increased, thereby increasing the overall cross-sectional area of the socket.[4] Contrary to the mechanics of the posterior-opening prosthesis, when end bearing is allowed within the medial window prosthesis, the magnitudes of the forces around the opening are reduced significantly.[3]

Components

The application of prosthetic feet to an ankle disarticulation socket is complicated by the minimal distance between the distal end of the limb and the floor. In the past, the solid ankle–cushion heel (SACH) foot was the only available option for this level of amputation to offer a smooth loading response, because of the heel cushion that absorbs some of the initial impact during the early stance phase of gait. Currently, several alternatives further improve ambulation. Flexible-keel feet with a SACH-type heel offer improved shock absorption over uneven terrain and are available in ankle disarticulation styles. Dynamic-response feet are also available in ankle disarticulation configurations, but because the leaf-spring keel of a dynamic-response foot requires increased force for deflection, the socket must be designed to distribute the increased forces that occur in terminal stance in a comfortable manner.

Biomechanics of Gait and Alignment

The ultimate goal for individuals with ankle disarticulations is to return to the highest level of function possible. A complete understanding of the mechanics and biomechanics of gait is necessary to achieve this goal.

Obtaining appropriate alignment, although somewhat difficult in the ankle disarticulation prosthesis, is critical to achieving an appropriate gait pattern. The complicating factor is that the limited space between the socket and the foot does not permit use of an adjustable alignment unit. This forces the practitioner to "cut and paste" the position of the foot until an appropriate socket/foot relationship is achieved.

Initial Contact to Loading Response

The lack of space (from residual limb to floor) inherent in the ankle disarticulation level of amputation precludes the use of certain feet, especially those with articulating ankles. At initial contact, the heel of the prosthetic foot must be soft enough to ab-sorb some of the impact of ambulation yet firm enough to provide adequate forward propulsion of the limb. The knee joint helps to compensate for some of the loss of normal shock absorption by flexing slightly more at initial contact than in normal gait. This increase in knee flexion also allows for a natural-appearing gait pattern.[4]

As the patient moves from initial contact through the loading response portion of the gait cycle, the center of mass will fall between the heel and the toe of the prosthetic foot, and the ground-reaction force will be posterior to the center of mass. This will cause a torque about the socket in a forward direction. In an effort to control this forward moment of the socket, the knee joint extends and the residual limb presses against the walls of the prosthesis in an attempt to slow the forward progression of the socket. In doing so, the forces on the residual limb are significantly higher in the area of the posterior proximal and the anterior distal aspects of the socket (Figure 5). The sagittal position of the prosthetic foot relative to the socket and the durometer of the prosthetic heel will have a significant impact on the gait pattern, the magnitude of force on the residual limb, and ultimately the long-term comfort and function of the device.

Loading Response to Midstance

After a period of knee flexion during initial contact, the knee begins to actively extend through loading response. At this phase of gait, because of the lack of true ankle plantar flexion in the prosthetic foot, the knee will extend fully to stabilize the system. This is contrary to normal gait, in which the knee continues to flex at this phase to act as a shock absorber.[8]

The horizontal pressures around the proximal posterior portion of the prosthesis at initial contact decrease during the loading response phase of gait and become more vertical. If the limb is end bearing, the pressures

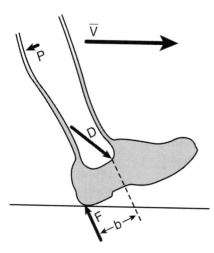

Figure 5 Initial contact. F = Ground-reaction force; b = Distance from the ground-reaction force to the center of mass; D = Approximate location of distal forces on the residual limb at this phase of gait; P = Approximate location of proximal forces on the residual limb at this phase of gait; V = Resultant vector force determined by the distance from the ground-reaction force to the center of mass, the speed of walking, the density of the heel of the foot, the density of the heel of the shoe, and the opposing forces at D and P. Should the proximal posterior wall be lowered, the pressure at D will increase significantly to attempt to compensate for the decreased control posteriorly.

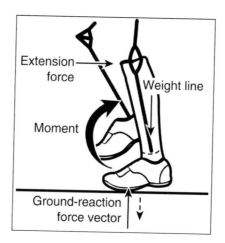

Figure 6 As the patient continues through midstance, the ground-reaction force vector moves anterior to the weight line. This provides an extension moment to the knee and redirects the socket pressures to the proximal anterior and posterior limb.

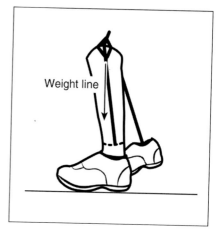

Figure 7 Vertical forces at midstance. Note the socket/foot angle in this example is approximately 85°.

around the distal end shift from anterior to straight distal and then to slightly distal posterior as midstance is completed. The actual location of the distal residual limb pressure when the foot is flat is determined by the foot/socket angular relationship and the amount of proximal anterior support given the residual limb inside the prosthetic device.[6] At this phase of gait, the body is moving forward over the prosthesis and the subsequent pressures within the device are changing considerably. Through loading response, the center of pressure under the prosthetic foot is moving forward as a result of load acceptance onto the prosthetic foot. Consequently, the vertical ground-reaction force is moving from behind the knee to the front of the knee, causing an extension moment at the knee joint (Figure 6). The effect of coronal-plane foot position is discussed below.

Midstance to Terminal Stance

As the gait cycle shifts from midstance to heel-off, the knee continues to play an active role in the continuation of a smooth gait pattern by compensating for the lack of range of motion at the ankle. The pressures on the residual limb shift to proximal anterior and distal posterior as the patient tries to overcome the knee extension moment from the ground-reaction force being anterior to the knee joint. The patient must use active knee flexion to overcome these pressures and ambulate comfortably. Peak pressures occur at the anterior proximal portion of the socket during this phase of gait and must be controlled by an appropriate proximal contour and enhanced socket construction. The peak knee extension moment occurs at the beginning of the terminal stance/preswing phase of gait. The greatest test of the socket's structural integrity will occur at this phase of the gait cycle (Figure 7).

Mediolateral Foot Placement, Angulation, and Toe-out

Mediolateral foot placement should be such that the plantar aspect of the

foot is parallel to the floor at midstance and creates a slight varus thrust at the knee. This foot position will keep the pressures of ambulation focused in the pressure-tolerant proximal medial and distal lateral regions of the socket and will result in a natural and comfortable gait pattern. When significant medial bowing of the tibia is present, the foot is placed at the most lateral aspect of the distal socket that is technically feasible. Transverse foot rotation should mimic that of the opposite side (Figure 8).

Ground-Reaction Forces and Energy Consumption

The pattern of ground-reaction forces, centralized in the prosthetic foot, supports the notion that the ankle disarticulation amputee has a normal lever arm for push-off at late stance that accounts for a smooth and energy-efficient gait pattern.[9] The ankle disarticulation amputation has been shown to be even more energy-efficient than midfoot amputations.[10-12] This surprising phenomenon seems to be due to the long limb length and adequate lever arm of the prosthetic foot with an ankle disarticulation prosthesis.

There is little functional disparity between an individual with an ankle disarticulation prosthesis and one with no amputation.[13] Patients with ankle disarticulation prostheses sel-

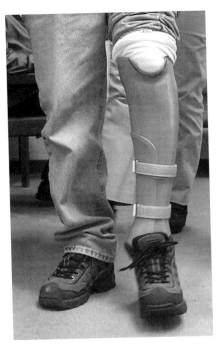

Figure 8 As the patient arrives at mid-stance and shifts the body weight over the prosthesis, the ground-reaction force through the foot will be medial to the weight line, causing a torque about the knee in a varus direction. This figure shows the typical coronal-plane foot placement on an ankle disarticulation prosthesis. Note the valgus appearance of the ankle during swing phase, and the lateral position of the foot on the distal socket.

dom require physical therapy and rarely require hospitalization for prosthetic gait training.[10]

Case Studies
Case Study 1

A 60-year-old man who had been a farm worker for nearly 35 years sustained a traumatic crush injury to his left forefoot after a 3,000-lb paper roll landed on his foot. After the accident, he underwent multiple procedures, including toe amputations, metatarsal amputations, neuroma resections, and a spinal nerve stimulator for pain. Despite these procedures, he continued to have severe pain and hyperesthesia suggestive of complex regional pain syndrome. The patient underwent an elective ankle disarticulation approximately 5 years after the initial injury. Following débridement

and reclosure of a small necrotic area on the lateral aspect of the scar line, the wound eventually healed well. At follow-up approximately 3 weeks later, the patient had no pain in the residual limb. A slight eschar was present on the lateral portion of an anterior scarline. The heel pad was centralized and stable, and the patient ambulated in a high-top tennis shoe with padding, requiring the use of bilateral axillary crutches for balance and comfort.

The patient had smoked 50 packs of cigarettes per year for the past 38 years. His past medical history included high blood pressure and coronary artery disease. He had two incidents of myocardial infarction and underwent cardiac bypass surgery 7 years ago. He was cleared for all activities by his cardiologist. At the time of presentation, he used no medication and appeared healthy.

The patient's goal was full-time community ambulation; he had no interest in high-impact activities. He was somewhat concerned about the appearance of his prosthesis, but overall he was ready to abandon crutches and resume fishing and gardening.

Physical examination revealed a rather bulbous ankle disarticulation amputation with full-width mediolateral malleoli. The distal heel pad was very stable and had slight abrasions from ambulation without a prosthesis. He had good range of motion at all joints proximal to the amputation.

After reviewing the alternatives with his prosthetist, the patient decided that the best option for him was a prosthesis with a medial door and straps to eliminate the bulk above the ankle that an insert or bladder type would require. The prosthesis was designed to maintain some proximal weight bearing but took full advantage of his end-bearing tolerance.

The patient was fitted with his prosthesis. On 1-week follow-up, the patient ambulated with only one crutch for security and could ambulate without an assistive device. He had no discomfort during ambula-

tion. Examination of the skin showed good total contact throughout the residual limb/socket interface, with no areas of significant redness or irritation. The previously scabbed area was improved with use of the prosthesis. He returned 1 month later, at which time he was ambulating without an assistive device. He had increased his sock ply to account for some limb shrinkage.

Case Study 2

A 25-year-old man sustained an open tibia and fibula fracture that required external fixation and several surgical interventions after a motorcycle accident 5 years ago. He had an avulsion injury to the dorsum of his foot that was nonsalvageable; he ultimately lost his foot, but the hindfoot was preserved. He elected to have a Syme procedure rather than a transtibial amputation at that time. Following a lengthy hospitalization, he was discharged home but returned to the clinic after falling onto the residual limb, opening the suture line approximately 2 cm on the medial side. The wound was allowed to heal by secondary intention and healed without further incident. The tibial fracture was not affected by the fall; however, it healed with a slightly larger medial bow than the contralateral limb. On presentation, the residual limb was well healed with a rather bulbous distal segment as a result of preservation of the medial and lateral aspects of the malleoli. A 2-cm area of adhered tissue on the medial scar line had not caused the patient any problems with prosthesis use in the past.

The patient was an extremely active young man who liked to participate in various sports, especially tennis and basketball. He weighed 200 lb, was in excellent physical condition, and was not taking any medications. Because strength of the prosthesis was a primary concern in this case, a bladder-type prosthesis was recommended. The socket was designed incorporating an expanded polyethylene foam liner for ease of donning and adjustability. The socket was made of carbon fiber throughout with an increase in laminate thickness around the anterior wall to help reduce the possibility of structural failure from compression forces during jumping and running. The design of the device allowed some weight bearing around the distal end; however, careful modification of the tibial shaft and proximal anterior contours were necessary to permit high-impact activities. Further relief around the area of adhered tissue was required, as was careful contour of the posterior distal aspect of the distal socket to prevent tension over the adhered tissue. Increased proximal weight bearing was needed in addition to the conservative distal modifications. A carbon-fiber dynamic-response foot, custom-made for the patient's weight, limb length, and activity level, was placed on the prosthesis. This foot was attached to the posterior wall of the socket with carbon fiber and allowed a natural gait pattern as well as enabling high activity function. The foot was placed as laterally as possible on the socket because of the increase in tibial bowing and was placed in a slight valgus position so that at midstance the foot was flat on the floor. This positioning allowed for a slight varus thrust at the knee during single-limb support. After 1 year of use, the liner and socket remained in excellent condition; however, the prosthetic foot had become delaminated and required replacement. No other prosthetic problems have been noted.

Summary and Conclusions

When fitting an ankle disarticulation prosthesis, a thorough understanding of the mechanics of the socket, limb, and gait is important. Patients often request a lower profile socket, but this compromises the gait pattern and comfort. Despite the limitations in cosmetic appearance and ankle-foot options associated with ankle disarticulation prostheses, the ankle disarticulation is a very functional level of amputation.

References

1. Marks GE (ed): *Manual of Artificial Limbs: An Exhaustive Exposition of Prosthesis.* New York, NY, AA Marks, 1907, p 37.

2. Berke GM: Amputations and prostheses of the foot and ankle: Partial foot prostheses, in Coughlin MJ, Mann RA (eds): *Surgery of the Foot and Ankle*, ed 7. St. Louis, MO, Mosby, 1999, vol 2, pp 995-1006.

3. Pritham CH: The Syme prosthesis, in Murdoch G, Donovan RG (eds): *Amputation Surgery and Lower Limb Prosthetics.* Oxford, England, Blackwell Scientific Publications, 1988, pp 87-93.

4. Radcliffe CW: The biomechanics of the Syme prosthesis. *Artif Limbs* 1961; 6:76-85.

5. LeBlanc MA: Elastic-liner type of Syme prosthesis: Basic procedure and variations. *Artif Limbs* 1971;15:22-26.

6. Iuliucci L, DeGaetano R (eds): *VAPC Technique for Fabricating a Plastic Syme Prosthesis with Medial Opening: Fabrication Manual.* New York, NY, Prosthetics and Orthotics, New York University Post-Graduate Medical School, 1969.

7. Cottrell-Ikerd V, Ikerd F, Jenkins DW: The Syme's amputation: A correlation of surgical technique and prosthetic management with an historical perspective. *J Foot Ankle Surg* 1994;33: 355-364.

8. Perry J: *Gait Analysis, Normal and Pathological Function.* New York, NY, McGraw-Hill Inc, 1992, pp 9-47.

9. Pinzur MS, Wolf B, Havey RM: Walking pattern of midfoot and ankle disarticulation amputees. *Foot Ankle Int* 1997;18:635-638.

10. Pinzur MS: Restoration of walking ability with Syme's ankle disarticulation. *Clin Orthop* 1999;361:71-75.

11. Waters RL: The energy expenditure of amputee gait, in Bowker JH, Michael JW (eds): *Atlas of Limb Prosthetics: Surgical, Prosthetic, and Rehabilitation Principles*, ed 2. Rosemont, IL, American Academy of Orthopaedic Surgeons, 2002, pp 381-387. (Originally published by Mosby-Year Book, 1992.)

12. Waters RL, Perry J, Antonelli D, Hislop H: Energy cost of walking of amputees: The influence of level of amputation. *J Bone Joint Surg Am* 1976;58: 42-46.

13. Pinzur MS, Littooy F, Daniels J, et al: Multidisciplinary preoperative assessment and late function in dysvascular amputees. *Clin Orthop* 1992;281: 239-243.

Chapter 38

Transtibial Amputation: Surgical Management

John H. Bowker, MD

Introduction

Among major amputations in the lower limb, amputations at the transtibial level are the most common. Many series report a ratio of at least two transtibial amputations to every transfemoral amputation.[1-6] The transtibial level is the most proximal level at which near-normal function can be expected for most patients. This is because preserving the knee joint allows transtibial amputees to consume much less energy than transfemoral amputees.[7-9] The relative ease of transtibial gait compared with transfemoral gait is borne out by several studies of prosthesis use. Combined data from 13 studies from 1943 through 1983 show an average rate of transtibial prosthesis use of 73.5%.[10-22] Analysis of four studies covering the same period shows prosthesis use by transfemoral amputees to average only 26.5%.[10,11,23,24] Most of the patients in these studies had peripheral vascular disease. A more recent retrospective review by Fletcher and associates[25] compared two local cohorts of unilateral dysvascular amputees, of whom 49% had diabetes mellitus. All were older than 65 years, with a median age at amputation of 79 years. The first group underwent amputations between 1956 and 1973, and the second group between 1974 and 1995. Of the combined 292 patients, only 78 (47%) with a transtibial and 15 (13%) with a transfemoral amputation were suc-

cessfully fitted with a prosthesis. There was no significant difference between the two groups in fitting success over the 40-year span, although significantly more transtibial amputations were performed in the later cohort.[25]

In contrast to these elderly patients, Purry and Hannon[26] made a detailed study of 25 unilateral amputees younger than 45 years at the time of amputation who had undergone transtibial amputation because of trauma. They were followed up at 2.5 years after surgery to assess function and lifestyle. Of the 25 patients, 21 (84%) wore the prosthesis more than 13 hours a day, 18 (72%) could walk 1 mile if necessary, and 21 (84%) drove an automobile. Eighteen (72%) played sports. The most notable finding was that 21 (84%) of these unilateral transtibial amputees regarded themselves as minimally disabled or nondisabled.[26]

In 2001, Dougherty[27] reported a 28-year follow-up of 72 unilateral transtibial amputees who had been injured by land mines or booby traps during the Vietnam war. The Medical Outcomes Survey Health Status Profile (MOS SF-36) is a 36-item self-report functional outcomes instrument describing physical functioning, role limitations due to physical and emotional problems, social functioning, general mental health, pain, health perception, energy, and fatigue.

In the 28 persons whose only injury was the amputation, SF-36 scores were close to those of age- and sex-matched controls. In contrast, the 44 amputees who sustained additional major injuries had significantly lower scores, and many required psychological help.

Another singular advantage of transtibial over transfemoral amputation is markedly reduced perioperative mortality. In three studies[1,10,16] the combined mortality associated with transtibial amputation was 9.5% compared with 29.7% for transfemoral amputation. Sarmiento and Warren[28] reported virtually the same findings. They noted a decrease in mortality rate from 24% to 10% that they related directly to the reversal of their transtibial-to-transfemoral amputation ratio from 1:2 to 2:1.

For many years, transfemoral amputations were preferred to transtibial amputations because primary healing was thought to be easier at the thigh level. Healing at that level, however, is far from certain. In a series of 171 amputations, Boontje[1] noted a 28% failure of transfemoral healing, compared with 35% for transtibial amputations. Pooling the data from eight reported series totaling 942 cases, each with at least 50 patients, showed that 70% of transtibial amputations healed primarily and 16% secondarily, for a total healing rate of 85%.[13,29-35] These series did not separate patients with diabetes mellitus who may or may not have had ischemia from patients with ischemic disease alone. Allcock and Jain[36] reported on 395 transtibial amputations performed using the Burgess technique between 1987 and 1996. They found that 80% healed primarily, 3% secondarily, and 13% after local wedge resection of a dehisced wound, for a success rate of 96%. Only 4% required revision to a transfemoral level.

Primary amputation at the transfemoral level was long recommended for patients with diabetes because of the supposed unlikelihood of healing at more distal levels in these patients. Data were combined from four series to compare the healing rate of transtibial amputations in patients with diabetes with that in patients with purely ischemic disease. Among 194 patients with diabetes, wounds healed in 92%. In contrast, wounds healed in only 75% of 188 patients with purely ischemic disease.[4,16,21,37] The authors of two additional series, each with 100 patients with diabetes, reported transtibial healing rates of 99% and 90%.[2,15] These studies strongly suggest the fallacy of the old notion that the best treatment of foot lesions in patients with diabetes is primary transfemoral amputation.

In ischemic conditions, unilateral transtibial amputation may be followed by loss of the opposite limb as vascular disease progresses. One study of 80 patients noted an average interval of 23 months between transtibial amputations.[38] The risk of contralateral limb loss is 10% per year.[3] With sufficient longevity, therefore, most transtibial amputees will face the prospect of loss of the opposite lower limb, and ambulation as a bilateral transtibial amputee thus becomes of major concern. Pooled data on 137 patients showed that 77% of bilateral transtibial amputees were able to attain functional ambulation.[21,24,38,39]

In summary, the importance of preserving the knee joint cannot be overemphasized. It allows younger patients to continue a vigorous lifestyle and elderly patients the opportunity to walk rather than be confined to a wheelchair. Because the risk of later contralateral amputation is high, every effort should be made to preserve at least a transtibial level at the first amputation and provide preventive care for the opposite foot over the long term.

Causal Conditions
Diabetes Mellitus

With aging of the population, trauma has been replaced by peripheral vascular disease with or without diabetes as the leading cause of lower limb amputation in developed countries. Smoking appears to be related to this increase.[40] In a review of 51 male lower limb amputees in the United Kingdom, Stewart[41] found a significantly higher rate of amputation in smokers (82.4%) than in the general population (55%). In another series, 58% of 110 transtibial amputees were smokers.[42] The precipitating cause of amputation may be gangrene, infection, or intractable claudication.[1] In diabetes mellitus, most amputations are related to various types of foot injury secondary to peripheral sensory neuropathy, often with minor foot damage providing a portal for infection. Infection in patients with diabetes may be difficult to combat at the tissue level because of decreased leukocyte activity in the hyperglycemic state.[43] Patients with diabetes often continue to walk on infected feet because they have lost deep pain sensation, thereby rapidly spreading infected fluids along tissue planes. Charcot neuroarthropathy, which can begin with minor trauma, may also lead to amputation if the bones of the foot and ankle become severely damaged. Although atheromatous disease often develops in patients with diabetes at an earlier age than in the general population, it may be difficult to determine the relative importance of occlusive changes seen in larger vessels and more peripheral small-vessel disease in the causation of gangrene.[44]

The population of patients with diabetes is growing rapidly, but it is unclear whether this is because of earlier detection, increased longevity because of better treatment, population growth, or other factors. It is certain, however, that an increasing percentage of lower limb amputations is being done in these patients. For example, a 1956 study showed diabetes as a factor in only 16% of lower limb amputations.[33] In contrast, combined data from 17 studies published between 1961 and 1988 showed that in an average of 52% of patients (range, 30% to 75%), diabetes mellitus was the primary or secondary cause of amputation.[1,3,13,14,17,19-21,23,29,37,45-50]

Infection

In Hansen's disease (leprosy), infection of peripheral nerves with *Mycobacterium leprae* causes foot insensitivity. Progressive loss of bone and soft tissues, aggravated by intractable deep infection following skin ulceration, may require transtibial amputation. Severe tissue destruction from fungal infection may occur in the presence of normal sensation, as in mycetoma, or "Madura foot." Other major infections that may result in lower limb amputation include chronic osteomyelitis and life-threatening forms of infectious gangrene, including clostridial myonecrosis (gas gangrene) and necrotizing fasciitis.

Indications

In general, transtibial amputation is indicated whenever the initiating disease or trauma cannot be treated effectively by more conservative procedures. In cases of severe foot infection, usually related to diabetes mellitus, much of the tibia can usually be spared even if the proximal spread of infection precludes a partial foot amputation or Syme ankle disarticulation. In peripheral vascular disease with distal gangrene, transtibial amputation is suitable if the level selected has enough vasculature. In cases of trauma to the foot and lower leg, an initial transtibial amputation should be done if there is such severe destruction of soft tissue and bone that reconstruction or a more distal amputation is not feasible. In addition, if warm ischemia of the leg and foot has been present for more than 6 hours following severe vascular injury to the lower limb, primary amputation should be considered.[51]

When reconstruction after trauma has resulted in an unsatisfactory limb because of deformity, pain, nonunion, or persistent infection, transtibial amputation is usually a good solution (Figure 1). The amputation should be done as soon as it becomes apparent that further attempts at salvage have little likelihood of success. This approach can spare the patient expense and distress and prevent chronic invalidism. Finally, transtibial amputation should be favored over transfemoral amputation whenever there is a reasonable possibility of prosthetic ambulation.

Contraindications

Several absolute and relative contraindications to transtibial amputation should be recognized. Inadequate vascularity for any reason at amputation sites between the knee and ankle is an absolute contraindication. Severe rest pain or gangrenous changes in the proximal portion of the calf may indicate the need for a primary transfemoral amputation. A patient with a knee flexion contracture severe enough to prevent use of a transtibial prosthesis may be best served by a knee disarticulation, provided that the skin at that level is viable. A relative contraindication to transtibial amputation is prolonged nonambulatory status, although Persson[34] maintains that the tibial portion of the limb can still be useful in transfer and wheelchair sitting activities, and he is reluctant to remove it based on nonambulation alone. If the patient is strictly bedbound, a knee flexion contracture will very likely develop, making knee disarticulation a good choice.

Several conditions are mistakenly thought of as relative contraindications to transtibial amputation. Patients with diabetes or Hansen's disease need not be denied a transtibial-level amputation based on insensate skin. With good prosthetic fitting and regular observation of the skin for areas of pressure, the transtibial amputee should do well long term. Even some patients with hemiparesis on the amputated side can accomplish household ambulation with a transtibial prosthesis. Poor knee control can often be managed with a hybrid "prosthosis" that combines a transtibial prosthesis with orthotic knee-control components, provided that flexion or extension patterning is not extreme and that reasonable balance is present. Patients who are able to comprehend and follow instructions can do quite well with a prosthesis. If patterning is extreme or if a knee flexion contracture is significant, a knee disarticulation should be considered, provided that hip control is present.

Even if patients are not candidates for prostheses, sitting and kneeling will be enhanced by salvaging as much of the leg as possible.

Children with congenital foot anomalies requiring revision to allow use of a prosthesis are not well served by transtibial amputation because it will interfere with the growth of the residual limb and make its relative length much less than ideal in adulthood. In these cases, disarticulation at the ankle joint, without disturbing the physis, will preserve end–weight-bearing capability and also allow a moderate increase in length over time.

Preoperative Care

Several important factors must be considered in the preoperative management of prospective amputees, largely related to the reason for amputation. For example, patients undergoing amputation for trauma often have concomitant injuries to other bones, soft tissue, or viscera. A careful evaluation is therefore manda-

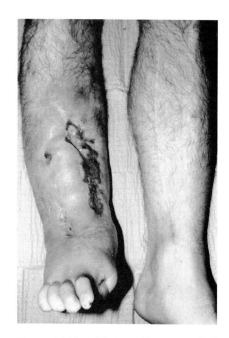

Figure 1 This 28-year-old man had chronic infected nonunion of the right tibia. He requested transtibial amputation 13 months after injury when it became apparent that further attempts at limb salvage would be futile.

tory to assess possible injuries to other areas.

When peripheral vascular disease with or without diabetes mellitus leads to amputation, the presence of associated diseases must be assumed. Barber and associates[10] found that 53 of 70 patients (76%) coming to transtibial amputation had degenerative diseases in addition to the primary disease that necessitated the amputation. Special attention must be directed to prompt and rapid preoperative control of congestive heart failure, arrhythmias, electrolyte imbalance, dehydration, hypertension, bronchitis, and diabetes.[20,41]

When diabetes mellitus–related infection has led to the need for amputation, serum glucose control will usually be markedly disrupted. Because the treatment of infection and of hyperglycemia are interdependent, they must be approached simultaneously for optimum effect. Following initial aerobic and anaerobic wound cultures, broad-spectrum antibiotic therapy should be started, pending bacterial sensitivity studies.

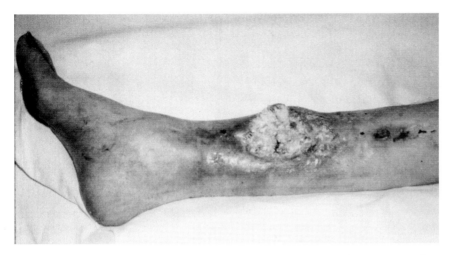

Figure 2 Right leg of man with chronic osteomyelitis of the tibia for 46 years after trauma. Squamous cell carcinoma had developed in the constantly draining sinus. There were no enlarged inguinal lymph nodes. A short transtibial amputation was performed and was curative.

Care should be taken to avoid nephrotoxic drugs whenever possible. If these drugs are needed, renal function should be closely monitored.

Icing of a necrotic or infected limb to control local and systemic effects of the infection is rarely, if ever, used today. Its use in selected cases had been suggested in the past by Kendrick,[33] but Pedersen and associates[52] have condemned this practice because after icing, they believe, a transfemoral amputation is unavoidable. Instead, they advocate prompt drainage of abscesses, followed by appropriate antibiotics and bed rest.[52]

In patients with diabetes, a wide range of bacteria may be associated with foot infections, including gram-positive, gram-negative, aerobic, and anaerobic organisms, occasionally occurring singly but more often in various combinations.[53,54] Hoar and Torres[15] found *Staphylococcus aureus*, *Streptococcus hemolyticus*, and *Proteus vulgaris* to be most common. Fearon and associates[2] cultured more than 15 different bacteria in a series of patients with diabetes-related gangrene. Systemic infection secondary to wet gangrene or infections independent of the foot must also be controlled preoperatively. Specifically, evidence of genitourinary and pulmonary infections should be sought. Assessments

of wound healing potential are also indicated. These include a serum albumin level of at least 3.0 g/dL as an indicator of adequate nutrition and a total lymphocyte count of at least 1,500/mm^3 as a measure of immunocompetence. If these values are abnormal, difficulties with primary wound healing may be expected.[55,56]

Adequate nutritional support to reverse the catabolic state associated with infection and bed rest should begin preoperatively, preferably by oral intake. Nutritional supplements such as multivitamins, ascorbic acid, zinc, and ferrous sulfate provide essential elements for collagen formation in wound healing.[57,58] Significant caloric enhancement will require corresponding increases in hypoglycemic agents to prevent iatrogenic hyperglycemia.

If time and the patient's condition allow, patients should be introduced to the team members who will be caring for them postoperatively. The physical therapist can start a whole-body conditioning program preoperatively to prevent contracture of the hip and knee on the side of the amputated limb and teach safe ambulation with a walker or crutches.[29,59]

Because the patient looks to the surgeon for guidance, the surgeon has a unique opportunity to influence pa-

tient compliance, which can lead to a better surgical outcome. The surgeon should give the patient a reasonably detailed account of the process, including the need for amputation, the proposed level and its implications, and the stages of prosthetic rehabilitation.[48,60] The surgeon should strongly discourage smoking perioperatively and postoperatively, as refraining from smoking will promote wound healing.[20] A Danish study showed 50% higher wound infection and reamputation rates in lower limb amputees who continued to smoke cigarettes before, during, and after hospitalization for amputation surgery. The investigators recommended smoking cessation 1 week before surgery, continuing throughout wound healing.[61]

The physical therapist and prosthetist should also meet with the patient preoperatively to outline their roles. A psychologist experienced in treating amputees can encourage patients to express their anxieties regarding both the surgical and prosthetic phases of care. A preoperative visit by a trained amputee peer counselor matched with the patient by age, sex, and level of amputation can also be very beneficial.

Level Selection

Level selection should be highly individualized. With tumor surgery, achieving adequate margins free of disease must be the surgeon's first concern, with preservation of limb length a secondary goal (Figure 2). With amputation after trauma, the length of reconstructible tissue distal to the knee is usually determined by the accident and previous treatment. In dysvascular patients, the surgeon should first determine if the limb can be salvaged by reconstructive vascular surgery, either entirely or with only partial loss of the foot. Consultation with the vascular surgeon has become increasingly important as vessel bypass and recanalization techniques have evolved. Ebskov and associates[62] found an inverse correlation between the rate at which vascular surgery services were used and the incidence of amputations for dysvascularity. A decrease in amputations from 34.5 to 25 per 100,000 population from 1983 to 1990 coincided with a 100% increase in peripheral vascular surgery procedures. Nonetheless, the enthusiasm for vascular salvage procedures generated by the high overall success rate must be tempered by comparative studies showing a higher rate of transfemoral amputation following failed infrainguinal bypass surgery. Van Niekerk and associates[63] conducted a prospective cohort study of 234 amputations in 219 patients performed for critical limb ischemia between 1994 and 1996. Patients were almost equally divided between those who had first undergone ipsilateral bypass surgery for limb salvage and those who had undergone primary amputation. The ratio of transtibial to transfemoral amputation was 2.05 following failed bypass surgery, compared with 5.05 for primary amputation at the indicated level, a statistically significant difference. These authors concluded that failed bypass surgery prejudices preservation of the transtibial level. They were unable, however, to identify those patients in whom amputation would be inevitable, indicating the advisability of primary amputation to avoid a futile and potentially harmful attempt at bypass surgery.[63,64] If vascular reconstruction is not feasible, it should then be determined what length of transtibial amputation has a reasonable chance of healing while providing a well-padded, durable soft-tissue envelope. In cases of foot infection, the proximal extent of infection along tissue planes may determine whether a ray, transmetatarsal amputation, or Syme ankle disarticulation is feasible. If purulence has extended proximally to the ankle, an initial open ankle disarticulation with fasciotomies and compartmental débridement is indicated to preserve length.[65]

Although level selection is multifactorial, many studies have tried to oversimplify the problem by basing success or failure solely on one criterion. Although both clinical evaluation and objective laboratory measurements of vascularity are reasonably predictive of success or failure at both the high and low ends of measurement spectra, an intermediate gray zone of unpredictability always remains. The best cluster of tests for level selection, which does not yet exist, would be that which predicts failure with 100% accuracy and thus guides the surgeon away from that level.[66,67] This would avoid amputation at higher levels in patients who could heal at the transtibial level but were excluded from transtibial amputation by overly strict application of criteria that include a built-in failure rate for reasons that are not determined by the study method. Until an infallible laboratory evaluation exists, surgeons should evaluate preoperatively factors other than tissue blood flow, such as poor nutritional status, tissue glycosylation secondary to chronic hyperglycemia, and infection. When failure occurs nonetheless, suboptimal surgical technique or poor postoperative wound management may be the cause.

The more traditional methods of level selection are considered in this chapter. For a detailed discussion of laboratory tests designed to give more objective measurements of limb and tissue blood flow, refer to chapter 3. In practice, level selection by either approach remains somewhat idiosyncratic and is based on the attitudes and prejudices of the surgeon as well as those of the prosthetist regarding the level under consideration. This is attested to by the varying ratios of transtibial to transfemoral amputations performed in similar institutions in different parts of the world and even in various parts of the same country or city.

Even with the development of more sophisticated tests, most surgeons continue to rely on factors that can be easily evaluated by touch and sight, including peripheral pulses, skin warmth and texture, color of the foot when dependent and elevated, hair growth, and the presence of indolent ulcers, tissue necrosis, gross infection, or lymphangitis.[1,2,12,16,19,29,30,31,52] Allcock and Jain[36] found that a skin temperature above 30.4°C at the proposed site of a long posterior transtibial flap correlated well with primary healing.

If peripheral pulses can be easily felt, they can be assumed to be present. If the pulses cannot be felt, however, they may still be present but obscured by edema, hypotension, or obesity. A significant number of transtibial amputations will heal despite the absence of palpable pulsation at any given site, including the superficial femoral level. In a series of 113 transtibial amputations,[21] 64 (57%) healed with only an aortic pulse present; the addition of a femoral pulse increased the success rate to 81%. When popliteal or pedal pulses were palpable, all the amputations healed. Combined data from six studies on the relationship of healing rate to the presence of a palpable popliteal pulse indicate that although 65% of these patients had no palpable popliteal pulse, 82.5% healed at the transtibial level.[10-13,47,68] These findings point out the difficulty in evaluation of collateral circulation by palpation. The profunda femoral artery, which may be the only major vessel providing collaterals to the calf, is, of course, inaccessible to the palpating finger.[46,69] Arteriography has been found to correlate as poorly with the healing potential of transtibial amputations as do palpable pulses.[34] Arteriography is now used chiefly to determine the feasibility of vascular reconstruction.[10]

Many surgeons have relied on the trial skin incision to decide at which level to amputate.[11,70,71] The presumption is that if the skin bleeds within 3 minutes after incision at the proposed level, it should heal at that level; if the skin does not bleed, the surgeon should immediately move proximally. Kendrick,[33] however, noted no correlation between bleeding of a trial skin incision and healing potential. Also, the basic question of how distally the initial trial skin incision should be made remains

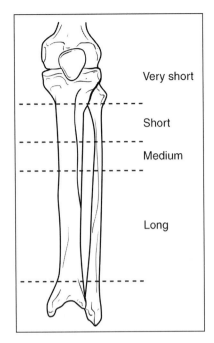

Figure 3 Levels of transtibial amputation. At the "very short" level, the fibular head is excised and the peroneal nerve is shortened. With sufficient vascularity and myodesis of the soleus to bone, preservation of two thirds to three quarters of tibial length can result in a very functional residual limb. *(Adapted with permission from Epps CH: Amputation of the lower limb, in Evarts CM (ed): Surgery of the Musculoskeletal System, ed 2. New York, Churchill Livingstone Inc, 1990.)*

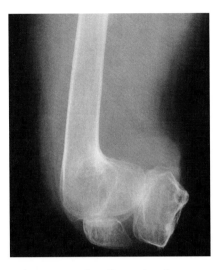

Figure 4 Lateral radiograph of a nonfunctional transtibial amputation transected proximal to the tibial tubercle. To preserve active knee extension, the tibial tubercle and patellar tendon must be saved.

unaddressed. A distal trial incision that bleeds, however, should encourage the surgeon to proceed at that level.

Once the decision has been made to amputate at the transtibial level, the equally important choice must be made as to the exact length to be retained (Figure 3). The shortest useful residual limb must include the tibial tubercle, to preserve knee extension by the quadriceps[16] (Figure 4). Flexion at this level is provided by the semimembranosus and biceps femoris. Beyond this basic universal agreement as to the shortest possible functional level, the ideal length for optimal prosthetic function has not been determined. The amputation method advocated by Burgess,[71] which results in a cylindrical residual limb, effectively limits length to approximately 15 cm because the leg be-

gins to taper beyond that point. Marsden[72] recommends limiting the length to 15 cm on the presumption that this length will be easier to fit with a prosthesis.

Over several decades, several authors have cast doubt on this certitude. Harris,[73] although recommending a short transtibial amputation in his article of 1944, noted that a long transtibial amputation is stronger than a short one. Despite this recognized functional advantage, he recommended a short residual limb because of the skin complications seen in longer amputations from wearing the prostheses with the plug-fit sockets and thigh corsets that were available at that time. Moore[69] stated that the greatest length compatible with healing should be retained, whereas Epps[74] stated that the basic rule was to save all length possible, correlating it to function and the prosthetic components to be used. McCollough and associates[75] did not specify an optimal length but flatly stated that the longer the residual limb, the better the gait. This position is supported by work showing that transtibial amputees with longer limbs require less energy to ambulate.[8]

In summary, there is no longer an *ideal* length or site of amputation. In dysvascular patients with an absent popliteal pulse, amputation in the proximal half of the leg seems reasonable, with a bony level as distal as the junction of the proximal and middle thirds. In patients with good blood flow to the ankle, bone length at the junction of the middle and distal thirds results in a strong lever arm and a broad interface with the prosthetic socket, providing better distribution of body weight during stance and improved suspension of the prosthesis during swing. Modern prosthetic components can be easily matched to these more distal levels.

Anesthesia

Various types of anesthesia are useful in transtibial amputation. The choice depends on the patient's condition, the skills and experience of the anesthetist, and, to the extent these factors allow, the patient's choice.

Local Anesthesia

An extremely ill or even moribund patient can undergo a transtibial amputation without pain under local anesthesia. The agent is injected along the proposed incision line with deeper tissues infiltrated as necessary. Nerves, especially the tibial nerve, are individually injected before any manipulation and section. Agents containing epinephrine should be avoided.

Regional Anesthesia

For patients with severe cardiopulmonary compromise, a sciatic-femoral block can be very effective. It can be supplemented, if necessary, with a local anesthetic agent.

Low Spinal Anesthesia

Low spinal anesthesia has little effect on the pulmonary system. Control of blood pressure, however, can be problematic. If hypotension occurs, it should be corrected with fluid administration and/or vasopressors.

General Anesthesia

In a healthy patient undergoing amputation for trauma, general anesthesia can be quite safe and effective. If the patient has severely compromised cardiopulmonary function, however, it may not be the best choice.

Surgical Technique

Amputation should no longer be considered as purely the ablation of a useless or debilitating part, but also a reconstructive procedure designed to restore optimum ambulatory function. As more functional goals for the transtibial amputee are realized, new surgical techniques have been developed to enhance function at that level.[76] To achieve optimum function, the surgeon must be willing at times to do staged procedures.[65] The ultimate goal is a residual limb that will interface well with a prosthesis. To achieve this, the amputation should be performed or directly supervised by an experienced surgeon and not performed unsupervised by the least experienced surgeon in training. A thigh tourniquet is recommended in cases of amputation for trauma. In dysvascular cases, a tourniquet may be put in place but inflated for only a short period of time if bleeding is problematic during surgery.

There are two criteria for the primary healing of transtibial residual limbs. First, as discussed above, is proper selection of level. A second and equally important criterion is the proper technical management of tissues during the procedure. The placement and measurement of flaps must be accurately related to the cross-sectional area of the leg at the bony level selected. Otherwise, either the bone will need to be shortened to avoid closure under tension or redundant soft tissue will have to be excised. Successful use of a variety of flap configurations has shown that incision placement is not crucial so long as the incisional scar does not adhere to the underlying bone. Transtibial amputations are listed in Table 1.

TABLE 1 Types of Transtibial Amputations

Closed Amputations	Open Amputations
Long posterior myofasciocutaneous flap	Guillotine
Equal anterior and posterior flaps	Open circumferential
Equal medial and lateral (sagittal) flaps	Open flap(s)
Skew sagittal flaps	
Medial flap	

End–weight-bearing amputations
    Distal tibiofibular synostosis
    Foot fillet	

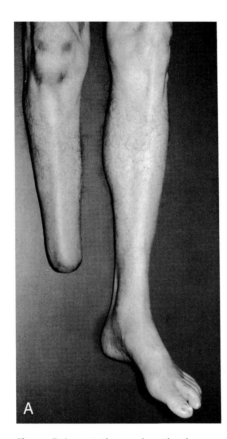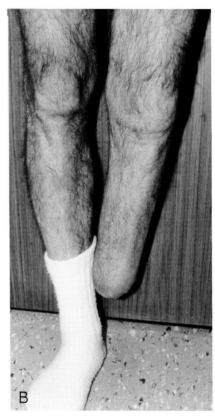

Figure 5 Amputations using the long posterior myofasciocutaneous flap technique. **A,** This 15-year-old boy underwent right transtibial amputation following severe foot trauma sustained in a motorcycle accident. Three quarters of the tibial length was retained, with distal padding provided by myodesis of the soleus to bone. The patient became an expert wrestler and handball player, and, eventually, a prosthetist. **B,** This 58-year-old man with diabetes underwent a transtibial amputation for ischemic gangrene of the foot. Two thirds of the tibial length was retained. Three years later, the right lower limb was amputated at the same level. The man remains an excellent walker with prostheses, using one cane for balance.

Closed Amputations

Long Posterior Myofasciocutaneous Flap

In 1943, Bickel[11] reported on the use of a long posterior myofasciocutane-
ous flap in 110 transtibial amputations. The educational efforts of Burgess,[71] however, were the major impetus for the acceptance of this concept (Figure 5). Provided that vascular perfusion is adequate, a poste-

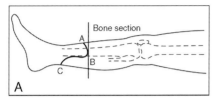

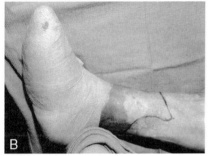

Figure 6 Long posterior myofasciocutaneous flap technique. **A,** Schematic diagram showing skin incision for very short anterior and long posterior flaps for transtibial amputation. Point A is 1 cm distal to bone section. The length AB is equal to two thirds the diameter of the calf. The length BC is equal to AB plus 1 cm. (*Adapted with permission from Wagner FW Jr: Resident Training Manual. Downey, CA, Rancho Los Amigos Medical Center.*) **B,** Intraoperative view of a long transtibial amputation. Note the very short anterior and long posterior flaps. The bone cut is made at the junction of the proximal two thirds and distal one third of the tibia in this patient with diabetes.

rior myofasciocutaneous flap can be formed down to the distal extent of the soleus muscle, with the technique becoming progressively easier in more distal amputations. There are several anatomic reasons for this. With distal tapering of the calf, the cross-sectional area of the leg decreases, resulting in a short, widely based posterior flap with good perfusion. Distal muscle bulk is minimal with less tendency for "dog ear" formation during wound closure. My technique, adapted from Wagner,[9] involves first marking reference points medially and laterally on the leg at the junction of the anterior two thirds and posterior third of the leg diameter at the level selected for bone section. Then, the two points are joined to form an anterior flap that is convex distally and no more than 0.5 to 1.0 cm long. The posterior flap is then drawn. Its

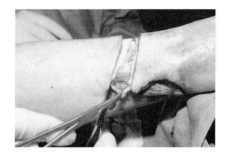

Figure 7 Intraoperative view of a long transtibial amputation. The superficial peroneal nerve is found in the sulcus between the anterior and lateral compartment muscles. It will be transected under slight tension.

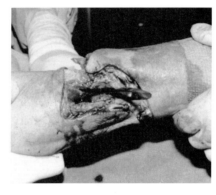

Figure 9 Intraoperative view of a long transtibial amputation. A long amputation knife is passed behind the tibia and fibula and then distally along the skin edges to create a tapered posterior myofasciocutaneous flap.

length should be equal to the distance from the original reference point to the anterior aspect of the tibia plus 1 cm. As this line starts distally, it goes slightly anteriorly from the reference point, and then gradually curves distally around the posterior aspect of the leg, where it meets a similar incision from the opposite side. The small medial and lateral half circles left at the junction of the anterior and posterior incisions eliminate "dog ears" on closure (Figure 6).

The subcutaneous tissue and investing fascia are cut in line with the skin incision. At this point, the greater saphenous vein is ligated and its companion saphenous nerve and the superficial peroneal nerve, lying laterally in the sulcus between the anterior and lateral compartment muscles, are

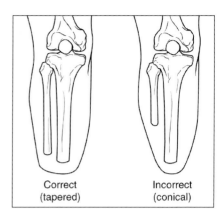

Figure 8 A naturally tapered residual limb results from cutting the fibula only minimally shorter than the tibia. If the fibula is cut too short, both the distal tibia and the distal fibula become unduly prominent and subject to painful pressure from the prosthetic socket. (*Adapted with permission from Moore WS, Malone JM (eds): Lower Extremity Amputation. Philadelphia, WB Saunders, 1989.*)

transected under slight tension, causing them to retract into the soft tissues (Figure 7). The anterior compartment muscles are carefully divided to expose the neurovascular structures. The artery should be doubly ligated, the veins ligated, and the deep peroneal nerve cut under slight tension. The tibia is stripped of periosteum only to the level of transection to reduce the chance of bone spur formation. It is then cut transversely with a saline-cooled power saw or a Gigli saw. The fibula is cleared with an elevator and cut obliquely with the power saw to form a facet facing posterolaterally. It should be made equal to or slightly shorter than the tibia to prevent undue distal tibial prominence, as seen in a conical, rather than a naturally tapered, residual limb (Figure 8). A long amputation knife is passed behind the tibia and fibula and drawn distally to create a tapered myofasciocutaneous flap (Figure 9). The peroneal and posterior tibial arteries are clamped, divided, and doubly ligated, and the veins are singly ligated. The tibial nerve may be ligated to secure its intrinsic vessels, then cut and allowed to retract proximal to the bone end (Figure 10). Alternatively, these vessels

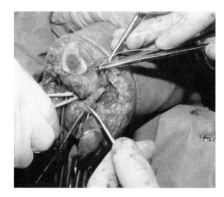

Figure 10 Intraoperative view of a long transtibial amputation. The tibial nerve is under slight tension as the suture ligature is placed to secure the vasa nervosum before sharp division. The posterior tibial vessels are clamped.

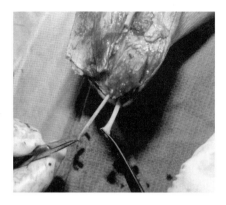

Figure 11 Intraoperative view of a long transtibial amputation. The sural nerve on the left will be sharply divided under tension, and the lesser saphenous nerve on the right will be ligated.

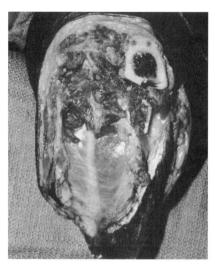

Figure 12 Intraoperative view of a long transtibial amputation. The deep posterior calf muscles have been excised, leaving the soleus as the only muscle in the posterior flap. Myodesis of the soleus to the drill holes, shown on either side of the anterior cortical bevel, will provide stable distal padding.

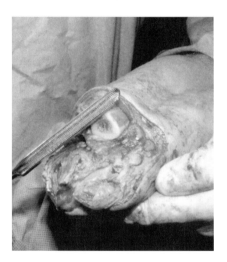

Figure 13 Intraoperative view of a long transtibial amputation. A fine offset bone file is used to smoothly contour the anterior tibial cortical bevel and distal fibular bevel to reduce potential pressure areas during prosthetic gait.

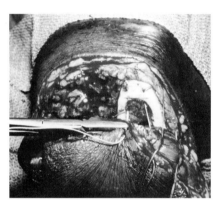

Figure 14 Intraoperative view of a long transtibial amputation. Reliable myodesis is effected by sewing the soleus myofascia and the posterior and anterior edges of the investing fascia to the tibia through two drill holes with heavy absorbable sutures, as shown. The remainder of the soft tissues are closed by myoplasty.

may be cauterized lightly before releasing the cut nerve. The lesser saphenous vein is found in the posterior flap and ligated, and the adjacent sural nerve is cut under tension and allowed to retract (Figure 11).

The deep calf musculature is excised to reduce the bulk of the posterior flap (Figure 12). An unusually bulky soleus may be tapered further to reduce the thickness of the distal tibial padding. If necessary, the medial and/or lateral flap edges can be trimmed further to obtain a good fit. The cooled power saw is then used to cut a bevel in the anterior cortex of the

tibia. All bone cuts are smoothly contoured with a bone file (Figure 13).

Transtibial wounds are best closed using a combination of myodesis and myoplasty techniques. Myodesis provides firm fixation of the posterior muscle padding to the distal tibia, thus preventing later retraction of the triceps surae from myostatic contracture. Although muscle fascia can be simply sewn to periosteum, this tissue is sometimes inadequate, in which case direct myodesis to bone is recommended. To best effect a secure myodesis to bone, a drill hole is placed on each side of the tibial crest

bevel. All bone detritus must be washed carefully from the wound after drilling. Following placement of an unsutured suction drain, the myodesis sutures are inserted. These sutures should be placed with minimal tension to avoid compromising blood flow to the flap. The tissues joined to the bone by these sutures include the anterior edge of the investing fascia, the soleus in the case of a long transtibial amputation (or the gastrocnemius in a short one), and the posterior edge of the investing fascia (Figure 14). A heavy absorbable suture works well for this. The medial and lateral portions of investing fascia and muscles are sutured with interrupted absorbable suture in a myoplasty technique. No subcutaneous sutures are necessary, and the skin is closed with interrupted, widely spaced, simple everting nylon sutures, placed without the use of skin forceps. The intervals are reinforced with adhesive paper strips (Figure 15).

A well-padded plaster or fiberglass cast is applied with the knee in 0° of extension. The drain tube is run between the layers of cast padding and

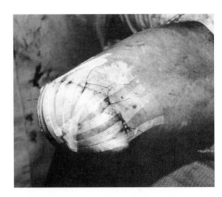

Figure 15 The skin is loosely closed with widely spaced, everting, simple sutures alternated with adhesive paper strips. This technique requires no subcutaneous sutures or use of forceps on skin, minimizing damage to cutaneous circulation.

out the top of the cast so that it can be removed after 24 to 48 hours without disturbing the cast (Figure 16). The cast is made as light as possible to allow the patient greater mobility in bed and on crutches.

Equal Anterior and Posterior Flaps

The absolute indication for equal anterior and posterior flaps, which conserves bone length, is when relatively little bone remains. In this technique, the length of each flap is equal to half the diameter of the leg at the level of bone transection. Starting from a midlateral apex on either side, the skin is cut to form equal anterior and posterior flaps (Figure 17). The anterior investing fascia and the muscles of the anterior compartment are then cut down to the neurovascular bundle. This bundle and the superficial peroneal nerve and saphenous vein

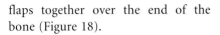

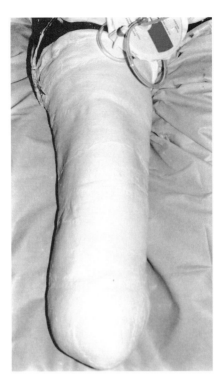

Figure 16 A lightweight immediate postoperative cast is applied with the knee in 0° of extension. The patella is heavily padded to prevent pressure ulcers. The drainage tube is led between the layers of padding to exit proximally for easy removal without disturbing the cast.

and nerve are managed as described in the previous section. The tibia and fibula are cut as before. The long amputation knife is used to create a posterior myofasciocutaneous flap. The vessels and nerves are dealt with as described above. The anterior tibial cortex is beveled and contoured with a bone file. The wound is irrigated and closed in a myoplastic manner by suturing the investing fascia and myofascia of the posterior and anterior

flaps together over the end of the bone (Figure 18).

Equal Medial and Lateral (Sagittal) Flaps

The advantages of equal medial and lateral (sagittal) flaps were outlined by Persson.[34] The flaps are less apt to become necrotic in dysvascular patients for two reasons. First, the configuration and placement of the medial and lateral flaps automatically reduce the amount of poorly vascularized anterior skin that is left. Second, the flaps are widely based and very short with reliable perfusion, thus enhancing their viability (Figure 19). Persson also stated that a side-to-side myoplasty covers the bone better and provides good spontaneous drainage. In trauma patients, another advantage is that the sagittal flap design allows the skin to be more easily cut proximal to any anterior or posterior areas of missing or damaged skin, thus helping to preserve bony length (Figures 20 and 21).

Skew Sagittal Flaps

Robinson,[59] a vascular surgeon, designed the technique using skew sagittal flaps to enhance transtibial wound healing in severely dysvascular patients in whom all major vessels are occluded. Thermography, oximetry, and vascular injection studies have shown that collateral circulation through small arteries accompanying the saphenous and sural nerves supplies blood to flaps served by these nerves.[77-80] On the basis of these studies, an anteromedial flap incorporating the saphenous nerve and artery and a posterolateral flap including the sural nerve and artery are recommended in severely dysvascular patients. The fasciocutaneous flaps are elevated from the muscles. If the posterolateral flap is noted to have very poor blood supply at the time of skin incision, it can be shortened. The anterior and lateral compartment muscles are divided at the same level as the bones, as are the deep posterior compartment muscles.

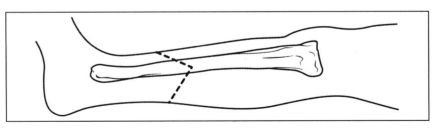

Figure 17 Drawing showing skin incision for equal anterior and posterior flap design. *(Reproduced with permission from Epps CH: Amputation of the lower limb, in Evarts CM (ed): Surgery of the Musculoskeletal System, ed 2. New York, Churchill Livingstone, 1990.)*

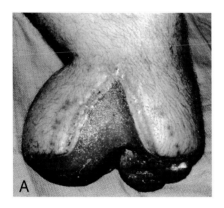
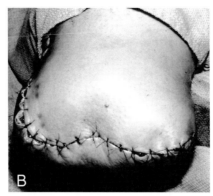
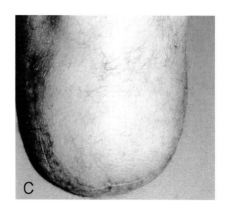

Figure 18 Application of equal anterior and posterior flaps to acute trauma in a 33-year-old man who sustained a gunshot injury to the superficial femoral artery. After three unsuccessful attempts to repair the injury, an open short transtibial amputation was performed. **A,** Lateral view just before closure 4.5 weeks after open amputation. Note the good granulation tissue formation and bulky posterior flap. **B,** Anterior view immediately after closure. Extensive trimming of posterior muscle tissue was required to achieve closure. Equal anterior and posterior flaps were used to preserve bony length. **C,** Anterior view 14 weeks after closure. Note the trim contour achieved with the use of a shrinker sock and prosthesis. Full knee extension was achieved, but flexion was limited to 90° because of the bulk of the posterior thigh muscles.

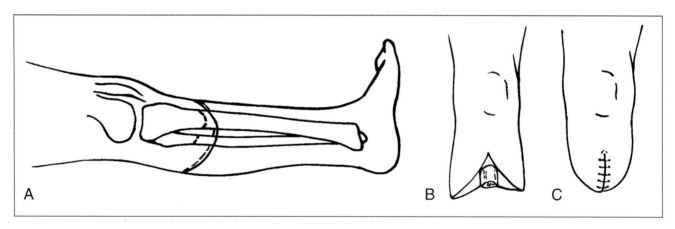

Figure 19 The technique for sagittal myofasciocutaneous flaps. **A,** Medial view showing the flaps in relation to the level of bone section in a short transtibial amputation. This method is easily adapted to any length transtibial amputation. **B,** Anterior view before wound closure. **C,** Anterior view showing midline closure. *(Reproduced with permission from Epps CH: Amputation of the lower limb, in Evarts CM (ed): Surgery of the Musculoskeletal System, ed 2. New York, Churchill Livingstone, 1990.)*

The gastrocnemius muscle is left long and fashioned into a flap that is sutured to periosteum over the tibial medullary canal as a myodesis. The fasciocutaneous skew flaps are then closed, with the resulting suture line passing obliquely between the tibia and the fibula, greatly reducing the chance of scarring to bone and damage from shear forces during prosthetic gait[81] (Figure 22).

In addition to enhancing healing in patients with only collateral circulation, this method is said to produce residual limbs that, because of their initial shape, require no shrinkage with elastic socks or wraps before prosthetic fitting. Using this technique, SK Jain and associates[82] reported satisfactory results in 28 dysvascular patients.

Ruckley and associates[83] reported on a randomized multicenter trial comparing the skew flap and long posterior flap method of Burgess in 191 patients with end-stage occlusive vascular disease. No statistically significant differences were found in early healing and revision rates or walking with a prosthesis. These investigators concluded that skew flaps offer an additional acceptable method for transtibial amputation in dysvascular patients. Robinson and Ward (personal communication, 2001) used skew flaps

in orthopaedic patients with a variety of diagnoses, excluding vascular disease, with satisfactory results in 48 of 54 patients (89%).

Medial Flap

In an effort similar to Robinson and Ward's work with skew flaps, AS Jain and associates[84] attempted to capitalize on the significant medial-to-lateral skin blood-flow gradient often seen in severely dysvascular patients by using a medially based flap. Using this technique, they were able to salvage a transtibial level in 27 of 34 patients who would otherwise have required a transfemoral amputation.

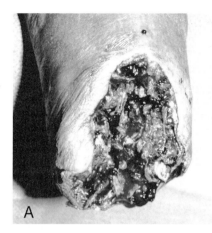
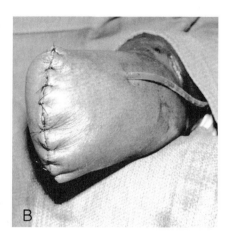

Figure 20 Application of sagittal myofasciocutaneous flaps to acute trauma in a 69-year-old woman. **A,** Open traumatic transtibial amputation 8 days after initial surgery. The tibia was fractured at the level of the wound apex. All soft tissue distal to the bone end was saved for secondary closure. **B,** Sagittal flaps were created by conservatively trimming the edges of the anterior defect and removing a narrow wedge of tissue posteriorly opposite the anterior defect. The flaps were trimmed to fit, and the wound was closed with minimal further loss of tibial length. Note the suction drain.

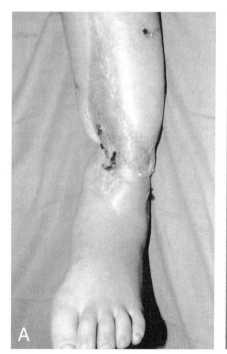
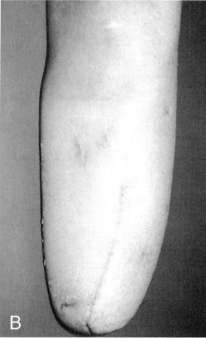

Figure 21 A 26-year-old woman sustained trauma to the left leg, resulting in draining painful nonunion of the tibia and fibula. **A,** Note the large anteromedial scarred and skin-grafted area. The patient requested transtibial amputation rather than further attempts at salvage. Amputation using sagittal myofasciocutaneous flaps was performed. **B,** Anterior view of the residual limb 8 weeks postoperatively. The large anteromedial skin defect was excised, and a narrow posterolateral wedge was removed, creating slightly skewed sagittal flaps, thereby saving considerable tibial length.

End–Weight-Bearing Transtibial Amputations
Distal Tibiofibular Synostosis

Distal tibiofibular synostosis by means of an osteoperiosteal bridge was first proposed by Bier in 1892.[85] This procedure was further developed by Ertl[86] and later by Dederich[87] for revision of inadequate transtibial residual limbs resulting from injuries in both world wars. Distal synostosis of the tibia and fibula is claimed to produce a residual limb with direct weight-bearing capability, thus enhancing prosthetic gait and comfort. Particularly in very short transtibial residual limbs or in cases where severe trauma has disrupted the interosseous membrane, this technique also prevents abduction of the fibula. Ideally, the bones fuse distally in a U shape. Direct weight bearing is said to prevent bone atrophy as well.

The original technique is as follows: Two osteoperiosteal flaps are elevated from the anteromedial and lateral aspects of the tibia, beginning approximately 10 cm distal to the proposed level of bone transection. The proximal attachments of these flaps are carefully preserved. Once the remainder of the amputation has been completed, the lateral osteoperiosteal flap is sewn to the medial aspect of the fibula, and the anteromedial flap is sutured to its lateral aspect. The flaps are then sewn to each other to form a tube joining the bone ends, which should then ossify to form a sturdy weight-bearing bony bridge (Figure 23). Distal coverage includes myoplasty. This method has been used in the US military, as reported by Deffer,[88] but to a much lesser extent in the civilian population. It has been recommended as a useful technique, especially in young traumatic amputees, both initially and as revision surgery.[72] The chief disadvantage of the original technique is the sacrifice of significant bone length, particularly where there is sufficient mobile soft tissue present to adequately cover a greater length of tibia.

Dederich[87] described an alternative method of creating an osteoperiosteal tube requiring resection of only 1.5 to 2 cm of bone. Osteoperiosteal flaps are raised medially and laterally from both the tibia and fibula, maintaining their proximal attachments. The exposed lengths of bone are excised. The lateral tibial flap is sewn to the medial fibular flap and the medial

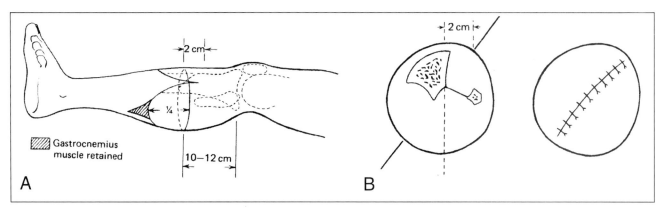

Figure 22 Skew flap technique. **A,** Anteromedial and posterolateral skew flaps as seen laterally. **B,** Distal end of left residual limb showing the orientation of the skew flaps in relation to the tibia and fibula as well as the axis of the sutured wound. *(Reproduced with permission from Robinson KP: Skew flap myoplastic below-knee amputation: A preliminary report.* Br J Surgery *1982;69:554-557.)*

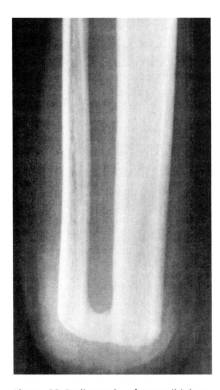

Figure 23 Radiograph of transtibial residual limb 5 months after Ertl osseoperiosteal tibiofibular synostosis.

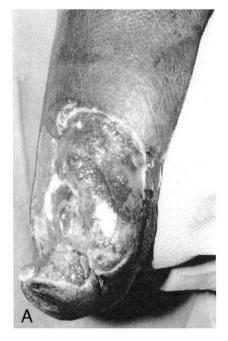

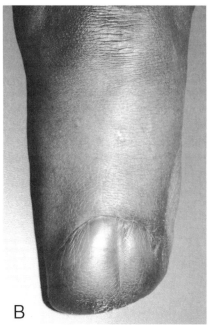

Figure 24 Application of long posterior myofasciocutaneous flap to acute trauma in a 60-year-old woman. **A,** Preclosure appearance of the transtibial amputation 10 days after the initial open procedure. All viable soft tissue distal to the bone ends was retained for secondary closure. **B,** The residual limb 28 months after closure. Considerable bone length was saved by use of the long posterior myofasciocutaneous flap retained at initial débridement. Scar placement caused no prosthetic problems.

tibial flap to the lateral fibular flap, completing the tube.[86]

Further modifications of the procedure include creation of a bridge from a salvaged distal portion of the fibula. The bone is cut, but the periosteum and attached musculature are left intact. The fibular fragment is placed between the bone ends, set into a slot in the tibia, and secured by sutures, a wire, or a screw.[85,89] There

has been a recent resurgence of interest in bone bridging, largely stimulated by amputees themselves. It is hoped that ongoing studies of this technique will provide some objective data to support the claims of its proponents.

Foot Fillet Procedures Foot fillet procedures represent another approach to end weight bearing in transtibial amputations for trauma. The

various techniques use the plantar soft tissues with or without a portion of the calcaneus in the form of an island pedicle flap based on the posterior tibial vessels and tibial nerve. The indications are limited but include unreconstructable tibial bone loss, massive circumferential skin loss between the knee and ankle from degloving or deep burns, and infected tibial nonunion with extensive skin

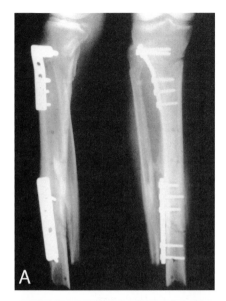

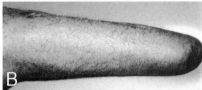

Figure 25 A 36-year-old man sustained segmental tibial fractures and a crushed foot. He underwent a transtibial amputation of the right limb. **A,** Lateral and AP radiographs of the residual limb. The wound was left open. **B,** Lateral photograph of the mature residual limb demonstrates that significant length was saved by the use of internal fixation rather than by amputating through one of the fracture sites.

loss.[90] The foot should be basically sound with protective plantar sensation and perfusion from the posterior tibial artery. As described by Singer,[22] the heel pad and remainder of the sole are dissected from the pedal skeleton, carefully preserving the neurovascular bundle. The nerve is separated from the vessels and folded into the soft tissues of the residual limb. A posterior tibial-popliteal arterial anastomosis is done, and the heel pad is sutured over the end of the tibia to provide direct weight bearing. Patterson and associates[90] described another method of achieving end bearing using an osteocutaneous flap derived from the sole and calcaneus. The sole is dissected proximally from the forefoot and midfoot skeleton,

carefully preserving the fibrous attachment of the heel pad to the calcaneus. The calcaneus is then divided between the posterior and middle facets. The intact neurovascular bundle is folded into the soft tissues with care to avoid kinking. The flap is then rotated so that the durable sole skin will fill any major skin defect. The calcaneal fragment is shaped and wired to the end of the tibia. The resultant residual limb is quite bulbous initially but assumes a suitable contour over time with wrapping and/or shrinker socks and prosthetic weight bearing.

Open Amputations

Open amputation is indicated whenever primary closure of the wound is likely to result in initial or continuing infection and/or necrosis. This applies equally to traumatic amputations and to cases of infection in which an attempt will be made to preserve maximum limb length below the knee to enhance prosthetic function. The "guillotine" amputation, in which all soft tissue and bone are transected at the same level, is rarely indicated and even then should be done only at distal levels to leave enough proximal tissue to create flaps for a functional transtibial amputation at the time of revision. The open circumferential technique, in which each successive layer is cut and allowed to retract before cutting deeper layers, has the advantage of minimizing exposure of the deeper soft tissues and bone and perhaps conserving some bone length. The technique does, however, require revision to allow good soft-tissue coverage over the end of the bones. A much better technique uses open flaps. In this case, all viable tissue is preserved by forming rough myofasciocutaneous flaps, the length and orientation of which are dictated by the trauma or infection. Although such flaps may appear excessively long initially, considerable shrinkage occurs by the time closure is feasible. If the flaps are so long that some distal viability is lost, this portion may be removed at the time of closure. Of these three techniques, the open flap

technique preserves the maximum amount of limb length (Figure 24).

In cases of irreparable loss of foot vascularity and sensation associated with segmental tibial fracture, fragments of tibial shaft may remain well attached to soft tissue. These bony fragments can be fixed to the proximal part of the shaft by internal or external fixation to provide a longer residual limb (Figures 25 and 26).

In some trauma patients there is enough muscle to adequately cover the bones but insufficient skin to completely close the wound. It is not necessary in these cases to shorten the bones to the level where full coverage by skin is possible. Available skin can be rotated to cover the anterodistal part of the tibia, the site where the greatest stress occurs during prosthetic walking. The remainder of the muscle is covered with a split-thickness skin graft (Figures 27 and 28).

In severe foot infection, an open ankle disarticulation is useful if the distal tibia is not involved. Otherwise, a supramalleolar amputation is required to remove infected bone.[91] If the leg compartments are involved, they may be easily opened medially and/or laterally for thorough débridement. Partial or complete closure is usually possible in 10 to 14 days[65] (Figure 29).

Special Considerations During Transtibial Amputation
Treatment of Skin

To have a successful amputation, the one tissue structure that must heal is the skin. The skin-subcutaneous incision should be made at 90° to the surface to avoid having portions of skin unsupported by subcutaneous tissue and, hence, making it more difficult to accurately appose these layers, making them more prone to necrosis. At no time should the skin be traumatized by grasping with forceps.[13,15,19,33,45,50] For the same reason, the use of staples is discouraged. Instead, skin edges can be everted for closure by the suturing needle, skin hooks, or gloved fingers. The skin must be precisely approximated without tension. Simple, widely spaced sutures can be alternated with adhesive paper strips to contain subcutaneous fat. In dysvascular patients, the sutures are kept in place for 3 weeks to allow for the slower healing that is common.[20] There should be no separation of layers in the creation of myofasciocutaneous flaps because this may interfere with the blood supply to the skin. The residual limb should not be left with inverted scars or redundant skin, or with "dog ears" that will not atrophy promptly.

Treatment of Fascia

The crural or investing fascia should be cut at the same level as the skin and subcutaneous tissue. It should never be separated from the surrounding soft tissues to prevent damage to any small perforating vessels serving the skin. In closing a myofasciocutaneous flap, care should be taken to ensure that the crural fascia is indeed found and firmly sutured both to ensure maximal wound strength and to take tension off the overlying skin. This, in turn, allows the use of fewer skin sutures, which may lessen skin necrosis. Complete closure of the investing fascia also prevents scarring of skin directly to bone, allowing dissipation of shear forces generated at the skin-socket interface.

Treatment of Muscle

Muscle is considered to carry at least some blood from the deep arteries of the leg to the skin. It is, therefore, generally accepted that muscle should not be dissected from its overlying investing fascia. Muscle may be trimmed, leaving sufficient padding for the end of the tibia without unnecessary bulk. Any ischemic or necrotic muscle, as determined by minimal stimulation with the electro-

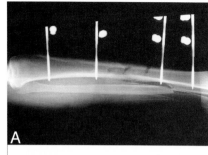
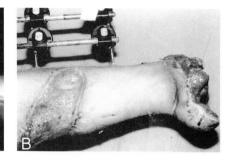
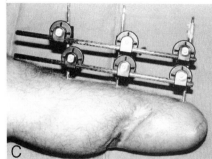
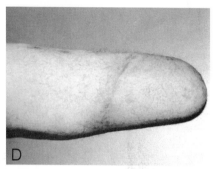
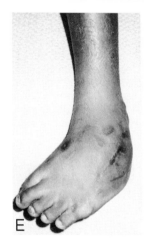
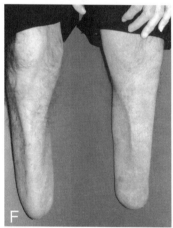
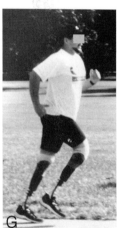

Figure 26 A 22-year-old man sustained bilateral lower limb injuries in an auto racing accident. **A,** Lateral radiograph of the right leg shows the open comminuted tibial and fibular fractures with external fixator in place. **B,** Medial view of the right open ankle disarticulation. The most distal pin has been removed and the frame shifted proximally to allow sufficient room for posterior flap development at the long transtibial level. **C,** Medial view showing distal closure and healing of the midcalf wound by contraction. **D,** Medial view 10 months after closure. The contracted scar of the calf wound was excised and closed directly. Note the excellent length and shape of the limb. **E,** Left lower limb with painful ankle/foot arthrosis and deformity. Two years later, the patient requested a second transtibial amputation rather than further attempts at reconstruction. **F,** Four years after the injury, the residual limbs are well matured. **G,** Patient training for a triathlon 4 years after the injury.

coagulator, should be excised. This condition appears most commonly in the anterior compartment. If muscle tissue is merely pale, it may be left because it will probably fibrose in time. Healing can occur following the complete removal of necrotic muscles so long as the skin remains viable.

Treatment of Nerves

Five nerves should be found and transected during transtibial amputation: the superficial peroneal, saphenous, deep peroneal, sural, and tibial nerves. The tibial nerve may present sufficient intrinsic vascular supply to

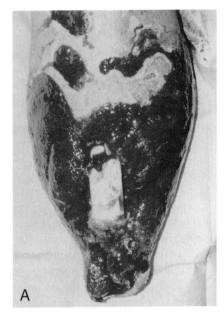
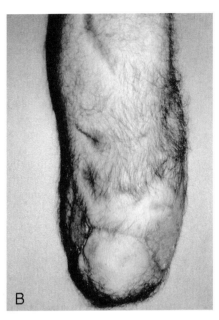

Figure 27 A 21-year-old man was injured in a farming accident. **A,** Open transtibial amputation. At initial débridement, the exposed tibia was retained as an internal splint to prevent contraction of posterior soft tissues. The wound is well covered with granulation tissue and ready for revision and closure. **B,** The residual limb 3 months after closure. Exposed bone was excised and the anterodistal tibia was covered with a sensate narrow posterior flap. The remaining medial and lateral defects were covered with split-thickness skin grafts. The patient was fitted with a prosthesis and returned to farm work without incident. (*Reproduced from Bowker JH: Surgical techniques for conserving tissue and function in lower-limb amputation for trauma, infection and vascular disease. Instr Course Lect 1990;39:355-360.*)

protected during prosthetic gait. Dellon and associates[92] demonstrated that nerve ends surgically buried in muscle show no tendency to form neuromas.

Treatment of Bone

Beveling of the tibia combined with careful smoothing of the bone edges will prevent damage to the skin in its position between the hard bone surface and the firm prosthetic socket. Various authors have suggested a bevel of 45° to 60° to be optimal.[11,16,21,93] All bone cutting with a power saw should be done with saline cooling to prevent thermal necrosis.[72] If the surgeon wishes to avoid fluid splattering, a Gigli saw may be used instead to cut the tibial shaft from posterior to anterior. As the saw enters the anterior cortex, it is directed proximally to cut the bevel.

The fibula should be no more than 0.5 to 1 cm shorter than the tibia if a conical shape of the distal residual limb with a prominent distal end of the tibia is to be avoided.[71] To prevent soft-tissue impingement during prosthesis use, the fibula may be cut with a bevel facing posterolaterally. Both bones should be carefully filed to remove all sharp edges and points. Before closure, the wound should be ir-

warrant ligation or cauterization of its vasa nervorum. A variety of methods have been advocated to inhibit neuroma formation by traumatizing the proximal cut end of the nerve.

The best approach appears to be simple sharp division following mild traction on the nerve.[71] The cut proximal end retracts into the soft tissues where the inevitable neuroma will be

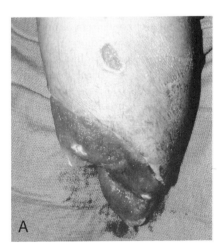
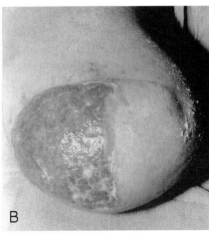
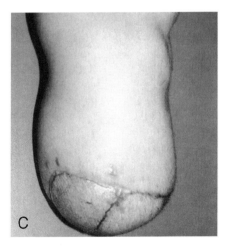

Figure 28 A 40-year-old woman sustained trauma to the left leg. **A,** Open left traumatic transtibial amputation ready for closure. Note the retained posterolateral soft tissue. At the time of initial débridement, this flap was considerably larger, but it contracted over the intervening 10 days. **B,** Residual limb 1 month after the tibia was covered by rotation of a local myofasciocutaneous flap. Coverage elsewhere is by muscle tissue only, which is ready for split-thickness skin grafting onto the granulation tissue base. **C,** Five weeks later, the graft is mature enough for application of a shrinker sock.

rigated generously to wash away bone detritus.

Total removal of the fibula may be required in cases of fibular osteomyelitis or bony necrosis caused by circumferential muscle loss or abscess formation. Removal may also be beneficial in a very short transtibial amputation at the level of the tibial tubercle where, if left in place, the fibular head may produce pain by its ball-like presence in the socket. After excision of the fibula, an intimate socket fit over the entire circumference of the tibia can be achieved (Figure 30). With the hip extended and the knee flexed, several centimeters of the peroneal nerve can be drawn gently into the wound, after which the neuroma will form in the thigh, away from socket pressure. Bleeding from the tibia or fibula can be controlled by electrocautery and closure of the wound. Bone wax should not be used because of its tendency to provoke a foreign-body reaction and its interference with firm healing of muscle to bone.

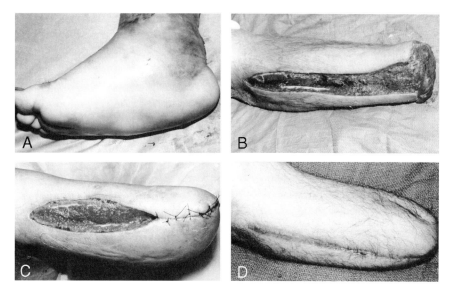

Figure 29 A 43-year-old man with type 1 diabetes mellitus required transtibial amputation. **A,** Severely abscessed foot and ankle before supramalleolar amputation and thorough débridement through extensile incisions of all crural compartments for ascending purulent infection. **B,** At time of definitive transtibial amputation 17 days later, all compartments and the distal portion of the wound had abundant granulation tissue. The wound edges and granulation tissue were excised in all areas that could be closed. **C,** Lateral view showing distal closure with myodesis of the soleus and partial closure of the anterior compartment wound. At the same time, partial proximal closure of the posterior compartment wound was done. **D,** Three months after initial open amputation, both remaining wounds had healed by secondary intention, and the limb was ready for prosthetic fitting.

Immediate Postoperative Management

A lightweight rigid dressing from the end of the residual limb to midthigh with the knee in full extension has several advantages. This prevents knee flexion contracture during the first few painful postoperative days, protects the wound from bed trauma, and limits edema formation. The patient is generally comfortable and, if the rigid dressing is light enough, can move about in bed quite easily. Another advantage of the rigid dressing is that it protects against falls onto the residual limb while the patient learns

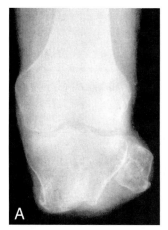
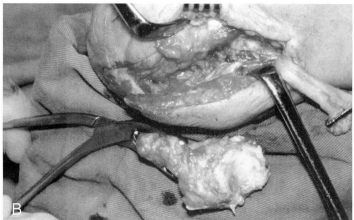
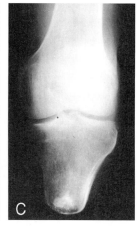

Figure 30 Very short transtibial amputation. **A,** Anterior radiograph of a very short traumatic transtibial amputation with a prominent residual fibula. **B,** Intraoperative view of the same limb shown in **A** demonstrating excision of the residual fibula to allow intimate, stable circumferential fit of the socket to the tibia. The peroneal nerve (in clamp) was shortened under moderate tension to ensure that the neuroma would form above the knee, well proximal to the socket brim. **C,** AP radiograph of another very short transtibial amputation following removal of the fibula, showing a smooth lateral tibial contour, allowing an intimate socket fit. (*A and B courtesy of Prof. Georg Neff, Berlin, Germany.*)

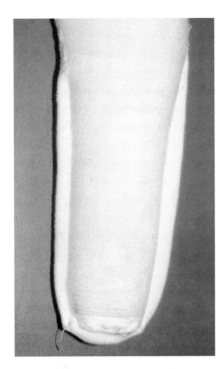

Figure 31 Shrinker sock applied to a residual limb after transtibial amputation was tightened twice within 4 weeks as the residual limb volume decreased. Lack of further atrophy in the previous week indicated readiness for prosthetic fitting.

to manage a walker or crutches. If necessary, the rigid dressing can be secured with a waist belt. The only disadvantage is that the wound cannot be readily inspected. Careful attention to the patient's general status, however, such as an otherwise unexplained fever or evidence of excessive drainage, will inform the surgeon of any indication for removal of the cast. The cast is worn for 3 weeks with weekly changes for wound inspection and full range of motion of the knee. A shrinker sock is then worn continuously, except for bathing, until residual limb volume has stabilized. The sock is tightened or changed as volume decreases (Figure 31).

A soft dressing, on the other hand, allows easy access to the wound for inspection and for motion of the knee with or without the guidance of a therapist. It does not, however, protect the wound from trauma, nor does it prevent knee flexion contracture if the patient does not move the knee regularly. One randomized study comparing soft and rigid dressings showed that rigid dressings resulted in less pain, an improved sense of well-being, and earlier prosthetic fitting.[10] In another series, hospital stay was reduced from 14 to 7 days.[46] A posterior plaster splint will keep the knee straight as long as the splint is not broken and the wrapping is firm. If it is necessary to look at the wound, however, a better plan is to make a strong posterior hemicylinder by removing the anterior half of a full cast.

An alternative method, used in a limited number of centers because it requires excellent patient compliance, is the immediate postoperative prosthesis (IPOP). The protocol developed by Smith and Fergason[94] can be summarized as follows. For diabetic/dysvascular patients and trauma patients with amputation above the zone of injury, the usual rigid dressing is applied on the operating table. If wound healing is seen to be progressing normally at 5 to 7 days postoperatively, a pylon and foot are attached to the second cast. Weight bearing starts at 20 to 30 lb. Following each weekly cast change, weight bearing is increased by 30 lb. When residual limb volume is no longer decreasing and the skin is wrinkled, a shrinker sock is applied and prosthetic fitting begun. If amputation for trauma has been done through the zone of injury, a more cautious approach is required to protect marginal tissue, split-thickness skin grafts, or open areas. Application of the IPOP is delayed until the wound is completely healed, at which point it may be considered unnecessary if residual limb edema has resolved during the interim. In this case, shrinker sock application and prosthesis fitting can be done without further delay.

The issue that most concerns patients during the immediate postoperative period is pain control. Patients should be given an amount of narcotics sufficient for good pain relief every 3 to 6 hours or by means of an on-demand machine for a maximum of 5 days, then switched to oral narcotics or nonsteroidal anti-inflammatory drugs. In this way, habituation should not occur. Avoidance of wound dependency should also help prevent pain.

A different approach to modulation of both immediate postoperative and phantom limb pain arose from observation of the similarities between preoperative limb pain and postoperative phantom pain. In 11 patients, Bach and associates[95] found that a lumbar epidural blockade with bupivacaine and morphine, given 72 hours preoperatively, greatly reduced the incidence of phantom limb pain at 7 days, 6 months, and 1 year after surgery compared with a similar control group of 14 patients. A second group of investigators then conducted a randomized, double-blind trial in 60 patients in whom the blockade or a saline placebo was begun 18 hours before surgery. The trial showed no significant difference in the incidence of phantom limb pain between the two groups at 1 week or at 3, 6, or 12 months postoperatively.[96]

Alternatively, a small Silastic catheter may be inserted at the time of surgery within or next to the tibial nerve sheath for administration of local anesthetic for the first 72 hours postoperatively, as advocated by Malawer and associates.[97] In another study of this technique, Elizaga and associates[98] found no effect on postoperative opioid requirements or phantom limb pain.

Preventing infection is an important goal of postoperative management that is usually met with perioperative intravenous antibiotics. If infection is an overriding factor in the amputation, however, one or more antibiotics chosen from organism sensitivity tests should be continued for 2 to 5 days postoperatively.[20,29] Further need for antibiotics can be determined by direct evaluation of the wound. Atelectasis can be prevented by positioning and by deep breathing exercises using various types of incentive respiratory devices.

The patient should be made mobile as soon as possible to prevent the deconditioning that may occur within just a few days. On the first postoperative day, the patient should be sitting in a chair with the residual limb elevated to the level of the chair seat. By the next day, the patient should be in the physical therapy department beginning ambulation on parallel bars. This should be followed by the use of crutches or a walker as conditioning and balance improve.

In recent years, introduction of the IPOP and its most commonly used component, the rigid postoperative cast, has enhanced early mobilization.[17,30,63] If an IPOP has been applied, limited weight bearing on the residual limb can start almost immediately, provided the patient demonstrates sufficient strength, balance, proprioception, and cognition to accurately determine the weight applied.

The cost of a hospital stay has become a major issue in recent years. In the past, many patients remained in the hospital or rehabilitation center following surgery until they had healed and had been fitted with a prosthesis and thoroughly trained in its use. In the United States, this is no longer financially feasible. Transtibial amputees are often discharged from the hospital 4 to 5 days after surgery unless they have failed to achieve their maximum level of independence in transfers and one-legged ambulation. In that case, they will stay until these goals have been achieved or abandoned as unrealistic. All further care, including prosthetic fitting and follow-up, is accomplished on an outpatient basis. Hospitalization for prosthetic gait training can be justified in cases of marked deconditioning, advanced age, bilateral concomitant lower limb amputations, or great distance from the center.

The psychological needs of the amputee must also be met. Counseling by various team members can help allay the patient's anxiety about the prosthetic phase of care. A trained amputee peer counselor matched with the patient's age, sex, and amputation level can be of inestimable help. Amputee/consumer peer support groups can also be extremely helpful in facilitating the amputee's transition to the community, especially by providing a comfortable social, educational, and recreational outlet.

Summary

Transtibial amputation, by saving the knee joint, provides the amputee with the possibility of near-normal ambulation and overall lifestyle. With the availability of new information on the efficacy of transtibial amputation and improved methods of determining potential healing levels in a limb, most major lower limb amputations are now being done at the transtibial rather than the transfemoral level. Diabetes mellitus is now the primary or secondary cause of amputation in at least 50% of patients in developed countries. Most patients with dysvascular limbs have one or more significant associated diseases calling for detailed preoperative management and skilled care in the immediate postoperative period.

The aim of amputation surgery is a well-healed, sensate, functional end organ that will interface well with a prosthesis. Selection of length is based on etiologic factors and on clinical and laboratory evaluation. As much length as possible should be preserved, compatible with eradicating disease and with good prosthetic function. Meticulous management of tissues will lead to preservation of the length obtained at surgery. Myodesis is advocated because it provides the most stable soft-tissue envelope. Postoperative rigid dressings are strongly recommended because of local protection of the wound and the prevention of edema and knee flexion contracture. Early mobilization prevents deconditioning, thereby allowing the early discharge to outpatient status. Early prosthetic weight bearing has great value in selected patients if they are closely monitored. Optimal amputee management is best achieved through a team approach, beginning even before surgery.

References

1. Boontje AH: Major amputations of the lower extremity for vascular disease. *Prosthet Orthot Int* 1980;4:87-89.

2. Fearon J, Campbell DR, Hoar CS, et al: Improved results with diabetic below-knee amputees. *Arch Surg* 1985;120:777-780.

3. Harris JP, Page S, Englund R, et al: Is the outlook for the vascular amputee improved by striving to preserve the knee? *J Cardiovasc Surg* 1988;29:741-745.

4. Kacy SS, Wolma FJ, Flye MW: Factors affecting the results of below-knee amputation in patients with and without diabetes. *Surg Gynecol Obstet* 1982;155:513-518.

5. Keagy BA, Schwartz Ja, Kotb M, et al: Lower extremity amputation: The control series. *J Vasc Surg* 1986;4:321-326.

6. Rizzo RL, Matsumoto R: Above versus below knee amputations: A retrospective analysis. *Int Surg* 1980;65:265-267.

7. Bard G, Ralston JH: Measurement of energy expenditure during ambulation, with special reference to evaluation of assistive devices. *Arch Phys Med Rehabil* 1959;40:415-420.

8. Gonzalez EG, Corcoran PJ, Reyes RL: Energy expenditure in below-knee amputees: Correlation with stump length. *Arch Phys Med Rehabil* 1974;55:111-119.

9. Wagner FW Jr: *Resident Training Manual.* Downey, CA, Rancho Los Amigos Medical Center.

10. Barber GG, McPhail NV, Scobie TK, et al: A prospective study of lower limb amputations. *Can J Surg* 1983;26:339-341.

11. Bickel WH: Amputations below the knee in occlusive arterial diseases. *Surg Clin North Am* 1943;23:982-994.

12. Block MA, Whitehouse FW: Below-knee amputation in patients with diabetes mellitus. *Arch Surg* 1963;87:682-689.

13. Chilvers AS, Briggs J, Browse NL, et al: Below- and through-knee amputations in ischaemic disease. *Br J Surg* 1971;58:824-826.

14. Cumming JGR, Jain AS, Walker WF, et al: Fate of the vascular patient after below-knee amputation. *Lancet* 1987;2:613-615.

15. Hoar CS, Torres J: Evaluation of below-the-knee amputation in the treatment of diabetic gangrene. *N Engl J Med* 1962;266:440-443.

16. Lim RC, Blaisdell FW, Hall AD, et al: Below-knee amputation for ischemic gangrene. *Surg Gynecol Obstet* 1967; 125:493-501.

17. Moore WS, Hall AD, Lim RC: Below the knee amputation for ischemic gangrene: Comparative results of conventional operation and immediate postoperative fitting technique. *Am J Surg* 1972;124:127-134.

18. Murray DG: Below-knee amputations in the aged: Evaluation and prognosis. *Geriatrics* 1965;20:2033-1038.

19. Perry T: Below-knee amputations. *Arch Surg* 1963;86:199-202.

20. Robinson K: Long-posterior-flap myoplastic below-knee amputation in ischaemic disease: Review of experience in 1967-1971. *Lancet* 1972;2:193-195.

21. Roon AJ, Moore WS, Goldstone J: Below-knee amputation: A modern approach. *Am J Surg* 1977;134:153-158.

22. Singer DI, Morrison WA, McCann JJ, et al: The fillet foot for endweight-bearing cover of below knee amputations. *Aust N Z J Surg* 1988;58:817-823.

23. Paloschi GB, Lynn RB: Major amputations for obliterative peripheral vascular disease with particular reference to the role of below-knee amputation. *Can J Surg* 1967;10:168-171.

24. Smith BC: A twenty year follow-up in fifty below-knee amputations for gangrene in diabetics. *Surg Gynecol Obstet* 1956;103:625-630.

25. Fletcher DD, Andrews KL, Hallett JW Jr, et al: Trends in rehabilitation after amputation for geriatric patients with vascular disease: Implications for future health resource allocation. *Arch Phys Med Rehabil* 2002;83:1389-1393.

26. Purry NA, Hannon MA: How successful is below-knee amputation for injury? *Injury* 1989;20:32-36.

27. Dougherty PJ: Transtibial amputees from the Vietnam War: Twenty-eight year follow-up. *J Bone Joint Surg Am* 2001;83:383-389.

28. Sarmiento A, Warren WD: A re-evaluation of lower extremity amputations. *Surg Gynecol Obstet* 1969;129: 799-802.

29. Castronuovo JJ, Deane LJ, Deterling RA, et al: Below-knee amputation: Is the effort to preserve the knee joint justified? *Arch Surg* 1980;115: 1184-1187.

30. de Cossart L, Randall P, Turner P, et al: The fate of the below-knee amputee. *Ann R Coll Surg Engl* 1983;65:230-232.

31. Ecker JL, Jacobs BS: Lower extremity amputation in diabetic patients. *Diabetes* 1970;19:189-195.

32. Fleurant FW, Alexander J: Below knee amputation and rehabilitation of amputees. *Surg Gynecol Obstet* 1980;151: 41-44.

33. Kendrick RR: Below-knee amputation in arteriosclerotic gangrene. *Br J Surg* 1956;44:13-27.

34. Persson BM: Sagittal incision for below-knee amputation in ischaemic gangrene. *J Bone Joint Surg Br* 1974;56: 110-114.

35. Yaramenko D, Andruhova RV: Below-knee amputation in patients with vascular disease and prosthetic fitting problems. *Prosthet Orthot Int* 1986;10: 125-128.

36. Allcock PA, Jain AS: Revisiting transtibial amputation with the long posterior flap. *Br J Surg* 2001;88:683-686.

37. Cranley JJ, Krause RJ, Strasser RS, et al: Below-the-knee amputation for arteriosclerosis obliterans. *Arch Surg* 1969;98:77-80.

38. Thornhill HL, Jones GD, Brodzka W, et al: Bilateral below-knee amputations: Experience with 80 patients. *Arch Phys Med Rehabil* 1986;67: 159-163.

39. McCollough NC, Jennings JJ, Sarmiento A: Bilateral below-the-knee amputation in patients over fifty years of age: Result in 31 patients. *J Bone Joint Surg Am* 1972;54:1217-1223.

40. Heller RF, Hayward D, Hobbs MST: Decline in rate of death from ischaemic heart disease in The United Kingdom. *BMJ* 1983;286:260-262.

41. Stewart CPU: The influence of smoking on the level of lower limb amputation. *Prosthet Orthot Int* 1987;11: 113-116.

42. Rush DS, Huston CC, Bivins BA, et al: Operative and late mortality rates of above knee and below knee amputations. *Am Surg* 1981;47:36-39.

43. Calvet HM, Yoshikawa TT: Infection in diabetes. *Inf Dis N Amer* 2001;15: 407-421.

44. Dwars BJ, Rauwerda JA, van den Brock TAA, et al: A modified scintigrafic technique for amputation level selection in diabetics. *Eur J Nucl Med* 1989; 15:38-41.

45. Alter AH, Moshein J, Elconin KB, et al: Below-knee amputation using the sagittal technique: A comparison with the coronal amputation. *Clin Orthop* 1978; 131:195-201.

46. Baker WH, Barnes RW, Shurr DG: The healing of below-knee amputations: A comparison of soft and plaster dressings. *Am J Surg* 1977;133:716-718.

47. Harris PD, Schwartz SI, DeWeese JA: Midcalf amputation for peripheral vascular disease. *Arch Surg* 1961;82: 381-383.

48. Murdoch G: Amputation surgery in the lower extremity. *Prosthet Orthot Int* 1977;1:72-83.

49. Pohjolainen T, Alaranta H: Lower limb amputations in southern Finland. *Prosthet Orthot Int* 1988;12:9-18.

50. Termansen NB: Below-knee amputation for ischaemic gangrene. *Acta Orthop Scand* 1977;48:311-316.

51. Lange RH, Bach AW, Hansen ST Jr, Johansen KH: Open tibial fractures with associated vascular injuries: Prognosis for limb salvage. *J Trauma* 1985;25:203-208.

52. Pedersen HE, LaMont RL, Ramsey RH: Below-knee amputation for gangrene. *South Med J* 1964;57:820-825.

53. Lipsky BA: Evidence-based antibiotic therapy of diabetic foot infections. *FEMS Immunol Med Microbiol* 1999;26: 267-276.

54. Lipsky BA, Berendt AR: Principles and practice of antibiotic therapy of diabetic foot infections. *Diabet Metab Res Rev* 2000;16(suppl 1):S42-S46.

55. Dickhaut SC, DeLee JC, Page CP: Nutritional status: Importance in predicting wound-healing after amputation. *J Bone Joint Am* 1984;66:71-75.

56. Pinzur MS, Smith D, Osterman H: Syme ankle disarticulation in peripheral vascular disease and diabetic infection: The one-stage versus two-stage procedure. *Foot Ankle Int* 1993; 16:124-127.

57. Sieggreen MY: Healing of physical wounds. *Nurs Clin North Am* 1987;22: 439-447.

58. Stotts NA, Washington DF: Nutrition. A critical component of wound healing. *AACN Clin Issues Crit Care Nurs* 1990;1:585-594.

59. Robinson K: Skew flap myoplastic below-knee amputation: A preliminary report. *Br J Surg* 1982;69:554-557.

60. Bowker JH: Questions to ask your amputation team members before surgery, in *First Step: A Guide for Adapting to Limb Loss*, ed 2. Knoxville, TN, Amputee Coalition of America, 2001, pp 10-11.

61. Lind J, Kramhoff M, Bodtker S: The influence of smoking on complications after primary amputations of the lower extremity. *Clin Orthop* 1991;267:211-217.

62. Ebskov LB, Schroeder TV, Holstein PE: Epidemiology of leg amputation: The influence of vascular surgery. *Br J Surg* 1994;81:1600-1603.

63. Van Niekerk LJA, Stewart CPU, Jain AS: Major lower limb amputation following failed infrainguinal vascular bypass surgery: A prospective study on amputation levels and stump complications. *Prosthet Orthot Int* 2001;25:29-33.

64. Ebskov LB: Hindsok, Holstein P: Level of amputation following failed arterial reconstruction compared to primary amputation: A meta-analysis. *Eur J Vasc Endovasc Surg* 1999;17:35-40.

65. Bowker JH: Surgical techniques for conserving tissue and function in lower-limb amputation for trauma, infection, and vascular disease. *Instr Course Lect* 1990;39:355-360.

66. Cheng EY: Lower extremity amputation level: Selection using noninvasive hemodynamic methods of evaluation. *Arch Phy Med Rehabil* 1982;63:475-479.

67. Lepantalo M, Isoniemi H, Kyllonen L: Can the failure of a below-knee amputation be predicted? *Ann Chir Gynaecol* 1987;76:119-123.

68. Eraklis A, Wheeler B: Below-knee amputations in patients with severe arterial insufficiency. *N Engl J Med* 1963;269:933-943.

69. Moore TJ: Amputations of the lower extremity, in Chapman M (ed): *Operative Orthopaedics*. Philadelphia, JB Lippincott, 1988.

70. Brodie IAO: Lower limb amputation. *Br J Hosp Med* 1970;4:596-604.

71. Burgess EM: The below-knee amputation. *Bull Prosthet Res* 1968;10:19-25.

72. Marsden FW: Amputation surgical technique and postoperative management. *Aust N Z J Surg* 1977;47:384-392.

73. Harris RI: Amputations. *J Bone Joint Surg* 1944;26:626-634.

74. Epps CH Jr: Amputation of the lower limb, in Evarts CM (ed): *Surgery of the Musculoskeletal System*, ed 2. New York, NY, Churchill Livingstone, 1990.

75. McCollough NC III, Harris AR, Hampton FL: Below-knee amputation, in *Atlas of Limb Prosthetics*. St. Louis, MO, Mosby-Year Book, 1981, pp 341-368.

76. Loon HE: Below-knee amputation surgery. *Artif Limbs* 1961;6:86-99.

77. McCollum PT, Spence VA, Walker WF, Murdoch GA: A rationale for skew flaps in below-knee amputation surgery. *Prosthet Orthot Int* 1985;9:95-99.

78. Towne JD, Condon RE: Lower extremity amputations for ischaemic disease. *Adv Surgery* 1979;13:199-227.

79. Gray DWR, Ng RLH: Anatomical aspects of the blood supply to the skin of the posterior calf: Technique of below knee amputation. *Br J Surg* 1990;77:662-664.

80. Haertsch P: The surgical plane in the leg. *Br J Plast Surg* 1981;43:464-469.

81. Robinson KP: Skew-flap below-knee amputation. *Ann R Coll Surg Engl* 1991;73:155-157.

82. Jain SK, Sanyal NC, Poonekar PD: An improved technique for below-knee amputation in ischemic limbs. *Med J Armed Forces India* 1988;44:191-195.

83. Ruckley CV, Stonebridge PA, Prescott RJ: Skew flap versus long posterior flap in below-knee amputations: Multicenter trial. *J Vasc Surg* 1991;13:423-427.

84. Jain AS, Stewart CP, Turner MS: Transtibial amputation using a medially based flap. *J R Coll Surg Edinb* 1995;40:263-265.

85. Weiss M: Bone treatment in amputations and reamputations, in *Myoplastic Amputation, Immediate Prosthesis and Early Amputation*. Washington, DC, US Government Printing Office, 1968, pp 61-65.

86. Ertl J: About amputation stumps. *Chirurgie* 1949;20:212-218.

87. Dederich R: Die muskelplastischen Amputationsstümpfe. *Orthop Techn* 1962;14:178.

88. Deffer PA: More on the Ertl osteoplasty. *Amputee Clin* 1970;2:7-8.

89. Pinto MAGS, Filho NA, Guedes JPB, Yamahoka MSO: Bone bridging in transtibial amputation. *Rev Bras Ortop* 1998;33:525-531.

90. Patterson BM, Smith AA, Holdren AM, Sontich JK: Osteocutaneous pedicle flap of the foot for salvage of below-knee amputation level after lower extremity injury. *J Trauma* 2000;48:767-772.

91. McIntyre KE Jr, Bailey Sa, Malone JM, et al: Guillotine amputation in the treatment of nonsalvageable lower-extremity infections. *Arch Surg* 1984;119:450-453.

92. Dellon AL, MacKinnon SE, Pestronk A: Implantation of sensory nerve into muscle: Preliminary clinical and experimental observations on neuroma formation. *Ann Plast Surg* 1984;12:30-40.

93. Harris WR: Below-knee amputation: A technical note. *Can J Surg* 1987;30:392-393.

94. Smith DG, Fergason JR: Transtibial amputations. *Clin Orthop Rel Res* 1999;361:108-115.

95. Bach S, Noreng MF, Tjellden NV: Phantom limb pain in amputees during the first 12 months following limb amputation, after preoperative lumbar epidural blockade. *Pain* 1998;33:297-301.

96. Nikolajsen L, Ilkjaer S, Christensen JH, Kronerk K, Jensen TS: Randomised trial of epidural bupivacaine and morphine in prevention of stump and phantom pain in lower limb amputation. *Lancet* 1997;350:1353-1357.

97. Malawer MM, Buch R, Khurana JS, et al: Postoperative infusional continuous regional analgesia (PICRA): A technique for relief of postoperative pain following major extremity surgery. *Clin Orthop* 1991;266:227-237.

98. Elizaga AM, Smith DG, Sharar SR, Edwards WT, Hansen ST: Continuous regional analgesia by nerve sheath block has no effect on postoperative opioid requirements and phantom limb pain following amputation. *J Rehab Res and Dev* 1994;31:108-115.

Chapter 39

Transtibial Amputation: Prosthetic Management

Susan L. Kapp, CPO
John R. Fergason, CPO

Introduction

Because transtibial amputation is so common, it is important to understand patient evaluation, biomechanical principles, prosthetic options, and component availability for this level. This chapter provides a framework to prescribe the most appropriate prosthesis. An appropriate prescription is based on a thorough physical examination, history, and interview, as well as follow-up to achieve a successful long-term outcome. Unless the patient has other significant physical limitations, prosthetic treatment of this level of amputation should generally restore a patient to his or her prior level of functioning.

Patient Evaluation

The clinic team should thoroughly analyze available patient information before considering specific socket designs, suspension systems, components, and the indications and contraindications for each. The prosthetic prescription should represent a consensus between the health care team and the patient. Several factors influence the prescription, as described below.

Activity Level

Although age partially correlates with activity level, age alone is not useful in determining the prescription. Active patients need a durable prosthesis that will function for many tasks, whereas less active patients generally require a lightweight prosthesis with a protective socket interface. A very athletic patient often requires not only a strong, durable prosthesis but also specialized components.

Geographic Location

The patient's geographic location may influence component selection. In an extremely hot, humid climate where perspiration is a concern, leather materials or rubber suspension sleeves may be contraindicated. If the patient will have difficulty returning for follow-up, components that require frequent maintenance are not practical.

Time Since Amputation

Time since amputation provides clues about the weight-bearing capability of the residual limb and the presence of postoperative edema. If the amputation is long-standing and the patient is an experienced user, the performance of the previous prosthesis should be discussed in detail as the new prescription is developed. Often, awareness of present problems or concerns can help avoid difficulties with the new prosthesis.

Medical Condition

Certain pathologies may influence the choice of components. For example, limited sensation in the residual limb could indicate the need for a protective interface such as a gel liner or thicker sock ply. Components that are simple to don and doff are indicated when upper limbs are also involved. The clinic team, in consultation with the patient and family, may decide against prosthetic fitting in certain cases. The energy requirements necessary for functional ambulation may prove too great a risk for those with severe cardiac conditions, for example.[1] In this context, a prosthesis intended strictly for safe transfers should suffice.

Employment

Although prostheses help patients return to normal activities, employers may need to make some accommodations in job tasks for physical restrictions associated with the amputation.[2,3] Standing time should be limited when feasible, and periodic rest may be necessary, particularly in the months immediately after amputation. Environmental barriers and unstable standing surfaces should be minimized.[4] Because prostheses need periodic maintenance, the patient may require time off from work while the component is being worked on, since most amputees cannot afford to have multiple well-fitting prostheses. Careful maintenance of the prosthesis will minimize the need for repairs and future time lost from work.

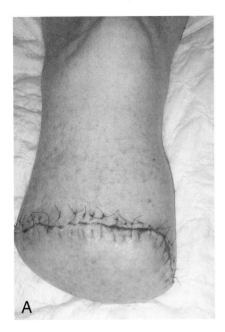 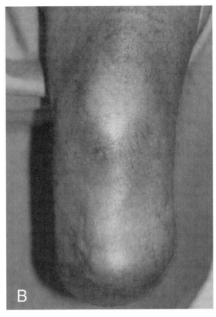

Figure 1 A, The bulbous distal end of this residual limb is typical in the early postoperative period. **B,** A muscle-balanced, cylindrical residual limb allows a greater distribution of weight-bearing forces.

Sports

Although some prostheses suitable for ambulation can also be used for some recreational sports, increasingly patients request a prosthesis specifically designed for sports. Specialized transtibial prosthetic components and techniques are available to facilitate swimming, skiing, jogging, and most other sports.[5] Exercise is key to good health, most especially for those with disabilities.[6] Walking to increase endurance can prevent further weakening for individuals with transtibial amputations, particularly in the geriatric population.[7] Dynamic-response feet and vertical shock pylons may help patients return to a more active lifestyle.

The goal of many rehabilitation programs is to help the patient become physically active and restore function to at least the level of activity before the amputation. This goal is especially important for the traumatic amputee.

Patient Goals

The prosthesis design should be tailored to meet the patient's personal goals. It is important for the prosthetist to help the patient establish realistic and attainable goals, given the patient's motivation and overall physical condition. Age should not be a factor because the elderly appear to have no greater difficulty in adjusting psychologically to physical activity with a prosthesis than adults as a whole. Transtibial amputees may be told that returning to their preamputation ambulatory level is a very reasonable goal, regardless of age.[8]

Shape of the Residual Limb

The shape of the residual limb may be an indicator of potential fitting problems. A bulbous residual limb, which is often present shortly after amputation, has a larger circumference distally than proximally. If this difference is large enough, the patient will find it difficult to don or doff the prosthetic socket (Figure 1, *A*). A conical residual limb is typical of an individual who is a long-term user and will generally not present a fitting problem, although the characteristic atrophied limb musculature may limit soft-tissue weight bearing. A cylindrical residual limb (Figure 1, *B*) is the ideal shape because pressure and stabilizing forces can be applied more evenly over the surface area.[9]

Soft Tissue

If soft-tissue coverage is limited distally, the depth of the socket and the fit of the distal pad are critical. If there is significant soft-tissue coverage distally, as is common with the long posterior flap amputation technique, it will likely reduce as the limb atrophies from normal prosthetic use. This is especially true with the preference of many surgeons to discontinue the traditional beveling of the gastrocnemius and soleus muscle bellies.[9] In this case, the limb may lose contact with the distal pad. If this occurs, distal contact must be restored to reduce limb edema in this area.

Skin Problems

Even areas of the residual limb that must bear weight in the prosthesis are unaccustomed to such large mechanical forces and need time to adapt to these new pressures. Persistent reddening is a warning sign that bruises, blisters, or excoriations may eventually develop. Without pressure relief, areas of excessive loading can develop into pressure ulcers that extend deep into the subcutaneous tissues. Many factors increase the risk of skin breakdown, including reduced elasticity of aged skin; moisture that tends to increase friction; heat, which will hasten blister formation; and skin that is directly over bone.

Skin problems result from an ill-fitting prosthesis and, therefore, can be resolved by socket or alignment modifications or by a new fitting. Allergic reactions can be remedied by switching to an alternate material. Skin tolerance for sustained pressure has been shown to increase over time in patients with spinal cord injury.[10] It is believed that gradually increasing the use of a new prosthesis will ease skin adaptations to pressure.

Condition of the Knee Joint

Ligamentous laxity in the coronal (frontal) or sagittal plane may necessitate modifications in prosthetic design to stabilize the joint and prevent further damage. A thorough physical examination, including the anterior drawer test and a knee varus/valgus stress test, is essential to determine the degree of clinical laxity. It is often possible to control mild laxity through prosthetic alignment. Increased laxity indicates the need to cross the knee joint to obtain adequate stability. This may be achieved by extending socket trimlines with a supracondylar design, a supracondylar-suprapatellar design for moderate instability, or steel joints and a thigh corset for severe knee laxity (Figure 2).

Range of Motion

Ideally, the patient should be able to achieve full knee extension and flexion. Normal knee range is approximately 145° of flexion. Although a patient with limited knee range can be fitted with a prosthesis, functional limitations should be anticipated. Normal gait requires a functional range of 0° to 70°, with the highest degree of flexion occurring during initial swing.[11,12] Although 70° is adequate for normal gait, Laubenthal and associates[13] observed that 83° of flexion was needed for stair climbing, 93° for sitting, and 106° for shoe tying. A knee flexion contracture can be accommodated in the prosthetic alignment, but a contracture greater than 25° may make prosthetic fitting difficult. The shorter the residual limb, the higher the degree of flexion contracture that can be accommodated.[14] Preventing joint contractures is advised because they are often difficult to treat once they have developed.

Condition of the Thigh Musculature

The transtibial amputee cannot achieve a smooth, controlled gait if the quadriceps muscles are weak. Knee extensor weakness can result in abrupt knee flexion, absent knee flexion, and an uneven step length. Physical therapy is an integral part of prosthetic management and may be required for strengthening.

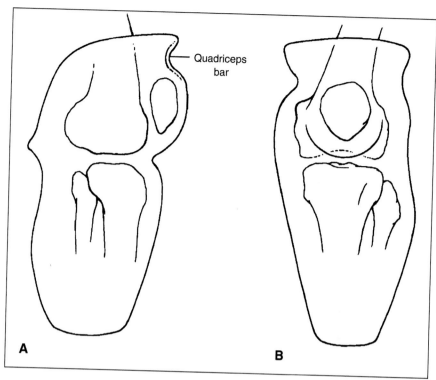

Figure 2 The PTB supracondylar-suprapatellar socket aids in sagittal and coronal knee stability. **A,** Medial view. **B,** Anterior view.

Staging of Care

Once the wound has healed adequately, rehabilitation focuses on shaping the residual limb for prosthetic fitting and increasing weight-bearing capacity. These goals are accomplished with the help of elastic bandages or prosthetic shrinkers, rigid dressings, postoperative prostheses, and preparatory prostheses. Coupled with gait training, physical therapy, and close supervision by the clinic team, these treatments prepare the limb for definitive prosthetic fitting. Elastic bandages are usually applied as the postoperative dressings are removed. These compression treatments help reduce limb edema, thereby promoting healing and decreasing pain. For patients with wound complications, delayed healing, or other circumstances that delay prosthetic fitting, an elastic bandage may be the most practical and economical form of residual limb conditioning. Residual limb shrinkers may be used in place of elastic bandages. They are provided by the prosthetist and fitted specifically to the patient's limb size. Easier to apply for both the patient and caregivers, these devices consist of a series of elastic bands sewn together to form a cylinder. The prosthetic shrinker is replaced with a smaller sized shrinker as the residual limb decreases in volume. Disadvantages of elastic bandages and shrinkers are that they do not protect the limb, must be reapplied several times each day, and do nothing to prevent knee flexion contractures. For the recent amputee, shrinkers or elastic bandages should be worn whenever the patient is not wearing the prosthesis, a rigid dressing, or some other compressive device (Figure 3).

Midthigh-length rigid dressings applied immediately after surgery control edema and reduce pain.[15] The removable rigid dressing was designed to allow frequent wound inspection and provide progressive limb shrinkage by the addition of socks (Figure 4). The removable rigid dressing may be particularly effective for patients with diabetes mellitus or delayed wound healing.[16]

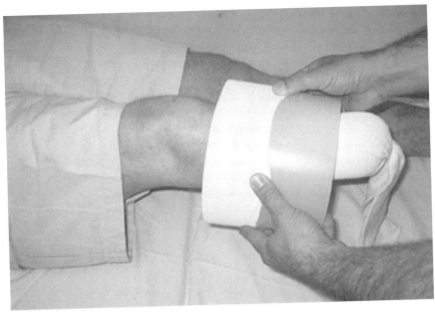

Figure 3 The residual limb shrinker can be applied using a donning ring to ease the discomfort of application.

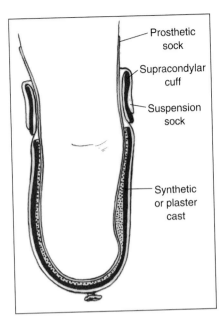

Figure 4 The removable rigid dressing is easily applied, protects the residual limb, and can be removed for suture line inspection.

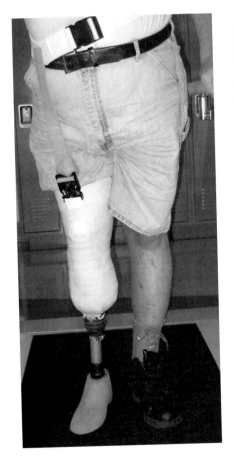

Figure 5 The immediate postoperative prosthesis allows early, supervised, touchdown weight bearing and ambulation.

Postoperative prostheses were introduced by Marian A. Weiss, PhD, of Poland and further refined in the United States by Ernest Burgess, MD, in the 1960s.[17] Immediate postoperative prostheses are applied immediately after amputation; "early" prostheses are applied within a few days after amputation. They offer all the benefits of rigid dressings and permit limited weight bearing and supervised early ambulation. The postoperative prosthesis is essentially a rigid dressing that extends to midthigh and is suspended by a waist belt to which a prosthetic pylon and foot are attached (Figure 5).

Given the possible complications of this treatment, success depends primarily on the skills of the clinic team. As the cast loosens, it must be removed and a new one applied after 7 to 10 days. Two or three cast changes may be needed until the patient is ready for a preparatory prosthesis.

Prefabricated postoperative devices are now available and are appropriate in many instances (Figure 6). They are adjustable and eliminate the need for recasting as limb volume decreases.[18]

A preparatory or intermediate prosthesis fitting can begin when the patient's residual limb has atrophied sufficiently to allow donning and doffing of a prosthetic socket (ie, when the circumference of the proximal limb at the tibial tubercle is larger than the distal limb circumference). Depending on the pace of residual limb atrophy, the preparatory prosthesis may be worn for a few months or as long as a year before the socket is replaced or definitive fitting is recommended. A preparatory prosthesis is generally constructed on an endoskeletal pylon, permitting alignment changes at any time. This is a considerable advantage because the needs of the patient can be constantly reassessed and accommodated as the ability to use the prosthesis improves.

Once fitted with a preparatory prosthesis, the patient should progress in physical therapy to full weight bearing. In addition to receiving gait training, the patient should be instructed in the use of prosthetic socks, the application of shrinkers or elastic wraps, residual limb hygiene, and how to inspect the limb for any sign of excessive pressure. The patient should also be educated about falls and how to reduce the risk of falling.[19] Alignment and socket fit are adjusted by the prosthetist as needed. It is not unusual for the patient to progress through several sockets within the first year following amputation.

A patient's readiness for a definitive prosthesis varies, depending on activity level, weight-bearing tolerance, and limb shrinkage. Atrophic changes may stabilize after 4 months in some cases but more typically continue for 12 months or more. The decision to proceed with definitive fitting is largely subjective and is based on the overall perception that the patient has reached a plateau in activity level, prosthetic wearing time, and residual limb volume. For example, young, active amputees who have worn a preparatory prosthesis are ready for definitive fitting when they can tolerate full weight bearing, wear the prosthesis all day, and have not had to add prosthetic socks to accommodate limb shrinkage for some weeks. In contrast, elderly patients with other health problems may use a walker and wear the prosthesis only 4 to 5 hours daily but may nevertheless be ready for definitive fitting because their activity level and residual limb volume changes have been stabilized.

The design and components of the definitive prosthesis are based on the goals of the patient. The definitive prosthesis may closely resemble the preparatory prosthesis that preceded it, or it may differ dramatically, depending on the goals established during rehabilitation.

A wide variety of prosthetic components, materials, and techniques is available, and every option has advantages and disadvantages that must be considered to provide the optimum combination for each patient's unique needs.

Socket Design
Patellar Tendon–Bearing Socket

To create a patellar tendon–bearing (PTB) socket, an impression is taken

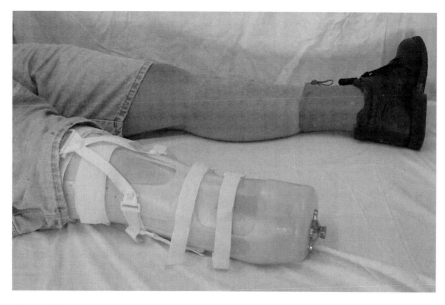

Figure 6 This prefabricated postoperative socket is removable for wound inspection and adjustable for volume fluctuations. A pylon and foot can be added.

of the patient's residual limb and then modified to achieve an intimate, total-contact fit over the entire surface of the residual limb. There is an inward contour or "bar" that uses the patellar ligament as a partial weight-bearing surface. The term "patellar tendon–bearing" can be misleading, however, because the patellar ligament is not the major weight-bearing surface used by this type of socket. The medial and lateral socket walls extend proximally to about the level of the adductor tubercle of the femur. Together, they control rotation, contain soft tissue, and may provide some mediolateral knee stability. The medial wall is modified with a slight undercut in the area of the pes anserinus on the medial flare of the tibia, providing significant weight bearing on this major, pressure-tolerant surface. The lateral wall provides a relief for the fibular head, supports the fibular shaft, and acts as a counterpressure to the medial wall. The posterior wall is usually designed to apply an anteriorly directed force to keep the patellar ligament on the bar. The posterior wall is flared proximally to allow comfortable knee flexion for sitting and to prevent excessive pressure on the hamstring tendons. The distal portion of the PTB socket may incor-

porate a soft, protective pad. The PTB total-contact socket is suitable for many transtibial amputations, except in some postoperative prostheses or when pathologic conditions require an alternative socket.

The total-contact techniques that were introduced with the development of the PTB socket were a radical change from the previous open-end socket designs. Total contact means that all areas of the limb are to have some contact, but weight bearing is limited to pressure-tolerant anatomy. Although the entire limb surface should have contact to prevent edema, not all surfaces carry weight or equal loads.[20]

Total Surface–Bearing Socket

Total surface–bearing (TSB) theory proposes that pressure can be distributed more equally across the entire surface of the transtibial residual limb than with a PTB socket. In principle, even the pressure-sensitive areas can carry some portion of the load. Increasing the pressure on the tissues around these areas can relieve bony ridges.[21,22] TSB advocates often suggest use of a special liner material to help disperse the forces applied to the residual limb.

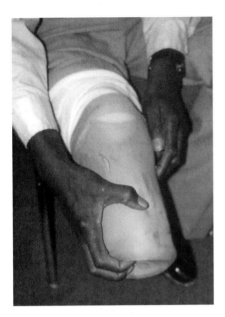

Figure 7 Polyethylene foam liners help protect the skin and provide shock absorption during ambulation.

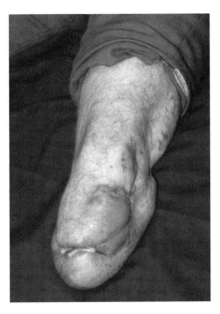

Figure 8 Residual limbs with skin that is susceptible to breakdown can be protected more effectively with a gel interface.

Hydrostatic Socket

In theory, a hydrostatic socket transmits pressure equally to every point within a socket to minimize localized weight-bearing areas.[23] The hydrostatic socket includes a gel liner to help reduce peak pressures. There is little statistical evidence to support any specific socket design theory, but there has been a clear evolution in thinking in recent decades to minimize local forces as much as possible.

Socket Variants

Hard Socket

The hard socket is made from rigid material and has specific advantages and disadvantages. This variant is indicated primarily for maximum durability when the residual limb has good soft-tissue coverage and no sharp bony prominences. It is not commonly used for residual limbs with thin skin coverage, scarring, skin grafts, or a predisposition to breakdown. The advantages of hard sockets include that they are perspiration resistant, less bulky than sockets with a soft insert, easy to keep clean, and durable. In addition, reliefs or modifications can be located with precision with these sockets. The disadvantages

of these sockets are that they require extra skill in casting and modification, are difficult to fit over sharp bony contours or sensitive residual limbs, and they are not as easily modified as a socket with a soft insert.

Soft Inserts

Soft inserts are fabricated over the modified cast to fit inside the socket. They act as an interface between the limb and socket to add comfort and protection by moderating impact and shear. They are often fabricated from a 5-mm polyethylene foam material (Figure 7). Soft inserts are recommended for patients with peripheral vascular disease; with thin, sensitive, or scarred skin and sharp bony prominences; or with peripheral neuropathy. Bilateral transtibial amputees may prefer inserts to protect the distal portion of the tibia when they rise from a chair or climb stairs and inclines. The added protection of a soft insert may also benefit the highly active patient. Liner materials are chosen based on their elastic properties and frictional characteristics with the skin.[24] A balance must be sought between the material's ability to reduce stress over bony prominences and

regulate shear stress on the skin. The advantages of soft sockets are that they provide a soft, protective socket interface, have "rebound" in the insert that may improve circulation by providing a "pumping action" and intermittent pressure over bony prominences, and are easily modified to adjust for atrophy in the residual limb. The disadvantages of these sockets are that the materials deteriorate over time, they are not as sanitary as hard sockets because the inserts tend to absorb fluids over time, they increase bulk around the residual limb, they may compress over time resulting in loss of fit, and they increase the overall weight of the prosthesis.

Gel Liners

Elastomeric liners, made of silicone or similar materials, are often recommended for patients whose skin is compromised by grafted areas or adherent scar tissue (Figure 8). Additional factors that limit the weight-bearing capability of the residual limb, such as short length or a conical shape, may also be indications for cushioning liner materials. These liners are usually worn directly against the skin and move with it, thus reducing friction and shear.[25,26] Several hygiene problems are associated with the elastomeric liners, specifically itching, perspiration, eruption, and odor.[27] These problems can be reduced by meticulous daily cleansing of the skin and liner, but elastomeric liners should be not considered if a patient is unwilling to maintain hygiene.

Distal Pads

To improve overall comfort and to help control edema, the distal portion of PTB sockets generally incorporates a soft pad made of silicone or polyethylene foam. These pads ensure total contact distally, provide increased comfort, protect the distal portion of the residual limb when it settles into the socket as a result of volume loss, and facilitate future modifications of the distal end of the socket. However, they also add fabrication time, increase overall weight of the prosthesis, and are considered less hygienic because they absorb fluids.

Flexible Inner Sockets With Rigid External Frames

Many patients prefer a flexible inner socket that is inserted into a rigid frame. The inner socket is fabricated from polyethylene or a similar material, and the frame is made from laminated plastic or a rigid thermoplastic material. The frame supports the socket over the primary weight-bearing areas, whereas the more pressure-sensitive areas, such as bony prominences and soft tissues not requiring rigid support, are enclosed only in the flexible socket. This technique often results in a more comfortable socket and can be used in endoskeletal or exoskeletal prostheses. These sockets decrease overall weight of the prosthesis, are considered more comfortable, improve heat dissipation, and can be replaced to accommodate anatomic changes. They are, however, difficult and time-consuming to fabricate and may lack the cosmesis of a hard socket.

Biomechanics of Prosthetic Feet

To ensure efficient ambulation, the prosthetic foot should mimic the functions of the human foot throughout the gait cycle to the degree that this is feasible. The function required of the prosthesis during each phase of the gait cycle is described below.

Initial Contact

During initial contact, the primary function of the foot is shock absorption. The prosthetic foot must absorb the impact of the heel contacting the ground and minimize the forces that are transferred to the residual limb. In the case of the transtibial amputee, too much shock absorption may fail to generate the normal knee flexion moment and result in an unnatural, straight-knee gait.

Loading Response

During the loading response phase, the foot must provide control of plantar flexion. Because the ground-reaction force vector is posterior to the ankle joint, a plantar flexion moment occurs during loading response. In the human foot and ankle, this moment is controlled by the ankle dorsiflexors. These muscles contract eccentrically and allow smooth, controlled plantar flexion of the foot to the floor. As the foot progresses to the floor, the tibia begins to advance forward, and limb progression is continued. Proper control of plantar flexion allows the tibia to advance at the proper velocity. Prosthetic plantar flexion can be affected by the stiffness of the heel portion of the foot component. Generally, the stiffer the prosthetic heel, the larger the plantar flexion moment that is generated.

Midstance

At midstance, the prosthesis must provide controlled advancement of the tibia. The momentum of the swing limb and forward fall of the body's weight create a dorsiflexion torque that takes the tibia from an 8° plantar flexed position to a 5° dorsiflexed position throughout the stance phase. Both the heel and forefoot remain in contact with the floor the entire time. The foot and ankle provide an ankle rocker that allows forward progression of the leg. The gastrocnemius and soleus muscles are active in controlling the speed of this progression and in maintaining stability.[11] The prosthetic foot simulates this muscle pattern by providing stance phase stability through a rigid, semi-rigid, or flexible keel within the foot.

Terminal Stance

During terminal stance, the foot must provide controlled heel rise and progression onto the forefoot. In this phase, the foot and ankle are essentially locked into position to provide heel rise as tibial advancement continues. The forefoot now becomes the rocker over which the tibia advances.

As the tibia continues to advance, body weight is transferred entirely onto the forefoot and the metatarsophalangeal (MTP) joints. The prosthetic foot must also support the terminal stance phase and should simulate MTP dorsiflexion.

Preswing

During preswing, the foot must provide support for transfer of body weight to the opposite side. After both limbs are supported, the weight of the body is taken off of the preswing leg and transferred to the opposite side. The prosthetic foot should provide enough support to help maintain balance and encourage smooth transfer of weight to the sound side. Ankle-foot function and prosthetic alignment during this phase will affect the degree of impact the contralateral foot experiences.[28,29] This may be particularly important for patients with compromised vascular and neurologic systems, putting the surviving foot at risk.

Rapid knee flexion at this point effectively shortens the leg and prepares it to have adequate clearance during swing phase. The toe-break area of the human foot is at the MTP joints. This allows the foot to roll over at the metatarsal heads instead of the tips of the toes. The prosthetic foot will also have a toe break to provide the same smooth rollover motion, or the design of the foot will allow forefoot flexibility to accomplish the same goal. This forefoot flexibility may also help reduce loading on the sound limb by minimizing the elevation of the center of gravity.[30]

Foot Selection

A thorough understanding of prosthetic foot biomechanics is essential because foot selection alone has a profound impact on the ultimate success or failure of a prosthesis. Five variables must be considered when selecting a prosthetic foot: alignment and length of the toe lever arm, width of the keel, flexibility of the keel, durometer of the heel cushion, and fit

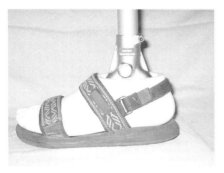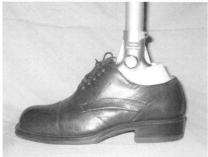

Figure 9 An adjustable-heel foot accommodates variations in the heel height of different shoes. This eliminates the need to change feet on the prosthesis.

of the prosthetic foot within the shoe.

The spatial relationship between the foot and socket is referred to as alignment and influences both the function and comfort of the prosthesis. Optimum foot position is determined during the fitting process with linear movements in the sagittal and coronal planes, inversion/eversion, dorsiflexion/plantar flexion, and foot rotation.

The manufacturer determines keel width. A wider keel provides greater mediolateral stability during stance phase by widening the base of support within the shoe. For example, external-keel feet and some flexible-keel feet have wider keels than do other feet. The difference, however, is rarely significant enough to be the sole rationale for prescription but may be significant in cases where coronal plane stability is a concern.

A flexible keel offers a smoother gait with a less pronounced transition at the toe break than does a rigid keel. To increase resistance of the forefoot during late stance phase, the flexible-keel/dynamic-response foot can be moved anteriorly or slightly plantar flexed during dynamic alignment of the prosthesis. Stiffer keels may offer greater stability during stance.

The heel cushion absorbs shock and helps initiate knee flexion during the loading response. Increasing heel stiffness increases the knee-flexion moment at loading response and decreases shock absorption. Conversely, decreasing heel stiffness results in a smaller knee-flexion moment and increased shock absorption during the loading response. Optimizing heel-cushion density requires balancing shock absorption against the moments acting to flex the knee. As in similar prosthetic decisions, the choice must be based on the patient's needs.

Heavier patients are more likely to require a firm heel cushion to provide a sufficient knee flexion moment during the loading response. Lighter patients will generally require medium- or soft-density heel cushions to avoid creating an excessive knee-flexion moment. Very active patients may prefer a firm heel cushion because more rapid cadences increase net loading on the foot. Elderly patients or household ambulators often require soft heel cushions to limit knee-flexion moment and maximize shock absorption.

The prosthetic foot is designed to function under the stress of ambulation. It compresses, rebounds, flexes, and extends as it operates throughout the gait cycle. With the exception of postoperative feet and those designed for barefoot ambulation, prosthetic feet are designed to fit inside a shoe. It should not be surprising, then, that the function of a prosthetic foot can be enhanced or decreased by the shoe it is fitted with. At times, it may be necessary to modify the foot or the shoe to ensure optimum function.

Heel height is the single most important factor in shoe fit related to foot function. It should match the built-in heel rise of the foot. This will ensure that socket alignment in the sagittal plane is not altered and that the keel of the foot maintains the correct position with respect to the floor. Once a prosthesis has been aligned and fabricated, the patient should not significantly increase the height of his or her shoe heel unless an appropriate wedge is added inside the shoe. Recently available ankle-foot assemblies that can be adjusted for different heel heights should be considered if frequent changes in heel height are anticipated (Figure 9).

The material and contours of the shoe heel can make a significant difference in the way the prosthetic wearer ambulates. For example, a soft crepe heel enhances the shock absorption qualities of a foot. In comparison, a hard leather or rubber heel will tend to increase knee-flexion moment during the loading response. If such heels present a problem, it is appropriate to round or bevel the posterior corner of the heel, thereby decreasing the knee moment at heel strike. Women's high heels may compromise stance phase stability and are not recommended for weak, debilitated patients.

Forcing a solid-ankle foot into a tight-fitting shoe diminishes the ability of the foot to compress and bend during ambulation. It is always better to fit the shoe slightly loose on the foot so that maximum flexibility is maintained.

Although function of the prosthetic foot is of primary concern to the prosthetist, the importance of appearance cannot be overlooked. The design of a particular foot may enhance or diminish its cosmetic appeal.

Socket and Alignment Biomechanics

Successful fitting of a transtibial prosthesis requires a thorough understanding of the biomechanical variables involved and the ability to achieve an appropriate compromise

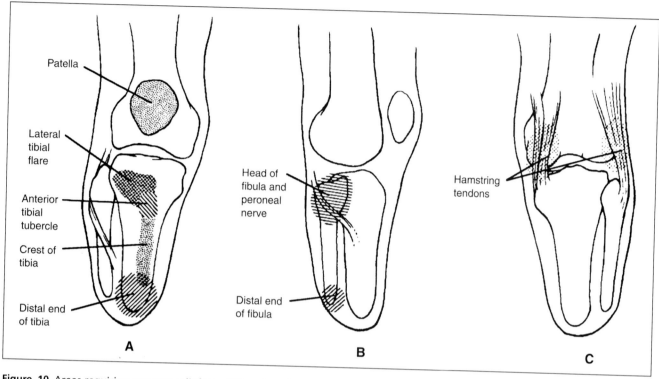

Figure 10 Areas requiring pressure relief in a PTB socket. **A**, Anterior view. **B**, Lateral view. **C**, Posterior view.

between these variables to meet the unique needs of each patient. Biomechanical factors can be divided into two broad categories—socket fit and alignment/foot function.

Socket Fit

The prosthetic socket is the primary connection between the residual limb and the prosthesis. It must bear the force of body weight and cushion the forces applied to the residual limb through contact with the socket. These forces are continually changing during dynamic use of the prosthesis. Successful distribution of these forces requires careful attention to detail during patient evaluation, casting, and socket modification.

Displacement and Pressure Tolerance of Residual Limb Tissues (Total Contact)

In theory, ensuring that every square centimeter of the residual limb is in contact with the socket and is sharing an equal portion of the load would maximally reduce the pressure between the residual limb and the socket. In actual practice, this is com-

plicated by differences in tissue displacement and tissue pressure tolerances. For example, some bony portions of the residual limb, such as the distal tibia or the fibular head, cannot be compressed as much as soft-tissue areas.

Most fitting problems can be resolved through appropriate socket design. To apply greater forces to pressure-tolerant areas and less to pressure-sensitive areas, tissues are selectively loaded over weight-bearing surfaces and relieved over sensitive areas. Areas within the socket that require relief may include the tibial crest, tibial tubercle, lateral tibial flare, distal tibia/fibular head, peroneal nerve, hamstring tendons, and the patella (Figure 10). Pressure-tolerant areas may include the patellar ligament, medial tibial flare, medial tibial shaft, lateral fibular shaft, and the anterior and posterior compartments (Figure 11).

Modification for Dynamic Forces

In normal human locomotion, ground-reaction forces produce mo-

ments at the joints of the lower limb. Forces are similar during ambulation with a prosthesis, but they are applied through the prosthetic socket to the residual limb. Forces on the residual limb, specifically anteroposterior and mediolateral forces, must be managed to achieve socket comfort and prevent skin breakdown. The greatest anteroposterior forces are generated from heel strike to foot flat while a powerful knee-flexion moment exists. Knee stability is maintained by contraction of the quadriceps. The resulting forces between the socket and residual limb are concentrated on the antero-distal portion of the tibia and postero-proximal soft tissue (Figure 12). The socket, therefore, must distribute pressure evenly in the popliteal area and relieve pressure anterodistally, as well as provide anterior, medial, and lateral counterpressures to prevent excessive pressure over the distal end of the tibia.

The greatest mediolateral forces occur during single-limb support on the prosthetic side. With normal foot inset, forces are generally increased over the proximomedial and distolat-

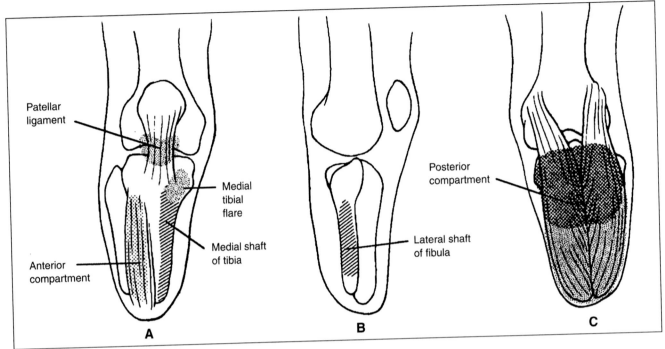

Figure 11 Pressure-tolerant areas in a PTB socket. **A,** Anterior view. **B,** Lateral view. **C,** Posterior view.

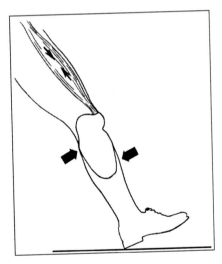

Figure 12 Areas of concentrated pressure during ambulation.

eral aspects of the residual limb. Although these forces can be reduced if the prosthetic foot is moved laterally, in most cases the prosthetic socket must accommodate these forces. Proximomedial forces are not a significant problem because they are focused on the pressure-tolerant medial femoral condyle and medial tibial flare. But distolateral forces can create excessive pressure on the transected end of the fibula. Socket modifica-

tions to prevent this problem include relief for the distolateral aspect of the fibula, lateral stabilizing pressure along the shaft of the fibula, and lateral stabilizing pressure over the anterior compartment (pretibial muscle group).

Torque and shear may also present prosthetic problems within the socket. If torque is excessive, the tendency of the socket to rotate in relation to the residual limb may cause discomfort, skin breakdown, or gait deviations.

A certain amount of shear is unavoidable because some motion between the socket and the underlying tissues will always occur. Shear occurs in all three planes whenever the socket moves in a direction opposite to residual limb motion. For example, if the suspension is too loose, the prosthesis tends to drop away from the limb during swing phase, only to be driven back to its correct position during loading response. This motion creates shear stress between the residual limb and the socket. These shear stresses can cause cell separation within the epidermal layer, leading to blisters and, if the epidermis is thin,

open wounds.[31] Patients with sensitive skin, such as burn patients or those with diabetes mellitus, may be especially susceptible.

A soft socket insert or a nylon sheath worn directly over the skin can reduce these forces. Rotation units or "torque absorbers" are another option to mitigate shear. These components are commonly used in transtibial prostheses if the patient wears the prosthesis during activities such as golfing that generate significant torque or if the patient has fragile skin.

Alignment/Foot Function

Correct dynamic alignment is determined by the prosthetist as the patient ambulates on an adjustable alignment unit. This unit allows anteroposterior foot positioning, anteroposterior tilting of the socket, mediolateral foot positioning, mediolateral tilting of the socket, height adjustment, and rotation of the prosthetic foot.

Proper anteroposterior positioning of the prosthetic foot will distribute weight evenly between the heel and toe portion. This will result in a smooth, energy-efficient gait, including controlled knee flexion after heel strike, smooth rollover without recurvatum, and heel-off before initial heel contact on the contralateral foot.

Proper anteroposterior socket tilt will load those areas that are pressure tolerant. Proper flexion not only improves the weight-bearing characteristics of the socket but also creates a smooth gait; places the quadriceps muscles "on stretch," giving them a mechanical advantage for controlling the prosthesis; and limits recurvatum forces during late stance.

Proper mediolateral foot positioning loads proximomedial and distolateral aspects of the residual limb. It helps create a normal genu varum moment at midstance and provides optimum loading of the medial tibial flare during stance phase. Optimum foot inset is related to the length and condition of the residual limb. A short residual limb may not tolerate as much because of the reduction in bony lever arm.

Foot inset loads the medial tibial flare appropriately, gives the gait a narrow base, and decreases energy expenditure but increases torque on the residual limb because of the normal genu varum moment created at midstance. It also gives the prosthesis a better cosmetic appearance. A wide gait increases energy expenditure but decreases torque on the residual limb because the genu varum moment is limited or eliminated.

The most convenient way to determine the correct height of the prosthesis is through clinical comparison of the iliac crests or the posterior superior iliac spines. This approach may not be appropriate if the patient exhibits pelvic obliquity, congenital limb-length discrepancy, or unilateral femoral shortening. Such cases must be considered individually, and often the best indicator of correct length is through gait analysis and patient feedback. Proper height will result in a smooth and symmetric gait without excessive leaning to either side.

Proper foot rotation is important both cosmetically and functionally.

Prosthetic toe-out refers to the angle between the line of net forward progression and the medial border of the prosthetic foot. A transtibial prosthesis is initially aligned so that the medial border of the foot is parallel to the line of progression. This results in a slight external rotation of the prosthetic foot, thereby approximating the 5° to 7° of normal anatomic toe-out. This position may need to be altered, however, during static and dynamic alignment so that foot position during ambulation visually matches that of the sound limb.

Foot rotation can also affect prosthetic function. The keel of the foot is a lever arm. During the stance phase the tendency of the body to fall over the foot is resisted by the counterforce of this anterior lever arm. Rotation of the foot, therefore, directly affects the length of the lever arm created and the direction of the force. The net effect of externally rotating the foot may be to increase stability by widening the base of support. Excessive foot rotation has been shown to adversely affect stance and swing time as well as step length.[32] Although slight external rotation of the foot may be beneficial, there is a cosmetic tradeoff if the toe-out attitude of the prosthesis does not match that of the contralateral limb.

Case Studies
Case Study 1

A 63-year-old woman 5 ft 6 in tall and weighing 145 lb underwent a transtibial amputation secondary to complications of diabetes mellitus 6 weeks earlier and at the time of presentation was wearing a prosthetic shrinker. Her preprosthetic physical therapy included training in transfers, use of a walker, maintenance of range of motion, and muscle strengthening. The distal limb circumference was 2 cm smaller than the proximal limb circumference. The suture line was well healed, and the woman was ready for prosthetic fitting. Range of motion in the lower limb and muscle strength in her hand were within normal limits. She had good upper limb strength

and no other complicating health problems. Before the amputation, the woman worked part time in the local library. Her goals were to ambulate unassisted and without limitation. She lived with her husband and one young grandchild and had a relatively sedentary lifestyle.

Prescription Recommendation

The woman received an initial transtibial prosthesis with a PTB socket design to load the weight-tolerant tissues and unload the weight-intolerant areas. It is a total-contact prosthesis to improve proprioception, with a custom silicone distal-end pad to encourage venous return and prevent distal edema. The soft silicone end pad will also accommodate some distal migration of the residual limb without undue end pressure. The socket is made of acrylic resin for reduced weight and increased strength and to facilitate socket adjustments. A neoprene suspension sleeve provides simple, effective suspension. A flexible keel foot will absorb some of the impact of walking and make rollover easier. The endoskeletal components are lightweight and adjustable for postfabrication alignment changes that will inevitably be necessary as the woman's gait improves. She received gel sheaths to wear directly against the skin to reduce shear on the residual limb and decrease the chances of skin breakdown. She was also given one-, three-, and five-ply prosthetic socks to accommodate volume fluctuations in the residual limb.

Case Study 2

A 26-year-old man 5 ft 10 in tall and weighing 160 lb was wearing an intermediate prosthesis 9 months after undergoing a midlength transtibial amputation of the right leg as a result of a crush injury incurred on a construction job site. The residual limb had a well-padded distal end because the gastrocnemius and soleus muscles were preserved in the long posterior flap. The surgical scar was not adherent, and the limb had a cylindrical shape. His right knee was stable in all planes of motion, 5/5 in strength, and within normal limits for range. His general health was excellent.

The man was in vocational counseling with the desire to return to work full time as a backhoe operator in a landscaping business. He had progressed to full-time ambulatory use of his preparatory prosthesis and was preparing to return to work. He also wanted to return to high-impact athletic activity and to train for running events. His PTB prosthesis no longer fit comfortably because of limb atrophy.

Prescription Recommendation

A TSB socket to distribute pressure evenly on the residual limb was recommended. The cylindrical shape of the residual limb is optimum for accommodating socket pressures. An elastomeric liner will absorb the shock and shear of high-impact activity and reduce shear stress on the residual limb skin. Suction suspension with an expulsion valve and gel sleeve will eliminate pistoning of the prosthesis on the residual limb and further decrease shear stress. A vertical shock- and torque-absorbing pylon will displace underloading conditions and absorb shock during high-demand activity, as well as allow transverse rotation of the socket when the foot is on the ground. A dynamic-response foot will offer energy return during high-demand activity. An endoskeletal structure will remain alignable and modular to allow changes in components or alignment as the amputee's activity level progresses.

Summary

Given the many prosthetic choices available to transtibial amputees, a thorough, objective evaluation and detailed discussions about the patient's functional level are vital. Some of the factors affecting component selection include time since the amputation; skin condition; medical conditions affecting sight, balance, and strength; and home environment, including the social support structure.

Proper socket and alignment biomechanics enable patients to function to their fullest potential. A knowledgeable rehabilitation team can help patients return to most or all of their preamputation activities. In the absence of other physical limitations, the prognosis for the transtibial amputee is good.

References

1. Moore WS, Malone JM: *Lower Extremity Amputation.* Philadelphia, PA, WB Saunders, 1989, pp 250-260.

2. Bruins M, Geertzen JH, Groothoff JW, Schoppen T: Vocational reintegration after a lower limb amputation: A qualitative study. *Prosthet Orthot Int* 2003; 27:4-10.

3. Schoppen T, Boonstra A, Groothoff JW, van Sonderen E, Goeken LN, Eisma WH: Factors related to successful job reintegration of people with a lower limb amputation. *Arch Phys Med Rehabil* 2001;82:1425-1431.

4. Girdhar A, Mital A, Kephart A, Young A: Design guidelines for accommodating amputees in the workplace. *J Occup Rehabil* 2001;11:99-118.

5. Fergason JR, Boone DA: Custom design in lower limb prosthetics for athletic activity. *Phys Med Rehabil Clin N Am* 2000;11:681-699.

6. Singh MA: Exercise to prevent and treat functional disability. *Clin Geriatr Med* 2002;18:431-462.

7. Van Heuvelen MJ, Kempen GI, Brouwer WH, de Greef MH: Physical fitness related to disability in older persons. *Gerontology* 2000;46:333-341.

8. Pinzur MS, Gottschalk F, Smith DG, et al: Functional outcome of below-knee amputation in peripheral vascular insufficiency: A multicenter review. *Clin Orthop* 1993;286:247-249.

9. Smith DG, Fergason JR: Transtibial amputations. *Clin Orthop* 1999;361: 108-115.

10. Yarkony GM: Aging skin, pressure ulcerations, and spinal cord injury, in Whiteneck GG, Charlifue SW, Gerhart KA, et al (eds): *Aging With Spinal Cord Injury.* New York, NY, Demos, 1993, pp 39-52.

11. Perry J: *Gait Analysis: Normal and Pathological Function.* New York, NY, McGraw-Hill, 1992, pp 61-69.

12. Soderberg GL: *Kinesiology: Application to Pathological Motion.* Baltimore, MD, Williams & Wilkins, 1986, p 208.

13. Laubenthal KN, Smidt GL, Kettelkamp DB: A quantitative analysis of knee motion during activities of daily living. *Phys Ther* 1972;52:34-42.

14. McCollough NC III, Harris AR, Hampton FL: Below-knee amputation, in *Atlas of Limb Prosthetics: Surgical and Prosthetic Principles.* St. Louis, MO, CV Mosby, 1981, pp 341-368.

15. Edelstein J: Pre-prosthetic management of patients with lower or upper-limb amputation. *Phys Med Rehabil Clin N Am* 1991;2:285-297.

16. Wu Y, Keagy RD, Krick HJ, Stratigos JS, Betts HB: An innovative removable rigid dressing technique for below-the-knee amputation. *J Bone Joint Surg Am* 1979;61:724-729.

17. Traub J: Immediate postsurgical prostheses past, present, and future. *Orthop Prosthet Appl J* 1967;148-152.

18. Schon LC, Short KW, Soupiou O, Noll K, Rheinstein J: Benefits of early prosthetic management of transtibial amputees: A prospective clinical study of a prefabricated prosthesis. *Foot Ankle Int* 2002;23:509-514.

19. Miller WC, Deathe AB, Speechley M, Koval J: The prevalence and risk factors of falling and fear of falling among lower extremity amputees. *Arch Phys Med Rehabil* 2002;82: 1031-1037.

20. Fergason JF, Smith DG: Socket considerations for the patient with a transtibial amputation. *Clin Orthop* 1999; 361:80-83.

21. Staats TB, Lundt J: The UCLA total surface bearing suction below knee prosthesis. *Clin Prosthet Orthot* 1987; 11:118-130.

22. Pearson JR, Holmgren G, March L, Oberg K: Pressures in critical regions of the below knee patella tendon bearing prosthesis. *Bull Prosthet Res* 1973; 10:53-76.

23. Goh JC, Lee PV, Chong SY: Stump/socket pressure profiles of the pressure cast prosthetic socket. *Clin Biomech* 2003;18:237-238.

24. Sanders JE, Greve JM, Mitchell SB, Zachariah SG: Material properties of commonly-used interface materials and their static coefficients of friction

with skin and socks. *J Rehabil Res Dev* 1998;35:161-163.

25. Heim M, Wershavski M, Zwas ST, et al: Silicone suspension of external prostheses: A new era in artificial limb usage. *J Bone Joint Surg Br* 1997;79: 638-640.

26. Narita H, Yokogushi K, Shii S, Kakizawa M, Nosaka T: Suspension effect and dynamic evaluation of the total surface bearing transtibial prosthesis: A comparison with the patellar tendon bearing transtibial prosthesis. *Prosthet Orthot Int* 1997;21:175-178.

27. Hachisuka K, Nakamura T, Ohmine S, Shitama H, Shinkoda K: Hygiene problems of the residual limb and silicone liners in transtibial amputees wearing the total surface bearing socket. *Arch Phys Med Rehabil* 2001;82: 1286-1290.

28. Pinzur MS, Cox W, Kaiser J, Morris T, Patwardhan A, Vrbos L: The effect of prosthetic alignment on relative limb loading in persons with trans-tibial amputation: A preliminary report. *J Rehabil Res Dev* 1995;32:373-377.

29. Pitkin MR: Mechanical outcomes of a rolling-joint prosthetic foot and its performance in the dorsiflexion phase of transtibial amputee gait. *J Prosthet Orthot* 1995;7:114-123.

30. Powers CM, Torburn L, Perry J, Ayyappa E: Influence of prosthetic foot design on sound limb loading in adults with unilateral below-knee amputations. *Arch Phys Med Rehabil* 1994; 75:825-829.

31. Sanders JE, Daly CH, Burgess EM: Interface shear stresses during ambulation with a below-knee prosthetic limb. *J Rehabil Res Dev* 1992;29:1-8.

32. Fridman A, Ona I, Isakov E: The influence of prosthetic foot alignment on trans-tibial gait. *Prosthet Orthot Int* 2003;27:17-22.

Chapter 40

Knee Disarticulation: Surgical Management

Michael S. Pinzur, MD

Introduction

In 1940, Rogers[1] described the evolution of knee disarticulation. Before the use of surgical anesthesia, the value of knee disarticulation was the speed of the surgery and the limited amount of associated bleeding, as this technique does not violate the medullary cavity or transect any muscle bellies. Surgical techniques have used a variety of surgical flap designs, including a circular flap, equal anterior and posterior flaps, a long anterior flap, a long posterior flap, and sagittal flaps. As originally described, these flaps consisted only of skin and subcutaneous tissue with no other padding between the skin and articular cartilage of the distal femur. The lack of additional cushioning, however, prevented some patients from comfortably using the distal femoral weight-bearing surface.

A disadvantage of knee disarticulation is that if the full length of the femur is retained, the mechanical axis of the prosthetic knee must be placed far distal to the contralateral anatomic knee center, which makes the thigh segment too long and the shank segment too short. Amputees often object to this appearance. In addition, the short shank can prevent a prosthetic foot from reaching the floor when the patient is seated. External knee joints can be used to mitigate these problems, but they add to distal bulkiness and can damage overlying clothing without providing control

during swing phase. Thus, despite the ease and safety of the surgery and the advantage of end-weight bearing along normal proprioceptive pathways, knee disarticulation had not gained wide acceptance in North America.

The reduction of femoral length and distal bulkiness while retaining end-weight bearing was first addressed in the 1800s by Stokes,[2] who advocated the use of a supracondylar amputation with fixation of the cartilage-denuded patella to the distal end of the femoral metaphysis.[3] The main problems of this procedure were pain from failure of bony union and inability to achieve functional end-weight bearing, probably because of the small area presented distally by the patella.

In 1966, Mazet and Hennessy[4] reduced distal bulkiness in the frontal plane by trimming the medial and lateral condyles. Bulkiness was reduced in the sagittal plane by trimming both condyles posteriorly and excising the patella. In 1977, Burgess[5] addressed the issue of excess length by removing the distal 1.5 cm of the condyles. This procedure provides the prosthetist with the ability to raise the knee joint center by this amount. Burgess also reduced the sagittal diameter by patellectomy.

In 1992, Bowker[6] reported the use of a combination of the techniques of Mazet and Burgess that produces a

weight-bearing residual limb with the appearance of a very long transfemoral limb. The first successful prosthetic method to reduce the inequality between the thigh and shank portions was introduced by Lyquist[7] in 1976. The Orthopaedic Hospital of Copenhagen prosthesis featured a four-bar-linkage polycentric knee that allowed the shank to fold under the socket when the patient was seated. This design reduced the distal protrusion of the thigh portion. Improved versions of this knee are still used.

Wagner[8] was the first to use the gastrocnemius muscle bellies to provide a cushion beneath the femoral condyles to enhance end-bearing comfort. This technique was successfully combined with sagittal flaps, leading to a resurgence of interest in knee disarticulation. In 1985, Klaes and Eigler[9] reported the use of a long posterior myofasciocutaneous flap, including the gastrocnemius muscle bellies. Excellent padding is provided, and the perforating vessels from muscle to skin are undisturbed. A complete description in English was provided by Bowker and associates.[10]

Advantages of Knee Disarticulation

Current prosthetic technology takes advantage of the weight-bearing properties of knee disarticulation.

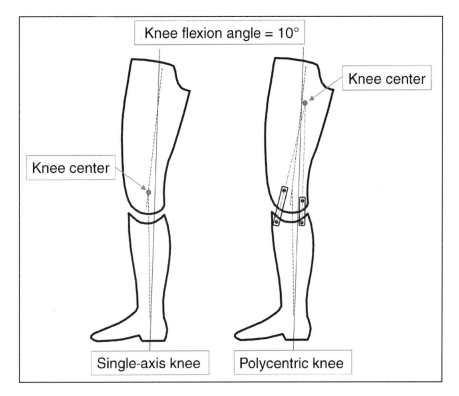

Figure 1 Whenever the ground-reaction force (weight-bearing line) falls posterior to the knee center, an external knee flexion moment is created and the prosthetic knee will flex abruptly under load. If the amputee steps onto the prosthesis with the knee slightly flexed, the typical single-axis knee will be unstable, as illustrated on the left. Many polycentric knees have an effective knee center similar to that shown on the right, resulting in an external knee extension moment during weight bearing even when the knee is slightly flexed. (*Reproduced with permission from Pinzur MS: Gait analysis in peripheral vascular insufficiency through-knee amputation. J Rehabil Res Dev 1993;30:388-392.*)

Knee disarticulation allows direct load transfer to the residual limb with enhanced walking independence and less energy consumption compared with transfemoral amputation. When combined with certain polycentric (four-bar-linkage) prosthetic joints, knee disarticulation can offer enhanced walking stability in the geriatric population. In growing children, knee disarticulation provides a durable residual limb that avoids the potential for appositional terminal bony overgrowth that is often observed after transosseous amputations. Surgical techniques designed to maximize function and the development of polycentric knee joints with fluid swing-phase controls have established knee disarticulation as an important component of a well-rounded amputation program.

Retention of all or a major portion of the weight-bearing surface of the distal femur allows distribution of the load over a large surface area.[6,11] The impact of initial loading during stance phase of gait is dampened by the biomechanical properties of the metaphyseal bone and the gastrocnemius-based end pad.

Walking stability is another key benefit of knee disarticulation. In the intact limb, the vertical ground-reaction force vector along the hip-knee-ankle axis of the lower limb passes posterior to the axis of the knee joint at initial contact (heel strike). This creates a knee flexion moment that can cause the knee to flex ("buckle") if not adequately counteracted by the action of the quadriceps. Some polycentric knee joint designs place the knee center

posterior to the ground-reaction force vector, thus acting to create an intrinsically stable knee joint during initial stance phase because a knee extension moment is created[12,13] (Figure 1).

The physiologic cost of walking with a knee disarticulation is midway between those of transfemoral and transtibial amputation levels with respect to walking speed and oxygen consumption per meter walked.[14-17] Transtibial amputees who are community ambulators increase the activity of the retained muscles to compensate for the lost muscles.[18] In contrast, household (limited) ambulators have no increase in muscle recruitment during gait.[19] This observation might explain the similarity of walking propulsion in sedentary patients to that of persons with transtibial amputations or knee disarticulations. Composite data suggest virtually no functional differences during walking in transtibial amputees who are marginally ambulatory and in patients who underwent knee disarticulation.[12,19] The enhanced stability of walking after knee disarticulation, as well as the population of unilateral transtibial amputees undergoing a second amputation, suggests an important role for knee disarticulation.[12]

Indications
Use After Trauma or in Patients With Infection
Forward propulsion during the terminal stance phase of gait is accomplished by knee extension against a stable foot and ankle. When foot salvage is not possible because of trauma or infection, every effort should be made to retain the forward propulsive capacity of the knee joint and proximal tibia. Transtibial amputation should be performed when the following structures can be retained: (1) a serviceable knee joint with no more than a 20° loss of full extension; (2) the proximal end of the tibia, including the patellar tendon attach-

ment; (3) an adequate soft-tissue envelope of mobile muscle to cover the distal end of the remaining tibia; and (4) full-thickness skin in areas of load transfer. If these criteria cannot be met or compensated for by creative reconstructive surgery or prosthetic adaptation such as a thigh corset and knee joints, these patients may be better served by knee disarticulation. Attempting to fit a transtibial amputation without an adequate soft-tissue envelope will often lead to repeated residual limb ulceration and pain.

A soft-tissue envelope covering the bone of the residual limb is essential for comfortable prosthetic fitting and weight bearing after any amputation or disarticulation. Pressure or shear loads are best accepted when the soft-tissue cover is composed of mobile muscle and full-thickness skin, which acts to both cushion direct pressure and dissipate shear forces. Split-thickness skin grafts in areas subject to pressure and/or shear will often break down in adults, especially if these grafts are adherent to bone. Although a knee disarticulation with an adequate soft-tissue envelope will function far better than a transtibial amputation performed with an inadequate soft-tissue envelope, the opposite has also been observed. Thus, the trauma surgeon should know that it may not be possible to create an adequately cushioned end pad for either a transtibial amputation or a knee disarticulation in patients who have severe soft-tissue injury. These amputees will ultimately function better if a muscle-balanced transfemoral amputation is performed to eliminate or reduce the discouraging cycle of discomfort, recurrent ulceration, and difficulties in prosthetic fitting.

Use in the Dysvascular Patient

The presence of viable tissue sufficient to provide an adequate soft-tissue envelope is the first consideration in patients who have peripheral vascular disease. The viability of tis-

sue at the proposed level of amputation can be determined preoperatively by noninvasive vascular testing. Intraoperatively, viability of tissue can be assessed by examining muscle color and consistency, skin and muscle bleeding, and muscle contractility when stimulated by electrocautery. Patients with amputations at the level of the tibial tubercle with an intact patellar tendon insertion retain the functional independence of transtibial amputees. If sufficient vascularity is present for a knee disarticulation to heal, it is also likely that amputation at a proximal transtibial level will heal.

A minor knee flexion contracture often improves with prosthetic limb fitting and walking, but when a contracture approaches 45°, the patient may not be able to use the quadriceps-powered tibial lever arm. These individuals may, therefore, achieve optimal functional independence after primary knee disarticulation. Hip flexion contracture causes the vertical ground-reaction force vector at initial contact (heel strike) to align posteriorly to the anatomic knee center, leading to knee instability and buckling with frequent falls. Placing the patient in the prone position for several periods daily can often reduce hip flexion contracture. Surgical release is rarely necessary to correct hip flexion contracture.

Some patients with ambulatory potential may benefit from knee disarticulation rather than transtibial amputation, even though they meet other accepted criteria for transtibial amputation. One group consists of patients who, after a cerebral vascular accident, have a spastic lower limb with a significant knee flexion contracture and an unsalvageable foot. If these patients retain reasonable voluntary control of the hip, they can be successfully fitted with and use a prosthesis after a knee disarticulation. In contrast, retaining a knee with spastic flexors will only lead to an increasing knee flexion contracture and the inability to fit a prosthesis.

Patients with poorly controlled congestive heart failure or those on dialysis for end-stage renal disease often have diurnal lower limb volume fluctuations that result in markedly increased distal pressures on the transtibial residual limb. Thus, the prosthetic socket does not fit intimately throughout the day. Patients with major volume fluctuations can do better with knee disarticulation and end bearing rather than total surface bearing. In these patients, the reduced requirement for intimate socket fit allows fabrication of a volume-adaptable socket (Figure 2).

Individuals who are morbidly obese are always difficult to fit for a prosthesis because the adipose tissues tend to displace proximally in the prosthetic socket under weight-bearing shear forces. This displacement results in unacceptable tension in the distal soft tissues over the bone at the end of the residual limb. In obese patients, end-bearing procedures such as a Syme ankle disarticulation or knee disarticulation may be more beneficial in terms of reduced pain and soft-tissue injury compared with a transosseous amputation.

Dysvascular unilateral transtibial amputees who are marginal walkers and require a contralateral amputation may benefit from knee disarticulation instead of transtibial amputation, although this is controversial. These patients can take advantage of the intrinsically stable polycentric knee joint of a knee disarticulation prosthesis during stance phase, and retain the forward propulsion of the knee joint on the transtibial side.[12,20,21] The functional effects of this approach on activities other than standing and level walking, such as stair climbing, walking on inclines, and rising from a chair or the floor, have not been investigated.

Use in Children

Knee disarticulation in children has generally been confined to the treatment of those with congenital deficiencies, malignant tumors, trauma, or

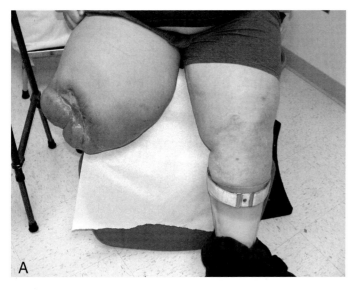
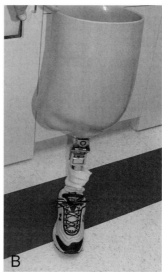
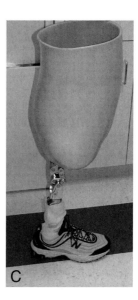

Figure 2 **A,** This patient with diabetes mellitus weighs more than 350 lb and would be difficult to fit with a conventional knee disarticulation socket. Using a volume-adaptable prosthetic socket (**B** and **C**), he was able to walk independently and comfortably bear much of his weight on the end of his residual limb.

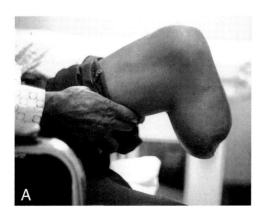
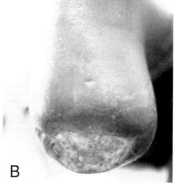

Figure 3 **A,** This transtibial amputee developed a knee flexion contracture because of muscle imbalance when using a wheelchair. **B,** Constant residual limb pressure on the patient's bedding led to the development of a large terminal ulcer, which could be resolved only by conversion to knee disarticulation. *(Reproduced with permission from Pinzur MS, Smith DG, Daluga DJ, Osterman H: Selection of patients for through-the-knee amputation. J Bone Joint Surg Am 1988;70:746-750.)*

infection. Femoral length in growing children is maintained by preserving the growth potential of the distal femoral physis. This procedure also avoids the risk of appositional bony overgrowth inherent with pediatric transosseous amputation.[22] The residual femur tends to grow at a slower rate than the contralateral femur. Such growth allows the prosthetic knee joint center to eventually approach the level of the normal contralateral knee and maintains the advantages of end-weight bearing.[23,24]

Use in Nonambulatory Patients

Knee disarticulation is most commonly indicated for nonambulatory individuals, such as those who are bed-bound in a skilled nursing facility. In general, these patients meet most criteria for transtibial amputation but do not have the real potential for prosthetic ambulation.[11,25-27] In addition, muscle imbalances can cause these patients to develop a knee flexion contracture after transtibial amputation or a hip flexion-abduction contracture

following transfemoral amputation. Knee flexion contracture in the nonambulatory transtibial amputee often leads to pressure ulcers on the distal residual limb (Figure 3).

The residual limb of the transfemoral amputee provides a small platform for sitting in a chair and a lever arm that is inefficient for use in transfers (Figure 4). A minimal sitting area decreases trunk stability and limits the ability of the bilateral transfemoral amputee to safely lean forward to perform tasks with the upper limbs, such as picking up a dropped object. Knee disarticulation, in contrast, provides a stable platform for sitting and a long, powerful, muscle-stabilized femoral lever arm to assist in positioning and transfers (Figure 5). In addition, knee disarticulation has the benefits of minimizing surgical blood loss and maintaining the cartilage barrier, which potentially reduces the risk of infection in this population of compromised patients.[10,11]

Surgical Techniques
Bone

The distal terminal femur is well suited to accommodate loading because of its large surface area. The metaphyseal bone of the distal termi-

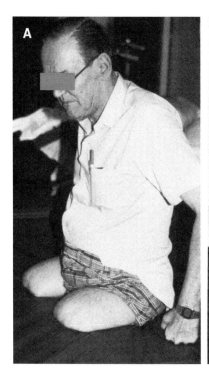

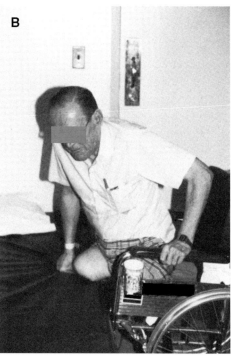

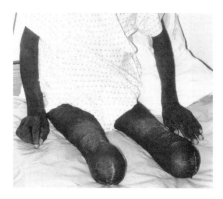

Figure 5 Knee disarticulation provides a stable platform for sitting and a strong lever arm to assist in transfers. (*Courtesy of JH Bowker, MD*)

Figure 4 Transfemoral amputation provides a small platform for sitting in a chair (**A**) and an inefficient lever arm to assist transfer from the chair (**B**).

nal femur is less stiff than cortical bone and thus dissipates the impact that occurs at initial distal loading. In contrast, loading must be distributed over the entire surface area of the residual limb and relieved from the distal end for the indirect load transfer after transosseous (transtibial or transfemoral) amputations; both of these criteria must be met for an intimate prosthetic fit. Knee disarticulation allows end bearing and minimizes the necessity for an intimate prosthetic fit, which makes suspension of the prosthetic socket the major requirement.

Rogers[1] elected to retain the entire distal femoral weight-bearing surface and recommended fusion of the patella to the anterior femur to enhance suspension. This procedure created a bulky but reasonably functional residual limb. Reduction osteoplasty can be used to decrease the bulk of the residual limb. The distal articular surface can be retained, however, by simply trimming the medial, lateral, and posterior protuberances as advocated by Mazet and Hennessy.[4] Burgess[5] re-

moved 1.5 cm from the condyles distally to keep the knee centers level but did not narrow them. Based on a series of osteoplasties by Mazet and Burgess, Bowker[6] showed that the weight-bearing characteristics of the distal femur are retained by shortening it by 2 cm and retaining the anterior cruciate ligament for quadriceps tenodesis. Shortening of the femur was perhaps more relevant before the development of the polycentric four-bar-linkage prosthetic knee joint. Although reduction of the distal femur improves cosmesis, this may impair suspension and rotational control.

Soft Tissues

Each of the aforementioned bony configurations has its proponents. Knee disarticulation, however, was not widely used, partly because of its limited ability to accept the load of weight bearing. Earlier flap designs had a high rate of wound failure and poor ability to act as the interface between the prosthetic socket and the residual limb because the soft-tissue envelope consisted only of skin and subcutaneous

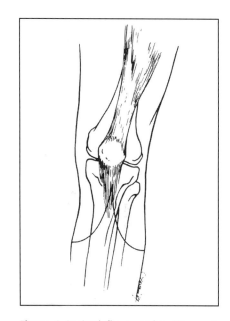

Figure 6 Sagittal flaps used in Wagner's version of the knee disarticulation. The apex of the skin flap is midway between the inferior pole of the patella and the tibial tuberosity. The length of each flap is one half the diameter of the limb at the level of the knee joint. (*Reproduced with permission from Pinzur MS, Smith DG, Daluga DJ, Osterman H: Selection of patients for through-the-knee amputation. J Bone Joint Surg Am 1988;70:746-750.*)

tissue. Wagner's[8] major contribution was the introduction of an end-bearing gastrocnemius cushion for amputations at this level. This refinement, combined with the development of the polycentric prosthetic knee joint, brought knee disarticulation to the forefront as a valuable com-

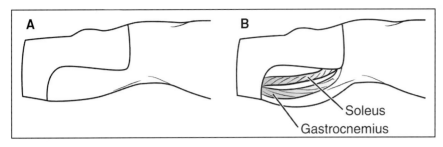

Figure 7 A, The posterior myofasciocutaneous flap is virtually identical to that used in performing a transtibial amputation. This illustration of the medial aspect of the knee shows the outline of the flap. **B,** This illustration shows the pendent posterior flap still attached distally. The plane has been opened between the soleus muscle anteriorly and the gastrocnemius muscle posteriorly. *(Adapted with permission from Bowker JH, San Giovanni TP, Pinzur MS: North American experience with knee disarticulation with use of a posterior myofasciocutaneous flap: Healing rate and functional results in seventy-seven patients. J Bone Joint Surg Am 2000;82:1571-1574.)*

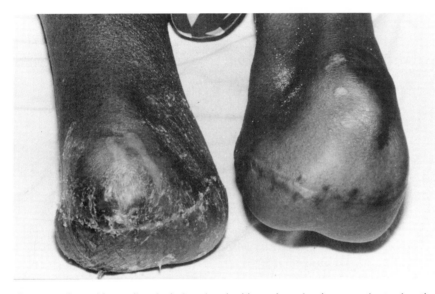

Figure 8 Bilateral knee disarticulations in a bed-bound nursing home patient using the posterior myofasciocutaneous flap of Klaes and Eigler. The left disarticulation is mature and the right one is recent. *(Courtesy of JH Bowker, MD.)*

ponent of a functionally oriented amputation program.

Sagittal Flap Technique of Wagner

Wagner[8] used sagittal flaps to minimize the length of the soft-tissue flaps in dysvascular patients (Figure 6). The use of a tourniquet is optional. The skin flaps begin at a point midway between the inferior pole of the patella and the tibial tuberosity and end at an opposite point in the popliteal fossa. The length of both medial and lateral flaps is half the diameter of the limb at the level of the knee joint plus 1 cm, which can be trimmed if redundant.

The flaps are raised in the interval between the skin and deeper structures. The patellar tendon is detached (skived) from the tibial tuberosity. The knee joint capsule is incised circumferentially at the level of the knee joint, leaving the menisci with the tibia. The cruciate ligaments are detached from the tibia. The gastrocnemius bellies are separated from the soleus. The posterior tibial and common peroneal nerves are gently drawn distally and divided. The popliteal vessels are doubly ligated. The quadriceps muscle is stabilized at a normal length by suturing the patellar tendon to the residual cruciate ligaments with nonabsorb-

able or heavy absorbable sutures. The distal pole of the patella should not extend beyond the distal femur. The cushioned end pad is created by suturing the posterior gastrocnemius fascia to the knee joint retinaculum without tension or redundant muscle. To ensure that the muscle flap is centered, the first suture should attach the muscle flap to the center of the patellar tendon. The skin is closed with sutures or staples.[8,11]

Posterior Myofasciocutaneous Flap of Klaes and Eigler

The posterior myofasciocutaneous flap has been adapted by Klaes and Eigler[9] for knee disarticulation.[10] This flap is familiar to amputation surgeons as it is virtually identical to that used for a midlength transtibial amputation. By avoiding dissection between the muscle and skin, this procedure lessens the potential for skin flap necrosis caused by division of the perforating vessels. A transverse anterior incision is made at the level of the knee extending to the midlateral line on each side. Longitudinal incisions extend from each end of the transverse incision to the distal limit of the gastrocnemius bellies, where they are joined with a transverse cut. The plane between the gastrocnemius bellies and the soleus is found medially and bluntly dissected to the lateral side (Figure 7). The gastrocnemius-soleus conjoined tendon is then divided transversely to free the flap distally. The rest of the procedure is similar to the Wagner technique. In addition to suturing the quadriceps tendon to the cruciates, the medial and lateral hamstring tendons should be sewn to the capsule to preserve their function as hip extensors. In a similar manner, the iliotibial band should be sutured to enhance abductor function and hip extension by the gluteus maximus. The resulting anterodistal transverse scar lies directly over the gastrocnemius muscle bellies, which cushion the scar from trauma (Figure 8).

In patients who are expected to use a prosthesis, the posterior condyles of the femur can be removed flush with the posterior femoral cortex to increase terminal flexion of the prosthetic knee. Any of these techniques can be modified, depending on the availability of viable soft tissue.

Immediate Postoperative Management

A rigid plaster or fiberglass dressing is preferable to a soft dressing to control swelling and protect the wound from soiling or trauma during the early postoperative period. The most simple technique is the addition of a pylon to a rigid dressing. Fitting of a prosthetic limb and weight bearing can be initiated as soon as the wound is secure. Once the patient becomes stable in walking, a knee joint can be added.

Summary

Knee disarticulation is most commonly indicated for patients in whom a surgical wound at the transtibial level will heal, but who will not be able to walk. The residual limb formed by this procedure provides an excellent platform for sitting and a powerful lever arm to assist in transfers and bed mobility. In patients who are able to walk, knee disarticulation provides a durable residual limb capable of direct load transfer. In children, it avoids the potential for bony overgrowth often observed after amputations at transosseous levels.

References

1. Rogers SP: Amputation at the knee joint. *J Bone Joint Surg* 1940;22: 973-979.

2. Stokes W: On supracondylar amputation of the thigh. *Proc Roy Med Chir Soc London* 1870;6:289.

3. Slocum DB: The end-bearing amputations, in *An Atlas of Amputations*. St Louis, MO, CV Mosby, 1949, pp 222-226.

4. Mazet R Jr, Hennessy CA: Knee disarticulation: A new technique and a new knee-joint mechanism. *J Bone Joint Surg Am* 1966;48:126-139.

5. Burgess EM: Disarticulation of the knee: A modified technique. *Arch Surg* 1977;112:1250-1255.

6. Bowker JH: Abstract: reduction osteoplasty of the distal femur to enhance prosthetic fitting in knee disarticulation, in *Proceedings of the Seventh World Congress of the International Society for Prosthetics and Orthotics*. Chicago, IL, International Society for Prosthetics and Orthotics, 1992, p 267.

7. Lyquist E: The OHC knee-disarticulation prosthesis. *Orthot Prosthet* 1976;30:27-28.

8. Wagner FW Jr: Management of the diabetic-neurotrophic foot: Part II. A classification and treatment program for diabetic, neuropathic, and dysvascular foot problems. *Instr Course Lect* 1979;28:143-165.

9. Klaes W, Eigler FW: Eine neue Technik der transgenikulären Amputation. *Chirurg* 1985;56:735-740.

10. Bowker JH, San Giovanni TP, Pinzur MS: North American experience with knee disarticulation with use of a posterior myofasciocutaneous flap: Healing rate and functional results in seventy-seven patients. *J Bone Joint Surg Am* 2000;82:1571-1574.

11. Pinzur MS, Smith DJ, Daluga DJ, Osterman H: Selection of patients for through-the-knee amputation. *J Bone Joint Surg Am* 1988;70:746-750.

12. Pinzur MS, Smith D, Tornow D, Meade K, Patwardhan A: Gait analysis of dysvascular below-knee and contralateral through-knee bilateral amputees: A preliminary report. *Orthopedics* 1993;16:875-879.

13. Greene MP: Four bar linkage knee analysis. *Orthot Prosthet* 1983;37: 15-24.

14. Fisher SV, Gullickson G Jr: Energy cost of ambulation in health and disability: A literature review. *Arch Phys Med Rehabil* 1978;59:124-133.

15. Waters RL, Perry J, Antonelli D, Hislop H: Energy cost of walking of amputees: The influence of level of amputation. *J Bone Joint Surg Am* 1976;58: 42-46.

16. Waters RL: The energy expenditure of amputee gait, in Bowker JH, Michael JW (eds): *Atlas of Limb Prosthetics: Surgical, Prosthetic, and Rehabilitation Principles*, ed 2. Rosemont, IL, American Academy of Orthopaedic Surgeons, 2002, pp 381-387. (Originally published by Mosby-Year Book, 1992)

17. Pinzur MS, Gold J, Schwartz D, Gross N: Energy demands for walking in dysvascular amputees as related to the level of amputation. *Orthopedics* 1992; 15:1033-1037.

18. Breakey J: Gait of unilateral below-knee amputees. *Orthot Prosthet* 1976; 30:17-24.

19. Pinzur MS, Asselmeier M, Smith D: Dynamic electromyography in active and limited walking below-knee amputees. *Orthopedics* 1991;14:535-538.

20. Pinzur MS: Gait analysis in peripheral vascular insufficiency through-knee amputation. *J Rehabil Res Dev* 1993;30: 388-392.

21. Pinzur MS, Cox W, Kaiser J, Morris T, Patwardhan A, Vrbos L: The effect of prosthetic alignment on relative limb loading in persons with trans-tibial amputation: A preliminary report. *J Rehabil Res Dev* 1995;32:373-377.

22. Epps CH Jr, Schneider PL: Treatment of hemimelias of the lower extremity: Long-term results. *J Bone Joint Surg Am* 1989;71:273-277.

23. Loder RT, Herring JA: Disarticulation of the knee in children: A functional assessment. *J Bone Joint Surg Am* 1987; 69:1155-1160.

24. Thomas B, Schopler S, Wood W, Oppenheim WL: The knee in arthrogryposis. *Clin Orthop* 1985;194:87-92.

25. Pinzur MS: New concepts in lower-limb amputation and prosthetic management. *Instr Course Lect* 1990;39: 361-366.

26. Pinzur MS: Current concepts: Amputation surgery in peripheral vascular disease. *Instr Course Lect* 1997;46: 501-509.

27. Pinzur MS, Bowker JH, Smith DG: Gottschalk f: Amputation Surgery in Peripheral Vascular Disease. *Instr Course Lect* 1999;48:687-692.

Chapter 41

Knee Disarticulation: Prosthetic Management

Donald R. Cummings, CP, LP
Rebekah Russ, CPO, LPO

Introduction

Knee disarticulation offers many advantages over transfemoral amputation, but the procedure is still somewhat uncommon in North America. The exception is in the pediatric population, in which knee disarticulation is preferred over procedures at higher levels because it retains both epiphyses and avoids bony overgrowth. For any amputee, the fact that knee disarticulation allows end bearing—the ability of the intact femoral condyles, articular surfaces, and overlying soft tissues to tolerate the patient's super-incumbent weight—is a significant advantage over amputation at the transfemoral level, which requires that pelvic structures provide most of the support. Through-knee surgery is also less traumatic because no bones or muscles are cut, so strength, muscle tone, and balance are generally excellent. The retained femoral condyles also enhance the patient's rotational control and ability to suspend the prosthesis.

Disadvantages of knee disarticulation are mostly associated with cosmesis, challenging socket design, and more limited options for prosthetic knees.[1] The often bulbous distal end requires prosthetists to use socket designs with more visible openings and straps or a bulky appearance. Because the full length of the femur is retained, the prosthetist may find it difficult or impossible to match the knee centers. Fewer than ten types of prosthetic knees designed specifically for knee disarticulations are commercially available, compared with well over one hundred for higher levels.

Despite the disadvantages associated with knee disarticulations, the procedure has significant benefits. After comparing patient satisfaction and functional outcome of knee disarticulation patients in Sweden, Hagberg and associates[2] concluded that knee disarticulation "should always be considered as the primary alternative to AK [above-knee] amputation when a BK [below-knee] amputation is not feasible."

Patient Evaluation

When the knee joint is disarticulated, the distal end of the femur, which is the largest horizontal load-bearing surface in the lower limb, is retained. In most cases, this diminishes or negates the need for weight bearing through the ischial tuberosity. This benefit should not be assumed, however. Hip joint pathology, femoral abnormality, compromised distal sensation or circulation, tenuous skin coverage, painful neuromas, patient preference, or other challenges may limit or rule out the patient's ability to bear weight successfully through the end of the femur. In such cases, the only advantages of knee disarticulation may be avoidance of bony overgrowth (in children), suspension over the condyles, and some improvement of rotational control of the prosthesis. In the absence of end-bearing capacity, deweighting of the distal femur is necessary, which requires extra space and padding as well as a proximal socket design similar to those used for transfemoral levels that emphasizes support through the ischial tuberosity and proximal soft tissues.

Patient evaluation should include an inventory of the multiple benefits that knee disarticulation can provide. When it is available, distal weight bearing transfers forces in a more physiologically normal fashion through the femur to the pelvis and trunk. As demonstrated by the ability of most people without amputations to kneel comfortably, the pressure-tolerant articular surface, soft tissues, and skin around the knee are well adapted to weight bearing. Many persons with a knee disarticulation can kneel with the prosthesis off. This is a significant advantage for amputees with bilateral knee disarticulations, many of whom can ambulate for short distances without prostheses. To maximize this potential, a second pair of short, protective sockets is often indicated in addition to full-length prostheses for such patients. In addition, the contours of the femoral condyles and patella (if present) enhance the patient's rotational control of the prosthesis and often provide an excellent means of suspending the device. Also, the

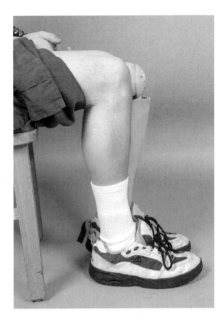

Figure 1 A polycentric knee disarticulation knee was used for this fitting, but the long femoral length, combined with a distal pad, attachment bracket, plastic, and hardware, resulted in a slightly longer thigh section on the prosthetic side. *(Courtesy of Texas Scottish Rite Hospital.)*

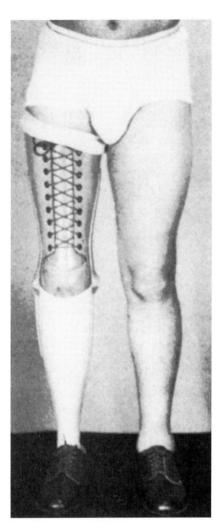

Figure 2 Photograph of a "traditional" molded leather socket with outside hinges. Modern versions may use more hygienic thermoplastic materials and Velcro closures rather than laces. Outside hinges enable the knee centers to match, but bulkiness is unavoidable. *(Reproduced with permission from Edwards JW (ed): Orthopaedic Appliances Atlas, Ann Arbor, MI, American Academy of Orthopaedic Surgeons, 1960, Vol 2, p 225.)*

long and powerful lever arm of the femur is retained. One obvious advantage for children is that the distal femoral epiphysis is retained, preserving 90% of femoral growth. Because no bones are cut, terminal osseous overgrowth, which is common among children with transdiaphyseal amputations, is avoided. Proprioception is better because the limb is longer; this is an advantage for both children and adults.

Even though these advantages generally translate into functional benefits and patient satisfaction, knee disarticulations have some obvious drawbacks.[2] When femoral lengths are equal, the prosthetist cannot match the knee centers exactly (Figure 1). Padding for the distal femur (which is generally recommended), socket thickness, attachment brackets, and the prosthetic knee itself all add additional length. Unless the patient is willing to accept a much longer prosthetic "thigh," options for knee mechanisms are limited.

To match knee centers, prosthetists traditionally used external, single-axis joints (Figure 2) that were inherently bulky. Most offered no friction or fluid control, so they were often noisy and wore out quickly in active patients. The development of modern polycentric knees has improved cosmesis, function, and durability for this level.

Another disadvantage is that the wide femoral condyles and resulting bulky appearance at the knee may not be acceptable to some patients. Finally, although rare, a hip flexion contracture combined with the long length of the thigh and the need to position the knee well behind it will create a poor cosmetic result.

History and physical examination details that should be reviewed for any level of amputation are pertinent for the knee disarticulation level as well. Before recommending a prosthetic design and treatment plan, the health care team should consider the following important questions specifically related to this level: (1) Are the femoral condyles intact or shaved? How wide are they, and how bulbous is the distal end of the limb? The size and shape of the distal femur relative to the thigh will determine socket and suspension options. Surgically reduced condyles may be less tolerant of pressure. The overall dimension of the reduced distal femur may not allow suspension of the prosthesis. (2) How long is the femur? If the affected femur is the same length as the opposite femur, either a prosthetic knee designed specifically for patients who have had a knee disarticulation or outside joints will offer the most cosmetic result. In children, an appropriately timed epiphysiodesis may be indicated so that more knee options are available by adulthood. (3) Does the patient have normal hip function, especially on the prosthetic side? The hip must be capable of tolerating forces translated from the distal end through the femur to the pelvis. Otherwise, a transfemoral amputation socket style must be used. (4) Are the muscles of the thigh in good balance? Hip flexion contractures are more cosmetically obvious in longer limbs. Also, control of the prosthesis and the degree of knee stability required are determined by hip strength. (5) Can the patient tolerate pressure distally? Has the scar healed well, and is the limb sensate? If distal pressure is not tolerated, more proximal structures will have to provide support. (6) Are other limbs involved? What other limitations or challenges does the patient face? (7) What are the patient's functional goals? A runner, for example, may require a fluid-controlled knee. A long limb and bulbous end will require some cosmetic compromises. (8) What are the patient's concerns regarding cosmesis?

Staging of Care

Immediate postoperative prostheses (IPOPs) or early postoperative prostheses can be applied following knee disarticulation, but additional challenges will be encountered compared with other procedures. Rigid dressings, with or without a pylon attached, may actually be easier to keep in place after a knee disarticulation than after a transfemoral amputation, but the cast may be more difficult to remove for wound access. The femoral condyles can be used to suspend the prosthesis, but they should be well padded, and the cast should include an auxiliary waist belt for safety and comfort. The wound closure is near the distal femur, where the patient will bear weight, so care should be given to padding and protecting this area. As with all amputations, the residual limb is sensitive to external pressure in the first weeks after the procedure. If the patella is retained, it may be especially sensitive to pressure or shear forces.[3]

Ideally, physical therapy should begin before prosthetic fitting to help build strength and range of motion. End bearing should be initiated gradually and cautiously through physical therapy within the first 4 to 6 weeks after surgery.[3]

If the patient does not begin with an IPOP or rigid dressing, soft dressings, elastic wraps, or shrinkers may be used immediately after surgery to reduce swelling and pain. Compressive dressings, wraps, or shrinkers also have the benefit of desensitizing the limb to outside pressure, which may help when fitting the prosthesis.[4]

Once the limb is ready for fitting with a more definitive socket, multiple options are available. If the femoral condyles are to transmit full weight onto the prosthesis, as they did on the tibial plateau before the amputation, the prosthetist will need to pay particular attention to the distal anatomy of the residual limb. Firm, supportive distal pads are generally preferred because they enable comfortable weight bearing and still protect tissues against trauma. Pads that are too thick may add bulk or lower the knee center. The entire lower surface of the femur may support the patient's weight, but the patella generally requires protection from external pressures. For this reason, some surgeons remove it.[3] Finally, when the prosthesis is being fabricated, care is required to minimize the distance between the distal end of the socket and the attachment to the knee (Figure 1).

Socket Design, Suspension, and Interfaces
Socket Design

Socket design for the patient who has had a knee disarticulation is often dictated by the degree to which distal weight bearing is tolerated and the size of the femoral condyles relative to the circumference of the thigh. Some of the most common approaches are described here, but multiple creative variations exist that are as unique as the patients who wear them and the prosthetists who design them.

Botta and Baumgartner[5] began their treatise on socket design by stating, "The bulbous shape of the residual limb and its full end-bearing quality requires a socket which has very little resemblance to above-knee sockets." They go on to describe the ideal requirements for a knee disarticulation socket: (1) total surface contact in both the sitting and the upright position; (2) total end-bearing quality (in normal anatomy the femoral condyles transmit full weight to the tibial plateau and vice versa); (3) no ischial seat and, therefore, free motion of the hip joint; (4) easy doffing and donning with the patient sitting, requiring no extra physical or intellectual effort; (5) no straps, laces, or suspenders; (6) minimal extra width or length compared with the normal anatomy of the thigh and knee; (7) ability to be fitted with every type of knee joint designed for knee disarticulations, including the possibility of knee locking or swing-phase control; (8) no special clothing adaptations required, and no extra wear caused by the prosthesis should be noticed; (9) easy to clean for effective residual limb hygiene; (10) light, but able to withstand the patient's activity; (11) adjustable for residual limb shape and volume changes; (12) capable of being fabricated by standard manufacturing techniques, requiring no extra skill from the prosthetist who is familiar with normal anatomy and current manufacturing techniques; and finally, (13) the socket should cost no more than conventional prostheses.[5]

Rarely will all of these lofty goals be realized in one design. However, multiple socket variations intended to meet the unique needs of a patient who has had a knee disarticulation are available.

Traditional anterior lacing sockets are rarely used in the United States today, but the design does have advantages (Figure 2). This type of socket is still commonly used in many countries where it is preferred because of material availability or familiarity with the technique. Whether made of flexible resins, thermoplastics, or leather, this socket has a lengthwise anterior opening that allows the passage of the wide femoral condyles. The prosthesis is then fastened around the residual limb using laces, Velcro straps, or some other form of closure. The molded flexible socket fits snugly over the bulbous distal femur, thus suspending the prosthesis.[6] Because the system is contoured directly against the atrophied thigh, it is rarely overly bulky in appearance. However, some patients have objected to poor durability or hygiene problems related to the leather, and others did not like the appearance of the anterior opening and

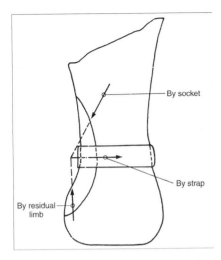

Figure 3 Illustration shows how a removable plate or "window" allows the bulbous condyles to pass through the socket; they are secured with a Velcro strap. This method is particularly advantageous for mature, atrophied limbs with wide and prominent femoral condyles. It may not work well when the condyles are buried in soft tissue, such as in obese or muscular patients. *(Reproduced with permission from Hughes J: Biomechanics of the through-knee prosthesis. Prosthet Orthot Int 1983;7:96-99.)*

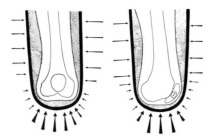

Figure 4 A soft distal pad and liner can both provide suspension over the femoral condyles and enhance comfort and protection of the residual limb. Once donned, the liner enables the limb to pass like a compressible cylinder through the socket. Compression of the liner between the socket walls, against the limb, and over the femoral condyles keeps the prosthesis in place. *(Reproduced with permission from Baumgartner RF: Knee disarticulation versus above-knee amputation. Prosthet Orthot Int 1979;3:15-19.)*

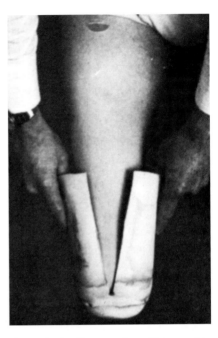

Figure 5 The liner can be split to enable the femoral condyles to pass through it so that children, geriatric patients, or bilateral amputees can don it easily. Many variations of such suspension pads are available. Materials include closed-cell polyethylene foams, foam and leather, silicon, and urethane. *(Reproduced with permission from Botta P, Baumgartner R: Socket design and manufacturing technique for through-knee stumps. Prosthet Orthot Int 1983;7:100-103.)*

visible laces or straps. Originally, this design was used with external metal hinges. When combined with modern knees, this socket design may still benefit some patients.

Suspension and Interfaces

A removable "window," which can be fastened back in place, allows the wearer to pass the femoral condyles through the socket comfortably (Figure 3). Traditionally, the opening is located medially, where it is less visible. When the plate is repositioned and fastened tightly, the prosthesis suspends over the condyles. A downside of this method is that it adds material to the thigh section and thus may have a less desirable appearance. Also, the design generally works best for a well-atrophied limb of stable volume with prominent femoral condyles.[7] If the distal femur is not bulky enough for suspension, some other form of socket may be preferable.

An internal pad or liner can also be used to secure the prosthesis over the femoral condyles (Figures 4 and 5). Botta and Baumgartner[5] advocated the use of an inner foam liner, either long or short, to suspend the knee disarticulation prosthesis and to facilitate donning and doffing. The short version extends up the thigh only to the point at which the thigh circumference is equal to the largest circumference of the bulbous distal femur. The liner includes a distal pad. Layers of foam are added to the liner and shaped until a cylindrical form of consistent circumference with tapered proximal edges is produced. A full liner extending to the proximal socket brim is another alternative. With either type of liner, a split can be made in the foam for easier donning. Usually, the patient dons the liner over a prosthetic sock and then steps into the prosthesis. A thin sock worn over the insert may reduce friction, making it easier for the patient to attach and remove the prosthesis.

A similar type of suspension involves the use of a split cylindrical suspension pad that the patient slips over the lower femur, converting it to a cylindrical shape. A distal pad is

built into the socket but is not part of the suspension device. Prosthetic socks are worn against the residual limb with an additional layer that is pulled on once the pad is positioned. Because this method does not require the use of a complete liner, no additional bulk is added around the bulbous distal end.

If the femoral condyles are not overly prominent, they can be pushed through an expandable inner elastic wall or flexible socket (Figure 6). Originally, this type of suspension consisted of a stretchy silicone "bladder" with a void between it and the outer socket to allow passage of the femur. This design, however, is quite difficult to make, and postfabrication adjustments to the socket are often not possible.[8] Similar designs are now made with flexible thermoplastic inner sockets or gel liners.

Suspension is often an inherent part of socket design, particularly for the patient with a knee disarticulation. Self-suspension over the condyles is generally the most desirable suspension for these patients. In pediatric patients, if a knee disarticulation is performed for congenital deficiency, the distal femur may be underdeveloped and unable to provide adequate suspension of the prosthesis. In such patients, transfemoral suspension methods such as a variety of waist belts or suction, Silesian, locking gel, or silicon liners may be indicated. Suction can be obtained by using a flexible inner socket and valve, housed within a rigid outer frame. Alternatively, if there is little or no flaring to the distal femur, a traditional suction socket may be used (Figure 7). When the femur on the prosthetic side is shorter than the opposite side, a gel locking liner might be used. Lanyard systems, which use a cord rather than a pin and lock to suspend the prosthesis, conserve space for the prosthetic knee. A relatively new option resembles a modified ski boot buckle that eliminates distal attachments through a locking mechanism mounted on the side of the gel liner and outer socket.[9] For patients with bilateral knee disarticulations, conserving space distally is less critical; thus there are more options for prosthetic knees and types of suspensions.

Components

The distance between the end of the socket and the anatomic knee center is usually a key determinant of which knee is most appropriate. There are often many options for pediatric patients and those with congenital limb deficiencies when an epiphysiodesis is performed or there is an existing femoral length discrepancy. However, these situations are rare in adult practice. Options for prosthetic knees are quite limited if approximating knee centers is a goal. Three general types of knees are appropriate for the typical

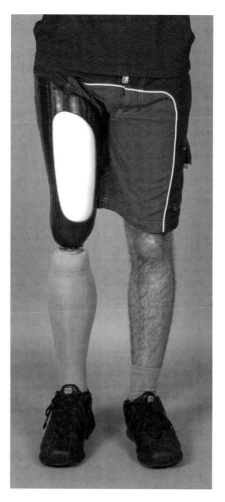

Figure 6 This young man underwent a knee disarticulation following a traumatic injury. The flexible socket stretches through the frame cutouts just enough to enable the femoral condyles to enter the socket. Voluntary muscle contraction also holds the prosthesis on more tightly. Although the prosthetic knee center is lower than the opposite side, the result is cosmetically acceptable. *(Courtesy of Texas Scottish Rite Hospital.)*

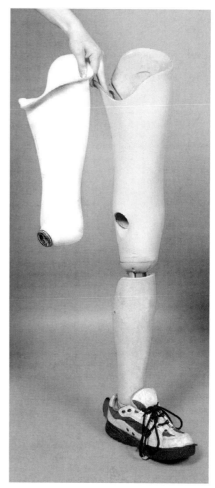

Figure 7 This socket uses both the elasticity of a flexible socket and a suction valve to suspend the limb. A slight circumferential void between the outer socket and the inner flexible socket enables the femoral condyles to slip into the prosthesis. A distal pad, not visible, is located inside the socket, below the flexible insert. The proximal brim is designed for some weight bearing on the ischial tuberosity. Although this is not usually necessary, it can help spread forces over a larger surface area. *(Courtesy of Texas Scottish Rite Hospital.)*

knee disarticulation: (1) outside joints, (2) knee mechanisms traditionally used for transfemoral amputees, and (3) knee disarticulation polycentric knees.

Outside Joints

Outside joints were used more frequently in the past. They consist of heavy-duty single-axis joints, often including ball bearings, that are mounted on the socket at the level of

the opposite knee joint. Distally, they attach to a prosthetic shin, usually of the exoskeletal type. One or two designs are suitable for active patients. They include a yoke and linkage system that enables a hydraulic or pneumatic cylinder to be placed inside the shin. Outside joints allow the prosthetist to match the knee center more closely, but they often have an uncosmetic appearance because of the added width at the knee.[10]

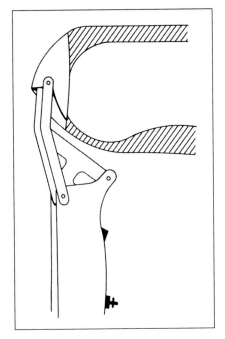

Figure 8 The knee-disarticulation four-bar-linkage is designed to fold up beneath the thigh segment when flexed to 90°, thus reducing the anterior protrusion of the knee when sitting. Only a few of the polycentric, or four-bar, knees on the market are designed to provide this advantage specifically for patients who have had a knee disarticulation. (*Reproduced with permission from Michael JW: Component selection criteria: Lower limb disarticulation. Clin Prosthet Orthot 1988; 12:99-108.*)

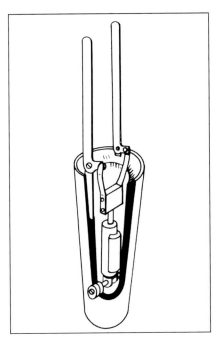

Figure 9 Cutaway view of a knee disarticulation shin and outside joints connected to a hydraulic unit through a special yoke. The hydraulic cylinder provides variable-cadence swing-phase control. The outside joints enable the prosthetist to match the knee center to that of the opposite side. Theoretically, the hydraulic swing-phase unit should also minimize noise and enhance the durability of the external hinges. (*Reproduced with permission from Michael JW: Component selection criteria: Lower limb disarticulation. Clin Prosthet Orthot 1988;12:99-108.*)

Transfemoral Knee Mechanisms

Another category includes most of the knee mechanisms traditionally used for transfemoral amputees. When used in conjunction with a knee disarticulation, nearly all of these will result in a lower prosthetic knee center as well as a thigh that appears longer than the opposite side. Nevertheless, these can be appropriate for bilateral amputees in whom the affected femur is shorter than the opposite side or for patients who are willing to accept a lower knee center to gain the benefit of a certain knee. This category includes single-axis, constant-friction knees; stance-control knees; manual lock knees; polycentric knees not designed specifically for knee disarticulations; hydraulic-controlled knees; and

the new class of microprocessor-controlled knees. These are discussed in detail in other chapters in this text.

Knee Disarticulation Polycentric Knees

The third class includes knee disarticulation polycentric knees (Figure 8). These are distinguished from other polycentric or multiaxis knees because they are designed specifically for patients with knee disarticulations, minimizing the space required to attach them below a socket. They also fold under the prosthetic socket during flexion, further minimizing the appearance of an overly long thigh section. As with most polycentric knees, these knees provide some benefits over single-axis knees. The advantages include enhanced

stance-phase stability, minimal knee protrusion when sitting, and acceleration-deceleration qualities inherent to a moving center of rotation. A few of these multiaxis knees also include hydraulic or pneumatic units, thus addressing the control needs of active patients who vary their walking speed (Figure 9). Michael[11] has eloquently described how a polycentric knee functions: "The point at which a polycentric knee prosthesis appears to be bending at a given moment is referred to as its instant center of rotation. Many polycentric knee prostheses have an instant center of rotation that is located in a very proximal and posterior location compared with the anatomic knee center. The more posterior the instant center of rotation is located with reference to the ground reaction force, the greater the knee extension moment developed in early stance and the more stable the prosthesis becomes."

Foot and ankle components for this level should be selected by the same criteria used for transfemoral prostheses. Because of the tendency of flexible keel feet to reduce stress on the relatively fragile knee units often used with this level, they may be preferable over more rigid designs such as the solid ankle–cushion heel (SACH) foot.[1]

Biomechanics

In general, the biomechanical challenges of fitting and aligning the patient with a knee disarticulation are similar to those encountered with transfemoral amputation. Yet there are some notable differences. Many of these, such as intact thigh musculature, distal weight-bearing capacity, rotational control, suspension over the condyles, and an extended lever arm, have already been discussed. Because of these advantages, individuals who have had a knee disarticulation can generally be expected to have an equal or greater degree of control over their prostheses than will patients with amputations at higher levels.[7]

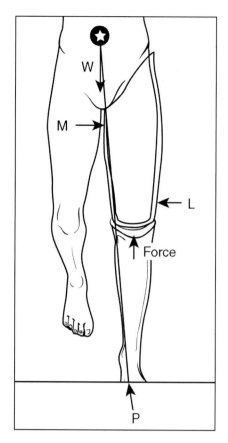

Figure 10 During single-limb support on the prosthesis, the body mass applies both vertical and rotary forces to the socket. The pelvis tends to drop away from the prosthesis, toward the opposite side. W = center of gravity, P = ground-reaction force, M (medial) and L (lateral) = force couple opposing the moment caused by P. *(Reproduced with permission from Hughes J: Biomechanics of the through-knee prosthesis.* Prosthet Orthot Int *1983;7:96-99.)*

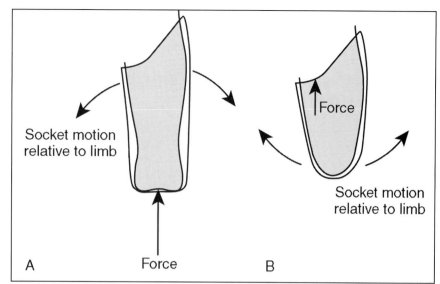

Figure 11 Center of rotation in a knee disarticulation socket and in a transfemoral socket. **A,** In a low-profile knee disarticulation socket, because of weight bearing on the end of the femur and the exclusion of the ischial tuberosity from the socket, the center of rotation of the socket about the limb is located distally. During midstance, the socket tends to rotate about this point and must be stabilized by counterpressure along the proximal aspect of the thigh. **B,** In a transfemoral socket, because of pelvic (ischial) bearing, the center of rotation of the socket about the limb is located proximally, at and around the ischium. As a result, the socket tends to rotate distally about the limb during midstance. Medial containment of the ischium may provide counterpressure to resist and decrease socket motion. *(Reproduced with permission from Hughes J: Biomechanics of the through-knee prosthesis.* Prosthet Orthot Int *1983;7:96-99.)*

One biomechanical distinction between transfemoral amputation and knee disarticulation is related to the forces generated on the residual limb by the socket during stance phase (Figure 10). A simplified discussion of these forces is presented here. The knee disarticulation prosthesis does not generally rely on ischial or gluteal support as does the transfemoral prosthesis. Thus the center of rotation in a knee disarticulation socket will be located at the distal end; that is, because the residual limb is end bearing during single-limb support on the prosthetic side, the socket will attempt to rotate in an external direc-

tion around the end of the residual limb in the coronal plane. The resultant pressures will be concentrated at the distal lateral femur and the proximal medial thigh. If this is not considered when the socket modifications are completed, the patient may have a resultant adductor roll at the proximal medial brim. With a transfemoral amputation, however, the distal end of the residual limb can tolerate only minimal pressure. Axial loading in the transfemoral socket is concentrated on the ischial tuberosity and proximal musculature (Figure 11). Thus the proximal posterior and proximal medial brim, and not the distal end, become the center of rotation of the transfemoral socket.[7]

Case Study

An 18-year-old man incurred thermal burns when he was 11 years old. Compartment syndrome developed in the lower left leg and the patient underwent a subsequent knee disar-

ticulation. Initially, he was fitted with a suspension pad and socks with a waist belt for auxiliary suspension. The suspension worked well, and he continued to use this method until he was 17 years of age. Initially, the femurs were of equal length, but in the first year postoperatively, the physician and family decided an epiphysiodesis should be performed to stop the growth of the left femur so that the difference in the length of the femurs would be approximately 6 cm. This difference would allow for more options for prosthetic components and would maintain the advantages of the knee disarticulation. After the growth was arrested, the prosthetist was able to place a hydraulic unit on the prosthesis and closely match the knee centers. The patient was interested in skateboarding and was quite successful at this activity for a few years. He later went on to be an active member of a local band. At 18 years of age, the patient transitioned to a prosthetic design with a flexible inner and rigid outer socket (Figure 7). He could tolerate end-weight bearing but wore a socket that allowed some weight to be supported by the ischial tuberosity. The inner socket is flexible enough for the residual limb to push through and get distal contact. The outer socket provides a void proximal to the femoral condyles so they can be pushed through easily. Suction and the contours of the femoral condyles provide suspension. The patient has also changed to a four-bar knee disarticulation knee on this prosthesis and a dynamic-response foot. The new design of the prosthesis has allowed the patient to be highly functional.

Summary

Knee disarticulation offers many functional advantages and a few cosmetic disadvantages compared with amputations at more proximal transfemoral levels. This procedure is preferred over transfemoral amputation for children because it preserves both femoral epiphyses, eliminates osseous overgrowth, and enables end-weight bearing. Among adults, knee disarticulation is generally considered to be functionally superior to amputation at transfemoral levels, but only if full distal weight bearing is achieved.[7] Many prosthetic sockets and knees have been designed to take advantage of the supracondylar suspension capacity, long lever arm, and distal load tolerance associated with knee disarticulation.

References

1. Michael J: Component selection criteria: Lower limb disarticulations. *Clin Prosthet Orthop* 1988;12:99-108.

2. Hagberg E, Berlin OK, Renstrom P: Function after through-knee compared with below-knee and above-knee amputation. *Prosthet Orthot Int* 1992;16:168-173.

3. Baumgartner R: Failures in through-knee amputation. *Prosthet Orthot Int* 1983;7:116-118.

4. www.aarogya.com/specialties/physiotherapy/amputationpost.asp. Accessed on July 16, 2004.

5. Botta P, Baumgartner R: Socket design and manufacturing technique for through-knee stumps. *Prosthet Orthot Int* 1983;7:100-103.

6. Gardner H: Basic steps in the fabrication of the through-knee socket, in *Report Workshop on Knee Disarticulation Prosthetics of the Subcommittee on Design and Development*. San Francisco, CA, National Research Council, Subcommittee on Design and Development, 1970.

7. Hughes J: Biomechanics of the through-knee prosthesis. *Prosthet Orthot Int* 1983;7:96-99.

8. McCollough NC III, Shea JD, Warren WD, Sarmiento A: The dysvascular amputee: Surgery and rehabilitation. *Curr Probl Surg* 1971:1-67.

9. www.coyotedandm.com. Accessed on July 16, 2004.

10. Oberg K: Knee mechanisms for through-knee prostheses. *Prosthet Orthot Int* 1983;7:107-112.

11. Michael JW: Modern prosthetic knee mechanisms. *Clin Orthop* 1999;361:39-47.

Chapter 42

Transfemoral Amputation: Surgical Management

Frank Gottschalk, MD, FRCSEd, FCS(SA)

Introduction

Transfemoral amputations are performed much less frequently than in the past, but they are often necessary in patients with very severe vascular disease and diabetes, in whom a lower level amputation is unlikely to heal. Most transfemoral amputees expend at least 65% more energy than normal for level walking at a regular walking speed.[1,2] Underlying medical conditions often contribute to this; for example, many dysvascular amputees lack the physical reserve required to be functional walkers and therefore often will be limited household walkers or unable to use a transfemoral prosthesis.[3] However, even individuals with no concomitant medical problems are unable to achieve normal gait in terms of velocity, cadence, or walking economy. Waters and associates[4] found that patients who had undergone a transfemoral amputation as a consequence of nonvascular causes also had limited ambulation and problems related to prosthetic use.

Many improvements have been made in prosthetic design and fabrication, but even the best prosthesis cannot provide a reasonable replacement for the limb following poor surgical technique that results in an inadequate residual limb. Too often the procedure is performed without thought for biomechanical principles or preservation of muscle function. One of the major goals of surgery is

primary wound healing, but biomechanical principles of lower limb function do not need to be sacrificed to achieve this.

When performing a transfemoral amputation, it is important to maintain a residual limb with as much length as possible. The longer the residual limb, the easier it is to suspend a prosthesis as well as to align it. The functional ability of the patient is also improved with a longer residual limb.

In some circumstances, the prevailing local pathology may require a more proximal transfemoral amputation. In these cases, a small portion of the femur at the trochanteric level should be left when possible. This allows for enhanced prosthetic fitting by providing additional contouring. The longest possible residual limb should be created because the longer limb provides a longer lever arm that can help with transfers and sitting balance. It can also reduce the potential for bone erosion through the soft tissues.

Biomechanics
Normal Alignment

The normal anatomic and mechanical alignment of the lower limb has been well defined[5-7] (Figure 1). The mechanical axis of the lower limb runs from the center of the femoral head through the center of the knee to the midpoint of the ankle. In normal

two-legged stance, this axis measures 3° from vertical and the femoral shaft axis measures 9° from vertical. Therefore, the normal anatomic alignment of the femur is in adduction, which

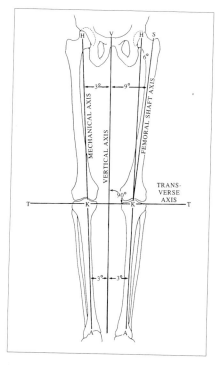

Figure 1 Mechanical and anatomic axes of normal lower limbs. H = hip; K = knee; A = ankle; S = shaft axis; T = transverse axis; V = vertical axis. (*Reproduced with permission from Gottschalk F, Kourosh S, Stills M, McClellan B, Roberts J: Does socket configuration influence the position of the femur in above-knee amputation? J Prosthet Orthot 1990;2: 94-102.*)

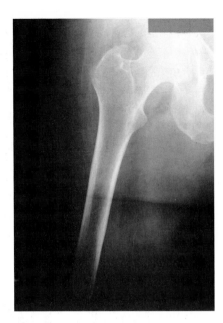

Figure 2 Radiograph showing abducted residual femur resulting from inadequate muscle stabilization. *(Reproduced with permission from Gottschalk F, Kourosh S, Stills M, McClellan B, Roberts J: Does socket configuration influence the position of the femur in above-knee amputation? J Prosthet Orthot 1990;2:94-102.)*

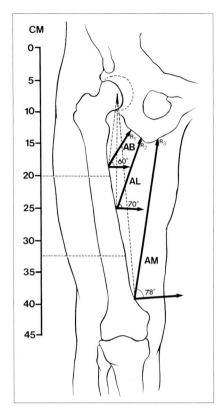

Figure 3 Moment arms of the three adductor muscles. Loss of the distal attachment of the adductor magnus results in a 70% loss of adductor strength. AB = adductor brevis; AL = adductor longus; AM = adductor magnus. *(Reproduced with permission from Gottschalk F, Kourosh S, Stills M, McClellan B, Roberts J: Does socket configuration influence the position of the femur in above-knee amputation? J Prosthet Orthot 1990;2:94-102.)*

allows the hip stabilizers (gluteus medius and minimus) and abductors (gluteus medius and tensor fasciae latae) to function normally and reduce the lateral motion of the center of mass of the body, thus producing a smoother and more energy-efficient gait.

In most transfemoral amputees, mechanical and anatomic alignment is disrupted because the residual femur is no longer in the natural anatomic alignment with the tibia, and the femoral shaft axis is in abduction compared with the contralateral limb. This is because in a conventional transfemoral amputation the major portion of the adductor muscle insertion is lost, especially the adductor magnus, which has an insertion on the mediodistal third of the femur.

During surgery, once this attachment is lost, the femur drifts into abduction because of the relatively unopposed action of the abductor system. The surgeon then sutures the residual adductors and the other muscles around the femur with the

residual femur in an abducted and flexed position. This abducted position leads to an increase in side lurch and higher energy consumption when the amputee walks.

Because the original insertions of the adductor muscles are lost, the effective moment arm of these muscles becomes shorter. Thus, the remaining smaller mass of adductor muscle would have to generate a larger force to hold the femur in its normal position. The muscles are unable to generate this force, so an abducted position results (Figure 2).

Prosthetists have recognized that residual femoral abduction compromises function. Newer prosthetic socket designs have tried to hold the

residual femur in a more adducted position by adjusting the socket shape[8] or using the ischium as a fulcrum.[9] However, a radiologic study of transfemoral amputees revealed that the position of the residual femur could not be controlled by the socket shape or alignment.[10] Positioning the soft tissues in adduction does not influence the position of the femur.

Of the three adductor muscles—the adductor magnus, the adductor longus, and the adductor brevis—the adductor magnus has a moment arm with the best mechanical advantage.[10,11] Figure 3 shows the directions of the components of force of the adductor muscles normal to the lines joining the points of attachment of the muscles. The adductor magnus is three to four times larger in cross-sectional area and volume than the adductor longus and brevis combined. Transsection of the adductor magnus at the time of amputation thus leads to a major loss of muscle cross-sectional area, a reduction in the effective moment arm, and a loss of up to 70% of the adductor pull.[11] This combination results in overall weakness of the adductor force of the thigh and subsequent abduction of the residual femur. In addition, loss of the extensor portion of the adductor magnus leads to a decrease in hip extension power and a greater likelihood of a flexion contracture.

Muscle Atrophy

Thiele and associates[12] showed that a reduction in muscle mass at amputation, combined with inadequate mechanical fixation of muscles and atrophy of the remaining musculature, was the major factor responsible for the decrease in muscle strength detected in transfemoral amputees. The decrease in strength of the flexor, extensor, abductor, and adductor muscles of the hip was most noticeable, which correlated with inadequate muscle stabilization.[13]

Jaegers and associates[14,15] documented muscle atrophy following transfemoral amputation. Three-dimensional MRI reconstructions of the hip muscles of 12 healthy transfemoral amputees were studied. Atrophy of 40% to 60% was noted in muscles that had been sectioned, whereas in the intact muscles, which included the iliopsoas, the gluteus medius, and the gluteus minimus, the atrophy ranged from 0% to 30% (Figure 4). The amount of atrophy of the intact muscles was related to residual limb length, with less atrophy in longer residual limbs. Despite the presence of muscle atrophy, fatty degeneration was not noted. The authors attempted to avoid abduction contracture of the hip by not reattaching the iliotibial tract. This strategy led to hip flexion contractures because of (1) the unopposed action of the iliopsoas muscle and (2) the large insertion of the gluteus maximus into the gluteal fascia, which continues into the iliotibial tract; thus, leaving the iliotibial tract unattached weakens the extensor mechanism.

The atrophy of the adductors also depended on the level of amputation. In none of the patients was the adductor magnus adequately reanchored. The more proximal the amputation, the greater the amount of muscle atrophy, and the more likely the development of an abduction contracture and atrophy of the glutei. The gluteus maximus was noted to be atrophied in all transfemoral amputees. Lack of fixation of the hamstrings resulted in up to 70% atrophy. Changes in muscle morphology after amputation are due to changes in volume and geometry (size and mass). Additional findings included reduced bone density, cortical atrophy, and increased volume of the femoral medullary cavity.[14]

Electromyographic Activity

Electromyographic studies during normal gait show activity of the adductor magnus at both the beginning and end of stance phase and into early swing phase.[16,17] A separate electromyographic study by Jaegers and associates[15] of transfemoral residual limbs showed that the intact muscles maintained the same sequence of ac-

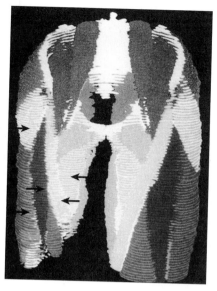

Figure 4 Three-dimensional MRI reconstruction of a residual limb following transfemoral amputation. Note the atrophy of the detached muscles (arrows). *(Reproduced with permission from Murdoch G, Wilson B (eds): Amputation: Surgical Practice and Patient Management. Oxford, England, Butterworth Heineman, 1996, pp 111-118.)*

tivity as a normal limb but for a longer time period. The activity of sectioned muscles depended on whether they had been reanchored and the level of amputation. Muscles that were reanchored correctly remained functional in locomotion, especially in a distal transfemoral amputation. The authors noted that alterations in muscle activity during walking were likely related to the altered morphology of once-biarticular hip muscles, the passive elements of the prosthesis, and the changed gait pattern of the amputee. The degree to which the gait was asymmetric was related to residual limb length. The greater the atrophy of the hip stabilizing muscles, the greater the lateral bending of the trunk to the prosthetic side.[18]

Surgical Approaches

The goal of surgery in a transfemoral amputation should be the creation of a dynamically balanced residual limb with good motor control and sensation. Preservation of the adductor magnus helps maintain the muscle balance between the adductors and

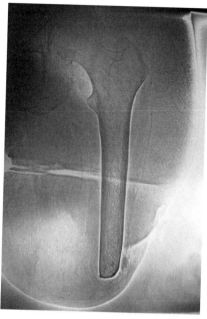

Figure 5 Xerogram of the thigh of a patient following transfemoral amputation shows the abducted residual femur and unattached medial soft tissue.

abductors by allowing the adductor magnus to maintain close to normal muscle power and a better mechanical advantage for holding the femur in the normal anatomic position. A residual limb with dynamically balanced function allows the amputee to function at a more normal level and use a prosthesis with greater ease.

Several authors[19-22] recommend transecting the muscles through the muscle belly at a length equivalent to half the diameter of the thigh at the level of amputation. Muscle stabilization has also been advocated as a means of controlling the femur, but in actuality this is infrequently achieved because the remaining muscle mass will have retracted at the time of transection (Figure 5). Reestablishing the normal muscle tension, as recommended in standard textbooks, then becomes more difficult. The authors attempted muscle stabilization either by myoplasty over the end of the femur or by myodesis to the femur just proximal to the end of the bone. Myoplasty, in which the agonist and antagonist groups of muscles are sutured to each other over the bone end, does not restore normal muscle tension, nor does it allow for adequate muscle control of the femur. The residual femur moves in the muscle envelope, producing pain and occasionally penetrating the soft-tissue envelope. Frequently a bursa develops at the end of the cut femur. The loss of muscle tension leads to some loss of control and reduced muscle strength in the residual limb. The soft-tissue envelope around the distal end of the residual limb is unstable and may compromise prosthetic fitting. Instead of myoplasty, a muscle-preserving technique is preferred whereby the distal insertions of the muscles are detached from their bony insertion and reattached to the residual femur under normal muscle tension. Once the myodesis has been done, any redundant tissue can be excised.

Indications for Transfemoral Amputation
Vascular Disease

Vascular disease, including vascular disease associated with diabetes, is the most common cause for transfemoral amputation in developed countries. Most patients who require a transfemoral amputation for vascular disease have widespread systemic manifestations of the disease, which has several implications. The disease may compromise the patients' postoperative rehabilitation. Their physical reserve is often insufficient to allow use of a prosthesis. Acute ischemia of the lower limb may result from thrombosis or embolism, and it may be difficult to determine which of the two conditions is the cause of the ischemia. Although embolism is the more likely diagnosis in older patients,[23] both systemic and local causes must be considered. Chronic ischemia necessitating amputation usually involves gangrene of the foot as a consequence of severe atherosclerosis. Van Niekerk and associates[24] have noted the association of failed bypass surgery with more proximal level amputations. Although success-ful vascular bypass surgery improves limb survival in patients with critical ischemia, failure of the procedure has resulted in more transfemoral amputations and residual limb complications. Infectious gangrene requiring amputation is most common in patients with diabetes mellitus. Patients with vascular disease associated with diabetes tend to be an average of 10 years younger at the time of amputation than those patients with purely vascular problems.[25] Patients with purely vascular disease are more likely to require transfemoral amputation than are patients with diabetes mellitus.[26]

Trauma

Most patients who require a transfemoral amputation as a result of trauma are younger than patients requiring amputation because of disease.[27] Usually, the indication for amputation is a combination of soft-tissue, vascular, neurologic, and bone damage so severe as to preclude satisfactory limb salvage or subsequent function. Foreign material may be embedded in the bone and soft tissues, requiring meticulous and at times repeated débridement.

Injuries from land mine blasts and other high-velocity penetrating wounds cause extensive tissue damage because of energy transfer to the tissues. Bullet wounds treated more than 24 hours after injury are four times more likely to require a transfemoral amputation than a transtibial amputation.[28] Any delay in treatment increases the risk of a more proximal amputation because of increased infection and greater soft-tissue damage. Depending on the severity of the initial injury, early intervention could minimize the risk of amputation or permit a lower level of amputation.

Maximum length should be retained, but it is also important to have a good soft-tissue envelope and avoid a split-thickness skin graft to bone. In these cases, at least a two-stage procedure is mandatory, leaving the wounds open at the initial stage to avoid wound infection and allow for additional débridement if necessary. On occasion, split-thickness skin grafts may be used on muscle to help preserve length. Revision surgery may be necessary and may require secondary skin expansion. Fractures of the femur should be stabilized by appropriate means rather than amputating through a proximal fracture site. The orientation of skin flaps is not critical, but closure must be without tension.

Infection

Amputation for severe soft-tissue infection or osteomyelitis should be done as a two-stage procedure at the minimum, with antibiotic coverage. In some situations, the placement of antibiotic-impregnated methylmethacrylate beads or absorbable antibiotic-impregnated substances is useful for controlling local infection. All infected tissue must be excised before definitive closure.

Tumor

With tumors, the level of amputation often is determined by the type, size, and location of the tumor. While observing the principles of tumor eradication, as long a residual limb as possible should be preserved so that maximum function can be maintained and restored.

Technique

Proper positioning of the patient on the operating table facilitates the surgery. The patient should be supine with the buttock on the side of the leg to be amputated elevated on folded sheets or blankets to allow for hip extension and adduction during the procedure.

A tourniquet is generally not used for most transfemoral amputations for vascular disease, but one may be used for traumatic amputations. When used, the sterile tourniquet should be placed as high on the thigh as possible and released before setting muscle tensions. Skin flaps should be marked before the skin incision (Figure 6). A long medial flap in the sagittal plane is recommended.[29] The flap

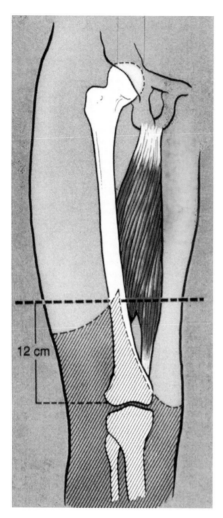

Figure 6 Proposed skin flaps and level of bone section before transfemoral amputation.

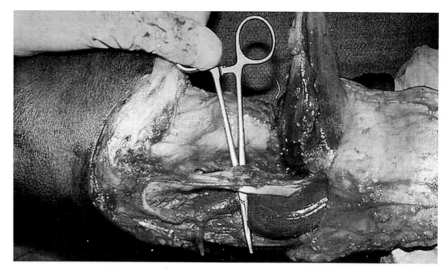

Figure 7 The adductor tendon is isolated before detachment from the adductor tubercle. The quadriceps tendon has been cut proximal to the patella. (Courtesy of John Bowker, MD.)

is developed as a myofasciocutaneous flap and sutured to the shorter lateral flap. In cases of trauma or tumor, however, any flap configuration that will best enhance the longest feasible residual limb is acceptable. Anterior skin flaps should not be longer than posterior flaps unless a long medial flap is not feasible. If anterior-posterior flaps are used, care should be taken to minimize the amount of subcutaneous tissue dissection to avoid damage to the perforating fascial vessels. Equal anterior-posterior skin flaps are unsatisfactory because this places the suture line under the end of the residual limb, which may lead to problems with prosthetic use. Another disadvantage of equal-sized flaps is the potential for increased skin

tension at wound closure because of inadequate flap length. The skin flaps should be made longer than may be initially thought necessary to avoid having to shorten the bone more than otherwise necessary because insufficient skin is available for closure.

After the medial skin flap is created, the adductor magnus tendon attachment to the adductor tubercle of the femur is identified[30] (Figure 7). The tendon is detached by sharp dissection, marked with a suture, and reflected proximally, exposing Hunter's canal. The femoral artery and vein are identified.

Once the major vessels have been isolated, they should be ligated and cut at the proposed level of bone section. The major nerves should be dissected 2 to 4 cm proximal to the proposed bone cut and sectioned with a new, sharp blade. The central vessel can be lightly cauterized or secured by a suture around the nerve. Local anesthetic infiltration of bupivacaine by means of a small catheter placed in the nerve is believed to decrease the severity of postoperative pain.[31]

Muscles should not be sectioned until they have been identified. The quadriceps is detached just proximal to the patella, retaining some of its tendinous portion. The adductor magnus is detached from the adduc-

tor tubercle by sharp dissection and reflected medially to expose the femoral shaft. It may be necessary to detach 2 to 3 cm of the adductor magnus from the linea aspera to increase its mobility. The smaller muscles, including the sartorius and gracilis, and the more posterior group of muscles should be transected approximately 2 to 2.5 cm longer than the proposed bone cut to facilitate their inclusion and anchorage. The biceps femoris is transected at the level of the bone cut.

The femur is exposed just above the condylar level and transected approximately 12 to 14 cm above the knee joint line with an oscillating power saw. The location of the cut may vary depending on the patient, especially with trauma. The blade should be cooled with saline. This level is recommended because it allows sufficient space for placement of the prosthetic knee joint. Two or three small drill holes for the purpose of anchoring sutures are made on the lateral cortex of the distal end of the femur 1 to 1.5 cm from the cut end. Additional cortical holes are drilled anteriorly and posteriorly at a similar distance.[27,29]

The femur is held in maximum adduction while the adductor magnus is brought across the cut end of the femur while maintaining its tension. The adductor magnus tendon is then

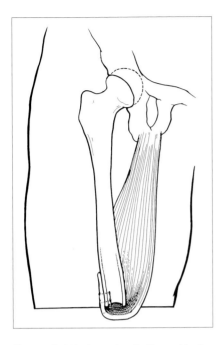

Figure 8 Attachment of the adductor magnus to the lateral part of the femur. *Courtesy of John Bowker, MD.)*

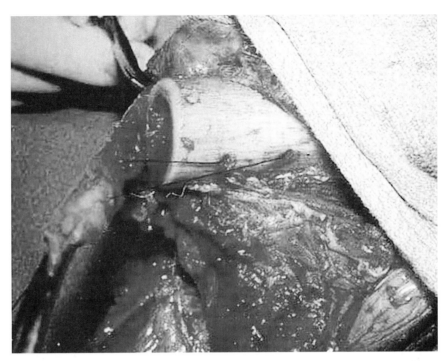

Figure 9 Intraoperative photograph showing the adductor tendon with sutures through drill holes on the lateral femur. *(Courtesy of John Bowker, MD.)*

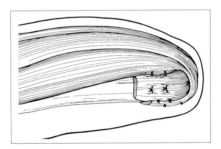

Figure 10 Attachment of the quadriceps over the adductor magnus.

sutured with nonabsorbable or long-lasting absorbable suture material to the lateral aspect of the residual femur via the drill holes (Figures 8 and 9). Additional anterior and posterior sutures are placed to prevent the muscle from sliding forward or backward on the end of the bone.

With the hip in extension to avoid creating a hip flexion contracture, the quadriceps is then sutured to the posterior aspect of the femur via the posterior drill holes (Figure 10). These sutures may also be passed through the adductor magnus tendon. The remaining hamstrings are then anchored to the posterior area of the adductor magnus or the quadriceps. The

investing fascia of the thigh is then sutured as dictated by the skin flaps. An adequate number of subcutaneous sutures to minimize skin tension may be used to approximate the skin edges, and fine nylon sutures (No. 3.0 or 4.0) or skin staples[29] are used to close the skin. They should be placed no closer than 1 cm apart, especially in dysvascular patients. The use of forceps on the skin edges is discouraged.

Figures 11 and 12 are postoperative radiographs showing the femur held in adduction by the adductor myodesis. Figure 13 shows a healed residual limb following transfemoral amputation.

Early Postoperative Care

Postoperatively, the residual limb should be wrapped with an elastic bandage, which may be applied as a hip spica with the hip extended. Although rigid dressings control edema and residual limb position better than soft dressings do, they are cumbersome to apply, do not offer any great advantage in the long term in trans-

femoral amputations, and have distinct disadvantages. The rigid hip spica restricts hip mobility, increases the risk of pressure sores over bony prominences, and makes postoperative management of patients more difficult. The use of rigid dressings for transfemoral amputations has been abandoned by many centers. A well-applied elastic bandage will not slip off the residual limb but should be removed and reapplied at least once daily for careful skin inspection because it can shift.

Another method of controlling swelling and reducing discomfort is to apply an elastic shrinker with a waist belt. The shrinkers are made of a one- or two-way stretch material that applies even pressure distally to proximally. The waist belt helps prevent the shrinker from slipping off. The shrinker may be applied at the first dressing change, at 48 hours postoperatively. The use of elastomer liners for control of edema may also be helpful in some patients.

Postoperative phantom limb pain immediately following surgery is not uncommon and can be reduced by infiltrating the sectioned nerve with bupivacaine at the time of surgery, as mentioned earlier. Local anesthetic can be administered directly to the nerve continuously or intermittently for 3 to 4 days and then discontinued. Two studies[31,32] have noted that this method may be beneficial for immediate relief of postoperative pain and showed that the amount of postoperative narcotic analgesic could be reduced in this way. It should be noted that neither of these studies was randomized or controlled. Continuous infusion does not prevent long-term residual or phantom limb pain, however. In addition, long-standing preoperative pain does not appear to be influenced significantly by any form of analgesic management. The use of perineural infusion does not prevent residual or phantom limb pain in patients who have had a lower limb amputation.

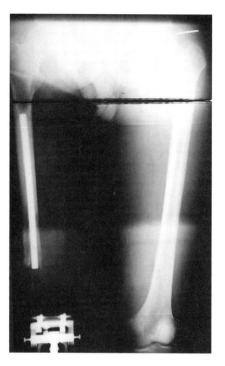

Figure 11 Weight-bearing radiograph of a patient wearing a prosthesis to show alignment of the residual femur.

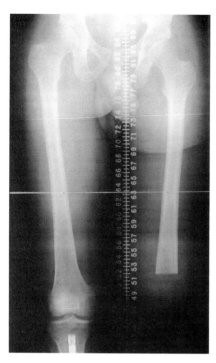

Figure 12 Radiograph of a residual femur held in normal anatomic alignment following adductor myodesis.

Late Postoperative Care

While the wound is healing, the patient should be mobilized in a wheelchair and on the parallel bars, and upper body exercises should be started, with the goal for the patient to have sufficient upper body strength to use crutches or a walker. Flexion contractures should be prevented by correctly positioning the patient in bed, as well as with initiation of muscle-strengthening exercises. In addition, conditioning of the contralateral leg is necessary. Most often, the sutures or staples can be removed approximately 2 weeks postoperatively for traumatic amputations and at 3 weeks postoperatively in the dysvascular amputee. During this time the patient will have been wrapping the residual limb or using a shrinker. After suture removal, a temporary adjustable plastic prosthesis can be fitted and gait training started.

With aggressive rehabilitation techniques and a motivated patient, early return to walking can be accom-

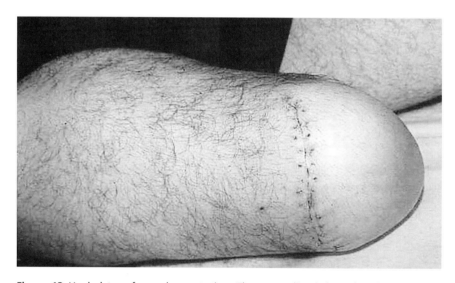

Figure 13 Healed transfemoral amputation. The suture line is lateral and proximal to the end of the residual limb.

plished in a short time. Patients who do not have the physical or mental ability to participate in a rehabilitation program designed to teach prosthesis use will be better off using a wheelchair. Transfer training is important in these cases. The decision whether to provide the patient with a wheelchair should be made early in the postoperative period.

The overall rehabilitation of the patient with a transfemoral amputation begins at the time of surgery and continues until the patient has achieved his or her individual maximum functional independence. Appropriate surgical techniques allow techniques for easier prosthetic fitting and facilitate physical therapy, helping the patient achieve the goals that have been set by the patient and the treating team.

References

1. Volpicelli LJ, Chambers RB, Wagner FW Jr: Ambulation levels of bilateral lower-extremity amputees: Analysis of one hundred and three cases. *J Bone Joint Surg Am* 1983;65:599-605.

2. Hagberg K, Branemark R: Consequences of non-vascular trans-femoral amputation: A survey of quality of life, prosthetic use and problems. *Prosthet Orthot Int* 2001;25:186-194.

3. Gonzalez EG, Corcoran PJ, Reyes RL: Energy expenditure in below-knee amputees: Correlation with stump length. *Arch Phys Med Rehabil* 1974;55:111-119.

4. Waters RL, Perry J, Antonelli D, Hislop H: Energy cost of walking of amputees: The influence of level of amputation. *J Bone Joint Surg Am* 1976;58:42-46.

5. Freeman MAR: The surgical anatomy and pathology of the arthritic knee, in Freeman MAR (ed): *Arthritis of the Knee.* Berlin, Germany, Springer-Verlag, 1980, pp 31-56.

6. Hungerford DS, Krackow KA, Kenna RV: (eds): *Total Knee Arthroplasty: A Comprehensive Approach.* Baltimore, MD, Williams & Wilkins, 1984, pp 34-39.

7. Maquet PGJ: (ed): *Biomechanics of the Knee.* Berlin, Germany, Springer-Verlag, 1976, p 22.

8. Long IA: Normal shape-normal alignment (NSNA) above-knee prosthesis. *Clin Prosthet Orthot* 1985;9:9-14.

9. Sabolich J: Contoured adducted trochanteric-controlled alignment method (CAT-CAM): Introduction and basic principles. *Clin Prosthet Orthot* 1985;9:15-26.

10. Gottschalk FA, Kourosh S, Stills M, McClellan B, Roberts J: Does socket configuration influence the position of the femur in above-knee amputation? *J Prosthet Orthot* 1989;2:94-102.

11. Gottschalk FA, Stills M: The biomechanics of trans-femoral amputation. *Prosthet Orthot Int* 1994;18:12-17.

12. Thiele B, James U, Stalberg E: Neurophysiological studies on muscle function in the stump of above-knee amputees. *Scand J Rehabil Med* 1973;5:67-70.

13. James U: Maximal isometric muscle strength in healthy active male unilateral above-knee amputees: With special regard to the hip joint. *Scand J Rehabil Med* 1973;5:55-66.

14. Jaegers SM, Arendzen JH, de Jongh HJ: Changes in hip muscles after above-knee amputation. *Clin Orthop* 1995;319:276-284.

15. Jaegers SM, Arendzen JH, de Jongh HJ: An electromyographic study of the hip muscles of transfemoral amputees in walking. *Clin Orthop* 1996;328:119-128.

16. Green DL, Morris JM: Role of adductor longus and adductor magnus in postural movements and in ambulation. *Am J Phys Med* 1970;49:223-240.

17. Inman VT, Ralston HJ, Todd F: (eds): *Human Walking.* Baltimore, MD, Williams & Wilkins, 1981, pp 102-117.

18. Jaegers SM, Arendzen JH, de Jongh HJ: Prosthetic gait of unilateral transfemoral amputees: A kinematic study. *Arch Phys Med Rehabil* 1995;76:736-743.

19. Bohne WHO: (ed): *Atlas of Amputation Surgery.* New York, NY, Thieme Medical Publishers, 1987, pp 79-112.

20. Burgess EM: Knee disarticulation and above-knee amputation, in Moore WS, Malone JM (eds): *Lower Extremity Amputation.* Philadelphia, PA, WB Saunders, 1989, pp 132-146.

21. Harris WR: Principles of amputation surgery, in Kostuik JP, Gillespie R (eds): *Amputation Surgery and Rehabilitation: The Toronto Experience.* New York, NY, Churchill Livingstone, 1981, pp 37-49.

22. Barnes RW: (ed): *Amputations: An Illustrated Manual.* Philadelphia, PA, Hanley & Belfus, 2000, pp 103-117.

23. McIntyre KE, Berman SS: Patient evaluation and preparation for amputation, in Rutherford RB (ed): *Vascular Surgery.* Philadelphia, PA, WB Saunders, 2000, pp 2181-2184.

24. Van Niekerk LJ, Stewart CP, Jain AS: Major lower limb amputation following failed infrainguinal vascular bypass surgery: A prospective study on amputation levels and stump complications. *Prosthet Orthot Int* 2001;25:29-33.

25. Jensen JS, Mandrup-Poulsen T, Krasnik M: Wound healing complications following major amputations of the lower limb. *Prosthet Orthot Int* 1982;6:105-107.

26. Christensen KS, Falstie-Jensen N, Christensen ES, Brochner-Mortensen J: Results of amputation for gangrene in diabetic and non-diabetic patients: Selection of amputation level using photoelectric measurements of skin-perfusion pressure. *J Bone Joint Surg Am* 1988;70:1514-1519.

27. Gottschalk F: Traumatic amputations, in Bucholz RW, Heckman JD (eds): *Rockwood and Green's Fractures in Adults,* ed 5. Philadelphia, PA, Lippincott-Williams & Wilkins, 2001, pp 391-414.

28. Molde A: Victims of war: Surgical principles must not be forgotten (again)! *Acta Orthop Scand* 1998;281(suppl):54-57.

29. Gottschalk F: Transfemoral amputation: Biomechanics and surgery. *Clin Orthop* 1999;361:15-22.

30. Gottschalk F: Above-knee amputation, in Murdoch G, Jacobs NA, Wilson AB (eds): *Report of ISPO Consensus Conference on Amputation Surgery.* Copenhagen, Denmark, International Society for Prosthetics and Orthotics, 1992, pp 60-65.

31. Malawer MM, Buch R, Khurana JS, Garvey T, Rice L: Postoperative infusional continuous regional analgesia: A technique for relief of postoperative pain following major extremity surgery. *Clin Orthop* 1991;266:227-237.

32. Pinzur MS, Garla PG, Pluth T, Vrbos L: Continuous postoperative infusion of a regional anesthetic after an amputation of the lower extremity: A randomized clinical trial. *J Bone Joint Surg Am* 1996;78:1501-1505.

Chapter 43

Transfemoral Amputation: Prosthetic Management

C. Michael Schuch, CPO
Charles H. Pritham, CPO

Introduction

The basic goals for fitting and aligning prostheses for transfemoral amputees are simple enough—comfort, function, and cosmesis. Achieving these goals, however, is a significant challenge because of the interrelationships among patient diagnosis, prognosis, medical history, residual and intact limb anatomy and kinesiology, and available prosthetic technology.

Review of Transfemoral Biomechanics
Analysis and Relevance of Residual Limb Range of Motion

Careful measurement and evaluation of residual and intact limb anatomy and kinesiology are essential for correct socket design and initial socket alignment. The necessity for measurement of length, circumference, and diameter is obvious. However, accurate evaluation of the range of motion of the residual limb in the sagittal and coronal (frontal) planes is perhaps more important and certainly less understood.

Range of motion in the sagittal plane consists of flexion and extension of the residual femur. Especially important is the ability to extend the residual femur fully. The normal hip is generally capable of a maximum of 5° of extension posterior to the vertical without anterior pelvic rotation or lordosis.[1] The inability to fully extend the residual femur usually indicates a hip flexion contracture. Because of their insertion, the hip flexors have a mechanical advantage over the hip extensors; therefore, hip flexion contractures are not uncommon and are especially likely to occur in shorter residual limbs. This range of motion in the sagittal plane should be documented along with other necessary measurements.

Range of motion in the coronal plane consists of abduction and adduction of the residual femur. Especially important is the amputee's ability to adduct the residual femur as much as the femur on the opposite side. Normal femoral adduction angles average about 6°.[2] The inability to fully adduct the residual femur usually indicates an abduction contracture. The adductors of the femur are at a mechanical disadvantage compared with the abductors because of their location and the fact that the most effective adductors have been severed at amputation. Abduction contractures, like hip flexion contractures, are not uncommon and are more prevalent in shorter residual limbs. This range of motion in the coronal plane should also be documented.

The analysis and measurement of the ranges of motion of the femur in the sagittal and coronal planes are important for establishing the initial angular alignment of the transfemoral prosthetic socket. Proper planning and incorporation of these angular measurements into the socket and overall prosthetic design will facilitate certain biomechanical and alignment advantages for the amputee during the various phases of gait.

Biomechanics of Knee Stability: Stance Phase of Gait

Knee stability in a transfemoral prosthesis is defined by the ability of the prosthetic knee to remain extended and fully supportive of the amputee during the stance phase of walking. Knee instability is the buckling or unintended flexing of the prosthetic knee during stance. Instability can be quite dangerous, causing unexpected falls. Excessive knee stability is a condition in which the knee of the prosthesis is so stable and resistant to flexing that it is difficult for the amputee to initiate the knee flexion required for toe-off and swing of the shank, resulting in high energy expenditure and an unnatural swing phase of the gait cycle. The distinction between knee instability and excessive knee stability is very fine. The key to avoiding these two undesirable characteristics and achieving optimum knee stability is an understanding of the biomechanics of prosthetic knee function.

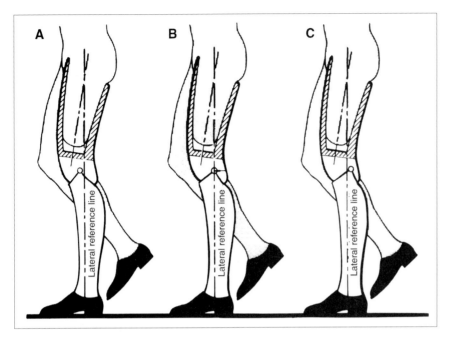

Figure 1 Transfemoral alignment variations and their effect on knee control. **A,** The knee axis is placed anterior to the lateral weight reference line to create a voluntary knee control alignment. This alignment has no inherent mechanical stability. **B,** The knee axis is placed directly on the lateral weight reference line to create a neutral knee control alignment. This alignment is stable during stance but requires voluntary control at heel strike. **C,** The knee axis is placed posterior to the lateral weight reference line to create an involuntary knee control alignment. This alignment is mechanically stable throughout stance phase, including heel strike. *(Reproduced with permission from Radcliff CW: Functional considerations in the fitting of above-knee prostheses. Artif Limbs 1955;2:35-60.)*

The two biomechanical descriptions of knee stability control are termed involuntary knee control and voluntary knee control[3-8] (Figure 1). With involuntary knee control, the control is not subject to the will of the amputee but is automatic. The degree of involuntary control varies in complexity. One form of involuntary knee control is alignment stability in which the prosthesis (when viewed laterally) is aligned so that the knee axis is posterior to the biomechanical weight line, which generally extends from the midpoint of the socket proximally to the midpoint of foot contact with the ground. With the weight line anterior to the prosthetic knee axis, increased weight bearing tends to force the knee into extension and locks it against the extension stop. Excessive knee stability occurs when the prosthetic knee joint is located too far posterior to the biomechanical weight line. Other forms of involuntary knee control are mechanical, including locking knees,

weight-activated stance-control knees, and certain hydraulic knee systems.

With voluntary knee control, the control is directly subject to the will of the amputee and is achieved and maintained through active participation of the hip extensor muscles. These muscles include the gluteal muscles (primarily the gluteus maximus) and the hamstring muscle group. When these muscles can exert enough force and are consciously fired at the proper time by the amputee, knee stability is achieved in the stance phase of gait. For the stronger and more physically fit amputee, voluntary control provides for a smoother and more energy-efficient gait because it takes less effort than involuntary knee alignment to initiate swing-phase flexion. Better muscle tone and coordination are achieved as well. Voluntary control is not always possible, however, particularly when amputees have muscle weakness or hip flexion contractures or fear falling, characteristics common in elderly and otherwise debilitated amputees.

Other factors that contribute to control of knee stability include initial socket flexion, the trochanter-knee-ankle relationship, and ankle-foot dynamics.[3-8] The hip extensor muscles contribute to knee stability by pulling the prosthetic knee into extension or by maintaining existing knee extension. The hamstring muscles, which are transected by transfemoral amputation, are believed to function best when stretched just beyond their resting length. The only fully intact hip extensor, the gluteus maximus, is not capable of exerting any significant force until the hip is flexed at least 15°.[3-5] To achieve some degree of stretching of the gluteus maximus, the prosthetic socket is designed for and aligned in a position of initial flexion. The amount of initial flexion increases as the amputee's ability to extend the hip decreases. The only limiting factor is the length of the residual limb. For longer residual limbs, some cosmesis has to be sacrificed as initial flexion is increased. In addition to enhancing voluntary control of knee stability, initial socket flexion decreases the tendency of the amputee to increase pelvic lordosis to compensate for weak hip extensors.

The trochanter-knee-ankle relationship is the most common reference for analyzing transfemoral alignment in the sagittal plane and is best understood as the socket-knee-ankle relationship. The more posterior the knee joint is placed with reference to the socket-ankle line, the more stable the knee becomes. In most transfemoral prostheses, the socket is mounted on an adjustable alignment device that permits multidimensional freedom of movement of the socket with respect to the knee-shank and ankle-foot components. (Such an alignment device may later be transferred out of the finished prosthesis.) In this ideal situation, the AP setting of the socket is determined under dynamic conditions as the amputee's gait is analyzed carefully. The goal is to align the prosthesis so that the amputee uses the least amount of alignment stability or involuntary knee control necessary, thereby optimizing voluntary knee control. A critical balance between these two biomechanical conditions must be maintained to achieve a safe yet efficient gait.

Ankle-foot dynamics are the shock-absorbing and stabilizing abilities of this prosthetic component system. The most unstable phase of gait for a transfemoral amputee is shortly after heel strike. During loading response, a moment or torque is created that tends to rotate the shin forward, flexing the knee and thus creating an instant of potential knee instability (Figure 2). In normal human locomotion, smooth and uninterrupted plantar flexion dampens the significant moment initiated at heel strike. In the transfemoral prosthesis, ankle-foot components that more closely replicate normal ankle-foot function enhance knee stability. If knee stability is of particular concern, such as in the case of isolated hip extensor weakness, foot components that reduce the induced knee flexion moment should be considered. Single-axis or multiaxial feet or those with a soft heel will serve this purpose well. The goal is inherent stability through early stance, followed by smooth, uninterrupted, gradually increasing flexion through initial swing phase.

Biomechanics of Pelvis and Trunk Stability: Stance Phase of Gait

When considering the gait of the transfemoral amputee, two specific goals are mediolateral pelvis-trunk stability and a narrow-based gait. These interrelated objectives are perhaps the most difficult challenges facing the prosthetist and the amputee.

In normal locomotion, the pelvis drops about 5° toward the unsupported side during midstance; this motion occurs around the hip joint of the weight-bearing limb.[3-8] The hip abductors, primarily the gluteus me-

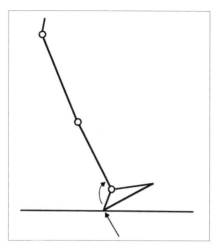

Figure 2 At heel strike, a moment or torque is created that tends to rotate the shin forward and flex the knee, creating an instant of potential knee instability. *(Reproduced with permission from Anderson MH, Sollars RE (eds):* Prosthetic Principles: Above-Knee Amputations. *Springfield, IL, Charles C Thomas Publishers, 1960, pp 129-146.)*

dius, prevent any additional drop through controlled eccentric contraction. This phenomenon is one of several gait determinants designed to provide energy efficiency in normal locomotion.[9] The pelvic shift that occurs helps maintain the center of gravity over the base of support, which is a primary goal of gait training for use of a transfemoral prosthesis.

In normal locomotion, weight bearing occurs through the bones of the leg, and contraction of the gluteus medius is effective in controlling pelvic tilt at the hip joint of the stance leg. In the case of the transfemoral amputee, the femur does not terminate in a foot planted firmly on the ground. The residual femur, now a lever no more than 40% of the normal length of the lower limb, floats in a mass of muscle, tissue, and fluid. The residual femur tends to displace laterally in the mass of residual muscle and tissue rather than maintain horizontal stability of the pelvis and trunk. This lack of support and ineffective pelvic stabilization results initially in pelvic drop away from the prosthetic support leg (positive Trendelenburg's sign), with concurrent

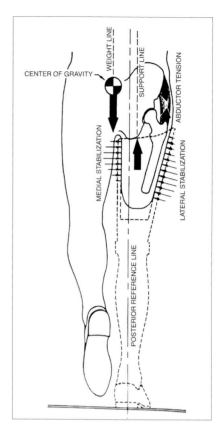

Figure 3 Hip abductors can be used to achieve lateral stabilization of the pelvis only if adequate lateral support is provided to the femur. *(Reproduced with permission from Radcliff CW: Functional considerations in the fitting of above-knee prostheses.* Artif Limbs *1955;2:35-60.)*

perineal or pubic ramus pressure and discomfort. The amputee will typically compensate by widening the base of the gait and using trunk sway over the wide-based point of support (compensatory Trendelenburg) to maintain a comfortable gait.

Effective pelvis-trunk stabilization and a narrow-based gait can be achieved in a transfemoral prosthesis only if adequate lateral support is provided to the femur (Figure 3). The femur must be maintained in a position as near as possible to normal adduction, thereby putting the gluteus medius and other abductor muscles in a position of stretch that allows them to function most effectively. This objective is accomplished through socket design and alignment, with particular attention to the medial and lateral walls of the socket.[3-8]

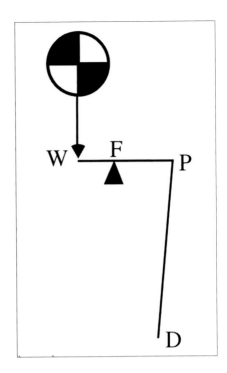

Figure 4 Illustration of the lever principle. W = weight, F = fulcrum, P = proximal part of femur, D = distal part of femur. *(Adapted with permission from Anderson MH, Sollars RE (eds): Prosthetic Principles: Above-Knee Amputations. Springfield, IL, Charles C Thomas Publishers, 1960, pp 129-146.)*

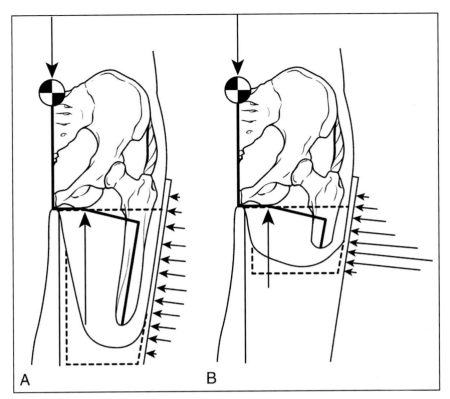

Figure 5 Relationship of femoral length to force distribution. **A,** The greater the femur length, the greater the ability to distribute pressure and forces. **B,** The short femur is subjected to a higher pressure concentration. *(Adapted with permission from Anderson MH, Sollars RE (eds): Prosthetic Principles: Above-Knee Amputations. Springfield, IL, Charles C Thomas Publishers, 1960, pp 129-146.)*

In the quadrilateral socket, the proximal medial wall is flat and vertical to help distribute stance-phase counterpressure forces; the lateral wall of the socket should be designed and aligned in a position of adduction that matches the adduction angle measurement obtained in the evaluation of residual limb range of motion. Restriction of adduction, such as an abduction contracture, will significantly limit the ability to control pelvis and trunk stability. Additional factors that affect mediolateral pelvis and trunk stability include the length of the residual limb, proximomedial tissue density, and proper alignment of the prosthetic components below the socket.

A longer residual limb provides a longer lever and greater surface area over which to distribute the inherent forces. In the simple lever system illustrated in Figure 4, the effective lever arms are W-F and P-D, and resulting forces or moments depend on weight and lever length. For example, if the lever W-F has an effective length of 4 in and the force or weight is 150 lb, the moment or torque around this lever system will be 600 in-lb. If the lever P-D is 10 in, only 60 lb of force need be exerted to equalize the moment or torque of 600 in-lb and thus stabilize the pelvis and trunk. However, if the femur length as simulated by lever P-D is only 5 in long, 120 lb of force is required to equalize the 600 in-lb of torque, thus subjecting the hypothetical femur to much greater levels of pressure.[3-5] The more evenly and broadly these pressures can be distributed, the more tolerable they become. If the force is distributed over a smaller area, pressure concentration may cause discomfort, pain, or skin breakdown (Figure 5). For this reason, the shorter the residual limb, the more difficult is the task of establishing and maintaining mediolateral pelvis and trunk stability. In these situations, the ideal gait is compromised to achieve the primary goal of comfort.

The biomechanical reaction to the contraction of the hip abductors and resultant femoral force against the lateral wall of the transfemoral socket is a laterally directed force or moment concentrated in the perineum by the proximomedial aspect of the transfemoral socket during midstance. When coupled with the normal and desirable gait determinant of lateral pelvic shift over the support limb, the forces generated at the perineum are significant. Firmer, denser, and more muscular residual limbs, which are often longer as well, are better able to tolerate this reaction force.[10-12] Soft, fleshy (and often shorter) residual limbs lacking muscle tone in the adductor region are very susceptible to tissue trauma and bruising and offer a less stable reaction point for support. In such cases, mediolateral pelvis-trunk stability will be compromised unless these reaction forces are directed

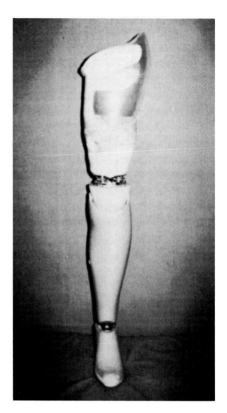

Figure 6 Alignment devices are between the transfemoral socket and the prosthetic knee component and between the shin and foot. The proximal alignment device allows angulation in both the sagittal and coronal planes (flexion-extension and adduction-abduction) as well as linear slide in the same planes of motion. The distal alignment device facilitates angulation changes of the foot, such as dorsiflexion or plantar flexion, eversion, and inversion.

against more stable anatomic features in this area such as the skeleton. The advent of the ischial-ramal containment transfemoral socket design provides a solution to this problem.

Prosthetic alignment contributes significantly to trunk and pelvis stability. Controversy exists over socket and foot relationships in the coronal plane.[13-15] Foot placement in the coronal plane is best determined dynamically with adjustable alignment devices within the prosthesis (Figure 6).

Biomechanics of Knee and Shank Control: Swing Phase of Gait

The goals of the swing phase of gait are normally easier for the transfemoral amputee to attain and the requirements are less demanding than those of the stance phase. However, significant deviations can result in greater energy consumption.

When the prosthesis has too much "alignment stability," excess energy and effort are required to initiate knee flexion. Overcoming such alignment stability takes effort and delays the initiation of swing phase. Vaulting, which is usually regarded as a deviation in response to a prosthesis that is too long, can also serve to subtly compensate for a delayed advancement of the prosthetic shank in mid-swing.

Swing-phase tracking refers to the smoothness of the pathway of the prosthetic limb during the swing phase of the gait cycle. Goals are to minimize vertical displacement of the prosthesis on the residual limb and to minimize deviations in the sagittal plane as the prosthetic limb advances during swing phase. Problems with vertical displacement stem from poor suspension and resulting piston action and/or inappropriate prosthesis length. Deviations in the sagittal plane include transverse plane "whips" during the swing phase that are caused by improper socket shape or improper knee axis alignment, as well as circumduction, which is usually caused by excessive prosthesis length or poor alignment.

Transfemoral Socket Designs: Variations and Indications

The total-contact quadrilateral socket, which has both US and European variations, was the socket of choice from the 1960s until the 1990s but has gradually been replaced by new designs and techniques.[16] In the early 1980s, innovative designs for transfemoral sockets began to emerge and were introduced under various acronyms. This basic socket design and philosophy has become known as the ischial containment socket. The origin is attributed to Ivan Long,

with further developments made by John Sabolich, Thomas Guth, Daniel Shamp, and Christopher Hoyt.[17] Techniques for fabricating this socket are similar to those of the quadrilateral socket; the chief difference is encasement of the ischiopubic ramus within the socket proper and related biomechanical and socket comfort enhancements.

Hall[18] described five principles of socket design. Although these were intended as design objectives of the quadrilateral socket, they apply equally well to any modern transfemoral socket. (1) The socket must be properly contoured and reliefed for functioning muscles. (2) Stabilizing pressure should be applied to the skeletal structures as much as possible, avoiding areas with functioning muscles. (3) Where possible, functioning muscles should be stretched to slightly greater than resting length for maximum power. (4) Properly applied pressure is well tolerated by neurovascular structures. (5) Force is best tolerated when distributed over the largest available area.

Regardless of the fitting method employed, the socket for any amputee must provide the same overall functional characteristics, including comfortable weight bearing, stability in the stance phase of gait, a narrow-based gait, and as normal a swing phase as possible consistent with the residual function available to the amputee.[19] These characteristics provide a context for the following description of transfemoral socket designs.

Quadrilateral Socket

The term quadrilateral refers to the appearance of the socket when viewed in the transverse plane (Figure 7) because there are four readily distinguishable sides or walls. The orientation of the four walls will vary according to the amputee's specific anatomy and the biomechanical requirements of the socket. According to Radcliffe,[20] "the socket is truly more than just a cross-section shape at the ischial level, it is a three-dimensional receptacle for the stump

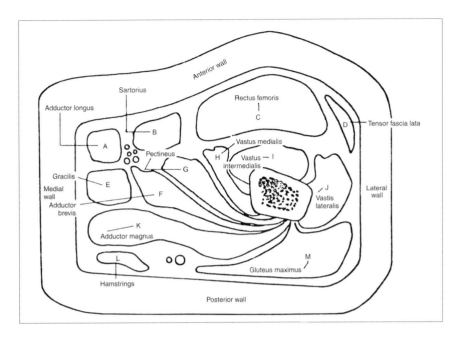

Figure 7 Transverse cross-section of the proximal aspect of a quadrilateral socket. *(Courtesy of Northwestern University, Evanston, IL.)*

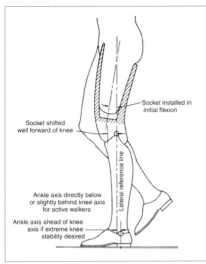

Figure 8 Socket aligned in initial flexion to avoid excessive pelvic rotation during the latter part of stance phase. *(Reproduced with permission from Radcliff CW: Functional considerations in the fitting of above-knee prostheses. Artif Limbs 1955; 2:35-60.)*

with contours at every level which are justifiable on a sound biomechanical basis."

Weight bearing in the quadrilateral socket is achieved primarily through the ischium and the gluteal musculature. This combination of skeletal and muscular anatomy rests on top of the posterior wall of the socket, which is formed into a wide seat parallel to the ground. Countersupport, intended to maintain the position of the ischium and gluteals on this posterior seat, is provided by the medial third of the anterior wall of the socket, which is carefully fitted against Scarpa's triangle. The AP dimension of these respective walls is based on anatomic measurements. A common error is to create deep, exaggerated Scarpa's triangle contours. As the concepts of total contact and total surface bearing became better understood, anterior counterpressure was deemphasized. Clinical experience with other socket designs has shown that enlarging this dimension of the socket often allows additional comfort in the perineum with no loss of comfortable weight bearing. This suggests that tissue and muscle loading occur as a supplementary weight-bearing mechanism. The

concept of total surface bearing suggests that weight bearing be as evenly distributed over the entire surface area as possible, with the forces and loads being evenly shared by skeletal anatomy, muscle, soft tissue, and hydrostatic compression of residual limb fluids.[21]

Incorporation of adduction into the quadrilateral socket depends on the range of motion available, generally a function of the length of the residual limb. The goal is to reestablish the normal adduction angle of the femur with respect to a level pelvis. The quadrilateral socket accomplishes this by contouring the lateral wall in the desired degree of adduction. The entire lateral wall is flattened along the shaft of the adducted femur with the exception of relief for the distal end of the femur. Proximal to the greater trochanter, the lateral wall is contoured into and over the hip abductor muscle group to discourage abduction. Midstance contraction of the hip abductor muscles leads to reaction forces occurring in the proximomedial aspect of the residual limb and socket. To provide counterpressure and distribute these reaction forces, the contour of the medial wall of the

socket is flat in the sagittal plane along the proximal 4 inches of the socket before reversing proximally at the brim into a smooth outward flare that is directed away from the residual limb and toward the perineum. Careful attention to this proximomedial socket contour is absolutely essential for stance-phase comfort in the perineum.

The quadrilateral socket should be designed with initial flexion to improve the ability of the amputee to control knee stability at heel contact and help minimize the development of lumbar lordosis at toe-off (Figure 8). If this is not done, the amputee will be unable to take a full-length stride on the sound side because of the limitation in hip extension on the prosthetic side.

The achievement of normal swing phase depends on several factors. Obviously, proper suspension enhanced by careful matching of residual limb and socket contours will aid in achieving a normal swing phase. Proper socket contours for actively functioning muscles (primarily the rectus femoris and gluteus maximus) also affect swing-phase tracking in the sagittal plane. The depth of the rectus

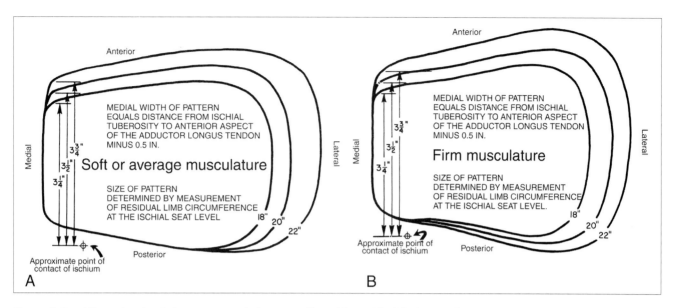

Figure 9 Quadrilateral socket brim pattern variations are affected by residual limb musculature, particularly the gluteals and rectus femoris. **A,** Pattern for a residual limb of soft or average musculature. **B,** Pattern for a residual limb of firm musculature. *(Reproduced with permission from Radcliffe CW: Functional considerations in the fitting of above-knee prosthetics.* Artif Limbs *1955;2:35-60.)*

femoris channel (in the transverse view) will vary depending on proximal circumference and muscular firmness of the residual limb, as well as femoral anteversion.[1] The posteromedial wall angle varies from 5° to 11°, depending on the muscular density of the proximoposterior aspect of the residual limb[1] (Figure 9). If the AP dimension of the lateral half of the quadrilateral socket viewed transversely is too tight, then muscle activity in the swing phase of gait can lead to undesirable socket rotations about the residual limb that appear clinically as swing-phase "whips."

The distal end of the socket must match the contour of the distal end of the residual limb and provide adequate distal contact in order to prevent development of edema and other skin problems.

The basic concept of the US-style quadrilateral socket was borrowed from Europe and refined through significant biomechanical analysis and research conducted in the United States.[20] The original concept also underwent simultaneous development in Europe. During the 1980s, several European-style quadrilateral casting brims became available in the United States. The transitions from the four socket walls were smoother and less

abrupt than the US-style quadrilateral brims. The medioproximal wall was slightly lower to increase comfort in the perineum. In the transverse view, these European brims featured a larger AP dimension balanced by a smaller mediolateral dimension than typical US-style quadrilateral shapes. Although the biomechanical principles remained the same, these subtle changes began to influence US quadrilateral techniques near the time when the ischial containment socket introduced new concepts in transfemoral socket theory.

Ischial Containment Socket

The term ischial containment is self-descriptive, referring to several similar concepts in socket design in which the ischium (and in some cases the ischial ramus) are enclosed within the socket. Pritham[22] described six objectives that would be achieved in the ideal ischial containment socket: (1) maintenance of normal femoral adduction and narrow-based gait during ambulation; (2) enclosure of the ischial tuberosity and ramus in the socket to varying extents medially and posteriorly so that forces involved in maintenance of mediolateral stability are borne by the bones of the pelvis medially and not just by the soft

tissues distal to the pelvis, ie, creation of a "bony lock"; (3) maximal effort to distribute forces along the shaft of the femur; (4) decreased emphasis on a narrow AP diameter between the adductor longus-Scarpa's triangle and ischium for the maintenance of ischial-gluteal weight bearing; (5) total contact; and (6) use of suction socket suspension whenever possible.

Weight bearing in the ischial containment socket is focused primarily through the medial aspect of the ischium and the ischial ramus.[19] The socket encompasses both the ischial tuberosity and the ramus; the specific contour depends on the musculature, soft tissue, and skeletal structure of the amputee.[11,12,23] Unlike the quadrilateral socket, in which the proximal contours are affected primarily by muscular variation, proximal contours of the ischial containment socket are affected by differences in pelvic skeletal anatomy. Of particular importance are the variations in the position of the ischium with respect to the trochanter (Figure 10). In females, the ischia are positioned more laterally, closer to the trochanter, to allow for childbearing. The posterior brim of the socket is proximal to and tightly posterior to the ischium. Countersupport, intended to keep the ischium and ramus

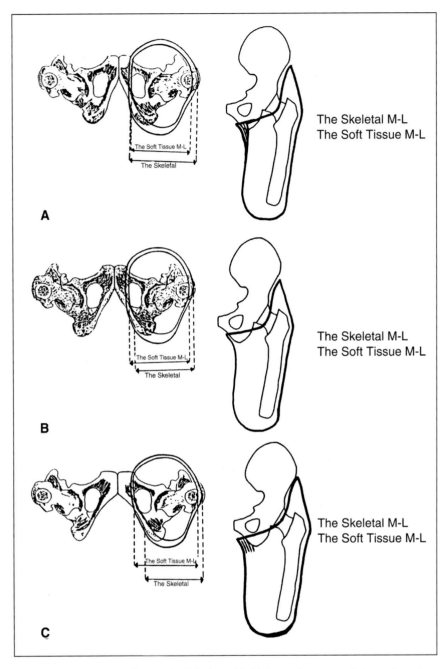

Figure 10 Variations in the proximal design of ischial containment sockets are based on pelvic structure and diameter and soft-tissue diameter just distal to the pelvis. Variations are individual and are most significant between males and females. M-L = medial-lateral diameter of the skeleton at the ischial level. *(Reproduced with permission from Hoyt C, Littig D, Lundt J, et al: The UCLA CAT-CAM Above-Knee Socket, ed 3. Los Angeles, CA, UCLA Prosthetics Education and Research Program, 1987, p 15.)*

sure from the trochanter anteriorly to the tensor fascia latae.[11,12,23] Additional weight-bearing support is thought to be provided by the gluteal musculature and the lateral aspect of the femur distal to the trochanter, as well as from pressures distributed as evenly as possible over the entire surface of the residual limb.[15,19] Because significantly more residual limb surface and volume are contained within the ischial containment socket than in the quadrilateral socket, identical residual limbs have greater force distribution and hence lower pressures with an ischial containment design.

One hypothesis is that the quadrilateral socket is displaced laterally during midstance and thus results in a shearing force on the perineal tissues. Secondarily, femoral abduction may occur and decrease the effectiveness of the gluteus medius. The solution provided by the ischial containment socket is to extend the medial brim of the socket proximally until pressure is brought to bear against the medial ischiopubic ramus. The resulting force couple between the ischium, trochanter, and laterodistal aspect of the femur is believed to provide a much more stable mechanism for acceptance of perineal forces, leading to increased comfort in the groin and better control of the pelvis and trunk[15] (Figure 11).

Stance stability may be enhanced by extensive contouring posterior to the femoral shaft; this allows more effective transmission of the movements of the femur to the prosthesis.[15]

Swing-phase suspension is critical and is usually achieved by suction. As with the quadrilateral socket, proper contours allow for smooth swing-phase tracking. Rotational control is provided by the proximomedial brim and its bony lock against the ischium, the shape and channels of the anterior wall, and the posttrochanteric contours of the lateral wall as seen in the transverse view[15,23] (Figure 12). Control of socket rotation for very fleshy residual limbs with poor muscle tone is best achieved with an ischial containment socket.

solidly against the medioposterior aspect of the socket, is produced in three ways. First, the skeletal mediolateral dimension—the distance between the medial aspect of the ischium and the inferolateral edge of the trochanter—must be carefully designed into the socket. Second, countersupport occurs through the distal mediolateral dimension, a soft-tissue measurement that reflects the diameter of the residual limb 1 to 2 inches distal to the skeletal mediolateral dimension. The third form of countersupport, most important in females because of their pelvic anatomy, is anterolateral counterpres-

Flexible Transfemoral Sockets

In 1983, Kristinsson of Iceland introduced the concept of the flexible socket design.[24] Known in the United States under various acronyms such as ISNY (Icelandic-Swedish-New York) and SFS (Scandinavian Flexible Socket), these techniques gained considerable favor.[22,25,26] The concept incorporates flexible thermoplastic vacuum-formed sockets supported in a rigid (or semirigid) fenestrated frame or socket retainer (Figure 13). The socket retainer may be made of laminated plastic or may be vacuum formed of thermoplastic material (Figure 14). Describing a flexible socket, Kristinsson[27] said, "To label a socket as flexible I would say that you should be able to deform it by your hands, and the material should not be elastic enough to stretch under the loads it will be subjected to." Kristinsson also indicated that when designing a flexible socket system, the most critical aspect for the comfort of the wearer is how the frame is designed. The frame must be capable of supporting the flexible socket, preventing permanent deformation, and the socket-frame combination has to be structurally strong and stable enough to counteract the reaction forces.[27]

According to Pritham,[22] the advantages of flexible wall sockets are increased comfort, improved proprioception, use of conventional fitting techniques, the ease with which minor volume changes are accommodated, temperature reduction, and enhanced suspension. He believes that the general indications for use of a flexible socket are a mature residual limb, for which socket changes would be infrequent, or a medium to long residual limb, where a significant portion of the wall can be left exposed and flexible.

Socket Indications: Current Trends

How is the clinician to sort out these conflicting philosophies?[16] Some of

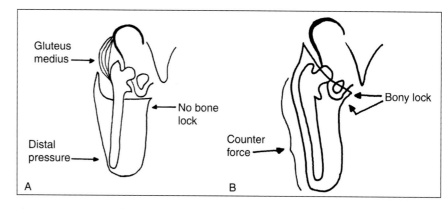

Figure 11 AP view of quadrilateral and ischial containment sockets. **A,** The quadrilateral socket lacks a proximal bone lock and hypothetically allows lateral socket displacement during stance phase. Pelvic stability is compromised. **B,** In the ischial containment socket, the ischial tuberosity is locked in the socket. The resulting bony lock between the ischium, trochanter, and lateral distal aspect of the femur provides a much more stable mechanism for acceptance of the perineal biomechanical forces. *(Reproduced with permission from Michael JW: Current concepts in above-knee socket design. Instr Course Lect 1990;39:373-378.)*

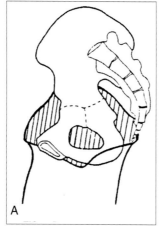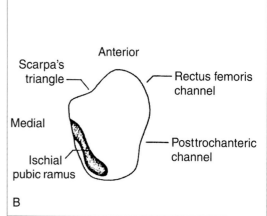

Figure 12 Rotational control of the ischial containment socket is provided by the proximomedial brim and its bony lock against the ischium, the shape and channels of the anterior wall, and the posttrochanteric contour of the lateral wall. **A,** Medial view, sagittal plane of the ischial containment socket. **B,** Transverse view, ischial containment socket. *(Reproduced with permission from Pritham CH: Biomechanics and shape of the above-knee socket considered in light of the ischial containment concept. Prosthet Orthot Int 1990;14:9-21.)*

the new socket designs introduced in the 1980s were associated with strident claims for their benefits, coupled with concurrent denigration of the quadrilateral design. According to Pritham and associates,[28] "most if not all of the major factors influencing the shape of the newer sockets can be explained in terms of the principle of ischial containment, and this principle is fully compatible with Radcliffe's biomechanical analysis of the function of the quadrilateral socket. The varying socket configurations are not

at odds but rather are separate but related entities in a continuum labeled above-knee sockets."

In a similar vein, Michael[16] contends that these new designs represent evolutionary, rather than revolutionary, advances. In reality, socket design indications can only be offered from shared clinical experience and workshops[10] because there are no impartial field tests or objective scientific studies produced to date to provide answers to this question. The following information can be summarized

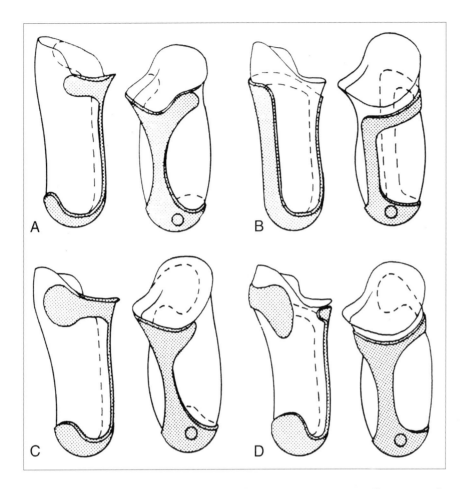

Figure 13 Flexible socket, rigid socket frame design variations. **A,** Durr-Fillauer's Scandinavian Flexible Socket (SFS) is shown from the posterolateral (left) and anteromedial (right) aspects. **B,** Sabolich-style frame with a totally flexible brim for use with an ischial containment socket. **C,** Frame for an ischial containment-style socket with a posterior seat, support pad posterior to the greater trochanter, and a distal support flange rotated posteriorly so that it supports the posterolateral end of the femur. **D,** Frame similar to that shown in **C** but with an anterior extension supporting the lateral support pad, thus providing total flexibility posteriorly. The frame is trimmed below the trim line of the socket and thus provides a totally flexible brim. *(Reproduced with permission from Pritham CH: Above-knee flexible sockets: The perspective from Durr-Fillauer, in Donovan R, Pritham C, Wilson AB Jr (eds): Report of ISPO Workshops, International Workshop on Above-Knee Fitting and Alignment. Copenhagen, Denmark, International Society for Prosthetics and Orthotics, 1989, pp 26-27.)*

from the work of a panel of physicians, prosthetists, and engineers who participated in an international workshop on transfemoral fitting and alignment:[11,12,16] (1) No specific contraindications were noted for any socket design; (2) some advocated no change for successful quadrilateral socket wearers; (3) quadrilateral sockets are most successful on long, firm residual limbs with firm adductor musculature; (4) ischial containment sockets are more successful than quadrilateral sockets on short, fleshy residual limbs; (5) ischial containment sockets are the better recommendation for high-activity sports participation; (6) no consensus was reached on the best recommendation for the bilateral transfemoral amputee; (7) flexible-wall sockets are not linked to any one philosophy of transfemoral socket design; and (8) total flexible brims are essential to the success of maximal ischial-ramal containment sockets. In general, clinical practice has borne out the efficacy of these guidelines.

Several additional factors should be considered. One concern regarding the ischial containment technique is the difficulty of efficiently obtaining a successful fit.[16] Initially, repeated test or trial sockets were the norm for this technique; in contrast, the quadrilateral technique rarely required more than one initial test socket. Increased experience among practicing prosthetists and the incorporation of instruction on the technique into prosthetic education program curricula has tended to level the differences between the two techniques. Today, ischial containment techniques have come to be widely accepted and are used to an ever-increasing degree.

The use of thermoplastics in prosthetic socket design is on the rise and offers some significant advantages over conventional laminated plastic sockets.[29] Flexible sockets are, however, less durable than rigid laminated sockets. Thermoplastic materials by their very nature will creep and change shape over time when subjected to continuous loads, particularly at body temperature. Amputees and others who advocate the use of flexible sockets must be prepared for the reality that the flexible socket will gradually lose its fit and require more frequent replacement.

Socket Fitting Techniques

The prosthetist must carefully measure and record a variety of data describing a patient's residual limb. This data is used to generate the specifications for production of a socket to meet the needs of the patient. A variety of methods are currently used for this purpose.

The introduction of laminated plastic, total-contact sockets (supplanting wood, open-ended sockets) also led to the adoption of the use of Plaster of Paris bandages to obtain a negative wrap cast of the patient's limb. A positive model is generated from this and the actual socket is formed about this model. A variety of casting aids is available to selectively mold the wrap cast during the casting process. These aids include a floor-

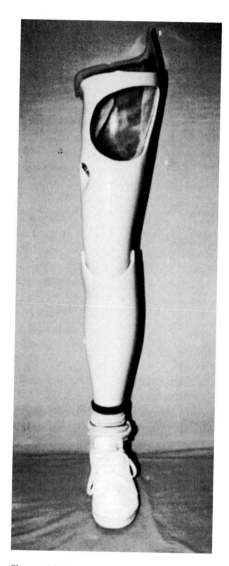

Figure 14 Anterior view of left transfemoral exoskeletal prosthesis with a flexible socket-rigid socket frame design.

socket template stored in the computer's memory can be selected. Design paradigms created by the software designer modify the template to reflect the patient's measurements. The resulting data are used to carve a positive socket model. This method is faster, cleaner, and less tiring for both prosthetist and amputee than the plaster cast methods described above. It has been hypothesized that consistent results are more readily obtained, particularly in achieving the more complex geometry of the newer socket configurations.

Regardless of how the positive model is obtained, in all likelihood it will be used to produce a check or test socket. Such trial sockets are used to refine the characteristics of the relationship between the socket and the patient and to ensure that both the patient and the prosthetist are satisfied with the result. The advent of ischial containment sockets with their more intimate fit about the structures of the pelvis weighs heavily in favor of using a test socket.

Test sockets and realignable endoskeletal components lend themselves to fabrication of prototype prostheses. A prototype prosthesis can best be described as a precursor to the prosthesis eventually intended for the patient's long-term use. It is fabricated in a temporary fashion using the test socket and endoskeletal components (knee, foot, etc) to dynamically assess the function of the socket and other components during gait as well as to complete the dynamic alignment process. If a component proves to be less than optimal, the prescription can be altered before the actual prosthesis itself is fabricated.

Suspension Variants

Improper suspension results in poor gait, decreased safety, and increased skin problems. Secure and dependable suspension enhances proprioception and control and creates the feeling that the prosthesis is more a part of the wearer.

Suction Suspension

Suction suspension is typically effected by an air expulsion valve in the distal end of the socket combined with a precisely fitted socket. Negative air pressure suspends the prosthesis during swing phase. The socket is sealed around the residual limb directly against the skin, without the use of prosthetic socks.

The prosthesis is typically donned by one of two methods. Most commonly, the amputee pulls the residual limb into the socket by applying a length of open-ended stockinette around the residual limb, putting the end of the stockinette through the valve hole at the distal end of the socket, and pulling the residual limb down into the socket. In the process of pulling the residual limb completely into the socket, the stockinette is gradually removed from the socket. This donning procedure requires some skill and effort. Balance problems, upper limb deficiencies, strength deficiencies, heart problems, and other conditions can contribute considerable difficulty to this method of donning, and at one time were considered contraindications for suction suspension.

An easier method of donning a suction socket is with the use of hand creams or lotions. A lubricating agent is spread either on the residual limb or inside the brim of the socket so that the amputee can push the residual limb into the socket. After the limb is completely in the socket, the valve is used to expel air and suction is achieved. Within a short period of time, the lotion is absorbed into the skin. This method of donning a suction socket has expanded the application of such suspension. Some patients, however, find the use of lotion messy and unappealing. In addition, soft tissues tend to be displaced proximally during the donning process. If the socket is too tight, this can create an adductor roll, a roll of flesh trapped between the medial brim of the socket and the bones of the pelvis. Adductor rolls can eventually cause considerable

mounted apparatus in which the amputee stands and simpler casting brims that are manually supported in place by the prosthetist and incorporated in the cast.

Alternately, the prosthetist can "hand cast" the patient's residual limb, without reliance on external aids. This course of action is most common when fitting ischial containment sockets.

The proliferation of computer aided design/computer aided manufacturing (CAD/CAM) technology in lower limb prosthetics has led to the introduction of yet another course of action. Data about the residual limb can be entered into a computer and a

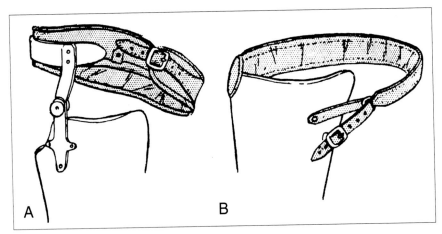

Figure 15 Two methods of suspension of the transfemoral prosthesis. **A,** Silesian belt. **B,** Hip joint, pelvic band, and waist belt. *(Reproduced with permission from Wilson AB Jr: Limb Prosthetics, ed 6. New York, NY, Demos Publications, 1989, p 58.)*

discomfort and are quite difficult to reduce once they have formed.

Suction suspension is usually indicated for amputees with smooth residual limb contours. Volume fluctuations such as weight gain or loss or fluid retention problems are contraindications for suction sockets. With the advent of ischial containment sockets, even very short amputation limbs can often be successfully fitted with suction as a primary suspension. Additional auxiliary belt suspension is generally prudent. Suction suspension can be used together with any of the other forms of suspension.

Suction suspension of transfemoral prostheses provides the best proprioception. The suspension is applied directly to the residual limb, rather than from belts around the waist; the skin is in direct contact with the socket; and the movements of the limb are transmitted to the prosthesis with minimal lost motion. Disadvantages include difficulty obtaining the required precise fit, occasional loss of suction in sitting or other positions, lack of a medium for absorbing perspiration, skin shear, and the requirement of weight and volume stability. Partial suction suspension, which uses the principles described above with a thin prosthetic sock or nylon sheath, sometimes eliminates or minimizes the disadvantages.

Suspension Liner

In recent years, prefabricated suspension liners and locking mechanisms have been used increasingly with transfemoral amputees. These devices afford many of the advantages of the traditional suction socket, while avoiding the primary disadvantage of the difficult donning techniques.

The various locking mechanisms do take up space distal to the socket. For longer residual limbs, this may result in displacement of the knee mechanism distally in the prosthesis and compromised cosmesis. Suspension liners demand meticulous hygiene to avoid undesirable odors and skin irritation.

Suspension is achieved through contact between the inside of the roll-on liner and the soft tissue of the residual limb. If the limb is fleshy, distal displacement of the prosthesis during swing phase can occur, making the prosthesis functionally too long during swing phase. This problem can be minimized with a tether system to elongate the residual limb during donning, or by employing a method to secure the liner proximally.

Soft Belts

Soft suspension belts may be used as either primary or auxiliary suspension. The traditional form of soft belt is the Silesian belt or bandage, a flexible, soft belt usually made of leather, cotton webbing, or Dacron. The belt is attached to a pivot point on the socket in the area of the greater trochanter and passes around the back and over the opposite iliac crest, where it achieves most of its suspension. Anteriorly, it attaches at either a single point or, in some cases, double attachment points (Figure 15). This belt provides a positive form of suspension of the prosthesis and is simple to use. The disadvantages of the Silesian belt are that it is usually not removable for washing, and there is sometimes discomfort associated with constrictive waist belts.

A number of simpler removable alternatives are now commercially available and have been well accepted clinically. These products were originally made of elastic neoprene material lined with a smooth nylon material but are also fabricated from lightweight open mesh fabric. This type of suspension belt fits around the proximal portion of the prosthesis and then around the waist and fastens anteriorly with Velcro (Figure 16). This belt is quite comfortable and forgiving because of its elasticity. It provides reasonably good suspension and enhances rotational control of the prosthesis. Disadvantages include body heat retention and limited durability; however, the open mesh fabric variations should dissipate heat more readily.

Hip Joint With Pelvic Band and Belt

The hip joint with pelvic band and waist belt provides rotational stability plus a significant degree of mediolateral pelvic stability. This is sometimes necessary in obese amputees or for those with significant redundant tissue that is difficult to stabilize. This suspension is particularly useful for the patient with weak hip abductors (Figure 15). Because most amputees object to the weight and bulk of this suspension, it is generally reserved for cases in which rotational control or mediolateral stability cannot be achieved in any other manner.

Case Studies

When recommending transfemoral prosthetic components, two sets of criteria may be applied. The first and most important set includes previous experience of the amputee, safety requirements, and functional requirements. Secondary considerations include the level of amputation, vocational and avocational needs, durability of components, weight of components, cosmesis, and cost. Prosthetic components that have been satisfactory in the past should not be changed without thorough discussion with the amputee. The longer an amputee has worn a specific system, design, or component, the less likely the success of a change.

The following case presentations include prosthetic recommendations and a rationale for each prescription element. These cases are intended to illustrate approaches commonly encountered in prosthetic practice; however, other prescriptions may well be successful in similar clinical situations.

Case Study 1

A 29-year-old woman presented with a long left transfemoral amputation at the supracondylar region of the femur. She had no other health problems, had normal range of motion and strength, and was athletically and socially active. Her preferred sports were tennis and racquetball. She was employed as an attorney's assistant.

Recommendation

Most prosthetists today would opt for the ischial containment socket design, usually with a flexible brim and suction suspension incorporating an expulsion valve. An endoskeletal component system including a transverse rotational torque absorber and dynamic response foot would also be appropriate. The critical component is the knee, which determines the range of normal activities of daily living that can be safely accomplished. The ideal knee would be a microprocessor-controlled hydraulic stance and swing control system with integrated force sensors in the shin tube component. A less desirable alternative would be a polycentric knee with hydraulic or pneumatic swing control.

Rationale

Suction suspension is ideal for active amputees and is enhanced by a long, muscular residual limb. A flexible socket is more forgiving for the active athlete and thus more comfortable. The cosmesis afforded by an endoskeletal prosthesis with soft cover meets the social and vocational needs of this amputee. A microprocessor-controlled hydraulic stance and swing control knee allows the most natural gait and the greatest stability. This knee facilitates functional activities such as descending stairs step over step, negotiating downhill inclines, and controlled knee flexion when seated. The 4-bar polycentric knee, if chosen, provides inherent stability during the critical stance phases of activity, is smooth in swing, and is compatible with long amputations. Either pneumatic or hydraulic knee control is essential for varying cadences, and the dynamic-response foot provides better propulsion and response during all activities.

Case Study 2

A 78-year-old man presented with a midthigh right transfemoral amputation and a history of peripheral vascular disease secondary to diabetes mellitus. His left lower limb had vascular disease involvement and was weak and insensate. He had decreased strength and range of motion of the residual limb. His eyesight was failing as well. He was retired and desired household ambulation for limited distances.

Recommendation

A semiflexible thermoplastic quadrilateral socket fit with thin prosthetic socks and a soft suspension belt of neoprene or spandex are suggested. Use of a roll-on locking liner could also be considered. A lightweight endoskeletal component system with

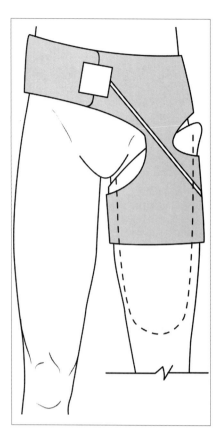

Figure 16 Total elastic suspension belt made of neoprene and Velcro. (Courtesy of Syncor, Ltd.)

weight-activated stance control knee and single-axis, flexible keel foot and ankle is also recommended.

Rationale

Stability is a primary concern because of the combination of weakness and poor vision. The weight-activated stance control knee provides safety and knee stabilization during stance, yet flexes quite easily for swing and sitting. The amputee's gait will be slow because of the comorbidities. The single-axis, flexible keel foot allows rapid footflat in early stance, thereby enhancing knee stability. The flexible keel permits smooth rollover with less effort in terminal stance. Minimization of weight reduces the effort involved in ambulation.

Case Study 3

A 15-year-old boy presented with a right transfemoral amputation at the proximal third of the femur secondary to cancer. The boy was very healthy and active, participated in junior varsity basketball and baseball, and was also an avid hunter and fisherman. He was described as "growing like a weed."

Recommendation

An ischial containment flexible socket with a rigid socket retainer and suction suspension is recommended, with the option of auxiliary suspension in a removable soft neoprene or spandex belt. An endoskeletal system with hydraulic knee control (preferably swing and stance control) is advised, along with a carbon fiber shank-ankle-foot for maximum dynamic response. A torque absorber should also be considered.

Rationale

An ischial containment suction socket is indicated by both the short residual femur and high activity level. The flexible socket enhances comfort and suspension, and the optional auxiliary suspension provides additional security for high-demand activities. The endoskeletal construction readily accommodates linear growth, and the swing-and-stance hydraulic knee control offers many options, including a knee-locking option for hunting and ambulating in rough terrain. The carbon fiber shank-ankle-foot provides maximum possible dynamic response for demanding sports activities in addition to dependable durability, and the torque absorber reduces shear stresses to the residual limb.

Case Study 4

A 38-year-old man presented with a muscular midthigh left transfemoral amputation. The cause of the amputation was a motor vehicle accident. He had worn several prostheses, all quadrilateral socket designs. He worked as a framing carpenter, climbing ladders and scaffolding. Because heat and perspiration are a chronic problem in the climate and his work, he requested a socket fit with prosthetic socks. He was very strong and agile and depended on the prosthesis for his work.

Recommendation

A quadrilateral socket and thin cotton sock fit with a valve for partial suction are advised. Silesian belt suspension is preferred. An exoskeletal design, swing-and-stance control knee, and a simple, maintenance-free, conforming foot such as a flexible keel foot should be considered.

Rationale

The quadrilateral socket is familiar to this amputee and, when properly fitted, is quite satisfactory for the muscular midthigh residual limb. The partial suction socket with a cotton sock provides a medium for absorption of perspiration and offers secure suspension when coupled with the Silesian belt. The exoskeletal construction is durable for repeated kneeling and similar occupational requirements. The swing-and-stance hydraulic knee provides stability and safety options that serve his vocational needs. The foot is simple and durable and conforms well to varying terrain.

Summary

The controversy created by the significant changes in the management of transfemoral amputees that occurred in the 1980s was largely resolved in the 1990s as a result of clinical experience and consensus. Through the use of new materials, components, and designs, the transfemoral amputee today can achieve a much higher activity level than was possible in the past. The fundamental goals of providing comfort, function, and cosmesis continue to guide clinical practice and the development of new techniques and components.

References

1. *Total Contact Socket for the Above-Knee Amputation* ed 5. Los Angeles, CA, UCLA School of Medicine, Prosthetics-Orthotics Education Program, 1976, p 19.
2. Moreland JR, Bassett LW, Hanker GJ: Radiographic analysis of the axial alignment of the lower extremity. *J Bone Joint Surg Am* 1987;69:745-749.
3. Anderson MH, Sollars RE (eds): *Prosthetic Principles: Above-Knee Amputations.* Springfield, IL, Charles C Thomas Publishers, 1960, pp 129-146.
4. Anderson MH, Sollars RE (eds): *Manual of Above-Knee Prosthetics for Physicians and Therapists,* ed 2. Los Angeles, CA, UCLA School of Medicine, Prosthetics Education Program, 1957, pp 86-104.
5. Anderson MH, Sollars RE (eds): *Manual of Above-Knee Prosthetics for Physicians and Therapists,* ed 2. Los Angeles, CA, UCLA School of Medicine, Prosthetics Education Program, 1957, pp 95-111.
6. Radcliffe CW: Biomechanics of above-knee prostheses, in Murdoch G (ed): *Prosthetic and Orthotic Practice.* London, England, Edward Arnold, 1970, pp 191-198.
7. Radcliffe CW: Functional considerations in the fitting of above-knee prostheses. *Artif Limbs* 1955;2:35-60.
8. Radcliffe CW: The Knud Jansen Lecture: Above-knee prosthetics. *Prosthet Orthot Int* 1977;1:146-160.
9. Saunders JB, Inman VT, Eberhart HD: The major determinants in normal and pathological gait. *J Bone Joint Surg Am* 1953;35:543-558.
10. International workshop on above-knee fitting and alignment, Workshop on teaching material for above-knee socket variants, in Donovan R, Pritham C, Wilson AB Jr (eds): *Report of ISPO Workshops, International Workshop on Above-Knee Fitting and Alignment (Appendix C).* Copenhagen, Denmark, International Society for Prosthetics and Orthotics, 1987.
11. Schuch CM: Modern above-knee fitting practice: A report on the ISPO Workshop on Above-Knee Fitting and Alignment Techniques. *Prosthet Orthot Int* 1988;12:77-90.
12. Schuch CM: Report from: International workshop on above-knee fitting and alignment techniques. *Clin Prosthet Orthot* 1988;12:81-98.
13. Long I: Allowing normal adduction of femur in above-knee amputations: Technical note. *Orthot Prosthet* 1975;29:53-54.
14. Long IA: Normal shape-normal alignment (NSNA) above-knee prosthesis. *Clin Prosthet Orthot* 1985;9:9-14.

15. Sabolich J: Contoured adducted trochanteric-controlled alignment method (CAT-CAM): Introduction and basic principles. *Clin Prosthet Orthot* 1985;9:15-26.

16. Michael JW: Current concepts in above-knee socket design. *Instr Course Lect* 1990;39:373-378.

17. Wilson AB Jr: Brief history of recent development in above-knee socket design, in Donovan R, Pritham C, Wilson AB Jr (eds): *Report of lSPO Workshops, International Workshop on Above-Knee Fitting and Alignment.* Copenhagen, Denmark, International Society for Prosthetics and Orthotics, 1987, pp 2-3.

18. Hall CB: Prosthetic socket shape as related to anatomy in lower extremity amputees. *Clin Orthop* 1964;37:32-46.

19. Radcliffe CW: Comments on new concepts for above-knee sockets, in Donovan R, Pritham C, Wilson AB Jr (eds): *Report of ISPO Workshops, International Workshop on Above-Knee Fitting and Alignment.* Copenhagen, Denmark, International Society for Prosthetics and Orthotics, 1987, pp 31-37.

20. Radcliffe CW: A short history of the quadrilateral above-knee socket, in Donovan R, Pritham C, Wilson AB Jr (eds): *Report of ISPO Workshops, International Workshop on Above-Knee Fitting and Alignment.* Copenhagen, Denmark, International Society for Prosthetics and Orthotics, 1987, pp 4-12.

21. Redhead RG: Total surface bearing self suspending above-knee sockets. *Prosthet Orthot Int* 1979;3:126-136.

22. Pritham CH: Biomechanics and shape of the above-knee socket considered in light of the ischial containment concept. *Prosthet Orthot Int* 1990;14:9-21.

23. Hoyt C, Littig D, Lundt J, Staats TB: *The UCLA CAT-CAM Above-Knee Prosthesis,* ed 3. Los Angeles, CA, UCLA Prosthetics Education and Research Program, 1987.

24. Kristinsson O: Flexible above-knee socket made from low density polyethylene suspended by a weight transmitting frame. *Orthot Prosthet* 1983;37:25-27.

25. Berger N: The ISNY (Icelandic-Swedish-New York) flexible above-knee socket, in Donovan RG, Pritham C, Wilson AB Jr (eds): *Report of ISPO Workshops, International Workshop on Above-Knee Fitting and Alignment.* Copenhagen, Denmark, International Society for Prosthetics and Orthotics, 1987, pp 20-23.

26. Fishman S, Berger N, Krebs D: Abstract: The ISNY (Icelandic-Swedish-New York University) flexible above-knee socket. *Phys Ther* 1985;65:742.

27. Kristinsson O: Flexible sockets and more, in Donovan R, Pritham C, Wilson AB Jr (eds): *Report of ISPO Workshops, International Workshop on Above-Knee Fitting and Alignment.* Copenhagen, Denmark, International Society for Prosthetics and Orthotics, 1987, pp 15-19.

28. Pritham CH, Fillauer C, Fillauer K: Experience with the Scandinavian Flexible Socket. *Orthot Prosthet* 1985;39:17-32.

29. Schuch CM: Thermoplastic applications in lower extremity prosthetics. *J Prosthet Orthot* 1990;3:1-8.

Chapter 44

Hip Disarticulation and Transpelvic Amputation: Surgical Management

Howard A. Chansky, MD

Introduction

Hip disarticulation is the surgical removal of the lower limb through the hip joint. Transpelvic amputation (hemipelvectomy) is the removal of the entire lower limb in addition to most of the pelvis. Although 85% of amputations are performed through the lower limb, few occur through the hip joint or pelvis. Nevertheless, the surgeon should become familiar with these high-level procedures as they are occasionally performed urgently for life-threatening infection or, rarely, for life-threatening hemorrhage in the case of massive pelvic trauma. In addition, elective amputations through the hip or pelvis are sometimes needed for the treatment of vascular disease, chronic infection with soft-tissue loss, and malignancies. In addition, congenital limb deficiencies are sometimes best treated by conversion to a hip disarticulation.

This chapter reviews the technical aspects of hip disarticulation and transpelvic amputation. Surgical indications as well as perioperative care are also discussed. Hip disarticulation and transpelvic amputation can be technically demanding procedures with the potential for catastrophic blood loss and injury to pelvic viscera. Although a surgeon will rarely perform these procedures, he or she should be versed in their technical and medical aspects. If the surgeon is unfamiliar with these techniques, and the patient can be safely transferred, then referral to a regional center skilled in the surgical and postoperative management of these proximal amputations should be considered.

Causal Conditions

Although most hip disarticulations are performed to treat the sequelae of peripheral vascular disease, trauma, and soft-tissue infections, most transpelvic amputations are undertaken to treat malignancies of the pelvis.[1,2] Even so, with the integration of adjuvant radiation therapy and chemotherapy, advanced imaging techniques and improved surgery have resulted in the ability to use limb-sparing procedures for many malignancies with local control rates equivalent to those of amputation. Similarly, a multidisciplinary approach to the care of those with paraplegia, vascular disease, or diabetes mellitus has lessened the need for ablative procedures to treat these conditions.[3,4] A mangled limb secondary to trauma remains an infrequent indication for hip disarticulation. Fortunately, transpelvic amputation to control massive bleeding due to trauma is needed only rarely.[5]

Indications and Contraindications

Preservation of life is the ultimate indication for amputation at these proximal levels. This often arises in patients with wet gangrene who are also debilitated from underlying disease, typically diabetes mellitus and severe vascular disease. Often these patients will exhibit profound systemic signs of sepsis although the peripheral white blood cell count may be normal. Necrotizing fasciitis is another condition in which emergent radical débridement or amputation may avert loss of life that occurs in up to 50% of cases.[6-9]

Many studies have documented the inverse relationship between the level of amputation and functional outcome. This is particularly true for patients undergoing amputation for ischemia, infection, and systemic disease as opposed to those often younger and healthier patients who are being treated for trauma or tumor. The need for these proximal ablations will most likely arise in patients who are bedridden or wheelchair bound because of paraplegia, previous amputation at a lower level, advanced ischemic disease, infection, or other systemic conditions. These patients are more likely to have lesions requiring proximal amputation but, fortunately, are less likely to have high functional demands. Nevertheless, these procedures are quite disfiguring and should not be undertaken lightly, regardless of the patient's preoperative functional status.

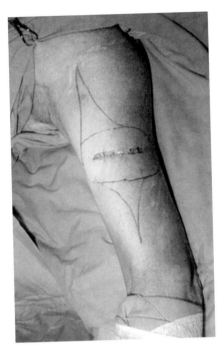

Figure 1 A transverse biopsy incision in the upper or lower limb severely compromises attempts at limb salvage or distal amputation. *(Reproduced with permission from Lawrence W Jr, Neifeld JP, Terz JJ: Diagnosis and staging of the soft-tissue sarcomas, in Egdahl RH (ed): Manual of Soft-Tissue Tumor Surgery. New York, NY, Springer-Verlag, 1983, p 28.)*

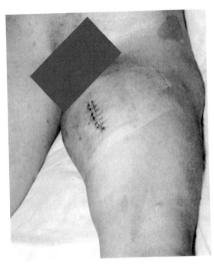

Figure 2 This patient has a soft-tissue sarcoma of the adductor compartment. The longitudinal incision is properly oriented, but the wide closure will require excision at the definitive procedure. Careful subcuticular closure is optimal. *(Reproduced with permission from Lawrence W Jr, Neifeld JP, Terz JJ: Diagnosis and staging of the soft-tissue sarcomas, in Egdahl RH (ed): Manual of Soft-Tissue Tumor Surgery. New York, NY, Springer-Verlag, 1983, p 28.)*

Hip disarticulation for treatment of a malignancy is performed less commonly than transpelvic amputation, limb-sparing procedures, or transfemoral amputation. Nonetheless, several clear indications exist for hip disarticulation when managing lower limb malignancy. These include soft-tissue sarcomas intimately involving the proximal sciatic nerve or femoral artery as well as distal femoral osteosarcoma with proximal intramedullary skip lesions or pathologic fracture through a proximal femoral osteosarcoma. Failed transfemoral amputation or progressive, life-threatening infection may also require hip disarticulation. Finally, childhood sarcomas adjacent to the proximal femoral epiphysis may be best treated with hip disarticulation if dramatic limb-length discrepancies will result from attempts at limb salvage.

The importance of a carefully planned biopsy of potentially malignant lesions in the thigh and pelvic area cannot be overstated. A poorly performed biopsy can lead to contamination of adjacent uninvolved tissues and can compromise or prevent possible limb salvage or lead to a more proximal amputation than might have been initially possible. Generally, biopsy incisions in the thigh should be longitudinal and in line with the eventual incision for definitive surgery, and only one anatomic compartment should be violated if possible. Also, prevention of postoperative hematoma with careful hemostasis is critical to prevent local dissemination of tumor cells. Incisions in the pelvis are usually oblique or transverse but always in line with the eventual incisions for either salvage or amputation. Figure 1 illustrates a poorly executed biopsy incision, and Figure 2 illustrates a more carefully planned incision.

Indications for transpelvic amputation include malignant tumors, severe infections, and the treatment of extensive decubitus ulcers. Transpelvic amputation is a disfiguring procedure that historically was the standard technique to remove sarcomas arising in and about the pelvis. The ability to achieve clear margins with a transpelvic amputation is offset by the functional impairment resulting from removing the entire leg, hemipelvis, and, often, part of the sacrum.

Most sarcomas that arise in the pelvis spare vital structures such as the pelvic viscera and iliac vessels and are thus amenable to treatment with neoadjuvant therapy and limb-sparing surgery. To be successful, limb-sparing protocols should yield a reasonably functional limb and tumor-free survival equivalent to that expected from amputation. For recurrent pelvic or hip tumors, limb-sparing resection should be undertaken only when wide surgical margins can be achieved. Involvement of pelvic viscera or the sciatic nerve or extension of tumor to the sacral neural foramina is generally considered a contraindication to limb-sparing surgery. Other contraindications are limited life expectancy or an inability to rehabilitate after limb-sparing surgery.

Fortunately, the indications for transpelvic amputation are decreasing with advances in imaging and multimodality preoperative adjuvant therapy. Similarly, aggressive multidisciplinary management of pressure sores associated with paraplegia, diabetes mellitus, and vascular disease has resulted in improved outcomes and fewer transpelvic amputations. Soft-tissue sarcomas that involve the pelvic viscera, the iliac vessels or the femoral vessels in the region of the inguinal ligament, and the bony pelvis may still require a radical amputation to achieve wide or even marginal margins. Extensive loss of soft tissue and disseminated osteomyelitis of the pelvis may also necessitate transpelvic amputation. In extreme cases, extensive involvement of the soft tissues and the anticipated location of flaps and suture lines may necessitate surgical diversion of the rectum. In these situations, a general surgeon should be consulted.

Patients who are candidates for transpelvic amputation to treat extensive decubitis ulcers and infection usually have significant medical comorbidities that jeopardize intraoperative and postoperative survival. With these patients, previous attempts at débridement and soft-tissue coverage have often failed. Reliance upon colleagues from internal medicine and physiatry before treating such patients is critical, but these colleagues may lack full appreciation of the limits of surgical technology and the effects of systemic disease on wound healing and tolerance of anesthesia and major surgery. These medical comorbidities are usually contraindications to transpelvic amputation and this must be discussed frankly with patients, family members, and medical colleagues—all of whom may have unreasonable expectations of surgical success and a tendency to minimize the risk of serious complications.

Preoperative Care

The orthopaedic surgeon is uniquely trained to coordinate the medical, surgical, and prosthetic needs of amputees. However, a multidisciplinary approach is often critical in caring for the amputee. The preoperative condition of the patient should be optimized by specialists in internal medicine. Because management of diabetes mellitus is often more difficult in the presence of an infection, consultation with an endocrinologist should be obtained to assist in the management of brittle diabetes or ketoacidosis. Treatment with broad-spectrum antibiotics can be instituted preoperatively, ideally after obtaining appropriate cultures. Intraoperative cultures are important, as this is usually the best opportunity to secure deep cultures through skin that has been sterilized during surgical preparation. Deep cultures are important, as there is poor correlation between

surface and deep cultures.[10] These infections are often polymicrobial, and adjustment of the dose, interval, and duration of multiple antibiotics is often complicated by renal insufficiency. Determination of appropriate antibiotics, monitoring of aminoglycoside or vancomycin levels, and checking for signs of ototoxicity and nephrotoxicity can be done by the infectious disease specialist.

In my experience, the specialist in rehabilitation medicine is often most helpful when predicting the potential for functional recovery after surgery. When the expected functional outcome is more precisely defined, the threshold for undertaking more complex tissue-sparing procedures may be lowered. For example, a patient expected to be confined to a bed postoperatively will not benefit from a more complex procedure with a greater risk of complications that is designed to preserve bone stock and soft tissue to enhance sitting balance. The physiatrist may also assist in customizing prostheses and wheelchairs and choosing the appropriate facility for postoperative rehabilitation.

Preservation of tissue and determination of the level of amputation is often best accomplished in consultation with both vascular and plastic surgeons. An orthopaedic surgeon usually performs a hip disarticulation, whereas a hemipelvectomy is often performed in conjunction with a general surgeon. Other consultants, including wound care specialists and social workers, may also play important roles in optimizing the postoperative care of these patients.

Level of Amputation

Once the decision has been made to perform a transpelvic amputation, the surgeon must decide how much of the hemipelvis and possibly the sacrum to remove. The level of the bony resection within the pelvis is determined primarily by disease management and much less by minor potential functional differences. Every attempt should be made to ensure the

removal of all diseased tissue while leaving adequate soft tissue for primary closure. Determination of the extent of osteomyelitis or malignancy has been improved by the combined use of plain radiography and other advanced imaging studies. However, especially for infection, no ideal single study exists that can perfectly delineate the extent of bone involvement. A three-phase technetium Tc 99m bone scan is supplemented at some institutions by an indium-111–labeled white blood cell scan. These studies assist in the differentiation of soft-tissue infection from osteomyelitis, but poor spatial resolution continues to limit their value when determining surgical margins in pelvic infections. Plain radiography cannot be used to detect early osteomyelitis with any reliability. CT is more sensitive to the presence of sequestra, loss of trabeculae, and cortical erosion. MRI provides detailed multiplanar anatomic information about both bone and soft tissue. The sensitivity of MRI is reported to be greater than 90%, and its specificity ranges from 75% to greater than 90%.[11] The reactive marrow changes seen on MRI scans can sometimes be difficult to distinguish from osteomyelitis.

The classification system initially described by Enneking and Dunham[12] to aid in the resection of pelvic sarcomas also has some use when conceptualizing the treatment of pelvic infection and soft-tissue necrosis. Pelvic tumor resections with preservation of the limb are divided into three types. Type I refers to resection of the iliac region, type II is resection of the periacetabular region, and type III involves resection of the ischiopubis. The Roman numerals can be combined to signify resection of multiple regions; for example, type II/type III resection.

Many patients undergoing ablative surgery for pelvic infection and soft-tissue loss are paraplegic, but situations arise when either the limb should be spared or amputation is performed in such a way as to remove the obturator ring and preserve the

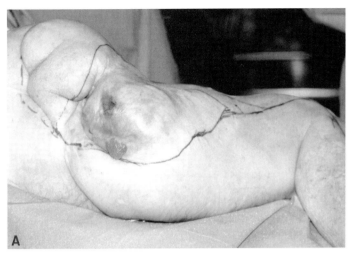

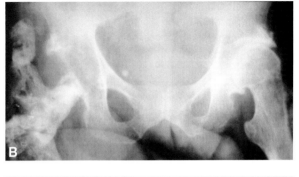

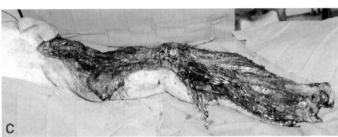

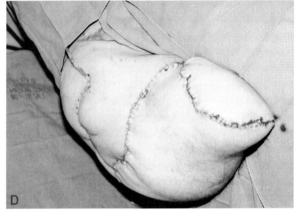

Figure 3 A 45-year-old man with longstanding paraplegia, severe pelvic osteomyelitis, and skin loss. **A,** The patient required frequent blood transfusions because of the erosive nature of this exposed bone and soft tissue. In previous operations, he had undergone transfer of all local rotation flaps. The only coverage available for transpelvic amputation was the thigh and calf fillet flap. **B,** Radiograph of the pelvis shows osteomyelitis and heterotopic bone formation. **C,** Following colostomy, a radical procedure was planned to remove the bony hemipelvis and all involved soft tissue but with preservation of the thigh and calf soft tissue for closure. The fillet flap is illustrated before rotation and closure. **D,** The flap was rotated and contoured to wrap over the sacrum, the ischium, and the defect from the hemipelvis resection.

ischial tuberosity. In addition, when other adequate local flaps are not available, a thigh or calf fillet flap can be used to treat end-stage extensive pressure sores involving the pelvis (Figure 3). This procedure entails resection of the involved pelvis, sacrum, femur, and tibia with filleting of the leg to provide a long, vascularized soft-tissue flap for reconstruction of the buttock and sacral areas.[13,14] As much of the bony pelvis is sacrificed as necessary. The goals of this procedure are to remove infected bone and soft tissues, bony prominences that may result in postoperative breakdown, and any bone necessary to reduce the area needing soft-tissue coverage. Cosmetic appearance can be enhanced by retention of the ileum. Sitting balance can be partially spared by preserving the ischial tuberosity.

Surgical Technique

Fortunately, a large, muscular soft-tissue envelope surrounds the pelvis and thigh. This permits a variety of incisions and flaps to work around quite extensive areas of skin necrosis and infection. The techniques described here are based on generally accepted principles and anatomic approaches, but at times, tissue required for reconstruction and closure of the amputation site is not available because of disease extent. Especially for cases involving malignant tumors, severe trauma, or necrotizing fasciitis, the surgeon may need to individualize the surgical approach and the reconstructive plan based on what tissues are salvageable. In these types of situations, considerable surgical ingenuity may be required to acheive a satisfactory result.

Hip Disarticulation

The standard technique for hip disarticulation is based on the procedure described by Boyd.[15] This procedure uses a racquet incision to create a durable posterior flap. Slocum[16] improved upon the initial technique by recommending a longer posterior flap to avoid weight bearing on the suture line (Figure 4). He also recommended dividing the sciatic, femoral, and obturator nerves as proximally as necessary to minimize irritation of the neuromas. For posterior decubitis ulcers or tumors, an anterior flap based on the rectus muscles and femoral artery can be used.

The patient is placed in a lateral decubitis or semisupine position on a beanbag with loose support that will allow 20° to 30° of both anterior and posterior additional mobilization to

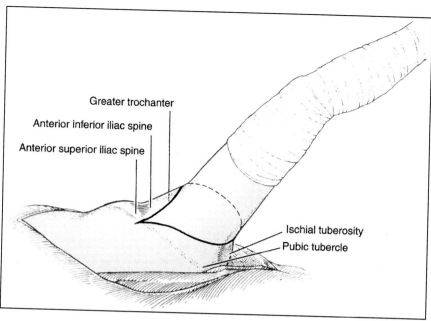

Figure 4 The typical racquet-shaped incision that is used for hip disarticulation. The incision is centered over the femoral triangle, and the femoral vessels are ligated and transected early in the procedure. *(Reproduced with permission from Malawer MM, Sugarbaker PH: Hip disarticulations, in Malawer MM, Sugarbaker PH (eds): Musculoskeletal Cancer Surgery: Treatment of Sarcomas and Allied Diseases. Boston, Kluwer Academic Publishers, 2001, p 340.)*

improve visualization as needed. The abdomen, groin, buttock, and leg are prepared for surgery, and the leg is draped free. The racquet-shaped incision begins just medial to the anterior superior iliac spine and descends nearly parallel and inferior to the inguinal ligament down to a point approximately 5 cm distal to the ischial tuberosity and gluteal crease. The posterior portion of the incision continues parallel to the gluteal crease, then curves anteriorly about 8 cm distal to the greater trochanter, and then runs obliquely across the anterior thigh to meet the apex of the original incision.

Medial and lateral flaps are created to expose the inguinal region and femoral triangle. Scarpa's fascia is incised, and the aponeurosis of the external oblique muscle is visualized. The spermatic cord (round ligament) is retracted medially. The superficial epigastric vessel is ligated. The femoral vessels and the femoral nerve are ligated at their exit from beneath the inguinal ligament. The sartorius and rectus femoris muscles are detached

from the anterior superior iliac spine and anterior inferior iliac spine respectively. The hip is flexed, and blunt dissection with a finger aided by an elevator is used to get around the iliopsoas muscle just proximal to its insertion into the lesser trochanter. The psoas is divided at its insertion. The plane between the pectineus and obturator externus muscles is identified, and the pectineus muscle is divided at its origin from the pubis. The obturator externus is transected at its insertion on the femur as opposed to its origin to avoid accidental division of the obturator artery and its retraction into the pelvis. The origins of the gracilis, adductor longus, adductor brevis, and adductor magnus muscles are divided with the electrocautery while the leg is held in extension and abduction. To complete the anterior portion of the procedure, the hip capsule is incised, and the ligamentum teres is divided with electrocautery.

The thigh is rotated internally, and the tensor fascia lata and gluteus maximus muscles are divided in line with the skin incision. Next, the glu-

teus medius and minimus muscles, as well as the external rotators, including the obturator externus, are detached at their insertions onto the greater trochanter. The sciatic nerve is divided at its exit from the sciatic notch and ligated; the nerve may be injected with bupivacaine to enhance postoperative analgesia. Finally, the hamstrings are divided from their origins on the ischial tuberosity. The incision of the posterior hip capsule completes the amputation.

The quadratus femoris and iliopsoas muscles can be approximated to cover and fill the dead space and the acetabulum. A saw and rasp can be used to smooth and lower the profile of the acetabular lip if this should be too prominent. Next, the obturator externus and gluteus medius muscles are sutured together over the acetabulum. Another alternative is to suture the stumps of the gluteus medius and minimus muscles to the free origins of the adductor muscles. The gluteus maximus fascia is placed over suction drains and anchored to the inguinal ligament and pubic ramus with a nonabsorbable suture. The skin is closed beneath a soft compressive dressing.

Hip disarticulation is better tolerated than transpelvic amputation, with wound complications being less frequent and potential for recovery of function and use of a hip disarticulation prosthesis much greater. Nevertheless, the complication rate remains significant, and mortality may actually be higher than with transpelvic amputation; this is likely related to the fact that most patients undergoing this procedure have severe vascular disease and coronary artery disease.[17]

Several modifications of the standard hip disarticulation have been described. One recent modification is a laterally based approach.[18] The approach is more familiar to most orthopaedic surgeons, and dissection of major blood vessels is easier, resulting in less blood loss. In addition, an anterior rectus femoris flap can be constructed in patients with posterior tu-

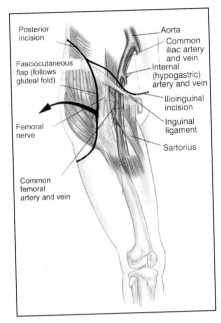

Figure 5 The utilitarian incision for pelvic resection or transpelvic amputation begins at the pubic tubercle and extends along the inguinal ligament and the iliac crest. Depending on the surgeon's preference, the incision is directed inferiorly somewhere between the anterior superior iliac spine and the posterior superior iliac spine. For transpelvic amputation, the incision is extended posteriorly behind the thigh and then along the inferior pubic ramus to the pubic tubercle. *(Reproduced with permission from Malawer MM, Sugarbaker PH: Overview of pelvic resections: Surgical considerations and classifications, in Malawer MM, Sugarbaker PH (eds): Musculoskeletal Cancer Surgery: Treatment of Sarcomas and Allied Diseases. Boston, Kluwer Academic Publishers, 2001, p 213.)*

mors or soft-tissue necrosis. Frey and associates[19] described the use of this femoral artery–based flap in transpelvic amputations, but it can also be used for hip disarticulation.

Transpelvic Amputation

The standard transpelvic amputation is performed with the patient positioned midway between the supine and the lateral decubitus position. This permits the pelvic viscera to move away from the ipsilateral pelvis, allowing easy surgical access to the anterior portion of the incision, thus

facilitating dissection. With the hip adducted and flexed, the perineal and posterior portions of the amputation can be performed. Enemas are used to empty the large bowel preoperatively. A Foley catheter is placed; the ipsilateral leg is draped free; and the skin of the abdomen, groin, buttock, abdomen, perineum, and leg is prepared for surgery. For tumor resection or complex cases of infection, a stent placed in the ipsilateral ureter at the beginning of the procedure may aid in safe dissection, especially after previous surgery or irradiation. The scrotum may be stitched to the opposite thigh to aid in retraction. The anus can be sutured or sealed with an impermeable dressing. If the tumor or infection does not involve the posterior soft tissues, a standard posterior flap is used. If the buttock muscles are involved, an anterior flap based on the rectus femoris is used.

The standard posterior flap for transpelvic amputation proceeds from the anterior dissection, designed to mobilize the parietal peritoneum and isolate the iliac vessels, to the posterior and perineal portions.[20,21] The incision begins at the pubic tubercle and extends along the inguinal ligament and the iliac crest. Depending on the surgeon's preference, the incision is directed inferiorly somewhere between the anterior superior iliac spine and the posterior superior iliac spine (Figure 5). The most posterior extent of the incision is not necessary unless the sacrum is involved, but the additional length affords easier access to the posterior dissection. The anterior portion of the standard transpelvic amputation proceeds by dividing the insertion of the rectus abdominus muscle and detachment of the inguinal ligament and abdominal muscles from the iliac crest. Unroofing the inguinal canal exposes the iliac vessels, the retropubic space, and the spermatic cord (round ligament). The bladder is retracted posteriorly away from the pubis. The inferior epigastric vessels are divided and ligated. The internal iliac vessels, ureter, and lumbosacral trunk are dissected free

from within the retroperitoneal space. At this point, division of the psoas muscle and obturator nerve may facilitate access to the common iliac and iliolumbar vessels. The external iliac vessels and the femoral nerve are divided and ligated. In the case of tumors, the vessels may need to be divided through the common iliacs. As the dissection proceeds posteriorly along the pelvis, the iliolumbar, lateral sacral, superior and inferior gluteal, and internal pudendal branches of the internal iliac artery are divided. At this point, the lumbosacral plexus and hypogastric vessels should be free to retract medially.

The incision for the posterior portion of the procedure passes either directly down the anterior border of the greater trochanter or anteriorly toward the trochanter and then down the leg, depending on how far the incision was carried posteriorly. The hip is sharply flexed and the incision is continued several centimeters distal and parallel to the gluteal crease. The larger the anterior-posterior diameter of the pelvis, the more distal this incision should be made. Mobilization of the intestines with exposure of the retroperitoneum often leads to an ileus. This can result in additional stress on the closure so the length of the flaps should be appropriately generous. For tumor cases, the posterior flap often consists solely of the skin and subcutaneous tissues; the gluteus maximus may be preserved in patients with nontumorous conditions. In this case, the aponeurosis of the gluteus maximus muscle is divided at its posterior and inferior edges.

The flap is retracted upward and elevated over the iliac crest and sacrum; the piriformis muscle and sciatic nerve are divided. The paraspinal muscles of the back must also be subperiosteally stripped from the posterior crest. For the perineal portion of the amputation, the limb is widely abducted by an assistant or suspended from a traction apparatus. The incision is continued from the pubic tubercle or symphysis down along the pubic and ischial rami to

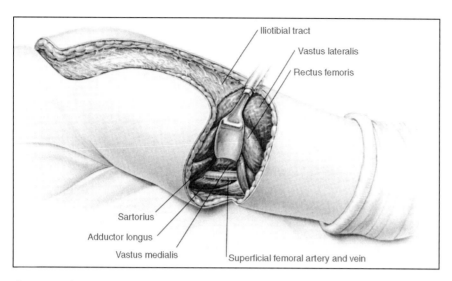

Figure 6 When posterior soft tissue is not available for coverage because of involvement by tumor or necrosis, an anterior myocutaneous flap based on the quadriceps and the blood supply from the superficial femoral artery is used. *(Reproduced with permission from Lawrence W Jr, Neifeld JP, Terz JJ: Diagnosis and staging of the soft-tissue sarcomas, in Egdahl RH (ed): Manual of Soft-Tissue Tumor Surgery. New York, NY, Springer-Verlag, 1983, p 28.)*

the ischial tuberosity. With the bladder and urethra protected by malleable retractors, the pubic symphysis is divided. The corpus cavernosum is stripped from the inferior pubic ramus. The division of the pelvic floor is completed from the ischial tuberosity to the coccyx, dividing the ischiococcygeus and iliococcygeus muscles as well as the sacrotuberous and sacrospinal ligaments. During these maneuvers, the rectum is mobilized from the muscles of the pelvic floor and protected. Returning to the inside of the pelvis, the sacral nerve roots are transected and ligated lateral to the foramina. The iliolumbar ligament is also divided. A Gigli saw is then passed through the sciatic notch or the sacroiliac joint, and the posterior pelvis is divided. An oscillating saw may also be used for this step. Closure is performed in a standard fashion over multiple large suction drains. Sutures may need to be left in place longer than the standard 10 to 14 days.

Occasionally, tissues that comprise the standard posterior hemipelvectomy flap may be contaminated by tumor or compromised by the presence of ulceration and necrosis. In

these situations, an anterior myocutaneous flap may be used that includes all or a portion of the quadriceps and is based on blood flow from the superficial femoral artery (Figure 6). This flap can be as long as necessary to obtain coverage posteriorly. In addition, the posterior coverage provided by the quadriceps muscle provides a durable cushion upon which the pateint may sit in a weight-bearing prosthesis.

There is a clinical role for what is referred to as a modified transpelvic amputation (modified hemipelvectomy). Preservation of the acetabulum and ischium will result in the best functional result with respect to sitting balance, and salvaging the iliac wing will allow for better suspension of a prosthesis and improved cosmesis.

Internal hemipelvectomy is used for treatment of bone tumors but is occasionally used for soft-tissue sarcomas and extensive pressure sores and infection. It is the technique performed when the bony pelvis and the bones of the leg are excised in the construction of a fillet flap.[13,22] An internal hemipelvectomy is usually done through an extended ilioin-

guinal incision, with an extension down the anterolateral thigh and even the leg as needed. Depending upon how far posterior or anterior across the midline this incision is carried, the entire internal and external bony pelvis can be exposed. An internal hemipelvectomy with a fillet flap extending nearly down to the ipsilateral ankle can be used to provide soft-tissue coverage of severe sacral and bilateral trochanteric decubitis ulcers.

Because these procedures often result in the creation of substantial dead space, suction drains should be used liberally and be sutured into place to prevent accidental removal. Soft compressive dressings are applied to encourage the different tissue planes to adhere, thus minimizing seroma and hematoma formation.

Transpelvic amputation is challenging for the surgical team and, of course, much more so for the patient. Complications are frequent, occurring in up to half of patients.[23] Wound complications are common regardless of surgical technique but are most common in those with a subcutaneous flap.[24] Postoperative death occurs in up to 6% of patients.[23] Rehabilitation is easiest for those with an internal hemipelvectomy with preservation of the sciatic nerve. For those with a standard transpelvic amputation, prostheses are mainly for cosmesis as they are heavy and provide only partial weight-bearing support. About one half of younger patients prefer to use a prosthesis. For many patients, crutch walking may actually be easier without the added weight of a prosthesis.[25] Special adaptive pillows can be fashioned to make sitting more comfortable.

Immediate Postoperative Management

If an ileus develops, insertion of a nasogastric tube should be considered in most cases. A general rule is to remove the suction drains when the output is less than 100 mL per day. Antibiotics are continued at least until the drains are removed, with the ultimate duration decided in conjunction with the infectious disease service. For prophylaxis against deep vein thromboses, at the University of Washington we typically use low-molecular-weight heparin and mechanical measures such as a foot pump or pneumatic sequential compression device on the contralateral leg. This regimen is resumed or begun 12 to 24 hours postoperatively but should be stopped with any sign of bleeding or hematoma formation.

Summary

Disarticulation of the hip and transpelvic amputation are technically challenging procedures that require careful planning to minimize the occurrence of intraoperative and postoperative complications. In addition, the broad spectrum of diseases leading to the need for hip disarticulation or transpelvic amputation, and the variable location of specific lesions, may demand a creative approach to develop adequate soft-tissue flaps. The patient is best served by a multidisciplinary team, including surgeons, internists, physiatrists, physical and occupational therapists, and prosthetists. Despite these efforts, the potential for functional rehabilitation following these procedures may be limited.

References

1. Hierton T, James U: Lower extremity amputation in Uppsala county 1947-1969: Incidence and prosthetic rehabilitation. *Acta Orthop Scand* 1973;44: 573-582.

2. Unruh T, Fisher DF Jr, Unruh TA, et al: Hip disarticulation: An 11-year experience. *Arch Surg* 1990;125: 791-793.

3. Larsson J, Apelqvist J, Agardh CD, Stenstrom A: Decreasing incidence of major amputation in diabetic patients: A consequence of a multidisciplinary foot care team approach? *Diabet Med* 1995;12:770-776.

4. Valdes AM, Angderson C, Giner JJ: A multidisciplinary, therapy-based, team approach for efficient and effective wound healing: A retrospective study. *Ostomy Wound Manage* 1999;45:30-36.

5. Smejkal R, Izant T, Born C, Delong W, Schwab W, Ross SE: Pelvic crush injuries with occlusion of the iliac artery. *J Trauma* 1988;28:1479-1482.

6. Brandt MM, Corpron C, Wahl WL: Necrotizing soft tissue infections: A surgical disease. *Am Surg* 2000;66: 967-971.

7. Elliott DC, Kufera JA, Myers RA: Necrotizing soft tissue infections: Risk factors for mortality and strategies for management. *Ann Surg* 1996;224: 672-683.

8. Francis KR, Lamaute HR, Davis JM, Pizzi WF: Implications of risk factors in necrotizing fasciitis. *Am Surg* 1993; 59:304-308.

9. Singh G, Sinha SK, Adhikary S, Babu KS, Ray P, Khanna SK: Necrotizing infections of soft tissues: A clinical profile. *Eur J Surg* 2002;168:366-371.

10. Sharp CS, Bessman AN, Wagner FW Jr, Garland D: Microbiology of deep tissue in diabetic gangrene. *Diabetes Care* 1978;1:289-292.

11. Unger E, Moldofsky P, Gatenby R, Hartz W, Broder G: Diagnosis of osteomyelitis by MR imaging. *AJR Am J Roentgenol* 1988;150:605-610.

12. Enneking WF, Dunham WK: Resection and reconstruction for primary neoplasms involving the innominate bone. *J Bone Joint Surg Am* 1978;60: 731-746.

13. Strinden WD, Mixter RC, Dibbell DG Sr: Internal hemipelvectomy as a treatment for end-stage pressure sores. *Ann Plast Surg* 1989;22:529-532.

14. Yamamoto Y, Minakawa H, Takeda N: Pelvic reconstruction with a free fillet lower leg flap. *Plast Reconstr Surg* 1997; 99:1439-1441.

15. Boyd HB: Anatomic disarticulation of the hip. *Surg Gynecol Obstet* 1947;84: 346-349.

16. Slocum DB: *Atlas of Amputations*. St Louis, MO, Mosby, 1949.

17. Endean ED, Schwarcz TH, Barker DE, Munfakh NA, Wilson-Neely R, Hyde GL: Hip disarticulation: Factors affecting outcome. *J Vasc Surg* 1991;14: 398-404.

18. Lackman RD, Quartararo LG, Farrell ED, Scopp JM: Hip disarticulation using the lateral approach: A new technique. *Clin Orthop* 2001;392: 372-376.

19. Frey C, Matthews LS, Benjamin H, Fidler WJ: A new technique for hemipelvectomy. *Surg Gynecol Obstet* 1976; 143:753-756.

20. King D, Steelquist J: Transiliac amputation. *J Bone Joint Surg Am* 1943;25: 351-367.

21. Sugarbaker PH, Chretien PB: Posterior flap hemipelvectomy, in Sugarbaker PH, Malawer MM (eds): *Musculoskeletal Surgery for Cancer: Principles and Techniques*. New York, NY, Thieme Medical Publishers, 1992, pp 121-137.

22. Lawton RL, De Pinto V: Bilateral hip disarticulation in paraplegics with decubitus ulcers. *Arch Surg* 1987;122: 1040-1043.

23. Apffelstaedt JP, Driscoll DL, Spellman JE, Velez AF, Gibbs JF, Karakousis CP: Complications and outcome of external hemipelvectomy in the management of pelvic tumors. *Ann Surg Oncol* 1996;3:304-309.

24. Capanna R, Manfrini M, Pignatti G, Martelli C, Gamberini G, Campanacci M: Hemipelvectomy in malignant neoplasms of the hip region. *Ital J Orthop Traumatol* 1990;16:425-437.

25. Sneppen O, Johansen T, Heerfordt J, Dissing I, Petersen O: Hemipelvectomy: Postoperative rehabilitation assessed on the basis of 41 cases. *Acta Orthop Scand* 1978;49:175-179.

Chapter 45

Hip Disarticulation and Transpelvic Amputation: Prosthetic Management

Kevin M. Carroll, MS, CP

Introduction

For hip disarticulation and transpelvic amputees, the path to functional prosthesis use can be long and challenging because of the inherent difficulty of ambulation when the entire lower limb has been lost. The energy requirements of prosthesis use in such situations have been shown to be as much as twice that of normal ambulation.[1] Historically, this level has the highest incidence of rejection of any lower limb prosthesis,[2,3] with uncomfortable sockets being mentioned by many amputees as one of the primary reasons for rejection.

Prosthetists who work with hip disarticulation and transpelvic amputees face a task that is daunting but not impossible. They must educate the patient about the unique design and fitting requirements of these high-level sockets. During the fitting process, both the prosthetist and the patient must be satisfied with slow, steady progress, remaining hopeful despite the inevitable frustrations that will arise. Good communication between the prosthetist and the hip disarticulation or transpelvic amputee is especially important to avoid discouragement.

Not only is the fitting of these amputees difficult, but because these high-level amputations are increasingly uncommon, most prosthetists have only limited personal experience fitting these patients. The principles discussed in this chapter should provide sufficient foundation to achieve a positive result. With proper attention to details in material selection and socket configuration, the fitting and fabrication of a comfortable, functional prosthesis can be achieved.

Historical Background

The original tilting table prostheses of the 1940s for hip disarticulation and transpelvic amputees were not very successful. These prostheses consisted of a molded leather socket with a laterally placed locking hip joint (Figure 1); shoulder straps were often required for suspension. The tilting table prosthesis always incorporated a locking knee joint, and the combination of a locked hip and knee resulted in a very awkward and ungainly gait.

Canadian researcher Colin McLaurin introduced the Canadian hip disarticulation prosthesis in 1954 (Figure 2). His design positioned the amputee's center of gravity posterior to the hip joint and anterior to the knee joint during weight bearing, using biomechanics to stabilize these joints without locking them.[4,5] Building on this concept, Lynquist[6] proposed a fitting concept for a Canadian-type plastic socket for a transpelvic amputee, which proved to be effective for achieving comfortable weight bearing via the soft tissues,

even though there is no bony structure on the involved side of these amputations.

In 1957, Radcliffe[7] presented a biomechanical analysis of the forces necessary for ambulation with the Canadian hip disarticulation prosthesis (Figure 3). This improved clinical un-

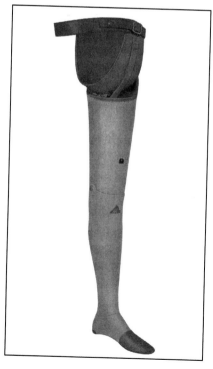

Figure 1 The tilting table prosthesis had a molded leather socket and a laterally placed locking hip joint. The center of gravity was positioned right through the prosthetic hip joint, making the design inherently unstable.

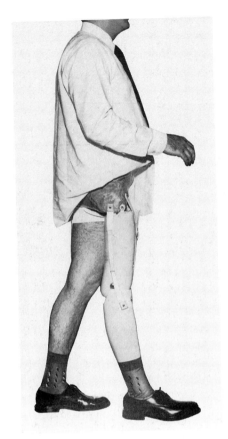

Figure 2 McLaurin's Canadian-style prosthesis was introduced in 1954. It demonstrated the feasibility of using unlocked hip, knee, and ankle joints that relied on biomechanics to achieve stance-phase stability while permitting flexion at the hip and knee during swing phase.

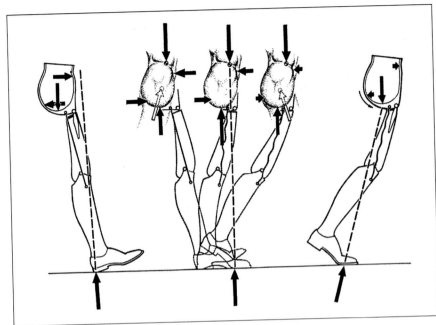

Figure 3 Biomechanical analysis of the forces necessary for ambulation led to development of the Canadian design, which demonstrated that locked joints were not necessary in hip disarticulation and transpelvic prostheses. *(Reproduced with permission from Radcliffe CW: The biomechanics of the Canadian-type hip-disarticulation prosthesis. Artif Limbs 1957;4:29-38.)*

derstanding of McLaurin's recommendations about alignment of these prostheses. Michael[8] further analyzed and endorsed the alignment of the Canadian-type prosthesis in 1988, noting the potential advantage of fluid-controlled knee mechanisms (Figure 4). McLaurin's alignment recommendations for hip disarticulation and transpelvic designs are now well accepted worldwide.

Patient Evaluation

The initial evaluation of a patient with a high-level amputation involves a thorough physical examination. This is an excellent opportunity to begin building a good rapport and open communication between the patient and the prosthetist. Listening to the amputee's frustrations and goals and providing factual information and encouragement are key elements of the prosthetist's role. The residual limb should be thoroughly palpated to ascertain the remaining bony architecture as well as pressure-tolerant and pressure-sensitive areas. Postoperative radiographs are helpful to refer to at this stage. Because of the lack of protective pelvic bone in transpelvic amputees, the prosthetist must determine how to prevent the socket from putting excessive pressure on the bladder or kidneys. This is accomplished by applying manual pressure at various angles on the residual limb. The skin surface must be examined carefully for adhered scar tissue and skin grafting. Some patients will have a colostomy bag or a catheter, which must be taken into consideration in the design of the socket. The patient is also examined carefully for compensatory scoliosis and other postural adaptations that may influence alignment of the prosthetic components.

Upper body strength is evaluated. The unaffected side is examined to detect any hip or knee flexion contracture. Physical therapy is an important part of recovery for these amputees, and it is often useful to invite a physical therapist to participate in the initial evaluation.

Socket Design and Interface

The component that merges the user with the prosthesis is the socket.[9] The fit of the socket is critical because it determines the comfort and functional capabilities of the prosthesis. Socket comfort is a major determinant of whether or not the user will wear the prosthesis long-term. Many hip disarticulation and transpelvic amputees who have a negative experience with the initial fitting give up on wearing a prosthesis altogether and opt to live life on crutches.[10]

Design

Modern endoskeletal prosthetic hip joints are typically placed somewhat more distally on the socket than were the exoskeletal joints of McLaurin's day (Figure 5, *A*). This often results in added bulk under the ischial tuberosity, causing the socket to lean toward the opposite side when the amputee sits. It is possible to place the endoskeletal hip joint lateral to the ischium and somewhat more proximally (Figure 5, B). This minimizes the socket thickness under the ischium and allows the amputee to sit more upright. This somewhat more anatomic placement of the hip joint results in a slightly longer thigh segment than if the joint were placed beneath the ischium, thereby better equalizing the thigh-shin length compared with the sound side.

The lateral socket contour can be shaped to match the opposite side, enhancing the cosmesis of the final result. The socket includes a platform inferior to the ischium that is parallel to the ground in standing; this helps keep the residual limb from slipping out of the socket as the patient ambulates. Suprailiac suspension can often be augmented by capturing the soft tissues in an intimately contoured socket, similar to the concept of a suction socket for the transfemoral amputee.[11,12]

Materials

The socket is commonly formed from a lightweight thermoplastic material such as polypropylene and copolymer that is durable yet permits areas of flexibility as needed.[13-15] Most sockets are positioned inside a rigid carbon-fiber–reinforced outer frame that adds stability and anchors the components securely. The socket should be custom designed to accommodate the weight of the individual user; accordingly, a lighter weight person should receive a lighter socket than would a much heavier individual. Because the primary weight of such prostheses derives from the components rather than the socket, lightweight materials such as titanium or carbon composites are generally indicated.

Containment

Weight bearing in the absence of pelvic bone on the involved side makes

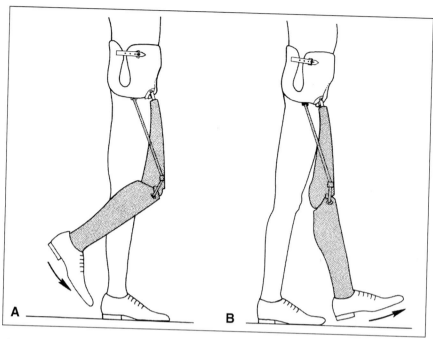

Figure 4 A, Canadian prosthesis in early swing phase. The hip joint remains neutral as the shank swings forward. **B**, Canadian prosthesis just after midswing. The hip joint does not flex until shank motion is arrested by the terminal extension stop. As a result, the prosthesis is fully extended at the instant of midswing, which makes toe clearance difficult. (*Reproduced with permission from Michael J: Component selection criteria: Lower limb disarticulations. Clin Prosthet Orthot 1988;12:99-108.*)

fitting a socket for the transpelvic amputee particularly challenging. The sound gluteus maximus should be captured within the socket as much as possible, and the trimline kept as close to the sound side as the patient can tolerate. Otherwise, the soft tissues tend to protrude distally under weight bearing as the socket pistons up and down on the patient's torso. This is sometimes referred to as an ischial shelf on the sound side,[16] but it is more likely peripheral weight bearing on the bulk of the gluteal musculature (Figure 6).

It is important to create a stable and secure weight-bearing surface in the socket, based on an accurate negative plaster impression. When the weight bearing is tenuous, controlling the prosthesis is very difficult, creating a feeling of uncertainty that is more pronounced for transpelvic amputees. When this occurs, patients sometimes try to compensate by tightening the proximal portion of the socket, increasing pressure directly underneath the rib cage. In ex-

treme cases, this can result in rib fractures.

Hip disarticulation sockets should incorporate ischial containment, which prevents the tuberosity from slipping out of the socket and enhances control over the prosthetic limb. Ischial containment stabilizes the prosthesis in the coronal and sagittal planes[11,12] (Figure 7). The lower portion of the pubic ramus is also contained within the socket, and the ascending portion exits the socket along the medial trim line. A thin piece of low-modulus material can be placed under the ischial tuberosity as a cushioning layer if necessary. If the ischiopubic ramus is not contained without causing discomfort, the patient will likely reject the prosthesis.

Casting, Fitting, and Suspension
Casting

The casting process for hip disarticulation and transpelvic sockets is very

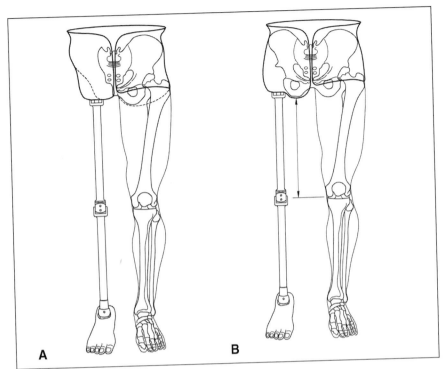

Figure 5 A, Transpelvic prosthesis demonstrates an outset hip joint, evenly aligned hips and knees, and the upper edge of the socket locked around the iliac crest and soft tissue. The dotted line on the unaffected limb identifies the key area of socket containment, defined as the gluteal ring. The dotted line on the amputated side indicates the weight distribution area where the residual limb contacts the socket. **B,** Hip disarticulation prosthesis demonstrates ischial containment, the outset hip joint, evenly aligned hips and knees, and the upper edge of the socket locked around the iliac crests.

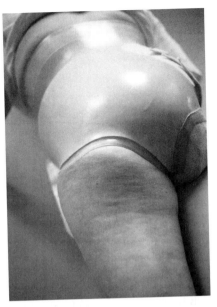

Figure 6 The gluteal ring on the unaffected side has been captured within this completed transpelvic socket, giving the user added stability and more even distribution of pressure.

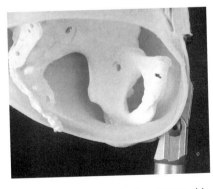

Figure 7 The anatomically correct hip disarticulation socket captures the ischium, allowing better stabilization of the prosthesis in medial-lateral and antero-posterior directions.

similar. The amputee dons a snug-fitting stockinette. If it has a vertical seam, this is positioned at the midline of the body, in contact with the coccyx and symphysis pubis. A simple device fashioned from clear plastic and soft tubing may be used to assist in the casting process. This casting apparatus is fitted to the patient before any plaster is applied, and the tubing is snugged over the ilium, particularly on the sound side. The tubing allows for a more accurate cast in this region, improving the suspension of the socket. In transpelvic amputees, the soft tissues on the involved side are contoured as if the iliac crest was still present. This improves suspension and provides a more normal appearance under clothing. Achievement of comfortable anterior/posterior compression during the casting process yields a socket that will offer the wearer good control over the prosthesis.

Measurements can then be taken and bony landmarks noted on the stockinette. The casting apparatus is then removed and up to 6 layers of 35-cm elastic plaster is wrapped snugly around the residual limb, beginning on the anterior, moving to the inferior, then up laterally around the sound hip above the iliac crest. It is important that the plaster mold extend to the midline anteriorly and posteriorly (Figure 8). Finally, the casting apparatus is donned again and the anterior and posterior impression plates are cinched tightly into place, contacting the cast directly and causing a slight flattening of the plaster (Figure 9). The hip joint placement can be identified at this time.

Fitting

After the positive model has been rectified, a clear, diagnostic test socket is created from a lightweight thermoplastic material. The transparency of the socket enables visual examination of the underlying tissue and its response when weight-bearing pressure is applied[16] (Figure 10). The test socket is modified until both the patient and the prosthetist are satisfied with socket comfort and security. Proceeding methodically at this phase of the fitting process helps to achieve the optimal result.

Suspension

The hip disarticulation socket is suspended by locking onto the waist just

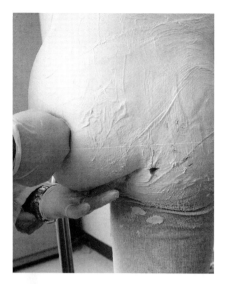

Figure 8 Lateral force applied to the gluteals is an important part of casting and fitting the socket.

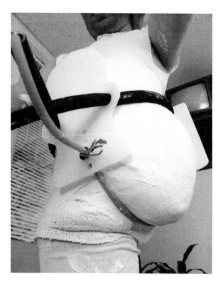

Figure 9 This casting apparatus employs anterior and posterior impression plates for compression, with a soft tube used for contouring above the iliac crests.

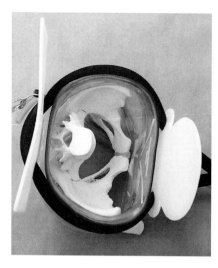

Figure 10 This view looking downward into a clear test socket shows how the skeletal structure of the pelvis is encased. The casting apparatus is positioned on the outside of the socket, demonstrating the anterior/posterior compression.

above the iliac crest on both sides. The upper border is usually trimmed just proximal to the iliac crests. The border can be an inch or so higher in some cases, if no rib impingement occurs during sitting. For the transpelvic socket, the distal trimlines are often so low that the anteroinferior border of the socket contacts the patient's thigh musculature during sitting (Figure 11). The best procedure is to start with extensive proximal and distal trimlines and trim in small increments, allowing both the patient and the prosthetist time to re-evaluate the fit during sitting, standing, and walking after each modification (Figure 12).

The final trimlines inevitably represent a compromise between socket control and patient comfort. The prosthetist must explain the fitting process to the patient, helping the patient understand the trade-offs that are required to achieve an effective final result.

Liners

Low-modulus gel liners may be used for both hip disarticulation and transpelvic amputees to protect the surface of the soft tissues. A large-sized prefabricated gel liner can usually be modified by cutting a hole for

the sound leg and then stretching the liner up around the user's trunk (Figure 13). This added layer between the skin and the socket absorbs some of the friction that occurs during ambulation.[17,18] The liner should reduce abrasions to the skin, and the elasticity of the material increases patient comfort and long-term use. Patients with notable areas of tissue breakdown are especially good candidates for a low-modulus gel liner.

Other Components

The foundation of a functional, properly aligned hip disarticulation/transpelvic prosthesis is a well-fitting, comfortable socket. Selection of the remaining components and determination of the functional length of the prosthesis are equally important, however (Figure 14). All elements of the prosthesis must work in harmony to achieve comfort and mobility at this level.

Hip Joint

The mechanical hip joint is attached directly to the socket or rigid frame, in a location sufficiently anterior to the acetabulum that the weight-bearing line falls posterior to the hip

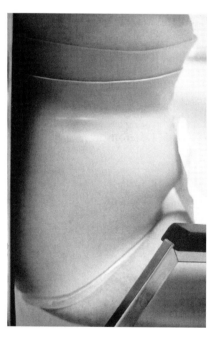

Figure 11 To capture the gluteal ring on the sound side, the anteroinferior edge of the socket extends quite low and may contact the proximal thigh during sitting. This improves the user's control over the limb.

axis during standing. Patients who require extra stability may prefer a locking hip joint with a stride limiter that allows only a short stride. Hip flexion bias systems, incorporating a spring-loaded hip that uses kinetic energy to

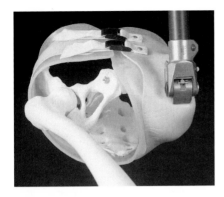

Figure 12 The socket must be comfortable when the patient sits as well as during standing and walking. The flat sitting surface on the anatomically correct hip disarticulation/transpelvic socket not only allows for good support while sitting but also prevents the soft tissue from slipping out of the socket.

flex the prosthetic thigh forward at toe-off,[8,19] result in more normal knee flexion timing, increasing midswing toe clearance (Figure 15).

Knee Joint

Knee joints are selected according to each user's activity level, just as with more distal amputation levels. The two basic categories of knees are single-axis and polycentric.[20] Single-axis knees work well for users with lower activity levels, while more active individuals often prefer polycentric designs,[21,22] particularly those offering increased stance-phase stability. Many polycentric knees also improve swing-phase clearance of the foot.[16,20] Motion studies conducted at Northwestern University confirmed that fluid-controlled knees (hydraulic or pneumatic) result in a more normal gait for the hip disarticulation/transpelvic amputee.[9] Gait analysis has demonstrated that for hip disarticulation users, hydraulic knees result in a more normal range of motion at the hip joint during ambulation and also contribute to a more rapid cadence.[23]

Rotators and Shock Absorbers

Positional rotators, torque absorbers, and vertical shock absorbers are often

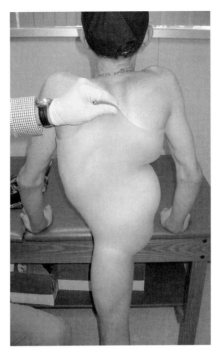

Figure 13 A low-modulus gel liner gives the user an immediate feeling of support and serves as a protective, shock-absorbing layer between the residual limb and socket.

useful for the hip disarticulation and transpelvic levels. The positional rotator allows the knee and shin to be rotated in relationship to the hip,[16] which is important when the user wants to change shoes, sit cross-legged, or get into or out of a car or similar confined space (Figure 16). The torque absorber allows the foot to rotate in relationship to the pelvis. The high-level amputee has lost all physiologic lower limb joints and hence has no way to compensate for the normal rotation of ambulation.[24] Use of a vertical shock absorber is believed to reduce ground-reaction forces on the torso in these amputees, increasing amputee comfort and acceptance of the prosthesis (Figure 17).

Foot Selection

The type of foot selected for the hip disarticulation/transpelvic prosthesis depends primarily on the user's activity level. In general, the more responsive the foot mechanism, the more important the resistance of the knee unit becomes.[9] Dynamic-response feet provide a sense of active push-off;

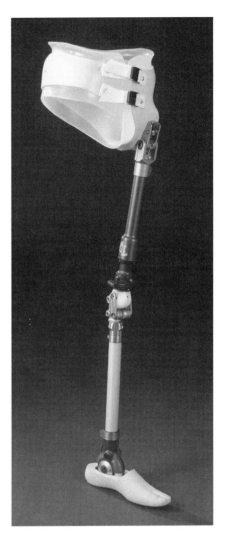

Figure 14 Complete hip disarticulation/transpelvic prosthesis—anatomically correct socket, anterior hip joint, torque- and shock-absorbing pylon, positional rotator, polycentric knee, and dynamic-response foot.

some hip disarticulation users report the ability to walk faster with such components.[25] When selecting any prosthetic component, the primary goals are minimizing component weight while facilitating a more normal and energy-efficient gait.[16]

Follow-up Care

Physical therapy is absolutely essential to the attainment of an optimal level of prosthetic function. The physical therapist ideally should have experience in gait training with hip disarticulation and transpelvic amputees.

After fitting the final prosthesis, follow-up visits should be scheduled at 2 weeks, 1 month, 3 months, 6 months, and 1 year. After the first year, an annual visit for inspection of the prosthesis and skin for any potential problems is prudent. Patients should also be encouraged to schedule an office visit whenever they experience pain or have any significant concerns related to their prosthesis.

Lifestyle Considerations

Numerous special lifestyle considerations should be discussed with hip disarticulation and transpelvic amputees, particularly if the limb loss is recent. Some of these topics are highly personal and include such concerns as toileting, sex, selecting the right undergarments, considering pregnancy and childbirth, controlling weight, and using assistive devices for balance.

Toileting

When urinating, men can leave the prosthesis in place, but women often need to remove it, particularly when the trimline is at the midline of the body. The prosthetist should consider trimming the socket, if possible, so the user can urinate without removing the prosthesis. This entails a trade-off—less weight-bearing support but greater convenience. For both men and women, it is almost always necessary to remove the prosthetic limb for a bowel movement. In the not unusual situation where the hip disarticulation or transpelvic amputee has a colostomy collection bag, a hole must be cut in the socket to allow access to the stoma. A small donut-shaped ring of soft, flexible plastic that encircles the stoma and positions the bag on the outside of the socket may be used. The ring also spreads socket forces away from the stoma region so that no pressure is placed around the collection bag (Figure 18).

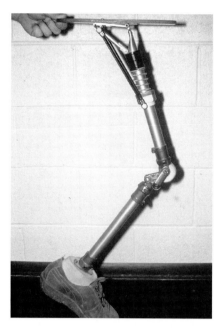

Figure 15 The hip flexion bias system has a spring-loaded hip that thrusts the prosthetic thigh forward at toe-off. This "shortening" of the leg allows for better ground clearance of the foot.

Undergarment Selection

Finding appropriate undergarments for use under a hip disarticulation or transpelvic socket can be another challenge. Commercial stockinettes and knitted body stockings are available, but many patients prefer to modify sports clothing for this purpose. Unitards, bicycle shorts with one leg sewn shut, and homemade cotton or Spandex garments are a few of the more common options.[26] Many women find it helpful to wear a long-line bra that extends into the proximal trimlines of the socket to prevent the tissue from forming rolls that are easily pinched by the socket edge.

Pregnancy and Childbirth

Female patients often have concerns related to pregnancy and childbirth.[26] Many hip disarticulation and transpelvic amputees can become pregnant, carry to term, and have a normal vaginal delivery. Although pregnant women can continue wearing a prosthesis, most eventually find crutches to be more practical by the second or third trimester, based on

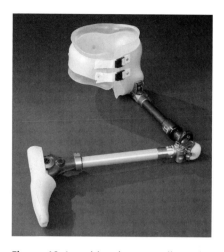

Figure 16 A positional rotator allows the knee and shin to be rotated in relationship to the hip, making it easier for the user to change shoes, sit cross-legged, or get into and out of a car.

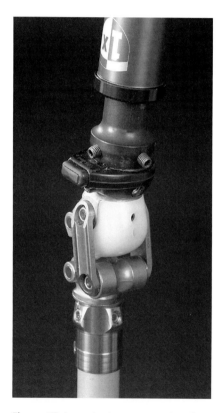

Figure 17 Important components often used in hip disarticulation/transpelvic prostheses include a torque/shock-absorbing pylon, positional rotator, and a polycentric knee.

comfort, energy expenditure, and other personal considerations. A supportive maternity sling that extends under the abdomen can be very help-

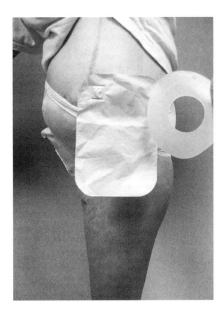

Figure 18 This soft plastic ring is positioned between the colostomy bag and the skin, distributing socket forces away from the stoma area.

ful when the patient is not wearing the prosthesis. Hip disarticulation amputees have the advantage of an intact pelvis, which supports the weight of the uterus during pregnancy. As the size of the abdomen increases, the socket can be trimmed and modified as needed. Significant alterations of the socket are required to accommodate the body changes during pregnancy, so that fabrication of a new socket is usually required after delivery.

Weight Control

Obesity can severely limit any amputee's ability to walk with a prosthesis, but it is particularly troublesome for hip disarticulation and transpelvic amputees. Excess weight adds stress to the sound leg, and adipose tissue on the trunk complicates creation of a comfortable socket. Swimming is an excellent and safe way for hip disarticulation and transpelvic amputees to exercise for weight control because less stress is put on the joints.

Considerations When the Prosthesis Is Not Being Worn

Just as many people like to take off their shoes when they come home,

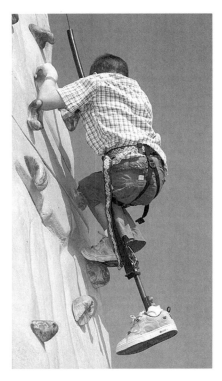

Figure 19 This young hip disarticulation amputee demonstrates high functionality, participating in rock climbing and other highly physical activities.

hip disarticulation and transpelvic amputees may prefer to remove the prosthesis after work. Sitting on the floor to play with young children, for example, is often easier without the prosthesis. Transpelvic amputees may benefit from use of a sitting socket when they are not wearing the full prosthesis,[27] particularly if they use a wheelchair part or all of the time. Sitting sockets are also recommended as a protective measure when hip disarticulation or transpelvic amputees participate in sporting activities without a prosthesis.

The hip disarticulation or transpelvic amputee must understand that hopping on the sound leg puts tremendous stress on the joints and foot. Proper use of crutches is far preferable to hopping for long distances.[26] Crutches that are not fitted correctly, however, can cause shoulder strain and problems with the joints and nerves in the arms and hands. A large percentage of hip disarticulation and transpelvic amputees find a cane to be

essential to their stability and balance while using the prosthesis.[26]

Summary

Clear communication and understanding between the prosthetist and the hip disarticulation or transpelvic amputee is critical to functional success. Both must be willing to overcome the inevitable frustration associated with creating a prosthesis for loss at these high levels. The efforts of a detail-oriented, methodical, communicative prosthetist in combination with optimally aligned components well suited to the patient's physical abilities and aspirations will result in significantly greater patient acceptance and long-term success with these prostheses (Figure 19).

References

1. Waters RL, Perry J, Antonelli D, Hislop H: Energy cost of walking of amputees: The influence of level of amputation. *J Bone Joint Surg Am* 1976;58: 42-46.
2. Steen Jensen J, Mandrup-Poulsen T: Success rate of prosthetic fitting after major amputations of the lower limb. *Prosthet Orthot Int* 1983;7:119-121.
3. Shurr DG, Cook TM, Buckwalter JA, Cooper RR: Hip disarticulation: A prosthetic follow-up. *Orthot Prosthet* 1983;37:50-57.
4. McLaurin CA: *Hip Disarticulation Prosthesis, Report No. 15.* Toronto, Canada, Prosthetic Services Center, Department of Veterans Affairs, 1954.
5. McLaurin CA, Hampton F (eds): *Diagonal Type Socket for Hip Disarticulation Amputees.* Chicago, IL, Northwestern University Prosthetic Research Center, 1962.
6. Lynquist E: Canadian-type plastic socket for a hemi-pelvectomy. *Artif Limbs* 1958;5:130-132.
7. Radcliffe CW: The biomechanics of the Canadian-type hip-disarticulation prosthesis. *Artif Limbs* 1957;4:29-38.
8. Michael J: Component selection criteria: Lower limb disarticulations. *Clin Prosthet Orthot* 1988;12:99-108.
9. van der Waarde T, Michael J: Hip disarticulation and transpelvic amputa-

tion: Prosthetic management, in Bowker JH, Michael JW (eds): *Atlas of Limb Prosthetics: Surgical, Prosthetic, and Rehabilitation Principles*, ed 2. Rosemont, IL, American Academy of Orthopaedic Surgeons, 2002, pp 539-552. (Originally published by Mosby-Year Book, 1992.)

10. Pitkin MR: Effects of design variants in lower-limb prostheses on gait synergy. *J Prosthet Orthot* 1997;9:113-122.

11. Sabolich J: Contoured adducted trochanteric-controlled alignment method (CAT-CAM): Introduction and basic principles. *Clin Prosthet Orthot* 1985;9:15-26.

12. Sabolich J, Guth T: The CAT-CAM-HD™: A new design for hip disarticulation patients. *Clin Prosthet Orthot* 1988;12:119-122.

13. Angelico J: Sockets for hip disarticulation and hemipelvectomy amputees. *In Motion* Sept/Oct 2001;19-20.

14. Imler C, Quigley M: A technique for thermoforming hip disarticulation prosthetic sockets. *J Prosthet Orthot* 1990;3:34-37.

15. Madden M: The flexible socket system as applied to the hip disarticulation amputee. *Orthot Prosthet* 1985;39:44-47.

16. Jeffries GE, Angelico J, Denison A, Kaier J: Prosthetic Primer: Fitting for hip disarticulation and hemipelvectomy level amputations. *In Motion* March/April 1999;38-45.

17. Haberman LJ, Bedotto RA, Colodney EJ: Silicone-only suspension (SOS) for the above-knee amputee. *J Prosthet Orthot* 1992;4:2:76-85.

18. Uellendahl J: Prosthetic socks and liners, in *First Step: A Guide for Adapting to Limb Loss*. Knoxville, TN, Amputee Coalition of America, 2001, vol 2, pp 56-58.

19. Haslam T, Wilson M: *Hip Flexion Bias, Concept 80*. Houston, TX, Medical Center Prosthetics, 1980.

20. Gard SA, Childress DS, Uellendahl JE: The influence of four-bar linkage knees on prosthetic swing-phase floor clearance. *J Prosthet Orthot* 1996;8:34-40.

21. Michael JW: Prosthetic knee mechanisms. *Phys Med Rehabil* 1994;8:147-164.

22. Oberg KET, Kamwendo K: Knee components for the above-knee amputation, in Murdoch G, Donovan RG (eds): *Amputation Surgery and Lower-Limb Prosthetics*. Oxford, England, Blackwell Scientific Publications, 1988, pp 152-164.

23. Van Vorhis RL, Childress DS: Kinematic aspects of the Canadian hip disarticulation prosthesis: Preliminary results, in Murdoch G (ed): *Amputation Surgery and Lower-Limb Prosthetics*. Oxford, England, Blackwell Scientific Publications, 1988, pp 245-249.

24. O'Riain M: Report: *Clinical Data on Floor Reaction Forces: Shear*. Ottawa, Canada, Royal Ottawa Rehabilitation Center, 1985.

25. Michael J: Energy storing feet: A clinical comparison. *Clin Prosthet Orthot* 1987;11:154-168.

26. Skoski C: HP/HD Help. http://hphdhelp.org/aboutthe.htm. Accessed January 29, 2002.

27. Moretto DF, Minkel JL, Cardi MD: Prosthetic/orthotic management after recent hemipelvectomy for a myelomeningocele patient. *J Prosthet Orthot* 1992;4:93-102.

Chapter 46

Translumbar Amputation: Surgical Management

Lawrence D. Wagman, MD

Jose J. Terz, MD

Introduction

Ablation of the caudal half of the human body described by the level of amputation is termed translumbar amputation (TLA); described by the extent of amputation, it is termed hemicorporectomy. TLA results in extensive loss of structure and function. Fortunately, advances in surgical reconstruction, physical and social rehabilitation, prosthetic materials and fitting, and functional aids can ameliorate the ravages of this surgical procedure. Unlike all other amputations, TLA involves the loss of structures used in functions other than mobility and manipulation. The sphincteric and storage functions of the anus and rectum and urogenital diaphragm and bladder are lost. Sexuality is severely diminished because both internal and external endocrine and reproductive organs are lost. Extensive postoperative problems are inevitable, charging the surgeon and the support team with the task of careful patient selection and preoperative patient and family education, including communicating with absolute clarity the risks and benefits involved. This operation is being performed with decreasing frequency and in a more carefully selected group of patients. The explanation for this is at once clear and arcane. Surgical procedures have, in general, trended toward a reduction in deformity and functional consequences. In addition, diagnostic modalities have improved analysis of nonlocal disease. Finally, the increasing success of chemotherapy and radiation is challenging the TLA, with its modest chance to cure disease and extraordinarily high morbidity.

Patient Selection

A TLA cannot be planned and accomplished within a short period of time. Patients must be gradually advised of the losses they will face and the relative benefit of the operation in arresting the disease process and alleviating the symptoms. Patients must be given latitude in deciding on the operation, and it may be anticipated that a patient will cancel or delay the planned TLA. The surgeon and rehabilitation team must be sensitive to this reluctance and respond with additional support and education. Coercion, intimidation, or incomplete discussion of the extent of the operation will undermine the team's ability to provide optimal patient care and endanger the requisite strong patient-physician relationship.

In general, patients who are eligible for TLA will have a local disease process that is recurrent or chronic. Recurrent conditions include low-grade, nonmetastasizing tumors with an excellent chance for long-term cure, such as low-grade chondrosarcomas, sacral chordomas, giant cell tumors, or vascular neoplasm (massive hemangiomas or arteriovenous malformations).[1] Only rarely will patients with significant spinal cord injury resulting in paraplegia, loss of potency, insensate anal sphincter, chronic urinary tract disease due to a neurogenic bladder, and severe pressure ulcers be candidates for TLA.[2] Patients with squamous cell carcinoma of paretic dysfunctional limbs have also been treated with TLA.[3,4] These tumors, however, may be quite aggressive, making them inappropriate for treatment by a surgical procedure with a recovery period that approaches 6 months to 1 year (Table 1). Also, despite the functional losses and significant structural distortion associated with this condition, few patients would consider loss of these cumbersome limbs and dysfunctional structures valuable or necessary. "Looking whole," even when the whole is defective, is psychologically important. The need for intactness of the body becomes one of the major driving forces in the patient's rehabilitation after TLA. The rehabilitation must be structural and functional.

An evaluation of the extent of the primary disease should include an exhaustive pre- and intraoperative search for metastases or proximal local tumor growth. Diagnosis of the intrathecal extension of sacral tumors includes MRI, which can differentiate between tumor and radiation therapy–induced changes.[5] MRI can also identify any infiltration of the

TABLE 1 Translumbar Amputations

Parameter	Patient 1	Patient 2	Patient 3
Age at surgery (years)	60	51	33
Years from primary diagnosis	4	0.25	20
Pathologic diagnosis	Sacral chordoma	Paraplegia, Marjolin's ulcer	Chondrosarcoma
Number of previous treatments	3	3	4
Extenuating circumstances	Pain, paresthesias	Septic wound	Left lower limb paralysis
Estimated blood loss (mm³)	3,500	8,700	3,000
Fluid replacement (mm³)			2,500
Blood	3,250	12,000	
Fresh-frozen plasma	1,000	3,800	
Complications	Renal dysfunction, acute respiratory distress syndrome, hypertension, flap necrosis, myocardial infarct	Wound separation, candida esophagitis, sepsis, small-bowel fistula	Wound infection, retained spinous process
Length of surgery (hours)	10.5	11.5	7.5
Hospital time (days)	65	133	52
Post-TLA survival (years)	6.5	0.5	2.0
Status	DOD	DOD	DOD

Parameter	Patient 4	Patient 5	Patient 6
Age at surgery (years)	26	23	29
Years from primary diagnosis	5	4	4
Pathologic diagnosis	Arteriovenous malformation	Giant cell tumor	Sacral chordoma
Number of previous treatments	3	2	2
Extenuating circumstances	Congestive heart failure, buttock necrosis	Pain, tumor, erosion to rectum	Pain, bowel dysfunction, bladder dysfunction
Estimated blood loss (mm³)	5,000	7,000	3,500
Fluid replacement (mm³)			2,500
Blood	5,000	3,750	2,500
Fresh-frozen plasma	1,250	1,500	800
Complications	Urinary leak, lobar collapse, renal cell carcinoma treated with left nephrectomy 9 years after TLA	Bleeding, wound separation, hypertension	Flap necrosis, urinary leak
Length of surgery (hours)	13	10.5	13
Hospital time (days)	90	66	31
Post-TLA survival (years)	7.0	2.7	10
Status	NED	NED	DOD

DOD = dead of disease; NED = no evidence of disease

paraspinal muscles by tumor and soft-tissue masses encroaching on the dural sac of the nerve roots. Patients in whom the disease cannot be encompassed completely are not candidates for TLA.

Surgical Technique

The strategy for the surgical portion of a TLA can be divided into three sections: soft tissue, bony and neural, and vascular. The latter two, once undertaken, commit the surgeon to completing the TLA, whereas the former can be undertaken as the preliminary portion of the operation and be used as a diagnostic as well as a therapeutic maneuver. The integrated surgical team includes an anesthesiologist, a neurosurgeon, an orthopaedic surgeon, a urologist, a reconstructive surgeon, and a surgical oncologist. The intraoperative findings will dictate the degree of involvement of each of these specialists. Adequate amounts of blood and blood products or a system for intraoperative blood loss collection and reinfusion should be prepared. Hemodynamic monitoring with arterial and central venous catheters is needed. The positioning of the patient after intubation will depend on the surgical plans for the individual patient. The surgery may be performed as a single-stage or two-stage procedure. The two-stage procedure consists of initial analysis of disease extent and diversion of fecal and urinary streams before the second, "clean" portion of the operation, which involves bony, vascular, and soft-tissue resection and reconstruction. The use of a two-stage procedure also distributes the surgical trauma, including tissue injury and blood loss.[6] If technically feasible, the first stage could be performed laparoscopically or with laparoscopic assistance, further reducing the surgical trauma. The incisions and/or placement sites must anticipate the resection incision, margins, and flaps for reconstruction.

In both a single- or two-stage TLA, the initial incision begins at the most posterior aspect of the iliac crest and extends anteriorly, along the inferior edge of the anterior abdominal wall at the level of the inguinal crease along the pubic bone to the pubic symphysis; the incision continues in a mirror image pattern on the contralateral side. The muscles of the anterolateral abdominal wall are divided from their bony insertions onto the pelvis. The inferior epigastric artery and vein are also divided at this time. In the male, the spermatic cords are left with the specimen. The abdomen is then opened. In the one-step procedure, an exploration can be performed to assess the intra-abdominal extent of the tumor and potential sites of metastases, including the periaortic nodes above the planned level of transection (L3-L4), paraspinal soft tissues, and the liver parenchyma. If any suspicious findings are noted, biopsies can be performed before any irreversible steps are taken. If there is any doubt regarding the level of tumor infiltration, a biopsy should be performed and evaluated with histologic procedures to ensure that the soft-tissue margin is adequate, with no evidence of pathology.

After the resectability of the tumor is confirmed, the anterior flap is reflected superiorly by dividing the balance of the anterior abdominal muscles, and attention can be directed toward division of the intra-abdominal vascular structures and soft tissues. The ureters are identified at or above the level of the common iliac vessels. Consideration of tumor location, previous radiation therapy, and planned urologic reconstruction will determine the level of ureteral division. Care is taken to preserve the entire length of the ureter with its enveloping blood supply. Because of the level of amputation, most of the blood supply to the ureters will descend in a caudal direction from the renal pelvis. At the time of ureteral division, a large clip or a tie is placed on the proximal portion of the ureter to allow dilation before reconstruction.

The aorta and vena cava are mobilized above their bifurcations and below the renal artery and veins. If necessary, the inferior mesenteric artery can be divided. Mobilization of the great vessels will invariably require division of one or two of the lumbar vessels and the right gonadal artery. After complete mobilization, the aorta is cross-clamped by placing a vascular clamp approximately 2 cm cephalad to the planned division site. Communication between the anesthesiologist and surgeon is required at this point to ensure precise evaluation of changes in arterial blood pressure, urine output, and central venous or left ventricular end diastolic pressure (pulmonary capillary wedge pressure). Because of the marked reduction in total vascular space, acute hypertensive changes may require stepwise clamping with the addition of peripheral vasodilators (nitroglycerine) and mild volume reduction (diuresis). It is best to have kept the patient euvolemic or slightly hypovolemic with a brisk urine output in preparation for this maneuver. Autotransfusion maneuvers—lifting the lower limbs or placing the patient in a Trendelenburg position—may be used with extreme caution and careful monitoring of central venous pressure, pulmonary artery pressure,

and arterial blood pressure. The aorta is transected sharply and the distal end is then oversewn. The proximal portion of the aorta is closed with a running 3-0 monofilament vascular suture. The vascular clamp is released one or two clicks and any additional hemostasis is secured with interrupted sutures. In rare instances, sutures and pledgets may be required because of atherosclerotic changes or injury from previous radiation therapy. Communication between the surgeon and the anesthesiologist is critical in anticipating and monitoring the sudden loss of venous return. The vena cava, which has been prepared and controlled, is clamped and divided in a similar manner. Often, a thinner suture material (4-0 monofilament) can be used for the closure. At the surgeon's discretion, vascular stapling devices may be used for these steps.

With the completion of mobilization and division of the aorta and vena cava, attention is turned to the right and left sides of the retroperitoneum. On the right side, the gonadal vein, and on the left side, the gonadal artery and vein are the primary remaining retroperitoneal vascular structures to be ligated and divided at the level of the planned muscular transection. The base of the small-bowel mesentery with the right and ileocolic vessels, cecum, and right colon are mobilized cephalad in a manner similar to that used in a right retroperitoneal lymph node dissection. The right colon and terminal ileum will be used to construct a continent reservoir for the urinary diversion (with loss of the ileocecal valve and most of the right colon), so preservation of maximum colonic length is important. Care must be taken in dividing the sigmoid colon at its most distal, viable extent. This is especially important if the inferior mesenteric artery has been ligated at its takeoff from the aorta. The paired structures of the retroperitoneum, including the sympathetic trunk, psoas muscle, and genitofemoral and femoral nerves, are divided. The musculature of the pos-

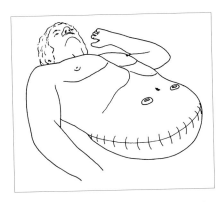

Figure 1 Standard flap technique. The anterior and posterior skin flaps are closed primarily. The paired stomas on the abdominal wall are at approximately the level of the umbilicus. The positioning of the stomas takes into account the planned design of a bucket prosthesis.

terior abdominal and lumbar areas is divided at a level selected to preserve the maximum amount of vascularized soft tissue for closure.

The division of the bony structures (vertebral bodies, transverse processes, and spinous process) and the dural sac with the spinal cord can be approached in one of two ways. In patients with neoplastic disease that extends proximally along the dura or meninges or in patients in whom preoperative evaluation suggests possible tumor extension intrathecally above a resectable level, the surgical procedure should begin with a posterior element laminectomy from approximately T11 to L3. This may have been done as the first stage of a two-stage approach. This initial exploration can be extended to include opening of the dura, division of the cauda equina (at the L1-2 level), and repair of the cephalad dura division. Caution should be exercised in dividing the cauda equina in patients with neurologically intact lower limb function, and functional bladder and anal sphincters. Spinal shock requiring volume expansion must be treated with consideration of the reduced vascular volume and risk of acute pulmonary edema.[7] Meticulous hemostasis is essential to prevent an epidural hematoma.

The patient can be turned supine to begin the anterior and intra-abdominal portions of the procedure. When the condition requires a primary anterior approach, such as in patients who require abdominal exploration or biopsy of retroperitoneal or anterior paraspinal musculature, the division of the bony and neural elements is the final step in the TLA. When this approach is used, the disk space is identified at the planned level of the TLA. The disk is removed or divided sharply with a knife and the dural sac is identified anteriorly. The sac is opened and the neural elements ligated and divided. The final division of the transverse process and spinous process is performed with an osteotome. Significant bleeding from the spinal artery and veins may occur at this step. If the bleeding is not easily controlled, packing with sponges can tamponade the vessels and allow for better exposure of these vessels by completing the soft-tissue division. The posterior skin and remaining musculature are rapidly divided. The specimen is removed from the surgical field and meticulous hemostasis is secured along the dura, in the paravertebral muscles, and along the skin edge. Care should be taken to resect any posterior elements (spinous or transverse processes) or residual vertebral bodies that may cause compression on the posterior flap.

Continent urinary diversion has been used more recently with creation of an Indiana pouch,[8,9] which is the formation of a detubularized reservoir from the right colon combined with plication of the terminal ileum and submucosally tunneled ureters. The result is a 350- to 700-mL continent reservoir that requires catheter drainage approximately every 5 to 6 hours. The stoma is created by using the plicated terminal ileum and is placed through the anterior body wall flap in the mid to upper right quadrant. After initial healing, no ostomy bag is required, and the difficulty in fitting the patient in a bucket prosthesis is reduced.

After adequate mobilization of the distal portion of the colon and reexamination of vascular integrity, an end colostomy is formed in a location that will be comfortable for the patient, usually in the center of the left upper portion of the anterior abdominal wall flap. Care must be exercised in planning a stoma that will not be compressed by the upper edge of the prosthetic bucket.

The flap closure is performed in layers, approximating the well-defined fascia of the anterior abdominal wall to the lumbodorsal fascia with interrupted, permanent suture material. The subcutaneous tissues are closed with interrupted absorbable suture and the skin with metal staples or monofilament suture. The colostomy and urinary pouch stomas can then be matured and all wounds covered with appropriate dressings or drainage bags. A net-type dressing covering the TLA stump helps in securing the dressings to the wound without placing tape on the skin of the tenuous flaps (Figure 1).

If large amounts of skin are to be removed, flap reconstruction with myocutaneous or fascial cutaneous flaps can be considered. Occasionally, tissue can be preserved from one or both of the lower limbs.[10] One such flap uses the skin, subcutaneous tissue, and muscle perfused by the femoral artery[11] (Figure 2). The use of free flaps has not been attempted but may provide an additional alternative for coverage of the soft-tissue defect and closure of the wound. This form of reconstruction would be best planned in a two- or even three-stage procedure, assuming that only soft-tissue/cutaneous coverage would be lacking. A temporary biologic dressing may be required while the patient recovers from the ablative stage of the procedure.

Complications

The complications of TLA are primarily related to flap formation, urinary reconstruction, and the extensive surgical procedure (Table 1). The ante-

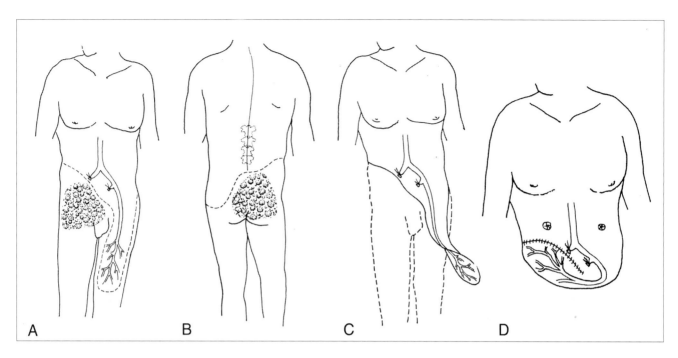

Figure 2 Condition requiring flap reconstruction. **A,** Anterior view. The tumor arises in the right true pelvis and extends across the midline to include the sacrum and lowest lumbar vertebrae. The tumor has penetrated the posterior pelvic wall and extends into the soft tissues of the buttock. The dotted line delineates the incision beginning at the right iliac crest and extending along the pubis and on the left thigh to create the myocutaneous flap. The aorta and left iliofemoral vessels are schematically outlined. **B,** Posterior view. The relationship of the tumor to the bone and soft tissues is shown. **C,** Anterior view. The area outlined by dotted lines represents the surgical specimen. The anterior thigh flap with its supporting vessel is shown. **D,** The completed resection with the anterior thigh flap transposed to cover the inferior defect is shown. The Indiana pouch urinary diversion stoma is seen in the right upper quadrant and the end colostomy in the left upper quadrant.

rior flap will have distal ischemia because of the division of the inferior epigastric artery and vein. In addition, the closure of the flaps may be performed under tension because of the reduction in the volume of the intra-abdominal space (loss of the false and true pelvis, or approximately 25% to 30% of the volume). The posterior flap will be relatively ischemic as a result of the division of the posterior musculature and because of prior treatments, especially radiation therapy for sacral malignancies and embolization for arteriovenous malformations. These factors may also contribute to the tenuous vascular supply to this myocutaneous or fasciocutaneous flap.

In the postoperative period, the patient can be placed in only the supine and lateral positions because of the new stoma, the need for respiratory support on the ventilator, and hemodynamic monitoring. This positioning increases the shear and compressive pressure on the posterior and lateral

aspects of the flap. It is important to remove all posterior bony elements to minimize pressure points on the flap. A variety of specialized beds have been designed to reduce pressure areas and shear effect. The beds are constructed as either a series of air cells that inflate in a cephalad-caudal and right-to-left sequence or as fluidized ceramic microspheres within a monofilament polyester filter sheet. These beds serve primarily to automatically shift the patient's position and prevent pressure, shear, and friction.

Hypertension is an unusual postoperative problem that occurs during the first postoperative week. This condition often requires a combination of diuretics, central α-adrenergic stimulators, peripheral α- and β-blockers, and angiotensin I-converting enzyme inhibitors. Although hypertension was thought to occur as a result of volume expansion during surgery, it may persist indefinitely even after a return to the correct preoperative volume status adjusted for the new body size.

Problems with the urinary diversion system occur in both the immediate and long-term postoperative period. The initial problems are related to urinary leaks from the conduit and the site of ureteral implantation. These are treated with diversion and drainage, and usually do not require formal revision. In the chronic phase, problems are related to urinary tract infections; chronic reflux (prevented by the nonrefluxing ureteral implantation in the Indiana pouch);[9] and metabolic problems related to pouch bicarbonate wasting that results in hyperchloremic metabolic acidosis. These metabolic problems are more common in patients with colonic-based conduits.

Postoperative Management

The early postoperative period is marked by redistribution of the large volumes of blood and other fluids re-

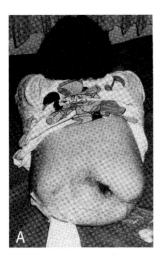 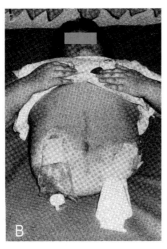 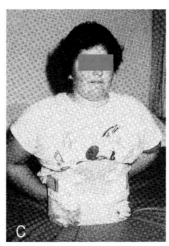 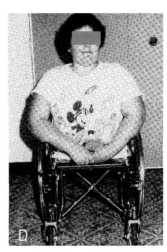

Figure 3 A patient who underwent TLA for arteriovenous malformation (patient 4 in Table 1) shown prone (**A**) and supine (**B**). Note that the flap has a major anterior component and the final suture line is on the posterior aspect. The upper aspect of the mons pubis is seen just to the right of the midline posteriorly. The stomas were placed in the lower portion of the flap (right-sided ileal conduit; left-sided end colostomy). **C,** The patient is independently supported in the bucket prosthesis with good access to the stomas and their appliances. **D,** The patient is prepared for mobility in a wheelchair.

placed intraoperatively. The blood loss may range from 3,000 to 8,500 mL, and replacement with packed red cells, whole blood, and fresh frozen plasma is required. Care is taken to prevent pulmonary overload and renal dysfunction by using volume assessment with central venous or pulmonary artery catheters. As mentioned, hypertension can be a problem and appropriate interventions are required. Following extubation, patients begin a slow readjustment to the upright position. They must overcome significant deficits in balance and transfer. The bed is initially equipped with a trapeze device to encourage the patients to pull the upper torso up enough to look around and to strengthen the upper part of the body. Preoperative upper limb strengthening may facilitate this phase of recovery and rehabilitation.[3] The sense of being able to move from side to side and arise from the supine position has psychological benefits. Sitting upright is accomplished by graduating through a series of sequentially increasing, semirecumbent positions. Care must be taken not to put excessive pressure or shear on the suture line. Upper limb strength-training exercises are required to develop adequate power for

transfer and locomotion. These exercises all begin in the bed with range-of-motion activities, lifting of light weights, and use of the trapeze. Patients gradually progress to self-mobilization in the wheelchair and use of a self-propelled gurney stretcher. Because of positioning requirements and pain, patients find it difficult to maneuver a wheelchair early in the postoperative period and instead use a gurney, which can be operated from a prone position. This is normally the first method of self-mobilization and travel outside of the room. Patients are generally able to carry out this activity 1 to 2 months postoperatively. With additional education in transferring, gain of self-confidence, and fitting in the bucket prosthesis, patients can begin to use a standard or motorized wheelchair as their primary means of mobility (Figure 3).

Maintenance of nutritional status in the preoperative and early postoperative periods can be difficult. Patients with severe pain or chronic infections may be malnourished when first evaluated because of decreased food intake and increased metabolic demands. Intravenous alimentation (either total or supplemental) may be started preoperatively and continued

through to the postoperative period. Although the rare patient may begin to have an adequate protein and calorie intake at 7 days postoperatively, most patients do not achieve this nutritional goal until about 3 to 4 weeks postoperatively. Patients who have already had a urinary diversion or colostomy formation performed in stage one are more likely to achieve nutritional goals early. The use of centrally administered glucose and amino acid mixtures with supplemental lipids can bridge the nutritional hiatus during the return of bowel function, healing of intestinal anastomoses that result from harvesting the urinary diversion conduit, and resolution of the noninfectious diarrhea related to the reduction in bowel length that is frequently required in these patients.

Pain is a significant component of the disease process in almost all patients who undergo TLA. In some patients, preoperative pain will have been a major motivating factor in deciding to undergo the surgery. Postoperative pain can be divided into two categories: incisional and phantom. Incisional pain is related to flap closure and ostomy formation. The sequential use of intravenous narcotics (morphine or other narcotics administered through patient-controlled an-

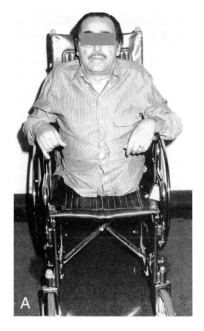
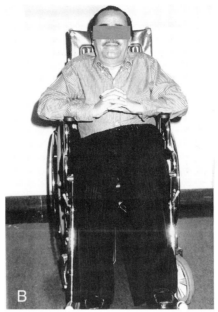
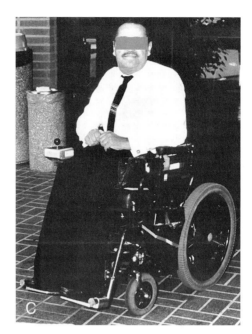
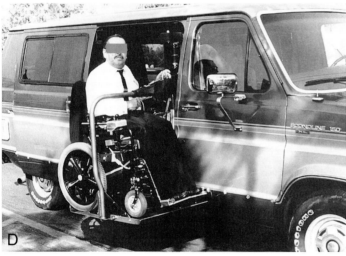
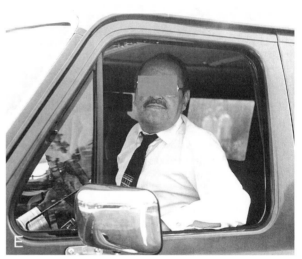

Figure 4   Patient who underwent TLA (patient number 1 in Table 1). **A,** Patient seated in bucket prosthesis in a wheelchair. The wheelchair in the photograph was used early in the rehabilitation process. It was later replaced with an automatic, self-propelled model as seen in **C** and **D. B,** Patient wearing cosmetic lower limb prostheses. **C,** Patient wearing complete (functional and cosmetic) prosthetic limbs. He is in a powered wheelchair outside the main hospital entrance and is heading to his specially equipped van. **D,** The patient on the hydraulic lift of his specially equipped van. **E,** The patient preparing to drive home in the van.

algesia devices), potent oral analgesics (oxycodone with acetaminophen, or hydromorphone), and then mild oral analgesics (acetaminophen with codeine) will be adequate for management of perioperative pain. Phantom pain is far more complex, and many patients require a variety of pharmacologic (oral and epidural agents), mechanical (changes in position and massage), and electrical stimulatory (transcutaneous electrical nerve stimulation) modalities for control.

Follow-up Evaluation

The primary surgical procedure and the initial recovery require about a 2-month hospitalization. During this period, the patient has the ablative surgery and care for any initial postoperative problems. Education regarding the care of the colostomy is provided and may include the use of stomal supplies, techniques of irrigation, and other aspects of care of the urinary diversion system, such as use

of the appliances or catheterization of the pouch. The basic techniques for bed-wheelchair transfers are mastered. The initial bucket and a cosmetic prosthesis for the lower limbs are fashioned. Muscular attrition, resolution of edema along suture lines and in flaps, and general redistribution of stomal location will likely require sequential modifications of the prosthesis.[12] The return to mainstream society requires that the patient be able to move not only within the home environment but also within the community. This may include modifying a car or van with the special apparatus necessary to load the wheelchair and to allow the amputee to be securely positioned in the vehicle (Figure 4). Of course, all controls must be designed for hand use, including those for acceleration and braking.

Even with all of these features, only a small number of translumbar amputees are able to be completely independent outside of home. Maneuvering on uneven surfaces and grass, across curbs, and in inclement weather is difficult and, at times, frightening for these patients. Psychological as well as physical problems are present. Early in the preoperative evaluation and throughout the postoperative convalescent and rehabilitative phases, the patient will need an advocate and support person. A social worker skilled in interpersonal and family dynamics is essential to provide support for the acute problems and during difficult transitions. For younger patients, counseling regarding employment options, education, and anticipated difficulties in social interactions is important. Patients in whom the operation was performed for malignant disease must be evaluated for recurrence according to standard methods. Unfortunately, in a significant number of patients, the tumor will recur with a likelihood of incurable metastatic disease. The risk and timing of recurrence of even low-grade malignancies must be empha-sized during the preoperative counseling sessions.

Summary

TLA is a structurally and functionally feasible ablative procedure. The preoperative preparation must include an extensive evaluation for metastatic disease. Discussions with the patient and family regarding the risks, expected benefits, and long-term results are essential.

The health care team includes nurses, social workers, physical and occupational therapists, a dietitian, and physicians. Surgical preparation includes measures to ensure that adequate blood and blood products will be available. Coordination of the multispecialty surgical team is also part of preoperative planning. Potential early postoperative problems include large fluid volume shifts, flap ischemia, and difficulties with the urinary diversion. Early involvement of the patient and family in the rehabilitative process, which includes mobilization, feeding, and socialization, is critical. Long-term goals of driving, education, employment, and interpersonal relations should be discussed and steps to achieve these goals should be initiated. The potential for recurrent disease and complications makes long-term follow-up evaluation essential.

References

1. Ahlering TE, Weinberg AC, Razor B: A comparative study of the ileal conduit, Kock pouch and modified Indiana pouch. *J Urol* 1989;142:1193-1196.

2. Ahlering TE, Weinberg AC, Razor B: Modified Indiana pouch. *J Urol* 1991; 145:1156-1158.

3. Aust JB, Page CP: Hemicorporectomy. *J Surg Oncol* 1985;30:226-230.

4. Larson DL, Liang MD: The quadriceps musculocutaneous flap: A reliable, sensate flap for the hemipelvectomy defect. *Plast Reconstr Surg* 1983;72: 347-354.

5. Ling D, Lee JKT: Retroperitoneum, in Stark DD, Bradley WG Jr (eds): *Magnetic Resonance Imaging.* St Louis, MO, Mosby-Year Book, 1988, pp 1141-1163.

6. Terz JJ, Schaffner MJ, Goodkin R, et al: Translumbar amputation. *Cancer* 1990;65:2668-2675.

7. Porter-Romatowski TL, Deckert J: Hemicorporectomy: A case study from a physical therapy perspective. *Arch Phys Med Rehabil* 1998;79:464-468.

8. Sanford EJ, Helal MA, Norman JG, Karl RC, O'Kelly K: Urological aspects of hemicorporectomy. *Br J Urol* 1993; 72:915-917.

9. Weaver JM, Flynn MB: Hemicorporectomy. *J Surg Oncol* 2000;73:117-124.

10. Shafir M, Abel M, Tausk H, Norton L, Miller TR, Aufses AH: Hemicorporectomy—perioperative management: A case presentation and review of literature. *J Surg Oncol* 1984;26:79-82.

11. Chang DW, Lee JE, Gokaslan ZL, Robb GL: Closure of hemicorporectomy with bilateral subtotal thigh flaps. *Plast Reconstr Surg* 2000;105: 1742-1746.

12. Smith J, Tuel SM, Meythaler JM, Cross LL, Schuch JZ: Prosthetic management of hemicorporectomy patients: New approaches. *Arch Phys Med Rehabil* 1992;73:493-497.

Chapter 47

Translumbar Amputation: Prosthetic Management

Greg Gruman, CP
John W. Michael, MEd, CPO

Introduction

Translumbar amputation (TLA; also called hemicorporectomy) represents a heroic effort to save the patient's life in the face of severe trauma, infection, or cancer.[1-9] These patients therefore require a special degree of care from the entire medical and prosthetic team. Success depends on the full cooperation of both the medical professionals and the amputee.

Prior to surgery, the surgeon will ensure that the patient understands both the outcome of the procedure and the potential for rehabilitation.[4,10,11] Ideally, the patient will have a good support system including family and friends and will have completed a realistic goal-setting process.[8] The purpose of preprosthetic therapy is strengthening of the entire upper part of the body because the upper limbs will be relied on for mobility following amputation.[8,10-12]

Because the TLA has been performed only since 1960 and is rarely encountered in clinical practice, prosthetists, therapists, and physicians tend to feel overwhelmed when faced with this challenge[6,8,11-16] (Figure 1). Prior experience with individuals with paraplegia is very good preparation for working with the TLA survivor. For individuals fitted with a sitting prosthesis, the loss of the nonfunctional body parts relieves the arms of the full body weight. The patient who is able to stand with a legged prosthesis may find that am-

bulation is easier after TLA because the weight of modern prosthetic limbs is but a fraction of the weight of the portions of the body that were amputated.[1,2,9,11,13,15,17,18]

A successful fitting can be with a sitting prosthesis with limbs for cosmesis only, or with a legged prosthesis used for upright ambulation. As described by Smith and associates,[4] a proper prosthesis will meet the following criteria: (1) stable upright posture and maximum upper limb freedom, (2) maintenance of soft-tissue support, (3) minimal weight bearing on the vertebral column, and (4) unimpeded respiratory and stomal drainage. The literature reports numerous cases of successful prosthetic fitting following TLA, including a few instances where patients achieved independent household and limited community ambulation.[2,5,6,8-17,19-22] However, some reports of legged household/community ambulation may be based on hopeful extrapolations from initial clinical demonstrations rather than long-term follow-up. Regardless of the patient's interest in ambulating with prostheses, it is always useful to direct prosthetic management toward optimizing the translumbar amputee's function while using a wheelchair for long-range mobility.

The prosthetic management of these patients involves several key decisions regarding expectations. A per-

son born without legs and pelvis will make good use of a prosthetic socket for upright balance and several different forms of mobility aids. Appropriate management may include a socket mounted on a caster cart for floor-level mobility and a standing-height frame. Floor-level mobility will phase into wheelchair use. The prosthetic socket should be lightweight and have a suspending shoulder strap so that it automatically moves with the user from place to place and from one piece of mobility equipment to the other. The bottom of the socket/platform will come into contact with the floor and with caster cart and wheelchair platforms. It should have a "footprint," or tread area, just large enough to provide hands-free stability.

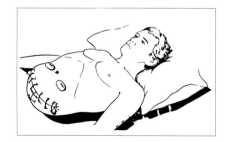

Figure 1 Typical appearance of the patient following translumbar amputation. Note the distal incision and dual stomas, both of which must be accommodated by the prosthetic socket. (*Reproduced with permission from Pearlman SW, McShane RH, Jockimsen PR, et al: Hemicorpectomy for intractable decubitus ulcers. Arch Surg 1976;111:1141.*)

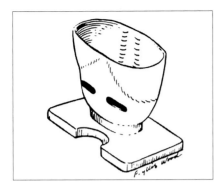

Figure 2 Typical sitting prosthesis with rectangular openings for bowel/bladder drainage bags and an extended platform for stability. A semicircular cutout in the platform allows the amputee to empty the drainage bags into the toilet without assistance. Base contours must be individualized to provide stability and yet permit hand walking. (*Reproduced with permission from Simons BC, Lehman JF, Taylor N, et al: Orthot Prosthet 1968;22:66.*)

The primary prosthetic challenges with translumbar or transpelvic amputations are adequate heat dissipation,[23] because these amputees will have almost 40% less skin area, and pressure management for prevention of ulcers caused by the unnatural weight-bearing areas of the prosthesis. Amputees with a paraplegic-level lesion are often very active, and the function of their arms and hands tends to cause significant shearing motions between the thorax and the proximal brim of the socket, requiring careful design of the socket in this region. All of these factors are important in developing a prescription and treatment plan and require close consultation with the prosthetist. One key factor is the amputee's interest in and physical potential for ambulation. Depression and significant medical complications are commonly encountered,[1,8,10,12] and both can preclude good function until resolved. Physical barriers to prosthetic fitting can include gross obesity,[12] inability to tolerate an upright posture, and poor upper limb strength. If upright weight bearing is not possible, a prone cart is usually the most practical alternative.

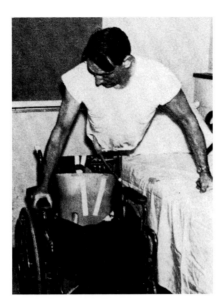

Figure 3 The limited body mass that remains following translumbar amputation facilitates independent transfer into a sitting prosthesis. (*Reproduced with permission from DeLateur BJ, Lehmann JF, Winterscheid LC, et al: Rehabilitation of the patient after hemicorporectomy. Arch Phys Med Rehabil 1969;50:15.*)

Sitting Prostheses

The traditional approach to prosthetic management for transpelvic and translumbar amputations considers a sitting prosthesis as preparatory to ambulation with a "legged" prosthesis. Carlson and Wood,[22] however, have recently suggested that ambulatory mobility is not as realistic a goal as wheeled mobility for this group.

Most authors advise provision of a sitting support system before consideration of ambulatory prostheses, and many variants have been detailed in the literature.[1,2,5,6,8-14,18-20,22] A sitting support system is used after primary healing is complete and while the rehabilitation options are being analyzed. The static sitting prosthesis is a good diagnostic tool for assessing amputee tolerance and cooperation. Greater acceptance will be achieved if the amputee is allowed to fully acclimate to the sitting device before the introduction of an ambulatory system. The sitting device can also be used as a permanent or final prosthesis. Indeed, some authors consider it

to be the best device for patient comfort and mobility.[4,22]

The initial design of the sitting device consists of a level distal surface to enhance safety and stability (Figure 2). Once comfort and a tolerance for sitting upright have been achieved, a rocker bottom can be added to allow for smoother forward progression by using the arms for a swing-through gait. The specific contour of the rocker depends on such factors as body weight, torso height, and arm length and is best determined by dynamic alignment of the prosthesis during hand walking. Dankmeyer and Doshi[14] have suggested that the proper height for the base is one that allows placement of the palms flat on the floor with slight elbow flexion. Ideally, it will provide sufficient stability to allow the amputee to pick up small objects without tipping over and yet allow an easy weight shift to initiate ambulation.

Prior to casting for the prosthesis, it is desirable to use a tilt table with varying degrees of elevation so that the amputee can develop a tolerance for the weight bearing required for the casting procedure. To allow the design of an accurate weight-bearing cast, it is generally recommended that the amputee be suspended vertically from a casting frame.[14,15,17] It is important to place the tissues carefully in the position they will occupy in the final prosthesis. An epoxy resin–based bandage can be used for the cast and reused later as a temporary prosthesis with the tilt table to increase the amputee's tolerance for weight bearing.

Socket Design

In designing the socket for the translumbar amputee, the prosthetist must precisely identify weight-bearing and relief areas by using multiple transparent test socket procedures. The major weight-bearing area is the thorax, assisted by containment of the abdominal tissues. Several areas need pressure relief, including the inferior borders of the scapulae, any promi-

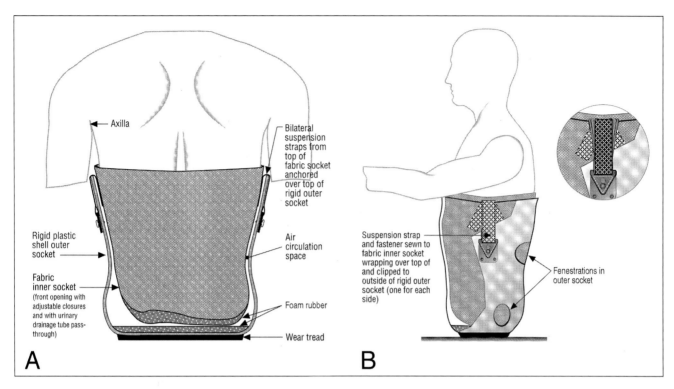

Figure 4 Cross section of Carlson and Wood's prosthesis. **A,** Posterior view. **B,** Lateral view.

nent spinous processes, the axillae, and the brachial plexus complex. A proximally adjustable socket can be used to accommodate weight loss or gain and allows the amputee to partially redistribute the weight-bearing forces to increase comfort. The socket design must also accommodate the ostomy stomas and allow free access to these sites for self care. The most common design uses rectangular openings to allow the collection bags to remain outside the socket, free of the pressures induced by weight bearing.[10,16] Any openings in the socket must be carefully limited, or the abdominal skin will protrude. In some cases, it is necessary to fashion a latex strap (fastened with Velcro) to cover rectangular openings and provide gentle pressure to reduce the soft-tissue herniation. With flat drainage bags, it may be possible to omit the colostomy opening, provided that the amputee can defecate daily when not wearing the prosthesis.[15]

Terz and associates[20] have summarized the goals of socket design for the translumbar amputee as follows:

1. Independent transfer into and out of the socket (Figure 3)
2. Sufficient stability to permit free use of the upper limbs and wheelchair mobility
3. Minimum socket tolerance of two 4-hour periods daily
4. Sufficient weight-bearing pressure distribution to prevent skin necrosis
5. Allowance for adequate respiratory exchange
6. No abdominal pain or nausea from pressure within the socket
7. Prevention of eversion of the colostomy and ileal bladder drainage bags
8. Easy access to drainage bags for self care
9. Pressure relief over the sternum and distal portion of the spine, even when leaning forward or back in the socket
10. Acceptable cosmesis
11. Ease in cleansing socket areas in contact with the body.[16]

Because of the limited surface area available for weight bearing, total contact is the best approach to reduce the pressure per square centimeter.[21] Although earlier reports speculated about the possibility of interfering with respiration, Grimby and Stener[19] noted only minimal change in vital capacity with a prosthesis designed to reduce rib contact. It is usually advisable for the amputee to unweight the prosthesis at frequent intervals by pushing up with the arms, similar to the technique used by individuals with paraplegia to avoid skin breakdown.[10] Over a period of weeks or months, the amputee can gradually increase the time spent wearing the prosthesis until an upright posture in the device can be tolerated for 8 hours or more daily.[10-12,15,16]

Carlson and Wood[22] emphasize the importance of focusing on basic goals, such as providing for heat dissipation and protection of skin from shear trauma, that are likely to positively affect patient acceptance and success. The loss sustained in TLA results in a decrease of 36% in total skin surface for heat release. When the thorax is contained inside a socket that is not permeable to air, the body is left with

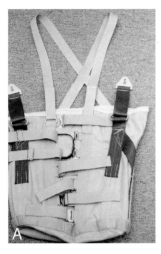
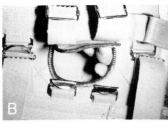
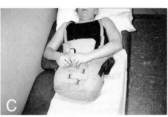
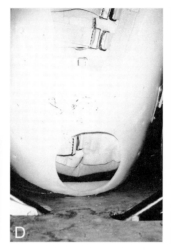
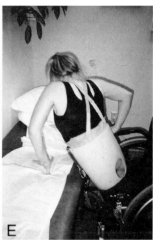

Figure 5 Features of Carlson and Wood's design. **A,** Flexible fabric inner socket. **B,** Detail of fabric inner socket showing opening for stoma site. **C,** Patient donning the flexible fabric inner socket. **D,** Distal relief area. **E,** Patient demonstrating transfer technique.

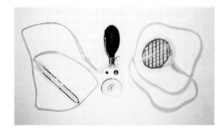

Figure 6 Pressure transducers for evaluation of socket fit.

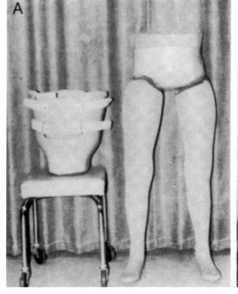
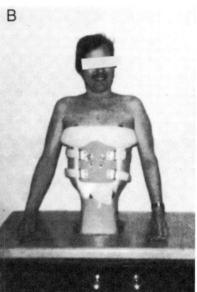

Figure 7 A, Dankmeyer and Doshi's endoskeletal prosthesis with a removable socket. Free hip joints, stance-control knees, and SACH feet provide good stability; transverse rotation units allow some reciprocal gait. **B,** The removable socket can be used as a sitting device.

only 45% of its original skin surface to dissipate heat by convection and evaporation. The translumbar amputee also faces potentially significant shear stress on the remaining thorax. The twisting, reaching, and bending motions involved in everyday activities can cause significant breakdown, especially in patients with sensory deprivation.[3] Therefore, the socket interface is of critical importance.

Carlson and Wood[22] favor a flexible fabric inner socket design that is flexibly suspended in a rigid frame (Figure 4). The design incorporates features that provide for heat dissipation, pressure and shear management, volume change, mobility, and cosmesis (Figure 5). It uses hydrostatic weight-bearing principles similar to the circumference tensioning used in transfemoral prosthetic socket design. Pressure transducers can be used to identify and correct at-risk locations (Figure 6).

Ambulatory Prostheses

Having accomplished the degree of independence afforded by a sitting prosthesis, some amputees will request prosthetic legs for cosmetic purposes or to permit limited ambulation. Davis and associates[12] have reported on long-term follow-up with two patients who remained ambulatory and gainfully employed for several years following prosthetic fitting and note

that "the appearance of body normality appeared to play an important part in motivating them toward seeking a life other than institutionalized hopelessness and helpless invalidism." Williams and Fish[16] concur and report that "when the patient was fitted with his final prosthesis, his attitude toward life changed dramatically... Legs, even in a wheelchair, apparently made a difference for which there was no substitute...." Although ambulation with crutches or a walker is feasible, trans-

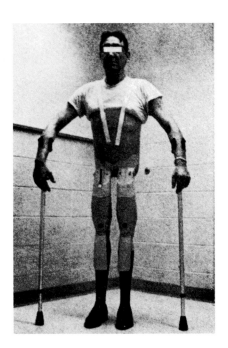

Figure 8 An exoskeletal prosthesis permits independent ambulation with forearm crutches. Note the shoulder straps for suspension.

fers will be more cumbersome with prosthetic legs attached. Rather than encumbering the sitting prosthesis, it may be preferable to prescribe a separate ambulatory prosthesis with a new socket. Dankmeyer and Doshi[14] have reported an alternative (Figure 7) that allows the ambulatory prosthesis to fasten on top of the sitting device, thus allowing the amputee to leave the legs behind in the chair when transferring.

Because of the small number of cases reported, it is not possible to recommend particular components. Each clinic team must make an individual determination based on its experience and judgment. Successful ambulation has been reported with either free[14] or locking[10] hip joints; polycentric, stance-control,[14] or locking[11] knees; and either articulated[15] or solid ankle-foot mechanisms.[14,16]

Although successful exoskeletal fittings have been reported in the past[6,10-12,15,16] (Figure 8), use of realignable endoskeletal componentry is more common now because of its versatility and light weight.[14] Endoskeletal designs with interchangeable components permit clinical verification of various foot, ankle, knee, and

hip joint combinations during gait training. It is also possible to add components sequentially. Initially, prosthetic feet may be added directly to the socket to create a "stubby" prosthesis similar to those used by bilateral transfemoral amputees. Length can be increased in increments as the patient's balance and strength permit, with hip and knee joints added as the amputee progresses.

Suspension of the prosthesis is critical if the stresses of swing-through ambulation are to be tolerated. Over-the-shoulder suspenders have proved to be the best option for this type of prosthesis.[6,11,12,14,16,22] Care must be taken not to pinch any protruding flesh where the suspenders cross the proximal edge of the socket.

Summary

Survival times for translumbar amputees sometimes may be limited, but they have increased steadily as medical care has advanced; survival for more than 20 years has been documented. Several reports of return to employment have been noted in the literature.[1,10,12,16,19-22] It is the mission of the clinic team to enhance quality of life during whatever time remains for the translumbar amputee. This is accomplished by providing the greatest possible independence and freedom, including ambulation to whatever degree the amputee is capable. The primary factors in the successful rehabilitation of the translumbar amputee are motivation and compliance: the highly motivated individual will succeed despite the difficulties.

Aust performed the first successful TLA in 1961; the amputee found work in a nursing home and survived until 1980. Aust summarized his long-term experience with this procedure as follows: "Freed of the nonfunctioning lower half, the patient is released from the dead weight holding him down, relieved of his chronic infection and/or cancer, and experiences a

new mobility, sense of well-being, and renewed enthusiasm for life."[13]

The loss of more than half of the body obviously presents enormous difficulties. However, numerous successful fittings following TLA attest to the potential for rehabilitation of individuals faced with this singularly difficult challenge.

References

1. Mackenzie AR, Miller TR, Randall HT: Translumbar amputation for advanced leiomyosarcoma of the prostate. *J Urol* 1967;97:133-136.

2. Miller TR, Mackenzie AR, Karasewich EG: Translumbar amputation for carcinoma of the vagina. *Arch Surg* 1966; 93:502-506.

3. Kennedy CS, Miller EB, McLean DC, et al: Lumbar amputation or hemicorporectomy for advanced malignancy of the lower half of the body. *Surgery* 1960;48:357-365.

4. Smith J, Tuel SM, Meythaler JM, et al: Prosthetic management of hemicorporectomy patients: New approaches. *Arch Phys Med Rehabil* 1992;73: 493-497.

5. Miller TR, Mackenzie AR, Randall HT: Translumbar amputation for advanced cancer: Indications and physiologic alterations in four cases. *Ann Surg* 1966;164:514-521.

6. Baker TC, Berkowitz T, Lord GB, Hankins HV: Hemicorporectomy. *Br J Surg* 1970;57:471-476.

7. MacKenzie AR: Translumbar amputation: The longest survivor. A case update. *Mt Sinai J Med* 1995;62:305-307.

8. Friedmann LW, Marin EL, Park YS: Hemicorporectomy for functional rehabilitation. *Arch Phys Med Rehabil* 1981;62:83-86.

9. Pearlman NW, McShane RH, Jochimsen PR, Shirazi SS: Hemicorporectomy for intractable decubitus ulcers. *Arch Surg* 1976;111:1139-1143.

10. DeLateur BJ, Lehmann JF, Winterscheid LC, Wolf JA, Fordyce WE, Simons BC: Rehabilitation of the patient after hemicorporectomy. *Arch Phys Med Rehabil* 1969;50:11-16.

11. Frieden FH, Gertler M, Tosberg W, Rusk HA: Rehabilitation after hemi-

corporectomy. *Arch Phys Med Rehabil* 1969;50:259-263.

12. Davis SW, Chu DS, Yang CJ: Translumbar amputation for nonneoplastic cause: Rehabilitation and follow-up. *Arch Phys Med Rehabil* 1975;56: 359-362.

13. Aust JB, Page CP: Hemicorporectomy. *J Surg Oncol* 1985;30:226-230.

14. Dankmeyer CH Jr, Doshi R: Prosthetic management of adult hemicorporectomy and bilateral hip disarticulation amputees. *Orthot Prosthet* 1981;35: 11-18.

15. Leichtentritt KG: Rehabilitation after hemicorporectomy. *Am J Proctol* 1972; 23:408-413.

16. Williams RD, Fish JC: Translumbar amputation. *Cancer* 1969;23:416-418.

17. Easton JKM, Aust JB, Dawson WJ Jr, Kottke FJ: Fitting of a prosthesis on a patient after hemicorporectomy. *Arch Phys Med Rehabil* 1963;44:335-337.

18. Miller TR, Mackenzie AR, Randall HT, Tigner SP: Hemicorporectomy. *Surgery* 1966;59:988-993.

19. Grimby G, Stener B: Physical performance and cardiorespiratory function after hemicorporectomy. *Scand J Rehabil Med* 1973;5:124-129.

20. Terz JJ, Schaffner MJ, Goodkin R, et al: Translumbar amputation. *Cancer* 1990;65:2668-2675.

21. The most radical procedure. *Inter-Clin Info Bull* 1966; 5:22-23.

22. Carlson JM, Wood SL: A flexible, air-permeable socket prosthesis for bilateral hip disarticulation and hemicorporectomy amputees. *J Prosthet Orthot* 1998;10:110-115.

23. Ferrara BE: Hemicorporectomy: A collective review. *J Surg Oncol* 1990;45:270-278.

Chapter 48

Physical Therapy

Robert S. Gailey, PhD, PT
Curtis R. Clark, PT

Introduction

As members of the rehabilitation team, the prosthetist and the physical therapist often develop a close relationship when working with lower limb amputees. The prosthetist is responsible for creating a prosthesis that will best suit the lifestyle of an individual patient. The physical therapist is involved in several steps of rehabilitation. Before the patient can be fitted with the prosthesis, the physical therapist helps the amputee become physically prepared for training in use of the prosthesis. Next, the amputee must learn how to use and care for the prosthesis. Prosthetic gait training can be the most frustrating, yet rewarding, phase of rehabilitation for all members of the team. The amputee must be reeducated in the biomechanics of gait as he or she learns to use the prosthesis. Once success in using the prosthesis is achieved, the amputee can look forward to resuming a productive life. Finally, the physical therapist should introduce the amputee to activities other than just walking. Although the amputee may not be ready to participate in recreational activities immediately, providing the names of support groups and recreational organizations will enable the amputee to seek involvement at the appropriate time.

Preoperative Aspects

At the initial contact, the physical therapist begins to establish rapport with the patient; this is important to earn the patient's trust and confidence. After introductions, the physical therapist should explain the timing of events during the rehabilitation process. The unknown can be extremely frightening to many patients. These fears can be addressed by explaining what the future holds and what will be expected of the amputee. Having another amputee visit and talk with the patient can often assist in this process. To this end, many hospitals have affiliations with local amputee support groups with members who visit prospective or new amputees to help them through the healing process. Visiting amputees should be carefully screened by appropriate personnel to discern whether they have a personality suitable for this task. If they do, they can be matched to the prospective or new amputee by level of amputation, age, gender, and avocational interests. Information on various prostheses or videos showing recreational activities may be useful to the patient. A sample prosthesis may be useful in answering the patient's questions. At all stages of rehabilitation, the physical therapist must consider the amount of information that the patient is psychologically prepared to absorb. The responsibilities of the physical therapist before surgery include advising the amputee about the possibilities of phantom limb sensation and phantom limb pain, discussing how to prevent joint contracture, describing the functional aspects of the prosthesis, and any other general issues.

Acute Postoperative Evaluation
General Factors

The acute postoperative evaluation consists of several significant components. First, baseline information must be obtained to establish the goals of rehabilitation and to formulate an individualized treatment plan. A complete medical history also should be obtained from the patient or from medical records to supply information that may be pertinent to the rehabilitation program. During the initial review of the medical record, the physical therapist should note any history of coronary artery disease, angina, myocardial infarction, congestive heart failure, arrhythmias, dyspnea, peripheral vascular disease, angioplasty, arterial bypass surgery, diabetes mellitus, hypertension, or renal disease. Any medications that may influence physical exertion or mental status should be recorded.

Throughout this process, the rehabilitation team (including the patient) must view the amputation in a positive light and as a reconstructive rather than as a destructive procedure. The goal is to return the amputee to his or her premorbid lifestyle and to prevent further adversity such as delayed healing, falls, or any other medical complications that could have been avoided. In preparation for prosthetic training, the amputee must be immediately taught functional skills and shown how to care for the healing residual limb, protect the sound limb, and avoid physical deconditioning. While the amputee is still in the hospital, the rehabilitation team must emphasize the totality of the rehabilitation process from the acute stages to completion of prosthetic training. The amputee should be advised about the entire rehabilitation process, including the incremental value of each step. Educating the patient in all aspects may reduce the anxiety associated with the uncertainty of what lies ahead and enhance compliance. As mentioned, amputee support groups, including peer visitation, can be a tremendous asset when support personnel are well informed and have views consistent with those of the rehabilitation team.

Cardiopulmonary Status

The heart rate and blood pressure of every patient should be closely monitored both during initial training and throughout the rehabilitation process as the intensity of training increases. If the amputee experiences persistent signs and symptoms such as shortness of breath, pallor, diaphoresis, chest pain, headache, or peripheral edema, further medical evaluation is strongly recommended. If the patient's cardiopulmonary status is a concern, relatively inexpensive and simple tools such as pulse oximetry, the Dyspnea Index,[1] and the Borg Perceived Exertion Scale[2] may be used to help monitor exertion or to assist the amputee with guidelines for effort during ambulation.

Mental Status

An accurate assessment of the patient's mental status can provide insight about the factors likely to affect future prosthetic care. The physical therapist should assess the patient's cognitive potential to perform activities such as donning and doffing the prosthesis, regulating prosthetic sock plies, bed positioning, providing adequate skin care, and ambulating safely. If the patient does not have the necessary level of cognition, family members and/or friends should become involved in the rehabilitation process to help ensure a successful outcome.

Range of Motion

The range of motion (ROM) of the upper limbs and the sound lower limb as well as the residual limb should be assessed. Joint contractures can hinder the amputee's ability to ambulate with a prosthesis, and steps should be taken to avoid this complication. The most common contractures in the transfemoral amputee are hip flexion, external rotation, and abduction. Knee flexion is the most commonly observed contracture in transtibial amputees. During assessment of ROM, the physical therapist should determine whether the patient truly has a fixed contracture or just muscle tightness from immobility; the latter can be corrected within a relatively short period of time. The presence of the contracture will affect the initial alignment of the prosthesis. This alignment must be adjusted over time as the contracture resolves.

Strength

Functional strength of the major muscle groups should be assessed by manual muscle testing of all limbs, including the residual limb and the trunk. This assessment will help determine the patient's potential to perform activities involving transfers, wheelchair mobility, and ambulation with and without the prosthesis.

Sensation

Evaluation of sensation is useful to the patient and physical therapist alike. Insensitivity of the residual and/or sound limb will affect proprioceptive feedback for balance and single-limb stance, which can lead to gait difficulties. The patient must be aware that decreased pain and/or temperature and light touch sensation can increase the potential for injury and soft-tissue breakdown. Thus, patients should be encouraged to monitor changes in sensation and use protective strategies to avoid injuries or tissue damage.

Bed Mobility

The importance of good bed mobility skills extends beyond simple positional adjustments for comfort or to get in and out of bed. These skills are necessary to maintain correct bed positioning to prevent contractures and to avoid excessive friction of the bedsheets against the suture line or frail skin. If the patient is unable to perform the skills necessary to maintain proper positioning, assistance must be provided. As with most patients, adequate bed mobility is a prerequisite skill for more advanced skills such as bed-to-wheelchair transfers.

Balance and Coordination

Balance while sitting and standing are of major concern when assessing the amputee's ability to maintain the body's center of mass (COM) over the base of support (BOS). Coordination makes moving easier and helps to refine motor skills. Both balance and coordination are required for shifting weight from one limb to another, thus improving the potential for an optimal gait. After evaluating mental status, ROM, strength, sensation, balance, and coordination, the physical therapist will have a good indication of the most appropriate initial choice of assistive device.

Transfers

Early assessment of a patient's ability to make transfers is essential, especially when the rehabilitation team is planning discharge from the acute care setting. Many elderly amputees can be discharged to home if they are able to complete transfers either independently or with limited help. If moderate to maximum assistance is needed for transfers, a facility that offers skilled physical assistance is often required until the amputee becomes more independent.

Potential for Ambulation With Assistive Devices

A comprehensive evaluation of the patient's potential for ambulation is necessary, including strength of the sound lower limb and both upper limbs, balance on a single limb, coordination, and mental status. The selection of an assistive device should match the amputee's level of skill, keeping in mind that the device required may change over time. For example, a patient may initially require a walker, but forearm crutches may be more beneficial for long-term use if proper training is completed. Some patients who have difficulty ambulating on one limb because of obesity, blindness, or generalized weakness can successfully ambulate with the additional support provided by a prosthesis.

Setting Goals

The rehabilitation team should establish realistic goals that are consistent with the amputee's desired outcomes for employment, social interactions, and recreational endeavors. Most amputees, regardless of age or the level of amputation, can return to their previous lifestyle with only minor accommodations.[3-5] Discussing the amputee's premorbid lifestyle and goals early in the rehabilitation process provides valuable information that helps to create a personalized treatment plan that is both appropriate and motivating.

Assessment of Functional Outcome

Instruments to help determine functional outcome can be categorized as (1) subjective or self-reported assessments or (2) more objective performance-based assessments. With a self-report instrument, the patient, family member, or clinician completes a questionnaire or survey from which a test score or descriptive profile is generated. For assessments of

individual activities of daily living (ADL) and overall functional capacity, self-rated instruments are more accurate and less biased than ratings by observers or reports by caregivers.[6] Several subjective instruments have been specifically designed for amputees. Instruments developed for general patient populations have also been used with amputees. Performance-based assessment tools are more objective and have the advantage of providing information regarding ambulatory ability by determination of the performance of specific tasks. With some of these instruments, the quality of the performance is graded by the clinician.

Several specific functional outcome instruments may be used by clinicians. Each instrument has advantages and disadvantages, depending on the information being collected. There appears to be no consensus among different rehabilitation centers regarding the selection of measurement tools used for lower limb amputees.[7] Often, a combination of assessment tools is required to obtain the appropriate information from an individual amputee or to provide a comprehensive evaluation of a particular group of amputees. Clinicians and clinical investigators need to understand the appropriateness of the information that a specific functional outcomes instrument will yield. The following sections review the most common self-report and performance-based instruments that have been used with amputees.

Self-Report Assessment Instruments
Amputee Activity Survey

The Amputee Activity Survey (AAS) is a 20-item questionnaire that allows the amputee to describe his or her average daily activity level.[8] A linear relationship between total AAS score and annual step rates of 21 subjects has been observed. No statistical analysis was completed, and the small

sample size limits any definitive conclusions with regard to correlation of score and step rate. The contention that amputees can fairly accurately assess their activity level, however, is supported by the finding that amputees with higher AAS scores walked farther. AAS scores also shared a reasonable distribution over the population group, and the preferred walking speed appeared to correlate with the AAS.[9]

Reintegration to Normal Living Index

The Reintegration to Normal Living (RNL) Index is designed to assess global functional status and measure the patient's perception of his or her own capabilities. Many of the 11 items focus on locomotion, self-care needs, perception of self, vocation, social aspects, and recreational activities. Thus, the RNL Index is a general indicator of physical, social, and psychological performance.[10]

Prosthetic Profile of the Amputee

The Prosthetic Profile of the Amputee (PPA), a 44-item closed- and semi-closed-ended questionnaire, is designed to evaluate and assess factors potentially related to prosthesis use after discharge from a rehabilitation center. Six broad categories are assessed, including physical condition, type of prosthesis, prosthesis use, environment, leisure activities, and general information. Multiple subcategories are included within each category. The PPA reflects the true prosthetic profile of the patient after discharge from a rehabilitation center and helps identify predisposing, enabling, and reinforcing factors. The predisposing factors are motivation, physical health, and type of rehabilitation program. Enabling factors are locomotor abilities, health services, accessibility to services, and physical environment. The reinforcing factors include satisfaction with prosthesis, social environment, and social interaction.[11-13]

Houghton Scale

The Houghton Scale is a six-item measure of performance designed to assess the amount of time and manner in which the prosthesis is used, whether a mobility device is required when walking outside, and the amputee's perception of stability while moving over a variety of terrains. One of the objectives for the Houghton Scale is to discriminate between prosthesis and wheelchair use in amputees with vascular conditions.[14-17]

Medical Outcomes Survey Short Form-36 Health Status Profile

In theory, patients will inherently accurately report their functional status when provided with the appropriate assessment instrument.[8,12,15,18] One of the most popular functional outcome measures is the Medical Outcomes Survey Short Form-36 (MOS SF-36) Health Status Profile.[19] This 36-item self-report instrument examines physical functioning, role limitations because of physical health and emotional problems, social functioning, general mental health, pain, health perception, energy, and fatigue.[20] The MOS SF-36 is, to date, perhaps the most widely applied self-report instrument used with amputees. This instrument was not specifically designed for amputees and, therefore, appears to have some weaknesses.[21] For example, MOS SF-36 scores in the physical functioning and role limitation categories are lower among amputees than among normal age-matched individuals because of problems with physical health and pain experienced by amputees.[18,22,23]

Prosthetic Evaluation Questionnaire

The Prosthetic Evaluation Questionnaire (PEQ) is a 16-item self-report instrument specifically developed for amputees with the intent of measuring small differences in prosthetic function and major life domains related to prosthetic function. The PEQ compares the effects of different types of prostheses and different methods of care. Responses are recorded along a linear analog scale with four topic headings: prosthetic function, mobility, psychosocial experience, and well-being.[24,25] The results of the PEQ correlate well with those of the PPA and the Houghton Scale.[17]

Sickness Impact Profile

The Sickness Impact Profile (SIP) is a commonly used patient-oriented measure that profiles functional problems using a 136-item self-report questionnaire. Items are divided into the following 12 categories designed to assess ADL: sleep and rest, emotional behavior, body care and movement, home management, mobility, social interaction, ambulation, alertness behavior, communication, work, recreation and pastimes, and eating. In addition to each subscale, there are two domain scores (physical and psychosocial) and one full-scale score of dysfunction.[26] Currently, more than 140 reports of its application in patients with more than 40 different diseases and impairments have been published.[27-30] SIP scores from amputees with diabetes mellitus show greater diversity in functional outcome compared with their preoperative functional abilities than from amputees who do not have diabetes mellitus. In most patients, functional abilities decrease after lower limb amputation.[31] Thus, lower limb amputees may appear quite disabled in all disability categories of the SIP scores.

Barthel Index

The Barthel Index[32] is a useful and popular measure of ADL for patients with a variety of impairments.[33,34] This performance test originally consisted of 15 measures but has been reduced to 10 measures of self care and mobility. Either two subscores for each measure or one combined score is generated. When administered to amputees, the overall index values are used to assess changes between admission and discharge.[35,36] The temporal change is a good indicator of prognosis and potential discharge placement to home, supervised care, or long-term institutionalization.[37,38] Lower Barthel scores indicate difficulties in ascending and descending stairs, walking on level surfaces, self-bathing, getting on and off a toilet, and bowel and bladder control.[36]

The Barthel Index does not detect subtle deficits in patients who are functioning at a high level. Therefore, it may be more applicable for the evaluation of self care and mobility of very impaired amputees but is probably not appropriate for assessing prosthesis use and mobility of more mobile amputees.[39]

Performance-Based Assessment Instruments
Electronic Step Counters

The use of step counters is not a new concept. Holden and associates[40] measured the extent of prosthesis use with electronic step counters during inpatient training and documented amputee walking habits for 2 years after discharge. Continuous monitoring provides data pertaining to the actual use of the prosthesis. In contrast, information provided by the patient or an observer is considered an estimate only. The activity levels correlated with functional independence are determined by a questionnaire. An amputee must be able to walk 600 steps a day to manage independently in a single-level house or apartment, with a moderate amount of support by family members or social agencies.[40] As discussed, Day[8] used step counters to validate the AAS.

The Prosthetic Research Study group[41] reported that gait styles and activity levels of amputees can be analyzed with the Step Activity Monitor, a device that continuously records steps during a specific time period. These data provide insight beyond that provided by simply counting steps because the time of day for each step is also recorded. Therefore, the data from a 2-week period can provide information concerning distance traveled per day, activity patterns such as standing versus walking time, and periods of day for high step activity versus low step activity. These data could assist with the interpretation of health status or the quality of prosthetic rehabilitation.

Functional Independence Measure

The Functional Independence Measure (FIM) was developed by a national task force in 1983 as part of a uniform data system.[42] The FIM measures the progress of rehabilitation in patients with multiple disabilities who are being treated on an inpatient basis and includes 18 items grouped in six categories: self-care, sphincter control, mobility, locomotion, communication, and social cognition. Improvement varied widely in amputees who scored low at admission, whereas improvement appeared to plateau in amputees who scored high on admission and had very little room to improve. Improvement in total FIM scores after rehabilitation depended on the ability to ambulate. Thus, the FIM score at admission appears to be a poor predictor of progress in rehabilitation because amputees who began at lower functional levels showed greater improvements.[43-45] Leung and associates[16] concurred, reporting that the admission FIM score was not useful in predicting successful prosthetic rehabilitation in lower limb amputees based on their study of prosthesis use in 29 amputees.

Functional Ambulation Profile

Nelson[46] developed the Functional Ambulation Profile (FAP) as a performance-based test of locomotor skills for a variety of neuromuscular and musculoskeletal disorders. This three-phase test assesses static standing, dynamic weight shifting, and basic ambulation efficiency. Although reported to be a valid instrument, there is no evidence of construct validity testing or reliability. The FAP, however, appears to be a very quick

and potentially informative tool for clinical use with amputees.[47]

Functional Reach Test

The Functional Reach (FR) test is performed by mounting a 48-in (1.2-m) stick on the wall at shoulder height. The subject stands parallel to the stick, raises an arm, and is directed to "Reach as far forward as you can without taking a step." The distance traveled by the tip of the finger from the start to finish position is recorded. Functional reach or the maximal safe standing forward reach is considered to be a precise, reliable, clinically accessible, and age-sensitive measure of balance that approximates COM excursion and estimates physical frailty.[48] In nonamputee subjects, the FR test can identify the risk of recurrent falls[49] and is sensitive to change over time.[49,50] Although standing reach with amputees has not been reported, Kirby and Chari[51] observed that sitting reach in transtibial amputees with and without a prosthesis and in transfemoral amputees without a prosthesis did not significantly differ. Only in the latter group was reach significantly decreased, probably the result of the anterior brim of the socket limiting hip flexion rather than a deficit in balance; this limitation is often observed with activities such as tying shoes.

Amputee Mobility Predictor

The Amputee Mobility Predictor (AMP) was designed to provide objective information on an amputee's potential ability to ambulate, thus assisting a clinician in prescribing the appropriate prosthetic knee and foot components. The AMP can be administered to patients with or without the use of a prosthesis. Therefore, the AMP can be given to an amputee before the initial fitting of the prosthesis or to an amputee who has used a prosthesis for years. The AMP is a 20-item functional measure that is relatively easy to administer in 15 minutes or less and uses a simple

scoring system requiring very little equipment or space. Each item addresses specific skills that contribute to overall function, such as sitting balance, standing balance, dynamic balance, coordination, agility, power, vestibular input, and vision. When an amputee cannot perform a specific test item, the clinician can select the appropriate exercises to address the functional deficit (Figure 1). To date, more than 30,000 reprints of this tool have been ordered.

Health care industry demands for mechanisms to classify patients for purposes of reimbursement have increased the need for valid, reliable measures of functional status. The reliability of the AMP suggests that with proper training caregivers from multiple disciplines can administer the test and results will be consistent over time.[52] In the case of amputees, Medicare and managed care providers use the Durable Medical Equipment Regional Carrier K Codes or Medicare Functional Classification Levels (MFCL) system to classify the amputee and determine the appropriate complexity of prosthetic prescription. The AMP can differentiate between MFCL categories and is strongly related to other measures of function in the amputee. In addition, the AMP can also predict the distance an amputee can walk in 6 minutes, when administered with or without a prosthesis, if the AMP score, age, time after amputation, and number of comorbidities are entered in a mathematical prediction equation. The AMP also shows the potential value of upgrading prosthetic feet and knees, as well as the effects of higher K code category components, on the distance an amputee can walk in 6 minutes.

The 6-minute Walk Test

Walking speed has long been suggested as a performance index because of its high correlation with oxygen uptake and sensitivity to the increasing age of subjects.[53] Improvement in walking speed is a useful predictor of independent mobility in

AMPUTEE MOBILITY PREDICTOR ASSESSMENT TOOL

Initial instructions: Testee is seated in a hard chair with arms. The following maneuvers are tested with or without the use of the prosthesis. Advise the person of each task or group of tasks prior to performance. Please avoid unnecessary chatter throughout the test. Safety First, no task should be performed if either the tester or testee is uncertain of a safe outcome.

The **Right Limb** is: PF TT KD TF HD intact   The **Left Limb** is: PF TT KD TF HD intact

1. Sitting Balance: Sit forward in a chair with arms folded across chest for 60s.	Cannot sit upright independently for 60s Can sit upright independently for 60s	= 0 = 1	_____
2. Sitting reach: reach forwards and grasp the ruler. (Tester holds ruler 12in beyond extended arms midline to the sternum)	Does not attempt Cannot grasp or requires arm support Reaches forward and successfully grasps item.	= 0 = 1 = 2	_____
3. Chair to chair transfer: 2 chairs at 90°. Pt. may choose direction and use their upper limbs.	Cannot do or requires physical assistance Performs independently, but appears unsteady Performs independently, appears to be steady and safe	= 0 = 1 = 2	_____
4. Arises from a chair: ask pt. to fold arms across chest and stand. If unable, use arms or assistive device.	Unable without help (physical assistance) Able, uses arms/assist device to help Able, without using arms	= 0 = 1 = 2	_____
5. Attempts to arise from a chair. (stopwatch ready): if attempt in no. 4. was without arms then ignore and allow another attempt without penalty	Unable without help (physical assistance) Able requires >1 attempt Able to rise one attempt	= 0 = 1 = 2	_____
6. Immediate Standing Balance (first 5s): begin timing immediately.	Unsteady (staggers, moves foot, sways) Steady using walking aid or other support Steady without walker or other support	= 0 = 1 = 2	_____
7. Standing Balance (30s) (stopwatch ready): for items nos. 7&8, first attempt is without assistive device. If support is required allow after first attempt	Unsteady Steady but uses walking aid or other support Standing without support	= 0 = 1 = 2	_____
8. Single limb standing balance (stopwatch ready): time the duration of single limb standing on both the sound and prosthetic limb up to 30s. Grade the quality, not the time. Sound side _____ seconds Prosthetic side _____ seconds	Non-prosthetic side Unsteady Steady but uses walking aid or other support for 30s Single-limb standing without support for 30s Prosthetic Side Unsteady Steady but uses walking aid or other support for 30s Single-limb standing without support for 30s	= 0 = 1 = 2 = 0 = 1 = 2	_____ _____
9. Standing reach: reach forward and grasp the ruler. (Tester holds ruler 12in beyond extended arm(s)midline to the sternum)	Does not attempt Cannot grasp or requires arm support on assistive device Reaches forward and successfully grasps item no support	= 0 = 1 = 2	_____
10. Nudge test (subject at maximum position #7): with feet as close together as possible, examiner pushes lightly on subject's sternum with palm of hand 3 times (toes should rise))	Begins to fall Staggers, grabs, catches self ore uses assistive device Steady	= 0 = 1 = 2	_____
11. Eyes Closed (at maximum position #7): if support is required grade as unsteady.	Unsteady or grips assistive device Steady without any use of assistive device	= 0 = 1	_____

Figure 1 Amputee Mobility Predictor. *(Copyright © Advanced Rehabilitation Therapy, Inc, Miami, FL, 2001.)*

			Prosthesis	Sound
12. Picking up objects off the floor: pick up a pencil off the floor placed midline 12in in front of foot.	Unable to pick up object and return to standing Performs with some help (table, chair, walking aid etc) Performs independently (without help from object or person)	= 0 = 1 = 2	_____	
13. Sitting down: ask pt. to fold arms across chest and sit. If unable, use arm or assistive device.	Unsafe (misjudged distance, falls into chair) Uses arms, assistive device or not a smooth motion Safe, smooth motion	= 0 = 1 = 2	_____	
14. Initiation of gait (immediately after told to "go")	Any hesitancy or multiple attempts to start No hesitancy	= 0 = 1	_____	
15. Step length and height: walk a measured distance of 12ft twice (up and back). Four scores are required or two scores (a & b) for each leg. "Marked deviation" is defined as extreme substitute movements to avoid clearing the floor. b. Foot clearance	a. Swing foot Does not advance a minimum of 12in Advances a minimum of 12in b. Foot does not completely clear floor without deviation Foot completely clears floor without marked deviation	= 0 = 1 = 0 = 1	_____ _____	_____ _____
16. Step Continuity.	Stopping or discontinuity between steps (stop & go gait) Steps appear continuous	= 0 = 1	_____	
17. Turning: 180 degree turn when returning to chair.	Unable to turn, requires intervention to prevent falling Greater than three steps but completes task without intervention No more than three continuous steps with or without assistive aid	= 0 = 1 = 2	_____	
18. Variable cadence: walk a distance of 12ft fast as possible safely 4 times. (Speeds may vary from slow to fast and fast to slow varying cadence.)	Unable to vary cadence in a controlled manner Asymmetrical increase in cadence controlled manner Symmetrical increase in speed in a controlled manner	= 0 = 1 = 2	_____	
19. Stepping over an obstacle: place a movable box of 4in in height in the walking path.	Cannot step over the box Catches foot, interrupts stride Steps over without interrupting stride	= 0 = 1 = 2	_____	
20. Stairs (must have at least 2 steps): try to go up and down these stairs without holding on to the railing. Don't hesitate to permit pt. to hold on to rail. Safety First, if examiner feels that any risk in involved omit and score as 0.	Ascending Unsteady, cannot do One step at a time, or must hold on to railing or device Step over step, does not hold onto the railing or device Descending Unsteady, cannot do One step at a time, or must hold on to railing or device Step over step, does not hold onto the railing or device	= 0 = 1 = 2 = 0 = 1 = 2	_____ _____	
21. Assistive device selection: add points for the use of an assistive device if used for two or more items. If testing without prosthesis use of appropriate assistive device is mandatory.	Bed bound Wheelchair Walker Crutches (axillary or forearm) Cane (straight or quad) None	= 0 = 1 = 2 = 3 = 4 = 5	_____	
	Total Score _____/47			

Abbreviations: PF, partial foot; TT transtibial; KD knee disarticulation; TF transfemoral; HD hip disarticulation; Pt, patient.

Test   no prosthesis   with prosthesis Observer _____ Date _____

Figure 1 continued

poorly mobile patients.[54] In addition, low gait speed is a significant indicator of falls in the elderly.[55]

Cooper[56] first introduced the 12-minute run performance test with his study of 115 US Air Force servicemen. He concluded that because of its high correlation with maximal oxygen consumption, the 12-minute field performance test is assumed to be an objective measure reflecting the cardiovascular status of an individual subject. Others have confirmed that the 12-minute walk test is a useful, measurable indication of exercise tolerance.[57-59]

Butland and associates[60] conducted 2-, 6-, and 12-minute walk tests on a group of elderly patients and concluded that length of the test was not critical, but a test that takes less time is easier for both patients and investigators. Results of all three tests are reproducible, but the longer the test, the greater the variation among patients within each test. As a result, the differences between the 2- and 12-minute tests were greater than the differences between the 6- and 12-minute tests. Thus, the 6-minute walk test was considered a sensible compromise.

The 6-minute walk test is strongly correlated with other functional measures in lower limb amputees wearing a prosthesis. Moreover, the 6-minute walk test can distinguish among the five MFCLs.[52] Although this test has yet to be evaluated in clinical trials with amputees, gait speed has been suggested as a useful measure of function and has been used to place patients when discharged from the hospital.[54] Faster ambulation in an elderly person is a good indicator of independence with regard to ADL.[61] For transtibial amputees, increased walking speed correlates with a more functional lifestyle.[9] Walking speed is an objective yet inexpensive method of monitoring gait rehabilitation.

Shorter walking tests have been used for amputees. The Timed Up and Go (TUG) Test, for example, has been suggested as a quick and easy measure of physical mobility for the lower limb amputee.[17,62] Although the 2-minute walk test is a questionable alternative to the 6-minute walk test as a measure of change over time, the correlation to other functional measures was moderate[9] and essentially equal to the TUG Test.[17]

Immediate Postoperative Treatment
General Management Principles

The goals of postoperative management in the new amputee are to reduce edema, promote healing, prevent loss of motion, increase cardiovascular endurance, and improve strength. Functional skills should be introduced as early as possible to promote independence in bed mobility, transfers, and ambulation techniques. Patient education concerning the self-care of the residual and sound limbs can prevent adverse effects such as contractures, excessive edema, delayed healing, or trauma to the sound limb from overuse. Moreover, each member of the rehabilitation team should be aware of the need to assist the patient with the psychological adjustment to the limb loss.

Postoperative Dressings

The selection of a postoperative dressing varies according to the level of amputation, surgical technique, healing requirements, patient compliance, and preference of the physician. The five major types used include soft dressings, nonremovable rigid dressings without an immediate prosthetic attachment, nonremovable rigid dressings with an immediate postoperative prosthesis (IPOP), removable rigid dressings, and prefabricated postoperative devices. Soft dressings are most often used for dysvascular patients so that regular dressing changes may be performed and alternative wound environments may be used. The disadvantage of soft dressings is that patients frequently decrease bed mobility because they are more hesitant to move the affected limb.[63] Rigid dressings, in addition to controlling edema and providing protection and support, help prevent knee flexion contractures and facilitate greater confidence with bed mobility.

IPOPs offer the benefits of rigid dressings and allow ambulation with limited weight bearing using an assistive device. These prostheses also afford the physiologic and psychological advantages of early walking with a limb. Some evidence exists that use of a strategy that incorporates a pylon and foot reduces the number of falls.[64] To date, IPOPs have not been associated with an increased number of falls or injury to the healing amputation wound. Providing additional support to the residual limb in amputees with a neuropathic opposite limb can potentially reduce foot pressures, improve balance, and reduce the effort required for ambulation with an assistive device. Removable rigid dressings were originally fabricated from plaster and suspended with a variety of supracondylar cuff systems. These dressings may now consist of a prefabricated copolymer plastic shell with a soft lining and, in some designs, will accept a pylon and foot to create an IPOP. The removable rigid dressing provides the protection and other benefits of the classic rigid dressing with the flexibility of removal for wound inspection or bathing. In addition, socks may be added or the system tightened for progressive shrinkage of the residual limb, which decreases the time to ambulatory discharge from the hospital with a temporary prosthesis.[65]

Positioning

When in a supine position, the transfemoral amputee should place a pillow laterally along the residual limb to maintain neutral rotation with no abduction. If the prone position is tolerable, then a pillow is placed under the residual limb to maintain hip extension. Transtibial amputees should avoid knee flexion for prolonged periods. A board will help maintain knee extension when in a wheelchair. All amputees must be advised that continual sitting in a wheelchair without any effort to promote hip extension may ultimately limit hip motion during prosthetic ambulation (Figure 2).

Transfers

Once bed mobility is mastered, the patient must first learn to transfer from the bed to a chair or wheelchair and then progress to more advanced transfer skills such as to the toilet, tub, or automobile. In patients who use an immediate postoperative or temporary prosthesis, weight bearing through the prosthesis can assist with transfers and provide additional safety. For transtibial amputees who are not candidates for ambulation, a lightweight transfer prosthesis may allow more independent transfers. A transfer prosthesis is typically fit when the wound is healed and the patient is ready for training. Bilateral amputees who are not fitted with an initial prosthesis transfer in a "head-on" manner in which the patient slides forward from the wheelchair onto the desired surface by lifting the body and pushing forward with both hands (Figure 3).

Wheelchair Propulsion

The primary means of mobility for most dysvascular amputees, either temporarily or permanently, is a wheelchair. The amount of energy conserved with wheelchair use compared to prosthetic ambulation is considerable with some levels of amputation.[66,67] Therefore, most amputees should be taught wheelchair skills as a part of their rehabilitation program. Bilateral and older amputees may use a wheelchair more often than unilateral and younger amputees; the latter are more likely to use other assistive devices when not ambulating with their prosthesis. Because of the loss of body weight anteriorly, amputees are prone to tipping backward while in a standard wheelchair. Amputee adapters set the wheel axle back approximately 2 in (5 cm), thus mov-

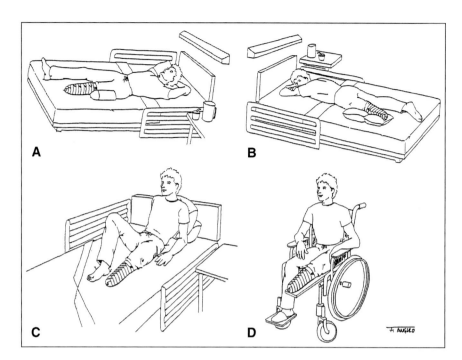

Figure 2 Proper positioning of the residual limb. **A,** Neutral hip rotation with no abduction. **B,** Hip and knee extension when prone. **C,** Knee extension when in bed. **D,** Knee extension when sitting. *(Copyright © Advanced Rehabilitation Therapy, Inc, Miami, FL, 1990. Illustrator Frank Angulo.)*

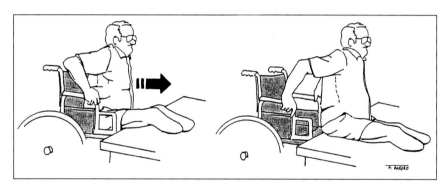

Figure 3 Head-on wheelchair-to-mat transfer. *(Copyright © Advanced Rehabilitation Therapy, Inc, Miami, FL, 1990. Illustrator Frank Angulo.)*

ing the COM anteriorly to prevent tipping, which is especially critical when ascending ramps or curbs. An alternative method is the addition of antitipping bars in place of, or in addition to, amputee wheel adapters. Transtibial amputees also require an elevated leg rest or board to maintain the knee in extension, thus preventing prolonged knee flexion and reducing the time the residual limb is in a dependent position, both of which control edema. Finally, wheelchairs should be fitted with removable arm-

rests to enable ease of transfer to or from either side of the chair.

Ambulation With Assistive Devices

All amputees need an assistive device for times when they choose not to wear their prosthesis or on occasions when they cannot wear their prosthesis secondary to edema, skin irritation, or a poor prosthetic fit. Some amputees require an assistive device while ambulating with the prosthesis.

Although safety is the primary factor for the selection of an appropriate assistive device, mobility is an important secondary consideration. The criteria for selection should include the following factors: (1) the ability for unsupported standing balance, (2) the degree of upper limb strength, (3) coordination and skill with the assistive device, and (4) cognition. A walker is appropriate for amputees with fair to poor balance, strength, and coordination. If balance and strength are good to normal, forearm crutches may be used for ambulation, with or without a prosthesis. A quad cane or straight cane may be selected if balance is questionable while ambulating with a prosthesis.

Patient Education
Skin Care

Patients must understand the importance of caring for the residual and sound limbs. The amputee must understand that proper care of skin and scar tissue on the residual limb is extremely important to prevent breakdown during prosthetic gait training, which would delay rehabilitation and lead to further deconditioning. Appropriate skin care is especially important for patients with diabetes mellitus and/or vascular dysfunction because these patients often have an increased wound healing time. Patients must also be taught the difference between the weight-bearing areas and pressure-sensitive areas of the residual limb in relation to the design and fit of the socket. Amputees should be familiar with the functions of the prosthetic components.

Amputees should be instructed to visually inspect the residual and sound limbs on a daily basis or after any strenuous activity. The residual limb is inspected for evidence of any abnormal pressures from the socket such as areas of persistent redness. Inspection of the sound limb has greater importance after amputation because the foot is subject to additional axial and shear forces to compensate for prosthetic weight bearing.

More frequent inspection of both limbs is necessary during the initial months of prosthetic training. A hand mirror may be used to view the posterior aspect of the residual limb and plantar aspect of the foot. Areas of redness should be monitored very closely as potential sites for abrasion or ulceration. Amputees with visual impairment should ask a family member to assist with these daily inspections. If a skin abrasion or ulcer develops, the amputee must understand that in almost all instances, the prosthesis should not be worn until healing occurs. In some circumstances, the patient may wear a protective barrier to avert additional skin insult while permitting continued use of the prosthesis. Without exception, any injury to the skin should be reported and closely followed to avoid further complications.

Desensitization

Many amputees experience postoperative skin hypersensitivity as a result of disruption of the neuromuscular system and associated edema. Progressive desensitization of the residual limb is often necessary for restoring normal sensation while using wound compression techniques to reduce edema. Desensitization involves gradually introducing stimuli to reduce the hyperirritability of the limb. For example, a soft material such as cotton cloth or lamb's wool is rubbed around the residual limb, followed by gradually more coarse materials such as corduroy. The amputee should progress as quickly as possible to tapping and massaging with the hand. Eventually, when the suture line has healed, pressure can be applied to the residual limb during transfers, mobility skills, and exercise. These measures will help expedite the ability of the residual limb to tolerate the prosthesis.

Care of the Prosthesis

The socket should be cleaned daily to promote good hygiene and prevent deterioration of prosthetic materials. The patient should be informed of the best cleansing agent for the specific materials of their socket or liners. In general, laminated plastic, copolymer plastic, silicone, and other composite materials are cleaned with mild soap on a damp cloth. Foam materials are cleansed with rubbing alcohol. Because some liner materials interact adversely with alcohol, manufacturers' recommendations should be followed. After a cleansing agent is applied, a clean, damp cloth should be used to wipe away any residue. To ensure maximum life and safety of the prosthesis, patients are reminded that routine maintenance of their prosthesis should be performed by the prosthetist.

Sock Regulation and Internal Suspension Sleeve Use

Sock regulation is of extreme importance to prevent excessive vertical motion or pistoning between the residual limb and the socket. The amputee should always carry extra socks to be added if pistoning or extreme perspiration occurs. A thin nylon sheath applied directly to the residual limb will help reduce friction at the interface between the skin and socket. Prosthetic socks are available in several thicknesses (plies), permitting the amputee to obtain the desired fit within the socket. Socks should be applied wrinkle-free with the seam horizontal and on the outside to prevent skin abrasion. Seamless socks are available to eliminate this problem.

Internal suspension sleeves and liners are made from a variety of material such as silicone, urethane, and gel composites. Some of the benefits of these materials include reduced pistoning, better management of unstable limb volume, improved cosmesis, and for some patients with impaired hand function, easier donning of the prosthesis. Liners not only reduce shear forces over scar tissue and bony prominences, but they also act as suspension devices.

Internal suspension sleeves and liners are widely accepted, but some amputees have problems with skin reactions from the materials used; some silicones and gels are not medical grade, and, therefore, are not hypoallergenic. Fortunately, a wide variety of materials is used, and many alternatives are available should a problem become evident. For example, a nylon sheath can be used as a protective layer beneath the sleeve or liner.

Lake and Supan[68] surveyed a group of amputees who used internal suspension sleeves and reported a lower incidence of perspiration, heat rash, and folliculitis among minimally to moderately active amputees and among older amputees with diabetes mellitus and/or vascular problems. The latter group also reported fewer problems with contact dermatitis and limb soreness. Although these results were not statistically significant, the differences were worth noting. The authors also reported that the longer an amputee used an internal suspension sleeve, the greater the likelihood of dermatologic problems. The authors summarized that silicone suction sleeves appear to offer amputees with diabetes mellitus and/or vascular problems a viable alternative to traditional suspension with less risk of dermatologic problems than reported by younger, traumatic amputees, who tended to wear their prostheses for longer periods of time each day.

Donning and Doffing of the Prosthesis

A wide variety of suspension systems is available for all levels of amputation. For example, the transtibial amputee has the option of a hard socket with or without a soft insert that could include various forms of auxiliary suspension such as a medial wedge or internal roll-on locking liner. The transfemoral amputee has the choice of a nonsuction external suspension or a suction suspension socket that can be donned with an elastic bandage, pull sock, nylon donning bag, or by wet fit, as well as internal suspension systems with or without pin and lock systems. The

methods of donning each of these combinations are too numerous to describe here; however, it is important to emphasize that amputees must become proficient in donning and doffing their particular prosthesis.

Compression Dressings for the Residual Limb

Early rigid or semirigid dressings, compression wrappings, or shrinker socks for the residual limb can have several positive effects: (1) decreased edema, (2) increased circulation, (3) assistance in shaping, (4) provision of skin protection, (5) reduction of redundant tissue, (6) amelioration of phantom limb pain/sensation, and (7) desensitization of the residual limb. Casting transtibial amputees in 0° of knee extension will prevent flexion contracture and provide greater confidence with early bed mobility.[63] For transfemoral amputees, there may be some value in counteracting contracture forces with specific compression wrapping techniques.

The use of traditional compression wrapping versus shrinker socks is controversial. Some institutions prefer commercial shrinkers because of the ease of donning. Advocates of compression wrapping, however, indicate that compression wrapping provides more control over pressure gradients and tissue shaping.[69] Condie and associates[70] observed that both transtibial and transfemoral amputees who used a shrinker sock within 10 days after amputation demonstrated a significantly reduced time from amputation to prosthetic casting versus those who used wrapping methods. Moreover, even shorter time to prosthetic casting has been observed with transtibial amputees receiving semirigid and rigid dressings.[69,70]

Many programs prefer to wait until the sutures or staples have been removed before using a shrinker sock. For amputees with diabetes mellitus, this period is often as long as 21 days. However, compression therapy can begin early with wraps or rigid dress-

ings and progress to shrinker socks after the suture line has healed. Compression therapy is a controversial topic and each rehabilitation team must determine the best course of treatment for their patients. All compression techniques must be performed correctly and consistently to prevent constriction of circulation, poor shaping, and edema (Figures 4 and 5). Likewise, compliance is an integral part of the compression program. All wrappings or shrinker socks should be routinely checked and/or reapplied several times each day. The application of a nylon sheath over the residual limb before wrapping or donning a shrinker sock may reduce shear forces to skin and thus provide additional comfort and safety.

Issues Pertaining to the Sound Limb

The loss of a limb and its substitution by a prosthesis clearly impact gait biomechanics in most amputees with diabetes mellitus. Therefore, when planning treatment for these patients, expert care of the sound limb is critical. Preservation of the sound limb may permit continued bipedal ambulation by delaying or preventing loss of the limb. One reason for concern is that the sound limb compensates for the amputee's inability to maintain equal weight distribution between limbs resulting in altered gait mechanics. Two known effects on the intact limb are altered forces on the weight-bearing surfaces of the foot and increased ground-reaction forces throughout the skeletal structures of the limb.[71-73]

Amputees with diabetes mellitus may have deviations from normal gait kinematics that increase vertical and shear forces in addition to the preexisting impaired sensation, dysvascularity, scar tissue, and any foot and/or ankle deformity of the sound limb. Collectively, these factors are associated with an approximately 50% incidence of amputation in the same or contralateral limb within 4 years of the primary amputation.[74-78] Accordingly,

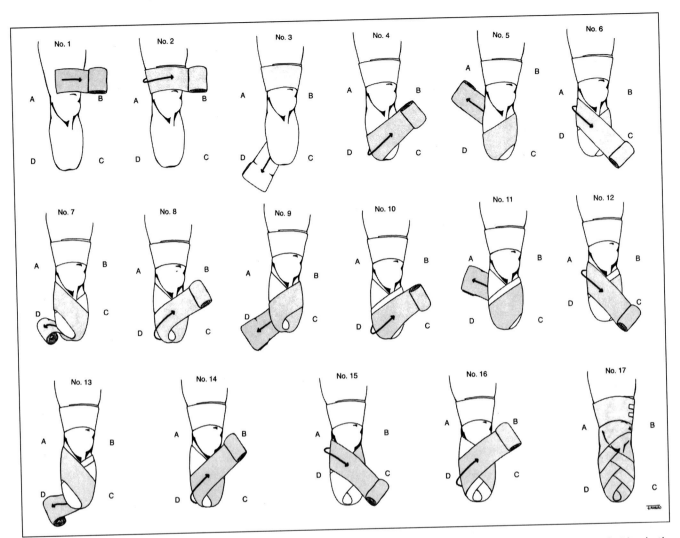

Figure 4 Wrapping of the transtibial residual limb using a figure-of-8 pattern guide. **1.** Begin by placing a double-length 4-in elastic bandage above the kneecap. **2.** Wrap around once to secure the bandage comfortably but not too tightly. **3.** Continue the bandage around the back and cross to corner D. **4.** Bring the bandage around corner D and cross up toward B. **5.** Continue around the back toward A. **6.** Wrap the bandage across and down to corner C. **7.** Continue to wrap around the end and cover corner D. **8.** Move the bandage up and across the front toward B. **9.** Continue to move the bandage across the back and down to corner D. **10.** Move up and across the front to B. **11.** Continue to move the bandage across the back to A. **12.** Move down and across the front to corner C. **13.** Continue to wrap across the end and cover corner D. **14.** Move the bandage up and across the front to B. **15.** Continue to wrap across the back and move down and across to corner C. **16.** Move around corner C to corner D and continue up and across the front to B. **17.** Continue with figure-of-8 pattern, moving the bandage higher on the residual limb until it is completely covered in a figure-of-8 pattern. Remember to apply less pressure as you move up. Complete the wrap by anchoring it with tape. *(Copyright © Advanced Rehabilitation Therapy, Inc, Miami, FL, 1989. Illustrator Frank Angulo.)*

expert care of the sound foot becomes even more critical after amputation for amputees with diabetes mellitus because their chances of achieving functional ambulation will decline if they become bilateral amputees.[79] From the onset of rehabilitation, therefore, the patient should be advised about the possible dangers to the opposite limb.

Strategies to Enhance Patient Education

Educating amputees about self care and home exercise programs is critical to the ultimate outcome of the rehabilitation process. The most difficult task is ensuring that the amputee retains the information and complies with instructions. An itemized checklist for the amputee to take home can

assist in achieving these goals. This list not only aids the amputee, but also provides the clinician with a format to prevent overlooking important points. A checklist designed specifically for amputees with diabetes mellitus also gives the clinician a systematic method of educating the amputee about preventive care of the insensate foot (Figure 6).

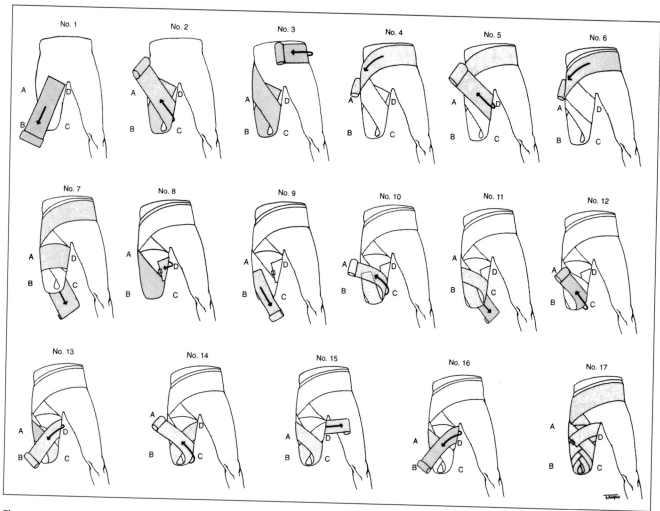

Figure 5 Wrapping of the transfemoral residual limb. **1.** Begin by placing a double-length 6-in elastic bandage at letter D and cross down to corner B. The pressure should be uniform throughout the first eight steps of the wrapping procedure. **2.** Wrap the bandage around corner C and cross up the front to A. **3.** Wrap the bandage around the waist with the thigh extended and then back to A. **4.** Continue wrapping the bandage around the back of the thigh to D. **5.** Cross to A and wrap the uppermost part of the inner aspect of the thigh. **6.** Wrap the bandage around the waist to A and then around the back of the thigh to D to cover the upper inner part of the thigh again. **7.** Return toward A, and wrap the bandage down and across to corner C and then return toward A. **8.** Wrap the bandage around the back and anchor with tape. This completes part 1 of wrapping with the 6-in bandage. **9.** Begin part 2 by placing a double-length 4-in elastic bandage on the residual limb between corners A and B. This part is the figure-of-8 pattern guide. Wrap the bandage diagonally around corners B and C. **10.** Cross up to A and anchor the wrap. **11.** Continue wrapping the bandage around the back and down to corner C. **12.** Wrap up and across to A and then around the back to D. **13.** Continue the bandage down and across to cover corners B and C. **14.** Continue wrapping the bandage up and across to A. **15.** Wrap the bandage around the back to D. **16.** Continue down and wrap corners B and C, but wrap slightly higher than the previous time around. **17.** Continue wrapping higher on the residual limb until the figure-of-8 bandage is completed. Remember to apply less pressure as you move up. Complete the wrap by anchoring it with tape. Note that the angle between the figure-of-8s should be 80° to 90° at the crossover point to avoid a tourniquet effect. (*Copyright © Advanced Rehabilitation Therapy, Inc, Miami, FL, 1989. Illustrator Frank Angulo.*)

Preprosthetic Exercises
General Conditioning

Decreased general conditioning and endurance often contribute to difficulties in learning functional activities, including prosthetic gait. Regardless of age or physical condition, amputees should begin a progressive general exercise program immediately after surgery, through the preprosthetic period, and eventually as part of a daily routine.

The list of possible general strengthening and endurance exercise activities is long. Examples include cuff weights in bed, wheelchair propulsion for a predetermined distance, dynamic exercises for the residual limb, ambulation with an assistive device before fitting of the prosthesis, lower and/or upper limb ergometry, wheelchair aerobics, swimming, aquatic therapy, lower and upper body strengthening at a local fitness center, and any sport or recreational activity of interest. One or more of these activities should be selected and performed to tolerance initially, pro-

Physical Therapy Diabetic Amputee Limb Care Check List	Date Completed
Topic Item	
Skin Inspection Education	
Daily inspection of skin with mirror for difficult to see areas	
Attention to bony prominences, between toes and scars	
Attention to problem areas	
Skin Care	
Daily cleansing techniques mild unscented soap	
Application of Moisturizer	
Avoid hot water	
Minimize exposure to perspiration and wet weather	
Minimize exposure extreme heat and cold	
Foot Care	
Toe deformity care (lamb wool between toes)	
Clean, dry socks without elastic bands	
Extra depth shoes with custom molded inserts	
Appropriate house slipper or shoes worn at all times in the home	
Never walk barefoot especially on beaches, hot surfaces or at night in the home	
Assistance with nail and callus trimming (if patient is independent use nail file for nails and pumice stone for corns & calluses, **NO Sharp Implements**)	
Friction Reduction	
Bed mobility avoid excessive sound limb use	
Posture and positioning	
Transfer techniques	
Equal weight-bearing during standing and ambulation	
Ambulation turning techniques, avoid pivoting on sound foot	
Appropriate shoe wear with socks	
Residual Limb	
Skin inspection (same as above)	
Skin care (same as above)	
Positioning	
Prosthetic Care	
Sock regulation (correct plys, sock application & main dry sock wear)	
Prosthetic wear schedule (discuss procedure if skin lesions appear)	
Daily socket cleansing	
Compression Therapy	
Wrapping or shrinker application techniques	
Precautionary signs (pain and swelling)	
Phantom Sensation and Pain	
Awareness and desensitization	
Support Group Participation	
Contact person and phone number	
Shoe Wear	
Suggest purchase of 2-3 pairs of proper shoes for daily rotation of shoes	
Change shoes with perspiration or when wet and soiled.	
Methods of assessment to insure proper fit of shoes	
Inspect the inside of shoes daily for foreign objects	
Inspect for excessive wear (sole wear, split in leather, holes etc..)	
Wear dry cotton or wool socks without elastic bands	
Wound Care	
Always follow prescribed treatment form your healthcare professional	
Insure that dressing always remain dry and clean	
Check for drainage of the wound into the sock or shoe, if this occurs have dressing changed	
Take all prescribed medication and never alter the dosage without consulting your physician	

Date item understood or mastered by amputee is signified in the "Date Completed" column.

(Adapted from Clark and Gailey. From One Step Ahead: an integrated approach to lower extremity prosthetics and amputee rehabilitation. Course workbook. Advanced Rehabilitation Therapy, Inc 1996 used by permission.)

Figure 6 Sample limb care checklist for amputees with diabetes mellitus. (*Copyright © Advanced Rehabilitation Therapy, Inc, Miami, FL, 1998.*)

gressing to 1 hour or more each day. The advantages of activity extend well beyond improving the chances of ambulating well with a prosthesis. Amputees have the opportunity to experience and enjoy activities that they may have thought were not possible. If the amputee experiences difficulties while still admitted to the hospital, resources such as a physical therapist or a fellow amputee who has mastered a particular activity will be available.

Cardiovascular Endurance

Because the average general physical and cardiac condition of amputees with vascular conditions is poor, cardiovascular endurance training can directly affect functional walking capabilities, particularly distance and the type of assistive device required for walking.[80-82] Aerobic training improves overall ambulation capabilities regardless of the level of amputation.[83]

Aerobic training typically begins immediately after surgery as the patient is increasing his or her tolerance for sitting. Training continues with early ambulation. Improving aerobic fitness should be incorporated into the rehabilitation program and remain a part of the amputee's general conditioning program long after discharge. Initially, most amputees can perform upper limb ergometry.[84-86] Once balance and strength return, lower limb ergometry may be performed with the sound limb first, progressing to the prosthetic limb when appropriate. As the amputee's level of fitness improves, other equipment such as treadmills, stair climbers, and rowing machines may be used. Remember that amputees enjoy the same activities as nonamputees, making swimming and walking the exercises of choice for general fitness, regardless of age or athletic ability.[87]

Strengthening

Eisert and Tester[88] first described dynamic exercises for the residual limb in 1954. Since then, their antigravity exercises have become the most favored method of strengthening. Dynamic exercises require little in the way of equipment. A towel roll or step stool is all that is required. In addition to increasing strength, these exercises offer benefits such as desensitization and increasing bed mobility and joint ROM. They are relatively easy to learn and can be performed independently, permitting the physical therapist to spend patient contact time on more advanced skills. Incorporating isometric contractions at the peak of the isotonic movement will help to maximize increases in strength. A 10-second contraction followed by 10 seconds of relaxation for 10 repetitions gives the patient an easily remembered mnemonic: the "rule of ten." The rationale behind a 10-second contraction is that a maximal isometric contraction can be maintained for 6 seconds; however, there is a 2-second rise time and a 2-second fall time. Thus, a 2-second rise plus a 6-second maximal contraction plus a 2-second fall equals a total time of 10 seconds.[89]

All amputees should consider performing abdominal and back extensor strengthening exercises to maintain trunk strength, decrease the risk of back pain, and assist in the reduction of gait deviations associated with the trunk. Figure 7 shows a basic dynamic strength training program for transfemoral and transtibial amputees.[90] Strengthening exercises should be performed in multiple planes of motion over time. For example, if a transtibial amputee were to strengthen just the knee flexors and extensors, which primarily control movement in the sagittal plane, control of the knee in the frontal and transverse planes would not be achieved. With a strengthening program that focuses on all three planes of motion, however, the ability to control excessive movement when walking in any direction or on uneven terrain will improve stability and confidence in control of the prosthesis. Exercises that promote strengthening in multiple planes while incorporating rapid movements with concentric and eccentric contractions can assist with prosthetic control and help the amputee respond to the demands of walking.[73] When possible, these exercises should be performed in a closed kinetic chain posture (Figures 8 and 9). Amputees who have access to isotonic and isokinetic strengthening equipment can benefit from using this equipment with a few modifications in positioning on the machines.

Range of Motion

Prevention of decreased ROM and contractures is a major concern in the rehabilitation of amputees. Limited ROM often results in difficulties with prosthetic fit, gait deviations, or the ability to ambulate with a prosthesis altogether. The best way to prevent loss of joint mobility and ensure full ROM in the joints is to remain active. Unfortunately, not all amputees have this option; therefore, proper limb positioning must be maintained long after amputation, especially in sedentary amputees (Figure 2). Amputees who have already lost ROM may benefit from traditional physical therapy such as passive ROM, contract-relax stretching, soft-tissue mobilization, myofascial techniques, joint mobilization, and other methods that promote increased ROM.

Functional Activities

Encouraging activity as soon as possible after amputation helps speed recovery in several ways. First, it offsets the negative effects of immobility by promoting joint movement, muscle activity, and increased circulation. Second, it helps amputees to reestablish their independence, which may be perceived as threatened because of the loss of the limb. Finally, the psychological advantages of activity and independence have an impact on patient motivation throughout rehabilitation.

Unsupported Standing Balance

In preparation for ambulation without a prosthesis, all amputees must learn to compensate for loss of the

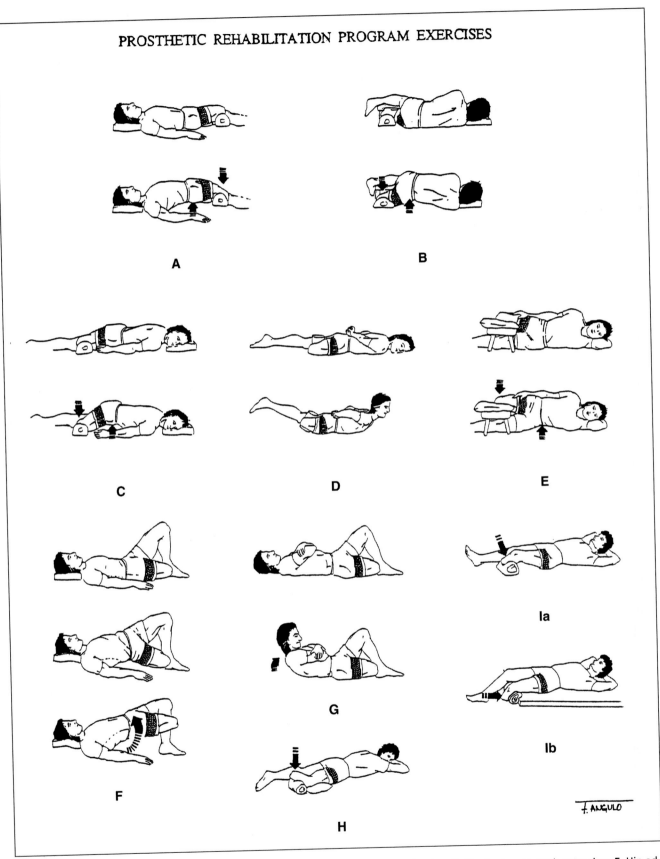

PROSTHETIC REHABILITATION PROGRAM EXERCISES

Figure 7 Strengthening exercises for the residual limb. **A,** Hip extension. **B,** Hip abduction. **C,** Hip flexion. **D,** Back extension. **E,** Hip adduction. **F,** Bridging. **G,** Sit-ups. **H,** Knee extension. **Ia,** Knee flexion, on table. **Ib,** Knee flexion, leg over table. *(Copyright © Advanced Rehabilitation Therapy, Inc, Miami, FL, 1989. Illustrator Frank Angulo.)*

weight of the amputated limb by balancing their COM over the sound limb. Although this habit must be broken when learning prosthetic ambulation, balance on a single limb must be learned initially to build confidence for stand-pivot transfers, ambulation with assistive devices, and hopping, depending on the amputee's level of skill. An amputee must be able to balance for at least 0.5 second to allow for the smooth and safe forward progression of an assistive device during ambulation.

One method of progression begins with the amputee standing in the parallel bars while using both hands for support[90] (Figure 10). Once the patient is able to stand in the parallel bars using both arms for support, the hand on the side of the amputation should be removed from the bars. Independent balance is achieved when both hands can be removed from the bars. To improve balance and righting skills, the patient is challenged by gently tapping the shoulders in multiple directions or by tossing a ball back and forth.[90] Enough time is allowed between taps or throws for the patient to regain a comfortable standing posture. Once confidence is gained within the parallel bars, the patient is permitted to practice these skills outside of the bars, eventually progressing to hopping activities.

Pregait Training
Balance and Coordination

After the loss of a lower limb, the decrease in body weight will alter the amputee's COM. To maintain the single-limb balance necessary during stance without a prosthesis, ambulate with an assistive device, or hop on a single limb, the amputee must shift the COM over the BOS, which is the foot of the sound limb. As the amputee becomes more secure in single-limb support, reorientation to maintaining the COM over both the sound and prosthetic limbs becomes more difficult. Ultimately, the amputee must also learn to maintain his or her COM and entire body weight over the

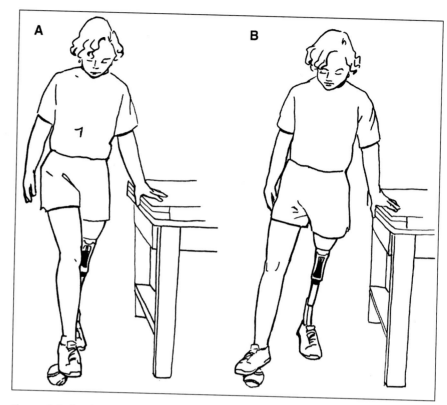

Figure 8 Ball rolls exercise. **A,** Place a tennis ball under the sound limb and hold onto an immovable object. **B,** Roll the ball quickly 10 to 15 times forward and backward and then side-to-side, followed by clockwise and counterclockwise movements. (Copyright © Advanced Rehabilitation Therapy, Inc, Miami, FL, 1994. Illustrator Frank Angulo.)

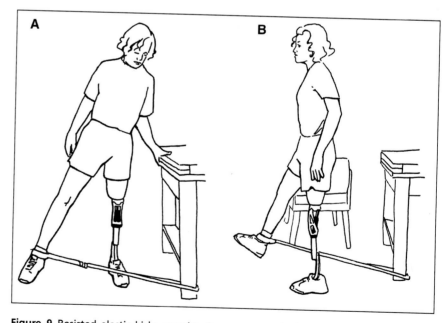

Figure 9 Resisted elastic kicks exercise. Secure one end of a rubber tubing band to a sturdy table leg and the other end around the sound ankle. Holding onto a chair, the amputee moves far enough away from the table so that the rubber tubing is slightly stretched. The amputee then (1) kicks the leg back, while facing the table; (2) kicks across the prosthetic limb and (3) away from the prosthetic limb while standing sideways to the table **(A)**; and (4) kicks forward, with his or her back to the table **(B)**. (Copyright © Advanced Rehabilitation Therapy, Inc, Miami, FL, 1994. Illustrator Frank Angulo.)

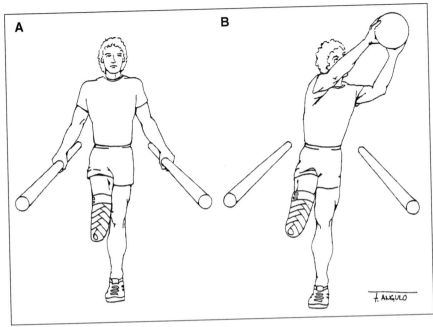

Figure 10 A, Standing balance using the parallel bars. **B,** Dynamic balance activities within the parallel bars. *(Copyright © Advanced Rehabilitation Therapy, Inc, Miami, FL, 1989. Illustrator Frank Angulo.)*

prosthesis. Once comfortable with bearing weight equally on both limbs, the amputee can begin to develop confidence with independent standing and eventually with ambulation.

Orientation to COM and BOS

Orientation of the COM over the BOS is necessary to maintain balance; thus the amputee must become familiar with these terms and their relationship. The COM is 2 inches (5 cm) anterior to the second sacral vertebra. Although the average person stands with his or her feet 2 to 4 inches (5 to 10 cm) apart, both the COM and the BOS vary according to height.[91,92] Various methods of proprioceptive and visual feedback may be used to help the amputee to maximize the displacement of the COM over the BOS. The amputee must learn to displace the COM forward and backward, as well as from side to side[93] (Figure 11). These exercises vary little from traditional exercises for shifting weight, with the exception that the emphasis is placed on the movement of the COM over the BOS rather than

weight bearing into the prosthesis. Increased weight bearing will be a direct result of improved COM displacement and will establish a firm foundation for weight shifting during ambulation.

Standing on a Single Limb

Bearing weight on the prosthesis is one of the most difficult challenges facing the physical therapist and amputee alike. Without the ability to maintain full single-limb weight bearing and balance for an adequate amount of time (0.5 second minimum), the amputee will exhibit several gait deviations including (1) decreased stance time on the prosthetic side, (2) shortened stride length on the sound side, or (3) lateral trunk bending over the prosthetic limb. Strength, balance, and coordination are the primary physical factors influencing single-limb stance on a prosthesis. Fear, pain, and lack of confidence in the prosthesis must be considered when an amputee appears to be extremely reluctant to bear weight on the prosthesis. Adequate weight bearing and balance on the

prosthesis before and during ambulation should be emphasized.

Balance on the prosthetic limb while advancing the sound limb should be practiced in a controlled manner so that when required in a dynamic situation such as walking, the amputee can do this with relatively little difficulty. The stool stepping exercise is an excellent method for learning this skill. The amputee stands in the parallel bars, or between two chairs when training at home, with the sound limb in front of a 4- to 8-in stool (or block); the height depends on level of ability. The patient is then asked to step slowly onto the stool with the sound limb while using bilateral upper limb support on the parallel bars. To increase these weight-bearing skills, the patient is asked to remove the hand on the sound side from the bars. Eventually, both hands are removed from the bars. Initially, the speed of the sound leg will increase when upper limb support is removed.[93] With practice, the movement will become slower and more controlled, thus promoting increased weight bearing on the prosthesis (Figure 12).

The amputee's walking speed and the ability to control sound limb advancement are directly related to the ability to control prosthetic limb stance.[94,95] The following three factors may help the amputee achieve adequate balance over the prosthetic limb: (1) control of the musculature of the amputated side; (2) use of the available sensation at the residual limb/socket interface; and (3) visualization of the prosthetic foot and its relationship to the ground. New amputees will initially have difficulty in understanding these concepts but will attain a greater appreciation of them with time.

Gait Training Skills
Sound and Prosthetic Limb Training

Another factor in adjusting to lower limb amputation is the restoration of the gait biomechanics that were unique to the amputee before amputation. That is to say, not everyone has the same gait pattern. The restoration of full function to the remaining joints of the amputated limb should be a goal of gait training. Prosthetic gait training should not alter the amputee's gait mechanics to suit the prosthesis; rather, the mechanics of the prosthesis should be designed to suit the gait of the amputee. Developments in prosthetics during the past decade have provided prostheses that closely replicate the mechanics of the human leg.

Pelvic Motions

The pelvis moves as a unit with the body's COM in four directions: (1) vertical displacement, (2) lateral shifting, (3) horizontal tilting, and (4) transverse rotation. Each motion can directly affect the amputee's gait, resulting in gait deviations with a concomitant increase in energy consumption during ambulation. If restoring function to the remaining joints of the amputated limb is a goal of gait training, then pelvic motion plays a decisive role in determining the final outcome of the amputee's gait pattern.

Vertical displacement is simply the rhythmic up and down motion of the body's COM. To reduce the metabolic cost of walking, the knee must flex 10° to 15° during loading response and be fully extended during midstance.[96,97] The transtibial amputee can flex and extend the knee during the stance phase of gait. The transfemoral amputee, unfortunately, is at a disadvantage because the knee must remain in extension throughout the entire stance phase to avoid collapse (buckling) (Figure 13). Evidence suggests that the contribution of stance phase knee flexion does not appreciably alter the amount of vertical movement during normal walking.[98,99]

Lateral shift occurs as the pelvis shifts from side to side approximately 2 in (5 cm) (Figure 14). The amount of lateral shift is determined by the width of the BOS, which is 2 to 4 in

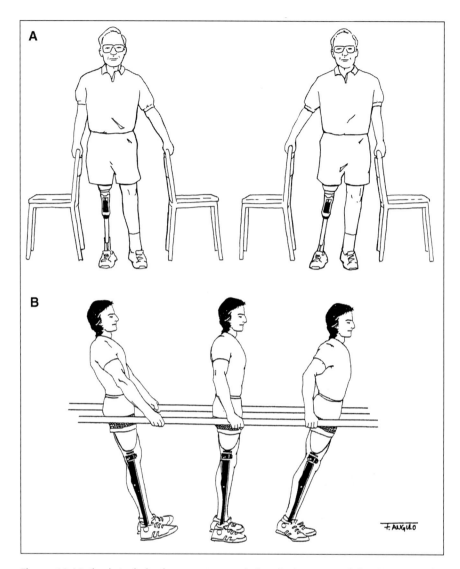

Figure 11 Methods to help the amputee maximize displacement of the COM over the BOS. **A,** Lateral shifting of weight and balance orientation. **B,** Forward and backward weight shifting and balance orientation. *(Copyright © Advanced Rehabilitation Therapy, Inc, Miami, FL, 1989.)*

(5 to 10 cm), depending on the height of the amputee. Amputees spend an inordinate amount of time in single limb stance on the sound limb, such as when they are on crutches, hopping without the prosthesis, or during relaxed standing. Therefore, they are adept at maintaining COM over the sound limb and have a habit of crossing midline with the sound foot. Thus, adequate space for the prosthetic limb to follow a natural line of progression is not available. The result is an abducted or circumducted gait with greater lateral displacement of the pelvis toward the prosthetic

side. More frequently, this is observed in transfemoral amputees; however, this altered BOS may also be seen with transtibial amputees.

Horizontal tilt of the pelvis is normal up to 5°, and any tilt greater than 5° is considered excessive. Usually, excessive horizontal tilt of the pelvis is directly related to weak hip abductor musculature, specifically the gluteus medius. Maintenance of the residual femur in adduction via the socket theoretically places the gluteus medius at the optimal length-to-tension ratio. If the limb is abducted, however, the muscle shortens in that posi-

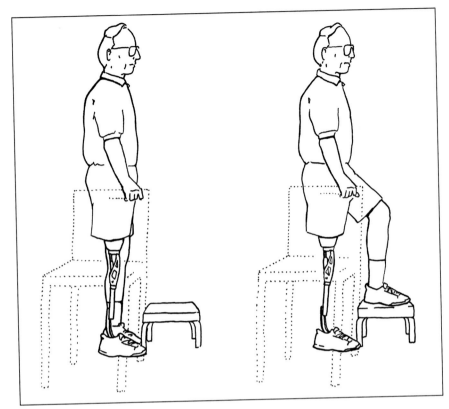

Figure 12 Stool stepping exercise. *(Copyright © Advanced Rehabilitation Therapy, Inc, Miami, FL, 1989. Illustrator Frank Angulo.)*

tion and is unable to function properly. The result is a Trendelenburg limp, or compensatory gluteus medius gait, in which the trunk leans laterally over the prosthetic limb in an attempt to maintain the pelvis in a horizontal position.

Transverse rotation of the pelvis occurs around the longitudinal axis approximately 5° to 10° forward and backward (Figure 15). This rotation assists in shifting the body's COM from one side to the other and helps to initiate the 30° of knee flexion during toe-off, which is necessary to achieve 60° of knee flexion during the acceleration phase of swing. Knee flexion during preswing is created by other influences as well, including plantar flexion of the foot, horizontal tilt of the pelvis, and gravity. No prosthetic foot permits active plantar flexion, and horizontal dip greater than 5° is abnormal. Therefore, restoration of transverse rotation of the pelvis becomes of great importance to obtain sufficient knee flexion. Normalization

of trunk, pelvic, and limb biomechanics can be taught to the amputee in a systematic way. First, independent movements of the various joint and muscle groups are developed. Second, these independent movements are incorporated into the functional movement patterns of the gait cycle. Finally, all component movement patterns are integrated to produce a smooth, normalized gait.

Sample Functional Prosthetic Training Program

In 1989, Gailey and Gailey[93] introduced a functional prosthetic training program that offers a systematic way to establish static and dynamic stability and promote single-limb standing balance over the prosthetic limb. Once the amputee has attained a basic level of strength and balance, resistive gait training techniques are implemented to reeducate the amputee in the normal gait movements necessary to maximize prosthetic performance and promote economy of gait. Ad-

vanced gait training exercises are offered to help the amputee negotiate a variety of environmental conditions that require multidirectional movements and superior dynamic balance. The time required to progress through the sequence and overall outcome varies, based on the amputee's physical ability, diagnosis, and motivation. The following sequence of steps is adapted from the Prosthetic Gait Training Program:[93]

1. Dynamic residual limb exercises are used to strengthen muscles (see Preprosthetic Exercises).

2. Proprioceptive neuromuscular facilitation, Feldenkrais techniques, or any other movement awareness techniques may be initiated for trunk, pelvic, and limb reeducation patterns. These exercises encourage rotational motions and promote independent movements of the trunk, pelvic girdle, and limbs.

3. Pregait training exercises are initiated (see Pregait Training).

4. Sound limb stepping within the parallel bars is initiated (Figure 16). The amputee steps forward and backward, heel rise to heel strike, with both hands on the parallel bars. The purpose of this activity is to familiarize the amputee and the physical therapist with the gait mechanics of the sound limb without having to be concerned about weight bearing and balance on the prosthetic limb. This activity also affords the physical therapist an opportunity to palpate the anterior superior iliac spines (ASISs) to gain a feeling for the amputee's pelvic motion, which in most cases is close to normal for the amputee.

5. Prosthetic limb stepping within the parallel bars is similar to sound limb stepping, except that the prosthetic limb is used. As the physical therapist palpates the ASISs, a posterior rotation of the pelvis may be observed in some patients. This posterior rotation is often a result of the amputee's attempt to kick the prosthesis forward with the residual limb, as it would when kicking a football. The amputee should feel the differ-

ence between the pelvic motion on the prosthetic side and the sound side.

6. To restore the correct pelvic motion, the amputee places the prosthetic limb behind the sound limb while holding the parallel bars with both hands (Figure 17). The physical therapist then blocks the prosthetic foot to prevent forward movement of the prosthesis. Rhythmic initiation is used, giving the amputee the feeling of rotating the pelvis forward as passive flexion of the prosthetic knee occurs. As the amputee becomes comfortable with the motion, he or she can begin to move the pelvis actively and progress to resistive movements when deemed appropriate by the physical therapist.

7. Once the amputee and physical therapist are satisfied with the pelvic motions, the swing phase of gait can be taught (Figure 18). The amputee is ready to step forward and backward with the prosthetic limb. The pelvic motions should be monitored so that the line of progression of the prosthesis remains constant without circumduction and the heel contact occurs within the boundaries of the BOS. As the amputee improves, the sound side and eventually both hands are released from the parallel bars. There should be little if any loss of efficiency with the motion; however, if there is loss of efficiency, the amputee may revert to the previous phase of training.

8. The next step is a return to sound limb stepping with both hands on the parallel bars. The physical therapist will determine if the mechanics are correct and that the sound foot is not crossing the midline with heel contact. When ready, the amputee will remove the hand on the sound side from the parallel bars. At this time, there may be an increase in the speed of the step, a decrease in step length, and/or lateral leaning of the trunk. These changes may occur as a direct result of the inability to bear weight or balance over the prosthesis. The amputee is verbally cued to remember the skills learned while performing the stool stepping exercise

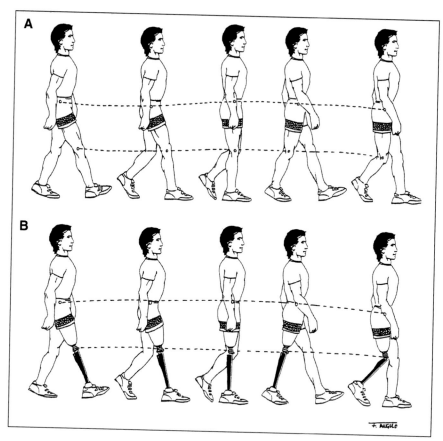

Figure 13 Vertical displacement of COM in a nonamputee **(A)** and in a transfemoral amputee **(B)**. *(Copyright © Advanced Rehabilitation Therapy, Inc, Miami, FL, 1989. Illustrator Frank Angulo.)*

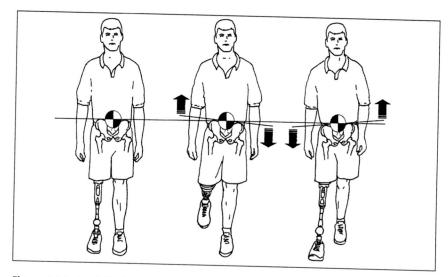

Figure 14 Lateral displacement of the body's COM is 5 cm, and horizontal tilt of the pelvis is approximately 5°. *(Copyright © Advanced Rehabilitation Therapy, Inc, Miami, FL, 1989. Illustrator Frank Angulo.)*

(see Pregait Training). After this skill is perfected, sound limb stepping without any hand support may be practiced until single-limb balance over the prosthetic leg is sufficiently mastered (Figure 19).

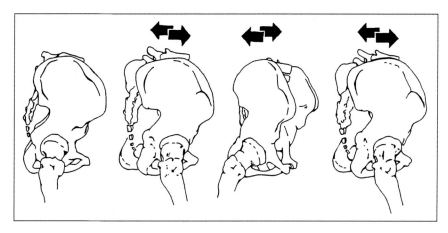

Figure 15 Transverse rotation of the pelvis is approximately 5° anterior and posterior to the neutral position. *(Copyright © Advanced Rehabilitation Therapy, Inc, Miami, FL, 1989. Illustrator Frank Angulo.)*

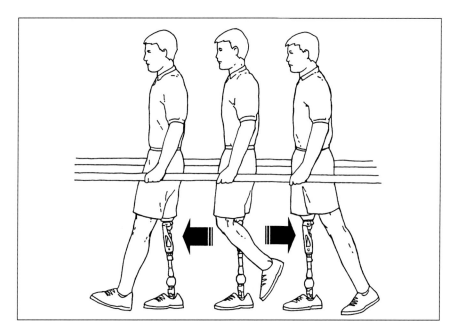

Figure 16 Sound limb stepping is designed to orient the amputee to gait biomechanics. *(Copyright © Advanced Rehabilitation Therapy, Inc, Miami, FL, 1990. Illustrator Frank Angulo.)*

9. When each of these individual skills has been performed to an acceptable level of competency, the amputee is ready to combine them and begin walking with the prosthesis. Initially, the amputee will walk within the parallel bars, facing the physical therapist. The physical therapist's hands are placed on the amputee's ASISs, and the amputee is holding onto the parallel bars. As the amputee ambulates within the parallel bars, the physical therapist applies slight resistance through the hips, providing proprioceptive feedback to the pelvis and the involved musculature of the lower limb.

10. When both the physical therapist and the amputee are comfortable with the gait demonstrated within the parallel bars, the amputee begins practicing outside the bars, with the amputee initially using the physical therapist's shoulders as support and progressing to both hands free when appropriate (Figure 20). The physical therapist may or may not continue to provide proprioceptive input to the pelvis. As the amputee begins to ambulate independently, verbal cueing may be necessary as a reminder to keep the sound foot away from the midline to maintain the proper BOS. Maintenance of equal stride length may not be immediately forthcoming because many amputees have a tendency to take a longer step with the prosthetic limb than with the sound limb. When adequate weight bearing through the prosthetic limb has been achieved, the amputee should begin to take longer steps with the sound limb and slightly shorter steps with the prosthetic limb. This principle also applies when increasing the cadence. As an amputee increases the speed of walking, a longer step is often taken on the prosthetic limb in compensation, thus increasing the asymmetry. By simply having the amputee take a longer step with the sound limb and a moderate step with the prosthetic limb, increased speed of gait is accomplished without increased asymmetry.

11. Trunk rotation and arm swing are the final components of restoring the biomechanics of gait. During locomotion, the trunk and upper limbs rotate opposite to the pelvic girdle and lower limbs. Trunk rotation is necessary for balance, momentum, and symmetry of gait. Many amputees have decreased trunk rotation and arm swing, especially on the prosthetic side, which may be the result of fear of displacing their COM too far forward or backward over the prosthesis. Normal cadence is 90 to 120 steps per minute or 67 to 82 meters per minute (2.5 to 3.0 miles per hour).[91] Arm swing provides balance, momentum, and symmetry of gait, and it is directly influenced by the speed of ambulation.[92] As walking speed accelerates, arm swing increases to permit a more efficient gait. Therefore, amputees who walk at slower speeds will initially have a diminished arm swing. Restoring trunk rotation and arm swing is easily accomplished by using rhythmic initiation or pas-

sively cueing the trunk as the amputee walks. The physical therapist stands behind the amputee with one hand on either shoulder (Figure 21). As the amputee walks, the physical therapist gently rotates the trunk. When the left leg is moved forward, the right shoulder is rotated forward and vice versa. Once amputees feel comfortable with the motion, they can actively incorporate this movement into their gait.

Amputees who will be totally independent ambulators and those who will require an assistive device can derive some benefit from this systematic rehabilitation program. Most patients can progress to the point of ambulating outside of the parallel bars. At that time, the amputee must use an assistive device to practice ambulating. Maintaining pelvic rotation, adequate BOS, equal stance time, and equal stride length all have a direct influence on the energy cost of walking. Trunk rotation will be absent in amputees using a walker as an assistive device. Those ambulating with crutches or a cane should be able to incorporate trunk rotation into their gait.

Variations for Syme and Hip Disarticulation Patients

The duration and degree of prosthetic training is unique to each amputee. Many factors influence training, such as age, general health, motivation, and cause and level of amputation. Patients who have had a Syme ankle disarticulation have a major advantage over transtibial amputees in that the former are able to bear some weight distally. The ability to bear weight distally provides better kinesthetic feedback for placement of the prosthetic foot. Because of this capability and the length of the lever arm, these amputees require minimal prosthetic gait training. Although patients who have had a Syme procedure can progress rapidly with weight shifting

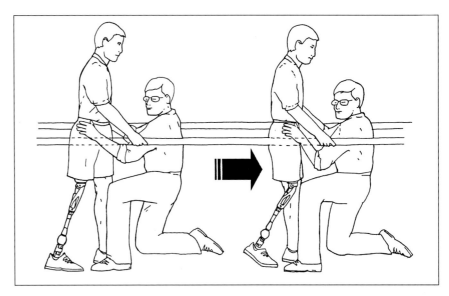

Figure 17 Rhythmic initiation is designed to promote transverse rotation of the pelvis. *(Copyright © Advanced Rehabilitation Therapy, Inc, Miami, FL, 1990. Illustrator Frank Angulo.)*

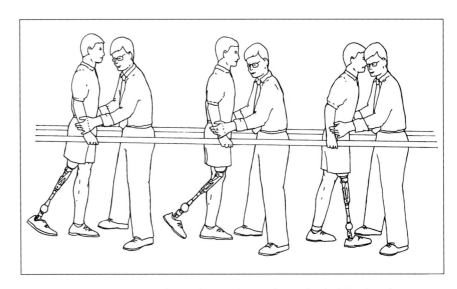

Figure 18 The swing phase of gait. *(Copyright © Advanced Rehabilitation Therapy, Inc, Miami, FL, 1990. Illustrator Frank Angulo.)*

and other gait skills, they may require practice to achieve equal stride length and stance time. Patients who have had a knee disarticulation also have several advantages over transfemoral amputees, such as a longer lever arm, enhanced muscular control, improved kinesthetic feedback, and greater distal end weight bearing. Although these advantages may decrease rehabilitation time, the knee disarticula-

tion amputee must learn the same prosthetic gait skills as a transfemoral amputee. Those who have undergone hip disarticulation and transpelvic amputees also need to master control of a mechanical hip joint as well as the knee joint and foot/ankle assembly. The gait training procedures are essentially the same as for the transfemoral amputee; however, in some patients the mechanical hip joint may

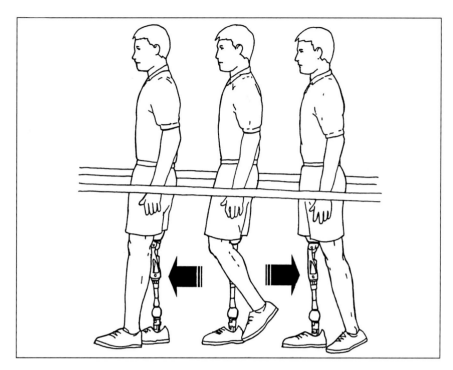

Figure 19 Sound side stepping to promote equal stride length of the sound limb and stance time of the prosthetic limb. *(Copyright © Advanced Rehabilitation Therapy, Inc, Miami, FL, 1990. Illustrator Frank Angulo.)*

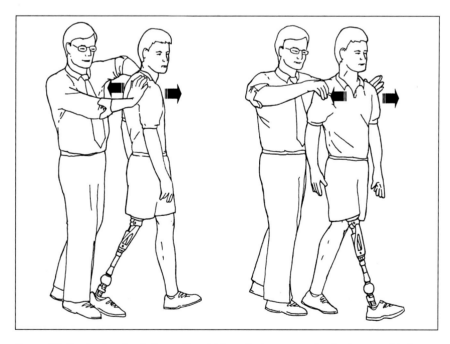

Figure 21 Passive trunk rotation will assist in restoring arm swing for improved balance, symmetry of gait, and momentum. *(Copyright © Advanced Rehabilitation Therapy, Inc, Miami, FL, 1990. Illustrator Frank Angulo.)*

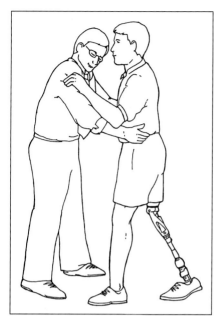

Figure 20 Once correct biomechanics are established within the parallel bars, resistive gait training may be performed in an open area to build confidence and independent gait skills. *(Copyright © Advanced Rehabilitation Therapy, Inc, Miami, FL, 1990. Illustrator Frank Angulo.)*

require a slight vaulting action for the foot to clear the ground.

Advanced Gait Training Activities
Stairs

Ascending and descending stairs is most safely and comfortably performed one step at a time (step-by-step). Using purely mechanical prostheses, only a few exceptional transfemoral amputees can descend stairs step-over-step, or by the "jack-knifing" method. A few very strong lower limb amputees can ascend stairs step-over-step. Most transtibial amputees have the option of either method. Transpelvic amputees or those who have had a hip disarticulation are limited to the step-by-step method.[93] Swing and stance hydraulic knees with yield rate control as well as some microprocessor-controlled knees can be adjusted to lower the amputee from step to step at a controlled rate. However, any step-over-step method requires some practice and confidence to perform safely.

Step-By-Step

This method is essentially the same for amputees at all levels of lower limb amputation. When ascending stairs, the body weight is shifted to the prosthetic limb as the foot of the sound limb is firmly placed on the stair tread. The trunk is slightly flexed over the sound limb as the knee extends, raising the body and the prosthetic limb to the same step. The process is repeated for each step. When descending stairs, the weight is shifted to the sound limb as the prosthetic limb is lowered to the step below by eccentrically flexing the knee of the sound limb. Once the prosthetic limb is securely in place, the body weight is transferred to the prosthetic limb, and the sound limb is lowered to the same step.

One of the primary goals for ascending stairs step-over-step is to increase the speed of ascent, but this comes at the cost of increased effort and decreased safety. A variation on the step-by-step method that counters these objections is to simply skip a stair with the sound limb and raise the body by placing the prosthetic limb on the same step (Figure 22). This technique, however, is usually reserved for the most physically fit amputees.

Transfemoral Amputees Step-Over-Step Stair Activity

Timing and coordination are critical in step-over-step stair climbing. As the transfemoral amputee approaches the stairs, the prosthetic limb is the first to ascend the stairs by rapid acceleration of hip flexion with slight abduction to achieve sufficient knee flexion to clear the step. Some transfemoral amputees will actually hit the approaching step riser with the toe of the prosthetic foot to achieve adequate knee flexion. With the prosthetic foot firmly on the step, usually with the toe against the riser of the next step, the residual limb must exert enough force to fully extend the hip

so that the sound foot may advance to the step above. As the sound side hip extends, the prosthetic side hip must flex at an accelerated speed to achieve sufficient knee flexion to place the prosthetic foot on the next step above.[93]

Descending stairs is achieved by placing only the heel of the prosthetic foot on the stair below, then shifting the body weight over the prosthetic limb, thus passively flexing the knee. The sound limb must quickly reach the step below in time to support the body weight. The process is repeated at a rapid rate until a rhythm is achieved. Most transfemoral amputees who have mastered this skill with mechanical knees descend stairs at an extremely fast pace, much faster than would be considered safe for the average amputee. With mechanical knees, both ascending and descending stairs step-over-step is so difficult and energy-demanding for transfemoral amputees that many who master these skills prefer the step-by-step method. As noted earlier, the use of swing and stance hydraulic knees and the recent availability of microprocessor-controlled knees appear to have made step-over-step mobility easier and less stressful for a broader range of amputees.[93]

Transtibial Amputees Step-Over-Step Stair Activity

When ascending stairs, the transtibial amputee who cannot dorsiflex the foot and ankle assembly must generate a stronger concentric contraction of the knee and hip extensors to successfully transfer body weight over the prosthetic limb. Descending stairs is very similar to normal descent except that only the prosthetic foot heel is placed on the step. This compensates for the lack of dorsiflexion within the foot and ankle assembly.[93]

Crutches

When climbing stairs with crutches, both crutches may be held in the hand opposite the handrail or can be used in the traditional manner.

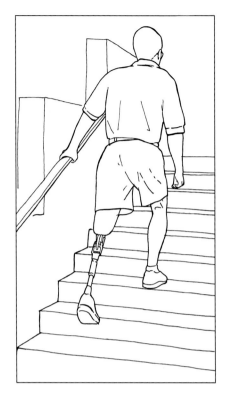

Figure 22 Transfemoral stair ascent by skipping a step for the purpose of increasing speed. (Copyright © Advanced Rehabilitation Therapy, Inc, Miami, FL, 1990. Illustrator Frank Angulo.)

Curbs

The same methods described for ascending and descending stairs are used for curbs. Depending on the level of skill, the amputee can step up or down curbs with either leg.

Uneven Surfaces

Good gait training practice requires that the amputee ambulate over a variety of surfaces such as concrete, grass, gravel, uneven terrain, and variable carpet thicknesses. Initially, the new amputee will have difficulty recognizing the different surfaces secondary to the loss of proprioception. To promote increased visual awareness of these differences, the amputee should spend time practicing on various surfaces. In addition, the amputee must realize that in many circumstances, it is important to observe the terrain ahead to avoid hazards such as slippery surfaces or holes that might cause a fall.[93]

Ramps and Hills

Ascending inclines presents a problem for lower limb amputees because of the lack of dorsiflexion in most prosthetic foot and ankle assemblies. For most lower limb amputees, descending inclines is even more difficult than ascending, primarily because of the lack of plantar flexion in the foot and ankle assembly. Transtibial amputees and amputees with prosthetic knees have the added dilemma of the weight line falling posterior to the knee joint, which results in a flexion moment. Advanced knee units with microprocessor-controlled stance phase automatically compensate by increasing knee stability, so descent is much easier to master. When ascending an incline, the body weight should be slightly more forward than normal to obtain maximum dorsiflexion with articulating foot and ankle assemblies or to keep the knee in extension. Depending on the grade of the incline, pelvic rotation with additional acceleration may be required to achieve maximum knee flexion during swing. Descending an incline usually occurs at a more rapid pace than normal because of the lack of plantar flexion, resulting in decreased stance time on the prosthetic limb. Amputees with prosthetic knees must exert a greater than normal force on the posterior wall of the socket to maintain knee extension unless they have a knee with a microprocessor-controlled stance phase, which automatically increases knee stiffness, reducing the effort to control the knee; however, pelvic control is still required. Most lower limb amputees find it easier to ascend and descend inclines with short, but equal, strides. This method is often preferred because it simulates a more normal appearance as opposed to a sidestepping or zigzag method.[93]

When ascending and descending hills, the amputee will find sidestepping to be the most efficient means. The sound limb should lead, providing the power to lift the body to the next level, while the prosthetic limb remains slightly posterior to act as a firm base by keeping the weight line anterior to the knee. During descent of a hill, the prosthetic limb leads but remains slightly posterior to the sound limb. The prosthetic knee remains in extension, again acting as a form of support so that the sound limb may lower the body. For transpelvic amputees or patients who have had a hip disarticulation, sidestepping is the most common alternative regardless of the grade of the incline. Ultimately, the most accepted method for use over a variety of inclines and conditions such as wet surfaces and ice, regardless of amputation level, is the use of another person's shoulder. For example, while descending an incline, the amputee will walk one step behind an assistant with a hand on the assistant's shoulder. As the two walk down the incline, the speed of decent is controllable, giving the amputee more confidence.[93]

Sidestepping

Sidestepping, or walking sideways, can be introduced to the amputee at various times throughout the rehabilitation program. The patient can begin with simple shifting of weight in the parallel bars. With practice, more complex activities can be performed such as unassisted sidestepping around tables or completing a small obstacle course that requires many small turns. During early rehabilitation, sidestepping provides the amputee with a functional exercise for strengthening the hip abductors; later in the rehabilitation process, it provides an opportunity to progress to multidirectional movements.[93]

Walking Backward

Walking backward is not difficult for transtibial amputees but poses a problem for those with a prosthetic knee because there is no means of actively flexing the prosthetic knee for adequate ground clearance. In addition, the posterior forces tend to cause the weight line to fall posterior to the knee, causing a flexion moment with possible buckling of the knee. The most comfortable method of backward walking for transfemoral amputees is to vault upward (plantar flex) on the sound foot to obtain sufficient height for the prosthetic limb to clear the ground as it moves posteriorly. In this maneuver, the prosthetic foot is placed well behind the sound limb with most of the body weight being borne on the prosthetic toe, which keeps the weight line anterior to the knee. The sound limb is then moved back, usually at a slightly greater speed for a somewhat shorter distance. The trunk is also maintained in some flexion to maintain the weight forward on the prosthetic toe. With a little practice, most amputees become quite proficient in walking backward.

Multidirectional Turns

Changing direction during walking or maneuvering within confined areas often increases an amputee's difficulty in controlling the prosthesis. Situations such as crowded restaurants, elevators, or simply turning around are often overcome by "hip hiking" the prosthesis and pivoting around the sound limb. This method is effective but hardly the most aesthetic means of changing direction. When turning to the sound side, two key factors for a smooth transition include maintaining pelvic rotation in the transverse plane and performing the turn in two steps. The prosthetic limb is crossed 45° over the sound limb, the sound limb is rotated 180°, and the turn is completed by stepping in the desired direction with the prosthetic limb, leading with the pelvis to ensure adequate knee flexion[93] (Figure 23).

Turning to the prosthetic side is performed in almost the same way except that slightly more body weight is maintained on the prosthetic toe to keep the weight line anterior to the knee, thus preventing knee flexion. The sound limb is crossed 45° over the prosthetic limb, automatically throwing the weight line forward. The prosthetic limb is rotated as close to

180° as possible without losing balance (135° is usually comfortable), and the turn is completed by stepping in the desired direction with the sound limb (Figure 24). If necessary, remind the transfemoral amputee to maintain knee extension by applying a force with the residual limb against the posterior wall of the socket.

One exercise that will reinforce turning skills is follow the leader, in which the amputee follows the physical therapist in making a series of turns in all directions with varying speed and degrees of difficulty.

The level of skill in turning varies among amputees. All functional ambulators should be taught to turn in both directions regardless of the prosthetic side. Lower limb amputees with poor balance, however, may be limited to unidirectional turns, requiring a series of small steps to complete the turn.

Tandem Walking

Walking with a normal BOS is of prime importance; however, tandem walking can assist with balance and coordination, as well as improve awareness of the prosthesis. After placing a 2- to 4-in wide strip of tape on the floor, the amputee is asked to walk in three ways. The amputee first walks with one foot to either side of the line, then along the line, heel to toe, with one foot in front of the other. Finally, the amputee walks with one foot crossing over in front of the other so that neither foot touches the line, with the left foot always on the right side and vice versa.[93]

Braiding

Braiding (cariocas or grapevine step) may be taught either in the parallel bars or in an open area, depending on the amputee's ability (Figure 25). Simple braiding consists of crossing one leg in front of the other. As the amputee's skill improves, the leg can alternate, first in front of and then behind the other leg. As ability improves, the speed of movement should increase. With improved speed, the arms will be required to as-

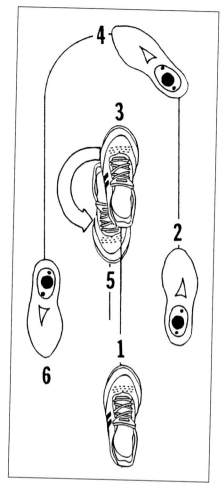

Figure 23 To turn to the sound side, the amputee completes the following sequence. **1** to **3**, Maintain normal gait biomechanics. **4**, Move the prosthetic limb over the sound limb 45°. **5**, Rotate the sound limb 180°. **6**, Complete the turn by stepping in the desired direction. *(Copyright © Advanced Rehabilitation Therapy, Inc, Miami, FL, 1990. Illustrator Frank Angulo.)*

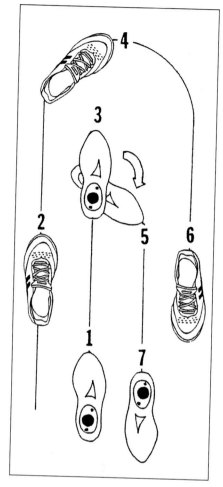

Figure 24 To turn to the prosthetic side, the amputee completes the following sequence. **1** to **3**, Maintain normal gait biomechanics. **4**, Move the sound limb over the prosthetic limb 45°. **5**, Rotate the prosthetic limb approximately 135°. **6** and **7**, Complete the turn by stepping in the desired direction. *(Copyright © Advanced Rehabilitation Therapy, Inc, Miami, FL, 1990. Illustrator Frank Angulo.)*

sist with balance and likewise, trunk rotation will increase, further emphasizing the need for independent movement between the trunk and pelvis.[93]

Single-Limb Squatting

Single-limb balance is taught during the early stages of rehabilitation for crutch walking, hopping, and other skills. Single-limb squatting is considerably more difficult but can help improve balance and strength. When first attempting this skill, half squats with a chair underneath the patient

are recommended in the event that balance is lost.[93]

Falling

Controlled falling and lowering to the floor are important skills not only for safety but also as a means to perform activities on the floor. During falling, amputees must first discard any assistive device to avoid injury and ensure they land on their hands with the elbows slightly flexed to reduce the force and decrease the possibility of injury. As the elbows flex, the amputee should roll to one side to further

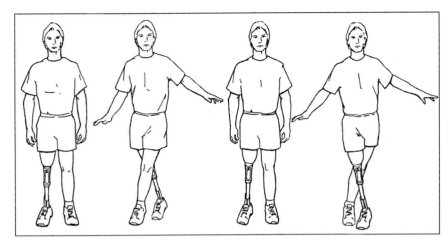

Figure 25 Braiding is an exercise designed to improve prosthetic control, balance, and coordination by crossing one leg in front of or behind the other leg in a continuous manner. (Copyright © Advanced Rehabilitation Therapy, Inc, Miami, FL, 1990. Illustrator Frank Angulo.)

decrease the impact of the fall. Lowering the body to the floor in a controlled manner is initiated by squatting with the sound limb followed by gently leaning forward onto the slightly flexed upper limbs. From this position, the amputee can remain quadruped or assume a seated position.[93]

Floor to Standing

Many techniques teach an amputee how to rise from the floor to a standing position and vary with the type of amputation and the skill level of the amputee. The amputee and physical therapist must work closely together to identify the most efficient and safe manner to successfully master this task. The fundamental principle, however, is to ensure that the amputee uses an assistive device for balance and the sound limb for power as the body begins to rise.

Conclusion

The physical therapist must work closely with the rehabilitation team to provide comprehensive care for the amputee. An individualized program must be constructed according to the abilities of each patient. The primary skills of preprosthetic training help build the foundation necessary for successful prosthetic ambulation. The degree of success with ambulation may directly influence how much amputees will use their prostheses and may be predictive of their overall level of activity. The primary goal of the rehabilitation team, therefore, should be to make this transitional period as smooth and successful as possible.

References

1. American College of Sports Medicine: *Guidelines for Exercise Testing and Prescription*, ed 4. Philadelphia, PA, Lea & Febiger, 1991, p 73.

2. Borg GV: Psychophysical basis of perceived exertion. *Med Sci Sports Exerc* 1982;14:377-387.

3. Brodzka WK, Thornhill HL, Zarapkar SE, Mallory JA, Weiss L: Long-term function of persons with atherosclerotic bilateral below-knee amputation living in the inner city. *Arch Phys Med Rehabil* 1990;71:895-900.

4. Medhat A, Huber PM, Medhat MA: Factors that influence the level of activities in persons with lower extremity amputation. *Rehab Nurs* 1990;13:13-18.

5. Pinzur MS, Gottschalk F, Smith D, et al: Functional outcome of below-knee amputation in peripheral vascular insufficiency: A multi-center review. *Clin Orthop* 1993;286:247-249.

6. Dorevitch M, Cossar R, Bailey F, et al: The accuracy of self and informant rating of physical functional capacity in the elderly. *J Clin Epidemiol* 1992;43:791-798.

7. Deathe B, Miller WC, Speechley M: The status of outcome measurement in amputee rehabilitation in Canada. *Arch Phys Med Rehabil* 2002;83:912-918.

8. Day HJB: The assessment and description of amputee activity. *Prosthet Orthot Int* 1981;5:23-28.

9. Hubbard W, McElroy G: Benchmark data for elderly, vascular trans-tibial amputees after rehabilitation. *Prosthet Orthot Int* 1994;18:142-149.

10. Wood-Dauphinee S, Opzoomer A, Williams J, Marchand B, Spitzer W: Assessment of global function: The reintegration to normal living index. *Arch Phys Med Rehabil* 1988;69:583-590.

11. Gauthier-Gagnon C, Grisé M: *Prosthetic Profile of the Amputee: Handbook of Documents Developed Within the Framework of a Prosthetic Follow-up Study.* Montreal, Quebec, Canada, École de Réadatation, Faculte de Médecine, Université de Montréal, 1992.

12. Gauthier-Gagnon C, Grisé M: Prosthetic profile of the amputee questionnaire: Validity and reliability. *Arch Phys Med Rehabil* 1994;75:1309-1314.

13. Grisé M, Gauthier-Gagnon C, Martineau G: Prosthetic profile of people with lower extremity amputation: Conception and design of a follow-up questionnaire. *Arch Phys Med Rehabil* 1993;74:862-870.

14. Houghton A, Allen A, Luff R, McColl I: Rehabilitation after lower limb amputation: A comparative of above-knee, through-knee, and Gritti-Stokes amputation. *Br J Surg* 1989;76:622-624.

15. Houghton A, Taylor P, Thurlow S, Rootes E, McColl I: Success rates for rehabilitation of vascular amputees: Implications for preoperative assessment and amputation level. *Br J Surg* 1992;79:753-755.

16. Leung EC, Rush PJ, Devlin M: Predicting prosthetic rehabilitation outcome in lower limb amputee patients with the functional independence measure. *Arch Phys Med Rehabil* 1996;77:605-608.

17. Miller WC, Deathe AB, Speechley M, Koval J: The influence of falling, fear of falling, and balance confidence on prosthetic mobility and social activity

among individuals with lower extremity amputation. *Arch Phys Med Rehabil* 2001;82:1238-1244.

18. Smith D, Horn P, Malchow D, Boone D, Reiber G, Hansen S: Prosthetic history, prosthetic charges, and functional outcome of the isolated, traumatic below-knee amputee. *J Trauma* 1995;38:44-47.

19. McHorney C, Ware J, Raczek A: The MOS 36-item short-form health survey (SF-36): II. Psychometric and clinical tests of validity in measuring physical and mental health constructs. *Med Care* 1993;31:247-263.

20. Stewart A, Hays R, Ware J: The MOS short-form general health survey. *Med Care* 1988;26:724-735.

21. Hart D: Orthotic and prosthetics national office outcomes tool (OPOT): Initial reliability and validity assessment for lower extremity prosthetics. *J Prosthet Orthot* 1999;11:101-111.

22. Schoppen T, Boonstra A, Groothoff JW, et al: Job satisfaction and health experience of people with a lower-limb amputation in comparison with health colleagues. *Arch Phys Med Rehabil* 2002;83:628-634.

23. Pezzin LE, Dillingham TR, MacKenzie EJ: Rehabilitation and the long-term outcomes of persons with trauma-related amputations. *Arch Phys Med Rehabil* 2000;81:292-300.

24. Harness N, Pinzur MS: Health related quality of life in patients with dysvascular transtibial amputations. *Clin Orthop* 2001;383:204-207.

25. Legro M, Reiber G, Smith D, del Angulia M, Larsen J, Boone D: Prosthetic evaluation questionnaire for persons with lower limb amputations: Assessing prosthesis-related quality of life. *Arch Phys Med Rehabil* 1998;79:931-938.

26. Granger C, Cotter A, Hamilton B, Fielder RC: Functional assessment scales: A study of persons after stroke. *Arch Phys Med Rehabil* 1993;74:133-138.

27. Bergner M, Bobbitt R, Carter W, Gilson B: The sickness impact profile: Development and final revision of a health status measure. *Med Care* 1981;19:787-805.

28. de Bruin AF, de Witte LP, Stevens F, Diederiks JP: Sickness impact profile: The state of the art of generic functional status measure. *Soc Sci Med* 1992;35:1003-1014.

29. Jurkovich G, Mock M, Mackenzie E, et al: The sickness impact profile as a tool to evaluate functional outcome in trauma patients. *J Trauma* 1995;39:625-631.

30. Patrick D, Deyo R: Generic and disease-specific measures in assessing health status and quality of life. *Med Care* 1989;27:s217-s232.

31. Greive A, Lankhorst G: Functional outcome of lower-limb amputees: A prospective descriptive study in a general hospital. *Prosthet Orthot Int* 1996;20:79-87.

32. Mahoney F, Barthel D: Functional evaluation: The Barthel index. *Md State Med J* 1965;14:61-65.

33. Collins C, Wade D, Davies S, Horne V: The Barthel ADL index: A reliability study. *Int Disabil Stud* 1988;10:61-63.

34. Wade D, Collins C: The Barthel ADL Index: A standard measure of physical disability? *Int Disabil Stud* 1988;10:64-67.

35. Goldberg R: New trends in the rehabilitation of lower extremity amputees. *Rehabil Lit* 1984;45:2-11.

36. Kullman L: Evaluation of disability and of results of rehabilitation with the use of the Barthel index and Russek's classification. *Int Disabil Stud* 1987;9:68-71.

37. O'Toole D, Goldberg R, Ryan B: Functional changes in vascular amputee patients: Evaluation by Barthel index, PULSES profile, and ESCROW scale. *Arch Phys Med Rehabil* 1985;66:508-511.

38. Stewart C: A prediction score for geriatric rehabilitation projects. *Rheumatol Rehabil* 1980;19:239-245.

39. Simpson M, Forster A: Assessing elderly people: Should we all be using the same scales? *Physiotherapy* 1993;79:836-841.

40. Holden J, Fernie G, Soto M: An assessment of a system to monitor the activity of patients in a rehabilitation programme. *Prosthet Orthot Int* 1979;3:99-102.

41. Coleman KL, Smith DG, Boone DA, Joseph AW, del Aguila MA: Step activity monitor: Long-term, continuous recording of ambulatory function. *J Rehabil Res Dev* 1999;36:8-18.

42. Davidoff G, Roth E, Haughton J, Ardner M: Cognitive dysfunction in spinal cord injury patients: Sensitivity of functional independence measure subscales vs. neuropsychologic assessment. *Arch Phys Med Rehabil* 1990;71:326-329.

43. Heinemann A, Linacre J, Wright B, Hamilton B, Granger C: Relationships between impairment and physical disability as measured by the functional independence measure. *Arch Phys Med Rehabil* 1993;74:566-573.

44. Heinemann A, Linacre J, Wright B, Hamilton B, Granger C: Prediction of rehabilitation outcomes with disability measures. *Arch Phys Med Rehabil* 1994;75:133-143.

45. Muecke L, Shekar S, Dwyer D, Israel E, Flynn J: Functional screening of lower-limb amputees: A role in predicting rehabilitation outcome? *Arch Phys Med Rehabil* 1992;73:851-858.

46. Nelson A: Functional ambulation profile. *Phys Ther* 1974;54:1059-1065.

47. Olney S, Elkin N, Lowe P, Symington DC: An ambulation profile for clinical gait evaluation. *Physiother Can* 1979;31:85-90.

48. Duncan P, Weiner D, Chandler J, Studenski S: Functional reach: A new clinical measure of balance. *J Gerontol* 1990;45:M192-M197.

49. Duncan P, Studenski S, Chandler J, Prescott B: Functional reach: Predictive validity in a sample of elderly male veterans. *J Gerontol* 1992;47:M93-M98.

50. Weiner D, Bongiorni D, Studenski S, Duncan P, Kochersberger G: Does functional reach improve with rehabilitation? *Arch Phys Med Rehabil* 1993;74:796-800.

51. Kirby R, Chari V: Prostheses and the forward reach of sitting lower-limb amputees. *Arch Phys Med Rehabil* 1990;71:125-127.

52. Gailey RS, Roach KE, Applegate EB, et al: The amputee mobility predictor: An instrument to assess determinants of the lower-limb amputee's ability to ambulate. *Arch Phys Med Rehabil* 2002;83:613-627.

53. Bassey EJ, Fentem PH, MacDonald IC, Scriven PM: Self-paced walking as a method for exercise testing in elderly and young men. *Clin Sci Mol Med Suppl* 1976;51:609-612.

54. Friedman P, Richmond D, Baskett J: A prospective trial of serial gait speed as a measure of rehabilitation in the elderly. *Age Ageing* 1988;17:227-235.

55. Wolfson L, Whipple R, Amerman P, Tobin J: Gait assessment in the elderly: A gait abnormality rating scale and its relation to falls. *J Gerontol* 1990;45: M12-M19.

56. Cooper K: A means of assessing maximal oxygen uptake. *JAMA* 1968;203: 201-204.

57. Dekhuyzen P, Kaptein A, Dekker F, Wagenaar J, Janssen P: Twelve-minute walking test in a group of Dutch patients with chronic obstructive pulmonary disease: Relationship with functional capacity. *J Respir Dis* 1986;69: 259-264.

58. McGavin C, Gupta S, McHardy G: Twelve-minute walking test for assessing disability in chronic bronchitis. *BMJ* 1976;1:822-823.

59. Mungall I, Hainsworth R: Assessment of respiratory function in patients with chronic airway disease. *Thorax* 1979;34:254-258.

60. Butland RJ, Pang J, Gross ER, Woodcock AA, Geddes DM: Two-, six-, 12-minute walking tests in respiratory disease. *BMJ* 1982;284:1607-1608.

61. Potter JM, Evans AL, Duncan G: Gait speed and activities of daily living function in geriatric patients. *Arch Phys Med Rehabil* 1995;76:997-999.

62. Schoppen T, Boonstra A, Groothoff JW, et al: The timed "up and go" test: Reliability and validity in persons with unilateral lower limb amputation. *Arch Phys Med Rehabil* 1999;80: 825-828.

63. Burgess EM: Immediate postsurgical prosthetic fitting: A system of amputee management. *Phys Ther* 1971;51: 139-143.

64. Schon LC, Short KW, Soupiou O, Noll K, Rheinstein J: Benefits of early prosthetic management of transtibial amputees. *Foot Ankle Int* 2002;23:509-514.

65. Wu Y, Keagy RD, Krick HG, Stratigos JS, Betts HB: An innovative removable rigid dressing technique for below-the-knee amputation. *J Bone Joint Surg* 1979;61:724-729.

66. DuBow LL, Witt PL, Kadaba MP, Reyes R, Cochran V: Oxygen consumption of elderly persons with bilateral transtibial amputations: Ambulation vs. wheelchair propulsion. *Arch Phys Med Rehabil* 1983;64:255-259.

67. Malone JM, Snyder M, Anderson G, Bernhard VM, Holloway GA, Bunt TJ: Prevention of amputation by diabetic education. *Am J Surg* 1989;158: 520-523.

68. Lake C, Supan TJ: The incidence of dermatological problems in the silicone suspension sleeve user. *J Prosthet Orthot* 1997;9:97-104.

69. May BJ: Stump bandaging of the lower limb amputee. *J Appl Toxicol* 1964;44: 808-814.

70. Condie E, Jones D, Treweek S, Scott H: A one-year national survey of patients having a lower limb amputation. *Physiotherapy* 1996;82:14-20.

71. Hongshen Z, Wertsch JJ, Harris GF, Loftsgaarden JD, Price MB: Foot pressure distribution during walking and shuffling. *Arch Phys Med Rehabil* 1991; 72:390-397.

72. Katoulis EC, Ebdon-Parry H, Vileikyte L, Kulkarni J, Boulton AJM: Gait abnormalities in diabetic neuropathy. *Diabetes Care* 1997;20:1904-1907.

73. Mueller MJ, Sinacore DR, Hoogstrate S, Daly L: Hip and ankle walking strategies: Effect on peak plantar pressures and implications for neuropathic ulceration. *Arch Phys Med Rehabil* 1994; 75:1196-1200.

74. American Diabetes Association: *Fact Sheet on Diabetes.* Alexandria, VA, 1991.

75. Ecker ML, Jacobs BS: Lower limb amputations in diabetic patients. *Diabetes* 1970;19:189-195.

76. Kucan JO, Robson MC: Diabetic foot infections: Fate of the contralateral foot. *Plast Reconstr Surg* 1986;77: 439-441.

77. McCollough NC, Jennings JJ, Sarmiento A: Bilateral below-the-knee amputation in patients over fifty years of age. *J Bone Joint Surg Am* 1972;54: 1217-1223.

78. Whitehouse FW, Jurgensen C, Block MA: The later life of the diabetic amputee: Another look at fate of the second leg. *Diabetes* 1968;17:520-521.

79. Isakov E, Burdoragin N, Shenhav S, Mendelevich I, Korzets A, Susak Z: Anatomic sites of foot lesions resulting in amputation among diabetics and non-diabetics. *Am J Phys Med Rehabil* 1995;74:130-133.

80. Cruts H, De Vries J, Zilvold G, Huisman K: Van Alste' J, Boom H: Lower extremity amputees with peripheral vascular disease: Graded exercise testing and results of prosthetic training. *Arch Phys Med Rehabil* 1987;68: 469-473.

81. Perry J, Shanfield S: Efficiency of dynamic elastic response prosthetic feet. *J Rehabil Res Dev* 1993;30:137-143.

82. Ward K, Meyers M: Exercise performance of lower-extremity amputees. *Sports Med* 1995;20:207-214.

83. Pitetti K, Snell P, Stray-Gundersen J, Gottschalk FA: Aerobic training exercise for individuals who had amputation of the lower limb. *J Bone Joint Surg Am* 1987;69:914-921.

84. Currie D, Gilbert D, Dierschke B: Aerobic capacity with two leg work versus one leg plus both arms work in men with peripheral vascular disease. *Arch Phys Med Rehabil* 1992;73:1081-1084.

85. Davidoff GN, Lampman RM, Westbury L, Deron J: Exercise testing and training of persons with dysvascular amputation: Safety and efficacy of arm ergometry. *Arch Phys Med Rehabil* 1992;73:334-338.

86. Finestone HM, Lampman RM, Davidoff GN, Westbury L: Arm ergometry exercise testing in patients with dysvascular amputations. *Arch Phys Med Rehabil* 1991;72:15-19.

87. Gailey RS: Recreational pursuits of elders with amputation. *Topics Geriatric Rehab* 1992;8:39-58.

88. Eisert O, Tester OW: Dynamic stump for lower limb amputees. *Arch Phys Med Rehabil* 1954;33:695-704.

89. Davies GJ: *A Compendium of Isokinetics in Clinical Usages and Rehabilitation Techniques*, ed 2. La Crosse, WI, S & S Publishing, 1985.

90. Gailey RS, Gailey AM: *Strengthening and Stretching for Lower Extremity Amputees.* Miami, FL, Advanced Rehabilitation Therapy Inc, 1994.

91. Murray MP: Gait as a total pattern of movement. *Am J Phys Med Rehabil* 1967;16:390-393.

92. Murray MP, Drought AB, Kory RC: Walking patterns of normal men. *J Bone Joint Surg Am* 1964;46:335-360.

93. Gailey RS, Gailey AM: *Prosthetic Gait Training for Lower Limb Amputees.* Miami, FL, Advanced Rehabilitation Therapy Inc, 1989.

94. Jones ME, Bashford GM, Biokas VV: Weight-bearing pain and walking velocity during primary transtibial amputee rehabilitation. *Clin Rehab* 2001; 15:172-176.

95. Jones ME, Bashford GM, Mann JM: Weight-bearing and velocity in transtibial and trans-femoral amputees. *Prosthet Orthot Int* 1997;21:183-186.

96. Inman VT, Ralston RJ, Todd F: *Human Walking*. Baltimore, MD, Williams & Wilkins, 1981.

97. Saunders JB, Inman VT, Eberhart HD: The major determinants in normal and pathological gait. *J Bone Joint Surg Am* 1953;35:543-558.

98. Gard SA, Childress DS: The effect of pelvic list on the vertical displacement of the trunk during walking. *Gait Posture* 1997;5:233-238.

99. Gard SA, Childress DS: The influence of stance phase knee flexion on the vertical displacement of the trunk during normal walking. *Arch Phys Med Rehabil* 1999;80:26-32.

Chapter 49

Bilateral Lower Limb Prostheses

Jack E. Uellendahl, CPO

Introduction

As medical care and rehabilitation techniques continue to improve, people are living longer, resulting in an increase in the number of patients with conditions that require bilateral amputations. The bilateral lower limb amputee presents unique challenges to the rehabilitation team. Most bilateral amputations are performed because of vascular disease with or without diabetes. The Centers for Disease Control and Prevention reports that between 1980 and 1996, the number of patients discharged from hospitals who had undergone diabetes-related lower limb amputations increased from 36,000 to 86,000 per year. In addition, peripheral vascular disease accounts for more than 30,000 lower limb amputations each year.[1]

In a review of 489 patients with end-stage peripheral vascular disease who required major amputation of a lower limb, Evans and associates[1] reported that 24% required amputation of the contralateral limb and that in 56% of the patients the second amputation was performed less than 1 year after the first. Esquenazi[2] reports that 50% of patients who undergo a lower limb amputation because of disease are at risk for amputation of the contralateral limb within 3 years. In light of these statistics, it is clear that health care professionals serving the needs of amputees should be well versed in the special needs of the bilateral amputee.

Patient Evaluation
Prior Experience Using a Prosthesis

Many dysvascular amputees will have had experience as a unilateral amputee before the second amputation. Prior experience using a unilateral prosthesis is a good indicator of future success with bilateral prostheses. In the absence of other concurrent disabilities, the patient with a second transtibial amputation could achieve a level of independence similar to that attained following the first amputation.[2] Evans and associates[1] report that in their series of bilateral transtibial amputees, where no selection criteria was used, 23 of 46 patients (50%) who were ambulators before contralateral amputation became bilateral prosthesis users. This is in contrast to only 4 of 59 patients (6.8%) who were not ambulators before contralateral amputation. The authors conclude that "successful prosthetic rehabilitation in the bilateral amputee appears primarily dependent on the use of a prosthesis before contralateral amputation and/or the preservation of at least one knee joint."

Atherosclerosis

In a retrospective assessment of 80 bilateral transtibial amputees, Thornhill and associates[3] found that 71% of the atherosclerotic patients achieved some function with bilateral prostheses. The authors conclude that most atherosclerotic bilateral transtibial amputees can use prostheses and that the high survival rate and low rate of residual limb revisions justify restorative efforts. Evans and associates[1] concluded that a high survival rate (60% at 2 years and 40% at 5 years) as well as the fact that a significant number of patients become independent and ambulatory justify an aggressive approach to the rehabilitation of the bilateral amputee. The demonstrated period of survival offers ample opportunity for rehabilitation professionals to improve the quality of these patients' remaining years. The life expectancy of these patients is limited, however, so rehabilitation that aims to reintegrate these patients into their places in society and to avoid unnecessarily lengthy periods away from their homes should be expedited.[3]

Traumatic Injury

Bilateral lower limb amputations resulting from traumatic injury are rare. Often the individuals who sustain traumatic injury resulting in bilateral loss are young and in otherwise good health, so the rehabilitation potential is excellent.

Knee Salvage

The importance of saving the knee whenever possible cannot be overemphasized. When a unilateral lower limb amputee loses the second limb, the chance of the patient achieving functional use of the prostheses is measurably higher if one or preferably both knee joints have been preserved. Most unilateral transtibial amputees who ambulated successfully with a prosthesis can also master bilateral amputee gait if the amputation performed on the contralateral limb is transtibial or more distal.[4] The success of rehabilitation decreases dramatically with transfemoral or higher level amputations.

General Health

Ambulation should be attempted only if the patient demonstrates adequate cardiac function, strength, balance, and endurance.[2] Coronary artery disease in an elderly, dysvascular transfemoral or bilateral amputee indicates a poor prognosis for ambulation with prostheses.[5]

Flexion Contractures

Flexion contractures at the hip and/or knee can seriously limit the patient's ability to ambulate with prostheses. Early attention to the prevention of such contractures is critical to the successful use of prostheses by the bilateral amputee.

Normal Human Locomotion and the Determinants of Gait

The more joints and muscles that are lost to amputation, the greater the loss of the normal locomotor mechanisms and therefore the greater the energy cost of ambulation and the degree of disability.[2] Loss of normal physiologic function at the various amputation levels leads to increased energy consumption, loss of shock absorption, and abnormal gait patterns. With higher amputation levels, the effects of these losses become more pronounced. To evaluate these functional deficits, it is useful to study the elements of normal human walking. The elements of walking, or determinants of gait, as described by Inman and associates[6] and Saunders

and associates[7] are (1) pelvic rotation, (2) pelvic list (dip), (3) knee flexion in stance phase, (4) plantar flexion/knee flexion (early stance), (5) foot/knee interaction (late stance), and (6) lateral displacement of the pelvis.

Acting in concert with these six determinants of gait is synchronous transverse rotation of the segments of the lower limb.[6] Through these six motion patterns, vertical and horizontal displacements of the center of mass are believed to be minimized, thereby reducing the muscular effort of walking and consequently saving energy. In addition, abrupt changes in direction of the center of mass are avoided, which also saves energy.[8]

During the initial contact and loading response phases of gait, shock absorption is a primary function of normal walking.[8] Controlled movements of the knee, ankle, and subtalar joints along with pelvic list dampen these forces.[6,8-11] The amputee's comfort will be enhanced to the degree this shock absorption is successfully replaced by the prosthetic components. This is especially true for the bilateral amputee, in whom the loss of physiologic shock absorption cannot be compensated for by the contralateral limb.

Energy Consumption

Energy consumption studies in bilateral amputees are limited. The available data suggest that walking with two prostheses of a particular level requires more energy than does walking with one prosthesis of that same level and that energy consumption increases as the amputation level becomes more proximal.[12] DuBow and associates[13] studied six bilateral dysvascular transtibial amputees walking at a natural pace and found that they required 123% more Vo_2 (mL/kg/m) and had a 26% higher heart rate and 36% slower velocity than a normal group during ambulation. Gonzalez and associates[14] found the energy expenditure of walking in bilateral transtibial amputees and unilateral transfemoral amputees was, respectively, 41% and 65% higher than nor-

mal. The authors concluded that the knee joint is a major determinant of the energy cost of ambulation and of successful rehabilitation of the older amputee.

Huang and associates[15] reported on four bilateral transfemoral amputees (mean age, 34 years) and found they expended 300% more energy per unit distance than did the able-bodied subjects. In a study of five otherwise healthy bilateral transfemoral amputees (mean age, 22 years), Hoffman and associates[16] found that the metabolic cost at the chosen walking speed for the amputees was 0.32 mL/kg/m. This was 88% higher than the value of 0.17 mL/kg/m for the able-bodied subjects. In light of the tremendous energy expenditures necessary to walk using bilateral transfemoral prostheses, Esquenazi[2] states that "Most transfemoral bilateral amputees over 50 years of age will find the wheelchair an easier and more practical means of locomotion." Certainly if the bilateral transfemoral amputee is to ambulate successfully, all possible means available should be used to reduce the energy expenditure.

To improve the chances for functional ambulation, it is of paramount importance that the knee joints be preserved. Retention of maximum limb length by amputation at the most distal level suitable is particularly important for the bilateral amputee, to provide maximum bony leverage to control the prosthesis.[4]

Lowering the Center of Gravity
Transtibial Amputees

For the bilateral amputee, lowering the center of gravity is believed to provide better balance and control of the prostheses. The optimal shin length for most bilateral transtibial prostheses is that which allows easy standing from a chair of typical height. In most cases, the prosthetic feet should be in full contact with the floor while the amputee is seated

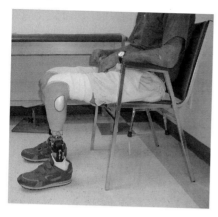

Figure 1 Prostheses with a medial tibial plateau height of approximately 18 inches facilitate getting out of a chair and allow the feet to rest on the floor when the amputee is seated.

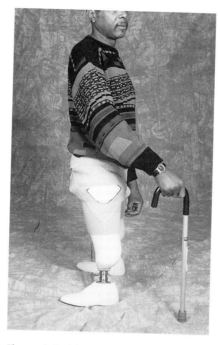

Figure 2 Stubbies with rearward-facing SACH feet are used during initial gait training.

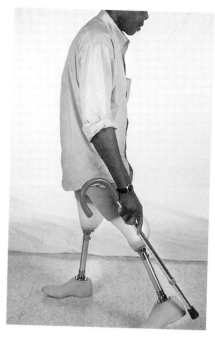

Figure 3 Length can be added to the endoskeletal stubby prostheses as the amputee gains confidence, strength, and balance.

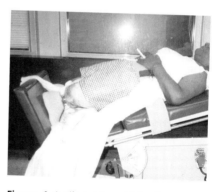

Figure 4 A tilt table, which allows controlled and graded weight bearing, is helpful when treating more debilitated amputees.

(Figure 1). A shin length that provides a medial tibial plateau height of 18 inches with the shoe on is therefore a good starting length for the shin. For individuals of short stature, these values do not apply, and it is usually preferable to match the patient's preoperative shin length.

Transfemoral Amputees and "Stubbies"

For the bilateral transfemoral amputee, the benefits of a lower center of gravity can be achieved through the use of "stubbies" (Figure 2), which offer potential advantages over conventional prosthetic devices in terms of safety, stability, and energy efficiency.[17] Stubbies are short prostheses that use rocker-bottom platforms attached directly to the end of the socket or close to it. The arc of the rocker is determined by using the hip as the center point. The rocker extends posteriorly to prevent the amputee from falling backward. This allows the user to sit back in the prostheses with the hips flexed, thereby maintaining a normal amount of lumbar lordosis. In discussing the use of stubbies for the infant or child with bilateral lower limb deficiencies, Kruger[18] states that the lower center of gravity provides a greater sense of stability, making it much easier for the child who is beginning to "cruise" to begin to walk in

the erect position without fear of falling. This feeling of security is even more important for adult amputees as they learn to balance on prostheses (Figure 3) because adults are more likely to be injured when they fall and therefore their fear of falling is greater.

For most bilateral transfemoral amputees, stubbies are recommended as a transitional phase of rehabilitation, in which case conventional prosthetic feet turned rearward can be used in place of custom-made rockers. Stubbies provide amputees with a means to become upright and to become confident in their ability to ambulate in a relatively safe and stable manner.

Training in the use of stubbies should begin on a tilt table. Initially, the amputee may be brought to an upright weight-bearing position on the tilt table (Figure 4). In this way, socket fit and comfort can be assessed, and graded weight bearing can be controlled. Once the amputee is comfortable in a fully upright position on the tilt table, training can proceed using parallel bars and then a walker or canes (Figure 5). Again, the minimum height should take into

consideration the height of a standard chair. The ischial height should be no less than 18 inches with shoes on; this minimizes the amount of lifting the amputee must accomplish to position the body in a chair. Obviously, upper limb conditioning is an important consideration for the bilateral lower limb amputee, especially when the amputations are at the transfemoral level.

As the amputee gains confidence in using stubbies, length can be added progressively to the endoskeletal prostheses. The rate of progression to full-

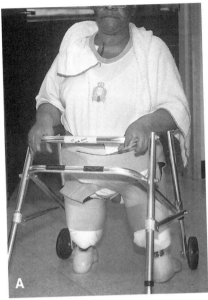
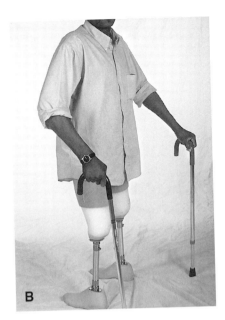

Figure 5 A, Initial gait training can be performed using a short walker for stability. **B,** The amputee can progress to the use of two canes as confidence is gained.

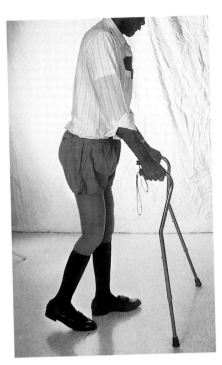

Figure 6 After the amputee is successful with stubbies, full-length prostheses can be provided. In this patient, one locked knee and one four-bar knee are used for stability.

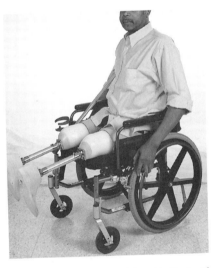

Figure 7 The functional length limit of stubbies is reached when negotiating tight spaces in the wheelchair becomes impossible.

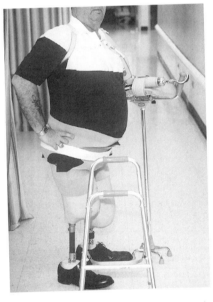

Figure 8 Definitive use of stubbies is sometimes desirable. This trilateral amputee enjoyed the security, stability, and reduced energy requirement of short prostheses. Note the posterior foot placement, which is required when using forward-facing feet.

length articulated limbs is determined by the success and confidence of the user (Figure 6). When the overall length has been increased to the point that the foot can be placed sufficiently posterior to prevent the amputee from falling backward, the feet should be turned to the normal, forward-facing position. Knees should be included when the limbs become too long for the amputee to easily negotiate doorways and restricted spaces while seated in a wheelchair (Figure 7). Locking knees may be used initially and unlocked to drop the feet out of the way while sitting, but progression to at least one free knee with sufficient inherent stability on the longer or dominant side is desirable. A more de-

tailed discussion of component selection is presented later in this chapter.

For some amputees, long-term use of stubbies is appropriate. If the amputee finds that full-length legs are unmanageable or create too much anxiety because of the possibility of falling, then definitive use of stubbies is indicated. Additionally, some amputees who use full-length prostheses choose to have a set of stubbies that are used primarily in the home or for outdoor recreational activities. These are usually patients who regard normal height to be important for psychosocial reasons when interacting with the public, yet at home they may enjoy the ease of use of the shorter limbs. The feet used on definitive stubbies can be either rockers, rearward-facing prosthetic feet, or forward-facing prosthetic feet that have been positioned sufficiently posterior to provide stability (Figure 8). The height of the definitive stubbies should take into account not only chair height but also the height of work surfaces and counters in the home.

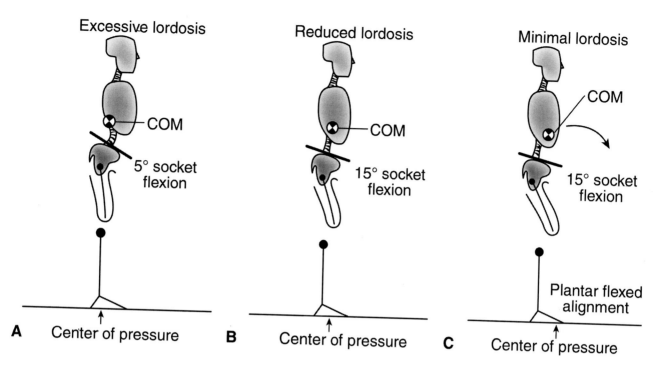

Figure 9 Excessive lumbar lordosis may result from improperly aligned prostheses. In the presence of an unaccommodated flexion contracture, the amputee must extend at the lumbar spine to position the center of body mass (COM) over the base of support. **A,** With socket flexion of 5° from vertical, excessive lordosis is required to position the COM over the center of pressure. **B,** Socket flexion of 15° lessens the amount of lumber lordosis required to maintain a stable posture. **C,** Dynamic response feet aligned in plantar flexion cause the amputee to lean forward over the flexible toe lever, further flattening the lumbar spine.

Crouse and associates[19] compared oxygen consumption and cardiac response in a bilateral transfemoral amputee using stubbies and full-length prostheses and found the stubbies to be 24% more efficient. They also recorded an interesting irregularity in expiratory flow waveforms found to be related to the stride frequency during use of the stubbies. This evidence indicates that when a subject wears prostheses, reactive forces associated with foot strike that are normally dissipated or stored as potential energy in elastic tissues are instead transmitted to the torso, affecting intrathoracic pressure and altering pulmonary ventilation patterns. The authors suggest that future prosthetic designs should include features that dissipate forces experienced during foot strike.

The primary disadvantage of stubbies is cosmetic, which makes them unacceptable to many individuals. Other problems include difficulty in transferring and in climbing stairs, curbs, and ramps.[20]

Minimizing Lumbar Lordosis

Bilateral transfemoral amputees commonly adjust their posture to position the center of body mass over the base of support, increasing lumbar lordosis. This abnormal posture is sometimes associated with low back pain. The amount of lordosis increases with increased hip flexor tightness (Figure 9, *A*). To avoid this, it is important to align the socket with sufficient initial flexion, which is best determined by measuring the flexion contracture using the Thomas test and then adding an additional 5° of flexion. Socket flexion alone may not be sufficient to reduce lumbar lordosis to normal values (Figure 9, *B*). Also, with a long residual limb, cosmetic considerations may limit the amount of socket flexion that can be achieved.

The new dynamic response feet make it possible to align the prosthetic feet in plantar flexion, reducing lumbar lordosis (Figure 9, *C*). Plantar flexed alignment with these feet, which provide an elastic or spring-like dorsiflexion action, causes the amputee to lean forward over the feet to find a point of stability. This shift of the center of pressure to a relatively anterior position and the accompanying forward lean as the amputee brings the center of body mass over that point will lessen the lordosis (Figure 9, *C*). As Radcliffe[21] noted, this plantar flexed alignment helps knee stability during early stance phase and affords improved knee control during late stance phase, allowing easier initiation of knee flexion. To achieve an appropriate amount of plantar flexion, a 6- to 10-mm space should be created under the heel, with the shoe on, during bench alignment (Figure 10). The amount of plantar flexion should be fine-tuned during dynamic alignment.

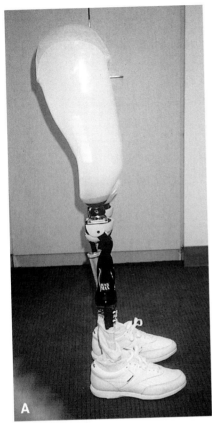
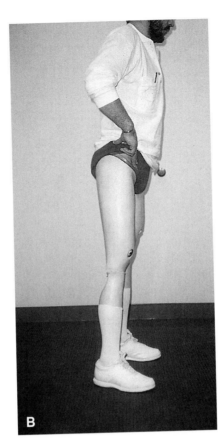
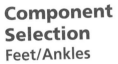

Figure 10 Prostheses with plantar flexed alignment. **A,** Prostheses aligned using a 10-mm spacer during bench alignment to achieve the desired plantar flexed alignment (shown without the spacers). **B,** Amputee standing in the prostheses with plantar flexed alignment. Note the slight forward lean and the resulting flattened lumbar spine. The patient is well balanced and standing unsupported.

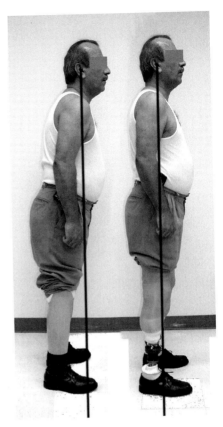

Figure 11 Bilateral transtibial amputee shown using exoskeletal prostheses with SACH feet. The vertical line has been added for reference. **A,** Note the forward lean required for balance because of the insufficient posterior lever arm, caused in this case by heel cushions that were too soft. **B,** Same patient using appropriately aligned prostheses with multiaxial dynamic response feet, vertical shock units, and vacuum-assisted suspension systems.

Component Selection
Feet/Ankles

Foot and ankle components that provide good shock absorption are generally indicated for bilateral amputees. As previously discussed, shock absorption is one of the primary functions of the physiologic foot and ankle complex, and replacement of this feature is critical to the comfort and normal and efficient ambulation of the amputee. Modern foot and ankle components that offer compliance and some measure of dynamic response should be considered for all bilateral leg amputees, regardless of the level of amputation. Because of the high energy cost of walking with two prostheses, it is advantageous to use dynamic response feet. A more flexible foot is generally preferred over one that is more rigid.

The goal of providing shock absorption through compliance will be compromised if the foot is too stiff. Appropriate prosthetic alignment of properly selected components is critical in achieving an optimal outcome (Figure 11). For the transfemoral amputee, the plantar flexion action of the foot must be soft enough to allow rapid transition to foot flat to enhance knee stability. Additionally, with the transfemoral prosthesis, it is necessary to select a foot with a spring-like dorsiflexion action for the recommended plantar flexed alignment to be successful. Dorsiflexion action that is too soft will fail to provide the necessary toe lever needed both for anterior support during standing as well as adequate knee control after midstance. In my experience, amputees who have used high-energy–storing feet report that not only do these feet provide a more

energy-efficient gait but they also improve speed control, especially during slow walking.

Knee Components

Radcliffe[21] documented the benefits of aligning the prosthetic knee to achieve voluntary control including (1) knee stability at heel strike through active control using the hip extensors, (2) ease of initiating knee flexion in late stance during double support, and (3) provision of a more natural gait that is energy efficient. For the active (unlimited community ambulatory) bilateral transfemoral amputee, use of voluntary control principles of alignment has proved advantageous.

Hydraulic swing and stance knee control units have been very successful in optimizing the gait of the active transfemoral amputee. These units offer good stance stability, can be locked for special circumstances, and are best aligned with the knee center in a relatively anterior position (compared with less inherently stable designs), which provides greater toe clearance than does a more posteriorly offset knee center (Figure 12). Less active transfemoral amputees who require a high degree of stability will benefit from knee mechanisms that are inherently more stable, including use of a locking knee on one side. In cases where one locking knee is found to be necessary, the locking knee should be fitted on the shorter or weaker side. In patients with one transtibial and one transfemoral amputation, it may be useful to shorten the transfemoral side up to 12 mm for added swing-phase toe clearance.

Polycentric knees

Polycentric knee designs offer several interesting features that may benefit

the bilateral amputee. Some linkage configurations place the instant center of rotation in a posterior and proximal location, providing excellent stability. In some cases, and particularly for the active walker, the instant center of rotation can be fine-tuned by the prosthetist to balance the need for stability at heel strike with the ease of knee flexion in late stance phase by adjusting the extension stop and thereby changing the position of the instant center of rotation within the zone of stability (Figure 13). Four-bar knee mechanisms also offer the advantage of greater toe clearance during swing phase (Figure 14) compared with single-axis hinges. This can be especially advantageous for bilateral amputees.

Stance-Phase Knee Flexion

Lack of stance-phase knee flexion is very noticeable in the gait of bilateral transfemoral amputees. This absence of one of the key determinants of gait results in an unnatural gait that lacks the normal shock-absorbing mechanism and is believed to require greater

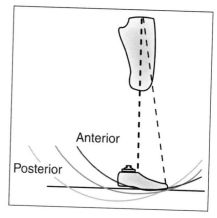

Figure 12 The effect of shifting the knee in the sagittal plane is shown. Anterior placement of the knee reduces the hip-to-toe distance during swing phase. The applicability of this approach depends on the inherent stability of the knee mechanism used. *(Courtesy of Steven A. Gard, Ph.D.)*

energy. Several prosthetic knee mechanisms that provide stance flexion using a compliant linkage are now available. Knee mechanisms that allow stance-phase knee flexion should not interfere with initiation of swing-phase knee flexion. Therefore,

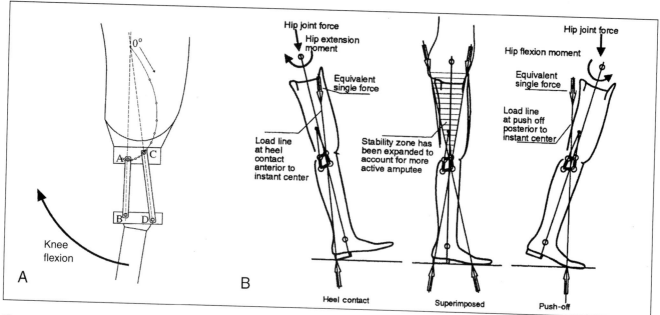

Figure 13 A, Four-bar knees with an adjustable extension stop allow the prosthetist to fine-tune the stability of the knee by selectively positioning the instant center of rotation along the arc shown. *(Reproduced with permission from Gard SA, Childress DS, Uellendahl JE: The influence of four-bar linkage knees on prosthetic swing. J Prosthet Orthot 1996;8:34-40.)* **B)** The zone of stability is described by superimposing the stability requirements during heel strike with those required at heel-off, which allow optimal voluntary knee control. *(Reproduced with permission from Radcliffe CW: The Knud Jansen lecture: Above-knee prosthetics. Prosthet Orthot Int 1977;1: 146-160.)*

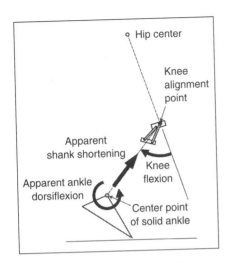

Figure 14 The effect of a particular four-bar knee on the trajectory of the foot is characterized by knee flexion, apparent ankle dorsiflexion, and apparent shank shortening. *(Reproduced with permission from Gard SA, Childress DS, Uellendahl JE: The influence of four-bar linkage knees on prosthetic swing.* J Prosthet Orthot *1996;8:34-40.)*

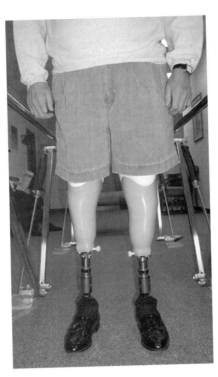

Figure 15 Vertical shock units afford greater comfort for the bilateral amputee. In this case, torque absorbers are incorporated into the same unit and are used in combination with low-profile dynamic response feet to maintain an acceptable overall length.

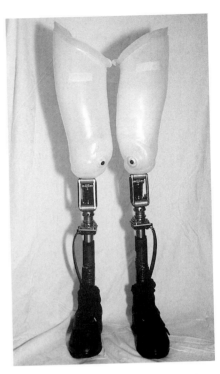

Figure 16 Vertical shock units replace some of the normal physiologic compliance lost by amputation. With such units, it can be beneficial to use four-bar knees that offer sufficient swing-phase shortening to make up for the reduced height during midstance on the weight-bearing side.

knees that rely on weight-activated braking should be avoided because they will hamper the ability of the amputee to initiate flexion late in stance during the preswing phase of double support.

Microprocessor-Controlled Swing and Stance

Perhaps one of the most important developments in prosthetic components in recent years was the introduction of microprocessor-controlled knee units. One such computerized knee uses real-time analysis of various parameters of gait to provide a high degree of stability during the loading response phase of gait and nearly eliminate resistance to flexion late in stance, lowering the energy requirements for walking. Because of the high resistance to flexion in early stance, the knee center can be placed in a relatively anterior position, affording greater toe clearance. Such anterior knee alignment also encourages use of the stance flexion feature, as the amputee allows the knee to flex against the high hydraulic resistance in response to loading. At least one commercially available microprocessor-

controlled knee also offers an optional flexion lock, which is useful for the bilateral amputee.

Vertical Shock Units

Vertical shock units offer another option for reduction of the impact forces experienced during normal gait as well as the peak forces that result from stepping down from a height (Figure 15). Vertical shock units increase compliance in the prosthesis, allowing body weight to be transferred to the prosthetic limb over a longer period of time, thereby decreasing the downward acceleration of the body and consequently reducing forces transmitted through the prosthesis to the body.[11] Because of the inherent shortening that occurs during stance phase with these units, sufficient contralateral toe clearance during gait must be ensured by carefully adjusting the amount of compression provided by the shock unit. When vertical shock units are incor-

porated into the transfemoral prosthesis, it may be beneficial to use a four-bar knee (Figure 16) to gain the additional toe clearance such knees offer.[22]

Torque Absorbers

When the foot is on the floor during the stance phase of gait, the biologic foot and ankle permit the leg to rotate externally while the foot remains stationary.[6] These capabilities are lost following amputation. Therefore, using a torque absorber to minimize the rotational shear forces that would otherwise be experienced at the socket interface is beneficial. Clinical observation and user feedback also suggest that torque absorbers allow greater step length because they facilitate external rotation between midstance and terminal stance. This is particularly significant in the transfemoral amputee with a flexion contracture because such limitations in hip range of motion restrict contralateral step length.

Interface Design

Socket design for the bilateral amputee is not significantly different than for the unilateral amputee. Sound prosthetic interface design principles should be used, including (1) total surface bearing, (2) close coupling of bony structures to the prosthesis, and (3) excellent suspension. Transtibial amputees benefit from soft interface materials such as silicone, urethane, or thermoplastic gel liners that, along with appropriate socket design, spread forces evenly over the greatest possible area (Figure 17). Bilateral transfemoral amputees have successfully used both ischial containment and quadrilateral sockets. If ischial containment designs are indicated, more aggressive containment on the weaker or shorter side and less containment on the stronger or longer side may be advisable because the different medial brim heights will reduce the tendency for pinching of the skin between the two sockets during ambulation.

To obtain an adequate impression of the limbs in the new bilateral transfemoral amputee, the amputee can be positioned either supine or lying on the side. At the time of the first socket change, casting can be accomplished with the amputee in the more conventional upright position by having the amputee alternately stand in first one and then the other initial prosthesis while supported between parallel bars.

Suspension

Suspension of a prosthesis is always critical and assumes even more importance for the bilateral amputee. Any amount of pistoning in the socket will increase the effective length of the prosthesis during swing phase, and the bilateral amputee cannot actively vault to compensate. Positive suspension will also provide better proprioception and will reduce shear forces and the perception of weight. Therefore, suction suspension

is recommended whenever possible, for all cases and levels of amputation. For the transfemoral amputee who may have difficulty donning a conventional suction socket, silicone suction suspension (3S) is a good alternative.[23] The benefits of 3S socket designs include (1) ease of donning while in a seated position, (2) maintenance of suction throughout the range of motion, and (3) easy accommodation of volume changes while maintaining suction. Belts can be added to the transfemoral prosthesis to enhance mediolateral stability. The belt should have a split design that allows the prosthetic legs to be separated from each other for prosthesis maintenance and other circumstances.

Other Considerations

Bilateral prostheses for ambulation are not the only option for bilateral amputees with transfemoral or higher limb loss. Nonprosthetic considerations include posteriorly offset wheelchair wheels to prevent flipping over backward because of the higher center of gravity. Additionally, amputees who are not candidates for ambulation may wish to be fitted with "sitting" prostheses for cosmetic reasons. In some cases, a prosthesis may be used solely for transfers. One example would be the transtibial/transfemoral amputee for whom ambulation is not feasible but for whom the unilateral use of a transtibial prosthesis improves independence and function. Even in patients who are not candidates for ambulation, amputation through the knee is preferable to bilateral transfemoral amputation because the longer residual limb provides more secure balance while seated in a wheelchair.[24] Although wheelchairs provide safe and efficient transportation, exclusive use of a wheelchair has many disadvantages because of environmental barriers such as stairs. Many bilateral lower limb amputees are best served by using prostheses in conjunction with a wheelchair.

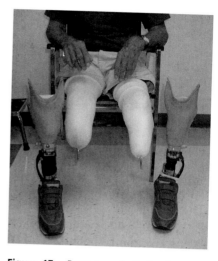

Figure 17 Because of their fluid-like characteristics, gel interfaces spread the forces of walking more evenly. The gel liners shown incorporate distal locking mechanisms for secure suspension.

Case Studies
Case Study 1

A 67-year-old man presented with bilateral transtibial amputations secondary to peripheral vascular disease with diabetes. The individual was otherwise in good physical condition. Both limbs had been amputated 5 inches below the knee. The left limb was amputated 18 months after the right, and the individual had successfully used a unilateral prosthesis before the second amputation. The left limb was managed with a rigid dressing immediately after the amputation. This was followed by a removable rigid dressing used in combination with the progressive addition of socks to encourage shrinkage, as described by Wu and Krick.[25] The individual has followed a strengthening and conditioning program as outlined by the rehabilitation team's physical therapist. A preparatory prosthesis was provided 3 weeks postoperatively, at which time the limb was well healed and only slightly bulbous. The socket was a total-surface–bearing design that used a gel-type roll-on liner with pin suspension, and a dynamic response foot with built-in multiaxial rotation was provided. These components matched those of the endoskeletal prosthesis the individual had been using. At the time of initial fitting, the prostheses were adjusted to reduce the individual's overall height 2 inches to provide greater stability and confidence. During the fitting, it became clear that the foot on the existing prosthesis would need to be more flexible because the activity level and the vigor of the man's gait would be reduced by the second amputation. Therefore, a new, softer foot to match the new anticipated activity level was provided. The man received gait training for the first 3 weeks after receiving the initial prosthesis and met his rehabilitation goals. Five months after he received the initial prosthesis, he was fitted with a pair of new prostheses of the same design and components as the initial prostheses with the addition of bilateral vertical shock units. The man has reported that the vertical shock units added comfort and were a definite improvement. The man is now an unlimited community ambulator and uses one cane for additional stability, especially when on uneven ground and in crowded places.

Case Study 2

A 34-year-old man presented with bilateral transfemoral amputations secondary to trauma from an automobile accident. His right leg had been amputated at the juncture of the distal and middle third of the femur, and his left leg had been amputated at midfemur. He was in good physical condition and had no other injuries. The man was first seen by the amputee rehabilitation team 4 months postoperatively, at which time the residual limbs were contained in elastic shrinkers and were well healed. He had a 10° flexion contracture on the left side and a 5° flexion contracture on the right side. Initially, stubby prostheses using rearward-facing feet attached with endoskeletal components were prescribed to allow easy adjustment of length and alignment. The sockets were ischial containment designs with suction suspension. The initial rehabilitation plan called for gait training, minimizing the flex-

ion contractures, and upper limb strengthening. After only 2 weeks of training, the man was able to manage prostheses that were 4 inches longer and was able to don the sockets independently using a nylon pull sleeve. He was also able to independently get into and out of his wheelchair, which has offset wheels for greater stability. The patient was eager to progress to articulated legs, so locking hydraulic knees with swing and stance control were installed and the Solid Ankle Cushion Heel (SACH) feet were replaced with forward-facing dynamic response feet of appropriate stiffness. The flexion contractures were still present, so the alignment was set to accommodate the contractures. With the added length, the patient became more tentative and cautious, preferring to stay within the parallel bars with the knees locked for the next few training sessions. The right knee was unlocked and training continued, with the patient progressing from the parallel bars to two canes. Next, the second knee was unlocked and training continued with two canes. After 3 months of prosthesis use, the patient was able to walk with one cane. Torque absorbers were added to the prosthetic systems, and the patient commented favorably about the ease of taking longer steps and reported generally improved comfort.

Summary

Numerous factors influence the successful rehabilitation of the bilateral lower limb amputee. A more distal level of amputation, particularly the preservation of the physiologic knee joints, and the general strength and health of the amputee are key predictors for successful use of bilateral prostheses. Careful attention by the prosthetist to the details of socket fitting, prosthesis alignment, and component selection following sound prosthetic principles, in addition to the services of an experienced rehabilitation team, will optimize the ambulation potential of the patient. Given these advantages and the deter-

mination of the amputee to succeed, a positive outcome is attainable. The rehabilitation team should remain open to new ideas. Thoughtful use of available assistive technologies including state-of-the-art prosthetic components can significantly benefit the bilateral lower limb amputee.

References:

1. Evans WE, Hayes JP, Vermilion BD: Rehabilitation of the bilateral amputee. *J Vasc Surg* 1987;5:589-593.

2. Esquenazi A: Geriatric amputee rehabilitation. *Clin Geriatr Med* 1993;9: 731-743.

3. Thornhill HL, Jones GD, Brodzka W, VanBockstaele P: Bilateral below-knee amputations: Experience with 80 patients. *Arch Phys Med Rehabil* 1986;67: 159-163.

4. Smith DG, Burgess EM, Zettl JH: Special considerations: Fitting and training the bilateral lower-limb amputee, in Bowker JH, Michael JW (eds): *Atlas of Limb Prosthetics: Surgical, Prosthetic, and Rehabilitation Principles*, ed 2. Rosemont, IL, American Academy of Orthopaedic Surgeons, 2002, pp 599-622. (Originally published by Mosby-Year Book, 1992.)

5. Moore TJ, Barron J, Hutchinson F III, Golden C, Ellis C, Humphries D: Prosthetic usage following major lower extremity amputation. *Clin Orthop* 1989;238:219-224.

6. Inman VT, Ralston HJ, Todd R: Human locomotion, in Rose J, Gamble JG (eds): *Human Walking*, ed 2. Baltimore, MD, Williams & Wilkins 1994, pp 1-22.

7. Saunders JB, Inman VT, Eberhart HD: The major determinants in normal and pathological gait. *J Bone Joint Surg Am* 1953;35:543-558.

8. Perry J (ed): Gait Analysis: *Normal and Pathological Function*. Thorofare, NJ, SLACK Inc, 1992.

9. Gard SA, Childress DS: The influence of stance-phase knee flexion on the vertical displacement of the trunk during normal walking. *Arch Phys Med Rehabil* 1999;80:26-32.

10. Gard SA, Childress DS: The effect of pelvic list on the vertical displacement of the trunk during normal walking. *Gait Posture* 1997;5:233-238.

11. Gard SA, Konz RL: The influence of prosthetic shock absorbing pylons on transtibial amputee gait. *Gait Posture* 2001;13:303.

12. Waters RL, Perry J, Chambers R: Energy expenditure of amputee gait, in Moore WS, Malone JM (eds): *Lower Extremity Amputation.* Philadelphia, PA, WB Saunders, 1989, pp 250-260.

13. DuBow LL, Witt PL, Kadaba MP, Reyes R, Cochran GV: Oxygen consumption of elderly persons with bilateral below-knee amputations: Ambulation vs wheelchair propulsion. *Arch Phys Med Rehabil* 1983;64: 255-259.

14. Gonzalez EG, Corcoran PJ, Reyes RL: Energy expenditure in below-knee amputees: Correlation with stump length. *Arch Phys Med Rehabil* 1974;55: 111-119.

15. Huang CT, Jackson JR, Moore NB, et al: Amputation: Energy cost of ambulation. *Arch Phys Med Rehabil* 1979;60: 18-24.

16. Hoffman MD, Sheldahl LM, Buley KJ, Sandford PR: Physiological comparison of walking among bilateral above-knee amputee and able-bodied subjects, and a model to account for the differences in metabolic cost. *Arch Phys Med Rehabil* 1997;78:385-392.

17. McCollough NC III, Harris AR, Hampton FL: The bilateral lower-limb amputee, in *Atlas of Limb Prosthetics: Surgical and Prosthetic Principles.* St Louis, MO, CV Mosby, 1981, pp 417-422.

18. Kruger LM: Stubby prostheses in the rehabilitation of infants and small children with bilateral lower limb deficiencies. *Rehabilitation (Stuttg)* 1990; 29:12-15.

19. Crouse SF, Lessard CS, Rhodes J, Lowe RC: Oxygen consumption and cardiac response of short-leg and long-leg prosthetic ambulation in a patient with bilateral above-knee amputation: Comparison with able-bodied men. *Arch Phys Med Rehabil* 1990;71: 313-317.

20. Wainapel SF, March H, Steve L: Stubby prostheses: An alternative to conventional prosthetic devices. *Arch Phys Med Rehabil* 1985;66:264-266.

21. Radcliffe CW: Above-knee prosthetics. *Prosthet Orthot Int* 1977;1:146-160.

22. Gard SA, Childress DS, Uellendahl JE: The influence of four-bar linkage knees on prosthetic swing-phase floor clearance. *J Prosthet Orthot* 1996;8: 34-40.

23. Trieb K, Lang T, Stulnig T, Kickinger W: Silicone soft socket system: Its effect on the rehabilitation of geriatric patients with transfemoral amputations. *Arch Phys Med Rehabil* 1999;80: 522-525.

24. Witso E, Ronningen H: Lower limb amputations: Registration of all lower limb amputations performed at the University Hospital of Trondheim, Norway, 1994-1997. *Prosthet Orthot Int* 2001;25:181-185.

25. Wu Y, Krick H: Removable rigid dressing for below-knee amputees. *Clin Prosthet Orthop* 1987;11:33-44.

Chapter 50

Prostheses for Sports and Recreation

John R. Fergason, CPO
David Alan Boone, CP, MPH

Introduction

Experts agree that physical and mental well-being are enhanced by exercise. The US Public Health Service and various public health organizations highly recommend regular physical activity to help combat health concerns. Physical activity promotes independence and increases self-confidence while decreasing the risk of many physical pathologies, such as cardiovascular disease.[1-7] Many amputees enjoy sports and recreational activities, and some with exceptional physical abilities excel in competitive sports, running 100 m in less than 11 seconds, climbing Mt. McKinley or Mt. Everest, traversing continents on foot and bicycle, or competing in professional baseball or boxing. Although the world-class amputee sprinter or marathon runner may attain the pinnacle of performance, most individuals with amputations do not aspire to this level of achievement. They simply want to enjoy sports and other recreational activities with family and friends.

A 1980 survey of lower limb amputees suggested both a strong desire to participate in sports and recreational activities and the need for a prosthesis that did not limit the amputee's ability to run or move quickly.[8] Evaluating the amputee patient and prescribing the right prosthesis for athletic activity must go well beyond the standard parameters associated with ambulation and vocational requirements. An artificial limb cannot offer the same complex integration of power and control as the natural limb, but a suitable prosthesis allows many amputees to enjoy participatory sports and other physical activities. Understanding the physical characteristics of the missing limb and how it functioned is the first step in determining what a prosthesis should offer. A high-quality, properly fitted prosthesis is critical to physical activity. This chapter presents principles to help guide the design of prostheses suitable for sports and recreational activities.

Initial Evaluation

As part of the physical evaluation and history, the cause of the amputation must be considered. For example, if the limb loss was due to complications of vascular insufficiency, the patient may not have engaged in any significant physical exertion for some time. It is equally important to recognize that increased physical activity can raise health risk levels in certain populations.[6] Pinzur and associates,[9] for example, suggest that dysvascular amputees with severe peripheral vascular insufficiency function at near-maximum capacity when simply ambulating. Patients with diabetes and peripheral neuropathy can develop potentially life- and limb-threatening ulcers because of excessive skin loading. When recommending exercise regimens and lifestyle choices, the prosthetist and amputee must balance the systemic benefits of activity with its potential health risks.

The prosthesis optimized for recreational use is finely tuned to both the specific function required and the user's capabilities. Realistic performance goals should be set in this context. It may be more encouraging for the amputee to reach lesser goals quickly and to then set more ambitious goals as incremental improvements in performance are attained.

Physical Preparation

Creation of a sports prosthesis should proceed in conjunction with the amputee athlete's general physical preparation and conditioning. Ideally, a comprehensive program of physical fitness should begin under the direction of a physical therapist who is familiar with the amputee's unique situation. It is important to communicate to the amputee that the prosthesis itself is not the sole means to attaining a higher activity level. Simply incorporating a sprinting foot into a lower limb prosthesis will not allow the individual to run; the prosthesis is merely an assistive device that will facilitate use of whatever strength and stamina the individual achieves through physical conditioning. When the amputee has developed the requisite physical capabilities, the prosthetist can opti-

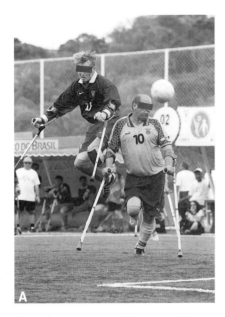
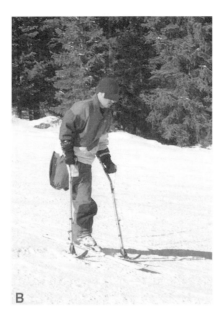

Figure 1 Many sports do not require use of a prosthesis. **A,** Bilateral forearm crutches worn in competitive soccer. **B,** Alpine skier using outriggers. *(Courtesy of Steve Wilber, Seattle, WA.)*

mize the prosthesis so the individual can increase speed and distance. Maximum sports performance may require modified or specialized components or significant deviations from standard alignment techniques to help improve interlimb symmetry and running velocity.[10]

Choosing Whether to Use a Prosthesis

An amputee can participate in sports without a prosthesis. Some amputee swimmers, for example, use a prosthesis only to reach the pool or shoreline, removing it before entering the water, whereas fly fishers may find that using a prosthesis is safer and makes wading less strenuous. Some organized sports for amputees, such as soccer, regulate the use of prostheses, requiring participants to use bilateral forearm crutches and forgo the use of a prosthesis on at least one residual limb (Figure 1, *A*). Amputee athletes participating in Alpine skiing in the Paralympic Games use single skis (for single-leg amputations), outriggers, or prostheses (Figure 1, *B*), and individuals with arm amputations forgo the use of poles.

An amputee who chooses not to wear a prosthesis may wear a residual limb protector, a thin plastic shell similar to the prosthetic socket, generally incorporating a simple belt or sleeve suspension that protects the limb from impact or abrasion. A simple flexible foam or rigid plastic shell is especially useful in high-speed sports, such as snow skiing, where high-impact falls are not uncommon.

Use of a prosthesis may be hazardous to others during some activities. For example, an amputee playing soccer or a competitive contact sport such as football may be required to cover the prosthesis with additional foam padding to protect the other players.

Design Considerations
Activity Level

Any sports prosthesis should be designed to withstand the level of demand the athlete will place on it. Recent long-term monitoring of ambulatory activity has demonstrated that some assumptions about activity levels may be inaccurate.[11] For example, running is commonly believed to

require a higher activity level than golf, but both are high-activity sports. Runners move quickly for a relatively short period of time, whereas golfers move more slowly over a period of several hours; each sport may require a similar number of steps.

Functional demands are more important in prosthesis design than activity level. The recreational jogger requires a prosthesis that will absorb the impact of initial contact and loading response, support the body weight through midstance to allow a long stride length on the sound side, and provide some measure of propulsive thrust at the end of stance. Golf has an entirely different set of functional demands. Although golf may not require the same cardiovascular demands as jogging, the golfer must be able to endure long periods of standing, maintain overall stability when twisting during swings, and ambulate safely over uneven terrain and inclines.

Alignment

Alignment is a key element for optimal functioning of lower limb prostheses. Socket and shank alignment critically affects the wearer's comfort and dynamic performance by altering the manner in which the weight-bearing load is transferred between the supporting foot and the residual limb. Alignment of the lower limb prosthesis for sports activities may differ significantly from that which is optimal for other activities of daily living. Water and snow skiing, for example, require increased ankle dorsiflexion (Figure 2). A prosthesis optimally aligned for these sports will not function well for general ambulation, so either a special-use prosthesis or interchangeable components will be required.

Dynamics of the Lower Limb

The human leg is a complex instrument offering dynamic shock absorption, adaptation to uneven terrain, torque conversion, knee stabilization,

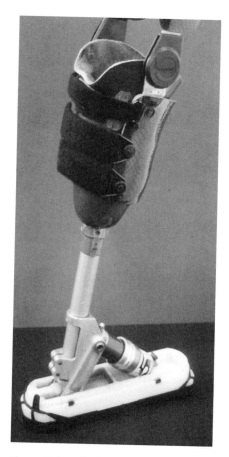

Figure 2 Prosthesis adjusted to allow increased ankle dorsiflexion for sports such as water and snow skiing. *(Courtesy of The Adaptive Sports Association, Durango, CO.)*

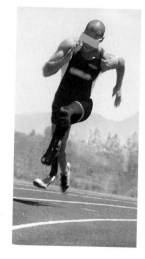

Figure 3 Competitive sprinter wearing foot configured without a heel. *(Courtesy of Ossur, Aliso Viejo, CA.)*

automatic limb lengthening and shortening to diminish the arc of the center of gravity, transfer of weight-bearing forces, and reliable weight-bearing support.[7] A lower limb prosthesis cannot fully replicate these critical functions, but a properly designed and fitted prosthesis will provide a reliable level of each.[12]

Impact Reduction During Loading

Impact on the residual limb begins when the foot contacts the ground. These forces are relayed through the structure of the prosthesis to the residual limb and are greatest during loading response while walking, during pushoff and landing on the prosthesis when jumping, and during the contact phase of a new stride while running. During sports activities,

these forces may become exponentially higher because of increased impact loads. The residual limb is subject to pressure and shear forces; both increase during high-impact activity. Shear stresses and/or pressure on the skin can cause occlusion of the blood flow.

The greater the shear forces generated with a prosthesis, the lower the pressure required to cause blood flow occlusion and resultant tissue breakdown.[13] The cyclic shear stress that inevitably occurs within a prosthetic socket can cause a blister to form within the epidermis or create an abrasion on the skin surface. Adherent scar tissue, common after traumatic amputations, can create shear stress adjacent to the area of amputation, resulting in skin tension that can cause blanching or even cell rupture.[14] One investigation of an instrumented patellar tendon–bearing prosthetic socket demonstrated that maximal pressure and resultant shear stresses shifted locations between the loading phase of stance and the latter phases of the gait cycle.[15] This is believed to be a result of the dynamic movement of the residual limb within the socket.

As an individual's activity level increases, both socket pressure and shear forces can easily rise to levels

that cause soft-tissue damage. For most sports and recreational activities, the prosthesis should be designed to reduce impact and its associated socket pressure and shear. The following discussion begins with the foot as the first contact with the ground and then considers the more proximal elements of the prosthesis.

Influence of the Foot on Impact Reduction

The heel of the foot can absorb some portion of the impact during ambulation and slow jogging, but this is speed dependent. Data show that in nonamputee athletes during normal ambulation, at a speed of 80 m/min, a full heel strike occurs during initial contact. As the ambulation speed increases to a fast walk or slow jog, at 140 m/min, the middle portion of the foot becomes the primary initial contact point and the heel has minimal effect. Once running speed (180 m/min) is achieved, heel contact is virtually eliminated.[16] Similar data have been demonstrated in studies of prosthetic limb kinematics.[17]

Clinical application of these data helps specify the durometer of the heel of the prosthetic foot for transtibial amputees. Shock absorption through compression of the prosthetic heel or plantar flexion bumper is very important for a recreational walker who has no intention of jogging or running; heel components also control the rate of foot plantar flexion during loading response in much the same way as does eccentric lengthening of the dorsiflexor group in the natural foot. When the amputee begins jogging or running, however, the heel component may not be loaded as fully, so its shock-absorbing value decreases. This explains why the amputee sprinter prefers a foot without a heel, even though this configuration is unsuitable for walking (Figure 3).

As the amputee enters midstance on the prosthesis, the foot should accommodate uneven terrain and help control advancement of the tibia. Tibial advancement that is too abrupt results in resistance to the knee flexion

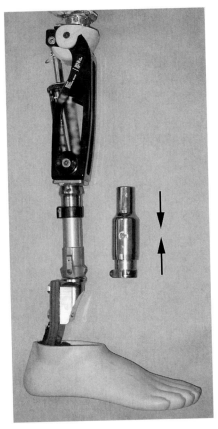

Figure 4 Shock-absorbing pylons reduce the forces transmitted to the residual limb and allow the prosthesis to continue to absorb impact after the foot has reached its limit.

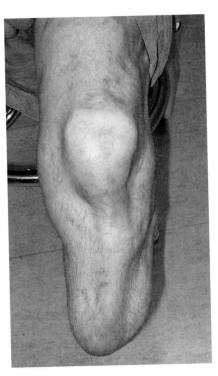

Figure 5 Skin grafts and lack of soft tissue reduce limb tolerance for shear.

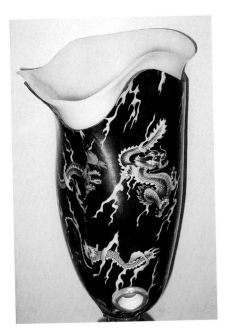

Figure 6 Flexible plastic inner socket supported by a rigid external frame. A flexible brim on the transfemoral prosthesis increases comfort during high activity.

moment, increasing the forces on the residual limb within the socket. A new prosthesis should be aligned and adjusted based on evaluation of its performance as the amputee uses it on surfaces similar to those that will be encountered in athletic activity. Activities such as hiking that include traversing uneven terrain may require use of a multiaxial ankle, which allows the prosthetic foot to conform to irregular surfaces, thus reducing the forces transferred to the residual limb. An articulated foot should be considered when reduction of the knee flexion moment on a transfemoral prosthesis is desirable. When the articulated foot plantar flexes rapidly to the ground during loading response, the ground-reaction force vector moves forward quickly and thereby prevents uncontrolled knee flexion under weight bearing.

Influence of the Shank on Impact Reduction

The prosthesis can continue to absorb impact after the foot has reached its limit if there is a shock-absorbing pylon between the foot and socket. These pylons may be integrated within the shin/ankle/foot component or added as independent structures separate from the foot (Figure 4). Most shock-absorbing pylons require adjustment by the prosthetist to provide the optimal amount of vertical travel for each individual.

Influence of the Interface on Impact Reduction

Amputees with conditions such as bony residual limbs, skin grafts, or adherent scars will have a reduced tolerance for shear (Figure 5). When athletic activity increases multidirectional forces that give rise to pressure and shear stresses, a socket liner made from an elastomeric gel is often recommended. For transfemoral amputees, special consideration should be given to the ischial tuberosity area and the proximal tissue along the

socket brim. The amputee's comfort can be increased by the use of a flexible plastic inner socket supported by a rigid external frame. This combination maintains the structural weight-supporting integrity of the socket while increasing the range of hip motion because of the flexibility of the proximal socket (Figure 6).

Reduction of Rotational Forces

Absorption of transverse plane rotary forces in the residual lower limb occurs when ankle pronation and supination allow lower limb rotation as the foot contacts the ground. A prosthetic torque absorber component can be provided that will allow internal and external rotation between the socket and the foot. Although multiaxial ankles offer some rotational movement, a separate torque-absorbing component does this most effectively. Some amputee golfers report that these components help them achieve a smooth swing and follow-through and also reduce the uncomfortable rotational shear that would otherwise occur between the

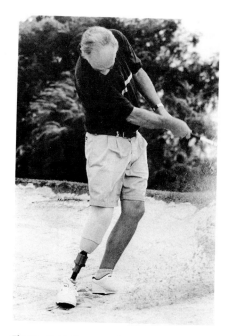

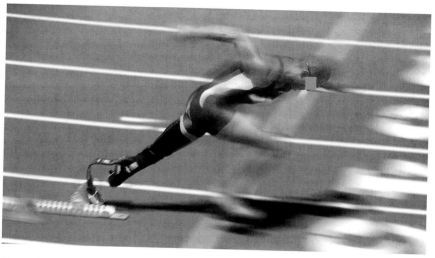

Figure 8 Competitive runner using dynamic-response foot with a spring keel extending into the shin region. The increased flexibility offered by this combination is generally preferred by advanced runners. (Courtesy of Ossur, Aliso Viejo, CA.)

Figure 7 Golfer wearing prosthesis with torque absorber component that allows internal and external rotation between the socket and the foot. Torque absorbers are particularly important for activities requiring transverse plane movements. (Courtesy of Ohio Willow Wood, Mt. Sterling, OH.)

skin of the residual limb and the socket (Figure 7).

Limb Acceleration for High Activity

The choice of foot affects the ability to propel the limb forward. Enoka and associates[18] studied the forces generated while running and jumping with a prosthesis. The large ground-reaction forces demonstrated during these activities led to the design of a prosthetic foot that could store the energy placed on it during weight bearing and release a portion of that energy later in the gait cycle to assist in propelling the limb forward during unweighting. Such dynamic-response feet vary widely in design, function, and cost. Fast-paced joggers and advanced runners often prefer a high-profile foot that incorporates a flexible shin portion. The longer spring length of these components has been shown to offer maximum capacity for energy storage and return (Figure 8).

General-Use Versus Activity-Specific Prostheses

One consideration is whether a prosthesis designed for sports activities can also double as an everyday limb. Some prostheses can be designed to allow the amputee to participate safely and comfortably in a relatively wide range of activity, including selected sports. Options like elastomeric gel liners that provide the socket comfort required during everyday tasks may suffice for some recreational activities. The use of an optimal prosthetic foot may allow the amputee to walk faster and achieve a more equal step length on both sides, facilitating recreational activity and routine walking.[19] Carefully selected dynamic feet, aligned for comfort and efficiency during walking, can sometimes function adequately for intermittent, moderately paced jogging.

A sports-specific prosthesis is usually necessary for maximum performance and personal safety. Despite strong evidence about the benefits arising from exercise as part of a healthy lifestyle, funding for sport-optimized prostheses is often denied, thereby limiting the amputee to the use of a general-purpose prosthesis for sports participation and sometimes forcing the amputee to refrain

from participation altogether.[20] An amputee planning to participate in downhill skiing on a regular basis requires a custom-designed ski prosthesis to ensure maximum personal safety and control on the slopes. Alpine skiing on a prosthesis intended only for walking is the functional equivalent of skiing in sneakers. The optimal design of an activity-specific prosthesis facilitates full participation in the desired activity.

In some instances a comfortable socket suitable for daily use can be coupled with interchangeable distal components that have been selected to facilitate different tasks. For example, a quick-release coupler can be provided to permit interchanging knee and foot/ankle components. This alternative, when appropriate, can be more economical than individual prostheses (Figure 9).

Other Considerations

Most amputees want to be more active and to participate in more vigorous activities.[21] Because of the lack of conclusive scientific evidence to support the choice of prostheses and components to permit such increased activity, the amputee and prosthetist must rely on their own experience.[22] The prosthetist must clearly under-

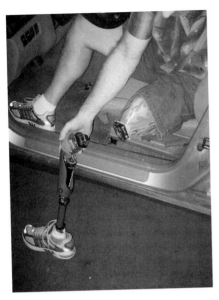

Figure 9 Amputee using a quick-release coupler to facilitate getting out of an automobile.

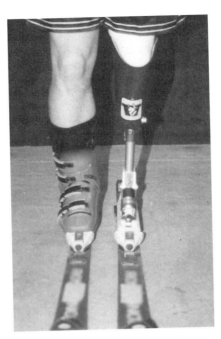

Figure 10 This single-purpose ski foot attaches directly to the ski binding, eliminating the need for a ski boot.

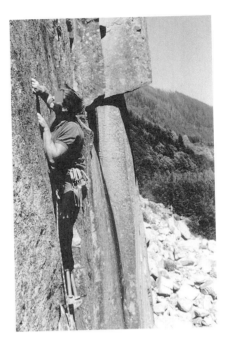

Figure 11 This athlete uses a custom foot designed for rock climbing. *(Courtesy of Prosthetic Research Study, Seattle, WA.)*

stand the functional and biomechanical demands of a specific sport when recommending a prescription to ensure that the functional characteristics of the components meet these demands.

The final weight of the prosthesis is another important consideration and is influenced by the desired activity. Prosthetic weight affects the duration of a demanding activity and has been demonstrated to be most important at higher velocities. The location of mass within the prosthesis is often more critical than the overall weight, with distally placed mass demonstrating more negative effects. The prosthetic design effort should therefore focus on keeping the necessary mass in a more proximal location whenever feasible.[23]

Single-Purpose Prostheses

Participation in most sports can be facilitated by adaptations of conventional socket designs combined with commercially available components, but some activities are best accomplished with unique custom-designed components. For example, amputee snow skiers may use a prosthetic "terminal device" modeled after the sole of a ski boot that can be directly at-

tached to the ski bindings. Cyclists may use a similar system of binding the prosthesis directly to the bike pedal. These single-purpose designs not only eliminate excess weight but, more importantly, also enhance energy transfer to the sporting equipment for more efficient performance (Figure 10).

Some sports have very specific demands that can be addressed only by unique custom components. Commercially produced prosthetic feet are unsuitable for rock climbing because the toe is not rigid enough to support the full body weight when only that portion of the prosthesis is in contact with the rock face. The shape and texture of a climbing foot can be customized to increase performance with added traction and the ability to fit in small cracks and crevices (Figure 11).

Design and fabrication of functional specialty items by prosthetists and amputees is sometimes the only practical option. Because of the lack of adequate facilities and professional expertise for clinical and practical evaluation of prototype devices, the current trial-and-error process can

result in adequate design but also present some risk to the amputee.

Waterproof Prostheses

Immersion of a prosthesis in water presents unique requirements for durability, comfort, and propulsion. Most prostheses will tolerate occasional, nominal exposure to moisture, particularly when protected under a layer of clothing. A specialized waterproof design is necessary when the amputee will have regular exposure to saltwater or fresh water, especially if complete immersion is possible, although many amputees participating in water sports may wear the prosthesis primarily to reach the water's edge. The recreational water-skier, for instance, may wear the prosthesis to ambulate safely on the dock and on the boat, then remove it to ski. It may be possible to modify the everyday prosthesis to make it resistant to splashes but not fully waterproof.

The simplest way to protect the prosthesis is to purchase a commercially available waterproof cover, such as those intended to be worn over leg

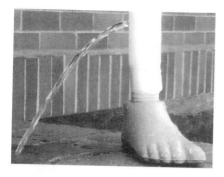

Figure 12 Prostheses used for water immersion should have neutral buoyancy. This model fills with water and drains automatically when the limb is no longer immersed. *(Courtesy of Prosthetic Research Study, Seattle, WA.)*

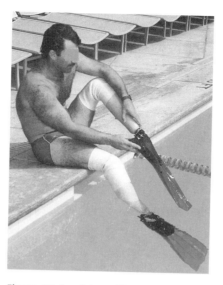

Figure 13 Specialty ankle with flipper attached to the limb locks in a plantigrade position to allow ambulation on land and locks in full plantar flexion for swimming. *(Courtesy of Rampro, Leucadia, CA.)*

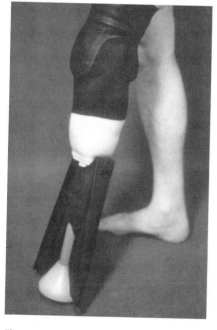

Figure 14 This waterproof peg-style leg is suitable for both ambulation and swimming. *(Courtesy of Prosthetic Research Study, Seattle, WA.)*

casts. These products are designed for short-term use and are not suitable for repeated use. A prosthesis completely covered with an airtight seal will tend to be buoyant, which can make some activities, such as swimming underwater, difficult. If swimming or snorkeling is anticipated, then the prosthesis should be designed to maintain neutral buoyancy (Figure 12). Adding a rubber suspension sleeve over the socket and distal

thigh is sometimes sufficient to keep water out of the interface between limb and socket. Knee sleeves aid suspension while still allowing adequate range of motion for swimming or wading.

Many options exist for a specialized prosthesis strictly for water use. Because metal, foam, and even plastic and composite materials may have adverse reactions to fresh water or saltwater, however, the prosthetist should consult with the component supplier's engineering department to avoid structural failure of water limbs.

Propulsion in the water is substantially enhanced by adding a flipper to the limb. Two primary methods provide this capability. First, some specialty ankles lock in neutral or in full plantar flexion, allowing regular ambulation when upright as well as use of the flipper when swimming (Figure 13). The second approach uses a modified flipper encasing the distal socket, which allows a more natural kick and reduces the torque on the residual limb. Incorporation of a waterproof peg-style foot allows reasonable ambulation out of the water or in shallows (Figure 14).

Summary

Prosthetic options for sports activities are rapidly evolving, and the prosthetist is generally the best source for up-to-date information. The amputee's needs and desires should be clearly understood and the functional demands of the activity determined before the prescription is developed. In some instances, the prosthetist can design a device that supports both everyday ambulation and less demanding athletic activities. At other times, the amputee will require a prosthesis optimized for a specific activity. Using a prosthesis for activities that it was not designed to accommodate can cause physical injury to the amputee as well as premature structural failure of the device. A properly designed prosthesis can substantially expand the opportunities for physical fitness and personal reward for many persons with amputations, allowing them to engage safely in a broader range of activities.

References

1. Pate RR, Pratt M, Blair SN, et al: Physical activity and public health: A recommendation from the Centers for Disease Control and Prevention and the American College of Sports Medicine. *JAMA* 1995;273:402-407.

2. *Healthy People 2000: National Health Promotion and Disease Prevention Objectives.* Washington, DC, US Public Health Service Department of Health and Human Services, 1991 DHHS Pub No PHS 91=50212.

3. Physical activity and cardiovascular health: NIH Consensus Development Panel on Physical Activity and Cardiovascular Health. *JAMA* 1996;276: 241-246.

4. Physical Activity and Health: A report of the Surgeon General. Atlanta, GA: U.S. Department of Health and Human Services, Centers for Disease Control and Prevention, National Center for Chronic Disease Prevention and Health Promotion, The President's Council on Physical Fitness and Sports, 1996. Available at http://www.cdc.gov/nccdphp/sgr/sgr.htm. Accessed May 19, 2004.

5. Williams MA: Cardiovascular risk-factor reduction in elderly patients with cardiac disease. *Phys Ther* 1996; 76:469-480.

6. Hahn RA, Teutsch SM, Rothenberg RB, Marks JS: Excess deaths from nine chronic diseases in the United States, 1986. *JAMA* 1990;264:2654-2659.

7. Kochersberger G, McConnell E, Kuchibhatla MN, Pieper C: The reliability, validity, and stability of a measure of physical activity in the elderly. *Arch Phys Med Rehabil* 1996;77: 793-795.

8. Kegel B: Physical fitness: Sports and recreation for those with lower limb amputation or impairment. *J Rehab Res Dev Clin Suppl* 1985;1:1-125.

9. Pinzur MS, Gold J, Schwartz D, Gross N: Energy demands for walking in dysvascular amputees as related to the level of amputation. *Orthopedics* 1992; 15:1033-1036.

10. Burkett B, Smeathers J, Barker T: Optimizing the trans-femoral prosthetic alignment for running, by lowering the knee joint. *Prosthet Orthot Int* 2001;25:210-219.

11. Coleman KL, Smith DG, Boone DA, Joseph AW, Del Aquila MA: Step activity monitor: Long-term, continuous recording of ambulatory function. *J Rehabil Res Dev* 1999;36:8-18.

12. Donatelli R: *The Biomechanics of the Foot and Ankle.* Philadelphia, PA, FA Davis, 1990, pp 9-27.

13. Bennett L, Kavner D, Lee BK, Trainor FA: Shear vs pressure as causative factors in skin blood flow occlusion. *Arch Phys Med Rehabil* 1979;60:309-314.

14. Sanders JE, Daly CH, Burgess EM: Interface shear stresses during ambulation with a below knee prosthetic limb. *J Rehabil Res Dev* 1992;29:1-8.

15. Sanders JE, Dickson L, Dralle A, Okumura R: Interface pressures and shear stress at thirteen socket sites on two persons with transtibial amputation. *J Rehabil Res Dev* 1997;1:19-33.

16. Lehmann JF, Price R, Fergason J, Okumura R, Koon G: Effect of prosthesis resonant frequency on metabolic efficiency in trans-tibial amputees. *J Rehabil Res Dev R&D Progress Reports* 1999.

17. Buckley JG: Sprint kinematics of athletes with lower limb amputations. *Arch Phys Med Rehabil* 1999;80: 501-508.

18. Enoka RM, Miller DI, Burgess EM: Below knee amputee running gait. *Am J Phys Med* 1982;61:66-84.

19. Mizuno N, Aoyama T, Nakajima A, Kasahara T, Takami K: Functional evaluation by gait analysis of various ankle foot assemblies used by below knee amputees. *Prosthet Orthot Int* 1992;10:174-182.

20. Carroll K: Adaptive prosthetics for the lower extremity. *Foot Ankle Clin* 2001; 6:371-386.

21. Burgess EM, Hittenberger DA, Forsgren SM, Lindh D: The Seattle prosthetic foot: A design for active sports. Preliminary studies. *Orthot Prosthet* 1983;37:25-31.

22. Hafner BJ, Sanders JE, Czerniecki J, Fergason J: Energy storage and return prostheses: Does patient perception correlate with biomechanical analysis? *Clin Biomech* 2002;17:325-344.

23. Lehman JF, Price R, Okumura R, Questad K, Lateur B, Níegretot A: Mass and mass distribution of below knee prostheses: Effect on gait efficacy and self selected walking speed. *Arch Phys Med Rehabil* 1998;79:162-168.

Chapter 51

Physical Therapy for Sports and Recreation

Robert S. Gailey, PhD, PT

Introduction

Advances in surgical procedures, postamputation rehabilitation, and prosthetic technology have afforded amputees of all levels more opportunities to participate in a variety of recreational and competitive sports. Surgical procedures have evolved, encouraging surgeons to consider optimum preservation of muscle function by myodesis, preserve bone length, and create end-bearing residual limbs when possible, improving patients' athletic capabilities. For example, athletes with knee disarticulations have repeatedly demonstrated greater speed in sprint racing than have transfemoral amputees. Now the consensus among those involved in track sports is that maintaining bone length and preserving or restoring muscle insertions, coupled with end-bearing capabilities, offers a sprinter with knee disarticulation a clear advantage. The same is true for a Syme ankle disarticulation compared with a transtibial amputation.

Rehabilitation methods have also progressed, including gait training techniques that have improved walking efficiency.[1,2] Moreover, functional progression techniques offer amputees the ability, through multidirectional strengthening exercises, to reeducate the neuromuscular system to better control movement in all planes. Closed kinetic-chain activities may also improve control of the prosthesis within the socket. Speed training permits amputees of all ages to vary their cadence and negotiate obstacles. Active amputees demand restoration beyond simple walking, embracing the goals of recreational and, occasionally, competitive sports. Rehabilitation must meet the challenge of restoring the amputee's physical capabilities to a level that permits maximum use of the prosthesis.

Prostheses available today easily eclipse the limited choices of the past. Improved socket designs permit improved muscular function within the socket. Socket interface systems reduce the compressive and shear forces, thereby increasing comfort and reducing the risk of skin irritation. More responsive knee systems permit increased mobility for transfemoral amputees. The wide variety of foot/ankle systems allows amputees a choice of components that have the potential to improve performance, whether the goal is to run faster, improve agility with multidirectional sports, or adapt to uneven ground with a firm footing for sports such as golf.

In addition, many specialty prostheses are available, either from manufacturers or on a custom basis for specific sports. Many amputees like to swim but have different needs for getting into and out of the water. For example, scuba divers do not need the ability to walk, whereas recreational swimmers may want to walk around the pool deck. Mountain climbers typically have needs specific to the type of climbing and level of amputation. Usually, the demand for these specialty devices is so small that custom prostheses must be fabricated. Fortunately, amputees new to a sport can access valuable print and electronic information about prosthetic designs that have worked for others.

Exercise Activities

Exercise activities can be divided into four distinct categories: (1) restorative, (2) regimented, (3) leisure, and (4) competitive. Many recreational sports enjoyed by amputees, such as walking, swimming, cycling, or golf, encompass all four exercise categories. As an example of a *restorative* exercise, walking is frequently used for rehabilitation after an injury or illness. Having a patient ambulate in the hospital room, down the hall, or in the rehabilitation center to increase strength and endurance are examples of walking as a restorative exercise. *Regimented* exercise is commonly performed after discharge from rehabilitation as a means to maintain fitness at home or a health club. Exercise walking may include work on a treadmill for 30 minutes, three times a week, at 60% to 70% of maximal oxygen uptake[3] or at a target heart rate to monitor progress or to maintain desired levels of physical conditioning.

Leisure exercise is often used to relax and reduce stress, often while simultaneously socializing with family and friends. An example is a group that walks together while chatting. *Competitive* exercise typically requires more intensive training than the previous three categories of exercise, and the participants have clearly established goals. Race walking is an example of competitive exercise.

To one degree or another, all amputees experience restorative exercise as they work through their rehabilitation. More motivated individuals will continue with some form of regimented exercise for a period of time after discharge from the hospital, whether at a rehabilitation center, a fitness center, or independently at home. The goal of the rehabilitation team should be to assist the amputee in the transition to leisure exercise or, in some cases, competitive sports. This does not mean that the team is involved every step of the way; rather, it is the team's responsibility to educate and motivate the amputee. Education includes the prescription of a personalized regimented exercise program that includes precautions about activities that could lead to injury as well as contacts for support groups and appropriate special-interest organizations. Equally important is motivating the amputees to meet long-term goals by inspiring them to pursue a lifelong program of leisure activities or recreational sports.

Younger amputees usually return more successfully to their premorbid level of activity than do elderly amputees. Health care workers tend to gain satisfaction from seeing a young person return to sports after a debilitating incident. Unfortunately, the same stimulus is not always present with older patients, even though these patients generally perceive their health to be good.[4] Preconceived notions about a particular age group's limitations and abilities are frequently an obstacle to be overcome by health care providers responsible for setting long-term rehabilitative goals. If the rehabilitation team establishes goals that fall short of the amputee's actual capabilities or exclude the amputee from higher-level tasks, the amputee's body image, activity level, or motivation to pursue healthful activities may be jeopardized.[5-7]

Recreational Pursuits of the Lower Limb Amputee

Gailey and associates[8,9] reported the results of a questionnaire exploring four topic areas: (1) the amputee profile, (2) prosthetic management, (3) degree of participation in recreational activities, and (4) the amputee's perception of rehabilitative needs and suggested improvements for the rehabilitation team. A total of 1,214 questionnaires were analyzed from 41 individuals with hip disarticulations, 592 transfemoral amputees, 492 transtibial amputees, 23 individuals with Syme ankle disarticulations, 43 bilateral transtibial amputees, and 23 bilateral transfemoral amputees. The mean age of the total sample population was 48 years. This population does not reflect the usual distribution of amputation etiologies in that 58% of all respondents lost their limb because of trauma, 20% from vascular disease, 13% from tumor, and 4% because of congenital deficiencies.[10-12] This differs from conventional estimates, which suggest that 70% to 90% of amputations in Western countries are related to vascular disease, 4% are tumor related, and 4% are congenital in nature, with the balance (up to approximately 20%) the result of trauma. Another bias in the study is that those who participated in recreational activities were more likely to complete the questionnaire, suggesting that traumatic amputees are more inclined to participate in recreational activities than are amputees who lose a limb because of vascular disease.

In this population, approximately 60% of previously active amputees returned to recreational activities within the first year after amputation. There was no appreciable difference between age groups. Thirty percent of patients attributed the delay in returning to activity to prosthetic fitting and comfort problems, prolonged recovery, phantom pain, and residual limb pain, although only 13% found that discomfort interfered with their return to activities. Only 20% of all respondents experienced no delay in their return to activities.

The recreational activities most commonly enjoyed by elderly amputees are golf, swimming, fishing, walking, dancing, boating, bowling, and bicycling. The most popular recreational activities for amputees younger than 49 years are almost identical. A comparison was made with the National Sporting Goods Association's (NSGA) annual survey of 20,000 Americans regarding their participation in sports.[13] The 1991 NSGA report indicates that Americans age 55 years and older ranked the following sports in order of popularity: walking, fishing, swimming, bicycling, golf, exercise with equipment, bowling, and camping (Table 1). Not surprisingly, amputees and nonamputees enjoy exactly the same recreational sport activities, regardless of the level of amputation. Running is not within the top 10 activities with either group, yet it is the one skill most amputees long to possess.

Participation by amputees in recreational activities across the life span varies only slightly from that of the total population, with 76% reporting participation and 20% reporting none. The total number of days per week that participation in recreational activities occurs indicates that, regardless of age, those who do participate maintain a weekly frequency similar to that of the general population, with 60% participating 1 to 4 days per week and 14% participating 5 to 7 days per week.

In most cases, these sports are not taxing to the residual limb and can be enjoyed by most younger and older amputees without placing the skin at risk. In some instances, minor adaptations by the amputee may be necessary, depending on the type of ampu-

TABLE 1 Recreational Activities in Order of Participation Popularity

All amputees	Amputees 0-19 years[9]	Amputees 20-29 years	Amputees 30-39 years	Amputees 40-49 years	Amputees 50+ years	All able-bodied[13]	Able-bodied 55+ years[13]
Swimming	Swimming	Swimming	Swimming	Swimming	Golf	Walking	Walking
Golf	Fishing	Dancing	Fishing	Golf	Swimming	Swimming	Fishing
Fishing	Walking	Fishing	Walking	Fishing	Fishing	Bicycling	Swimming
Walking	Bicycling	Boating	Dancing	Dancing	Walking	Camping	Bicycling
Dancing	Bowling	Bicycling	Boating	Walking	Dancing	Fishing	Golf
Boating	Dancing	Walking	Bicycling	Boating	Boating	Bowling	Exercise with equipment
Bicycling	Boating	Golf	Golf	Bicycling	Bowling	Exercise with equipment	Bowling
Bowling	Basketball	Snow skiing	Snow skiing	Snow skiing	Bicycling	Basketball	Camping

tation and the level of athleticism at which the sport is played. The reasons for limiting participation in recreational activities were similar across all age groups. The inability to run and to jump, decreased endurance, increased fatigue, decreased balance, and reduced speed of locomotion were also problems found to impede competition on an equal basis with nonamputees, as was the inability to regain the level of skill achieved before amputation.

The results from the amputee survey suggested that older amputees may be more willing to return to prior activities than are younger amputees. The amputee survey also noted that three responses were given with similar frequency: embarrassment, lack of instruction, and lack of supportive organizations to join. These results go on to suggest that middle-aged amputees may find recreational activities intimidating, but that they acquire a degree of comfort through instruction and working with others in groups. Older amputees, however, may be more willing to return to prior activities independently, with less fear of embarrassment.[8,9]

One common problem for all amputees, especially the elderly, is difficulty with their prosthesis during physical activity. Thirty-seven percent of amputees experience prosthetic problems all of the time during activity. As amputees age, this percentage increases to approximately 50%. Only 13% of amputees never experience any prosthetic problem during physical activity.[8,9] Many amputees view their prosthesis as part of their athletic equipment and learn to anticipate problems. Persistent prosthetic problems, however, can often be reduced with a variety of adaptations or ingenious modifications to meet the demands of a particular sport.

The most common prosthetic problem is skin irritation or breakdown. Approximately 55% of all amputees experience skin problems with activities of daily living or during rigorous activity, the only difference being the frequency with which the problems occur. Interestingly, 26% of amputees experienced a decrease in skin irritation when they changed from a traditional to a contemporary socket design. This may indicate that improved socket design is having a positive effect on the superficial shear force at the limb-socket interface.[8,9]

Support and motivation are obviously key ingredients for getting people involved in leisure activities. Sixty percent of the amputees reported that family and friends were encouraging about their activity level. Unfortunately, when participants were asked how informative members of the medical profession were about recreational activities, the results were disappointing. Only 6% of physicians were perceived by the respondents to be extremely informative, 19% somewhat informative, and 51% uninformative. Prosthetists were perceived as more knowledgeable, with 15% being extremely informative, 32% somewhat informative, and 31% uninformative. Amputees who received physical therapy reported that only 6% of physical therapists were extremely informative, 14% were somewhat informative, and 24% were uninformative.[8,9]

Of all the questions asked, the one that may best represent the positive attitude of many amputees is: When participating in organized sports with nonamputees, should allowances be made? Fifty-four percent responded no, and 30% said yes. This response may be extrapolated to mean that amputees do not want the rules changed, they just want quality prostheses, instructional training, and local athletic organizations that permit them to compete or participate on an equal footing. In fact, the suggestions from the amputees to improve functional activity included better prostheses (60%), amputee instructors (35%), instructional literature (24%), and additional supportive sports organizations (18%).[8,9]

Running

Although running is a lower ranked activity, amputees list the inability to run well as the single most common

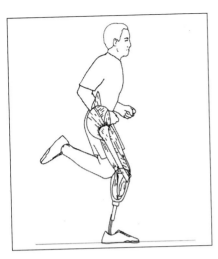

Figure 1 Transtibial amputee in the absorption phase of running. (Copyright © Advanced Rehabilitation Therapy, Inc, Miami, FL, 2002. Illustrator Frank Angulo.)

factor limiting participation in recreational activities; it is their most desired skill. That running is a prerequisite skill for sports is a misconception, however. Most sports either require very little running or can be participated in if some minor adaptation is made. Many amputees who do not have a strong desire to run for sport or leisure may have an interest in learning how to run simply for the peace of mind that comes with the knowledge that they can move quickly to avoid a threatening situation.[14] Rarely, if ever, is running taught in rehabilitation. Running, as with all gait training and advanced skills, takes time and practice to master. Amputees should be exposed to basic running skills during rehabilitation so that they can pursue running if they wish.

Learning to run is not an easy task for the lower limb amputee, whether or not the person is athletically inclined. Most nonamputee runners intuitively link running mechanics and the economy of running. As a result of training, most nonamputee runners are able to adopt a running style that is most economical for their own personal needs. The amputee runner, however, is at a disadvantage when attempting to develop an efficient running style because learning to use a prosthesis is not as intuitive as running with the anatomic limb. It therefore becomes important for clinicians and coaches as well as amputee athletes to become familiar with the biomechanics of running for able-bodied runners as well as for amputee runners.

Running is most often described in terms of speed, but the skills are much more complex. Because describing every type of running would be too comprehensive for this text, the focus will be on the skills for the novice amputee runner and present some insight into the techniques used by accomplished amputee runners.

Biomechanics of Running

The running cycle is divided into stance and swing phases. During stance phase, the period from initial contact to midstance is referred to as the absorption phase, when the body decelerates as the runner contacts the ground. From midstance to toe-off is known as the acceleration or propulsion phase, when the body's acceleration carries over to initial swing as the limb enters the swing phase. From midswing to terminal swing, the limb begins to decelerate as it returns to the absorption phase. The beginning and end of each swing phase has a period of double-float, when neither limb is in contact with the ground while the body is moving through space. As a result, the stance phase accounts for less than 50% of the running gait cycle. As speed increases, the percentage of the cycle represented by the stance phase decreases, becoming as little as 20% in sprinters.[15-17]

Absorption Phase

From initial contact to midstance is regarded as the absorption phase (Figure 1), when the lower limb acts as a shock absorber for the body, thereby reducing the considerable ground-reaction forces passing upward through the limb, which can be two to three times greater than body weight.[18] As the foot strikes the ground, a backward force is generated by the strong contraction of the hip extensor muscles while the hip abductors provide the necessary pelvic stability.[19] Muscular stabilization, coupled with joint motion, creates a biomechanical spring that reduces the effects of the ground-reaction forces.[20,21]

When amputees run, there is no peak in ground-reaction force for the prosthetic limb. This reduction in ground-reaction force suggests that amputees both absorb and generate less energy with their prosthesis than do runners with intact limbs. The reduction in energy generated by the prosthetic limb could be the result of a more passive use of the limb, the absorption of forces by the soft tissue encapsulated within the socket, or the presence of an isometric or stabilizing contraction by the muscles.[22]

As the transtibial amputee strikes the ground with the prosthetic limb, a backward force is instantly created by the prosthetic side hip musculature. This generates two to three times more work than the contralateral limb, partly to help move the body over the stationary foot as well as to compensate for the loss of active plantar flexion at the ankle.[23,24]

One notable difference between novice and well-trained transtibial amputee runners is that novice runners have a reduction in knee flexion during the absorption phase. With proper training, strength, and adequate residual limb length, knee flexion comparable to that with an intact limb can be achieved with the prosthetic limb.

The length of the residual limb and the amount of muscle mass retained play important roles in determining the transfemoral amputee's running potential. This has become most apparent in recent years as knee disarticulation amputee runners have become extremely successful in competition. The additional power potentially available to knee disarticulation runners should not overshadow the need for athletic ability and training.

Acceleration Phase

From midstance to terminal stance and through initial swing is referred to as the acceleration phase of the running cycle (Figure 2), when the body moves from stance phase energy absorption to acceleration or generation of speed. At this point, most of the forward propulsion of the body comes from the contralateral swing limb and the arms.

The well-trained transtibial amputee can achieve flexion-extension patterns similar to those of nonamputee runners during stance. Contracting of the quadriceps and the calf muscles creates adequate knee stability. Many believe that the J-shaped design of the Flex-Foot (Ossur, Aliso Viejo, CA), which permits controlled dorsiflexion, assists significantly with control of knee flexion. In fact, the Flex-Foot has been found to provide a more normal pattern of muscle activity in the hip and knee extensors throughout the stance phase.[25]

The transfemoral amputee's hip remains in a neutral position and is related to the extended prosthetic knee. To continue advancement over the prosthetic stance limb, the hamstrings and gluteus maximus promote rapid hip extension.[25] The amount of ankle dorsiflexion present is a direct result of prosthetic foot design and alignment. To date, the Flex-Sprint (Ossur, Aliso Viejo, CA) design has delivered the maximum mechanical energy return for transfemoral runners.

As the hip reaches maximum extension, all movements are passive during terminal stance except for those of the hip adductors, which contract to stabilize the pelvis. The peak plantar flexion is the result of the rapid movement of the tibia over the foot, creating a rigid lever in the foot to release the elastic energy. During nonamputee running, more than half the elastic energy is stored in two springs, the Achilles tendon and the arch of the foot.[26]

The elastic energy found in the anatomic foot has been replicated to

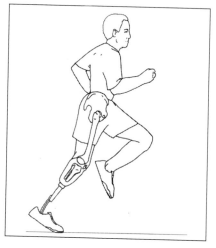

Figure 2 Transtibial amputee in the acceleration phase of running. *(Copyright © Advanced Rehabilitation Therapy, Inc, Miami, FL, 2002. Illustrator Frank Angulo.)*

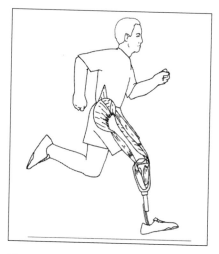

Figure 3 Transtibial amputee in the deceleration phase of running. *(Copyright © Advanced Rehabilitation Therapy, Inc, Miami, FL, 2002. Illustrator Frank Angulo.)*

varying degrees in prosthetic feet. Dynamic feet have been found to generate two to three times more elastic energy than a solid ankle-cushion heel (SACH) foot.[22] In 1991, Czerniecki and associates[22] defined spring efficiency as the amount of energy generated divided by the amount of energy absorbed. The spring efficiency of the SACH foot was found to be 31%, whereas that of the Seattle foot (Seattle Systems, Inc, Poulsbo, WA) was 52% and that of the Flex-Foot was an impressive 82%. In comparison, the human foot has 241% spring efficiency because of the additional concentric plantar flexion contraction of the triceps surae.

At terminal stance, the transtibial amputee runner's total muscle work on the prosthetic side is half that measured in the intact limb and in nonamputee runners. This is not too surprising, considering that the plantar flexors are absent. To compensate, the amputee's intact swing-phase leg increases energy transfer by about 75%.[27]

Hip flexion is initiated by a powerful contraction of the hip flexors. Stability with a steady line of progression of the limb is maintained by stabilizing contractions of the hip abductor and adductor muscles. The mechani-

cal work of the hip, or the energy generated by the intact hip flexors, was found to be more than twice the magnitude of that generated in nonamputee runners, with the work of the hip on the prosthetic side being somewhat greater than normal but not as great as on the intact side.[23]

Deceleration Phase

In the deceleration phase (Figure 3), as the foot prepares to strike the ground, the thigh muscles are preparing to propel the body forward while also absorbing the ground-reactive forces. The hip extensors work eccentrically to decelerate the thigh and leg during late swing and extend the hip prior to, and immediately upon, initial contact. The hip abductors and adductors contract to stabilize the pelvis as the foot approaches initial contact.[20]

Transtibial amputee runners tend to have lower angular velocities at peak flexion and extension as well as maximal hip and knee flexion angles. In addition, premature extension of the knee during swing is commonly observed. Socket designs, coupled with suspension requirements, have been identified as probable causes for the reduction in peak knee flexion, which, in turn, limits hip flexion.[25]

Creating a transtibial socket that provides both stance-phase stability and swing-phase mobility has been a difficult task.

The transtibial amputee contracts the muscles of the lower limb in a pattern identical to the nonamputee during terminal swing. The knee should be slightly flexed, and, as stated earlier, there will be a reduction in forces as the foot prepares to strike the ground.[23]

The transfemoral amputee must land with the prosthetic knee extended. Initiating a backward force before initial contact will not only accelerate the body forward but also ensure that the knee remains in extension. Although it is unnecessary, many transfemoral amputee runners also adopt an extended trunk posture as the prosthetic foot prepares to strike the ground.

Trunk and Arm Swing

For amputees, symmetry of arm movement is extremely important, yet often difficult to master. They must make a concentrated effort to restore a symmetric arm swing, especially as speed increases, when the legs have a tendency to lose symmetry of movement.

Transfemoral amputees have a tendency to increase abduction of the prosthetic side arm, especially when the prosthetic lower limb is abducted. The adverse positions of both the leg and the arm create opposing forces that tend to impede forward momentum and increase the metabolic requirement. Likewise, poor medial/lateral socket stability will require additional effort by the prosthetic-side arm and facilitate unwanted trunk movement.

Running Skills

Individuals with Syme ankle disarticulations and transtibial amputees can achieve the same running biomechanics as able-bodied runners if they emphasize the following: (1) At ground contact the prosthetic limb hip should be flexed when moving toward extension, the knee should be flexed, and the prosthetic foot should be dorsiflexed. Knee flexion not only permits greater shock absorption but also creates a backward force between the ground and the foot to provide additional forward momentum. (2) As the center of gravity is transferred over the prosthesis during stance phase, the ipsilateral arm should be fully forward (shoulder flexed 60° to 90°) while the contralateral arm is back (shoulder extended). Extreme arm movement can be difficult for the amputee concerned with maintaining balance. (3) During the acceleration phase, the hip should be forcefully driving down and back through the prosthesis as the knee extends. If the prosthetic foot has dynamic elastic response, the force produced by hip extension should deflect the keel so that the prosthetic foot provides additional push-off. (4) During the forward swing and float phase, the hip should be rapidly flexing, elevating the thigh. The arms should again be opposing the advancing lower limb, with the ipsilateral arm backward and the contralateral arm forward. (5) During the late deceleration phase or foot descent, the hip should be flexed and beginning to extend as the knee is rapidly extending and reaching forward for a full stride.

Traditionally, transfemoral amputees and individuals with knee disarticulations run with a period of double support on the sound limb during the running cycle, commonly referred to as the hop-skip running gait. The typical running gait cycle begins with a long stride with the prosthetic leg, followed by a shorter stride with the sound leg. To give the prosthetic leg sufficient time to advance, the sound leg takes a small hop as the prosthetic limb clears the ground and moves forward to complete the stride. The speed that a transfemoral amputee can achieve will be limited because every time either foot makes contact with the ground, the forces of the foot are traveling forward, and the reaction force of the ground must be in a backward or opposite direction (Newton's third law). The result is that each time the foot contacts the ground, forward momentum is decreased. In other words, with every stride, the amputee is slowing down when running with the hop-skip gait.

Most transfemoral amputees achieve the ability to run leg-over-leg through training and working with knowledgeable coaches. The transfemoral amputee takes a full stride with the prosthetic leg, followed by a typically shorter stride with the sound leg. With training, equal stride length and stance time may be achieved. This running pattern is a more natural gait in which the double support phase of the sound limb is eliminated and forward momentum may be maintained by both legs. Initially, other problems that may occur include excessive vaulting off the sound limb to ensure ground clearance of the prosthetic limb, decreased pelvic and trunk rotation, decreased and asymmetric arm swing, and excessive trunk extension. Again, with training, many of these deviations will decrease and possibly be eliminated.

The leg-over-leg running style does permit the transfemoral amputee to run faster for short distances but at a greater metabolic cost. Although leg-over-leg is preferred, the hop-skip method is often more easily taught and is less demanding physically. When the sole purpose of running instruction is to teach the individual to move quickly in a safe and sure manner, the hop-skip method is most frequently suggested.

The Five Basic Steps of Amputee Running

Learning how to run using a prosthesis can be very challenging, yet when simplified into a series of basic elements it can be much easier to learn. Table 2 describes the five basic steps that have made it possible for hundreds of amputees with all levels of amputation to relearn the skill of running and have enabled them to benefit from the ability to move rapidly when necessary.

TABLE 2 The Five Basic Steps of Amputee Running

Step 1

Prosthetic Trust

The runner must first gain trust in the prosthesis and develop confidence that the prosthetic limb will be there and will not collapse when it strikes the ground. This is accomplished by reaching out with the prosthetic limb and landing squarely on the foot. The runner is taught to ignore everything else, knowing that the prosthetic limb is reliable.

Step 2

Backward Extension

The runner reaches out with the prosthetic foot during swing. Just as the prosthetic limb strikes the ground, the runner pulls the prosthetic leg back forcefully, creating a backward force which propels the runner forward. The ground also produces a forward accelerating force on the body. This movement has two effects: First, it propels the body forward with increased speed. Second, it produces the power to shift the body's weight over the prosthesis and fully load the prosthetic foot, resulting in maximum prosthetic foot performance as the forefoot is loaded

Step 3

Sound Limb Stride

The focus shifts to the sound limb. The runner concentrates on taking a longer stride with the sound limb, easily accomplished by continuing to pull down and back through the prosthetic limb. Pulling back during the prosthetic foot's initial contact with the ground initiates the movement pattern. The runner continues to extend the hip by pulling down and back into the socket. This generates more power and a stronger push-off with the prosthetic limb, which enables the sound limb to reach out to complete a full stride.

Step 4

Stride Symmetry

This phase is designed to decrease the enormous effort being exerted, and to simply relax and jog a little. The runner chooses a comfortable jogging pace that produces an equal stride for both limbs. There is no concern for the arms. Attention is focused on maintaining stability over the prosthetic limb using the muscles of the hips to create equal and relaxed strides.

Step 5

Arm Carriage

The runner focuses on arm swing. The arms and legs move in opposition to each other during gait, so as the right leg moves forward, so will the left arm. The elbows should flex to about 90° and the hands should be loosely closed and rise to just below chin level when brought forward. Just as in walking, arm swing is the result of trunk rotation as the trunk and pelvis rotate in opposition to each other for balance, momentum, and economy of effort.

Adapted with permission from Gailey RS: The Essentials of Lower Limb Amputee Running and Sports Training. Miami, FL, Advanced Rehabilitation Therapy, Inc, 2004.

Initially, for safety reasons, it is strongly suggested that amputees work with skilled clinicians and use a gait belt to soften the impact of a fall.

After mastering the five basic steps of running, amputees should be ready to put all the individual elements of running together. They should relax and think about only a couple of elements of running with each pass. Many long distance runners augment their endurance training program with low-impact activities, such as swimming, stationary biking, or stair climbing. In time, runners will develop their own comfortable running style, depending on the sports or recreational activities chosen.

Running can be learned on just about any type of prosthesis. Initially, the type of prosthetic foot is not critical. However, if amputees decide that running is going to be a part of their lifestyle, they should discuss the available options with their prosthetist. The same principles of running apply, regardless of the prosthetic foot and knee systems; however, prosthetic feet

and knees designed for running can reduce effort and improve performance.

Prostheses for Athletics
Prosthetic Components for Sports

The prosthetic options for recreational and competitive athletes have grown tremendously through the years. Unfortunately, the literature offers very little insight into the functional differences between appliances and the impact that they have on performance. Part of the process of training is learning how to maximize the use of prosthetic components. In particular, prosthetic knees and feet can be tremendous assets to an athlete but, unfortunately, their influence is often overlooked. Once a foundation of strength and endurance is established and use of a prosthesis is understood, a training program to improve or maintain athletic performance should be designed to meet the specific needs of each athlete.

Socket Design and Suspension Systems

The use of secondary suspension systems is common among athletes. Suction is the primary suspension system used today. Suction suspension can be created through a variety of components including pull-in suction sockets, internal roll-on locking liners, and one-way suction valves. No specific method of suspension has been shown to be superior, so this remains a clinical decision while materials and fitting techniques continue to evolve.

Socket design and suspension choice are frequently determined through trial and error until a comfortable fit is achieved. Generally speaking, most recreational athletes will find that the socket design used for their walking prosthesis will serve them well for most sports. It certainly is appropriate to use the walking prosthesis as a starting point when designing an athletic prosthesis. After

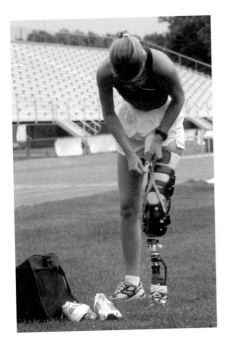

Figure 4 A transtibial athlete who has incorporated a rigid knee orthosis into a prosthesis to protect against excessive medial/lateral or rotation motion. (*Courtesy of Advanced Rehabilitation Therapy, Inc, Miami, FL.*)

the athlete participates in the chosen sport, modifications may be made according to comfort and performance. For example, transfemoral amputees who are recreational cyclists characteristically prefer to have the proximal brim trimmed down, especially medially, to reduce rubbing along the groin. They require little additional suspension, as losing the prosthesis is not likely because they are in constant contact with the foot pedal. Likewise, transtibial amputee cyclists reduce the brim and use a minimum of suspension to permit maximal knee flexion. Transfemoral amputees who are competitive cyclists do not wear a prosthesis during races because, if a prosthesis is used, they would have to compete against transtibial amputee cyclists.

Other sports may require an extremely tight fit for prostheses. For instance, some competitive sprinters choose a socket design that is extremely tight to prevent unnecessary motion within the socket and reduce the need for secondary suspension. This type of prosthesis can be worn

for only a short period of time and is not very comfortable. Fortunately, roll-on suspension sleeves and better suction have dramatically reduced the need for such a tight fit for most athletes.

Socket design should also include consideration of volume changes over time. Long-distance runners, depending on the individual, may experience residual limb swelling, loss of volume, or very little volume change. Stopping to add socks or change liners during a race may not be feasible; therefore, experimenting with socket size and liner materials may be necessary. Secondary suspension systems can augment socket designs by preventing excessive pistoning and controlling unwanted movement that could result when volume changes occur.

The type of secondary suspension selected is often unique to each athlete. As a rule, most athletes prefer to wear as few additions as possible because of weight and restriction of movement. External suspension sleeves have become very common for transtibial amputee athletes because they assist with suction suspension. They can be excessively warm, however, increasing perspiration within the socket as well as restricting knee flexion as the material bunches in the popliteal area. Supracondylar cuffs are still worn by many athletes as a lightweight secondary suspension, but these cuffs can also feel somewhat restrictive. Occasionally, transtibial amputees wear waist belts with inverted Y-straps more for psychological security than actual suspension. Transtibial amputee athletes who have knee instability may want to add a rigid knee orthosis to protect against excessive medial/lateral or rotation motion (Figure 4). Rigid knee orthoses have replaced the thigh corset with metal uprights in most cases because of the reduced weight, stronger material, improved ventilation, ease of donning, and increased freedom for muscle contraction.

Transfemoral amputee athletes will typically use a flexible Silesian belt to aid in suspension and rotational con-

trol. The other alternative is a total elastic suspension (TES) belt, which can be used as needed because it simply slips over the socket and around the waist. The TES belt tends to be warmer and a little more restrictive than the Silesian belt, but it can be removed.

Socket Stability

Stability in the socket may be established surgically with combined myoplasty/myodesis procedures that stabilize the muscles by suturing muscle to muscle and muscle to bone. In addition to creating anatomic stability, some prosthetic socket designs not only create stability but also help maintain normal bony alignment, thereby placing the residual muscles in a functionally tensioned position so they can provide maximal contraction to aid prosthetic control in everyday activities. Although the benefits of surgical procedures and socket designs are frequently debated, most authorities agree that anatomically sound surgery and a well-designed socket will be of some advantage to the amputee. Nonetheless, unless the amputee learns to use the muscles effectively within the socket, there will be no benefit from advances in surgery and socket design.

Stability within the socket is essential to quality performance. Stability requires not only strength but also the ability to control movement in all directions and at varying speeds. Learning to use the remaining muscles within the socket in a way that allows control of forces placed on the prosthesis from any direction will assist tremendously in all activities requiring speed, power, and agility. A training program designed to improve stability within the socket should focus on joint proprioception, where the speed of contraction, not the maximal force of the contraction, becomes the emphasis of the exercises.

The following exercises are designed to build strength and power in multiple directions in a low-impact fashion, thereby reducing the stress on the residual limb and the chance

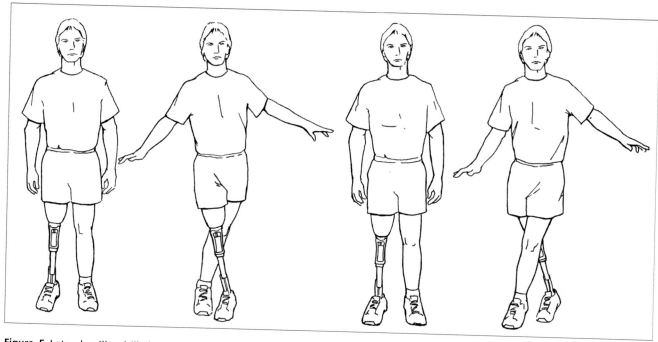

Figure 5 Lateral agility drill. *(Copyright © Advanced Rehabilitation Therapy, Inc, Miami, FL, 1989. Illustrator Frank Angulo.)*

of injury. The exercises can improve the overall abilities of amputees of any functional level and allow them to get the most benefit from their surgical procedure and socket design.

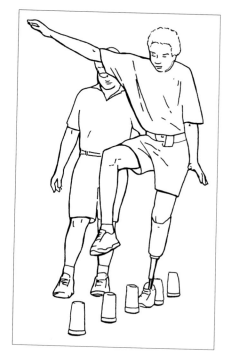

Figure 6 Cup walking drill. *(Copyright © Advanced Rehabilitation Therapy, Inc, Miami, FL, 2002. Illustrator Frank Angulo.)*

Exercises for Maximizing Stability Within the Socket

Lateral Agility Drills

Lateral agility drills[28] are one of the strategies necessary for moving in different directions. The amputee simply moves sideways for a predetermined distance, starting with slow steps and picking up speed as the movement becomes easier. Athletes who participate in sports that require lateral movements regularly, such as tennis, basketball, and softball, should practice at speeds consistent with their sport. Once speed and balance have been established, the drills can include the use of a racquet or ball, adding more complex skills such as swinging the racquet or passing the ball during each repetition.

Crossing one leg in front of the other also assists in learning movement strategies in multiple directions (Figure 5). Care must be taken not to bump the prosthetic knee with the sound limb, which can cause the prosthetic knee to collapse. Rapidly creating a backward force within the socket with hip musculature will help

to maintain stability. As skill level improves, braiding or placing one leg in front of the other and then behind on the subsequent step will help the athlete develop the speed of residual limb movement and stability necessary to move confidently in any direction. To improve dynamic balance, the athlete should perform braiding with trunk rotation in which the trunk moves in opposition to pelvic motion. As agility improves, the athlete can vary the speed during the lateral agility drills to approximate game conditions and further improve prosthetic control in multiple directions.

Cup Walking Drills

A cup walking drill[28] is a challenging, low-impact exercise that has been shown to be extremely beneficial in helping amputees learn to control their prosthesis. Five to 10 disposable cups should be placed in a row approximately 12 to 18 in apart. Paper cups are a good choice because they crush more easily than plastic if stepped on (Figure 6). Starting at one end of the row of cups, the athlete slowly raises one leg while stepping forward so that the knee is waist high, or so that a 90° angle is formed at the hip, and then slowly returns the foot to the floor while stepping over the cup. Using the alternate leg, the procedure is repeated over the next cup.

When balancing over the prosthetic limb as the sound limb advances, the athlete should focus on three key elements: First, for the transfemoral amputee, only the muscles within the socket, the buttocks, and the thigh muscles on the prosthetic side are contracted. The transtibial amputee should also contract the buttocks and thigh muscles in addition to those within the socket. Second, a downward force through the socket creates maximal weight bearing within the socket. Third, the weight of the body must pass over the prosthetic foot to maintain weight over the great toe of the prosthetic foot.

One of the major benefits of this exercise is the heightened awareness of the prosthetic foot. Feeling the body weight over the foot and learning how to balance over the foot will enhance prosthetic control in a variety of activities.

A number of variations can be introduced into the cup drill. For instance, walking on a compliant or foam surface increases the need for stability within the socket of the prosthetic limb to execute the exercise exactly the way it is performed on a solid floor. The athlete needs to maintain knee stability in all directions and therefore must react faster with the muscles of the knee and hip to maintain balance. Sideways walking will further challenge the residual limb musculature and improve balance.

Backward walking is another skill that helps develop prosthetic control. Athletes should focus on the same key elements: contracting the muscles, exerting a downward and backward force within the socket, and feeling the weight progress over the prosthetic foot. Limiting any unnecessary movement from the trunk will also help.

Sports and Prosthetic Ankle/Foot Options

The choice of prosthetic feet for sports remains a clinical decision, and there are very few sports-specific prosthetic feet. The most popular sports feet are designed primarily for running. Fortunately, most sports do not require extensive running, so an everyday prosthesis with appropriate components and suspension may allow recreational amputee athletes to participate. Some people who are comfortable with their socket and/or knee system will elect to change just their prosthetic foot for certain sports. A small adapter can be prescribed to provide athletes with a quick-changing, self-aligning device to permit amputees to quickly swap prosthetic feet or knee-shin systems. Competitive athletes may have a sport-specific prosthesis, particularly for high-impact activities that accelerate wear and tear on the components.

When selecting a prosthetic ankle/foot system, it is important to discuss recreational and sports interests thoroughly because amputees will likely try to participate in their favorite sport in the first year after amputation. If the prosthetic components do not respond to the demands of the sport, chances of success will diminish, resulting in frustration and embarrassment that may keep the person from ever participating in that sport again. Many prosthetic feet are suitable for walking but are not dynamic enough for sport. As a result, when higher loads are placed on the foot, the energy is absorbed without any energy release, resulting in performance unacceptable to the amputee. Therefore, it is very important to prescribe a foot that not only permits a natural gait but also allows the amputee to participate in recreational sports. In other words, components should be prescribed that are suitable for the highest level of activity anticipated by the amputee.

During the initial evaluation, the prosthetist should explore the recreational sports in which the amputee

might develop an interest. Not all sports require ultradynamic prosthetic feet. In fact, many amputees participate in sports such as golf, bowling, shuffleboard, and boating, which require more mobility than dynamics.

Multiaxial foot systems with dynamic keels provide the advantages of a moveable ankle, whereas the elastic keel offers the benefits of a dynamic-response foot. Because of the mobility at the ankle, it is believed that some of the "energy release" generated in dynamic-response feet with moveable ankles is not as great. But a multiaxial foot/ankle system should be strongly considered for persons who walk on hills or uneven terrain, such as golfers, or those who need movement in all planes of motion, such as bowlers and shuffleboarders, or those who require motion at the ankle for standing balance, such as boaters.

The source and the degree of mobility available in prosthetic feet have changed tremendously through the years. No longer does motion come only from the ankle, although multiaxial ankles are still very popular. Other options include the "split-toe"—a divide running the length of the foot plate—permitting motions that replicate ankle inversion and eversion without absorbing as much elastic energy as rubber bumpers in an ankle joint. The advantage is motion without much loss of dynamic properties. Another design that has become very popular uses elastomer or other types of hard rubber sandwiched between primary and secondary foot plates. Once again, frontal plane and some transverse plane ankle motion can be mimicked while maintaining foot dynamics. Other foot designs incorporate shock absorbers and rotators in the shin above the traditional ankle location, providing long-axis rotation. These shock absorbers and rotators can be coupled with any number of foot designs.

The degree of motion required should be determined by the everyday environment that an amputee must negotiate and the recreational activities in which he or she chooses to participate. A golfer who lives in a hilly part of the country will need a fairly large degree of motion in all planes to negotiate hills when walking, adopt a stance on uneven terrain, or permit some rotation during the swing. In contrast, a bowler may require a significant degree of sagittal plane movement, with dorsiflexion and plantar flexion, but may not want to have much frontal plane motion. A dynamic-response prosthetic foot meeting these guidelines would allow for a rapid approach, whereas the sagittal flexibility would permit the requisite lower limb motion as the bowling ball is released. Boaters, however, want to keep the prosthetic foot flat on the deck of the boat and would therefore prefer some motion at the ankle to adapt to the rocking motion of the boat. If the prosthetic ankle moves slightly to accommodate the rocking motion, similar to the sound limb's motion, the muscular effort at the proximal joints will be reduced, decreasing the fatigue of standing while on the boat. Too much motion may have an opposite effect and result in greater muscular effort to control balance on the prosthetic foot, so the stiffness of the motion-limiting elements must be individualized for each amputee.

There are far too many variables to try to match a sport with a particular prosthetic foot. Suffice it to say that a wide variety of dynamic feet is available today to meet almost everyone's activity level. What is most important is that the amputee's recreational interests be explored at the time of prosthetic prescription and an appropriate choice be made.

Prosthetic Sprinting Foot Options

Sprinting feet are designed, selected, and aligned to maximize sport performance but are neither safe nor effective for normal walking. When combined with a sprinting-specific socket and suspensions, these specialized limbs have enabled well-trained am-

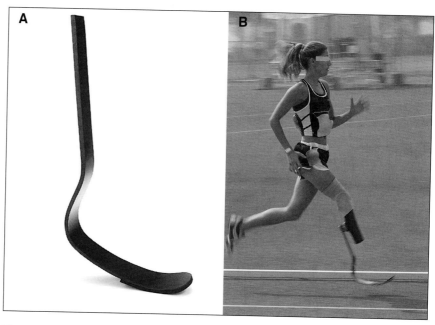

Figure 7 A, Cheetah running foot. *(Courtesy of Ossur, Aliso Viejo, CA.)* **B,** Transtibial amputee sprinter competing with a Cheetah running foot.

putee athletes to run almost as fast as able-bodied Olympic medalists.

Cheetah

Designed primarily for unilateral and bilateral transtibial amputees, Cheetah foot components (Ossur, Aliso Viejo, CA) are inherently plantar flexed to keep sprinters on their toes. The distal posterior pylon is bowed, lengthening the foot plate to increase the moment arm for maximal deflection so that, as the material energy is returned, it will propel the athlete's limb into the acceleration phase of swing (Figure 7). Because of the forces applied to the foot during sprinting, the height of the prosthetic limb is typically 1 to 2 in higher than the sound limb, allowing for the decreased height when the foot is compressed. The goal is to have the pelvis level during midstance and to eliminate any unnecessary trunk or head movement. Spring stiffness also plays a significant role in foot compression. A number of athletes believe that they perform better when the foot is not too stiff.

The manufacturer provides the initial alignment setup for the running foot, but individual alignment changes must be made at the track under train-

ing conditions. The forces generated during sprinting cannot be recreated in the office or parking lot. Using a video camera to film the athlete at competitive speeds from multiple angles and then reviewing the footage at slow speeds is the only effective method to align a running prosthesis.

Trimming the distal end of the foot plate should be done only to reduce the sharp edges. The longer the foot plate, the longer the stance phase, giving the sound limb time to achieve full hip flexion. This of course may be individual to each athlete, but any reduction in length should be done only after the athlete has achieved final alignment or feels that the length is a consistent hindrance. Otto Bock HealthCare (Minneapolis, MN) manufactures the Sprinter foot, which has a similar design to the Cheetah.

Flex-Sprint

The Flex-Sprint (Ossur), an inverted J-shaped prosthetic foot, is popular with transfemoral amputee sprinters. There is no posterior bow, which moves the ground-reaction force anteriorly, making the prosthetic knee a little more stable. An optional heel module is available for transtibial am-

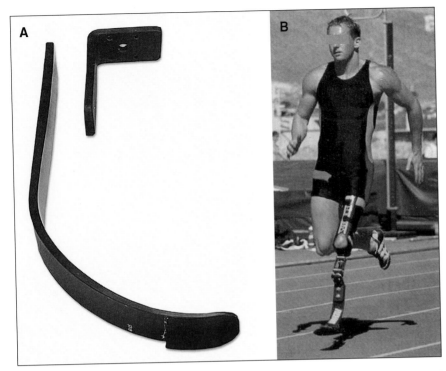

Figure 8 A, Flex-Sprint running foot. *(Courtesy of Ossur, Aliso Viejo, CA.)* **B,** Transfemoral sprinter competing with a Flex-Sprint foot.

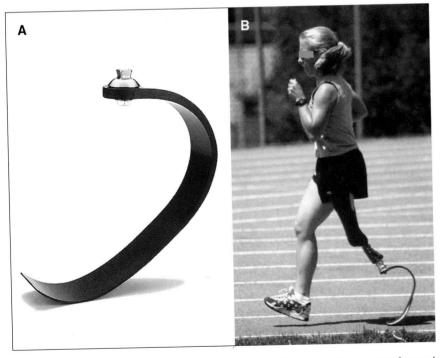

Figure 9 A, C-Sprint running foot. *(Courtesy of Ossur, Aliso Viejo, CA.)* **B,** Transfemoral distance runner competing with a C-Sprint foot designed for long-distance running or jogging.

foot and the knee moments, where there is just enough stability to ensure that the knee will not buckle but not so much that knee flexion becomes difficult (Figure 8).

Sprinting feet typically provide no medial/lateral mobility, so all motion occurs only in the sagittal plane. Although novice runners do not need these specialized feet to start training, no elite track athletes have competed over the past decade without using these specialized designs.

C-Sprint

C-Sprint feet (Ossur) are designed for long-distance running or jogging. Because of the exaggerated posterior bow shape, its vertical compliance is much greater than in any other running foot design (Figure 9). C-Sprint feet have been used successfully by transtibial amputees, transfemoral amputees, and bilateral amputees who want to run longer distances. To take full advantage of this design, the athlete lands on the prosthetic toe, extending the hip throughout the support phase and achieving maximal deflection of the foot. As the prosthetic limb is about to enter the acceleration or swing phase, the effort for jogging is minimized by allowing the foot to initiate the upward motion. Then, as the spring effect reaches a peak, upward acceleration is continued by flexing the hip as the limb moves into the float phase. Runners perceive less muscular effort after they gain a sense of the foot's compression and release, allowing the foot to initiate upward momentum while they use the hip flexors to continue the forward progression of the limb. There is no evidence to support claims of reduced work while running with C-Sprint feet. Nevertheless, the "bouncy" sensation that amputee runners experience with a little training seems to result in a more rhythmic running pattern. This may increase the chance that they can reach a steady state. The benefit of being able to establish a comfortable pace is that the amputee runner can then develop muscular and cardiopulmonary endurance using the prosthesis while al-

putees wearing this style of foot who want the security of knowing they will not hyperextend the knee if their weight falls posterior to the shin. Transfemoral amputee sprinters tend

to bounce off the prosthetic foot and have a marked reduction in hip flexion with both the prosthetic and sound limb. An alignment balance must be made between the prosthetic

lowing the residual limb to gradually develop a tolerance to the high forces being applied within the socket. Although few amputees choose to run for long distances as a method of endurance training, this option is possible for many individuals, particularly those with unilateral limb loss.

Maximizing Ankle/Foot Performance

The functional ability of the amputee is the primary consideration when selecting the appropriate foot/ankle components. A rehabilitation plan designed to match the specific requirements of the prosthetic components fitted will optimize the effectiveness of the prescription. Matching the right exercises to the ankle/foot assembly permits optimal use of the prosthesis and improves athletic performance.

Dynamic-response prosthetic feet can allow the amputee to run faster with greater ease and agility. They are typically designed for amputees who have the ability to vary their walking speed or change directions quickly, or who want to run. The advantages of dynamic-response feet are realized only if the transition of weight over the foot is of the magnitude and duration to permit the deflector system to work as designed. In other words, to take full advantage of a dynamic-response foot, full body weight must pass over the foot long enough for the deflector plate to bend fully and store the energy and then allow the elastic properties to release the stored energy. Athletes should spend time learning how to properly land, load, and change direction with the prosthetic foot in order to maximize athletic performance.

Exercises to Maximize Performance
Toe-Box Jumps

For toe-box jumps,[28] four pieces of tape are placed 2 ft apart, forming a square. The athlete stands with both

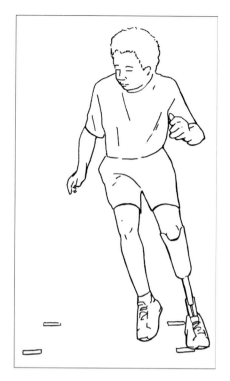

Figure 10 Toe-box jumps. *(Copyright © Advanced Rehabilitation Therapy, Inc, Miami, FL, 2002. Illustrator Frank Angulo.)*

feet together, then jumps diagonally to the opposite mark, landing on the toe of the prosthetic foot and using the unaffected limb for balance. The body weight loads the prosthetic foot; then, as the deflector plate releases its stored energy, the athlete quickly pushes off, using the quadriceps muscle to extend the knee to the next mark to the lateral side. Again landing on the toe of the prosthetic limb and balancing with the unaffected limb, the athlete jumps diagonally to the last remaining mark. Initially, a spotter should be present for safety. Timing of foot release and knee extension is the focus of this exercise, as well as learning how to take advantage of the prosthetic foot's energy return (Figure 10).

Lateral Speed Weave

For the lateral speed weave,[28] four to five cones are placed approximately every 4 ft with another alternating set of cones set halfway between and 2 to 3 ft across (Figure 11). The lateral speed weave is designed to promote

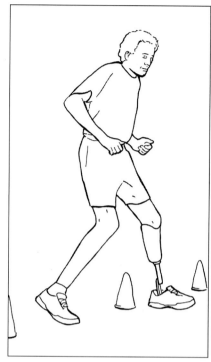

Figure 11 Lateral speed weave. *(Copyright © Advanced Rehabilitation Therapy, Inc, Miami, FL, 2002. Illustrator Frank Angulo.)*

speed, power, and agility in all directions by having the amputee run forward to the side, backward to the side, and forward again.

Because of the differences in knee control, the transtibial amputee and transfemoral amputee should perform this exercise slightly differently. When transtibial amputees run in and out of the cones, they should emphasize staying on the toe of the prosthetic foot for quick acceleration and deceleration. Again, it is important to focus on the time between the deflection of the prosthetic foot plate and extension of the knee to achieve maximal power. This exercise prepares the athlete for multidirectional movements that include starting, stopping, and changing direction. Transfemoral amputees should concentrate on learning to control the flexion and extension of the prosthetic knee. As the prosthetic limb moves forward, a full-length step is achieved as the knee flexes and reaches the forward cone with a natural step length. The lateral and backward movements re-

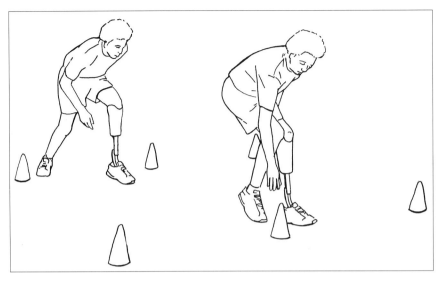

Figure 12 Agility drill. *(Copyright © Advanced Rehabilitation Therapy, Inc, Miami, FL, 2002. Illustrator Frank Angulo.)*

quire that the prosthetic knee remain straight. The athlete can keep the knee straight by maintaining hip extension force against the back wall of the socket, even as the sound limb is taking a step backward.

Agility Drills

For agility drills,[28] several cones or cups should be lined up in two rows approximately 6 ft apart (four to six cones on either side). The athlete should move quickly from one cone to another, squatting down to touch each cone while zig-zagging from one cone to another. The key to this exercise is maintaining speed by staying on the toe of the prosthetic foot and using the quadriceps and hip extensor muscles to rapidly extend the prosthetic limb while coming up from the squatting position (Figure 12).

Prosthetic Knee Options

Transfemoral amputees have additional considerations when learning to run with a passive prosthetic knee. To date, no knee system provides sufficient controlled knee flexion during the prosthetic support phase of running, so the residual limb must absorb the ground-reaction forces during initial ground contact. The transfemoral amputee must also achieve and maintain cadence speed during the swing phase. Hydraulic knee units offer the ability to adjust the hydraulic resistance of knee flexion and extension to keep pace with the runner. During running, lowering the hydraulic extension resistance permits faster knee extension, while increased flexion resistance decreases the amount of heel rise for novice runners. Seasoned runners set the resistances to achieve symmetry between limbs. Knee flexion resistance should be set low enough to allow sufficient time for the hip to achieve full flexion. If there is too little resistance, the knee will flex too quickly, resulting in insufficient time for the hip to generate maximal power to move body weight over the contralateral limb, thus reducing running speed. Extension resistance is optimized when the limb comes forward smoothly into the float phase.

A transfemoral amputee can learn the basics of running on almost any type of knee system. However, friction-control knees are too slow to respond to any speed greater than a fast walk, and prosthetic knees without some type of stance control are not recommended to teach running as they are not designed for running and are not safe. Pneumatic systems are also not sufficiently cadence-responsive for the demands of run-ning or agility sports. The two preferred knee systems for athletes are the Mauch Swing'N'Stance (SNS) type hydraulic or S-type Swing Only hydraulic knee (Figure 13) (Mauch Laboratories, Dayton, OH) or the Otto Bock 3R55 modular polycentric axis joint with hydraulic swing-phase control (Otto Bock HealthCare) (Figure 14). The Mauch hydraulic cylinder uses a single-axis frame, and the SNS offers athletes a wide range of resistance adjustment to stance control. Most competitive athletes, however, use the S-type Swing Only hydraulic unit because stance control is no longer necessary with athletes who are successful runners. The Otto Bock 3R55 polycentric axis joint is a favorite for knee disarticulation athletes because of the instantaneous center of rotation capabilities of a four-bar design, providing increased toe clearance and greater stride symmetry.

Learning how to maximize knee performance during running requires transverse rotation of the pelvis to generate a full stride length and to strike the ground with a backward force during the support phase (as described in Table 2). For lateral movements, keeping the prosthetic limb slightly posterior to the sound limb will keep the weight line anterior to the knee joint, ensuring a knee extension moment to decrease the risk of knee buckling.

Ancillary Components

Shock absorbers are thought to reduce ground-reaction forces. This can be a tremendous benefit for athletes who run long distances or participate in high-impact sports. Because shock absorbers also absorb an undetermined quantity of energy, they do not return much stored energy, which reduces acceleration as the athlete moves into the swing phase. As a result, many athletes who participate in high-speed sports elect not to incorporate a shock absorber into their sport prosthesis.

Torsion adapters are often chosen by athletes who participate in multidirectional sports such as tennis or who generate rotation about the long axis, as in swinging a golf club. Theoretically, torsion adapters reduce the shear forces within the socket and permit greater rotation for improved performance. Not all individuals who participate in tennis or golf find the added motion beneficial. Some find the additional motion difficult to control or conclude that the benefits do not outweigh the additional weight and maintenance.

Knee rotation adapters allow the amputee to move the foot and shin components into a variety of positions that would otherwise be impossible. For example, to facilitate recreational activities that involve sitting, such as gardening, just being able to move the foot out of the way is very helpful. Knee rotators also facilitate greater ease with dressing, changing shoes, and similar routine tasks.

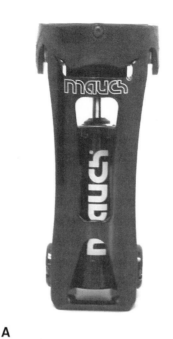
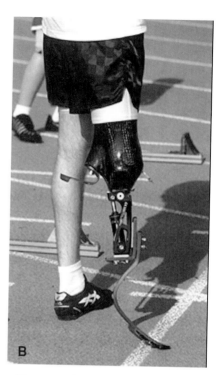

Figure 13 A, Mauch SNS type hydraulic knee. *(Courtesy of Ossur, ALiso Viejo, CA.)* **B,** Mauch SNS type hydraulic knee used with transfemoral amputee runners. *(Courtesy of Advanced Rehabilitation Therapy, Inc, Miami, FL.)*

Specific Sport Considerations

Swimming

Swimming is both a competitive and recreational sport enjoyed by amputees of all ages. The freedom of the water, cardiovascular benefits, and muscular endurance gained from swimming make it a nearly ideal activity. Competitive swimmers are not permitted to wear a prosthesis while competing, so these athletes learn to swim extremely well unaided. When first learning to swim, lower limb amputees may experience some difficulties, such as drifting toward the amputated side when kicking with the sound limb. Others describe difficulty in maintaining their trunk and shoulder parallel to the water surface, thus reducing their speed and requiring additional exertion to propel through the water. On the whole, however, most amputees young and old learn to swim easily.

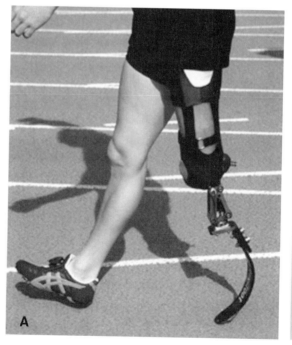
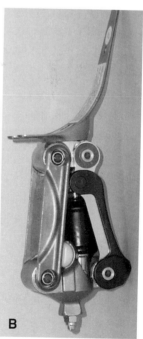

Figure 14 A, Otto Bock 3R55 modular polycentric axis joint with hydraulic swing phase. *(Courtesy of Otto Bock HealthCare, Minneapolis, MN.)* **B,** Otto Bock 3R55 used with transfemoral and knee disarticulation runners. *(Courtesy of Advanced Rehabilitation Therapy, Inc, Miami, FL.)*

Advantages to wearing a prosthesis during swimming include having two limbs to enter and exit the water and shower facilities and to facilitate poolside activities. In addition, the prosthesis can add propulsion during

TABLE 3 Considerations for Golf for Amputees

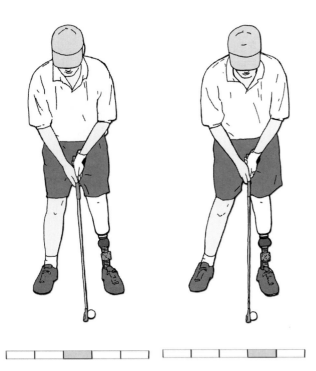

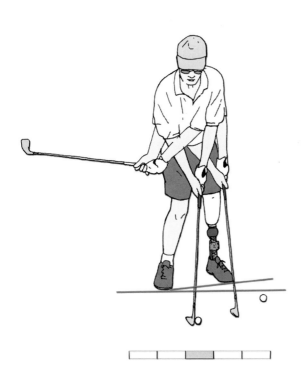

Putting

There are countless aspects to putting, from stance to club selection. For the purpose of this exercise, the classic pendulum-type stroke has been selected.

Stance

The golfer should set up with a comfortable, wide stance, with the knees slightly bent. Transfemoral amputees should keep the prosthetic knee straight with the sound limb slightly flexed, if possible. Weight should be balanced over the center of the feet, with a little more weight on the front foot. The upper arms should rest lightly on the trunk, and the eyes should be directly over the ball.

Stroke

Hands, arms, and shoulders all work together to create a pendulum-type stroke. Shoulders and arms create a triangle that moves an equal distance on both the backswing and the through-swing, with the head remaining still at all times.

Prosthetic foot

The golfer should feel the points of the heel, little toe, and great toe on the prosthetic foot. This will help balance the weight over the foot. Starting with weight distributed equally over both feet, the weight should move slightly toward the forward foot, whether it is the prosthetic foot or the sound foot.

Exercises

A helpful exercise is to start with short, 3-ft putts and progress to longer and longer putts. Golfers should focus on maintaining the same swing while creating a stable base within the lower body.[28] As shown in the illustration, most of the golfer's body weight should be over the shaded box on the lower scale.

Benefits

Besides improving the putting game, this exercise helps the amputee work on prosthetic weight bearing, develop a sense of how the weight is distributed over the prosthetic foot, connect the body and foot to the ground, and challenge standing balance. This exercise also begins the process of differentiation of the trunk from the pelvis, which aids in arm swing during walking and other sports.

Chipping and Pitching

Getting on the green and close to the hole can reduce any golfer's score dramatically. Chipping and pitching is all about balance and repeating the same stance and stroke over and over.

Stance

The golfer should set up with a narrow, open stance, positioning the feet fairly close together. The forward foot is slightly back and the body is aligned slightly left of the target. The ball is positioned toward the back foot with a fair amount of weight on the forward foot. Knees are slightly flexed with the back straight and the hips flexed a little.

Stroke

The hands move ahead of the ball, with wrists firm (no bending) and with the body's weight moving toward the forward leg. The distance the ball goes is dictated by the distance of the backswing and through-swing. Both movements are usually equal in distance. A short chip requires only a short backswing and through-swing, whereas if the ball needs to fly farther to reach the green, a more complete stroke is required, along with a little wider stance.

Prosthetic foot

Getting the weight down into the prosthetic foot is essential for consistently successful chipping and pitching. A prosthetic foot that permits vertical as well as rotational shock absorption can make this stroke much smoother and more comfortable, especially when the prosthetic limb is forward.

Exercises

After getting comfortable with motion and weight-shifting without using a golf club, golfers should practice using a sand wedge and perform the same motion. They should hold their finished position with the club raised and their body weight well forward. Because golf courses are neither flat nor firm, it is helpful to create a practice condition using the same stroke with a golf club and with a foam cushion under both feet while holding the finished position.[28] As shown in the illustration, most of the golfer's body weight should be over the shaded box on the lower scale.

Benefits

This exercise allows golfers to start getting the ball in a better position to reduce the number of putting strokes. They will also notice improved weight shifting, stability, and balance over the prosthetic limb in various positions. As leg strength and balance improve, bigger swings will become easier.

TABLE 3 Considerations for Golf for Amputees (Cont.)

Full Swing
A smooth, full swing will add distance and accuracy to any golfer's game.

Stance
Setup should be with feet shoulder-width apart and turned outward slightly. The knees should be bent slightly until weight is over the center of the feet. Transfemoral amputees will need to keep their prosthetic knee straight and, as a result, the sound knee will be straighter as well. Hips should be slightly flexed, keeping the lower back straight and chin up.

Stroke
The classic backswing is a smooth, seamless turn, moving the club, hands, arms, chest, and shoulders together, sweeping the club head back and low with a full and wide swing. Weight should be maintained on the inside of the back foot with the front foot firmly on the ground. For the downswing, the lower body should initiate the movement as the body unwinds, and the hands should remain soft as the club head moves through the ball. Golfers should shift their body weight smoothly from the back foot to the front foot. The body should rotate all the way through the shot, with most of its weight finishing over the front leg.

Prosthetic foot
As the magnitude of the golf swing increases, the need to have a sense of where the prosthetic foot is also increases. The more golfers can "feel" where the weight is distributed over the prosthetic foot, the better their balance and swing control will be. Also, the greater the forces that are generated throughout the prosthetic limb, the more a shock absorber or torsion control device will reduce the forces and offer greater mobility and comfort.

Exercises
To practice for full swings, golfers should start with a half swing and progress to a three quarters swing and then a full swing. They should focus on shifting the weight between the feet. Weight should be kept toward the inside of the back foot during the backswing, allowing the weight to move to the front foot during follow-through. Golfers should hold the follow-through position for a couple of seconds.[28] As shown in the illustration, most of the golfer's body weight should be over the shaded box on the lower scale.

Benefits
Maintaining a stable base not only improves the amputee's golf game, but also improves prosthetic control during everyday activities and walking. Controlling both the backswing and follow-through will build eccentric or deceleratory strength throughout both lower limbs, especially within the socket. As club head speed improves, the need for greater strength and balance will also increase.

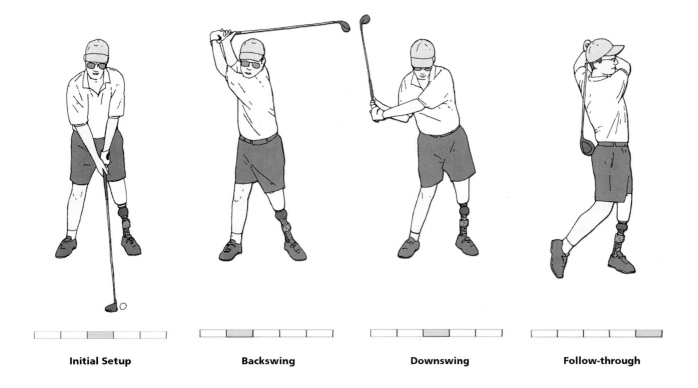

| Initial Setup | Backswing | Downswing | Follow-through |

(Copyright © Advanced Rehabilitation Therapy, Inc, Miami, FL, 2002. Illustrator Frank Angulo.)

swimming or wading. Amputees who have problems with limb volume fluctuations may also have difficulty donning the prosthesis after swimming and may therefore benefit from wearing a prosthesis while in the water. Wheelchair-mobile amputees may require assistance to get into and out of the pool if they are unable to perform floor-to-chair transfers independently. Many public and private pools are being equipped with Hoyer lifts as a result of increased public awareness and public policy such as the Americans With Disabilities Act.

Golf

Good balance and the ability to shift weight are two key skills necessary to play golf well. Training for both of these skills can begin early during rehabilitation and continue at home until the amputee is ready to return to the driving range. Consistently practicing trunk rotation and weight shifting will help develop balance and ambulation skills to prepare the amputee to return to the golf course.

The mechanics of the golf stroke are relatively individual to each golfer. The amputee will invariably lose distance on the swing; however, if the swing keeps the ball in play or on line, then the golfer's objective has been met. The key to teaching amputees to golf is that they play within their own individual limitations; this means that they need to learn to maintain balance and weight shift whether they are standing or swinging from a wheelchair.

Assistive devices in golf and the manner in which golfers choose to play are almost as varied as their golf strokes. Many amputees prefer not to wear a prosthesis; others use a wheelchair, tripods, or other devices to lean on as they swing. Some amputees who do wear their prosthesis and stand independently prefer some type of rotator or swivel device, but others find the additional weight or rotational movement to be a disadvantage. A number of golfers will take the spikes out of their golf shoes so that the shoes will be able to rotate directly on the ground.

Golf is one of the most popular sports enjoyed by amputees of all ages, levels of amputation, and functional abilities. Very few recreational activities encourage people to get outside, compete within their comfort level, and enjoy social exchange with friends the way golf does. Interestingly, golf is also one of the most beneficial activities that anyone can use to improve balance, coordination, range of motion, strength, and endurance. In many ways, golf is the perfect rehabilitation therapy. Being able to control all the movements with an activity as complex as a golf swing will make everyday activities seem simpler. Using prosthetic components that assist with shock absorption and torsion control can reduce the shear forces within the socket and help create a more stable base of support between the foot and the ground. Considerations for golf for amputees are outlined in Table 3.

Cycling

Cycling affords the amputee a chance to enjoy speed and cover great distance. Many amputees choose cycling as a form of exercise because it offers excellent aerobic conditioning without the high impact on the residual limb that occurs during running. Another advantage is that little is required in the way of adaptive equipment for any level of lower limb amputation.

Amputee cyclists of all levels may have difficulty in achieving maximum power when they push downward on the pedal. Biomechanically, the best way to achieve optimum power is to place the prosthetic shank directly over the pedal, unlike the intact side, where the metatarsal heads are centered on the pedal. Recreational riders should simply place the midfoot directly over the pedal. Competitive cyclists who desire to use the power of the residual limb during both downward and upward strokes will use a toe clip to hold the prosthetic foot in place. To fit the forefoot into the toe clip and still position the shank over the pedal, amputee cyclists may cut the prosthetic forefoot off or use a toe clip that provides extra depth.

Transtibial amputees generally experience minimum difficulty in riding with a prosthesis, but additional suspension may be needed, for which there are many alternatives. For transfemoral amputees who ride with their prosthesis, seating and hip range of motion present the greatest problems. The transfemoral amputee cyclist requires a saddle that is wide enough to balance upon yet narrow enough so that the upper thigh is not pinched between the socket and the saddle. A racing saddle is generally used for this reason because of its narrow design. Some riders initially choose a woman's saddle for the added balance obtained by a wider posterior portion. Soft-tissue pinching may be greatly reduced with the addition of a padded seat cover and a well-padded pair of cycling shorts. The thinner, more flexible polyethylene plastic sockets also aid in maintaining balance on the bike and reducing pinching.

Although most competitive cyclists prefer to ride with their prosthesis for the added power of using both legs, many transfemoral amputees find it more comfortable to ride without it. They simply remove the pedal on the prosthetic side and use a toe clip on the sound side to apply power on both downward and upward strokes of the pedal.

Preparing the Amputee for Recreational and Competitive Sports

Clinicians, such as physical therapists and prosthetists, often play the role of coach early in the rehabilitation process as the athlete with a disability prepares to return to athletics. One of the most common obstacles to success is the lack of knowledge among athletes, coaches, therapists, prosthetists, and parents about how to encourage amputees with athletic potential to improve their performance or to begin participating in a particular event. Often the easiest and most frequently used approach is "Just get out there and try it!"

Ideally, a qualified coach would instruct the athlete in the proper skills necessary for a given event, and with time and training the athlete would comfortably return to the sport. Unfortunately, this is rarely the case. Because of the small number of amputee athletes in any one region, coaches rarely have the opportunity to work with them enough to develop any real

TABLE 4 Tips for Coaching the Novice Disabled Athlete

Listen to the athlete.

Training with disabled athletes must be a cooperative effort. No absolute system of training has been developed, so novice coaches should listen to the athlete and discuss and develop technique variances together.

Seek out other disabled athletes competing in the same sport.

Most of the development in equipment and performance techniques has been achieved through the experiential knowledge and efforts of the athletes themselves. Many of the top coaches are disabled athletes, either retired or still competing. In addition, a training partner can also help to make the practices easier.

Recruit able-bodied coaches.

Disabled coaches are often difficult to find. Many elite disabled athletes train with able-bodied sport teams and athletes under the direction of able-bodied coaches. Often, the coordinated efforts of a coach and a therapist who are aware of the abilities and constraints of the athlete's physical capabilities work well when the disabled athlete wants to improve technique.

Read texts and publications pertaining to both able-bodied and disabled athletics.

In recent years, there have been a number of significant contributions to the body of literature concerning disabled sport. Unfortunately, there is still is a tremendous void in many particular sports and for many specific disability groups. However, reading and learning about able-bodied training methods and techniques is still an excellent way to gain insight into how to train a disabled athlete in a particular sport.

Call the appropriate disabled sports organizations for information and names of people to assist with training.

All disabled sports organizations maintain some form of database for a variety of topics, including athletes and coaches. Disabled sports organizations are generally underutilized as resources and should be contacted to assist with providing athletes and coaches direction in the training process.

Videotape practices and competitions.

Viewing videotapes of practice sessions and competitions for immediate visual feedback or for more detailed critique later is an excellent method of instruction. Moreover, videotapes of elite competitors with similar disabilities help the athlete visualize the biomechanics of accomplished performance. Coaches should caution athletes not to imitate other athletes, however. No two athletes perform the same way; therefore, young athletes should be wary of imitating movements of even celebrated elite athletes.

Consult with technical experts about adaptive equipment.

Many disabled athletes use adaptive equipment such as wheelchairs, prostheses, orthoses, and other assistive devices. Prosthetists, orthotists, biomedical engineers, and other adaptive equipment specialists can provide specially designed equipment to meet the athlete's individual needs and enhance performance. Only a few clinical professionals specialize in disabled athletic adaptive equipment because of the infrequent demand. Because poorly fitting equipment can be more harmful than helpful and in some cases even dangerous, the coach and athlete should make an effort to seek out and collaborate with one of these clinical professionals.

Use motivational techniques to help maintain the athlete's interest in training and the sport.

Maintaining an athlete's level of intensity when training for a sport can sometimes be a real challenge. A wide variety of literature, motivational tapes, and other resources is available to coaches who are interested in the inspirational aspects of coaching. As with any athlete, maintaining a balance between level of difficulty and level of frustration is important. Continuing to experience success with training and competition is positive reinforcement that will ensure that the athlete continues in the sport.

Become familiar with the rules or rule changes that may influence performance techniques.

As disabled sports evolve, classifications, rules, and competition formats will continue to change. Athletes and coaches alike must keep abreast of these changes to prevent any last-minute confusion and alterations in competition strategies.

Attend conferences for coaching both able-bodied and disabled athletes.

Conferences and seminars are excellent forums in which to exchange ideas and learn innovative approaches to sport techniques.

Experiment with new techniques.

Experimenting with new and unique techniques may help overcome a particular obstacle or enhance performance. Be careful of new styles that emerge from a single athlete as they may lack mechanical advantages and provide only a psychological edge. Keep an open mind, however.

Maintain written records.

Keeping journals of training sessions and competitions provides a log that may be reviewed by the coach and the athlete to determine trends that may enhance or hinder performance. There is also a tremendous need for the publication of positive and negative outcomes with regard to athletic performance to assist other athletes who are in similar situations.

expertise. There are several excellent coaches for amputees in the United States, many of them current and former competitive athletes, but only a small number of developing athletes have the opportunity to work with them. As a result, most amputee athletes must rely on themselves, other athletes, parents, interested able-bodied coaches, and clinicians.

Most coaches of athletes with disabilities have to become extremely resourceful in working toward enhancing the athlete's performance. Because little information is available specific to sports performance in persons with disabilities, coaches must build on several sources of knowledge and synthesize them for practical application to the athlete's training. This problem-solving approach to training can be the most exciting and rewarding aspect of coaching disabled athletes. The coaching tips outlined in Table 4 approach can be used to successfully coach the novice disabled athlete.[28]

Conclusion

A person who is interested in participating in sports typically maintains enthusiasm for athletics long after losing a limb. Health care professionals and athletic coaches can assist amputee athletes to return to sports with a few minor adaptive modifications and relatively little special training. Providing the opportunities and assistance to return to recreational sports activities should be a part of the standard rehabilitation program. Although it can be difficult to predict how long it will take an amputee to heal and adjust to the loss of a limb, proper training should be available to all amputees when they are ready. Therefore, clinicians should either be able to assist the amputee directly or have the necessary information to refer the amputee to a suitable program that will return the amputee to sports.

Manufacturer List

Mauch Laboratories
3035 Dryden Road
Dayton, OH 45439

Ossur USA
27412 Aliso Viejo Parkway
Aliso Viejo, CA 92656
800-233-6263

Otto Bock HealthCare
3000 Xenium Lane N.
Minneapolis, MN 55441
800-328-4058

Seattle Systems, Inc.
26296 Twelve Trees Lane, NW
Poulsbo, WA 98370
360-697-5656

References

1. Yigiter K, Sener G, Erbahceci F, Bayar K, Ulger OG, Akdogan S: A comparison of traditional prosthetic training versus proprioceptive neuromuscular facilitation resistive gait training with transfemoral amputees. *Prosthet Orthot Int* 2002;26:213-217.

2. Gailey RS, Gailey AM: *Prosthetic Gait Training Program for Lower Extremity Amputees.* Miami, FL, Advanced Rehabilitation Therapy, Inc, 1989.

3. American College of Sports Medicine: *Guidelines for Exercise Testing and Prescription,* ed 4. Philadelphia, PA, Lea & Febiger, 1990.

4. Linn BS, Linn MW: Objective and self-assessed health in the old and very old. *Soc Sci Med* 1980;14A:311-315.

5. Goldberg G, Shephard RJ: Personality profiles of disabled individuals in relation to physical activity patterns. *J Sports Med* 1982;22:477-484.

6. Lamb KL, Roberts K, Brodie DA: Self-perceived health among sports participants and non-sports participants. *Soc Sci Med* 1990;31:963-969.

7. Bernstein LC: *Aging: The Health Care Challenge,* ed 2. Philadelphia, PA, FA Davis Co, 1990.

8. Gailey R: Recreational pursuits for elders with amputation. *Top Geriatr Rehabil* 1992;8:39-58.

9. Gailey R, Gershon S, D'Esposito T, Warby-Marsh G: A Survey of Recreational Activities Participated in by Lower Extremity Amputees. Coral Gables, FL, University of Miami, 1992.

10. Armstrong DG, Lavery LA, Harkless LB, Van Houtum WH: Amputation and reamputation of the diabetic foot. *J Am Pod Med Assoc* 1997;87:255-259.

11. Isakov E, Budoragin N, Shenhav S, Mendelevich I, Korzets A, Susak Z: Anatomic sites of foot lesions resulting in amputation among diabetics and non-diabetics. *Am J Phys Med Rehabil* 1995;74:130-133.

12. Glattly HW: Statistical study of 12,000 new amputees. *S Med J* 1964;57:1373-1378.

13. National Sporting Goods Association: *Sports Participation in 1990.* Mt. Prospect, IL, NSGA, 1991.

14. Kegel B: Physical fitness: Sports and recreation for those with lower limb amputation or impairment. *J Rehabil Res Dev* 1985;(suppl 1):125.

15. Cavanagh PR (ed): *Biomechanics of Distance Running.* Champaign, IL, Human Kinetics, 1990.

16. Alexander RM: *Elastic Mechanisms in Animal Movement.* Cambridge, England, Cambridge University Press, 1988.

17. Ounpuu S: The biomechanics of walking and running. *Clin Sports Med* 1994;13:843-863.

18. Cavanagh PR, Lafortune MA: Ground reaction forces in distance running. *J Biomech* 1980;13:397-406.

19. Hay JG: *The Biomechanics of Sports Techniques,* ed 3. Englewood Cliffs, NJ, Prentice-Hall, 1985.

20. Mann RA, Moran GT, Dougherty SE: Comparative electromyography of the lower extremity in jogging, running, and sprinting. *Am J Sports Med* 1986;14:501-510.

21. Nuber WN: Biomechanics of the foot and ankle during gait. *Clin Sports Med* 1988;7:1-12.

22. Czerniecki JM, Gitter A, Munro C: Joint moment and muscle power output characteristics of below knee amputees during running: The influence of energy storing prosthetic feet. *J Biomech* 1991;24:63-75.

23. Czerniecki JM, Gitter A: Insights into amputee running: A muscle work analysis. *Am J Phys Med Rehabil* 1992;71:209-218.

24. Sanderson DJ, Martin PE: Joint kinetics in unilateral below-knee amputee patients during running. *Arch Phys Med Rehabil* 1996;77:1279-1285.

25. Buckley JG: Sprint kinematics of athletes with lower-limb amputations. *Arch Phys Med Rehabil* 1999;80:501-508.

26. Adelaar RS: The practical biomechanics of running. *Am J Sports Med* 1986;14:497-500.

27. Czerniecki JM, Gitter AJ, Beck JC: Energy transfer mechanisms as a compensatory strategy in below knee amputee runners. *J Biomechs* 1996;29:717-722.

28. Gailey RS: *The Essentials of Lower Limb Amputee Running and Sports Training.* Miami, FL, Advanced Rehabilitation Therapy, Inc, 2004.

Chapter 52

Research in Lower Limb Prosthetics

Saeed Zahedi, OBE, FIMechE

Introduction

Rapid technologic advances in lower limb prosthetics have occurred since the early 1990s. Paradoxically, these advances have been concurrent with an estimated 20% reduction in funding for amputee care. Despite the technologic improvements in components and materials, studies from Europe and the United States suggest that overall amputee satisfaction with prostheses has remained relatively constant, varying from 70% to 75% of those polled.

In the second edition of this *Atlas*, Charles Pritham postulated that pending decreases in academic research in prosthetics might force commercial component manufacturers to divert profits into increased product research to fill the void. The accuracy of that prediction was borne out during the 1990s when published research from universities and government research organizations dropped dramatically. Since the early 1950s, virtually all applied research has come out of the commercial sector—new suspension options, innovative socket configurations, advances in knee mechanisms, and guidelines for prescription and reimbursement of prostheses.

Increased understanding of the biomechanics of locomotion combined with clinical experimentation have led to a steady evolution in lower limb socket design. Modern sockets generally emphasize diffuse rather than localized weight bearing to re-duce peak pressures and increase amputee comfort. Advances in material technology have led to the use of novel polymers in the manufacture of socket liners and to the creation of ever thinner, lighter, and stiffer sockets for transmission of weight-bearing loads. Alternatives such as direct skeletal attachment via osseointegration and limb transplantation are being explored as alternatives to the use of external prostheses.

In the 1990s, the combination of amputees' expectations and industrial competition resulted in many new developments in lower limb components. US companies combined advanced prosthetic feet with various shock-absorbing systems, while European firms took the lead in developing novel components such as a rotary hydraulic knee and microprocessor-controlled knee mechanisms. Rapid growth and consolidation of prosthetic component manufacturers worldwide also characterized this decade, often through the purchase of young and innovative companies by established and better funded firms. This consolidation has created several major multinational competitors with sufficient sales to privately fund ongoing research activities.

Current Developments

Before 1990, most information about socket-limb interface pressures was based on static measurements. The availability of low-cost dynamic transducers combined with an increased understanding of soft-tissue mechanics has resulted in new concepts in amputation surgery, prosthetic socket design, and the use of new materials to enhance control of the prosthesis by the amputee. Increased control of the prosthesis requires and facilitates improvements in prosthetic components and has refocused efforts on enabling the amputee to engage in a full range of normal activities of daily living.

The recent growth of regulatory requirements and the development of International Organization for Standardization (ISO) testing protocols for endoskeletal lower limb prosthetic components have enhanced the standards for the manufacture of high-quality products that are safe and reliable yet economically competitive.

Centralized fabrication—the use of technology to provide an economic and professional advantage—has been suggested as one strategy for coping with diminishing health care funding for rehabilitation. More extensive use of computer-aided design and manufacturing has also been offered as a method to deliver care with fewer financial resources. Although both trends have increased in clinical practice, further integration of these two concepts into one cohesive alternative to current on-site manual fabrication can be anticipated.

Computer-Aided Prosthetic Laboratory Concepts

The concept of the computer-aided prosthetic laboratory (CAPL) was first described in the 1990s but has not yet been fully realized in practice. Potential applications for such knowledge-based concepts in routine clinical service include the routine scanning of both limbs as the amputee enters the clinic and assessing the amputee's gait; CAPL could then suggest the appropriate type of ankle, foot, knee control, and alignment. Once the residual limb geometry is scanned, the amputee's ability to voluntarily control the prosthesis could be assessed. CAPL of the future could make a diagnostic socket using rapid prototyping methods with integrated sensors, ready for fine adjustments by the prosthetist. A custom protective-cosmetic system could then, in theory, be manufactured while the amputee's socket is being fitted.

CAPL of the future would record all data and deliver the completed limb in one session and would be capable of making exact replicas at any later time. CAPL might also control central inventory, arranging just-in-time delivery of required components and materials. Furthermore, because the need for casting is eliminated, amputee perception of the prosthesis might be enhanced, and labor costs would be reduced compared with the present reality.

Limb-Socket Interaction

The primary requisite for successful use of an artificial limb is a comfortable, secure, and well-fitted socket. Secondary requirements to gain full benefit from functional components are the amputee's willingness for rehabilitation and optimum biomechanical alignment of the selected components. Proprioceptive feedback and sensations of comfort/discomfort largely determine whether the prosthesis feels as if it is an integral part of the body. These issues are all functions of the limb-socket interface and illustrate the importance of this subjective aspect of prosthetic care.

The desire for the best possible fitting has led to widespread acceptance of the use of a clear test socket. Test sockets are used to evaluate the accuracy of casting and rectification performed by the prosthetist before the final socket is manufactured and to obtain sufficient information on present methods of casting and rectification. This information is then used to improve methods of casting and rectification. Furthermore, the use of test sockets is intended to produce accurately and correctly fitting sockets with very close tolerances so that the fitting of hard sockets can be facilitated.

Limitations to this method include the largely static nature of most test sockets, as well as the qualitative nature of the data used to evaluate socket fit. These limitations have led investigators to examine pressure magnitudes and variations at the limb-socket interface, particularly under dynamic walking conditions.

Early studies were of limited value because of the shortcomings in available measurement technology. Early investigations measured dynamic forces at the interface using a pneumatic transducer that measured pressure over a relatively large area of 25 cm.[2] Boni[1] developed an improved transducer in the 1960s that comprised silver electrodes bonded to a conductive rubber; the transducer had a 9/16-in diameter and was approximately 1 in thick.

In their extensive studies on interface pressures, Appoldt and associates[2-5] used strain gauges of various configurations and manufacture before finally opting for diaphragm-mounted semiconductor strain gauges wired in a full bridge configuration. This transducer, only 0.02 in thick, was encapsulated in a droplet of silicone rubber for improved dynamic response. As with earlier studies, modifications to the socket were required to accommodate the transducer. Maximum dynamic values of approximately 175 kN/m[2] were obtained at the brim of transfemoral sockets. Corell[6] selected a similar yet less expensive sensor but reported problems with repeatability. Rae and Cockrell,[7] Pearson and associates,[8] and Burgess and Moore[9] reported studies using strain gauge transducers. Redhead[10] used silicone-etched diaphragm transducers that required extensive modifications to the socket. Meier and associates[11] used capacitance transducers of relatively large dimensions (20-mm diameter, 2-mm thickness) to investigate the interface pressure in transtibial prostheses. Other investigators have used hydraulic pressure transducers and hybrid electronic transducer systems.[12,13]

The current generation of pressure transducers and miniature force strain gauges offers new opportunity for dynamic measurements of the skin-socket interface. Only recently have transducers using electrotextile materials been developed, facilitating pressure-force measurements at the interface without modification to the existing socket. Various studies focusing on the dynamics of interface measurements are currently underway in North America and Europe.

The acquisition of limb-socket interface pressure data has important implications for improving socket design, especially in computer-aided design/computer-aided manufacturing (CAD/CAM) applications. In the future, in vivo data might be programmed to control socket design and manufacturing.

Testing of Interface Pressures During Locomotion

In an effort to evaluate interface pressure transducers under dynamic conditions and concurrently determine the quality of fit between residual limb and socket, I carried out tests on

TABLE 1 Average Peak Interface Pressures (kN/m²) for Transtibial Amputees

Patient	1* Test A	1 Test B	2* Test A	2 Test B	3*	4	5	6	7
Transducer position									
Patella bar	375	223	189	180	204	214	124	266	104
Fibula head	40	110	51	20	20	215	38	26	83
Medial hamstring	93	43	31	Fail	52	151	95	23	25
Lateral hamstring	49	15	40	18	Fail	108	55	N/R+	58
Distal end of tibia	0	24	0	0	0	0	0	50	0
Midposterior calf	201	108	121	130	94	45	119	253	138
Subpopliteal fossa								88	
Lateral tibia crest	123	160	156						
Suprapatellar bar					74				

* These results were recorded using a hardwire method. All other measurements were made via the 8-channel amplifier and MT8 telemetry system.

+ Subpopliteal site selected instead of lateral hamstring

The run-to-run variation in pressure at the various transducer sites was a maximum of ±11% but was less than ±6% at five of the sites, thus within the standard deviation of the mean of the Force Sensing Resistor transducer.

nine healthy male amputees ranging in age from 30 to 60 years. Day's[14] amputee activity assessment forms were used. Results showed a range of reported activity from moderately to highly active. The socket designs of this group of transtibial and transfemoral amputees varied.

Selection of Socket Transducer Sites

Transducers were placed in the socket around those areas considered as pressure-sensitive and pressure-tolerant. The rationale was that unusual pressures in these areas would indicate a potentially poor fit of the socket in that region. With the transducer-fitted prosthesis donned and the associated pointer and telemetry equipment worn on a waist belt, the patient was instructed to walk normally along a defined walkway incorporating two Kistler (type 92651A) force plates.

Results From Transtibial Testing

Interface pressures and ground-reaction forces were measured and recorded. Peak pressures at each transducer site for the seven transtibial subjects are shown in Table 1. Although the range in peak pressure values was wide, the temporal pattern of pressure buildup was similar for all patients.

Results From Transfemoral Testing

Interface pressures and ground-reaction forces were measured and recorded for two transfemoral subjects. The average peak pressures at the various transducer sites are shown in Table 2.

TABLE 2 Average Peak Interface Pressures (kN/m²) for Transfemoral Amputees

Transducer site	Patient 8	Patient 9
Ischial tuberosity	325	345
Lateral ischial seat	238	Fail
Scarpa's triangle	72	70
Midvastus lateralis	108	80
Distal anterior femur	0	68
Anterior medial brim	255	120
Greater trochanter	N/A	350

The run-to-run variation in pressure at the various transducer sites was a maximum of ±11.37%; at five of the sites it was less than ±10%, within the standard deviations of the mean of the Force Sensing Resistor transducer.

As expected, the highest interface pressures were recorded at the ischial tuberosity transducer site, with only 20 kN/m² difference between the two patients. For both patients, the ischial tuberosity transducer indicated loading throughout the gait cycle, with a constant load of approximately 140 kN/m² registered throughout the swing phase.

Discussion of Interface Measurements

Two patients had peak pressures at the fibular head transducer site in excess of 150 kN/m²; one of these was 215 kN/m², higher than the pressure recorded at the patellar bar site. The implication is that the fibular head is providing a horizontal reaction force as the body weight is transferred from the sound to the prosthetic side, consistent with the maximum peak mediolateral shear force measurements of the force plates.

An alternative reason for this anomalous result might stem from mediolateral instability. As a consequence of this subject's short residual limb length, lateral stabilizing forces applied by the socket may be less effective in controlling mediolateral instability. This patient showed consistently high interface pressure readings (> 100 kN/m²) at the proximal sites within the socket but low interface pressure readings (< 50 kN/m²) at the more distal sites.

Interface pressures measured at the medial hamstring transducer site, another proximal-pressure sensitive area, were less than 90 kN/m² for the two patients mentioned above. The cause of the high pressure values could be the lack of knee stability inherent with short residual limbs.

The interface pressure developed at the patellar bar transducer site shows a characteristic double peak. The initial peak, occurring shortly after heel strike, is a result of the deceleration of the center of gravity relative to its position during the latter part of the swing phase. During midstance, there is zero acceleration of the center of gravity; the axial load, and hence the patellar bar interface pressure thus falls to a value corresponding to that produced by body weight alone. Upon rollover and push-off, the absence of active plantar flexor muscle action causes the amputee to apply active knee extension.

The reaction force that is due to acceleration of the center of gravity in an upward direction results in increased pressure at the patellar bar interface. This is likely to be further increased by the anatomic change to the patellar tendon when, because of the extensor action of the rectus femoris

muscle, it is put into tension relative to the underlying skeletal structures. This combination of effects results in the push-off phase developing a higher peak pressure than that occurring during the initial shock-absorbing phase. This characteristic pattern of interface pressure at the patellar bar is consistent with those recorded by Isherwood,[13] Pearson and associates,[8] and Rae and Cockrell.[7] Active knee extension at push-off increases force on the anterior distal area and decreases pressure on the patellar tendon.

My study illustrates the importance of looking at socket interface pressures as a dynamic entity. In fact, assumptions made based on static models of tissue mechanics now seem to be incorrect. Most areas of the residual limb can tolerate much higher loads than expected if for a short duration only. Tissue injury and discomfort probably arise primarily from prolonged application of pressure, presumably due to incorrect distribution of pressures within the socket.

Role of Osseointegration in Future Lower Limb Prosthetic Research

Brånemark and associates[15] described the use of implants for direct connection of external prostheses to the skeleton via an internal prosthesis. Brånemark and his associates have been developing this idea for many years. Recently they published fairly successful results in both lower and upper limb fitting. This concept of osseointegration is based on the use of pure titanium implants that, after a systematic healing and weight-bearing protocol, provide very good load-bearing properties. These implants have been tried in different sizes, varying from partial finger to femoral sizes.

This interface requires routine daily cleaning to reduce the risk of infection. Many transfemoral amputees using osseointegrated prostheses demonstrate a wider range of walking speeds than individuals walking with

a conventional prosthesis.[16] Despite more than 30 years of success in developing dental and maxillofacial implants and fitting more than 450,000 patients with a 95% success rate, Brånemark is being cautious in the use of osseointegration to attach lower and upper limb prostheses.

The potential for osseointegration to provide more control over the prosthesis and increase the power transfer between amputee and limb is great enough to provide significant new challenges for prosthetic component design. More sophisticated designs might include special mechanisms for absorption of shock load and axial rotational torque to avoid direct transmission of these stresses to the bone interface. Future research advances in prosthetics technology could involve the use of a microprocessor to provide closed-loop control of knee and ankle movement and the possibility of electromagnetic control and biofeedback, potentially leading to electromechanical suspension for heavier prostheses.

Limitations still exist, however. A mechanical fail-safe mechanism, adjustable to different levels of activities, is essential to avoid loosening or breakage of the implant. The cosmetic appearance and psychological issues associated with osseointegration require specialized training. The reliability and limited scope for repair, significant cost of the initial surgery and possible subsequent surgeries, and feasibility of reverting to wearing conventional prosthetic devices remain barriers to more widespread use of this method.

Increased Use of Soft Tissues for Force Transmission

In recent years, clinical exploration of the ability of the soft tissues to serve as a medium for force transmission has resurged. This renewed interest is based on the similarity of the soft tissues to fluids; both are incompressible and can therefore transmit forces

TABLE 3 Typical Daily Activities of Lower Limb Amputees

Activity	Times per day
Changes walking speed	437
Stumbles	108
Stops and stands	1,450
Sits	48
Descends stairs	23
Descends ramps	38

when properly constrained within a container.

Prior studies have demonstrated a longitudinal internal piston action of the skeletal elements in the socket. In theory, longitudinal movement of the skeleton into the socket could be prevented by the incompressible nature of the residual limb tissues contained within a rigid socket.

To transmit force in this manner, the soft tissues of the residual limb must be contained in a vessel that accurately matches the volume of the residual limb. Various pressurized casting systems have been developed in an effort to achieve this match. A combination of pressure casting with a silicone liner that is distally fixed to the socket has been proposed as one method to achieve an efficient connection between the skeleton and the socket.

Vacuum casting has also been advocated, but its effect differs from pressurized casting. When a vacuum is created only between the surfaces of the residual limb and the casting apparatus, no load is applied to the soft tissues even though the replication of the unloaded surface shape and volume are accurate. With pressurized casting, the shape and volume of the residual limb are influenced by the load applied to the soft tissues. The soft tissues displace and stabilize the limb; the degree of displacement depends on the load applied, which is determined by the casting pressure. Pressurized casting is believed to produce a volume-matched and surface-matched impression. At least

in the casting situation, the soft tissues change shape in response to the equal pressure being applied. However, the shape of the socket needs to be adjusted in order to minimize pressure peaks that may occur in the dynamic situation, by either conventional relief or building a silicone pressure pad into the surface of the socket where a pressure peak is likely to occur.

Review of Prosthetic Component Developments
Application of Microprocessor Control to Lower Limb Prostheses

Research conducted in the early 1970s at the Massachusetts Institute of Technology (MIT) demonstrating the feasibility of using a computer to control the prosthetic knee was dismissed as impractical at the time. In 1986, when Nakagawa[17] of Hyogo Rehabilitation Center in Kobe, Japan, described a simpler application of microprocessor technology based on concepts developed at Osaka University, significant doubt still existed as to the clinical acceptability of such technology. It was not until the 1990s that the first commercial application of microprocessor control to prosthetic knee mechanisms was described.[18]

The traditional viewpoint was that the knee joint should be designed to provide stance control during the weight-bearing phase of locomotion and swing control during the non–weight-bearing phase. The swing phase was perceived as a simple pendulum action, which required a limited damping control during normal walking activity that also enabled the amputee to sit down. More recent research has demonstrated that this simplistic view of prosthetic knee function is inadequate.

My recent investigations have shown that, during a typical day, a lower limb amputee undertakes a number of standard repetitive mo-

tions (Table 3). Interestingly, stopping and standing with a stable knee is one of the most frequent functions required. The need to change walking speed occurs more often than descending stairs and ramps. The data in Table 3 are from 15 amputees who wore an electronic knee that recorded these activities over a period of 3 months.

Data such as these suggest that future prosthetic knee joints must provide stumble control—usually before the amputee is aware of the need—as well as support during stance to facilitate slowing down. In addition, the knee joint must alter the swing characteristics for slow, preferred, and fast walking speeds and provide stable support when standing. Additional stability during stair and ramp descent is also required. The specific type of mechanism for achieving these requirements was created through development of an adaptive prosthesis.[18] If microprocessor controls or mechatronic solutions provide the most reliable and cost-effective solution, then prosthetic component design will continue to evolve in those directions.

Microprocessor Control of Hydraulic and Pneumatic Knee Resistances

All currently available prosthetic components are passive systems—energy-dissipating replacements for human limbs. Current power sources and actuators have far too low a ratio of mass to energy capacity to actively power lower limb components under weight-bearing loads. Microprocessor-controlled passive prosthetic knees are now clinically available worldwide; they offer a wider range of walking speeds than earlier fluid-controlled systems that could be set by the prosthetist only for a fixed range of resistances.

The requirements for prosthetic knee function during level walking (Figure 1) are considerable. At heel strike the prosthetic knee must be stabilized as the foot begins plantar flex-

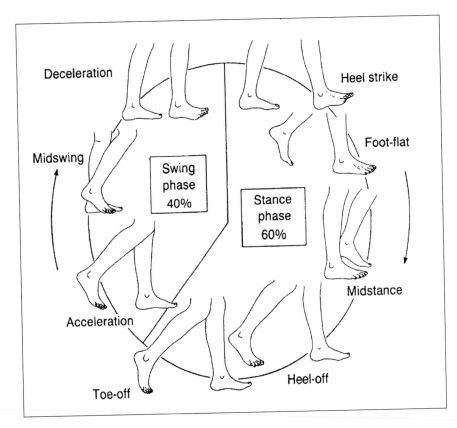

Figure 1 Phases of level walking.

ion. During this load-bearing period, the prosthesis has two major functions—support of the body weight and reduction in the impact of heel strike. This is achieved by a yielding flexion of the knee joint, which requires high flexion resistance. During the single-support phase, the body moves over the stabilized leg like an inverse pendulum. During this phase, the ground-reaction force vector changes its position from heel to forefoot. Because the flexed knee tends to extend rapidly, an appropriate extension resistance is also necessary to prevent abrupt extension of the knee. This resistance should adapt to different gait speeds. At the end of single-leg support, the maximum vertical load is generated and knee flexion begins shortly thereafter to prepare the limb for swing phase. Therefore, the knee resistance to flexion should be minimal.

The swing phase begins with the knee already flexed 30°; the maximum knee angle is 55° to 65°, and the time during which this range of knee motion must occur is very short. The prosthetic knee should start with minimal flexion resistance and adapt automatically to a wide range of gait speeds. At midswing, the shank changes the direction of rotation because of mass-reaction forces and the knee starts to extend. The terminal swing phase begins when the shank is vertical and ends when the extended leg hits the ground again. It is important that the knee joint extends quickly so that the leg is fully extended, but the terminal impact should be minimal.

This complex dynamic procedure can be best handled with an electronically controlled knee joint that provides hydraulic resistance during the extension elements of the swing and stance phases (Figure 2). The basic principle of this system is the detection of the current state of the amputee's gait by integrated sensors and the immediate adaptation of the flexion and extension resistances of the pros-

thetic knee. Key input signals are the knee flexion angle, the angular speed of the knee joint, and the anteroposterior bending moment of the shank. A hydraulic cylinder generates the required resistances for flexion and extension control.

I have documented recent developments providing microprocessor-controlled pneumatic swing-phase control.[18] Clinical experience with nearly 10,000 such devices has demonstrated that microprocessor control can optimize knee resistance over the entire range of the amputee's walking speed and result in a more energy-efficient gait. The Intelligent Prosthesis Plus (Charles A. Blatchford & Sons, LTD, Hampshire, England) uses microprocessor control to optimize pneumatic resistance to knee flexion and extension during swing phase.

In 1996, my associates and I began work on the next generation of microprocessor control by analyzing the activities that amputees undertake. Earlier research and development focused only on the primary function of walking. Real-time monitoring demonstrated that amputees undertake many activities in a day, including standing, slowing down, walking at various speeds, and descending ramps and stairs. The project goal was to create a prosthetic knee capable of adapting to different modes of locomotion while optimizing the amputee's voluntary muscle control and hip joint strength.

This development provides stance control ranging from minimal resistance to a yielding lock and is capable of detecting level walking, ramp descent, stair descent, sitting, standing, and stumble conditions. The stance resistance is set to a preprogrammed level for these different modes, which the prosthetist matches to the amputee's level of voluntary muscle control.

Rapid detection of different modes of locomotion is accomplished by the use of microprocessor technology and a range of sensors detecting kinetic and kinematic parameters around the knee. The prosthetist uses a remote programming device to adjust and fine-tune motor valve controls and to adjust the resistance to flexion in stance and swing in order to individualize the function for specific amputees.

The central concept in this knee design is the creation of a prosthesis that is accurately matched to an amputee's hip strength and ability to control the limb in all modes of ambulation. Clinical results suggest that most active amputees are able to control the prosthesis during level walking but may need additional support from the device when stopping or during ramp and stair descent. Amputees with limited hip power may need stumble control during the initiation of level walking. Most amputees seem to benefit from the standing mode, which allows them to relax without concern that the prosthetic knee may collapse.

The Adaptive Knee (Charles A. Blatchford & Sons, Ltd) combines the proven swing-phase control from the earlier Intelligent Prosthesis with a novel microprocessor-controlled hydraulic cylinder that provides variable stance stability for standing, stopping, stumble recovery, sitting, and stair or ramp descent.

Future of Microprocessor Technology

The widespread clinical acceptance of the integration of microchips into prosthetic knee mechanisms sets the stage for an exciting future. The immediate challenge is to increase processing power in order to create a prosthetic leg that can manage balance, stability, and comfort on its own. Work on the third generation of "smart" prostheses has already been initiated by the main companies that provide commercial microprocessor-controlled knee prostheses. MIT's Leg Laboratory, a research facility dedicated to studying locomotion and reproducing it robotically, is working on a knee that will automatically adapt as the amputee's gait changes, eliminating the need for the prosthe-

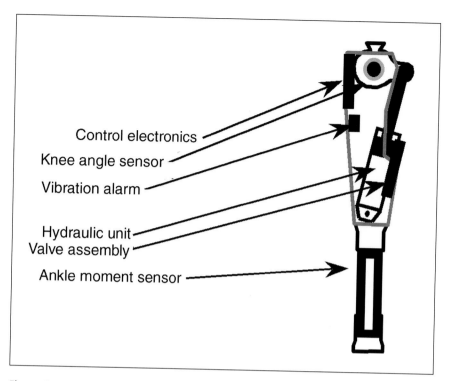

Figure 2 Sensors and electronic elements of the C-Leg system (Otto Bock HealthCare, Minneapolis, MN).

tist to make continual minor adjustments. Sensors generate a digital snapshot of the wearer's gait, which is analyzed by onboard software. Damping of knee motion is performed by metal plates that are separated by an iron-rich substance called magnetorheological fluid. The microprocessor switches the magnetic field around the fluid on and off, altering the way the plates move past each other and thus adjusting the resistance in the knee.

Funded by the US Department of Energy, Sandia National Laboratories has teamed with a group of Russian nuclear scientists to develop a microchip-embedded knee. German, Japanese, and British companies are working on future versions of their own computer-controlled prosthetic componentry. In another project, the Seattle Orthopaedic Group Inc (Seattle, WA; a private prosthetic component manufacturer) and Sandia National Laboratories—again working with Russian researchers—are collaborating to create a smart integrated lower limb that will be entirely digi-

tally controlled. Not only the knee, but also the ankle, foot, and leg socket will gather information from sensors and receive instructions from a software-guided microchip.

The intelligent hip joint described by Nakagawa[17] and a microprocessor-controlled prosthetic foot described by Zahedi[18] represent the short-term future of microprocessor control to complement available knee controls. Use of Bluetooth technology for communication between the ankle, knee, and hip will make interactive control on a commercial scale feasible. Formulation of a standard protocol would enable prescription of different feet, knees, and hip joints, regardless of manufacturer.

Intelligent Prosthetic Hip Joint

Hip disarticulation prostheses could be improved by controlling the swing of the hip joint. Careful observation and gait analysis have demonstrated that hip flexion angular velocity of current prostheses is far slower than in normal gait, and mechanical means

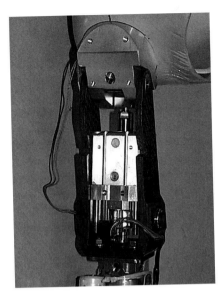

Figure 3 Intelligent hip joint. This prototype microprocessor-controlled pneumatic hip joint allows hip disarticulation amputees to walk at varying speeds with less effort than is required with a mechanical hip.

to accelerate hip flexion have been used clinically with some success. In one prototype (Figure 3), a pneumatic cylinder is compressed by the body weight of the user during stance phase. This air spring then accelerates thigh flexion in early swing phase. The compression varies depending on walking speed and is controlled by microprocessor positioning of the valve. This component allows hip disarticulation amputees to vary their cadence with less effort than that required with simpler mechanical hip joints.

Microprocessor-Controlled Ankle-Foot Complex

One concept for a prosthetic foot uses space frame technology for load structures and air muscles as primary stiffeners (Figure 4). The power ball pump provides controlled ankle movement and generates the air pressure needed to provide correct stiffness to the structure. This assembly can be loaded to absorb and restore energy at correct points in the gait cycle and to respond to changes in ca-

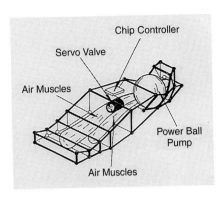

Figure 4 Microprocessor-controlled foot.

dence. The ability of the frame to absorb shock loads and provide axial rotation in a very low profile design makes this concept potentially suitable for many lower limb prostheses.

Cosmesis Developments

For many amputees, a prosthesis with a lifelike appearance is as important as its mechanical functionality. Today's patient often demands an external covering that in addition to protecting the components is lifelike, durable, lightweight, feels like normal skin, and is shaped and colored to closely match the contralateral leg.

Several manufacturers have developed elastomeric coverings, often made from silicone resins, that increase both the durability and cosmesis of artificial limbs. Patient acceptance has been excellent, particularly for transtibial prostheses. Unfortunately, when such coverings cross the knee joint, they tend to restrict flexion, so additional research is required to overcome this limitation.

Summary

Commercially funded research appears to be on the verge of significant technical advances that will improve the comfort, control, function, and appearance of lower limb prostheses in the coming decade. Whether this pace of development is sustained will depend largely on continued funding for prosthetic rehabilitation. If the current trend of reduced support for modern prostheses continues or in-

tensifies, commercial funding for research will also decline. Because governmental support for prosthetic research has been quite limited for several decades, a significant reduction in privately funded research will have a profound effect on the pace of innovation in future years.

References

1. Boni G: Socket fit studies: An investigation of the pressure patterns between stump and socket. Biotechnology Laboratory Technical Note No 25, Los Angles, CA, University of California, Los Angeles, May 1962.

2. Appoldt FA, Bennett L: A preliminary report on dynamic socket pressures. *Bull Prosthet Res* 1967;10:20-55.

3. Appoldt FA (ed): *Pressure and Force Measurement: A Report of a Workshop Sponsored by the Committee on Prosthetics Research and Development of the Division of Engineering and National Research Council.* Washington, DC, National Academy of Sciences, 1968.

4. Appoldt FA, Bennett L, Contini R: Socket pressure as a function of pressure transducer protrusion. *Bull Prosthet Res* 1969;10:20-55.

5. Appoldt FA, Bennet L, Contini R: Tangential pressure measurements in above-knee suction sockets. *Bull Prosthet Res* 1970;10:70-86.

6. Corell EB (ed): *Normal Pressure Distributions Applied by Total Contact Below-Knee Prostheses.* Ann Arbor, MI, University of Michigan, Medical School, Department of Physical Medicine and Rehabilitation, Orthotics Research Project, 1969.

7. Rae JW, Cockrell JL: Interface pressure and stress distribution in prosthetic fitting. *Bull Prosthet Res* 1971;10: 64-111.

8. Pearson JR, Grevsten S, Almby B, Marsh L: Pressure variation in the below-knee patellar tendon bearing suction socket prosthesis. *J Biomech* 1974;7:487-496.

9. Burgess EM, Moore AJ: A study of interface pressures in the below-knee prosthesis: Psychological suspension. An interim report. *Bull Prosthet Res* 1977;14:58-70.

10. Redhead RG: Total surface bearing self-suspending above knee sockets. *Prosthet Orthot Int* 1979;3:126-136.

11. Meier RH III, Meeks ED Jr, Herman RM: Stump-socket fit of below-knee prostheses: Comparison of three methods of measurement. *Arch Phys Med Rehabil* 1973;54:553-558.

12. Naeff M, van Pijkeren T: Dynamic pressure measurements at the interface between residual limb and socket: The relationship between pressure distribution, comfort, and brim shape. *Bull Prosthet Res* 1980;17:35-50.

13. Isherwood PA: Simultaneous PTB Socket Pressure and Force Plate Values. Preliminary Report, BRADU [Biomechanical Research and Development Unit] Report, 1978, pp 45-49.

14. Day HJB: The assessment and description of amputee activity. *Prosthet Orthot Int* 1981;5:23-28.

15. Brånemark R, Brånemark PI, Rydevik B, et al: Osseointegration in skeletal reconstruction and rehabilitation: A review. *J Rehabil Res Dev* 2001;38: 175-181.

16. Bergkvist R, Johansson S, Karlsson D: Gait analysis of amputee with osseointegrated lower limb prosthesis. *Proceedings of XIII International Interbor Congress.* Oslo, Norway, 1996.

17. Nakagawa A: Abstract Microprocessor control of hip joint functions. *Book of Abstracts.* 10th World Congress of the International Society for Prosthetics and Orthotics, 2001.

18. Zahedi S: Bewertung und Biomechanik der intelligenten Prothese: Eine Zwei-Jahres-Studie. *Orthop Tech* 1995;46:32-40.

Section IV

Management Issues

Future Developments: Osseointegration in Transfemoral Amputees

Kingsley Peter Robinson, MS, FRCS
Rickard Brånemark, MD, MSc, PhD
David A. Ward, FRCS Orth

Introduction

The possibility of attaching a prosthesis directly to the bone of a residual limb has long been anticipated. What was required was technology that enabled bone to incorporate a foreign material and allowed the material to safely penetrate the external surface of the body.

The first application of metal penetration of both skin and bone was by Malgaigne in 1843, when he used an external screw to engage a fractured tibia in an early form of external fixation. Since then, the Steinmann pin has been used routinely to control bone position by temporary transfixion of soft tissue and bone. Today, treatment by external fixation is well accepted. Over a long period of time, however, intraosseous foreign material may loosen and could remain an infection risk. Despite the extensive research and progress that has allowed prosthetic implants in bone to become part of routine orthopaedic practice, this problem still exists.

Experimental work on bone fixation of limb prostheses in the past has been sporadic and limited in scale.[1] A project to develop this in the United States in 1942 was rejected. In 1946, Dummer of Pineberg in Germany studied implanted metal limb extensions in sheep and extended the study to human patients, four of whom had prostheses attached to metal implants. When infection developed in one patient, the study was discontinued and all implants were removed. Cutler and Blodgett[2] also studied skeletal attachments experimentally.

In the United States, Mooney and associates[3] fitted a prosthesis to the humerus of a triple amputee; because of leakage, the implant was removed after a few months. Further study of penetrating implants to attach prostheses in a dog model was conducted by Esslinger.[4] Hall and Rostoker[5] reported a considerable degree of success with implants into the hind limb of Spanish goats; of 20, only two implants failed over a period of 14 months, during which time some of the goats were very active. Ling[6] reviewed the problems inherent in these procedures.

These data provided little encouragement for further studies until an unrelated observation by Brånemark[7] revealed the possibility of long-term tolerance of a metal implant connected to the exterior. To study microcirculation within bone, Brånemark inserted a titanium observation tube into the bone marrow of rabbit tibia. The device was almost impossible to remove after several weeks of study. The titanium appeared to have integrated with the bone, despite the transit through the skin and soft tissue.

In later studies, Brånemark and others[8-12] showed that commercially pure titanium was well tolerated within living bone and relatively resistant to infection. Titanium forms a resistant surface oxide layer. In living tissue this can be augmented by a peroxide layer, which is thought to be a hydrated titanium peroxy matrix. This layer does not tolerate surface pathogenic activity, nor does it inhibit endothelial cells or osteocytes. At the same time, however, it does inhibit macrophages, thus allowing the material to be tolerated in the living bone without the interposition of a fibrous tissue layer. This close contact has been termed osseointegration with the implanted material.[13] Research continues to investigate the benefit from surface additives or treatment of the machined titanium surface. The biomechanical effects of an intraosseous implant have been studied in California, Sweden, and the United Kingdom.[9,11,14,15] Jacobs and associates[16] investigated the sensation derived from the prosthesis in amputees with conventional and bone-fixed prostheses. Nerve endings in proximity to the intraosseous titanium implant and the role of neuropeptides were demonstrated in work by Ysander and associates.[17]

The interface between the skin and the penetrating metal has been the subject of a large number of studies. Acrylate adhesives provide only temporary attachment to a metal surface. A considerable degree of cellular invasion into mesh materials, including titanium gauze and textile meshes of

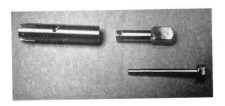

Figure 1 Titanium components of the Brånemark prosthetic attachment system. The threaded implant is on the left; the skin-penetrating abutment is on the right, with the retaining screw below it. (*Courtesy of Rickard Brånemark, MD, MSc, PhD.*)

various polymers, has been observed, but these materials have not yet been shown to provide any advantage over the simple skin perforation of the Brånemark method. One case of osseointegrated attachment of a prosthesis in a male transfemoral amputee was reported by Staubach and Grundei.[18] They used titanium mesh and reported on surface treatment of the titanium.

The Brånemark System for Bone Attachment of Limb Prostheses

The implant that is inserted into the medullary cavity of the residual long bone after an amputation consists of a tubular component with a surface self-tapping screw thread that engages the inner aspect of the cortex of the shaft of the bone (Figure 1). The connecting component, called the abutment, is attached to the lower end of the implant. The abutment penetrates the skin at the most distal part of the residual limb and protrudes to permit the attachment of the prosthesis with a screw-tightened clamp.

The abutment is located in the lower end of the implant in a hexagonal recess and is retained by a long bolt that passes through the abutment to engage an internal threaded section in the lower part of the implant. The head of the retaining bolt thus forms the lowest point of the protruding abutment when in place. This arrangement enables the abutment to

be changed without disturbing the implant. A damaged abutment can be replaced painlessly without anesthetic. If use of the system has to be discontinued, only the abutment need be removed, after which the penetration site heals rapidly.

All of the components facing the biologic environment are fabricated from commercially pure titanium to avoid electrolytic corrosion. For this reason, the stronger titanium alloys are avoided in the system. The instruments used to handle these components are also made of the same titanium.

Time is required for the living bone to develop tolerance to the titanium. At present this period is considered to be 6 months in the residual femur, 3 months in a digit, and less in a dental implant. A two-stage surgical procedure is necessary to establish the system in limb amputees. During the first stage, the implant is placed in the bone, and the skin and soft tissues are closed. In the second stage, the scar is reopened, the skin penetration formed, and the abutment placed, in preparation for attachment of the training aid that precedes the use of the limb prosthesis.

The Brånemark system has been used extensively for dental prostheses, maxillofacial reconstructions, prosthetic ears, and hearing aids. Phalangeal and metacarpal implants are particularly effective for thumb prostheses. Radial and ulnar implants have been used for transradial amputees, and humeral implants for higher levels. All of these amputees have been treated by custom-designed implant systems.[19]

In the lower limb, the most common use is for implants in the residual femur for transfemoral amputees, with the system available "off the shelf." The system is not yet available for other lower limb levels. Because of the high loading imposed by lower limb prosthesis use, the load is slowly and progressively applied. The time from commencement of loading to unrestricted use of a prosthesis without aids may be 6 to 12 months, de-

pending on body weight and initial bone quality.

Clinical Management

Management of the transfemoral amputee is in accordance with the guidelines of Malchau[20] for the stepwise introduction of new implant technology. These guidelines have now been used in Gothenburg, London, and Melbourne with minor variations.

Amputees interested in the Brånemark system at present must appreciate that the procedure remains in an early stage and must therefore be prepared to be recruited as volunteers for participation in the clinical study. They must sign an in-depth informed consent document that incorporates the widest ethical considerations and is approved by the appropriate authorities.

Comprehensive information is provided to each candidate in an initial pamphlet and during a preliminary clinic consultation, after which the candidate's medical advisors are consulted to obtain their approval and referral. Further consultation and discussion is undertaken to determine if the patient should proceed to a 3- to 5-day residential assessment. During this period each member of the multidisciplinary team can contribute, and the amputee can obtain all the available information on which to base a decision to take part in the clinical study. The opportunity to meet others using the system for the same amputation level is an important factor in establishing realistic expectations. In addition, because 18 months is such a lengthy time commitment to a clinical program, the amputee must be confident that the benefit will justify participation. Outside employment may not be possible during the training period after the second-stage operation.

Recruitment to the osseointegrated prostheses study is intended to exclude those amputees with factors that interfere with bone healing, such as steroid use, immunosuppression, diabetes mellitus, chemotherapy medication, neoplastic disease, and age older

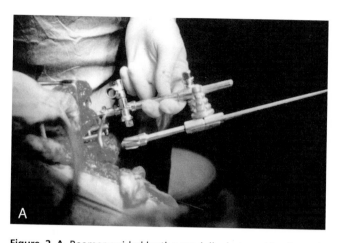
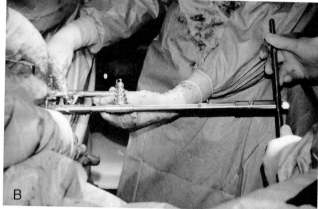

Figure 2 A, Reamer guided by the specially designed jig. **B,** Implant being introduced into the prepared medullary cavity of the femur.

than 70 years, as well as adverse factors such as heavy smoking, weight greater than 100 kg, or psychiatric disorders that could interfere with maintenance of the treatment protocol.

Local factors in the residual limb may also be adverse, such as osteopenia, residual bone infection, and local or general bone disease. Residual bone length that is too short to contain the implant, degenerative hip joint disease, and fixed flexion deformity of the hip are also contraindications.

The amputees who are likely to benefit most are those who are unable to tolerate a conventional socket prosthesis, either entirely or to the extent that the use of a prosthesis is limited significantly. Individuals with short residual limbs and bilateral transfemoral amputees are good candidates. A survey of transfemoral amputees indicates that many of them accept discomfort and poor function from their socket prostheses.[21] As experience with the technique expands, indications for the system may also grow.

Preoperative Preparation

Prior to the first operation, the implant is selected or manufactured on the basis of 1:1-scale CT scans of the residual femur. The spiral CT scan on skeletal setting is calibrated for 1-mm cuts over the length of the proposed site of the implant and 3-mm cuts over the remainder of the femur. The limb must be immobilized securely during

the scan, and the axis must be maintained constantly at 90° to the plane of the scan cuts. Three-dimensional reconstruction may be helpful with deformed or abnormal bones. The implant is placed where it has optimum contact with the compact cortical bone of the femoral shaft; this location is where the self-tapping screw thread must engage to a depth of 1.5 mm over the maximum surface area of the implant. The typical diameter in an adult male amputee is 16 to 20 mm.

The surgical preparation is the same as for any other major orthopaedic procedure in which a prosthesis is implanted. Low-molecular-weight heparin prophylaxis is initiated, and perioperative intravenous antibiotics are administered. The patient's blood type should be known, and a transfusion capability should be available on-site; however, transfusion is rarely required.

Surgical Procedure
First-Stage Operation

Either epidural or general anesthesia is satisfactory. The patient should be in the prone position, with the residual limb isolated and mobile. The operating room should be equipped with image intensifier capability. Mono- and bipolar diathermy are used, and saline irrigation with suction is required. Free blood and bone material are collected to provide lubrication for insertion of the implant and as a source of bone cells.

Usually the existing terminal scar of the residual limb is excised and the original full-thickness skin flaps are raised. The muscle in the vicinity of the bone end is cleared. The optimum length of the residual femur will already have been determined from radiographs; any necessary shortening will be performed at this stage. Ideally, space of at least 25 cm will be available from the end of the femur to the level of the opposite knee joint line for the attachment of components. The minimum length of residual femur should be 5 to 8 cm below the lesser trochanter. Bone graft to the intertrochanteric bone might be indicated where poor-quality cancellous bone is present. The periosteum will be stripped proximally to facilitate the necessary resection. Any required reconstruction of the residual limb is normally delayed until the second-stage procedure.

The bone end is exposed, the femoral medullary cavity is identified, and the muscles are split proximally to expose the femoral shaft 5 to 10 cm proximal to the bone end. In this exposed area, the clamp of the introducer jig is applied, and a provisional alignment with the bone end is fixed (Figure 2, *A*). Using the jig, the femoral canal is entered and the alignment checked with the image intensifier. With this alignment, the femoral medullary cavity is bored out with hand reamers to the diameter planned from the CT scan. Slow rotation and fre-

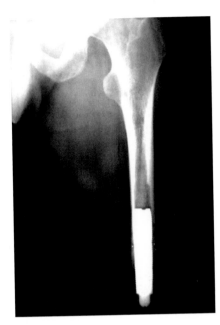

Figure 3 Postoperative radiograph of the residual femur with the implant in place. Ideally, reaming should coincide with the top of the implant.

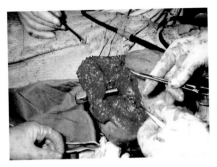

Figure 4 The second-stage surgery, showing the abutment penetrating the prepared skin flap and connected to the implant, which is within the femur on the right.

quent saline irrigation are used to avoid bone heating. The hazards of bone damage from heating have been described by Krause and associates.[22] The alignment is checked repeatedly until the implant is inserted.

Any bone residues and the filtrate of any blood collected are introduced into the marrow cavity above the implant site. The implant is mounted on its introducer, which is placed in the guide used for the reaming process (Figure 2, *B*). The introducer acts as a shaft to drive the implant mounted on its proximal end, powered by the "T" handle at the other end. Some skill and strength are required to screw the implant into its planned position. If the rotation is stopped, the implant may bind, despite lubrication with blood and saline. When the implant is in place, the position is checked again, and the image intensifier images are recorded for future reference (Figure 3).

The lumen of the implant is thoroughly cleansed with saline irrigation. The closing screw and stage-one temporary cylinder are then inserted from below to close the lower part of the lumen of the implant and pre-

serve the internal thread, which later will accept the abutment-retaining bolt. The displaced muscle and soft tissue are sutured into place, and the skin is closed with suction drainage in place. A normal dressing is applied.

The amputee usually makes a rapid recovery. The residual limb is rested until the suction drain is removed at 24 hours. At this time, when full activity is resumed, most amputees who have been unable to use a prosthesis will recommence crutch walking. A conventional prosthesis can be worn if this was possible before the operation. However, a supervised exercise program should be initiated promptly so that a hip flexion contracture does not develop.

In the 6 months until the second stage, maintaining a high level of physical fitness is encouraged. Weight gain must be avoided, and anything that compromises bone healing is discouraged, including smoking, substance abuse, and excessive alcohol consumption. A normal varied diet with calcium and vitamin supplements is recommended. During this period, radiographs and isotope scans should be avoided if possible.

Second-Stage Operation

The preoperative management is the same as for the first-stage operation, with administration of antibiotic prophylaxis and low-molecular-weight heparin. The previous surgical scar is excised or reopened to allow full-thickness skin and subcutaneous tis-

sue flaps to be raised. The estimated site for the penetration of the abutment would have been marked when the formation of the flaps was planned. The important considerations are the need for healthy skin, a blood supply uncompromised by previous scars, and a flap design that, if possible, avoids excessive tissue separation. The dissection is carried to the bone end and the closing screw is revealed.

If the first-stage operation did not produce an effective myoplasty or myodesis, this procedure must now be performed to retain the function of the residual muscles. Redundant soft tissue is trimmed and muscle is securely sutured to the distal periosteum and the opposing muscle to effect a strong myoplasty located at, but not covering, the bone end. In some early cases the muscles were secured by sutures through multiple small drill holes at the bone end (myodesis), but this impaired healing at the penetration site. The bone end should be flat, smooth, and clear of periosteum, with rounded edges to produce the largest possible area of living bone for adhesion to the skin at the penetration site.

The position of the penetration mark is checked when the flap is placed over the bone end. The inside of the flap at this site is thinned over an area corresponding to the bone end, in the manner of a full-thickness skin graft. This can be safely achieved by using the edge of a glass slide as a scraper. The closing screw and cylinder are removed and the selected abutment checked for size and fit. Considerable cleansing and irrigation are required to clear the lumen of the lower portion of the implant. The penetration of the skin for the transit of the abutment is made with a single stab incision or with a puncture by a dermatology biopsy punch. The abutment is passed through the penetration in the skin flap and seated in the hexagonal socket at the lower end of the implant (Figure 4). The abutment-retaining bolt is then introduced into the lower end of the abutment and advanced to engage the threaded part of the lumen of the implant. It is finger-tightened at this stage, and the soft tissue is lightly sutured to locate the flap without any tension on the penetration site.

The skin closure is accomplished in a conventional fashion, with suction drainage if required (a hematoma could compromise the viability of the skin at the penetration site). The abutment bolt is tightened to a torque value of 12 N·m, and its security is once again checked. The penetration site is dressed with paraffin gauze, and the residual limb with a fluffed gauze light-pressure bandage. A dressing cylinder is provided to fit on the stem of the abutment and retain the penetration dressing. This 10-cm-diameter cylinder is secured by a slide to the abutment shaft; this allows easy removal for dressing changes. The pressure exerted by the dressing must be monitored to avoid skin necrosis of the penetration site over bone end.

After the operation, close supervision is necessary to ensure rapid healing with adhesion of the skin to the bone end. Close approximation of the skin to the abutment shaft and stable healing of the skin onto the bone end appear to provide the best chance of a trouble-free penetration (Figure 5). Because daily hygiene is also critical, the amputee is instructed in the care of the penetration. Each day the site should be wiped with sterile saline solution and any crusting or discharge removed. After the first week, no dressing is required; a polyethylene foam disk or a twist of dry gauze is all that is required. Ventilation and cleanliness are the only necessities.

Postoperative Management

The patient is discharged home 2 to 3 weeks after the second-stage operation, when the skin around the penetration is satisfactory and the tissue reaction to the surgery has resolved. A gentle exercise program that avoids resisted or rotational movements is

started. The prevention of hip flexion contracture is of great importance. The patient is reviewed weekly until the sixth postoperative week, when the training program begins.

The torque of the abutment-retaining bolt is checked at regular intervals. Some tightening may be required to regain the 12-N·m torque. Any loosening at the abutment-implant interface will cause micromotion, with component wear and black discharge of titanium oxide particles.

A short training prosthesis is provided to facilitate the exercise program and to apply measured force to the abutment and thus to the implant. The training prosthesis is a tubular extension 35 to 40 cm long, which is clamped to the abutment. This corresponds to the length of the opposite femur, measured from the opposite knee joint line. The prosthesis has a platform end on which the amputee can apply measured vertical loads to the abutment, initially 20 kg, by pressing onto spring bathroom scales. The axial weight load is increased by 10 kg each week. After 3 weeks, the load is applied for 10 to 15 minutes each day. When 40-kg weight bearing is achieved, resisted exercise is commenced with a 1-kg weight attached to the end of the short training prosthesis. The amputee may then proceed to prone kneeling. Once 60-kg loading is achieved, upright kneeling can be initiated. By 12 weeks, full weight bearing may be reached. If at any stage the residual limb becomes painful, the loading program is interrupted until the pain has resolved. Full weight bearing should be achieved 3 to 6 months after the second-stage operation. At this time, the amputee can be supplied with a full-length temporary prosthesis with a knee and foot mechanism.

Standing weight bearing is commenced between parallel bars with a progressive increase in load until 6 weeks of partial weight bearing enables the patient to start walking with crutches. The patient progresses to walking with canes until unrestricted

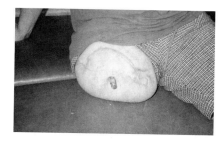

Figure 5 The healed residual limb, with the abutment projecting from the penetration site.

walking is possible. The amputee learns to recognize that pain in the vicinity of the implant represents overloading and that this resolves quickly with load reduction or rest. Persistent pain must be investigated to exclude the possibility of deep infection. Repeated overstress pain will delay progress, especially if the pain takes several weeks to resolve. This will determine the time required until full weight bearing and activity can be achieved. From our experience, we have found that the amputee should be prepared for the loading program to take up to 1 year from the second-stage operation, but usually it is achieved in 3 to 6 months.

Prosthetic Management

When the initial assessment is conducted, the amputee is asked to provide his or her latest lower limb prosthesis, even if it has not been used for some years. To assess gait, a dynamic video recording is made of the amputee walking while wearing the prosthesis in the gait laboratory; force plate gait studies are also conducted. The knee mechanism is first replaced with the Swedish Total Knee (Ossur, Reykjavik, Iceland), which is the standard for the study. Records (including video) are then made of the amputee's gait in the preoperative state.

As described earlier, a short training prosthesis is provided after the second-stage operation for loading of the abutment before the first full-length training prosthesis is made. This is a temporary endoskeletal prosthesis, constructed from standard components with the exception of the

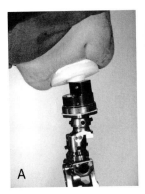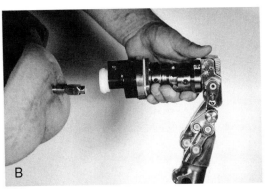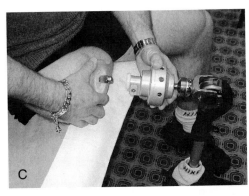

Figure 6 The prosthetic attachment system. **A,** The top clamp conceals the abutment and incorporates the Mark 1 fail-safe device, above the universal knee mechanism attachment. **B,** The clamp released to show the relationship to the abutment. **C,** The later Mark 2 fail-safe device (Rotasafe) provides protection against excessive rotational and bending forces in the event of accidental trauma.

securing clamp at the upper end. This screw-tightened clamp closes around the squared lower end of the abutment. The screw is operated by an Allen wrench, which is carried by the amputee. The clamp is incorporated into an abutment protection device with a rotational fail-safe mechanism. Below this is the alignment device for angular and axial adjustment. These devices require a large range of movement and a high degree of security. Beneath this assembly is a standard adaptor for attachment of the knee joint mechanism. The length of the residual limb must allow a minimum distance of 25 cm for these components.

The basic knee mechanism for the clinical trial, the Swedish Total Knee, allows 160° of flexion and has a mechanical stance-phase control; a hydraulic swing-phase control is an alternative. When the amputee is able to assess the qualities of the knee mechanism, other units are offered to meet individual preferences. Some have preferred the Otto Bock 3R80 mechanism (Otto Bock HealthCare, Vienna, Austria), which allows 140° of knee flexion with both hydraulic swing-phase control and stance-phase control. Without a socket, the full range of knee flexion is possible. This has great value to the osseointegration project amputees because they are able to pedal a cycle without difficulty and can squat or sit cross-legged on the ground. Amputees also have the opportunity to try other

devices to suit their individual requirements.

Below the knee mechanism, a standard shank is connected to a Dynamic Foot (Otto Bock). The interposition of a torque control and shock-absorbing unit at ankle level has proven to be of value. The characteristics of the prosthetic heel and the compliance of the system are quite obvious to the amputee, who will select the degree of shock absorption that provides the maximum comfort during and after walking activities. The degree of comfort appears to be strongly related to the accuracy of the alignment and the way in which it is matched to the individual's gait pattern. This seems to be more critical in amputees with bone-fixed prostheses than in those with a conventional socket that provides a degree of compliance and tolerance.

The implant and abutment are in line with the femoral shaft, which anatomically meets the axis of the lower leg at 7° of valgus. However, if this angulation is incorporated into the alignment, it is poorly tolerated, and the gait remains abnormal with a lateral movement in each step. Currently the alignment is set by a process of trial and adjustment, to produce the best gait for the individual amputee. The gait is satisfactory for the individual yet appears abnormal to an observer. Although not required by the amputee, use of a cane will improve the gait. A general weakness in the

muscles of the residual limb, in particular the hip adductors, and/or myostatic contracture of the abductor muscles will favor an abducted stance with the prosthesis and a resulting lurching gait. Amputees with well-developed muscles walk with an almost normal gait.

A cosmetic cover can be supplied. Caution must be exercised, however, to avoid changes in the functional characteristics of the knee and ankle mechanisms.

The most salient problem with the prosthesis is protection of the implant and abutment from abnormal stress and trauma. Although the implant within the femur is largely protected, the femur could fracture above the implant. Fracture or bending of the abutment and its retaining bolt are more likely. The damaged abutment can be removed and replaced by unscrewing the bolt and extracting the abutment under sterile conditions. This procedure is best performed in a minor operating room; however, no anesthesia is required. The penetration and the screw thread are carefully cleansed with saline before the new abutment and bolt are inserted. When correctly seated, the bolt is set to the correct torque of 12 N·m and the prosthesis is then reattached.

Because this is a costly and troublesome complication, incorporation of a fail-safe device in the prosthetic system is desirable (Figure 6). This device should be immediately below the abutment clamp at the upper end of the prosthesis to protect against excessive rotational and angulation stress. One sophisticated and complex component is available, the Rotasafe device (Integrum AB, Gothenburg, Sweden), which can be placed between the clamp and the knee mechanism. This device can be set to release when stressed to a predetermined value. It will then stabilize to prevent uncontrolled collapse or detachment of the prosthesis.

The prosthetic system gives the amputee a feeling of security. In addition, because the prosthesis is attached to the body, the amputee will experience some sensory feedback from ground contact, enabling recognition of differences in the walking surface. Termed osseoperception, this phenomenon has been studied in relation to the awareness of vibration. Some patients comment that the prosthesis feels like a part of them; as a result, they feel more normal. The prosthesis is worn without time limitation and incorporated into a normal lifestyle. Opportunities to participate in sporting activities expand, including cycling and swimming in clean water. The ability to perform manual labor, drive vehicles, and operate machinery has enabled return to employment in the British group. Swedish amputees have returned to farming and animal husbandry. The prosthesis can be attached and removed readily with the Allen wrench, and full hip and knee flexion yields an increase in agility.

Clinical Application

The clinical application of the osseointegration technique in amputees followed the experimental work in Gothenburg, after considerable experience had been acquired in the use of implants for dental restoration and maxillofacial reconstructions. The application was extended to digital, metacarpal, and arm implants for prosthetic attachment. Thumb prostheses mounted on metacarpal implants are particularly successful in restoring function to the damaged hand. Radial and ulnar implants transmit pronation and supination to the prosthesis, and the stability of the prosthesis allows precise myoelectric control of hand function. Humeral implants also enhance arm prosthetic function. Although these have been under progressive development since 1991, the number of users remains small. Brånemark and associates[19] reviewed these various aspects of osseointegration in 2001.

The first application of lower limb implants was in a bilateral transfemoral amputee with short residual limbs who was unable to wear prostheses and was limited to wheelchair mobility. Her implants show no change after 11 years. In the early part of the series, while the procedure and instrumentation were being developed, the implants were performed on an individual volunteer basis. The design of the implant was then refined, the surgical procedure modified, the abutment improved, and the duration of the healing phase and the loading program altered. Because of all these changes, it was difficult to choose a starting point for the collection of clinical evidence to evaluate the procedure. A formal clinical trial for lower limb amputees called Osseointegration Prosthesis Rehabilitation for Amputees began in May 1999. Although 50 lower limb amputees have undergone the procedure, only 16 have been formally enrolled in the research trial.[23] The trial was extended to London and Melbourne, in addition to the Swedish subjects.

The Swedish lower limb amputees include three at transtibial level, two with very short residual limbs. These procedures failed as a result of poor bone quality at the site, with resulting lack of stability. The third transtibial amputee had a long residual limb (27 cm from the tip of the greater trochanter) and has successfully used the system for more than 5 years. The other trial participants were all at the transfemoral level. Some episodes of minor superficial infection occurred, and deep infection or loosening necessitated the removal of the implant

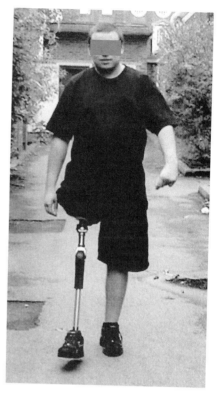

Figure 7 One of the London amputees during a prosthetic review 2 years after the second-stage operation.

from eight amputees. In two of them, the implant was later replaced, with satisfactory results. One amputee fell, fracturing the femur, but went on to full recovery. Several required abutment replacement because of damage from falls; these incidents preceded introduction of the Rotasafe device.

The Melbourne experience includes two transfemoral amputees who have used the system for 2 years. The male amputee had one abutment change, and the female amputee has had no problems.

The London experience is of 11 male amputees, aged 25 to 41 years. The longest period of use is 6.3 years (cumulative use, 33 years). Two amputees had the implant removed because of deep infection; one may have been a recurrence of a past infection. Both now have satisfactory socket prostheses. The remaining nine amputees are all effective prosthesis users with active lifestyles; one is undergoing job retraining, and the rest have returned to employment (Figure 7).

Superficial infections at the penetration site, which have been infrequent, have been treated initially with amoxyl and flucloxacillin replaced as indicated by the microbiology swab culture result. However, the active lifestyles enjoyed by the group have resulted in the replacement of 11 abutments. In one patient the appearance of black discharge indicated some micromotion in the titanium attachment of the abutment. This was not controlled by maintaining the specified torque, and a customized new abutment solved the problem.

The groups were assessed by a clinical psychologist both by interview and questionnaire. The positive findings were enjoyment of increased activity, greater mobility, and a more normal lifestyle. Several commented that they no longer felt disabled by their amputation. The quick and easy connection and removal of the prosthesis were appreciated, together with the sensory awareness of the type of ground contact. The appearance of the abutment was accepted by close family, and a cosmetic cover was not always requested. Pain was an issue only after severe overload or trauma and cleared spontaneously. Pain that did not clear could be an indication of a deep infection.

The primary negative aspect that emerged was the long period of commitment to the program, with the attendant domestic, social, and employment problems. The previously healthy amputees found it difficult to assume the role of patient; involvement with the hospital included frequent supervision and adjustments. The hygiene requirements were only slightly inconvenient. All amputees felt that the advantages outweighed the disadvantages, however.

Summary and Conclusions

Osseointegration provides a new and original method for the direct attachment of prostheses to the skeleton. Although the concept provides stability and improved function for upper limb prostheses and a valuable replacement for a missing thumb, application in the lower limb offers the opportunity for full prosthetic use to transfemoral amputees who have been unable to achieve rehabilitation and walking function with a conventional socket prosthesis. In the future, osseointegration may play a role in forequarter and transpelvic amputations as well as transtibial amputations. Perhaps one day the technique will have developed to the point where it could be used as a primary treatment.

Acknowledgments

We wish to acknowledge the contribution made to this work by the multidisciplinary teams of the Orthopaedic Departments and Rehabilitation Services in Gothenburg and Kingston Hospital with the Rehabilitation Centre of Queen Mary's Hospital, Roehampton, London. We are grateful for the support of the Institute of Applied Biotechnology, the University of Gothenburg, the University of Surrey, the Douglas Bader Foundation, the Remedi Foundation, and the Norman Rowe Trust.

References

1. Murphy EF: History and philosophy of attachment of prostheses to the musculo-skeletal system and of passage through the skin with inert materials. *J Biomed Mater Res* 1973;7: 275-295.

2. Cutler E, Blodgett JB: Skeletal attachment of prostheses for the leg (final report of Harvard University). Contract OEM cmr-214. Washington, DC, 1945, Committee on Medical Research of the Office of Scientific Research and Development.

3. Mooney V, Predecki PK, Renning J, Gray J: Skeletal extension of limb prosthetics attachment problems in tissue reaction. *J Mater Res Symp* 1971; 2:143-159.

4. Esslinger JO: A basic study in semi-buried implants and osseous attachments for application to amputation prosthetic fitting. *Bull Prosthet Res* 1970;10:219-225.

5. Hall WC, Rostoker W: Permanently attached artificial limbs. *Bull Prosthet Res* 1980;17:98-100.

6. Ling RS: Observations on the fixation of implants to the bony skeleton. *Clin Orthop* 1986;210:80-96.

7. Brånemark PI: Vital microscopy of bone marrow in rabbit. *Scand J Clin Lab Invest* 1959;11(suppl 38): 1-82.

8. Brånemark PI: Osseointegration and its experimental background. *J Prosthet Dent* 1983;50:399-410.

9. Brånemark PI, Rydevik BL, Skalak R: *Osseointegration in Skeletal Reconstruction and Joint Replacement*. Chicago, IL, Quintessence Publishing, 1997.

10. Albrektsson T, Brånemark PI, Hansson HA, Lindstrom J: Osseointegrated titanium implants: Requirements for ensuring a long-lasting direct bone-to-implant anchorage in man. *Acta Orthop Scand* 1981;52:155-170.

11. Brånemark RA: *A Biomechanical Study of Osseointegration: In-vivo Measurements in Rat, Rabbit, Dog and Man*. Gothenburg, Sweden, Gothenburg University. 1996. Dissertation.

12. Hansson HA, Albrektsson T, Brånemark PI: Structural aspects of the interface between tissue and titanium implants. *J Prosthet Dent* 1983;50: 108-113.

13. Linder L, Albrektsson T, Brånemark, PI, et al: Electron microscopic analysis of the bone-titanium interface. *Acta Orthop Scand* 1983;54:45-52.

14. Skalak R: Biomedical considerations in osseointegration prostheses. *J Prosthet Dent* 1983;49:843-848.

15. Xu W, Crocombe AD, Hughes SC: Finite element analysis of bone stress and strain around a distal osseointegrated implant for prosthetic limb attachment. *Proc Inst Mech Eng* 2000; 214:595-602.

16. Jacobs R, Brånemark R, Olmarker K, Rydevik B, Van Steenberghe D, Brånemark PI: Evaluation of the psychophysical detection threshold level for vibrotactile and pressure stimulation of prosthetic limbs using bone anchorage or soft tissue support. *Prosthet Orthot Int* 2000;24:133-142.

17. Ysander M, Brånemark R, Olmarker K, Myers RR: Intramedullary osseointegration: Development of a rodent

model and study of histology and neuropeptide changes around titanium implants. *J Rehab Res Dev* 2001;38: 183-190.

18. Staubach KH, Grundei H: The first osseointegrated percutaneous prosthesis anchor for above-knee amputees. *Biomed Tech* 2001;46:355-361.

19. Brånemark R, Brånemark PI, Rydevik B, Myers RR: Osseointegration in skeletal reconstruction and rehabilitation:

A review. *J Rehabil Res Dev* 2001;38: 175-181.

20. Malchau H: *On the Importance of Stepwise Introduction of New Hip Implant Technology.* Gothenburg, Sweden, Gothenburg University, 1995. Thesis.

21. Hagberg K, Brånemark R: Consequences of non-vascular trans-femoral amputations: A survey of quality of life, prosthetic use and problems. *Prosthet Orthot Int* 2001;25:186-194.

22. Krause WR, Bradbury DW, Kelly JE, Lunceford EM: Temperature elevations in orthopaedic cutting operations. *J Biomech* 1982;15:267-275.

23. Gunterberg B, Brånemark PI, Brånemark R, Bergh P, Rydevik B: Osseointegrated prostheses in lower limb amputation. *Proceedings of IXth World Congress of the International Society for Prosthetics and Orthotics.* Amsterdam, The Netherlands, 1998, pp 137-139.

Chapter 54

Musculoskeletal Complications

John J. Murnaghan, MD, MSc, MA, FRCSC
John H. Bowker, MD

Introduction

One of the primary aims of any surgical procedure, apart from obtaining rapid, sound wound healing, is the prevention of surgical complications. Amputation has the additional possibility of complications related to the residual limb–prosthesis interface. In general, the frequency and severity of complications associated with amputations can be minimized if the surgeon is interested in the challenge of accomplishing a properly designed and executed amputation and keeps abreast of innovations. A casual or defeatist attitude toward amputation surgery as a treatment modality may contribute to many of the problems discussed in this chapter.

Musculoskeletal complications in amputees can occur early (within days or weeks postoperatively) or late (months or years after amputation). Early complications include delayed wound healing, limb-fitting problems related to residual limb shape, joint flexion contractures, and impaired motor control of the residual limb. Late complications include painful bursitis, chronic sinus formation, pain, adherent scar, damage to insensate skin, volume changes, and bony spurs. In addition, several regional phenomena are associated with lower and upper limb amputations. Optimal management of musculoskeletal complications requires the knowledge and skills of the entire rehabilitation team. Systematic follow-up will ensure early identification and timely management of complications.

Early Complications
Delayed Wound Healing

Delayed wound healing can result from marginal necrosis, infection, malnutrition, or direct trauma to the residual limb from falls. These factors may be present alone or in various combinations. Delayed wound healing is reported to affect from 19% to 40% of transtibial amputations.[1,2] Careful preoperative assessment of transcutaneous oxygen tension (> 20 to 30 mm Hg) and Doppler pressures (ankle-brachial index > 0.5), combined with a comprehensive clinical assessment, should identify the appropriate biologic level for amputation that would result in a greater than 75% probability of healing.[3] The correct rehabilitation-related level for the amputation is affected by other factors as well, discussed in the chapters on particular amputation levels.

Marginal Necrosis

Wound necrosis may be due to suboptimal surgical technique. In an attempt to save length, surgeons sometimes retain marginally viable tissue. Such tissues must be handled and retracted gently, using the hands rather than instruments whenever possible. The bone should be beveled appropriately to prevent soft-tissue injury during prosthesis use (Figure 1). By using atraumatic technique during skin closure, the surgeon can to a large extent avoid producing local ischemic areas. Such techniques include using widely spaced, simple sutures placed in well-everted skin edges and supplementing them with paper su-

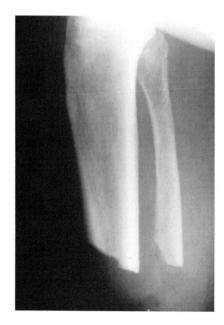

Figure 1 Lateral radiograph of a transtibial amputation shows inappropriate beveling of the tibia and fibula. The chisel-shaped tibia caused severe pain on attempted weight bearing while wearing the prosthesis. The tibial bevel should be confined to the anterior cortex. A posterolateral fibular bevel conforms to the shape of the socket, avoiding a painful bony prominence.

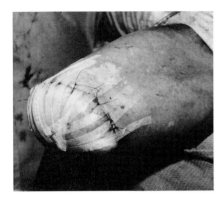

Figure 2 Transtibial amputation closed with minimal tension. Note the widely spaced simple skin sutures reinforced with adhesive paper strips.

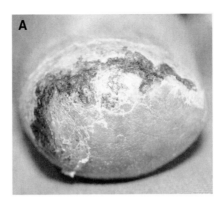
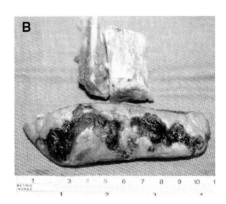

Figure 4 A, Marginal wound necrosis overlying the distal tibia. **B,** An elliptical area of necrotic skin was excised, and 2 cm of the tibia and fibula was resected to allow primary closure without tension.

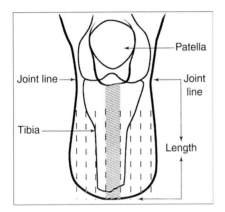

Figure 3 The likelihood of a revision is high when delayed healing or marginal necrosis occurs in the shaded area overlying the tibia, especially distally. *(Adapted with permission from Sunnybrook Centre for Independent Living, Toronto, Canada.)*

ture strips (Figure 2). In addition, the use of mattress sutures, staples, and forceps on the skin should be avoided. Subcutaneous sutures are rarely necessary if a good myofascial closure has been obtained. Removal of skin sutures should be delayed until wound healing has progressed well (usually 3 to 4 weeks). This is especially important in nutritionally depleted or immunocompromised patients.

If wound necrosis occurs, the principal decision relates to the timing and extent of revision surgery. In turn, this depends on the location, depth, and extent of the necrosis, as well as the health of the limb and overall condition of the patient. McCollough[4] recommends revision if the band of necrosis extends more than 1.2 cm from the wound edge. Treatable conditions such as malnutrition should be addressed by caloric and nutritional supplementation. Underlying medical conditions (eg, diabetes mellitus or renal failure) should be managed to the extent possible. If the surgeon decides to proceed with revision, the choices are local wound revision in the same limb segment or revision to the next more proximal level.

In lower limb amputations, the location of the wound necrosis relative to the tibia is a key consideration (Figure 3). Small areas of marginal wound necrosis not overlying the distal tibia can be locally débrided and allowed to close by secondary intention. If the area of necrosis overlies the distal tibia, however, shortening of the bone is required (Figure 4). If this central area of necrosis is not resected, the soft tissues frequently adhere to bone and are either painful with weight bearing or tend to break down later because of tension from shear forces. The surgeon should consider a local revision in this situation.

Trauma

Amputation wounds that have dehisced because of trauma and have minimal evidence of infection can usually be treated with thorough excisional débridement and primary closure.[5] If débridement reveals deep necrosis, the dead tissue should be resected, followed by a trial of dressings for 7 to 10 days. Occasionally the necrosis may continue to extend despite wound débridement, warranting revision to a more proximal level. Often this revision can be done within the same limb segment, but sometimes amputation at the next proximal level is required.

Rigid, semirigid, or soft postoperative dressings can be used for transtibial amputations. The benefits of a rigid or semirigid postoperative dressing include support for the posterior soft tissues (thereby diminishing tension across the wound), control of edema, and reduction in pain during postural repositioning. In addition, a rigid dressing protects the wound from direct trauma such as might be sustained from a fall and also prevents knee flexion contracture. Every possible method should be used to minimize the risk of falling in this patient population.

Infection

Another cause of delayed wound healing is infection, which affects approximately 16% of transtibial amputation wounds.[4] Treatment includes débridement, irrigation, dressings, and antibiotics. Closure techniques can be selected after the infection has been controlled. Techniques include delayed primary closure, healing by secondary intention, skin grafting, or

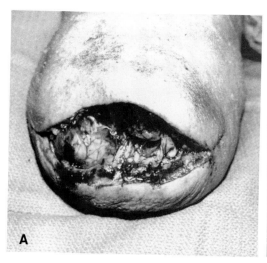

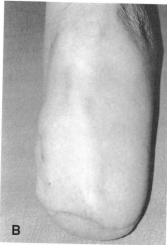

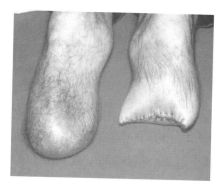

Figure 5 A, An 87-year-old woman with severe vascular compromise sustained major dehiscence from a direct fall onto the end of a transtibial amputation wound. **B,** The residual limb 4 months after immediate closure with myoplasty. Healing was enhanced by a series of 11 hyberbaric oxygen sessions starting on the day of closure. The woman became a successful household ambulator with a prosthesis.

Figure 6 Short left transtibial amputation with excessive, unstable soft tissue; large "dog ears"; prominent distal tibia; and distal scar placement. Frequent socket changes over several months were required to improve the contour of the residual limb and achieve definitive fitting. In contrast, the amputation of the right limb has a well-tailored posterior myofasciocutaneous flap, stabilized by gastrocnemius myodesis.

revision to a more proximal level. Delayed primary closure may work if healthy granulation tissue is present 7 to 10 days after débridement. Although healing by secondary intention is excellent in theory, it often creates a significant delay (2 to 6 months) in all other aspects of the patient's rehabilitation, especially if the affected area is large. This is not a useful technique if necrosis overlies the distal tibia because the soft tissues usually adhere to underlying bone and become painful or break down with subsequent weight bearing. Split-thickness skin grafting may significantly shorten the healing time of a débrided wound, but the surgeon must be very selective in applying this technique. Skin grafts do not hold up well to the tension or shear forces of weight bearing over subcutaneous bone, particularly in adults.[6] Surgical revision to a more proximal level may result in the best tissue coverage.

Ancillary treatments such as hyperbaric oxygen therapy have been advocated for healing of chronic ulcers and marginal necrosis of amputation wounds. Although some reports[7] support its use, we have found that hyperbaric oxygen treatments have not obviated the ultimate need

for surgical treatment. Two recent reviews indicate equivocal benefits.[8,9] One clinical report of 56 problem lower extremity wounds found that none of the patients experienced complete healing.[10] The potential role of hyperbaric oxygen therapy in promoting healing after adequate surgical treatment can be evaluated before revision. Baseline transcutaneous oxygen measurements, with the subject breathing room air, are taken on skin just proximal to the area of necrosis. If values are less than 30 mm Hg, the measurements should be repeated after inhalation of 100% oxygen by mask for 15 to 20 minutes. If these values exceed 30 mm Hg, postoperative hyperbaric oxygen treatment may be beneficial. This approach may allow preservation of the knee joint in selected cases (Figure 5).

Malnutrition

Preoperative screening for malnutrition should include determination of the serum albumin level as an indicator of wound healing potential. Levels greater than 3.0 to 3.5 g/dL have been shown to correlate well with healing.[11,12] Lower levels should be corrected aggressively perioperatively with oral hyperalimentation.

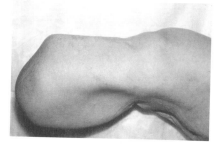

Figure 7 Transtibial amputation with grossly excessive soft-tissue envelope. The amputee had poor rotational control of the prosthesis because of an unstable skin-socket interface.

Residual Limb Shaping
Surgical Techniques

A great deal can be done during surgery to create a residual limb that readily accepts prosthetic fitting. The ideal tapered shape results from a proper balance between skeletal and soft-tissue elements. To achieve this, care must be taken to avoid redundant soft tissue and corner flaps (dog ears) (Figure 6). Floppy soft tissues are slow to shrink and can interfere with optimal prosthetic gait because of an unstable skin-socket interface that causes poor rotational control of the prosthesis (Figure 7). Excessive tension in wound closure, which can result from a disproportion between

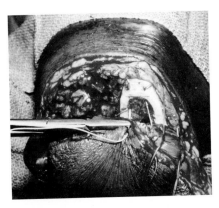

Figure 8 Myodesis in which the posterior myofascia and the anterior and posterior investing fasciae are sutured to the tibia through drill holes on either side of an anterior cortical bevel. The lateral musculature is closed by myoplasty.

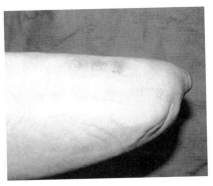

Figure 9 Lateral view of a long transtibial amputation done with myoplasty alone. After a few years, the distal tibia became subcutaneous because of myostatic contracture of the triceps surae. To correct painful local pressure and prevent ulceration, 3 cm of bone was removed, and the soleus was myodesed to the tibia.

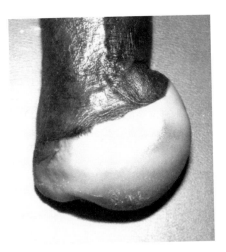

Figure 10 Right Syme ankle disarticulation with fixed medial shift of heel pad. Reduction required removal of 1.5 cm of the distal ends of the tibia and fibula and elliptical resection of medial scar tissue. There was no contracture of the triceps surae or posterior tibial muscles in this case.

bone length and flap length, must also be avoided. Careful design of the skin incision, trimming of the muscle flap, correct relative bone length, myodesis, and elimination of redundant skin will all contribute to a good initial shape of the residual limb.

To further ensure an optimal configuration, proper shaping of the bone end and soft tissues is also very important. In a large series of transfemoral revisions for World War II veterans, Dederich[13] was among the first to demonstrate the value of stabilizing the soft tissues by suturing agonists to antagonists over the end of the bone in a balanced, physiologically tensioned manner. The benefits included improved circulation and decreased pain, allowing the patients their first comfortable prosthetic fitting. If this construct becomes too mobile, however, a distal bursa with painful crepitance may form. The most structurally stable residual limb, therefore, is achieved with myodesis in which the surrounding muscles and their fasciae are sutured directly to bone through drill holes or firmly to periosteum (Figure 8). The advantages of adductor magnus myodesis for transfemoral amputation, as described by Gottschalk,[14] include stabilization of the femur in adduction, which enhances the function of the physiologically tensioned gluteus me-

dius. Myodesis of the quadriceps to the posterior femur provides excellent distal padding. The gluteus maximus, through its iliotibial band insertion, and the hamstrings are reattached by myoplasty, restoring strong hip extension. Firm attachment of all these muscles is of particular importance for patients who are candidates for a prosthesis.

Myodesis without suture to bone can be effective in short to midlength transtibial amputations where the fascia of the triceps surae is firmly sutured to the deep fascia/periosteum of the anterior tibia. This provides adequate soft-tissue stability and padding to the distal end. In long transtibial amputations, however, myodesis of the soleus directly to bone may be preferred because myostatic contracture of the triceps surae may leave the distal tibia in a subcutaneous position if periosteal myodesis alone is used (Figure 9).

Postoperative Management

Following amputation, the residual limb often swells. Control of this swelling will reduce the tendency for wound complications. Rigid or compressive postoperative dressings of plaster or fiberglass or a combination of plaster and flannel are effective in limiting swelling. As the postoperative

swelling decreases, the rigid dressing may slip distally and produce local pressure on the skin or circumferential constriction with choking. The cast should be changed at least weekly and even sooner if there are any signs of loosening, foul odor, increased pain, or fever.

In amputations performed for malignancy that must be treated with postoperative chemotherapy, nonabsorbable sutures should be used to appose the fasciae and other deep structures to minimize their tendency to retract in the presence of chemotherapeutic drugs. These drugs may also delay skin healing, so in these cases it is advisable to leave sutures in place for 3 to 4 weeks.

Syme ankle disarticulation presents unique surgical issues. If the heel pad is secure and well centered, the patient will be able to tolerate a great deal of end bearing. If, however, the heel pad is not properly anchored to the distal end of the tibia and/or the socket is loose, the heel pad may migrate posteriorly or to one side in the prosthetic socket (Figure 10). If the heel pad can be repositioned passively, it can be held with a carefully fitted prosthesis. If the heel pad becomes fixed by contracture or scar and cannot be passively positioned, it should be surgically repositioned by division of the contracted tissue, including the Achilles tendon, and removal of a horizontal ellipse of excess skin opposite the contracture, including that portion of the surgical scar. It may be necessary to remove a wafer of distal tibia and fibula to allow proper positioning of the heel pad. The plantar fascia of the heel pad may then be firmly sutured to the distal anterior portion of the tibia and fibula with drill holes.

Vascular surgery scars provide a distinct challenge to the surgeon and the prosthetist (Figure 11). Lower abdominal and inguinal scars can be irritated by the socket, and surface depressions in the residual limb from scar contracture can create difficulty in achieving suction suspension.

Traditionally, shrinking and shaping of the residual limb have been achieved by repeated application of elastic bandages. Less than expert application of these bandages can produce a poorly shaped residual limb with distal edema. The bandages should be applied on the bias with gradually decreasing pressure as the wrapping proceeds proximally. Because layers of bandage tend to shift with movement, frequent rewrapping is necessary to avoid circumferential constriction and distal edema. As a result, many surgeons and prosthetists now recommend the use of an elastic shrinker sock. The sock is easy to don and doff and provides a proper pressure gradient from distal to proximal. The shrinker sock should be snug when first fitted. A tuck may be sewn in the sides of the sock every 7 to 14 days to keep the fit snug as the limb decreases in volume (Figure 12). Depending on limb shape and activity level, the sock may need to be fitted with a waist belt to keep it in place. To prevent distal edema, the patient must keep the end of the sock firmly against the end of the residual limb by pulling it proximally as often as required throughout the day. The sock is worn continuously except for short

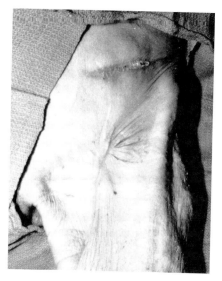

Figure 11 Scar from prior vascular surgery crosses the left inguinal crease and causes discomfort from the anterior socket brim and difficulty in achieving suction suspension.

breaks every few hours as needed for comfort, bathing, and skin care. Two socks should be supplied so that a clean one can be worn each day.

Decrease in residual limb volume is caused by loss of edema fluid as well as muscle atrophy. The most rapid decrease in volume occurs during the first 6 weeks of prosthesis use. This process may continue at a slower pace for up to 1 year. When a definite plateau in shrinkage has been reached, as indicated by no further need for shrinker sock tightening or by stable weekly circumferential measurements, a definitive prosthesis may be fitted. The attained volume can be maintained by applying the snug shrinker sock every night and whenever the prosthesis is removed during the day.

The residual limb of a very muscular or obese amputee may show little or no change in volume when an elastic wrap or shrinker sock is used. In these cases, a temporary prosthesis should be fitted as soon as the wound is strong enough to tolerate weight bearing. This will cause the calf or thigh muscles to shrink most rapidly. The technique can also be used routinely after amputation, with an im-

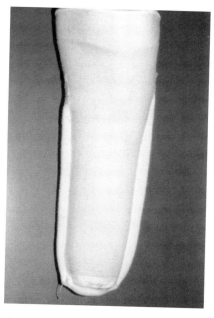

Figure 12 Elastic shrinker sock used to shape a transtibial residual limb. Some patients experience significant pain relief with a shrinker sock because of the contact pressure against the limb. Note the tucks that were sewn in the sock as volume reduction occurred over several weeks.

mediate postoperative prosthesis. Because this requires frequent wound checks, it may be impractical in many situations.

Joint Contractures

Joint contractures can significantly affect prosthesis fit and function. It is important to recognize any contractures preoperatively (Figure 13). If a patient with a significant knee flexion or extension contracture is definitely not a prosthetic candidate, a knee disarticulation or transfemoral amputation should be the primary procedure even if a transtibial level is achievable. (Figure 14). On the other hand, if the patient is a possible prosthetic candidate, a concerted effort should be made perioperatively to minimize the contracture by stretching, splinting, and quadriceps strengthening.

Transtibial Level

Various techniques can be used to avoid postoperative knee flexion contractures in transtibial amputees, including a rigid dressing (cast), semi-

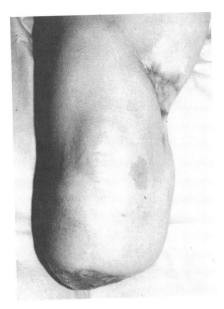

Figure 13 Knee extension contracture in a young woman following traumatic transtibial amputation and open femoral fracture. The femur healed with scarring of the quadriceps to the fracture site. The contracture did not improve with 3 months of therapy. At the time of knee disarticulation, dense scarring was found throughout the knee joint.

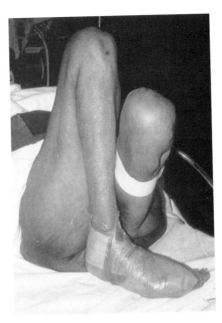

Figure 14 Bed-bound nursing home resident with dementia who has gangrene of the right foot and a severe knee flexion contracture. A knee disarticulation, as done on the left side, was the best and safest solution for the patient.

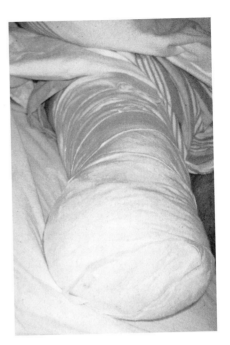

Figure 15 Semirigid dressings can be used following transtibial amputation. A posterior slab is applied over a well-padded dressing with the knee in full extension and then left in place for 3 to 5 days before wound inspection. A removable backslab is then used until the patient regains full quadriceps strength.

rigid dressing, and knee immobilizer. Lightweight casts are effective but can cause pressure sores over the patella if adequate padding is not applied. A semirigid dressing consists of a padded backslab placed from the proximal thigh over the end of the residual limb, coming anteriorly to the level of the tibial tubercle. This is wrapped snugly with flannel, holding the knee in full extension (Figure 15). The dressing is left in place for 3 to 5 days and changed in the clinic. If the patient does not have a quadriceps lag, a removable backslab can be used. Limb supports should be used until full active knee extension is regained. Amputee boards are supplied to patients using wheelchairs in the early postoperative period to support the knee and residual limb while seated. Because they are difficult to fit accurately, knee immobilizers are probably the least effective means of preventing knee flexion contractures.

Transtibial amputees with a short tibial segment are very likely to develop knee flexion contractures (Fig-

ure 16). A circumferential rigid dressing (cast) with the knee in full extension is recommended until the wound heals sufficiently to allow the removal of sutures. This is replaced weekly for 3 weeks with full, active-assisted range of knee motion between cast applications. Care must be taken to adequately pad the thin skin over the tibial crest, tibial tubercle, and patella to prevent pressure necrosis. Pillows should not be placed under the casted limb because this can contribute to hip flexion contracture. Patients should also be encouraged to lie prone and actively extend the hips two or three times a day to minimize this risk.

Severe knee flexion contractures are virtually impossible to eliminate once they become fixed. The dysvascular patient with a short, contracted residual limb may require fitting with a bent-knee prosthesis, which is functionally no better and cosmetically inferior to that used for a knee disarticulation (Figure 17). Occasionally, a moderate knee flexion contracture may be improved by aligning the

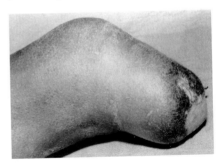

Figure 16 A knee flexion contracture occurred postoperatively in a patient not treated with a rigid or semirigid dressing following transtibial amputation.

prosthesis with the foot in slight plantar flexion (equinus) to provide a knee extension moment on forefoot contact. Consideration should be given to hamstring and capsular release for contractions in limbs that are not dysvascular.

Partial Foot Amputations

Patients with partial foot amputations between the transmetatarsal and Syme ankle disarticulation levels are likely to develop a plantar flexed

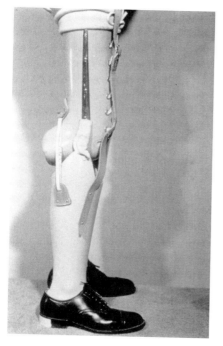

Figure 17 An amputee with severe knee flexion contracture fitted with a "bent-knee" prosthesis that functions as a knee disarticulation device.

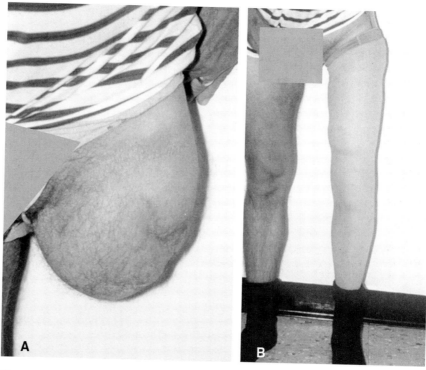

Figure 18 A, Left transfemoral amputee with abduction contracture of the hip. **B,** Although socket adduction aligned the prosthesis with improved cosmesis, shortening of hip abductors resulted in an energy-consuming lateral shift of the trunk over the prosthesis during stance phase.

(equinus) ankle and hindfoot varus deformities due to the unopposed action of the triceps surae. These may be prevented after tarsometatarsal (Lisfranc) and midtarsal (Chopart) amputations by preserving and/or reattaching the anterior extrinsic muscle-tendon units of the forefoot to more proximal bone structures in a balanced fashion, combined with percutaneous lengthening of the Achilles tendon.[15] A postoperative cast applied with the foot in neutral or mild dorsiflexion will prevent contracture until a prosthesis is fashioned. An ankle-foot orthosis with an anterior ankle stop to stabilize the distal tibia can also be used. If a flexion contracture develops despite these preventive measures, percutaneous Achilles tendon lengthening can be performed or the amputation can be revised to a Syme ankle disarticulation.

Transfemoral Level

At the transfemoral level, a flexion-abduction contracture of the hip can markedly increase the already high-energy requirement for ambulation (Figure 18). An adductor magnus myodesis, as part of a muscle-balanced transfemoral amputation as described by Gottschalk,[14] is the best prevention. Active adduction exercises should be performed as soon as they can be tolerated postoperatively. Active extension of the residual limb while flexing the opposite limb to the chest, in addition to lying prone for 15 minutes 3 times a day, will minimize the chance of developing a hip flexion contracture. Placing a pillow under the residual limb or excessive sitting should be avoided for the same reason. Efforts should be directed toward early upright balance exercises and walking with a walker or crutches.

At the short transfemoral level, a flexion contracture of up to 25° may be accommodated by prosthetic alignment. It is important to realize that this flexed position limits hip extension power needed for prosthetic knee stability. It is increasingly difficult, both mechanically and cosmeti-

cally, to accommodate hip flexion contractures by prosthetic modification in more distal transfemoral amputations. More than 15° of hip flexion contracture will require a marked compensatory increase in lumbar lordosis that may lead to or aggravate low back pain.

Prosthetic Considerations

When a prosthesis is prescribed for patients with a significant flexion deformity of the hip and/or knee, the patient and the family should be informed about the relatively unattractive appearance of the socket needed to accommodate the physical deformity. If they do not understand the rationale for the initial fitting and the fact that prosthesis use will tend to decrease the contracture, they may be very dissatisfied with the appearance of the prosthesis and reject it. Children with knee and hip flexion contractures are fitted using conventional alignment techniques. Spontaneous use of the prosthesis will usually

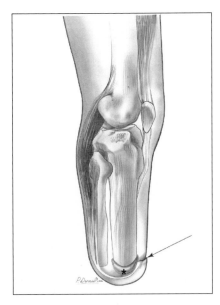

Figure 19 In this transtibial amputation, the sinus overlying the subcutaneous portion of tibia (arrow) may communicate with the bursa (*) at the distal end of the tibia. The bursa is adherent to the distal end of the tibia, and minimal bone resection will remove the deep portion of the bursa. A preoperative sinogram can clarify the location and extent of the bursa. Intraoperative injection of methylene blue through a small catheter helps to ensure its complete removal.

stretch the contractures without special treatment.

Upper Limb Amputations

Contractures also occur in upper limb amputations. Limitation of glenohumeral abduction and forward flexion is common in short transhumeral amputations. If these contractures are severe, the patient may best be fitted with a shoulder disarticulation-type prosthesis. Elbow flexion contracture occurs readily in a short transradial amputation. Early range of motion with adequate analgesia is the best prevention and should commence 5 to 7 days postoperatively. Gentle muscle strengthening exercises can begin 2 to 3 weeks postoperatively. If contractures become fixed, even an extensive program of stretching may be ineffective. Selective release of contracted muscles may be required to allow fitting of a prosthesis.

Motor Control of the Residual Limb

Some patients have significant difficulty coordinating muscle activity of the residual limb after a lower limb amputation. Some of these problems may be due to the physiologic effects of losing part of the limb. Provided there is no underlying neuromuscular disease, a physical therapist can assist in retraining the quadriceps, hamstrings, and hip musculature by using several modalities such as muscle stimulation and biofeedback. Patients should not proceed to weight bearing in a prosthesis until adequate control of knee and hip extension is restored.

Late Complications

Late complications are those that occur or become apparent after definitive prosthetic fitting. They include bursitis; chronic sinus drainage; epidermoid cysts and inflamed sweat glands; bone spurs; ulceration of adherent, insensate, or burn-scarred skin; phantom pain; bony overgrowth in children; fractures; degenerative arthritis; and back pain. Attention should be directed initially to diagnosing the condition accurately. Because many of these problems are caused or aggravated by a poorly fitting prosthesis, optimizing the prosthetic fit and minimizing shear forces at the skin-socket interface are paramount. Local modification of the socket or use of a more compliant interface material may decrease these forces sufficiently to enable full activity.

Bursitis

Amputees with bursitis have residual limb pain localized either within the socket or at the edge of the socket. Careful clinical examination should eliminate other possible causes, such as infection (infected hair follicle or cellulitis), phlebitis, skin ulceration, or abrasion. Bursae can form in areas of chronic friction such as over the distal tibia, deep to the myofascial sleeve that covers the bone. If the lin-

ing of a bursa becomes inflamed, swelling and tenderness may occur. Initial treatment includes rest, ice, and nonsteroidal anti-inflammatory drugs. If symptoms persist, the bursa can be aspirated under local anesthesia and injected with 20 to 40 mg of long-acting corticosteroid medication. Excision of the bursa and the redundant skin often associated with it is sometimes required.

Chronic Sinus Formation

In some patients, persistent serous or synovial fluid drainage may come from a bursa at the end of the tibia or other long bone (Figure 19). A small adhesive bandage on an outpatient's residual limb showing minimal drainage may be the only indication of an underlying problem such as a superficial suture abscess, a bursal sinus caused by a bone spur, or a low-grade localized osteomyelitis. A good way to determine if a sinus is present is to probe the opening. A malleable metal probe, a cotton-tipped applicator, or a flexible polyethylene intravenous catheter may be safely introduced after adequate skin preparation. Sinus tracts are unlikely to heal with rest and frequently become colonized or infected. They are best excised during a noninflamed interval. Complete excision of the sinus tract can be guided both by a preoperative sinogram and an intraoperative injection of methylene blue (Figure 20). Plain radiographs of the residual limb may demonstrate underlying bone spurs or localized osteomyelitis. The latter can be confirmed by MRI or a positive bone scan. These lesions must be excised completely to effect a cure and allow the patient to proceed with rehabilitation.

Epidermoid Cysts/Inflamed Sweat Glands

Epidermoid cysts and inflamed sweat glands are seen most often in the

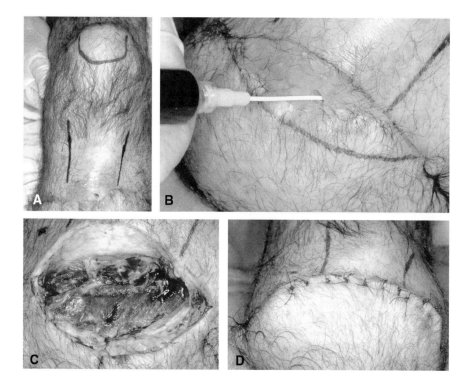

Figure 20 Management of a bursa in a transtibial residual limb **A,** Preoperative view showing the sinus in a central area overlying the tibia. **B,** Ellipse of skin marked for excision of bursa. A local injection with methylene blue will stain the full extent of the bursa and sinus tract. **C,** Wound after excision of skin, subcutaneous tissue, and stained bursa. **D,** Wound closure. The wound healed promptly, and the patient was weight bearing in 3 weeks.

popliteal and inguinal areas secondary to irritation from the prosthetic socket. They may respond to adjustments of prosthetic fit combined with warm soaks and antibiotics. Recurrence and chronicity are common. The usual pattern is of increasingly painful inflammation followed by spontaneous drainage. Once thick cyst walls form, excision is usually necessary. Daily cleaning of the residual limb and socket liner with an antibacterial soap may be helpful in prevention.

Residual Limb Pain

All amputation wounds are painful in the early postoperative phase. The acute discomfort settles over 24 to 48 hours, and the discomfort further decreases gradually as the wound heals. Some patients experience significant pain relief by compression of the residual limb in an elastic bandage or a shrinker sock. This de-

creases swelling and promotes proper shaping to enhance early prosthetic fitting. A variety of conditions can cause residual limb pain, including severe preamputation pain from trauma, adherent skin, bone spurs, a prominent fibula, excessive localized pressure from the socket, neuromas, or claudication from vascular disease.

Preamputation trauma involving tissues adjacent to the level of amputation can give rise to late pain. Disruption of the tibiofibular interosseous membrane and the proximal tibiofibular joint ligaments can cause painful instability of the fibula. Review of the initial radiographs may show wide displacement of the fibula, indicative of interosseous membrane disruption. Pain relief may be obtained by stabilization of the fibula either proximally, by fusion of the tibiofibular joint, or distally, by an Ertl procedure between the fibula and the tibia.[16]

Occasionally, patients may experience pain in the residual limb during walking. In patients with peripheral vascular disease, this may be due to intermittent claudication. A careful history should reveal that the onset of the pain occurs quite regularly after walking a specific distance. The pain of claudication usually resolves after standing or sitting for several minutes. This pattern may indicate borderline ischemia in the muscles of the posterior flap, but cessation of smoking, even at this late stage, may relieve the symptoms. The patient should be urged to continue walking exercise in an attempt to develop collateral circulation. Evaluation by a vascular surgeon for the presence of treatable proximal iliac and femoral artery obstructions is encouraged. The amputee should also be assured that modification of the prosthesis or fabrication of a new socket will not help his or her symptoms.

Whenever late pain occurs following an amputation for tumor, local recurrence must be suspected. Clinical assessment with appropriate imaging (plain radiographs, bone scan, or MRI) should complete the workup. The appropriate treatment will depend on the type of tumor and its staging. Collaboration with an oncologist experienced with management of the underlying tumor is essential.

Problematic Bony Prominences

Another late complication is created by bone spur formation or appositional bone growth at the cut end of a long bone in a child (Figure 21). Pain is due to localized pressure often associated with an inflamed bursa. Although prosthetic modification may relieve some local symptoms, localized surgical excision of the bursa and underlying bony spur may be required. Minimal periosteal stripping and copious lavage after bone cuts during the initial surgery are believed to minimize the occurrence of spur formation.

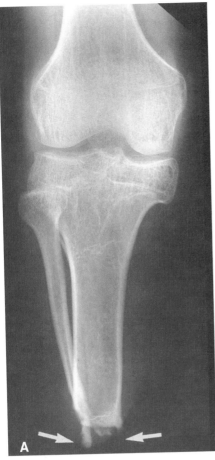

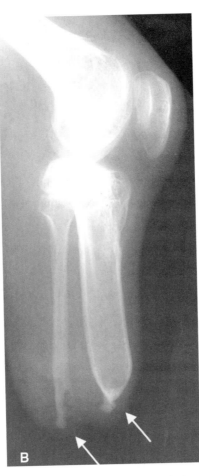

A prominent distal fibula or fibular head can cause pressure-related pain within the socket. If the fibula is left longer than the tibia, tenderness associated with bursitis frequently occurs over the distal prominence (Figure 22). Prosthetic modification may be successful, but a surgical revision is usually necessary. Care should be taken to shorten the fibula 0.5 to 1.0 cm more than the tibia and cut a posterolateral bevel at the time of the initial amputation or revision. For very short transtibial amputations (within 5 cm of the tibial tubercle), the proximal shaft and head of the fibula should be excised. When excising the proximal fibula, the peroneal nerve can be easily identified locally and drawn distally with the knee flexed, allowing excision of several centimeters of the nerve. The resultant neuroma forms well proximal in the thigh. If this is a secondary procedure, the peroneal nerve should be identified beside the biceps tendon above the knee joint and a generous section excised, thus avoiding an unnecessary and possibly problematic scar in the residual limb.

Figure 21 A, AP radiograph shows bony spurs (arrows) of both the tibia and fibula in a 24-year-old man who underwent an amputation at age 11 years. The patient had extreme tenderness over the distal fibula. **B,** Lateral radiograph of the same residual limb. Local excision of distal 2 cm of fibula alone led to complete resolution of symptoms.

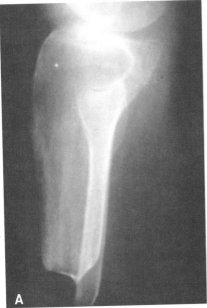

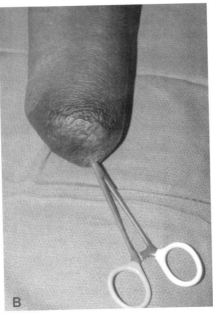

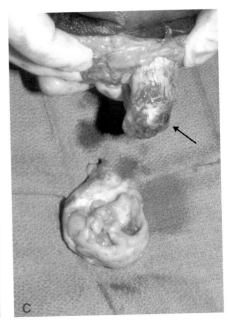

Figure 22 A, Lateral radiograph of a transtibial amputation with an excessively long fibula, causing localized pain on weight bearing. **B,** The same residual limb with a hemostat in a sinus leading to a chronic bursa over the fibula. **C,** Intraoperative view shows excised bursa and overly long fibula (arrow), which was resected to 0.5 cm above the level of the tibia with a posterolateral bevel.

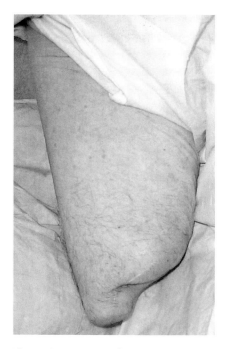

Figure 23 Because of inadequate deep soft-tissue coverage, this femur became prominent and painful 1 year after transfemoral amputation.

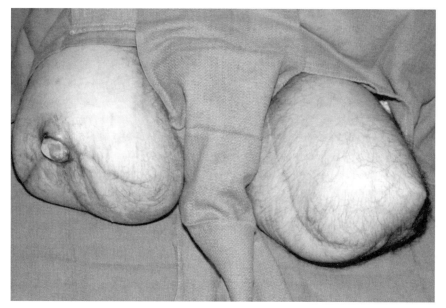

Figure 24 Bilateral transfemoral amputations in a nonambulatory patient. The muscle groups were simply closed over the ends of the femurs rather than being sewn to bone. Note that the right femur protrudes from the skin and the left femur is in a subcutaneous position.

Pain from prominent bone may also occur in transfemoral amputations. This pain is not usually caused by formation of a bone spur; rather, the femur may become prominent anterolaterally because of poor soft-tissue coverage associated with a hip flexion abduction contracture (Figure 23). This situation generally results from failure to perform a myodesis. Forces generated at the skin/socket interface during weight bearing and walking can lead to pain and skin breakdown. In the absence of breakdown, prosthetic modification may be effective for ambulatory patients, but surgical revision with a myodesis may still be required. Adductor magnus and quadriceps myodesis with myoplastic reattachment of the hamstring tendons and iliotibial band, as described by Gottschalk,[14] may correct this problem in ambulatory patients with distal transfemoral amputations. In nonambulatory patients, a simple overlapping myoplasty of the quadriceps and hamstrings may be sufficient to contain the femur; however, a simplified myodesis of the deep quadriceps layer to bone will still help prevent subcutaneous migration of the femur (Figure 24).

Neurogenic Pain

In transfemoral amputees using a quadrilateral socket, burning dysesthesia was once common in the early weight-bearing phase. This was likely due to excessive pressure on the posterior cutaneous nerve of the thigh. The zone of irritation could include the buttock, perineal region, and posterior thigh. The increased use of ischial containment sockets, which provide a better distribution of weight-bearing forces, has reduced the incidence of this complication.

Neuroma formation is a natural response to nerve section because all cut nerves form neuromas to a greater or lesser extent. If nerves are cut at a level that avoids both inclusion in the wound scar and significant pressure from the prosthesis, the resulting neuromas should not cause symptoms. If a tender nodule is found at the end of a cut nerve and local tapping causes the tingling pain typical for that patient (Tinel's sign), it is likely to be a symptomatic neuroma. The first step

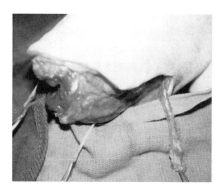

Figure 25 Exploration of a painful left transtibial residual limb. The amputee had a positive Tinel's sign over each of the neuromas held in the hemostats—saphenous medially (left), sural posteriorly (center), and superficial peroneal laterally (right).

is to modify the socket to minimize pressure over the area. If this approach is unsuccessful, local anesthetic and corticosteroid should be injected adjacent to the painful nodule. If symptoms persist, excision of the neuroma by proximal division of the nerve as well as burying the nerve end within muscle may provide relief (Figure 25). In areas such as the fibular neck or metacarpal heads, where the neuroma is directly over a bony prominence, surgical treatment is rec-

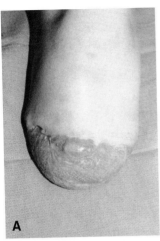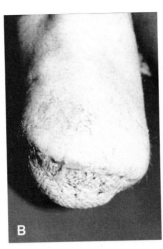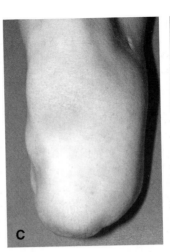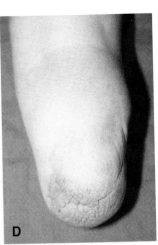

Figure 26 A, Very short transtibial amputation in a 21-year-old trauma patient. A split-thickness skin graft was placed over the myodesed muscle to salvage 9.5 cm of tibial length. Note the central area of painful blistering over the distal tibia that required the use of a thigh corset and knee joints for 9 months. **B,** The same residual limb following circumferential advancement of redundant skin to cover the anterodistal part of the tibia 9 months after the skin graft. The end of the tibia is now covered with sound skin. The patient was subsequently fitted with a supracondylar-suprapatellar prosthesis. **C,** Anterior view 10 years after injury. The grafted area is no longer visible. **D,** Posterior view (patient prone). Note that the grafted area has displaced posteriorly. The patient leads an active life, including snow skiing and running while wearing a prosthesis.

ommended. With a peroneal neuroma, excision of a generous portion of the nerve well proximal to the fibular head in the thigh, where it lies adjacent to the biceps tendon, usually relieves the symptoms. This approach avoids a potentially painful scar over the fibular head and neck in the residual limb and allows a rapid return to prosthesis use.

Adherent Skin

Adherence of skin to bone can lead to pain and/or ulceration when a prosthesis is used. This condition occurs because the adherent skin either does not possess enough compliance to shear or direct forces or becomes ischemic because of tension in the skin, preventing blood flow. Appropriate beveling of bones will reduce closure tension by removing a bony prominence. Careful soft-tissue closure, providing a resilient myofascial layer to cover the bone deep to the skin, can also help avoid this problem. If adherence occurs early after surgery, local skin mobilization by daily gentle, persistent fingertip massage may prevent breakdown. The use of a low-shear prosthetic interface, such as a silicone gel liner, may reduce local

shear to a tolerable level. Partial unloading of forces by the addition of a thigh corset and knee joints also may be beneficial. Some patients do not respond to these conservative measures and may require surgical revision.

After a transtibial amputation, scar can become adherent to bone following localized wound necrosis over the distal tibia. A relatively aggressive approach to prompt removal of necrotic tissue over the tibia is therefore justified. After scarring has occurred, the surgical approach is to excise an elliptically shaped adherent zone of skin and advance a fascial layer to cover the bone, allowing separate closure of skin with its subcutaneous tissue.[5] If enough muscle atrophy has occurred, the necessary tissue advancement may be achieved without resecting bone. If the closure will be under significant tension, some of the distal tibia should be resected. In this situation, distal bony prominence can be prevented by removing a proportionate length of fibula as well. Revision to a transfemoral amputation level is rarely indicated.

Adherence to bone and/or ulceration is the reason that split-thickness skin grafts usually fail over bony

prominences, especially in adults. The skin graft may heal, but it remains thin and insensate. When subjected to weight-bearing loads, the tissue often breaks down, leading to a frustrating cycle of dressings and prolonged periods of non-weight bearing followed by recurrent breakdown. Consequently, the use of skin grafts over bony prominences in weight-bearing areas should be avoided whenever possible. When faced with this situation, it is worth trying a low-shear interface such as a silicone gel liner with a thigh corset and knee joints to offload the grafted area. If redundant skin is present or develops over time, a small area of graft can be excised and local tissue advanced (Figure 26). When larger areas are involved, consultation with a plastic surgeon may allow the use of a local sensate fasciocutaneous graft. If no such flap is available, the options are abandoning prosthesis use or revising to a more proximal level.

Other sites where split-thickness skin grafts are unlikely to stand up to prosthesis use are the adductor tendon region in the groin, the biceps tendon in the antecubital fossa, and the anterior axillary fold. Some areas of full-thickness skin defect may be covered in two stages by the insertion of a tissue expander under normal adjacent skin. The expanded skin can then be mobilized to cover the area of skin graft to be excised. A plastic surgeon should be consulted and involved in this type of treatment. The challenge is determining when the tissue has expanded enough to cover the defect. A rotation flap of full-thickness skin and subcutaneous tissue from the abdomen is the best way to cover defects in the groin or the adductor tendon area.

The ideal surgical closure following an amputation includes an adequate soft-tissue envelope for the enclosed bone or bones. Myodesis or myoplasty are the two techniques available to both provide distal padding and prevent adherence of the incisional scar to underlying bone. If the skin cannot slide over the underlying bone, it will not be able to tolerate the shear forces applied during use of a prosthesis. If wound closure is to involve split-thickness skin grafting, this should be applied only over deeper soft tissues such as muscle. The exceptions to this rule occur in upper limb amputations, which are not weight bearing, and in children, who generally do very well with split-thickness skin grafts.

Insensate Skin

Diminished sensation in the residual limb is common, especially in diabetic patients with sensory neuropathy. Sensory neuropathy is also seen in patients with myelomeningocele, Hansen's disease (leprosy), alcoholic neuropathy, syphilis, congenital indifference to pain, and spinal cord or peripheral nerve trauma, among others. These patients lack the normal protective sensation to warn them of local excess pressure or impending skin breakdown, so they continue to walk, either on the residual limb or the remaining foot, despite local pathology such as abrasions or ulcerations. These patients must understand that serious soft-tissue infection can result from a small skin abrasion. They must be taught to remove the prosthesis and inspect their limbs on a regular basis, especially during the early phases of prosthesis use. If the patient's eyesight is poor, the limb must be inspected by someone else.

Poor Prosthetic Fit

The volume of a residual limb decreases most rapidly during the first year following amputation. Some volume loss can be accommodated by additional socks or socket padding. Poor prosthetic fit can lead to abrasions, bursitis, and thickening of the skin in areas of increased or insufficient pressure. These skin changes are often due to loss of suspension and rotational control of the prosthesis or shear forces as the residual limb "pistons" in the socket. The signs of increased friction and/or pressure on the skin from poor fit include persistent erythema of the skin in weight-bearing areas, erythema in areas of skin not usually weight bearing, tenderness under an erythematous area, and callus or bursa formation. All members of the rehabilitation team must watch for signs of poor socket fit.

Socket looseness can cause increased friction and/or pressure over the tibia and fibula, including the fibular head and tibial tubercle as well as the lower pole of the patella. The additional pressures on these areas are caused by the residual limb sinking too far into the socket because of a decrease in volume of the residual limb from atrophy or weight loss, which makes the socket liner loose. The sinking is visually evident as weight is transferred to the prosthesis after heel contact. Although mild decreases in volume can be accommodated with an increase in the thickness of socks and/or strategically placed partial socket padding, once 10 to 15 plies of socks are needed, a new socket and liner are usually required for definitive management.

Socket tightness can cause tenderness at the socket brim due to direct pressure on the tibial tubercle or adjacent structures. This pressure is usually generated by an increase in volume from weight gain, peripheral edema, or application of too many socks. On attempted donning, the patient is unable to fully insert the limb with liner into the socket. The concentrated pressure and shear forces can result in local skin irritation or ulceration. This also may be associated with a chronic skin change over the distal residual limb called verrucous hyperplasia, which is caused by loss of skin contact with the distal end of the socket. This edematous, thickened skin can crack and become painful, leading to local breakdown and serous weeping with or without infection. If the clinical cause of the socket tightness is potentially reversible (eg, fluid retention in congestive heart failure or renal insufficiency), temporary relief (1 to 2 weeks) can be provided with a shrinker sock or a compression dressing. The same socket is reapplied, and a support stocking is provided for the remaining limb. If the edema is not reversible, a new socket will be required; however, the extra weight of the edematous limb may limit the patient's ability to walk. When weight gain is the cause of socket tightness, the most practical solution is fabrication of a new socket to accommodate the increased volume of the residual limb.

A third variant of poor fit is more subtle and usually presents as an ill-defined discomfort in the residual limb. Examination reveals no evidence of pistoning with weight bearing, and the limb seats fully within the socket. Checking the fit with only the liner on may reveal excessive distal liner volume, especially in the sagittal plane. Subtle signs of pressure over the distal subcutaneous portion of the tibia, such as erythema and abrasion, may be present after weight bearing. In other words, the residual limb has good proximal fit inside the brim but excessive motion distally. The distal tibia behaves like the clapper inside a bell, slapping back and forth against the liner each time the

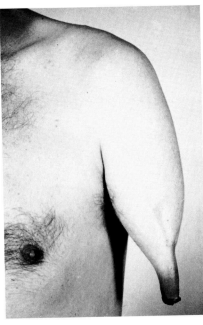

Figure 27 Appositional overgrowth of the humerus that occurred after amputation in childhood. The amputee did not seek medical attention until the humerus had penetrated the skin.

knee is extended in swing phase. A weight-bearing radiograph of the residual limb-liner-socket interfaces may reveal a distal void that allows this motion and also some distal swelling as a result of proximal "choking" from the relatively tight socket inlet. These problems may sometimes be corrected by padding the socket void posteriorly. A new socket may be required if this modification does not fully correct the problem.

The recent emergence of computer-based measurements of limb and socket parameters has made the identification of volume changes more objective. It is possible to scan the initial shape of a patient's residual limb, calculate its volume, and store these data. Future measurements can then be compared with the original and used as the basis for the fabrication of a new socket.

Bony Overgrowth in Children

Amputations in children may be complicated by appositional bony overgrowth that can tent the skin and even penetrate it (Figure 27). This phenomenon is seen in the humerus, fibula, tibia, and femur, and ceases when the growth plates close. This can be managed by the resection of sufficient bone to allow adequate soft-tissue coverage and closure, but overgrowth may recur several times before skeletal maturity. Caps, plugs, bone wax, chemical cautery, or electrocautery have not proved useful in controlling overgrowth. The one exception appears to be the capping procedure developed by Pfeil and associates[17] to treat and prevent terminal osseous overgrowth in both congenital transverse deficiencies and amputations. A cartilage-osseous graft, including a physis, is salvaged from a long bone or the posterior iliac crest. After removal of the overgrowth, this graft is fixed firmly with a screw or Kirschner wires to the distal diaphysis. Good incorporation of the grafts has been demonstrated, with the added benefit of end–weight-bearing in selected patients.[17] Proximal epiphysiodesis is contraindicated because it will leave the child with an unnecessarily short limb and not affect the distal overgrowth.

Degenerative Arthritis

Some patients will have preexisting degenerative changes in joints proximal to the amputation. Ambulation with a prosthesis may exacerbate arthritic symptoms because of altered gait mechanics. Routine medical management may provide significant relief. Arthritis of the hip joint may be alleviated to some extent in a transfemoral amputee because some body weight is transferred through the ischium to the socket. Hip joint compressive forces can be minimized by using light materials and by use of a cane in the opposite hand to decrease muscular effort across the affected joint. If pain is not adequately relieved, a total hip arthroplasty should be considered to maintain walking function in a prosthesis user. Transtibial amputees with significant degenerative arthritis of the hip may also benefit from a total hip arthroplasty.

Weight-bearing pain from degenerative arthritis in the knee of a transtibial amputee may be partially relieved by the addition of a thigh corset and knee joint. This will allow partial load transfer through the corset and joints to the thigh and thus relieve some of the forces across the joint. Patellofemoral joint pain has not proved to be a major concern except in cases of recurrent lateral dislocation of the patella, seen in amputees with excessive genu valgum. If slight varus realignment of the prosthesis with padding of the lateral supracondylar extension is ineffective, surgical correction may be necessary. This usually includes release of the lateral capsule, separation of the vastus lateralis from the intermuscular septum, and advancement of the vastus medialis (Figure 28). In cases of internal derangement of the knee, arthroscopic evaluation and treatment can provide significant relief. If these measures prove inadequate, a total knee arthroplasty should be considered.

Low Back Pain

A significant percentage of adults in the general population experiences low back pain. In ambulatory transfemoral and transtibial amputees, the forces through the lower lumbar region are markedly increased because the low back and pelvis help carry the weight of the prosthetic limb and propel it forward with each step. Any preexisting low back pain would be expected to increase with time and the aging process. In amputees without preexisting pain, back symptoms are likely to develop over time. In addition, many transfemoral amputees develop a postoperative hip flexion contracture, further increasing lumbosacral stress. The best approach is prevention by maintaining general physical fitness, including daily back

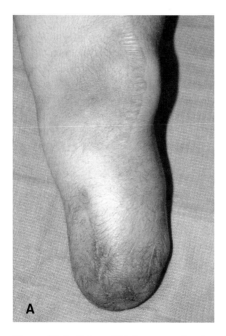
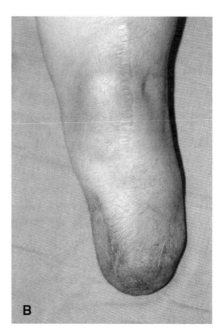

Figure 28 Left transtibial amputation in a 26-year-old woman who reported frequent painful lateral dislocations of the patella despite a previous realignment procedure. **A,** Under anesthesia, the patella was dislocated laterally with ease. **B,** Patella in reduced position. Following release of the lateral capsule, separation of the vastus lateralis from the intermuscular septum, and advancement of the vastus medialis, a new prosthesis was aligned in slight varus with padding of the lateral supracondylar extension.

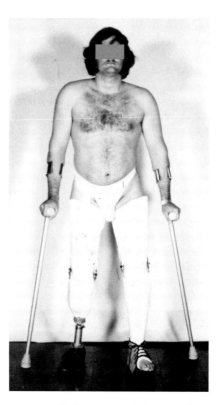

Figure 29 Patient with right transtibial amputation and comminuted, short oblique right supracondylar fracture and left femoral shaft fracture. After 8 weeks of bilateral skeletal traction, the patient was treated with a bilateral cast-brace technique for 5 months.

flexibility and strengthening exercises, and avoiding weight gain. Acute episodes of low back pain may be managed with analgesics, anti-inflammatory medication, stretching, and strengthening. If significant leg pain develops in a dermatomal distribution, appropriate investigation should be conducted to rule out the possibility of disk herniation. Care should be taken to maintain optimal prosthetic fit and alignment so that limb-length inequality or gait abnormalities do not contribute to low back pain.

Fractures

Appropriate management of fractures in the residual limb following amputation can enable return to prosthesis use. The general principles of fracture care apply equally to amputees: obtain and maintain fracture reduction. Some modifications of treatment are necessary because of the decreased distal limb mass and the associated diminution in forces causing displacement of fracture fragments.[18] The most common mechanism of in-

jury is a fall while wearing the prosthesis. The injuries of greatest concern here are those involving the residual limb. The use of a knee joint and thigh corset does not protect against supracondylar fractures of the femur in transtibial amputees, nor does the use of a pelvic belt with a metal hip joint protect transfemoral amputees from hip fractures.[18]

Restoration of the anatomic neck-shaft angle in displaced intertrochanteric hip fractures is very important to facilitate optimal function of the hip abductors.[15] Amputees are best served by open reduction and internal fixation and early return to weight bearing. Displaced femoral neck fractures may be managed by multiple screws, a sliding screw with sideplate, or endoprosthetic replacement (hemiarthroplasty or occasionally a total hip arthroplasty). Excision of the femoral head alone will cause an unstable gait, which could prevent a previously ambulatory patient from walking. Nondisplaced fractures in the intertrochanteric region and shaft in transfemoral amputees can be

managed by non-weight bearing or use of lightweight casts. The mass of the residual limb is small and the muscular forces across the fractures are significantly diminished.

For transtibial amputees, preservation of knee motion and restoration of limb alignment are crucial.[18] Patients with stable supracondylar fractures should be treated surgically to allow early range of motion at the knee. Severely comminuted supracondylar fractures may be managed with immobilization for 4 to 6 weeks followed by cast bracing (Figure 29). Adjustment of the prosthesis can compensate for moderate malunion or loss of limb length. All efforts should be made to minimize flexion contracture of the hip or knee joint. For displaced intra-articular distal femoral or proximal tibial fractures, open reduction and stable internal fixation followed by early range of

TABLE 1 Regional Considerations for Lower Limb Amputations

Level of Amputation	Problems	Prevention/Treatment
Metatarsophalangeal first toe	Migration of sesamoids	Leave 1 cm proximal phalanx or suture flexor hallucis brevis tendons to capsule
Metatarsophalangeal second toe	Hallux valgus	Prevention: second ray resection initially Treatment: resection with fusion base first toe
Transmetatarsal	Painful metatarsals	Long plantar flap Bevel bone cuts plantarly Do not skin graft plantarly
Tarsometatarsal (Lisfranc)	Plantar flexion and varus	Release Achilles tendon at time of surgery Splint/cast in dorsiflexion
Midtarsal (Chopart)	Plantar flexion and varus	Release Achilles tendon at time of surgery Transfer dorsiflexors to talus Splint/cast in dorsiflexion
Ankle disarticulation (Syme)	Migration of heel pad	Postoperative casting Maintain good prosthetic fit Consider soft-tissue revision
Transtibial	Delayed wound healing	Long posterior myofasciocutaneous flap Bevel anterior tibial cortex
	Symptomatic neuromas	Identify and resect nerves proximal to expected socket pressure areas, including superficial peroneal, sural, tibial, and saphenous nerves
	Bursitis	Check prosthetic fit Inject with steroid if resistant to conservative measures Excise if persistent or sinus develops
Transfemoral	Flexion-abduction contracture of hip	Myodesis for ambulatory patients Modified myodesis/myoplasty for nonambulatory patients
Transtibial or transfemoral	Bone spurs	Rinse wound well after bone cut Trim edges of periosteum
	Back pain	Tends to increase with time Prevent flexion contractures Back exercises often effective

motion will help minimize the occurrence of knee flexion contractures. Careful assessment of the quality of bone available for internal fixation is necessary before commencing treatment. Special techniques using pin or wire fixation or bone cement may be required to augment screw fixation in osteoporotic bone. Threaded plates may also be beneficial in maintaining alignment. With these devices, the screws thread into the plate as they are tightened, effectively locking the bone into position. If bone quality is judged too poor to hold screws, closed management may be the best choice. Ankle fractures in partial foot

amputees should be managed as in other patients: unstable fractures should be reduced and stabilized by internal fixation. If the bones are osteopenic, closed treatment may yield better results. Remember that the blood supply is often compromised, and wound healing may be poor if there is tension on the soft tissues.

Fractures of a residual upper limb are rare.[18] Falls are less frequent than in lower limb amputees. In general, humeral fractures are treated by splinting. If delayed union or malunion occurs, surgical stabilization with bone grafting should be performed. Fractures about the elbow

should be managed so as to maintain range of motion. This may be achieved with closed or open techniques depending on the fracture pattern. Fractures of the forearm should be managed as with other patients. Fractures of both the radius and the ulna should be treated by open reduction and internal fixation. Fractures at the wrist should be treated to maintain both stability and range of motion.

Amputations Associated With Burns

Three major types of burns lead to amputations—electrical, chemical, and flash fire. Electrical injuries cause tissue necrosis at both the entry and exit areas. The electrical charge is transmitted preferentially along the blood vessels and nerves, leading to tissue necrosis that gradually manifests itself over 4 to 7 days. Despite this slow process of demarcation, indicated amputations and débridements should not be delayed; the patient's condition may deteriorate rapidly. Stimulation of muscle tissue with the electrocoagulator on a low setting will help identify necrotic muscle for excision. All wounds should be left open because secondary débridement will be necessary in 1 to 3 days. Amputation wounds can be slow to heal, aggravated by poor arterial inflow, venous congestion, tissue edema, and continuing or undetected muscle necrosis.

A small percentage of patients with electrical burns of the upper limbs develop ankylosis of the elbows from heterotopic ossification. The heterotopic bone typically forms in a plane deep to the triceps muscle and tendon along the distal humerus and may extend to the proximal ulna, creating a pain-free extracapsular ankylosis. The new bone may encase the ulnar nerve where it passes behind the elbow. Plain radiographs of the elbow usually reveal the posterior bony bridge. Supplemental information may be obtained by CT or MRI. The bone mass is frequently mature within 6 months of the burn injury and usually does not recur after surgical removal. Adjunctive measures such as nonsteroidal anti-inflammatory medication or radiation are not necessary. A functional range of motion is restored in most cases.

Chemical burns also present difficulties with respect to wound healing because, as in electrical burns, the area of injury is often more extensive than initially appreciated. Aggressive lavage of adjacent tissues with an appropriate diluent is essential. In contrast to electrical burns, with chemical burns the biologic level of amputation should be clear following initial débridement. Once this is established, wound healing should progress normally.

Flash fires can cause full-thickness skin damage and permanently impair sensation and function of small joints, especially in the hand. These injuries are not prone to spread proximally as in electrical burns. Amputations performed proximal to the zone of injury heal promptly. Flash fire burns do not have the same propensity to form heterotopic bone as do electrical injuries.

Regional Considerations and Recurrent Unexplained Problems

In addition to the general complications described above, many regional problems are specific to certain amputations. Table 1 describes problems and management techniques for lower limb amputations, and Table 2 focuses on upper limb amputations.

On rare occasions, an amputee will have recurrent skin problems that do not fit the usual patterns of abrasion or ulceration. There may be a range of problems—excoriations, sores, abscesses, or deep infections. When these events occur in an immunocompetent individual, self-injury could be a possible cause. Clearly, appropriate treatment should be provided for the medical condition. If

TABLE 2 Regional Considerations for Upper Limb Amputations

Level of Amputation	Problems	Prevention/Treatment
Phalanx to metatarsal	Neuroma	Careful attention to level of nerve division
Wrist	Reduced pronation-supination	Avoid injury to distal radioulnar joint Early movement
Transradial	Joint contractures	Early movement
	Limited pronation-supination	Early movement
	Symptomatic neuromas	Identify and resect nerves proximal to expected socket pressure areas
Transhumeral	Symptomatic neuromas	As in transradial
	Shoulder contracture	Early movement
	Shoulder pain	Early movement
	Neck pain	Gentle manipulation Traction with management of degenerative disk disease if present

over time there are recurrent episodes with varying etiologies, the underlying problem may be psychological in origin. A pattern of unexplained problems, often requiring surgical treatment, is characteristic in these individuals. Repeated surgical revisions will not be successful.[19] These individuals may benefit from psychiatric assessment and treatment.

Summary

Early complications after amputation are due to inappropriate selection of amputation level, delayed wound healing, infection, trauma, and malnutrition. These can be minimized by comprehensive preoperative assessment, careful surgical technique, and postoperative splinting or casting. Minor areas of wound necrosis can be treated with débridement and dressings. Full-thickness wound necrosis over the tibia requires local excision and possibly local revision if a sinus exists. Major wound healing problems may require revision to a more proximal level. Joint flexion contractures and initial shaping of the residual limb to obtain optimal prosthetic rehabilitation also deserve close attention.

Late complications after amputation include bursitis, skin problems, neuromata, and fractures. These require comprehensive assessment and usually nonsurgical treatment. Some

neuromata and bone spurs are best treated by surgical excision. Fractures are managed as they are in the nonamputee population. Unexplained recurrent wound problems may be a presentation of psychiatric illness.

Effective management of musculoskeletal complications after amputation requires early recognition of developing problems and prompt review. The nonsurgical members of the rehabilitation team—the diabetes nurse, home care aide, physiotherapist, physiatrist, or prosthetist—are often the first to encounter and report problems. Open communication of concerns among all members of the full rehabilitation team will lead to early problem identification and treatment.

References

1. Jensen JS, Mandrup-Poulsen T, Krasnik M: Wound healing complications following major amputations of the lower limb. *Prosthet Orthot Int* 1982;6: 105-107.

2. Lexier RR, Harrington IJ, Woods JM: Lower extremity amputations: A 5-year review and comparative study. *Can J Surg* 1987;30:374-376.

3. White RA, Nolan L, Harley D, et al: Noninvasive evaluation of peripheral vascular disease using transcutaneous oxygen tension. *Am J Surg* 1982;144: 68-75.

4. McCollough NC III: Complications of amputation surgery, in Epps CH (ed): *Complications in Orthopaedic Surgery*, ed 2. Philadelphia, PA, JB Lippincott Company, 1986,vol 2, pp 1335-1367.

5. Hadden W, Marks R, Murdoch G, Stewart C: Wedge resection of amputation stumps: A valuable salvage procedure. *J Bone Joint Surg Br* 1987;69:306-308.

6. Wood MR, Hunter GA, Millstein SG: The value of stump split skin grafting following amputation for trauma in adult upper and lower limb amputees. *Prosthet Orthot Int* 1987;11:71-74.

7. Kalani M, Jorneskog G, Naderi N, Lind F, Brismar K: Hyperbaric oxygen (HBO) therapy in treatment of diabetic foot ulcers: Long-term follow-up. *J Diabetes Complications* 2002;16:153-158.

8. Wang C, Schwaitzberg S, Berliner E, Zarin DA, Lau J: Hyperbaric oxygen for treating wounds: A systematic review of the literature. *Arch Surg* 2003;138:272-279.

9. Wunderlich RP, Peters EJ, Lavery LA: Systemic hyperbaric oxygen therapy: Lower-extremity wound healing and the diabetic foot. *Diabetes Care* 2000;23:1551-1555.

10. Ciaravino ME, Friedell ML, Kammerlocher TC: Is hyperbaric oxygen a useful adjunct in the management of problem lower extremity wounds? *Ann Vasc Surg* 1996;10:558-562.

11. Dickhaut SC, DeLee JC, Page CP: Nutritional status: Importance in predicting wound-healing after amputation. *J Bone Joint Surg Am* 1984;66:71-75.

12. Pinzur MS, Morrison C, Sage R, Stuck R, Osterman H, Vrbos L: Syme's two-stage amputation in insulin-requiring diabetics with gangrene of the forefoot. *Foot Ankle* 1991;11:394-396.

13. Dederich R: Technique of myoplastic amputations. *Ann R Coll Surg Engl* 1967;40:222-226.

14. Gottschalk F: Transfemoral amputation: Biomechanics and surgery. *Clin Orthop* 1999;361:15-22.

15. Wagner FW Jr: Amputations of the foot and ankle, in Moore WS, Malone JM (eds): *Lower Extremity Amputation*. Philadelphia, PA, WB Saunders, 1989, pp 93-117.

16. Ertl J: About amputation stumps. *Chirurg* 1949;20:218-224.

17. Pfeil J, Marquardt E, Holtz T, Neithard FU, Schneider E, Carstens C: The stump capping procedure to prevent or treat terminal osseous overgrowth. *Prosthet Orthot Int* 1991;15:96-99.

18. Bowker JH, Rills BM, Ledbetter CA, Hunter GA, Holliday P: Fractures in lower limbs with prior amputation: A study of ninety cases. *J Bone Joint Surg Am* 1981;63:915-920.

19. Hunter GA: Limb amputation and re-amputation in association with chronic pain syndrome. *Prosthet Orthot Int* 1985;9:92-94.

Chapter 55

Skin Problems in the Amputee

S. William Levy, MD

Introduction

Skin lesions in the amputee must always be taken seriously. A neglected lesion can lead to an extensive skin disorder that may be mentally, socially, and economically disastrous to the amputee. It is best to view any skin irritation, however minor, as potentially dangerous and to treat it as early as possible. This is especially true in patients with diabetes.[1] A skin problem should never be ignored in the hope that it will heal of its own accord. Early attention to skin problems avoids the frustrating situation in which a person with a lower-limb amputation must remain off the prosthesis or use crutches because a neglected minor skin eruption or trauma has become severe.

Some amputees will be free of skin problems for months or even years. In others, the skin is a weaker tissue, and frequent difficulties arise. The orthopaedic surgeon, prosthetist, dermatologist, and other medical personnel who work with amputees should be aware of the conditions and danger signals that are frequently forerunners of seriously incapacitating skin problems. Once an amputee has begun to use a lower limb prosthesis, the amputee will want to continue to ambulate on the limb, so the physician and the prosthetist should do their best to prevent any disorder that might return the amputee to crutches, bed rest, or wheelchair.

Numerous advances in the development of prostheses for transtibial and transfemoral amputees have occurred in the past few decades. At the strong urging of amputees wishing to participate in sports with unusually high physical demands, lighter weight, stronger prostheses with more dynamic action have been developed. Many new designs are now reported to store energy during stance phase and release energy as the body weight progresses forward, thus helping to passively propel the limb. Numerous innovations in prosthesis suspension have been developed, and a variety of modifications are now available to fit individuals of differing physical characteristics and lifestyles.[2]

The skin of an amputee who wears a prosthesis on a lower limb is subjected to numerous abuses. Most prostheses have a snugly fitting socket in which air cannot circulate freely, thereby trapping perspiration. The socket provides for weight bearing; uneven loading may cause stress on localized areas of the skin of the residual limb, such as intermittent stretching of the skin and friction from rubbing against the socket edge and interior surface. With some prostheses, stump socks are worn to reduce the friction. Nylon sheaths, Teflon sheets, and gel liners have been used in recent years to reduce the shearing action. In the transfemoral amputee, pressure may be exerted on the adductor region of the thigh, the groin, and the ischial tuberosity, all points of contact with the socket rim. If suction is used for suspension, the skin of the residual limb is subjected to both positive and negative pressure. The transtibial amputee usually has at least the upper third of the tibia remaining, and areas of pressure occur over the anterior portion of the tibia, as well as the sides and sometimes the end of the residual limb. Mechanical rubbing over the prepatellar and infrapatellar areas also occurs. With the older conventional transtibial prostheses, constriction of soft tissues of the thigh by a thigh corset can cause significant obstruction to venous and lymphatic drainage of the residual limb. In addition, the skin of the residual limb may become irritated or experience an allergic reaction to the material used in the manufacture of the prosthesis or to topical agents applied by the patient or by a therapist.

Healthy skin on the residual limb is of utmost importance to the successful use of a prosthesis. If the normal skin condition cannot be maintained despite the daily wear and tear the residual limb sustains, then the prosthesis cannot be worn, no matter how accurate the fit of the socket.

This chapter describes the common skin problems and danger signals associated with the wearing of a lower limb prosthesis. Many of the is-

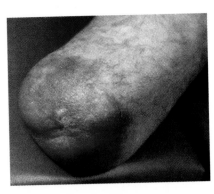

Figure 1 Distal stump edema and hemorrhage in the residual limb of a transtibial amputee.

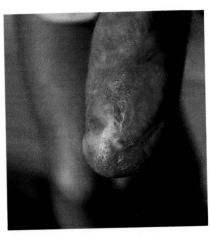

Figure 2 Erosion and ulceration of skin on a residual limb from continued mechanical rubbing and injury.

sues addressed here are relevant to the care of the upper limb amputee as well. In working with numerous amputees over the years, I have assembled and correlated specific information regarding various clinical problems. Because residual limb and socket hygiene is important in relation to several clinical disorders of the skin, a specific hygiene program for care of the residual limb and socket is described here.

Skin Hygiene

In the absence of a consensus as to what hygiene measures should be used routinely, amputees have varied and sometimes strange ideas about hygiene. If either the residual limb or the socket is not washed adequately, maceration and malodor can result. Poor hygiene may be an important factor in producing some pathologic conditions of the skin of the residual limb, such as bacterial and fungal infections, eczema, intertrigo, and persistent infected epidermoid cysts. I suggest a simple hygiene program using a bland soap or sudsing detergent, which has often had a preventive or therapeutic effect on a skin disorder. For example, this simple regimen has been curative for some persistent eruptions of eczema on the residual limb. Soaps or detergents containing bacteriostatic or bactericidal agents can help to reduce the possibility of subsequent infection.

Amputees should be educated in hygiene. As part of the instruction, they should be asked to purchase a plastic squeeze container of a liquid detergent containing chlorhexidine gluconate, triclosan, or other antiseptic agent. These solutions are relatively inexpensive and are available in drugstores throughout the world, often without a prescription. Alternatively, a cake or bar soap may be used. The amputee should be instructed in how to clean both the skin of the residual limb and the wall of the socket. The cleaning routine should be followed nightly or every other night, depending on the rate of perspiration, the degree of malodor, the bathing habits of the person, and the climate. The residual limb should not be washed in the morning unless a stump sock is worn because the damp skin may swell, stick to the socket, and become irritated by friction during walking. For the same reason, the best time to clean the inner wall of the socket is also at night. Some amputees prefer to use witch hazel or rubbing alcohol compounds for cleansing the wall of the socket. If a stump sock is worn, it should be changed daily and should be washed as soon as it is taken off, before perspiration is allowed to dry in it. If the sock becomes wrinkled while drying, a plastic or rubber ball inserted into the base of the sock during drying will give it the correct shape.

Edema

When a transfemoral amputee first starts to wear a prosthesis with suction suspension, the skin must adapt to an entirely new environment. Similarly, a transtibial amputee wearing a total contact socket must adapt to the heat, rubbing, and perspiration generated within the socket. Mild edema and a reactive hyperemia, or redness, should be expected at first. These changes are the inevitable result of the altered conditions that are now forced on the skin and subcutaneous tissues of the residual limb. In most instances, they are relatively innocuous and do not require significant therapy, and they can be minimized by gradual compression of the tissues of the residual limb postoperatively with an elastic bandage or shrinker sock. Compression can be begun before the amputee begins wearing the prosthesis; after prosthesis use has begun, it can be used at bedtime, when the prosthesis is off. An incorrectly fitted socket can contribute to edema and redness by imposing a pressure distribution that can disturb local circulation.

Continued use of a poorly fitting prosthesis can cause edematous portions of the skin of the distal part of the residual limb to become pinched and strangulated within the socket, which may cause ulceration or gangrene as a result of the impaired blood supply. The pigmentary changes so often seen on the distal portion of the residual limbs of amputees are due to deposits of hemosiderin, or blood pigment (Figure 1). This temporary disorder is thought to be vascular in origin, a venous and lymphatic congestion producing edema and hemorrhage. Superficial erosion of the skin in this area is uncommon, in rare instances, deep ulcers can result from continued mechanical injury and poor skin nutrition (Figure 2). In such cases, for treatment to be successful, a dermatologist must work with the orthopaedic surgeon and the prosthetist to eliminate all mechanical factors contributing to the edema, such as strangulation by the socket or lack of total contact distally.

Continued uneven mechanical rubbing can produce thickened, lichenified areas on the skin or weeping, superficial erosions (Figures 3 and 4). Occasional use of an oral diuretic in the morning and a shrinker sock at night can be advantageous. Excessive negative pressure in a socket can also contribute to circulatory congestion and edema. Treatment should be directed toward better support of the distal soft tissues by restoring distal tissue contact, perhaps by inserting a pad or raising the bottom of the socket.

The interface of human tissue and synthetic material is unavoidable in the wearing of a prosthesis. Every amputee who wears a prosthesis experiences skin adaptations and problems incidental to this intimate interface because much of the involved skin is not designed physiologically to withstand the environment and the variety of pressures that are inherent in wearing a prosthesis. The disorders described here are seen not only in lower limb amputees but also in upper limb amputees. I have classified common skin problems in lower limb amputees and have described and evaluated the treatment of numerous patients.[3] Out of these studies, improved methods of treatment are continuing to evolve. In addition, newer plastics, laminated carbons, titanium, and other metals developed through the United States National Aeronautics and Space Administration program are presently being used in the manufacture of many prostheses. Despite these improvements in technology, computerization, and treatment, certain skin problems associated with the wearing of a prosthesis continue to persist.

Contact Dermatitis

Acute and chronic skin inflammatory reactions can result from contact with an irritant or allergen.[4] The irritant form of contact dermatitis, which is the most common, can result from

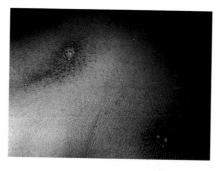

Figure 3 Lichenified skin secondary to mechanical rubbing on the residual limb of a 9-year-old boy with a transtibial amputation.

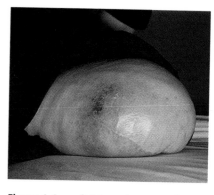

Figure 4 Superficial erosion secondary to mechanical rubbing on the residual limb of a 50-year-old woman with a transfemoral amputation.

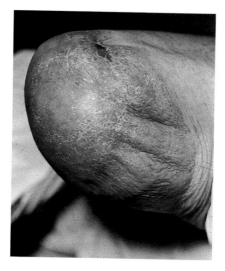

Figure 5 Contact dermatitis secondary to the use of a new plastic pad on the bottom of the socket.

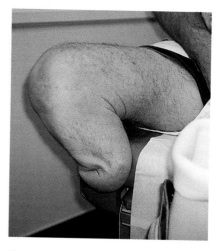

Figure 6 Contact dermatitis secondary to the use of a silicone suspension sleeve.

contact with strong chemicals or other known irritants. Allergic contact dermatitis can arise from the application of topical agents by the patient or the physician or from agents used in the manufacture of the prosthetic socket. The socket wall itself can also produce allergic contact dermatitis. Amputees may experience delayed hypersensitivity to a variety of substances that come into contact with the skin. Although older patients have been found to be less readily sensitized to experimental allergens than are younger patients, in my own experience, allergic contact dermatitis develops in many from a variety of agents, resulting in intense itching or

burning when using a prosthetic socket, sock, or suspension sleeve. Common sensitizers include nickel; chromates (used in leathers); wool fats, especially lanolin, which is found in many moisturizers and skin creams; rubber additives; topical antibiotics such as neomycin; and topical anesthetics such as benzocaine or lidocaine. Areas of itching eczema appearing at the site of contact with an irritant or allergen may be acute, with small blisters, swelling, or oozing of the skin, or more often chronic, with scaling and mild erythema.

In many patients with contact dermatitis of the residual limb, the disorder is caused by contact with chemical substances that act either as a

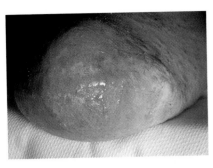

Figure 7 Acute eczematization of the distal residual limb.

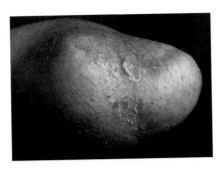

Figure 8 Chronic nonspecific eczematization of the distal residual limb.

primary irritant or drying agent or as a specific allergic sensitizer to the skin (Figures 5 and 6). Knowledge of the materials used in the manufacture of prostheses is necessary to understand and treat the problem adequately. Analysis of the heat, humidity, and friction within the socket is also important because these factors affect the intensity of the reaction. For example, varnishes, lacquers, plastics, and resins are frequently used in finishing the inner lining of the prosthesis socket. Incompletely cured plastic resins and cements can produce a primary irritant reaction or even cause specific allergic sensitization. Foam rubber cushions and plastic-covered pads used by some amputees on the bottom of the socket can also produce allergic sensitization over time. In addition, some cements and volatile substances used to repair prostheses (eg, plastics and epoxies) can produce either an irritant reaction or allergic sensitization. Any of these agents can produce contact dermatitis after weeks, months, or even years of continued use. When contact dermatitis is suspected or diagnosed, every attempt should be made to identify the substance that is responsible to avoid future problems. In some patients, only a careful history will reveal that the use of a new cream, lotion, lubricant, or cleansing agent coincided with the onset of the dermatitis. In other patients, over-the-counter topical antibiotics or "skin-toughening" agents can produce a dermatitis. Patch tests are most informative in pinpointing specific substances as the

cause of a given dermatitis. Because patch testing with strong concentrations of known primary irritants will cause a reaction on almost any skin, solutions of such substances are first diluted according to standard specifications to prevent a false-positive reaction and possible continued injury to the skin.[5] I have investigated several cases of contact dermatitis in amputees and have found some to be due to neomycin, epoxy resins, various cements, Naugahyde, waxes and polishes, and even certain adhesive tapes; in these cases, removing the suspected contactant resulted in a cure, and patch testing after the acute process subsided confirmed the identity of the offending agent. In instances of contact dermatitis in which the irritant was not obvious and patch test results were inconclusive, temporary therapy directed at the symptoms was always successful. Cool or cold compresses, soothing anti-itch lotions, and the application of topical corticosteroids or similar preparations have been beneficial in controlling the process and allowing for improvement or cure. Of course, once an agent has been identified as the cause of a given reaction, it should be avoided as much as possible. All documented skin allergies should be noted carefully on the patient's record because systemic exposure to compounds related chemically to the contact allergen may result in systemic allergic reactions.

Eczema of the residual limb is an acute or chronic, persistent, weeping, itching area of dermatitis over the

distal portion of the residual limb. The lesions can be dry and scaly at times, whereas at other times they become moist without apparent reason (Figures 7 and 8). The condition often fluctuates in severity, alternating from a moist to dry state between active and latent phases over a period of weeks or months, and may cause the patient much anxiety. In some patients the eczema appears to be seasonal, and in others it appears to be related to periods of poor hygiene, continuous standing, or unusually intense physical activity.

A complete history, physical examination, laboratory tests, and subsequent observation of the clinical course of the condition is almost always required to identify the cause of recurrent eczema. One must ascertain the correct fit and alignment of a new or old prosthesis to determine whether the eczema may be related to a fitting problem. In some patients, the onset of the eczema corresponds to the use of a new drug taken orally or some unusual dietary changes. Other patients have been found to have a significant history of recurrent allergic eczema or have active eczematous lesions on other portions of the body. When eczema is secondary to the poor fit or alignment of the prosthesis or to edema and congestion of the terminal portion of the residual limb, the fitting problems must be resolved before the condition will improve. Symptomatic topical therapy with immunomodulatory agents, hydrocortisone, or other corticosteroid preparations can be temporarily effective, but the condition frequently recurs unless its cause can be identified and eliminated.

Epidermoid Cysts

Many authors have described an association between wearing a prosthesis and the appearance of multiple cysts, frequently called posttraumatic epidermoid cysts, in the skin of residual limbs.[6] These cysts occur most frequently in the areas covered by the upper medial margins of the prosthesis in transfemoral amputees, but they

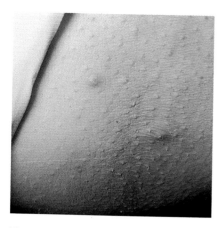

Figure 9 Early epidermoid cysts over the adductor portion of the thigh on a 16-year-old girl with a transfemoral amputation.

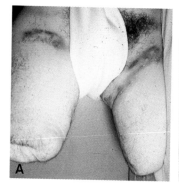
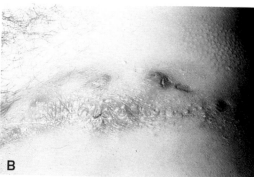

Figure 10 A, Epidermoid cysts and sinuses over the adductor area of the thigh on a 29-year-old transfemoral amputee. B, Close-up of the same patient.

have also been seen in other areas and in transtibial amputees. Usually the cysts do not appear until the patient has worn a prosthesis for months or even years (Figures 9 through 11).

In the transfemoral amputee, small follicular keratin plugs characteristically develop in the skin of the inguinal folds and/or the skin of the adductor region of the thigh, along the brim of the prosthesis. Similar plugs can occur over the inferior portion of the buttock, where the posterior brim or ischial seat of the prosthesis rubs. Through the process outlined below, some of these plugs may become deeply implanted and develop into nodules and cysts, with some lesions becoming as large as 5 cm in diameter. The lesions appear as round or oval swellings deep within the skin. As they gradually enlarge, they become sensitive to touch or pressure, and the skin may break down and erode or ulcerate. If irritation by the prosthesis continues, the nodular swelling may suddenly break and discharge a purulent or serosanguineous fluid. The sinus discharge may become chronic, making effective use of the prosthesis impossible. These ruptured nodules can be exceedingly tender and painful, and frequently scars remain after the cysts have eventually healed. If the break occurs within the deeper portion of the skin, subcutaneous intercommunicating sinuses may develop.

I have found that epidermoid cysts arise when the surface keratin and the epidermis become invaginated and act as a foreign body. With continued friction and pressure from the prosthesis, the keratin plug and its underlying epidermis are displaced into the corium, resulting in nonspecific inflammation and implanted epidermoid cysts. These cysts can remain quiet and asymptomatic for a long period or can, with secondary bacterial invasion by *Staphylococcus* or *Streptococcus*, become abscessed and produce the characteristic clinical picture.

Incision and drainage of an infected nodule or excision of a chronic, isolated, noninfected nodule may give temporary relief, but no method of treatment is completely satisfactory. With acute infection, hot compresses and topical or oral antibiotics, selected through bacterial studies and sensitivity tests of the cystic fluid, are indicated. As the cyst localizes, incision and drainage may be temporarily beneficial. Chronic epidermoid cysts can sometimes be minimized or even eliminated by improving the fit and alignment of the prosthesis.

At my institution, we use various topical preparations such as 1% to 2.5% hydrocortisone lotions in an effort to prevent or retard the inflammation that follows formation of the keratin plug that may be the precursor of the epidermoid cyst. We have also developed a stump sock or adductor rim sock for use with the

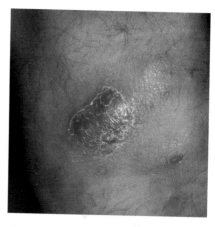

Figure 11 Popliteal epidermoid cysts in various stages on the residual limb of a 50-year-old man with a transtibial amputation.

suction-suspension prosthesis to prevent cyst formation. We have tried various gel socks and suspension sleeves as socket liners to reduce friction over the pressure areas, especially over the brim of the socket. Polytetrafluoroethylene (Teflon) film, which allows for a gliding action and prevents continued rubbing and pressure, has been found satisfactory for this purpose. Teflon patches provide a similar adhesive interface, designed to reduce friction over areas of maximum rubbing and pressure, and can be effective whether the surface environment is wet or dry. When these newer liner materials are used, cysts are generally less common, and when they do occur, they are smaller and less irritated. We have injected cortisone or its derivatives into the cysts and their channels to reduce the in-

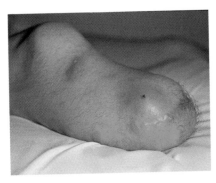

Figure 12 Acute bacterial infection and abscess on the skin of the distal residual limb of a 28-year-old patient with a transtibial amputation.

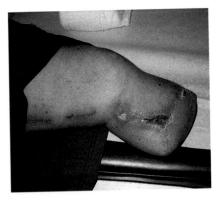

Figure 13 Edema, cellulitis, and a pyogenic ulcer from bacterial infection on the residual limb of a 50-year-old female diabetic patient with a transtibial amputation.

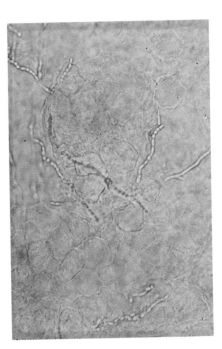

Figure 14 Fungal filaments seen on direct microscopic examination of scales removed from the skin of an amputee with a superficial fungal infection.

flammatory reaction. Topical application of corticosteroids to areas of maximum friction have been found to reduce inflammation, but this provides only temporary, symptomatic relief. No method of treatment has been found to be completely satisfactory, and each patient presents unique therapeutic and prosthetic challenges.

Bacterial and Fungal Infections
Bacterial Folliculitis

Bacterial folliculitis is seen in amputees with hairy, oily skin. The condition is aggravated by sweating and by rubbing from the socket wall. Bacterial folliculitis is usually more severe in the late spring and summer, when increased warmth and perspiration promote skin maceration within the socket, favoring bacterial invasion of the hair follicle. In most patients the resulting condition is not serious, but sometimes, especially in diabetic patients, it can progress to furuncles, cellulitis, or an eczematous weeping, crusted, superficial impetiginized pyoderma (Figures 12 and 13). Folliculitis and furuncles, or boils, can also result from poor residual limb and/or socket hygiene, though the environment within the socket can encourage bacterial growth despite a conscientious hygiene routine. Allende and associates[7] compared the bacterial flora of the skin of the residual limb with the flora of the opposite, normal

limb. All subjects wore prostheses and followed a satisfactory routine of skin hygiene. The skin of the residual limb was found to harbor more abundant bacterial flora than did the skin of the intact leg. In some patients, chronic recurrent folliculitis can be cured by adherence to the routine hygiene program described earlier. In other patients, therapy may require a wet compress, incision and drainage of boils after localization, oral or parenteral use of antibiotics, and local application of bacteriostatic or bactericidal agents. Topical application of oily or lanolin-containing preparations should also be avoided, as their use has been found to be associated with bacterial folliculitis.

Superficial Fungal Infections

Superficial fungal infections, such as tinea corporis and tinea cruris, can appear on any part of the residual limb enclosed by the socket. A nonspecific, scaling, erythematous eruption can be diagnosed through culture and/or microscopic evidence of the fungus filaments in scales or tiny blisters or vesicles removed from a given lesion (Figure 14). Chronic recurrent fungal infections are especially common in amputees who perspire heavily. Therapy consists of fungistatic creams and powders applied over an extended period of

time. Once-nightly application of the newer antifungal agents can be curative. In patients for whom topical antifungal agents are not effective, oral antifungal antibiotics can be helpful and curative. Griseofulvin, ketoconazole, fluconazole, itraconazole, or terbinafine taken orally for several weeks can be curative in resistant cases. Superficial fungal infections of the skin of the residual limb may be difficult to eradicate completely, however, because of continued moisture, warmth, and maceration within the socket. Although some patients have reported anecdotally that socket liners must be discarded to prevent recurrence of a fungal infection, there is no scientific basis for this, any more than a pair of shoes must be thrown away to prevent recurrence of athlete's foot. The fact is that a fungal infection is not completely eradicated by treatment. Rather, the fungus is kept in a nonactive state by using an antifungal cream at bedtime and perhaps an antifungal powder after bathing daily to keep the area dry. Active bacterial and fungal infections are usually short-lived if the diagnosis is made early and correct therapy is administered. Fortunately, most such infections respond to topical medications.

Intertriginous Dermatitis

Intertriginous dermatitis, or intertrigo, occurs in skin surfaces that are in constant apposition and where there is hypersecretion and retention of perspiration. The condition usually occurs in the inguinal or crural areas. On occasion, however, it occurs in the folds at the end of a residual limb, where two surfaces of skin rub against each other and where the protective layer of keratin is removed by friction. Continued friction and pressure from the socket may result in lichenified or pigmented skin. The thickened skin may subsequently itch or burn, depending on the severity of the rubbing. A chronic disorder may develop, characterized by deep, painful fissures and secondary infection along with eczematization. Careful cleansing of the opposing folds and the use of drying powders or mild drying lotions can be beneficial. Frequently, this dermatitis can be relieved by proper prosthetic fit and alignment.

Other Skin Disorders

Several chronic dermatoses have been observed to localize on the skin of the residual limb. Patients with acne vulgaris of the face and back sometimes have acne lesions on the residual limb as well. Similar localization has been seen in patients with seborrheic dermatitis, folliculitis, and atopic eczema. Localization on the skin of the residual limb following a general eruption is not unusual. Psoriasis, as well as lichen planus, has been known to develop on the skin of the residual limb, with a few lesions being present elsewhere on the body.[3] To improve the local eruption, it is important to treat the generalized cutaneous disorder, so an accurate diagnosis is critical. To establish an accurate diagnosis, a careful history and physical examination are of utmost importance. To establish a diagnosis of acne, the skin of the face, neck, back, and chest should be examined for pustules, fol-

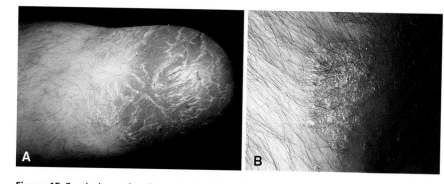

Figure 15 Psoriasis on the distal residual limb **(A)** and elbow **(B)**.

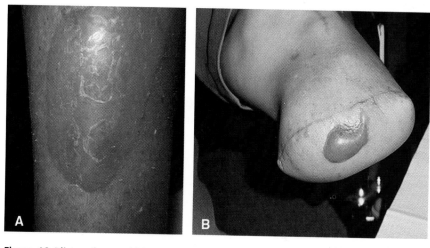

Figure 16 Blisters from rubbing of the prosthesis in patients with diabetes. **A**, Pretibial blister. **B**, Blister on the distal residual limb.

licular nodules, and comedones. Psoriasis usually presents as pink to red plaques on the skin of the residual limb with similar lesions on the elbows, knees, and trunk (Figure 15). Even a small skin biopsy can corroborate the correct diagnosis.

Skin Disorders in Individuals With Diabetes

The skin of individuals with diabetes is especially prone to chronic disorders that can be serious and disabling. Bacterial and fungal infections are common in amputees with uncontrolled diabetes. A high blood glucose level can lead to folliculitis on the residual limb or elsewhere on the body. Ulcerations and erosions of the skin must be diagnosed and treated early to prevent serious infection or osteomyelitis. Painful deep ulcers and edematous processes can become

chronic and disabling. Candidal, or yeast, infections are not uncommon in the groin and on the residual limb following a course of antibiotics for some other disorder. Diabetic dermopathy, which presents as bullae, or blisters, from the rubbing of the prosthesis against the skin, requires several weeks for complete healing (Figure 16).

Growths

Viral verrucae, or warts, on the skin of the residual limb are common and are treated by cauterization. Simple cutaneous papillomas (Figure 17) are easily removed. Cutaneous horns and warty keratoses are also common. All of these can be treated by using a local anesthetic and superficially removing the lesion. This seldom requires a large surgical excision. Healing is usually by secondary inten-

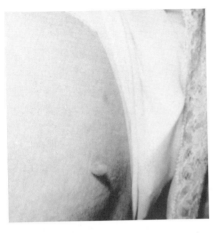

Figure 17 Cutaneous papilloma on the residual limb. To avoid irritation, cutaneous papillomas can be excised and the base cauterized.

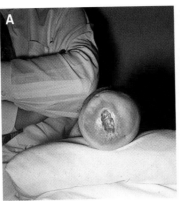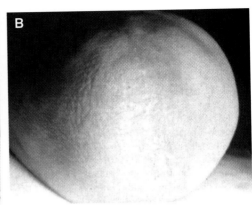

Figure 18 **A**, Chronic ulcer of 2 years' duration on the distal residual limb on a 42-year-old man with a transtibial amputation, secondary to edema and a poorly fitting prosthesis. **B**, Healed ulcer 6 weeks after reduction of edema and correction of the prosthetic socket fit.

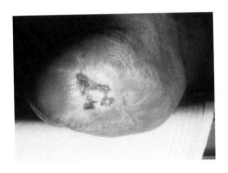

Figure 19 Short transtibial residual limb with an adherent scar and traumatic ulcerations.

tion and occurs within a short period of time. Skin cauterization following removal of a lesion usually heals within 2 to 3 weeks.

Tumors of the skin of the residual limb can be benign or malignant. I have removed small basal and squamous cell carcinomas without incident, and healing has been successful and without recurrence. When excision of skin of the distal residual limb is indicated for squamous cell carcinoma associated with verrucous hyperplasia, a well-planned plastic procedure that will ensure complete removal of the malignancy and prevent recurrence of the hyperplasia is crucial. The goal is to maintain a well-formed and well-padded distal residual limb that will tolerate significant compression within the distal socket. However, I have had two patients who

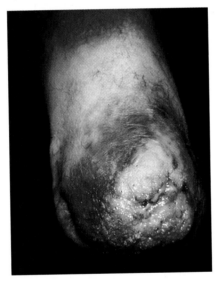

Figure 20 Squamous cell carcinoma secondary to verrucous hyperplasia with ulceration on the residual limb of a transtibial amputee. The patient died from metastases to bone and lung.

required amputation because of lymphangioma; the condition recurred, with subsequent lymphangiosarcoma developing and death. In such cases, an early, accurate diagnosis is of utmost importance.

Chronic Ulcers

Chronic ulcers of the residual limb may result from bacterial infection, from radiation therapy, or from poor cutaneous nutrition secondary to edema or to an underlying vascular

disorder. Somtimes localized pressure from a poorly fitting prosthesis produces erosion, followed by ulceration (Figure 18).

Persistent edema must be corrected early to avoid ulceration. Malignant ulcers can develop within chronic ulcerations; therefore, every effort should be made to treat the process before it becomes chronic. Also, with repeated infection and ulceration of the skin, the amputation scar may adhere to the underlying subcutaneous tissues, inviting further erosion and ulceration (Figure 19). Surgery to free the scar in the bound area may then be necessary to allow effective prosthesis use. The cause of the stump ulceration must always be identified and corrective therapy discussed with the orthopaedic surgeon and prosthetist.

Verrucous Hyperplasia

A verrucous, or warty, condition of the skin of the distal portion of the residual limb is common (Figure 20). Some describe the disorder as an invasion of the common wart virus into the skin, while others believe that the condition is always associated with malignancy.[8,9] I have treated many cases of verrucous hyperplasia in amputees; in most patients, the process has been entirely reversible[3,10] (Figure 21).

Verrucous hyperplasia of the skin of the residual limb can be associated with ulceration, in addition to edema

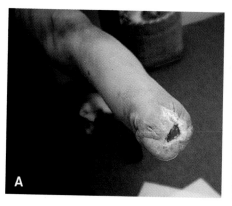
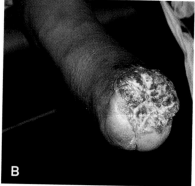
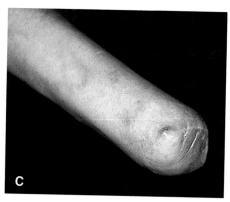

Figure 21 Squamous cell carcinoma in a 55-year-old man with a Syme ankle disarticulation who presented with verrucous hyperplasia of many months' duration. Excision of the skin of the distal residual limb proved successful, and the patient had no recurrence on 5-year follow-up. **A,** Early ulceration with verrucous hyperplasia. **B,** Appearance of the limb several months later, when the patient presented with infection, fever, ulceration, and malodor. **C,** Appearance of the limb 3 months later following excision of skin of the distal residual limb and correction of the fit of the distal prosthesis socket. There has been no evidence of recurrence of the carcinoma.

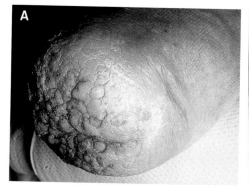
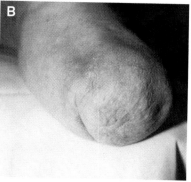
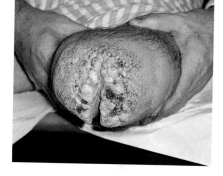

Figure 22 Reversible verrucous hyperplasia of 2 years' duration on the residual limb of a 54-year-old transtibial amputee. **A,** Before compression, the limb has a warty appearance. **B,** After partial end-bearing compression and correction of the fit of the prosthesis socket, the skin is completely clear.

Figure 23 Severe verrucous hyperplasia on the residual limb of a 34-year-old man with a transfemoral amputation secondary to proximal strangulation from a poorly fitting prosthetic socket.

(Figures 22 and 23). Many patients endure this condition for months or even years, seeking help from various health professionals and being treated with topical preparations and other forms of therapy without effect, or, at best, realizing only temporary benefit. My colleague and I found that external compression, in combination with adequate control of bacterial infection and edema, is the best method of treatment.[10] In the transtibial amputees with verrucous hyperplasia we treated, the distal part of the residual limb was edematous, and it dangled without sufficient distal support in the socket. Once the end of the limb was compressed by means of a temporary platform in the socket built up with cushions, the warty condition

slowly resolved. The greater the compression, the more immediate and lasting was the improvement. As a result of our investigation, the engineers and prosthetists modified the prosthetic design to provide compression of the tissues at the end of the residual limb. After several weeks, the verrucous condition gradually disappeared and did not recur, as long as the compression was continued. The successful treatment of this disorder is an example of the need for cooperation among various professionals to provide the maximum benefit to the individual amputee.

Verrucous hyperplasia appears to be secondary to a vascular disorder related to poor prosthetic fit and alignment and, possibly, bacterial in-

fection. Although these factors may be present in combination, it is clear from our studies that a poor pressure gradient, which tends to drive fluids into the distal tissues, plays an especially important role. This occurs whenever the proximal tissues experience greater pressure than do the distal tissues. Edema is likely to develop in the redundant, unsupported tissues of the residual limb before prosthetic treatment because of the lack of support for and pressure on the terminal tissues and the absence of any pumping action by the muscles.[11] A shrinker sock used continually until prosthetic fitting and thereafter, whenever a prosthesis is not worn, is distinctly advantageous. If the amputee is then fitted with a prosthesis that distributes pressure properly, the edema will subside. However, if the prosthesis produces greater proximal than distal pressures, the edema will increase and verrucous hyperplasia can result.

Summary

Through the combined efforts of orthopaedic surgeons, prosthetists, engineers, and dermatologists, the many skin problems of the amputee can be treated effectively. The importance of early recognition and treatment of the common skin disorders of residual limbs cannot be overemphasized.[12-14]

References

1. Jelinek JE: (ed): *The Skin In Diabetes.* Philadelphia, PA, Lea & Febiger, 1986.

2. Wirta RW, Golbranson FL, Mason R, Calvo K: Analysis of below-knee suspension systems: Effect on gait. *J Rehabil Res Dev* 1990;27:385-396.

3. Levy SW (ed): *Skin Problems of the Amputee.* St Louis, MO, WH Green, 1983.

4. Lyon CC, Kulkarni J, Zimerson E, Van Ross E, Beck MH: Skin disorders in amputees. *J Am Acad Dermatol* 2000; 42:501-507.

5. Fisher AA (ed): *Contact Dermatitis,* ed 3. Philadelphia, PA, Lea & Febiger, 1986.

6. Allende MF, Levy SW, Barnes GH: Epidermoid cysts in amputees. *Acta Derm Venereol* 1963;43:56-67.

7. Allende MF, Barnes GH, Levy SW, O'Reilly WJ: The bacterial flora of the skin of amputation stumps. *J Invest Dermatol* 1961;36:165-166.

8. Gillis L (ed): *Amputations.* London, England, W Heinemann Medical Books, 1954.

9. Schwartz RA, Bagley MP, Janniger CK, Lambert WC: Verrucous carcinoma of a leg amputation stump. *Dermatologica* 1991;182:193-195.

10. Levy SW, Barnes GH: Verrucous hyperplasia of amputation stump. *Arch Dermatol* 1956;74:448-449.

11. Golbranson FL, Asbelle C, Strand D: Immediate postsurgical fitting and early ambulation: A new concept in amputee rehabilitation. *Clin Orthop* 1968;56:119-131.

12. Persson B: Lower limb amputation: Part 1. Amputation methods: A 10 year literature review. *Prosthet Orthot Int* 2001;25:7-13.

13. Geertzen JH, Martina JD, Rietman HS: Lower limb amputation: Part 2. Rehabiliation: A 10 year literature review. *Prosthet Orthot Int* 2001;25:14-20.

14. Cochrane H, Orsi K, Reilly P: Lower limb amputation: Part 3. Prosthetics: A 10 year literature review. *Prosthet Orthot Int* 2001;25:21-28.

Chapter 56

Chronic Pain Management

Dawn M. Ehde, PhD
Douglas G. Smith, MD

Introduction

Pain after limb amputation is unfortunately an all too common consequence. Amputation-related pain can become chronic and, for some individuals, limit quality of life and functional capacity. Living with chronic pain can change one's outlook, one's personality, and one's relationships. As the French philosopher Marcel Proust said, "To kindness and to knowledge we make promises only. Pain we obey."

In the past quarter century, research, particularly that on phantom limb pain, has advanced our understanding of chronic pain in individuals with limb loss. In this chapter we summarize what is currently known concerning the nature, scope, and treatment of chronic pain with acquired limb loss. We discuss the prevalence, severity, and impact of pain as well as the factors that contribute to, or are associated with, adaptation to chronic pain in this population. Pharmacologic and rehabilitation approaches to pain management are also discussed. Answers to the research and clinical questions that grow out of this knowledge will contribute to our long-term goal of reducing pain and suffering in persons with limb loss.

Conceptual Issues
Definitions

The International Association for the Study of Pain (IASP) defines pain as "an unpleasant sensory and emotional experience associated with actual or potential tissue damage or described in terms of such damage."[1] The IASP defines chronic pain as recurrent or persistent pain that is present for more than 6 months. This includes pain that persists beyond expected healing time. There are at least three subtypes of chronic pain. One is the result of an identified, ongoing disease process, such as chronic pancreatitis or cancer, that results in pain. Another subtype is that with clear evidence of injury to the peripheral or central nervous system; phantom limb pain is one example of this subtype. The third is chronic pain whose pathophysiology is either undetectable by current diagnostic procedures or is of a degree that does not fully explain the symptoms or apparent disability. Examples of this third subtype include chronic back pain and fibromyalgia. This subtype is the most perplexing to health care professionals and to persons experiencing this type of pain. As will be discussed, it is likely that some amputees may have pain that fits into this third category.

Although not the focus of this chapter, acute pain warrants definition because severe acute pain is a risk factor for the development of chronic pain.[2] Acute pain may be defined as that elicited by activating nociceptive transducers at the site of local tissue damage because of trauma, surgical procedures, or disease.[3] By definition, acute pain lasts for a limited time and remits as the underlying injury or disease heals. Thus, it differs from chronic pain in both duration and etiology. As will be discussed later, the two pain types also differ in their optimal treatment.

Multidimensional Construct of Pain

In the clinic, pain is often thought of as a one-dimensional construct, with patients typically asked to rate pain on a numeric rating scale ranging from absence of pain to severe pain. In contrast, pain researchers and clinical specialists view pain as a multidimensional construct with several relevant dimensions, including, but not limited to, location, frequency, duration, intensity, effect, and pain-related disability.[4]

Pain location specifies the site where pain is experienced. In individuals with acquired amputation, the phantom limb and the residual limb are the areas typically assessed. The frequency and duration of pain are also commonly assessed and involve when and how long pain is experienced. To a lesser extent, pain intensity, which involves the severity of the pain, is also assessed in studies of postamputation pain and is also commonly evaluated clinically. Pain intensity is typically assessed using a numeric rating scale. The literature varies widely as to the type of pain intensity studied (eg, worst, average, least, usual).[5] The affective component of pain has received the least attention in the amputation literature. Pain affect is defined as the emotional arousal and disruption produced by pain (the "bothersomeness"). It is important to note that pain affect is distinct from pain intensity; for example, one may have intense pain but not be upset or bothered by it. Finally, pain-related disability refers to the degree that chronic pain interferes with activities and quality of life. Few studies have examined the disability attributable to chronic pain in patients with limb loss.

Conceptual Models of Pain

In addition to understanding the multiple dimensions of the pain experience, it is also important to understand the conceptual models of chronic pain that have influenced thinking and research over time. These models include the biomedical model, the gate-control theory of pain, and the biopsychosocial model.

The biomedical model assumes that pain results from a specific disease process and that it is synonymous with tissue injury and nociceptive stimulation. In this model, diagnosis is confirmed by objective tests, with treatment directed toward correcting the organic dysfunction. Psychosocial factors are viewed as reactions to pain rather than as contributors. This dualistic model assumes that symptoms are either psychogenic or organic, despite no empirical evidence for this dichotomy. This model has long been criticized for failing to recognize psychosocial variables in chronic pain or the interaction of these variables with pathophysiology.[3,6]

The gate-control theory of pain[7,8] conceptualizes pain as a multidimensional phenomenon with motivational-affective, cognitive-evaluative, and sensory-physiologic components, all of which can potentiate or moderate pain perception. This model includes psychological factors as well as central nervous system mechanisms and provides a physiologic basis for psychological factors in pain perception. After its introduction into the field, this model radically changed the way that researchers and clinicians thought about pain. It spurred physiologic research on pain, including research-identified psychological variables, and demonstrated how they modulate pain perception. The model also emphasized that pain is not exclusively sensory, and, hence, simply measuring pain intensity is inadequate. Most significantly, the gate-control theory emphasizes that there is not a one-to-one relationship between injury or disease severity and pain symptoms.

The biopsychosocial model, often considered an extension of the gate-control theory, conceptualizes chronic pain as the result of the complex interaction of biologic, psychological, and social variables. Within this model, these factors interact in a dynamic process, affecting a person's experience of pain. This model acknowledges that biologic factors are central to the experience of pain for most, if not all, persons with pain.[9] It also argues that psychosocial factors, such as the responses of family and significant others to pain behaviors[10] and pain-related cognitions, beliefs, and coping behaviors[11] influence adjustment to chronic pain, including psychological distress, pain-related disability, and health care utilization.[12,13] This model accounts for the diversity in the expression of and responses to pain. It has also significantly advanced our understanding of some of the variability in individuals' adjustment to chronic pain[11,14] and has provided a useful theoretical framework for treatment.[15] Finally, this model incorporates rehabilitation approaches with medically based treatments.

Additional Concepts That Distinguish Pain

In addition to these conceptual models, several prominent pain researchers[4,10,16] have argued for the importance of distinguishing among nociception, pain, suffering, and pain behavior. Nociception is defined as the activation of A-delta and C-fiber axons by mechanical, thermal, or chemical energies that are capable of damaging body tissues. Nociception typically leads to pain, which is defined as the perception of a noxious stimulus. Pain involves conscious awareness, appraisal, ascription of meaning, and learning and, thus, is seen as a perceptual process comprising the integration and modulation of a number of afferent and efferent processes. Pain often leads to suffering, defined as a negative affective or emotional response generated in the brain in response to pain and other stressors associated with the pain experience, such as anxiety, fear, distress, occupational problems, interpersonal disruption, and economic distress. Suffering is a personal experience that can only be observed indirectly if the person engages in a behavior that is attributable to the suffering. Specifically, suffering may lead to pain behavior, which is defined as "the things people do when they suffer or are in pain."[17] Pain behaviors are verbal or nonverbal behaviors that serve to communicate that pain is being experienced. Examples of pain behaviors include moaning, grimacing, limping, lying down, rubbing the affected area, feeling unable to work, seeking health care, and taking pain medications. All pain behaviors are observable and quantifiable. Nociception, pain, and suffering are individual, private, internal events, the existence of which in another person can only be inferred.[16]

An important caveat to this concept is that an individual does not necessarily experience all four aspects of this model (nociception, pain, suffering, and pain behavior) simultaneously and, in fact, may experience one or more without the others. For example, an athlete may fracture a bone in his hand during a crucial play of a football game and thus have nociception without experiencing any pain or suffering or exhibiting pain

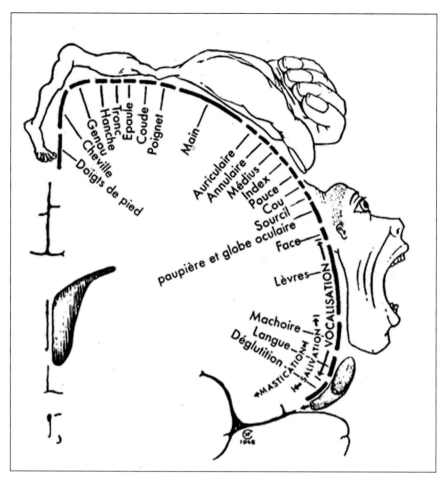

Figure 1 The historic illustration from Penfield and Rasmussen of the amount of cortex dedicated to different anatomic areas. *(Reproduced with permission from Penfield W, Rasmussen T: Homunculus moteur in* The Cerebral Cortex of Man: A Clinical Study of Localisation of Function. *New York, NY, Hafner Publishing Co, 1957.)*

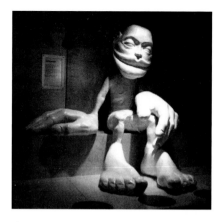

Figure 2 A more modern sculpture of the homunculus from the Glasgow Science Centre (Glasgow, Scotland) representing a human being modified in proportions that correspond to the brain's cortical map. *(Courtesy of Glasgow Science Center, Glasgow, Scotland.)*

chological or personality disorder. More recently, phantom limb pain has been viewed as a natural and common response to limb loss with a physiologic, rather than psychological, basis.[18,19] Interestingly, during the last few decades, as theories of phantom limb pain have evolved from a primarily psychological to a physiologic focus, models of other chronic pain problems have broadened from an almost exclusively biomedical approach to incorporate psychosocial variables.[20,21] Thus, for the purposes of this chapter, we will examine chronic pain secondary to limb loss from a biopsychosocial model that views chronic pain and suffering as a complex phenomenon with multiple dimensions and factors.

Types of Phantom and Residual Limb Pain and Sensation
Nonpainful Phantom Limb Sensations

In addition to phantom limb pain, nonpainful phantom limb sensations are typical.[22] For example, an amputee may have a feeling that a missing foot is wrapped in cotton or that a missing limb is actually present. These sensations can take a variety of

behavior until he leaves the game and realizes that he is injured. Similarly, an individual may walk on hot coals without feeling pain or suffering. In contrast, an amputee may perceive phantom limb pain without nociception. Alternatively, a stoic person may experience nociception, pain, and suffering without exhibiting any pain behaviors.

Individuals with limb loss often report that phantom pain is most intense in the hand or foot. Over time, as the phantom feeling lessens, they often describe a telescoping or shortening of the limb, with the phantom hand or foot moving closer to the amputation site. The cortex of the brain has areas dedicated to all parts of the body. The amount of brain cortex that represents each part is not proportional to the size of the part. For example, the thigh has very small representation, whereas that of the hand is very large. The homunculus is a way to illustrate the body according to the amount of cerebral cortex devoted to each area. This may, in part, explain why individuals report more intense and vivid phantom sensation and phantom pain in the hand and foot compared with the knee or elbow (Figures 1 and 2).

To summarize, the literature views chronic pain as a multidimensional experience that involves not only sensory and physiologic processes but also psychosocial, behavioral, and environmental factors. This is in contrast to the traditional phantom limb pain literature, which presented phantom limb pain as a symptom of a psy-

forms, such as touch, pressure, temperature, itch, posture, or location in space.[22,23] They can also involve feelings of movement in the phantom limb. For some, an occurrence referred to as "telescoping" can happen when the amputee senses that the distal part of the phantom limb is moving progressively closer to the residual limb over time.

The methodology of much of the research on nonpainful phantom sensations has varied so greatly that the prevalence of the experience remains unclear. For example, prevalence varies with the sample studied: the clinic versus community, inpatient versus outpatient, lower limb versus upper limb. In addition, nonpainful phantom sensations have not always been well differentiated from phantom limb pain.[23,24]

When distinguished, some estimates suggest that phantom limb sensations are experienced by virtually all amputees,[25] whereas others have reported high but somewhat lower rates (eg, 80%).[26] In one prospective study of nonpainful phantom limb phenomena, 90% of the 58 patients reported phantom limb sensations at some time during the 2-year follow-up period.[27] Although the prevalence of these sensations did not decline over time, the frequency and duration of the sensations did. More recent cross-sectional research also suggests that nonpainful phantom sensations are common years after the amputation. In a sample of 92 adults with lower limb amputations, 80.4% reported experiencing nonpainful phantom limb sensations in the 4 weeks preceding the study.[28] Time from amputation did not correlate with the occurrence of nonpainful sensations ($r \cong 0.02$); in fact, participants had lived with their amputation an average of 18 years (SD = 17.2, range of time from amputation = 1 to 53 years). Similarly, Ehde and associates[29] reported that 79% of their community-dwelling sample of 255 adults with lower limb amputations experienced nonpainful phantom limb sensations. Similar to the study

by Smith and associates,[28] participants in this community-dwelling sample had lived with their amputations a long time, an average of 14.2 years (range = 6 months to 74 years), and described their sensations as intermittent (71%). Thus, nonpainful sensations cannot be assumed to remit after surgery; rather, they appear to be chronic for many individuals with limb loss.

Less is known about the prevalence of phantom limb sensations in upper limb amputations. In one of the few studies to specifically address nonpainful sensations after upper limb amputation, Kooijman and associates[30] reported the prevalence of nonpainful phantom sensations to be 76% in a sample of 72 adults with acquired amputation. Similar to what has been reported in adults with lower limb amputations, the sensations tended to be intermittent. Interestingly, the authors also reported that the risk of phantom sensations was higher (a relative risk of 1.2) for those experiencing residual limb pain than in those with no residual limb pain. No other factors were associated with phantom limb sensations in this group.

Little is known about the effect of chronic nonpainful phantom limb sensations on the lives and functioning of individuals who experience them. Because by definition these sensations are not perceived as painful, one might assume that they do not negatively affect the individuals who experience them. To our knowledge, however, no studies have examined this hypothesis.

Phantom Limb Pain

One of the most commonly discussed consequences of amputations has been phantom limb pain. Phantom limb pain refers to painful sensations in the missing portion of the amputated limb. Although earlier reports suggested that the incidence of chronic phantom limb pain was low, it is now thought that most amputees, possibly as many as 55% to 85%, experience phantom limb pain from

time to time.[26,31-34] Recent studies conducted in large nonclinical samples have confirmed its high prevalence.[28,29,35] For example, in a random sample of 526 British veterans with amputations, 55% had phantom limb pain.[36] Other recent studies have reported even higher rates. In one large study of 255 community-dwelling adults with lower limb amputations (mean years since amputation = 14), 72% of these respondents had phantom limb pain (most commonly described as sharp, tingling, shooting, and stabbing).[29] The prevalence of phantom limb pain was 75% in another large sample of 478 community-dwelling adults with acquired lower limb amputations.[37] A similar prevalence of phantom limb pain was reported (69.2%) in a sample of 104 adults in Ireland with lower limb amputations.[35]

It is important to note that prevalence estimates likely vary not only because different populations are studied (eg, clinic versus community) but also because of how phantom limb pain is defined. For instance, studies that ask amputees whether they have "unrelenting phantom limb pain" will likely show very different prevalences from studies that ask amputees whether they have had "any phantom limb pain." We suspect that many of the studies in which phantom limb pain was found to be quite prevalent included persons for whom phantom limb pain, although episodically present, was not problematic. Thus, it is important for researchers not only to specify how phantom limb pain is defined but also to examine the prevalence of pain that is bothersome and disabling, that is, the proportion of persons who suffer as a result of phantom limb pain.

In addition to its prevalence, phantom limb pain has been characterized in terms of onset, frequency, duration, intensity, and quality.[19] Onset of phantom limb pain is early, with several studies suggesting that it develops within the first few days after the amputation.[19,26,38] Phantom limb pain tends to be intermittent or episodic, with only a few individuals reporting constant pain.[28,29,32,34,35] Using a prospective diary design uncommon in the amputation literature, a British study of 89 adults with phantom limb pain after lower limb amputation reported the episodic and variable nature of phantom limb pain.[39] Study participants recorded, among other things, the intensity of their pain (using a numeric rating scale) on an hourly basis for 7 days. The investigators found that 84% of participants reported pain on each of the 7 study days, and 16% reported pain on 3 to 5 days of the study period. In terms of the frequency of episodes within a day, 71% of participants reported episodes of phantom limb pain on more than one occasion per day, and of these, 75% reported 4 to 5 episodes per day. Regarding duration of episodes, 80% of participants experienced phantom limb pain for 6 to 10 hours each day, with only 11% reporting an average of 12 or more hours of phantom limb pain each day.

Typically, most patients describe phantom limb pain to be moderate in intensity, for example, an average pain intensity of 5 on a numeric rating scale of 0 to 10.[19,29,32] Through the use of hourly pain diaries, Whyte and Niven[39] reported that the average intensity across the 7-day study period ranged from 3 to 8 on a scale of 0 to 10 (mean = 4.5, SD = 4.6). Sixty percent of their sample reported average pain intensity in the lower half of the scale (3 to 4), and 40% reported pain intensity in the higher end (5 to 8). These investigators also found great variation both among and within individuals in intensity, frequency, and duration of painful episodes. Patients use various words to describe phantom limb pain. For example, it was most commonly described as "squeezing," "burning," "knife like," and "throbbing" in one sample[26] and as "sharp," "tingling," "shooting," and "stabbing" in another.[29]

Most of the research on phantom limb pain described thus far has been conducted on samples mostly or completely consisting of lower limb amputees. Given that upper limb amputation is less common than lower limb, few studies have specifically focused on phantom limb pain in individuals who have lost an upper limb. A recent survey found that 41% of a sample of 99 adults with upper limb amputations had phantom limb pain.[31] In a sample of 72 adults in the Netherlands with upper limb amputations, mostly because of trauma, Kooijman and associates[30] reported that 51% had phantom limb pain, with 48% of those experiencing it daily. Age and time since amputation were not associated with the phantom limb pain in their sample, although having sensations of a phantom limb was (relative risk = 11.3). Sixty-nine percent of a clinic sample of 76 patients with upper limb amputation reported phantom limb pain.[40] More research is needed on the prevalence of phantom limb pain as well as its characteristics in those with upper limb amputation.

A number of mechanisms, both central and peripheral, have been hypothesized to explain the development of phantom limb pain.[22,25,41] Although persistent peripheral nerve discharges have been recorded after amputation,[42] most evidence suggests a central abnormality in patients with phantom limb pain. Some authors have postulated, on the basis of clinical data, that hyperirritable foci develop in the dorsal horn of the spinal cord after peripheral nerve transection, possibly a result of the loss of high-threshold input to the dorsal horn neurons.[25,43] There may also be more rostral central factors as well, because severe phantom limb pain has been reported to be unresponsive to cordotomy[25] and can also be unmasked by spinal anesthesia.[44] Whatever central changes exist, the initiating event in the development of phantom limb pain is probably peripheral. It is thought that the massive afferent barrage at the time of injury or amputation may establish central processes that generate later pain, or alternatively, that the sudden loss of peripheral input may trigger central changes that result in differentiation pain.

Residual Limb Pain

Until recently, less was known about residual limb pain, although it was generally believed that most residual limb pain resolved with wound healing.[25,32] This type of pain occurs in the portion of the amputated limb that is still physically present. There is considerable discrepancy in the reported prevalence of chronic residual limb pain. For example, in their thoughtful review of phantom limb pain, Nikolajsen and Jensen[45] contended that residual limb pain persists in only 5% to 10% of patients. This contrasts starkly with several other studies of adults with lower limb amputations. For example, 74% of a community-dwelling sample of 255 adults with lower limb amputations had residual limb pain.[29] Similar rates have been reported in other community-based samples.[28,37] Other studies report rates of 48% to 56%.[34,35] This variation in rates is likely affected by differences in study populations (clinic versus community) as well as methodology (definition of residual limb pain). Longitudinal epidemiologic studies that clearly define residual limb pain are needed to clarify the problem.

Similar to phantom limb pain, residual limb pain appears to be episodic. Gallagher and associates[35] found that, of the 48% of their sample of 104 patients who reported residual limb pain, 13% experienced an episode once or twice in the week preceding the survey, 63% experienced an episode more than twice, and 13% experienced constant residual limb pain. Only 7% reported no residual limb pain during the 1-week period (4% did not specify). Other studies have also reported residual limb pain to be intermittent.[19,28,29] With the exception of frequency and duration, other characteristics of residual limb pain have received considerably less attention in the literature. When these factors have been examined, studies suggest that residual limb pain is typically of moderate intensity for most, although a notable subset (15% to 35%) describe it as severe.[28,29,46] In a study by Gallagher and associates[35] residual limb pain was described as "distressing" by 26% and as "horrible" or "excruciating" by 13% of their sample.

Chronic residual limb pain is also thought to be common after upper limb amputation, although less research has been done in this population. In one study, Kooijman and associates[30] reported that 48.6% of their sample of 72 Dutch adults with upper limb amputations reported chronic residual limb pain. In one of the few studies to focus exclusively on chronic pain following upper limb amputation,[40] 55% of the patients reported current residual limb pain, with 75% of those describing their pain as intermittent and 25% as continuous.

Other Sources of Pain

In addition to phantom sensations and phantom pain, many other sources of pain and discomfort affect individuals with limb loss. Some of the more common problems include back pain and pain in other regions, neuromas, bone spurs, heterotopic bone, chronic wounds/cysts, musculoskeletal overuse, and prosthesis-related pain.[47]

Back Pain

Although the focus of amputation pain research has primarily been on the amputated limb, back pain has recently been identified as a significant problem among lower limb amputees, affecting 71% in an initial survey[28] and 52% in a follow-up study in a different sample.[48] In both of these studies, the reasons for amputation included trauma, vascular disease, congenital deficiencies, or cancer. In an investigation of the health-related quality of life of 97 adults with unilateral transfemoral amputations because of nonvascular causes, Hagberg

and Brånemark[49] reported that 47% of their sample had back pain. These rates are considerably higher than those reported in the general population, where it has been estimated that the point prevalence of back pain is 15% to 25%.[50] More important, the existing studies suggest that back pain was significantly more bothersome to lower limb amputees[28] and interfered more with activities[51] than either phantom limb pain or residual limb pain. It has been hypothesized that, for some amputees, back pain results from altered gait patterns developed to accommodate a prosthesis; this hypothesis awaits experimental confirmation, however. In upper limb amputees, biomechanical factors, such as shoulder hiking and positional scoliosis, may place them at risk for neck, shoulder, and back pain, although whether these changes lead to chronic pain remains unstudied.

Pain in Other Regions

Recent studies suggest that amputees experience pain in regions other than the amputated limb and back. For example, Ehde and associates[29] surveyed 255 amputees and found that pain occurred in locations other than the back, including the contralateral sound leg or foot (43%), the buttocks/hips (37%), and the neck/shoulders (31%). More than one third of this sample reported pain in three or more locations. Forty-six percent of a Swedish sample of transfemoral amputees (for nonvascular causes) reported pain in the sound limb.[44] In a well-designed epidemiologic study of outcomes of persons with traumatic amputations, Pezzin and associates[46] reported that 16.9% of their sample of patients with trauma-related amputations experienced severe pain in the joints of the contralateral limb. Thus, like many other groups with disability, persons with limb loss may experience pain in multiple locations and from different causes (eg, phantom limb pain may be neuropathic; back or contralateral pain may be musculoskeletal).

Neuromas

Every time a nerve is transected, the axons within the nerve will attempt to regenerate and grow. For lacerations of nerves, this can be productive because if the nerve sheath (epineurium) is repaired in proper alignment, the axons can grow down the nerve and eventually reinnervate the distal limb. If there is no epineural sheath, as after an amputation, the axons start to grow but then stop after forming an intertwined mass of scar and nerve tissue, which can become painful to pressure, stretching, and other types of physical manipulation. This is called an amputation neuroma. Even when completely undisturbed, electrical potentials may arise within the neuroma, causing negative local and distant sensory and motor phenomena. These sensations can be bothersome and painful to the person with limb loss.

In a transtibial amputation, five major nerves (tibial, superficial peroneal, deep peroneal, saphenous, and sural) and countless smaller sensory and fine motor branches are transected. Although surgeons have devised numerous techniques to minimize neuroma formation, none has proved uniformly successful. The traditional method applies longitudinal traction, divides the nerve simply, and then allows it to retract. Other methods have included cauterization of the nerve ends with chemicals or heat, burying the nerve in bone or muscle, encasing the nerve in impervious material, ligating the nerve, or injecting it with a variety of chemicals. Additional methods include sewing the sectioned nerves to other nerves or sewing them back onto themselves, thereby creating a nerve loop.

Because neuroma formation is inevitable to some degree, the generally accepted method to correct the problem is still drawing the nerve distally, sectioning it, and allowing it to retract away from areas of pressure, scarring, and pulsating vessels. Clinical experience suggests that neuromas that form in very scarred areas are the most symptomatic. When working in these areas, the surgeon should apply moderate tension to the nerve and section it cleanly, allowing it to retract away from the site of amputation and into proximal soft tissues free of scarring. This circumvents the problem of the distal end of the nerve scarring to the surgical site where traction and pressure are more likely. Traction on the nerve at the time of sectioning should not be excessive because too much tension can lead to proximal pain and neuropathy. Knowledge of prosthetic designs and regions or areas of contact and pressure will aid the surgeon in nerve placement. Thus far, none of the other methods cited above has been shown to lower the rate of symptomatic neuromas or phantom pain.

Bone Spurs and Heterotopic Bone, Chronic Wounds and Cysts

When the bone is transected, a small slip of periosteum can ossify into spurs of bone, which can cause pressure and pain when weight bearing in the prosthetic socket pushes tissues against the bone spurs. In individuals with trauma and burns, the damaged muscle can also form areas of heterotopic bone. Typically, this bone has a very irregular surface and edges and can cause undue pressure and pain. It is usually diagnosed with plain radiographs. Initial treatment consists of prosthetic modification to minimize the pressure in this area. If this approach is unsuccessful, then resection of the bone spur or heterotopic bone is indicated.

Small wounds, which can often start as inflamed hair follicles or sweat glands, can become chronic and painful.

Overuse Musculoskeletal Pain

Amputees have lost anatomic structures that were designed specifically for interacting with the environment; after amputation, the residual limb tissues are exposed to the tremendous

forces and stress of walking several thousand steps per day. Although the tissues do accommodate and become more durable over time, they were never designed for this use; thus, they naturally experience overuse wear and tear and cause some pain. In addition, gait patterns may change, and overuse of the contralateral limb may occur. These are all potential sources of pain following limb loss.

Prosthesis-Related Pain

A prosthetic socket must be carefully constructed not only to fit the shape of the residual limb but also to apply pressure in areas that can tolerate it. It also must be designed to relieve and protect more sensitive areas. An exact mold of the residual limb does not make a good socket because it does not differentiate among these anatomic regions or areas. The skilled prosthetist modifies the socket by indenting tolerant regions to increase their share of the load, relieving other areas. Inevitably, as a residual limb changes shape by normal maturation, muscle atrophy, or weight loss or gain, the location and distribution of forces and loads change. The patient can experience severe local pain, bruising, redness, blisters, or skin ulceration from these forces.

Impact of Amputation-Related Pain on Functioning and Quality of Life

Chronic pain is frequently accompanied by changes in physical, emotional, social, and vocational functioning. For example, individuals with chronic pain often experience changes in lifestyle, such as deconditioning and decreased participation in social activities. In the general population, chronic pain is also a major cause of unemployment because of pain-related disability. Chronic pain has also been associated with psychiatric disorders. For example, in a sample of 200 adults with chronic low back pain, 59% had current symptoms of,

and 77% met lifetime criteria for, at least one psychiatric diagnosis.[52] Major depressive disorder, substance abuse, and anxiety disorders were the most commonly experienced disorders in this sample.

Although many authors have speculated that chronic pain negatively affects functioning and quality of life in those with limb loss, only a few studies have examined this hypothesis. In addition to a lack of research, the field has also tended to focus on only a few outcomes and to use nonstandardized measures of functioning and quality of life, which make comparisons to other populations, including the general population, difficult. Thus, although it is suspected that chronic pain likely contributes to suffering and disability and affects quality of life for many individuals with limb loss, the nature and magnitude of this impact have not been quantified or adequately explored.

A few studies have included general questions regarding the impact of chronic pain (typically phantom limb pain). Gallagher and associates[35] reported that phantom limb pain interfered "quite a bit or a lot" for 11% of their sample. Kooijman and associates[30] reported that 64% of a sample of patients with upper limb amputations described suffering "moderately to very much" from phantom limb pain; 60% of those with residual limb pain reported suffering "moderately to very much." Pezzin and associates[46] reported that 24.4% of their sample of 78 persons with limb loss secondary to trauma reported severe problems with phantom limb pain in the month before completing an interview; a severe problem was defined as being "extremely" or "very" bothered by phantom limb pain in the past month.

Living with chronic pain caused by an amputation may also affect vocational functioning. One study[53] found that, compared with employed amputees, unemployed amputees reported higher levels of pain and lower levels of prosthesis use. Both phantom limb pain and residual limb pain have been negatively associated with return to work.[54,55]

Only a few studies have examined pain-related disability using standardized measures. Marshall and associates[56] reported on the Sickness Impact Profile,[57,58] a standardized measure of physical and psychosocial well being frequently used in the rehabilitation field. In this study, amputees with high levels of pain showed higher levels of overall disability (physical and psychosocial) than did participants with lower levels of amputation pain. In the first study using a standardized measure of pain-specific disability, the Chronic Pain Grade,[59] nearly one fourth (23%) of the subjects reported moderate to severe disability because of phantom limb pain.[29] However, this study did not examine the disability associated with residual limb pain and was limited to lower limb amputations. In another study of 205 persons with lower limb loss, the degree to which pain interfered with activities varied with pain type.[51] That is, at the same level, back pain interfered more significantly with daily function than phantom limb pain did after pain levels reached 5 or more on a pain intensity scale of 0 to 10. To our knowledge, pain-related disability in upper limb amputees has not been examined.

Risk and Biopsychosocial Factors

Although a number of risk factors for chronic pain have been identified in the literature, less is known about the risk factors for chronic pain following limb loss.

Biological Risk Factors

Severe acute pain has been shown to be a major risk factor for chronic post-amputation pain in several samples.[2] Within this category, the duration of preamputation limb pain of longer than 1 month and more severe pain (eg, burn injury, gangrene, thrombo-

sis) has been associated with a greater risk of chronic pain.[32,60] Other biologic factors that have been examined include level of amputation, amputation etiology, and comorbid medical problems. No consistent risk factors have been found, however, and this area requires further epidemiologic study.

Psychosocial Risk Factors

Only a few studies have examined the role of psychosocial factors such as pain coping, cognitions, and social environmental variables in phantom limb pain. In one study, Hill[61] found strong associations between a measure of pain catastrophizing (having excessively negative and unrealistic thoughts about pain, such as "this pain is awful" or "I can't stand this") and measures of both pain severity and psychological distress (R = 0.50 and 0.51, respectively). In a follow-up study of phantom limb pain in 228 patients, Hill and associates[62] reported that catastrophizing was again significantly associated with pain severity, physical disability, and psychosocial dysfunction, accounting for an additional 26%, 11%, and 22% of the variance in these variables, respectively, even after amputation-related and demographic variables were controlled. These two cross-sectional studies also showed that pain coping strategies (eg, diverting attention away from pain, increasing activity levels) were significantly associated with adjustment to chronic phantom limb pain. Using a longitudinal study design to test the utility of a biopsychosocial model for understanding chronic phantom limb pain, Jensen and associates[63] reported that pain coping, pain cognitions, and social environmental variables predicted both concurrent (1 month after amputation) and future (5 months later) functioning in a group of 61 lower limb amputees. Specifically, the investigators found that psychosocial factors contributed significantly to concurrent pain interference and depression (28% and 46% additional variance accounted for after control-

ling for pain intensity), as well as changes in pain interference and depression (39% of the variance accounted for in both criteria after controlling for pain intensity). Higher levels of catastrophizing predicted poorer concurrent functioning, whereas lower levels of catastrophizing and family solicitousness (eg, offers of assistance, taking over a task) and higher levels of family support predicted improvement in functioning over time. Catastrophizing was the single most important predictor of pain, pain interference, and depressive symptoms in this sample. Thus, these three studies are consistent with what is known about adjustment in populations where pain is the primary disability: persons who think negatively (catastrophize) about their pain show greater physical and psychosocial dysfunction than those who do not.[11,14,64]

Chronic Pain in Youth With Amputations

A 1993 review of phantom limb pain suggested that youth (ie, children and adolescents) with limb loss or limb deficiency may not experience chronic phantom limb pain.[65] This conclusion may have been premature, however, because there had been few, if any, empirical tests of this assumption at that time.[66] More recent research suggests that the prevalence of chronic phantom limb pain in youth with acquired amputations is no less frequent than that for adults.[67-69] Many questions remain regarding chronic pain in youth with limb loss, however. No studies have examined whether such youth experience pain in other regions or what impact pain may have on activities and participation.

Pain Management
Clinical Assessment

A first and important step in the treatment of chronic pain secondary to limb loss is an accurate assessment of the pain problem. This includes assessment of the biologic, psychological, and environmental factors that contribute to nociception, pain, suffering, and pain behavior.[4]

Medical Assessment

The physician must conduct a complete physical examination with an open mind to the differential diagnosis of musculoskeletal pain in patients with limb amputation. The proximal nervous system is, unfortunately, the easiest to overlook during this examination. The examination should include tests for neurologic signs and symptoms that may indicate radicular pain radiating from the neck or low back or nerve compression. Cervical stenosis, disk herniation, or thoracic outlet syndrome can be present in an upper limb amputee who describes a change in severity of phantom pain. Likewise, lumbar disk herniation or spinal stenosis can present with pain or dysesthesia in an amputated foot. Traditionally, the physical examination attempts to identify focal changes in motor units or changes in sensation in the hand or foot; in patients with amputated limbs, these signs and symptoms might not be present in the physical examination. Likewise, traditional nerve traction tests, such as the straight leg raise test for sciatic nerve irritation, are certainly more difficult to perform and interpret in an individual with limb loss.

The physical examination of the amputation site itself is designed to identify for mechanical or local pain that can be reproduced with direct palpation. Neuromas, local nerve compression, bone spurs, heterotopic bone, muscle herniation, and muscle compression are all possible direct local causes of pain. Neuromas can often be diagnosed by deep palpation of a nodule and Tinel's sign (tingling or distinct reproduction of "electrical" pain with tapping of the end of the nerve).

Imaging studies, specifically MRI, can assist in the diagnosis of neuro-mas. Care must be exercised because every transected nerve will form a neuroma, but not all neuromas will be irritated and symptomatic. Because MRI scans might reveal neuromas that are not necessarily symptomatic, the imaging study and physical examination must be correlated to confirm that the pain is emanating from the entrapped, scarred, or irritated nerve end. Local nerve compression can occur where the peroneal nerve wraps around the fibular neck or where the ulnar nerve passes behind the medial epicondyle of the elbow. The prosthetic socket can occasionally be a major contributor to nerve irritation, and even with modification of the socket, the irritated nerve might remain symptomatic for some time.

Mechanical pain from bone spurs or heterotopic bone can be suspected from the discomfort that accompanies tissue crepitus as tissue is moved over the end of the irregular bone surface or compressed onto a bone spur. These suspicions can often be supported by radiologic findings of irregular bone in an area that directly correlates to the physical finding. Diagnostic imaging can be a mixed blessing. It is not unusual for radiographs to show irregular bone formation near the amputation site. Sometimes it is asymptomatic, so it needs to be correlated with physical findings before intervention. Modification of the prosthetic device is often tried first in an attempt to remove pressure or transfer load from that area. Only if the physical examination correlates with the imaging study and nonsurgical treatment has failed should surgical excision be considered.

Finally, ischemia from peripheral vascular disease may be causing claudication or rest pain in the amputated limb. Typically, patients report that the pain ceases immediately when they stop walking or when they remove the prosthesis. If the pain began after a change to a new type of socket or suspension system, ischemia must be considered. Once again, the physician must realize that, because tradi-tional examinations of distal pulses and capillary refill of the toes cannot be done, the diagnosis is more difficult. The proximal pulses and the texture and temperature of the residual limb must be examined. Occasionally, the prosthetic socket or suspension system can induce venous congestion or arterial occlusion with static or dynamic use of the device. Patients with transtibial amputation, for example, may get popliteal compression only when sitting, and the pain is relieved with standing, removal of the device, or even simple release of a distal locking mechanism.

Prosthetic and Orthotic Assessment

The general examination must also include observation of gait in the prosthetic device. With the patient standing, limb length equality and pelvic level are assessed. Improper prosthesis length can lead to gait deviations that may be improved with adjustment of the device.[70]

Gait assessment also includes observation of symmetry, balance, proportion of time in the stance and swing phases on each limb, and deviations of the trunk, hips, knees, and feet. Some deviations may be related to prosthesis alignment and can be improved with changes in rotation, varus, valgus, and translational position of the foot. Chronic gait deviations may aggravate or contribute to back pain, although this assumption has not been tested empirically.

As mentioned previously, if the patient has localized pain, the prosthesis must be examined in that area to determine whether the socket or suspension system might be causing undue pressure or irritation there. How the device contacts the body at rest, with sitting, and when moving must be considered. A device that appears to cause no local pressure may, in fact, piston and cause repeated friction or irritation at a particular site during gait. With transfemoral amputation, insufficient socket flexion may result in excessive lordosis during ambulation as the patient compensates for this imbalance. An upper limb prosthesis that looks benign at rest can change contact areas and loading when it is used to carry a weight or when it is used in a specific position or activity.

Assessment of Pain

Although only a few measures are specific to or include assessment of amputation pain (eg, Prosthesis Evaluation Questionnaire [PEQ],[71] Trinity Amputation and Prosthesis Experience Scales [TAPES][72]), a number of good standardized measures of pain are available in the chronic pain literature.[4] We encourage the use of standardized instruments to assess pain because such measures are reliable and valid and allow populations to be compared.

To fully understand the pain experience, multiple dimensions of pain should be assessed, including pain location, intensity, frequency, duration, affect, and pain-related disability. Which dimensions should be measured obviously depends on the purpose of the assessment. Whatever measures are chosen, we encourage even the busiest of clinicians to ask not only about pain severity (intensity), location, and frequency but also about pain-related interference with activities.

Several assessments, two specific to lower limb amputation and two general measures, are available. The PEQ[71] is a 43-item tool developed to measure prosthesis function and quality of life of lower limb amputees. The PEQ comprises 10 scales that have been shown to have high internal consistency, temporal stability, content validity, and criterion validity. Although developed to measure constructs other than pain, the PEQ has 12 items that assess the frequency, intensity, and "bothersomeness" of nonpainful phantom sensations, phantom limb pain, residual limb pain, and back pain. To do this, it uses a visual analog scale that is a 100-mm line bounded by two anchor phrases describing the extremes of possible answers (never and all the time). Respondents indicate their answer to the questions by making a mark across the line. The PEQ has been shown to be useful in assessing both chronic pain and nonpainful phantom sensations in adults with lower limb loss,[28] so it is a valuable clinical and research tool.

The TAPES[72] are a multidimensional self-report measure (54 items) designed to assess the experience of amputation and adjustment to a lower limb prosthesis. Like the PEQ, it is not limited to measurement of pain. It assesses a number of dimensions of the postamputation experience, including psychosocial adjustment, activity restriction, and satisfaction with the prosthetic device. The TAPES tool specifically assesses the presence, frequency, duration, and intensity of phantom limb pain and residual limb pain. It also asks respondents to rate the extent to which pain interferes with their daily lives (not at all, a little bit, moderately, quite a bit, a lot). The TAPES tool appears to have good internal consistency and validity.[72] Like the PEQ, it is limited to persons with lower limb amputations, so it merits consideration as a clinical or research tool.

The Chronic Pain Grade (CPG)[60,73] is a simple, reliable, and valid measure that has been used to grade the severity of chronic pain in a variety of pain populations. This measure consists of the following: (1) three ratings (present, worst, and average) of pain intensity as described above; (2) a question concerning the number of days in the past 3 months that the respondent was kept from usual activities because of pain ("disability days"); and (3) three interference items that ask how pain has interfered with daily activities, social activities, and work over the past 3 months. The first interference item asks respondents to rate how their pain interferes with daily activities on a scale of 0 to 10 where 0 = no interference and 10 = unable to carry out activities. The second item asks respondents to rate how much pain has changed their ability to take part in recreational, social, and family activities (0 = no change, 10 = extreme change). The third interference item asks how much pain has changed their ability to work (including housework), using the same scale (0 = no change, 10 = extreme change).

The CPG then combines the intensity items, disability days, and interference items to classify individuals with pain into one of five grades: grade 0 (no pain problem), grade I (low disability, low pain intensity), grade II (low disability, high pain intensity), grade III (high disability that is moderately limiting), and grade IV (high disability that is severely limiting). In this scale, the term disability refers to pain-related disability and not to the disability associated with actually having an amputation. This measure has been useful in at least one sample of persons with limb loss[29] and has the advantage of being brief while yielding information about pain on several dimensions. Thus, although not specific to amputation-related pain, it is a strong candidate for clinical and research use in the limb loss population.

One other measure that we think is particularly worthy of mention is the Pain Interference Scale from the Brief Pain Inventory (BPI).[74] This scale provides a broad-based assessment of the impact of pain on a variety of activities, including sleep, work, self-care, recreational activities, as well as mood and relationships. It is a simple assessment because it can be done quickly and is easily self-administered. As such, it is a potentially valuable tool for examining the impact of chronic pain on individuals with limb loss.

Assessment of Psychological Distress

Unfortunately, depressive disorders are common among persons with chronic pain. Major depressive disorder is a psychological disorder characterized by depressed mood or loss of

TABLE 1 Measure and Scoring Instructions of the PHQ-9

Over the last 2 weeks, how often have you been bothered by any of the following problems?	Not at all	Several days	More than half the days	Nearly every day
a. Little interest or pleasure in doing things	❏	❏	❏	❏
b. Feeling down, depressed, or hopeless	❏	❏	❏	❏
c. Trouble falling or staying asleep or sleeping too much	❏	❏	❏	❏
d. Feeling tired or having little energy	❏	❏	❏	❏
e. Poor appetite or overeating	❏	❏	❏	❏
f. Feeling bad about yourself—or that you are a failure or have let yourself or your family down	❏	❏	❏	❏
g. Trouble concentrating on things, such as reading the newspaper or watching television	❏	❏	❏	❏
h. Moving or speaking so slowly that other people could have noticed? Or the opposite—being so fidgety or restless that you have been moving around a lot more than usual	❏	❏	❏	❏
i. Thoughts that you would be better off dead or of hurting yourself in some way	❏	❏	❏	❏

Major depressive syndrome is indicated if answers to a or b and five or more of a through i are at least "More than half the days" (count i if present at all).

(Adapted from Spitzer RL, Kroenke K, Williams JB: Validation and utility of a self-report version of PRIME-MD: The PHQ primary care study. Primary care evaluation of mental disorders: Patient health questionnaire. JAMA 1999;282:1737-1744.)

interest or pleasure that is not directly caused by a general medical condition. It is associated with a variety of emotional and physical symptoms, such as weight loss or gain, insomnia or hypersomnia, psychomotor retardation or agitation, loss of energy and concentration, feelings of worthlessness and hopelessness, and thoughts of suicide or death.[75] Emotional distress may also include subclinical levels of depressive symptoms, anxiety, psychosocial stress, and other mood complaints.

Approximately one third of persons who have chronic pain also experience a major depressive disorder.[76] This is much higher than rates of depressive disorders in the general population (prevalence 3% to 9%)[75] or primary care populations (prevalence 10% to 15%).[77] Among persons with acquired amputation, the point prevalence for depression appears to be somewhere between 25% and 35%.[78] Although less is known about rates of depression in persons with both acquired amputation and chronic pain, it is probably safe to assume that depression is a common problem in this group.

Psychological distress, including depression, is often underdiagnosed and undertreated. Because it may be missed, depressive symptoms should be screened for and evaluated routinely by clinicians working with persons with limb loss. A number of tools are available for use that are easy to administer and useful as initial screens.[79] One that we particularly recommend is the Patient Health Questionnaire-9 (PHQ-9)[80] (Table 1). The PHQ-9 is the 9-item depression screening scale from the larger Patient Health Questionnaire, a recently developed measure for making criteria-based diagnoses of depressive and other mental disorders commonly encountered in medical settings.[81] The PHQ-9 scale is half the length of most other depression screens, has comparable sensitivity and specificity, and comprises the nine criteria upon which DSM-IV diagnoses of depressive episodes are based. Thus, the PHQ-9 can not only provide an index of depressive symptom severity but can also establish depressive disorder diagnoses. In addition to its good reliability and validity, the PHQ-9 is also easily self-administered, taking only a few minutes to complete. The larger

PHQ has been well accepted and perceived to be useful by both patients and clinicians.[81] Thus, although the clinical utility of this measure has not been studied in the limb loss population or clinic, its strong performance in other medical settings suggests that it warrants consideration for these patients.

If substantial depressive symptoms are detected, referral to a mental health provider can be made for a more complete evaluation and for treatment. Aggressive treatment with pharmacotherapy or psychotherapy should be considered. Depression has been shown to negatively affect physical, cognitive, social, and work functioning in other medical populations.[82] Thus, treatment of depression has the potential not only to reduce suffering but also to minimize this additional disability.

Treatment of Chronic Pain

The treatment of pain in amputees has received considerable attention in the literature, most of which is focused on the treatment of phantom limb pain. In his review of the history of treatments for phantom limb pain, Sherman[19] reported that more than

60 different treatments have been suggested, including a variety of medical, surgical, psychological, and alternative options. For example, conventional treatments such as opioids[83] have been suggested, as have less conventional treatments such as therapeutic touch[84] and electroconvulsive therapy.[85] Unfortunately, the success rates of these treatments have rarely exceeded the expected placebo response rate of 25% to 30%. In addition, most studies of the treatments for phantom limb pain suffer from significant methodologic weaknesses; the published literature has consisted primarily of single-group designs, clinical commentaries, and case studies, with randomized clinical trials absent.

One exception was a randomized clinical trial of transcutaneous electrical nerve stimulation, but it proved it to be ineffective in treating chronic phantom limb pain.[86] In addition, a recently published randomized controlled trial found amitriptyline to be ineffective in treating chronic phantom and residual limb pain in adults with lower or upper limb amputations.[87] Given the lack of controlled trials for postamputation pain, it is evident that we are far from establishing standards of care for managing chronic phantom limb pain, and even less is known about treating residual limb pain and other amputation-related pain.

One novel line of research is developing strategies to prevent chronic phantom limb pain. Several studies have examined the use of perioperative epidural anesthesia provided at the time of amputation.[38,88-90] This approach is based on the theory that phantom limb pain is, in part, mediated centrally at the spinal cord at or around the time of the amputation. It is thought that administering epidural anesthesia perioperatively may reduce the massive afferent discharge entering the central nervous system as a result of preamputation disease or trauma, the amputation itself, and the immediate postoperative processes. Results of at least one of the studies

have been positive,[88] whereas other studies have not shown any long-term prophylactic effects.[38,89,90] These studies vary considerably in their methodologies, sample sizes, anesthesia techniques, and reasons for amputation, so it is too early to draw conclusions about the efficacy of this approach. More randomized clinical trials are needed.

Although there is a lack of controlled treatment studies for phantom limb pain, we know even less about the types of treatment sought by persons with phantom limb pain or their perceptions of treatment. A few studies have suggested that persons with phantom limb pain may have difficulty accessing treatment for pain, and even when they do, they find such treatment unsatisfactory. For example, among 149 British veterans with amputations who discussed their phantom limb pain with their physician, 49 were told there was no treatment to help their pain and only 17 were referred to a pain clinic.[34] In this same study, the type of treatment that was most frequently administered was acetaminophen (53%) or an acetaminophen/opioid combination (37%). The only treatments that satisfied more than half of the respondents were acetaminophen/opioid medication, nonsteroidal anti-inflammatory drugs, and alcohol. Similarly, a study of 2,694 American veterans reported that 54% of the sample had discussed phantom limb pain with their physician, but only 19% were offered treatment.[91] Only 8% of respondents reported being helped to any real extent by treatment. In another large study of 764 American veterans, the only treatments that reportedly produced permanent effects were noninvasive corrections of problems in the residual limb, such as desensitization.[92] Short-term benefits were reported from pain medications such as hypnotics and analgesics. The authors concluded that most of the treatments surveyed were generally ineffective.

Pain Interventions

Given the limitations in the treatment literature, we will briefly summarize the more common interventions for pain.

Pharmacologic

Tricyclic antidepressants have long been used to treat phantom limb pain.[19] Nevertheless, until recently, no clinical trials evaluated their efficacy for phantom limb pain. In a meta-analysis of 39 controlled trials, antidepressants were found to be beneficial in the treatment of a variety of types of chronic pain.[93] None of the clinical trials included in this meta-analysis, however, focused on pain after limb loss. A number of studies have also suggested that tricyclic antidepressants are beneficial in treating painful peripheral polyneuropathies.[94] Given that amputation often includes the severing of multiple peripheral nerves, it is plausible that these medications may be helpful in treating phantom limb pain. Nevertheless, only one randomized controlled trial has examined the efficacy of tricyclic antidepressants for relieving chronic phantom limb pain. In this randomized trial of 39 adults with chronic phantom limb pain and/or residual limb pain, amitriptyline was compared with an active placebo (benztropine mesylate), and was found not to be efficacious.[87] More research is needed.

Antiseizure drugs, which can be effective in calming excited nerves, have been used for years to combat phantom limb pain, with gabapentin emerging most recently as a first-line medication. Clinical reports suggest that these drugs may minimize the number of episodes of phantom limb pain, although this hypothesis has not been tested empirically. Recently, a crossover randomized controlled trial of gabapentin revealed that it was effective for some, but not all, patients (DG Smith, MD, DM Ehde, MP Jensen, et al, unpublished data).

Opiates and narcotics have been used since ancient times to treat pain. Although we use narcotics extensively around the time of surgery, we usually try to avoid long-term use because, although they calm the reaction to phantom limb pain, they do not make it disappear. Unfortunately, some patients may need a low level of chronic narcotic therapy but typically only as a last resort, when other strategies have not helped. Narcotics do not act at the source of the pain. Instead, they work in nerve centers and the brain. The pain is still there, but it is not as bothersome. The opiate forms a cloud-like barrier that diminishes pain signals being transmitted between the injury site and the brain, making the person more indifferent to pain. Traditional narcotics have a very fast onset and a high initial peak effect, but that effect wears off quickly, and the pain recurs. As tolerance for opiates increases, often more of the narcotic is needed to produce the same effect, and it may be needed more frequently. An array of safety risks accompanies the use of narcotics, including decreased reaction time, clouded judgment, and drowsiness. In large doses, narcotics can inhibit respiration, making breathing difficult or even impossible.

Newer, longer-acting narcotics linger in a person's system for more extended periods. They do not have the rapid, high peak and fast wear-off of traditional opiates. Instead, they take effect more slowly and maintain a steadier state. Such drugs do have dangers, however. Misuse of these newer drugs, such as oxycodone hydrochloride, is increasingly common. On the street, these drugs can be manipulated to remove their long-acting nature. This creates a tremendous dilemma for physicians and providers who must balance improving a person's life while minimizing the risk of abuse to society. Some states limit the number of pills that can be dispensed in a single prescription or closely scrutinize physicians who prescribe these drugs. Addiction risks, for both psychological and physical dependencies, mean that narcotics are not a path of treatment that we want to stay on for long, if we venture onto it at all.

Rehabilitation Interventions

At this time, there is no single curative treatment for chronic pain. For individuals whose chronic pain significantly interferes with mood, functioning, and participation in activities, rehabilitation is recommended. The most commonly accepted and empirically supported approach in the chronic pain literature is interdisciplinary and based on a biopsychosocial model of chronic pain. Interventions grounded in this model address the pathophysiologic processes as well as the psychological, social, and behavioral factors that have been associated with pain, distress, and pain-related disability. Treatment goals typically involve modifying affective, behavioral, cognitive, and sensory symptoms associated with the person's disability and suffering and, ultimately, increasing the functioning of the person with pain. Treatment goals may be met by participating in any of several rehabilitation therapies, including, but not limited to, physical therapy, occupational therapy, vocational rehabilitation, and psychotherapy. For example, if a person is identified as using maladaptive coping strategies to deal with pain, such as catastrophizing (thinking negatively), he or she might participate in psychotherapy (group or individual) aimed at decreasing negative thoughts about pain and increasing reassuring, positive thoughts.

Considerable evidence supports the efficacy of interdisciplinary pain programs in improving psychological and physical functioning when pain is the primary disability,[95] although the efficacy of such programs for persons with amputation-related pain is not known, nor is it known how often amputees participate in such rehabilitation programs. We suspect that they commonly participate in only physical therapy. For some, this may be sufficient. However, for those who are suffering and/or very disabled by their amputation-related pain, more comprehensive assessments and treat-

ment approaches are recommended. Unfortunately, amputation patients often do not have access to such multidisciplinary services.

Summary

Pain following amputation remains a frequent and very bothersome issue for many individuals with limb loss. Phantom pain, phantom sensation, residual limb pain, back pain, neck pain, and general musculoskeletal overuse pain all occur. Pain also has many different characteristics, qualities, and patterns and can present in various ways. Measuring and treating pain is by no means straightforward or routinely successful. Great strides have been made over the last decades in our understanding of the different types and sources of pain. We have also advanced in our ability to define and measure different types of pain. Nonetheless, there is still much work to be done. We simply cannot at this time eliminate or even minimize all types of pain. The scientific and medical communities realize that many individuals suffer from chronic pain, and we continue to seek new treatments to improve the quality of life for anyone who has pain.

The American Pain Foundation publishes the following *Pain Care Bill of Rights*.[96] These are notable goals for all who treat pain to review and strive to achieve. This is what our patients hope for and expect from health care professionals.

As a person with pain, you have the right to:

• have your report of pain taken seriously and to be treated with dignity and respect by doctors, nurses, pharmacists, and other healthcare professionals.

• have your pain thoroughly assessed and promptly treated.

• be informed by your healthcare provider about what may be causing your pain, possible treatments, and the benefits, risks, and costs of each.

• participate actively in decisions about how to manage your pain.

• have your pain reassessed regularly and your treatment adjusted if your pain has not been eased.

• be referred to a pain specialist if your pain persists.

• get clear and prompt answers to your questions, take time to make decisions, and refuse a particular type of treatment if you choose.

References

1. Merskey H, Bogduk N (eds): International Association for the Study of Pain Task Force on Taxonomy, in *Classification of Chronic Pain*. Seattle, WA, IASP Press, 1994, pp 209-214.

2. Dworkin RH: Which individuals with acute pain are most likely to develop a chronic pain syndrome? *Pain Forum* 1997;6:127-136.

3. Bonica JJ: *The Management of Pain*, ed 2. Philadelphia, PA, Lea & Febiger, 1990.

4. Turk DC, Melzack R (eds): *Handbook of Pain Assessment*, ed 2. New York, NY, Guilford Press, 2001, p 760.

5. Ehde DM, Jensen MP, Engel JM, Turner JA, Hoffman AJ, Cardenas DD: Chronic pain secondary to disability: A review. *Clin J Pain* 2003;19:3-17.

6. Engel GL: The need for a new medical model: A challenge for biomedicine. *Science* 1977;196:129-136.

7. Melzack R, Wall PD: Pain mechanisms: A new theory. *Science* 1965;150: 971-997.

8. Melzack R, Wall PD: *The Challenge of Pain*. New York, NY, Basic Books, 1982.

9. Abdi S, Lee DH, Chung JM: The antiallodynic effects of amitriptyline, gabapentin, and lidocaine in a rat model of neuropathic pain. *Anesth Analg* 1998;87:1360-1366.

10. Fordyce WE: *Behavioral Methods for Chronic Pain and Illness*. St. Louis, MO, Mosby-Year Book, 1976.

11. Jensen MP, et al: Coping with chronic pain: A critical review of the literature. *Pain* 1991;47:249-283.

12. Jensen MP, et al: Patient beliefs predict patient functioning: Further support for a cognitive-behavioural model of chronic pain. *Pain* 1999;81:95-104.

13. Jensen MP, et al: Relationship of pain-specific beliefs to chronic pain adjustment. *Pain* 1994;57:301-309.

14. Boothby JL, et al: Coping with pain, in Gatchel RJ, Turk DC (eds): *Psychosocial Factors in Pain*. New York, NY, The Guilford Press, 1999, pp 343-359.

15. Gatchel RJ, Turk DC, Dennis C (eds): *Psychological Approaches to Pain Management: A Practitioner's Handbook*. New York, NY, The Guilford Press, 1996, p 519.

16. Loeser JD: What is chronic pain? *Theor Med* 1991;12:213-225.

17. Fordyce WE: Pain and suffering: A reappraisal. *Am Psychol* 1988;43: 276-283.

18. Melzack R: Phantom limbs and the concept of a neuromatrix. *Trends Neurosci* 1990;13:88-92.

19. Sherman RA: *Phantom Pain*. New York, NY, Plenum Press, 1997, p 264.

20. Gatchel RJ, Turk DC: *Psychosocial Factors in Pain: Critical Perspectives*. New York, NY, The Guilford Press, 1999, p 510.

21. Novy DM, et al: Perspectives of chronic pain: An evaluative comparison of restrictive and comprehensive models. *Psychol Bull* 1995;118:238-247.

22. Melzack R: Phantom limbs. *Sci Am* 1992;266:120-126.

23. Davis RW: Phantom sensation, phantom pain, and stump pain. *Arch Phys Med Rehabil* 1993;74:79-91.

24. Jensen T, Rasmussen P: Phantom pain and other phenomena after amputation, in Wall P, Melzack R (eds): *The Textbook of Pain*. London, England, Churchill Livingstone, 1994.

25. Loeser JD: Pain after amputation: Phantom limb and stump pain, in Bonica J (ed): *The Management of Pain*. London, England, Churchill Livingstone, 1994, pp 224-256.

26. Jensen TS, et al: Phantom limb, phantom pain and stump pain in amputees during the first 6 months following limb amputation. *Pain* 1983;17: 243-256.

27. Jensen TS, et al: Non-painful phantom limb phenomena in amputees: Incidence, clinical characteristics and temporal course. *Acta Neurol Scand* 1984; 70:407-414.

28. Smith DG, et al: Phantom limb, residual limb, and back pain after lower extremity amputations. *Clin Orthop* 1999;361:29-38.

29. Ehde DM, Czerniecki JM, Smith DG: Chronic phantom sensations, phantom pain, residual limb pain, and other regional pain after lower limb amputation. *Arch Phys Med Rehabil* 2000;81:1039-1044.

30. Kooijman CM, Dijkstra PU, Geertzen JH, Elzinga A, van der Schans CP: Phantom pain and phantom sensations in upper limb amputees: An epidemiological study. *Pain* 2000;87: 33-41.

31. Dijkstra PU, et al: Phantom pain and risk factors: A multivariate analysis. *J Pain Symptom Manage* 2002;24: 578-585.

32. Jensen TS, et al: Immediate and long-term phantom limb pain in amputees: Incidence, clinical characteristics and relationship to pre-amputation limb pain. *Pain* 1985;21:267-278.

33. Sherman RA, Sherman CJ, Parker L: Chronic phantom and stump pain among American veterans: Results of a survey. *Pain* 1984;18:83-95.

34. Wartan SW, et al: Phantom pain and sensation among British veteran amputees. *Br J Anaesth* 1997;78:652-659.

35. Gallagher P, Allen D, Maclachlan M: Phantom limb pain and residual limb pain following lower limb amputation: A descriptive analysis. *Disabil Rehabil* 2001;23:522-530.

36. Houghton AD, et al: Phantom pain: natural history and association with rehabilitation. *Ann R Coll Surg Engl* 1994;76:22-25.

37. Ehde DM, Smith DG, Czerniecki JM, et al: *Chronic Pain and Pain-related Disability Following Lower Limb Amputation*. Phoenix, AZ, American Pain Society, 2001.

38. Nikolajsen L, et al: Randomised trial of epidural bupivacaine and morphine in prevention of stump and phantom pain in lower-limb amputation. *Lancet* 1997;350:1353-1357.

39. Whyte AS, Niven CA: Variation in phantom limb pain: Results of a diary study. *J Pain Symptom Manage* 2001; 22:947-953.

40. Fraser CM, et al: Characterising phantom limb phenomena in upper limb amputees. *Prosthet Orthot Int* 2001;25: 235-242.

41. Postone N: Phantom limb pain: A review. *Int J Psychiatry Med* 1987;17: 57-70.

42. Nystrom B, Hagbarth KE: Microelectrode recordings from transected

nerves in amputees with phantom limb pain. *Neurosci Lett* 1981;27: 211-216.

43. Howe JF: Phantom limb pain: A re-afferentation syndrome. *Pain* 1983;15: 101-107.

44. Mackenzie N: Phantom limb pain during spinal anaesthesia: Recurrence in amputees. *Anaesthesia* 1983;38: 886-887.

45. Nikolajsen L, Jensen TS: Phantom limb pain. *Br J Anaesth* 2001;87: 107-116.

46. Pezzin LE, Dillingham TR, MacKenzie EJ: Rehabilitation and the long-term outcomes of persons with trauma-related amputations. *Arch Phys Med Rehabil* 2000;81:292-300.

47. Czerniecki JM, Ehde DM: Pain after lower extremity amputation. *Crit Rev Phys Med Rehabil* 2003;15:309-332.

48. Ehde DM, et al: Back pain as a secondary disability in persons with lower limb amputations. *Arch Phys Med Rehabil* 2001;82:731-734.

49. Hagberg K, Brånemark R: Consequences of non-vascular trans-femoral amputation: A survey of quality of life, prosthetic use and problems. *Prosthet Orthot Int* 2001;25:186-194.

50. Andersson GBJ, et al: Epidemiology and cost, in Pope MH, et al (eds): *Occupational Low Back Pain: Assessment, Treatment, and Prevention*. St. Louis, MO, Mosby-Year Book, 1991, pp 95-113.

51. Jensen MP, et al: Pain site and the effects of amputation pain: Further clarification of the meaning of mild, moderate, and severe pain. *Pain* 2001;91: 317-322.

52. Polatin PB, et al: Psychiatric illness and chronic low-back pain: The mind and the spine--which goes first? *Spine* 1993;18:66-71.

53. Whyte AS, Carroll LJ: A preliminary examination of the relationship between employment, pain and disability in an amputee population. *Disabil Rehabil* 2002;24:462-470.

54. Millstein S, Bain D, Hunter GA: A review of employment patterns of industrial amputees: Factors influencing rehabilitation. *Prosthet Orthot Int* 1985;9:69-78.

55. Sheikh K: Return to work following limb injuries. *J Soc Occup Med* 1985; 35:114-117.

56. Marshall M, Helmes E, Deathe AB: A comparison of psychosocial functioning and personality in amputee and chronic pain populations. *Clin J Pain* 1992;8:351-357.

57. Bergner M, et al: The Sickness Impact Profile: Conceptual formulation and methodology for the development of a health status measure. *Int J Health Serv* 1976;6:393-415.

58. Bergner M, et al: The Sickness Impact Profile: Validation of a health status measure. *Med Care* 1976;14:57-67.

59. Von Korff M, et al: Grading the severity of chronic pain. *Pain* 1992;50: 133-149.

60. Weiss SA, Lindell B: Phantom limb pain and etiology of amputation in unilateral lower extremity amputees. *J Pain Symptom Manage* 1996;11:3-17.

61. Hill A: The use of pain coping strategies by patients with phantom limb pain. *Pain* 1993;55:347-353.

62. Hill A, Niven CA, Knussen C: The role of coping in adjustment to phantom limb pain. *Pain* 1995;62:79-86.

63. Jensen MP, Ehde DM, Hoffman AJ, Patterson DR, Czerniecki JM, Robinson LR: Cognitions, coping and social environment predict adjustment to phantom limb pain. *Pain* 2002;95: 133-142.

64. Sullivan MJ, et al: Theoretical perspectives on the relation between catastrophizing and pain. *Clin J Pain* 2001;17: 52-64.

65. Wesolowski JA, Lema MJ: Phantom limb pain. *Reg Anesth* 1993;18: 121-127.

66. Katz J: Children do experience phantom limb pain. *Reg Anesth* 1997;22: 291-293.

67. Krane EJ, Heller LB: The prevalence of phantom sensation and pain in pediatric amputees. *J Pain Symptom Manage* 1995;10:21-29.

68. Smith J, Thompson JM: Phantom limb pain and chemotherapy in pediatric amputees. *Mayo Clin Proc* 1995;70: 357-364.

69. Wilkins KL, et al: Phantom limb sensations and phantom limb pain in child and adolescent amputees. *Pain* 1998;78:7-12.

70. Lee RY, Turner-Smith A: The influence of the length of lower-limb prosthesis on spinal kinematics. *Arch Phys Med Rehabil* 2003;84:1357-1362.

71. Legro MW, et al: Prosthesis evaluation questionnaire for persons with lower limb amputations: Assessing prosthesis-related quality of life. *Arch Phys Med Rehabil* 1998;79:931-938.

72. Gallagher P, Maclachlan M: Development and psychometric evaluation of the Trinity Amputation and Prosthesis Experience Scales (TAPES). *Rehabil Psychol* 2000;45:130-155.

73. Korff MV, et al: Grading the severity of chronic pain. *Pain* 1992;50:133-149.

74. Cleeland CS, Ryan KM: Pain assessment: Global use of the Brief Pain Inventory. *Ann Acad Med Singapore* 1994;23:129-138.

75. American Psychiatric Association: *Diagnostic and Statistical Manual of Mental Disorders*, ed 4. Washington, DC, American Psychiatric Association, 1994.

76. Robinson ME, Riley JL III: The role of emotion in pain, in Gatchel RJ, Turk DC (eds): *Psychosocial Factors in Pain*. New York, NY, The Guilford Press, 1999, pp 74-88.

77. Coyne JC, Fechner-Bates S, Schwenk TL: Prevalence, nature, and comorbidity of depressive disorders in primary care. *Gen Hosp Psychiatry* 1994;16: 267-276.

78. Rybarczyk B, et al: Limb amputation, in Frank R, et al (eds): *Handbook of Rehabilitation Psychology*. Washington, DC, American Psychological Association, 2000, pp 29-47.

79. Mulrow CD, et al: Case-finding instruments for depression in primary care settings. *Ann Intern Med* 1995;122: 913-921.

80. Kroenke K, Spitzer RL, Williams JB: The PHQ-9: Validity of a brief depression severity measure. *J Gen Intern Med* 2001;16:606-613.

81. Spitzer RL, Kroenke K, Williams JB: Validation and utility of a self-report version of PRIME-MD: The PHQ primary care study. Primary care evaluation of mental disorders: Patient health questionnaire. *JAMA* 1999;282: 1737-1744.

82. Katon W: The impact of major depression on chronic medical illness. *Gen Hosp Psychiatry* 1996;18:215-219.

83. Huse E, et al: The effect of opioids on phantom limb pain and cortical reorganization. *Pain* 2001;90:47-55.

84. Leskowitz ED: Phantom limb pain treated with therapeutic touch: A case report. *Arch Phys Med Rehabil* 2000;81: 522-524.

85. Rasmussen KG, Rummans TA: Electroconvulsive therapy for phantom limb pain. *Pain* 2000;85:297-299.

86. Finsen V, et al: Transcutaneous electrical nerve stimulation after major amputation. *J Bone Joint Surg Br* 1988;70: 109-112.

87. Robinson LR, Czierniecki JM, Ehde DM: Trial of amitriptyline for relief of pain in amputees: Results of a randomized controlled study. *Arch Phys Med Rehabil* 2004;85:1-6.

88. Bach S, Noreng MF, Tj'ellden NU: Phantom limb pain in amputees during the first 12 months following limb amputation, after preoperative lumbar epidural blockade. *Pain* 1988;33: 297-301.

89. Jahangiri M, et al: Prevention of phantom pain after major lower limb amputation by epidural infusion of diamorphine, clonidine and bupivacaine. *Ann R Surg Engl* 1994;76: 324-326.

90. Lambert AW, et al: Randomized prospective study comparing preoperative epidural intraoperative perineural analgesia for the prevention of postoperative stump and phantom limb pain following major amputation. *Reg Anesth Pain Med* 2001;26:316-321.

91. Sherman RA, Sherman CJ, Parker L: Chronic phantom and stump pain among American veterans: Results of a survey. *Pain* 1984;18:83-95.

92. Sherman RA, Sherman CJ: Prevalence and characteristics of chronic phantom limb pain among American veterans: Results of a trial survey. *Am J Phys Med* 1983;62:227-238.

93. Onghena P, Van Houdenhove B: Antidepressant-induced analgesia in chronic non-malignant pain: A meta-analysis of 39 placebo-controlled studies. *Pain* 1992;49:205-219.

94. McQuay HJ, Tramer M, Nye BA, Carroll D, Wiffen PJ, Moore RA: A systematic review of antidepressants in neuropathic pain. *Pain* 1996;68: 217-227.

95. Turk DC: Okifugi, Akiko: Treatment of chronic pain patients: Clinical outcomes, cost-effectiveness, and cost-benefits of multidisciplinary pain centers. *Phys Rehabil Med* 1998;10: 181-208.

96. American Pain Foundation: *Pain Action Guide*. Baltimore, MD, American Pain Foundation, 2001.

Chapter 57

Psychological Adaptation to Amputation

John C. Racy, MD

Introduction

Amputation represents a triple loss. It involves loss of function, loss of sensation, and loss of body image. That so many patients adapt so well is attributable to their resilience and the ingenuity and dedication of those who care for them. The experiences of many such people, including the eight members of a Tucson-area self-help group and patients at the University of Arizona College of Medicine, have been incorporated into this chapter (D Atkins, personal communication, 1984; S Kohl, personal communication, 1984).

Determinants of Psychological Response

The psychological response to amputation is determined by many variables, which can be categorized as either psychosocial or medical. These variables reflect the premorbid health and the medical and surgical management of the amputee.

Psychosocial Variables
Age

In general, the greatest challenges for the young amputee are those relating to identity, sexuality, and social acceptance. For the elderly, the greatest challenges relate to livelihood, functional capacity, and relationships.[1-5] Infants with a congenital limb defi-

ciency adapt well, learning to use their remaining faculties in a compensatory manner. Children also adapt well to the loss of function, and they manipulate prostheses with great dexterity. They are, however, particularly sensitive to peer acceptance and rejection.[3,6] Amputation in preadolescents or adolescents complicates issues of emerging sexual identity.[7] For example, a 13-year-old member of the Tucson self-help group interviewed for this report, when told that an amputation was necessary to treat the osteogenic sarcoma in her leg, reacted with the statement, "No boy is going to look at me."

In a sensitive review of amputation in teenagers, Lasoff[8] addressed two areas that may lead to resistance to care: autonomy and modesty. Lasoff recommended that resistance to care be mitigated by allowing the teenager to make as many decisions as possible. Modesty is best protected by sensitivity of the health care team to the patient's feelings when inspecting and examining the body. Among young adults, the response to limb loss depends largely on its causes and the extent of disability and disfigurement. Because young adults enjoy the advantages of an established identity, physical resilience, and social confidence, these individuals tend to adapt well to amputation.

Among the elderly, ill health, social isolation (especially after the death of

a spouse), financial constraints, and occupational limitations may all complicate adjustment to the loss of the limb. The correlation between age and the long-term emotional consequences of amputation remains controversial. Several early studies suggested that elderly amputees were at greater risk for psychiatric disturbances, such as depression, than were younger patients. More recent studies, however, report just the opposite.[9]

Personality Style

Individuals who are narcissistically invested in their physical appearance and strength tend to react negatively to the loss of the limb. They see it as a major assault upon their dignity and self-worth. Conversely, dependent individuals may cherish the role of patient and find in it welcome relief from pressure and responsibility.

Those with a history of depression are more susceptible to dysphoria following amputation.[4] The loss of a limb serves to crystallize notions of a basic defect, sometimes expressed in self-punishing behaviors.[10]

Portions of this chapter have been adapted with permission from Racy JC: Psychological aspects of amputation, in Moore WS, Malone JM (eds): *Lower Extremity Amputation.* Philadelphia, PA, WB Saunders, 1989.

Timid and self-conscious individuals who are excessively concerned about their social standing are more likely to suffer psychologically from limb loss than are self-assured individuals.[11,12] Individuals tending toward a pessimistic or paranoid outlook are likely to feel that their worst expectations have been confirmed, and their rehabilitation may be colored by much bitterness and resentment. Kolb and Brodie[13] reported that a rigid personality style may be associated with a greater risk of postoperative complications, including phantom pain, but a more recent literature review by Sherman and associates[14] did not reveal any relationship between such a personality and phantom pain.

Unexpected reactions may arise from secondary gain. If disability results in improved financial or social status, psychological adjustment may be easier. If the amputation brings about the resolution of a conscious or unconscious psychological conflict, the individual may indeed be happy that it occurred.

Coping Strategies

Coping strategies can take several forms and are a vital component of the adjustment to amputation. Livneh and associates[15] suggested four basic categories: (1) active problem-solving, including seeking support, reframing the event, and planning; (2) emotion-focusing, such as social withdrawal, wishful thinking, or self-blame; (3) problem disengagement, such as turning to alcohol or drugs or to religion; and (4) cognitive disengagement, or denial. As expected, active problem-solving appears to be the most effective strategy. The other strategies mentioned (emotion-focusing, problem disengagement, and cognitive disengagement) are more likely to be associated with depression, anxiety, and internalized and externalized hostility, and they therefore lead to an overall poorer level of adjustment and acceptance. Sociodemographic factors (eg, age, marital status) and disability-related factors

(eg, site of amputation, time since amputation) influence coping to a lesser extent.[15]

In a study of 104 lower limb amputees, Gallagher and MacLachlan[16] found a similar correlation between the discovery of a positive meaning in the amputation and facile adjustment. Specifically, they described the positive effect of "making favorable social comparisons [ie, comparing oneself to those less fortunate], reevaluating the event as positive, redefining the amputation in one's life, finding side benefits, and imagining worse situations or forgetting negative aspects of their situation."

Economic and Vocational Variables

Individuals who earn their living from motor skills that are lost with the amputation are especially vulnerable to adverse reactions. Those who have a wide range of skills or whose main line of work is not particularly dependent on the function of the lost limb may experience less emotional difficulty. Of course, no amputee is completely insulated from discriminatory practices, subtle or otherwise, in the workplace, despite their prohibition by federal law. Unemployment is associated with a greater degree of psychological stress and may be a predictor of phantom pain.[17]

Psychosocial Support

All human beings require a support system throughout life to maintain emotional health. However, not all are so blessed, and many find themselves in a transient or permanent state of isolation. Single, widowed, and isolated individuals suffer more psychological distress and difficulty in adapting to amputation than do those who are married or are actively connected to family or friends. Particularly helpful in the adjustment of the adult amputee is the presence of a supportive partner who assumes a flexible approach, takes over functions when needed, cuts back when the amputee is able to manage, and at all times supports the amputee's self-esteem.[18,19]

Parents are the major source of support for children and adolescent amputees.[7,20] One study by Tebbi and associates[21] emphasized the importance of a supportive hospital staff for the adolescent undergoing amputation. But peer acceptance beyond the family and hospital staff is critical in the successful adaptation of all amputees, especially children and adolescents. The effect of traumatic amputation on the person's family is worth noting. In a sensitive case report, White[22] described the development of "hidden post-traumatic stress disorder" in the mother of a child who lost both upper limbs secondary to electrical injury. This affected her care of the child and her relationship to the rest of the family.

Medical Variables
Health

Healthy young individuals who lose a limb traumatically have many advantages over older, frail individuals. Most amputees are elderly, in whom the surgery usually occurs after a prolonged period of treatment for peripheral vascular disease.[3,4,23] These patients often have at least two other comorbid medical disorders. These disorders are likely to limit restoration of function and the return to an active lifestyle.

Mental health problems can easily arise through a complicated series of psychosomatic and somatopsychic responses to the loss. Shukla and associates[24] studied 72 amputees prospectively in India and found that nearly two thirds manifested postoperative psychiatric symptoms, the most common of which was depression, followed by anxiety, crying spells, insomnia, loss of appetite, and suicidal ideation. In this regard, depression—with its attendant loss of energy, pessimism, and psychomotor retardation—may delay rehabilitation, a delay that in turn exerts a depressing effect on the individual. Furthermore, anger often underlies the depressive reaction. In a study of 46 amputees seen in London, Parkes[11] found that among the 38 amputees who were thought to have some overall limitation of function attributable to psychological origin, factors inculpated, in order of frequency, were depression, timidity, fear of further self-injury, self-consciousness, low intelligence, senility, anger, resentment of the need to rely on others, and secondary gain.

Reason for the Amputation

Much of the earlier work on amputation in the 20th century centered on wartime casualties.[2,13,25] The current situation in the United States is quite different in that amputations affect a much older age group and follow either accidents or chronic illness rather than combat. The situation in which the injury to the limb is sustained during combat and leads to evacuation, honorable discharge from the service, and return to civilian life is not often seen today.[2] Adults who sustain a traumatic or accidental limb loss tend to react with varying forms of denial and bravado.[3,26] They are also more likely to experience symptoms of posttraumatic stress disorder.[27] Those who undergo an elective amputation for the cure of a malignancy benefit from the availability of time for preparation and exploration of alternatives. Not surprisingly, amputation appears easier to accept when the affected body part is the site of a malignant lesion or is a source of substantial pain or hindrance to normal functioning.[28] The reaction is usually one of realistic acceptance and cooperation with the treatment team.[3,29] Such individuals seem to make an excellent adjustment, assuming of course that the malignancy has been cured and the pain has been relieved.

For the elderly, surgery usually occurs after a long period of suffering resulting from diabetes mellitus and peripheral vascular disease. Most accept the surgery with relief because it often signals the end of suffering and the return to improved functioning. Some react indifferently or negatively and view the surgery as proof of failure.[3,29] Amputation necessitated by

the negligent or malicious behavior of others is likely to produce persistent feelings of resentment and self-doubt.[13] Litigation can easily complicate the process of psychological rehabilitation and recovery.

Preparation for the Amputation

Individuals who have had adequate time to prepare for an amputation fare better in the immediate postoperative period than those who do not receive such preparation. Individuals who are unprepared tend to react negatively or with massive denial. It is not certain whether these differences persist, given that adaptation is ultimately governed by many other variables preceding and following the amputation.[30-32]

In general, the greater the loss, the greater the difficulty in adjustment to the amputation.[12] There are, however, instances of massive psychological reaction to small physical losses such as the loss of a toe or a thumb as well as minimal reaction to the loss of several limbs.[33] Transhumeral amputation brings with it great anxiety and frustration, and bilateral transhumeral amputation is perhaps the most difficult situation of all. In contrast, amputation of one leg below the knee allows relatively good adjustment, with restoration of both function and body image.[12] In a study comparing amputation and limb salvage in the treatment of extremity sarcoma, there were surprisingly no significant differences in psychological response and functioning between the two groups.[34]

Surgical Complications

Individuals with postoperative pain or infection or who require residual limb revision tend to develop despair and withdrawal to a greater degree than those who do not.[11] This observation highlights the importance of surgical skill in the performance of

the amputation. As Bradway and associates[30] noted, "A poorly performed amputation almost guarantees poor rehabilitation. Although a well-performed amputation does not guarantee a successful rehabilitation outcome, it certainly makes successful rehabilitation more possible."

Prosthetic Rehabilitation

The earlier a prosthesis is applied after amputation, the less the psychological distress observed. Conversely, if application of the prosthesis is delayed or a prosthesis is not provided at all, greater degrees of anxiety, sadness, and self-consciousness are noted. The crucial elements appear to be the integration of the prosthesis into the body image and the concentration of attention on future function rather than on past loss.[5,30]

Extremes of age are by no means absolute contraindications for prostheses. Among the elderly, however, preexisting illness may compound the difficulties of adjusting to such devices. Elderly amputees with chronic obstructive pulmonary disease, for example, will already have compromised strength and endurance. Nonetheless, they deserve a trial period of rehabilitation with a prosthesis, albeit under close supervision.[35]

The Team Approach

Adaptation to amputation is a multifaceted and evolving process requiring different kinds of attention at each stage. Thus, the team approach has emerged as the standard approach to rehabilitation.[3,18,28,30,36-41]

Having a wide range of skills and approaches represented on the rehabilitation team increases the probability that all aspects of rehabilitation will be addressed and none overlooked. The team may include members of the amputee's family as well as amputees who have been successfully treated. Self-help groups for amputees are extensions of the team approach.[42,43]

Vocational Rehabilitation

Restoration of the capability for gainful employment is an integral part of successful rehabilitation. Kohl[18] notes that amputees may regard unemployment as a "denial of their 'right' to participate in the family's decision-making processes" and says that "the success of rehabilitation efforts should not only be measured by return to income-producing work, but rather the return to the person of his decision-making abilities to choose the lifestyle that would be most fulfilling to him."

Stages of Adaptation

The psychological reactions to amputation are clearly diverse, ranging from severe disability at one extreme to a determined and effective resumption of a full and active life at the other.[44] In general, the process of adaptation can be viewed as occurring in four stages: the preoperative stage, the immediate postoperative stage, in-hospital rehabilitation, and at-home rehabilitation.[18,30,34,45-48] With the exception of the clearly demarcated preoperative and postoperative stages, most adjustment occurs along a gradual continuum. A division into four stages, however, allows for the highlighting of issues that arise most critically at each point in time.

Preoperative Stage

In amputees who have ample opportunity to be prepared for surgery, approximately one third to one half welcome the amputation as a signal that suffering will be relieved and a new phase of adjustment can begin. Along with this acceptance, there may be varying degrees of anxiety and concern. Such concerns fall into two main groups. Perhaps for most persons, the more important issues are practical ones such as the loss of function, loss of income, pain, difficulty in adapting to a prosthesis, cost of ongoing treatment, and disposal of the limb. The second group of concerns are more symbolic, such as changes in appearance, losses in sexual intimacy, and perception by others. Most individuals informed of the need for amputation go through the early stages of a grief reaction, which may not be completed until well after their discharge from the hospital. Dise-Lewis[10] suggests that the death and dying paradigm may be applied to the impending loss of a body part, a loss that may threaten the amputee's core identity. One young patient, for example, found significant relief of preoperative anxiety by writing a farewell letter to her leg, much like addressing the loss of a loved one.[28]

The manner in which the surgery is presented by the surgeon can have much bearing on the magnitude and kind of affective response. Mendelson and associates[40] recommended that the surgeon paint a realistic picture of the immediate and long-term goals for the patient and the family. Labeling the amputation as a reconstructive prelude to an improved life is much different from implying that it is a mutilation and a failure. Furthermore, a hopeful attitude, a detailed explanation of all aspects of the surgery and the rehabilitative process, and a full response to all questions (especially those that seem trivial) appear to diminish anxiety, anger, and despair.

Several members of the self-help group interviewed for this report eloquently described the consequences of failed communication. One who regarded her impending amputation as "losing a member of my family" felt scared "out of my wits" and was repeatedly "horrified." She reported that her surgeon had described her as his "failure" and told her very little about the details of the surgery and the process beyond. Another, when informed that she would lose her leg, reacted with the thought, "They might as well take off my head."

A useful part of preoperative preparation is talking with an age-matched amputee. One physician told of an adolescent girl who spoke with a boy of similar age who had previously undergone the same procedure. He stated, "The boy told her about his experience and took off his prosthesis to show her how it worked. She, thereafter was much more amenable to the operation and to rehabilitation; she saw that she was not alone in having to face the specific problem."[28]

Group members who received adequate preparation before the surgery indicated that the preparation contributed to their peace of mind after the event. The process of acceptance, however, required time and effort. One member of the group described her reaction as one of ambivalence and oscillation. She switched repeatedly from acknowledging that the amputation was expected and even desirable, to having feelings of great fear and dread. "Like a ghost in my closet," she said, "I took it out now and then to scare myself with it."

Immediate Postoperative Stage

The period between the surgery and the start of rehabilitation may last a matter of hours or days, depending, among other things, on the reason for the amputation, the extent and condition of the residual limb, and the kind of rehabilitation thought to be feasible. Psychological reactions noted in this phase are concerns about safety, fear of complications and pain, and, in some instances, loss of alertness and orientation.[31] In general, patients who undergo an amputation after a period of preparation react more positively than those who sustain it suddenly, after assault or accident. Most individuals are, to a certain degree, numb, partly as a result of the anesthesia and partly as a way of handling the trauma of loss. For those who have suffered considerable pain before the surgery, the amputation may bring much-needed relief. This was true for four of the eight members of the self-help group interviewed for this report.

In-Hospital Rehabilitation

In-hospital rehabilitation, in many ways, is the most critical phase and presents the greatest challenges to the patient, the family, and the rehabilitation team. It calls for a flexible approach addressed to the rapidly evolving needs of the individual. Initially, the patient is concerned about safety, pain, and disfigurement. Later, the emphasis shifts to social reintegration and vocational adjustment.[3,18] In this phase, some individuals experience and express various kinds of denial shown through bravado and competitiveness. A few resort to humor and minimization. They might make wisecracks such as, "You see more when you walk slowly." Mild euphoric states may be reflected in increased motor activity, racing through the corridors in wheelchairs, and talking excessively.[26]

Eventually, sadness sets in. The grief response to limb loss is probably universal and time limited.[4,44,49] Parkes[29] describes the response as similar to that seen in widows. He lists four phases: (1) "numbness," in which outside stimuli are shut out or denied, (2) "pining" for what is lost, (3) disorganization, in which all hope of recovering the lost part is given up, and (4) reorganization. The degree and rate at which individuals go through these four phases varies from individual to individual, and indeed, the process often lasts well beyond the period of in-hospital rehabilitation. During this time, some patients experience phantom limb sensations and phantom pain, which are discussed later.

Depression of varying severity has been shown to affect approximately 40% of amputees.[12] Schubert and associates[50] observed a decrease in depression during in-patient hospital rehabilitation and attribute the decrease to "diminishing life crises effects, increased functional ability, general psychotherapeutic milieu effects, and nonspecific effects." A decrease in depression was correlated significantly with an increase in functional ability, suggesting that increasing functional ability may be one of the most important factors in postamputation rehabilitation with regard to depression.

Factors that facilitate adjustment and rehabilitation in this phase are early prosthetic fitting, acceptance of the amputation and the prosthesis by family and friends, and introduction of a successfully rehabilitated amputee to the recovering patient.[3,18,31,39,40,45,51] Almost all the members of the group interviewed for this report agreed that early prosthetic introduction was of the highest importance. Two women who sustained transtibial amputations reported that awakening to find that they had two "legs" in bed was most reassuring. The 13-year-old girl delighted in throwing back the bedclothes and flaunting her artificial leg to her adolescent visitors. Those who did not, for one reason or another, obtain a prosthesis looked forward to it and often fantasized about it. One young man who lost his arm at the high transhumeral level as a result of an electrical injury dreamed of becoming a "bionic man."

Sadness, although keenly felt, may be concealed. A young mother who lost her hand in a paper shredder tried to put on a happy face for her family. "Sometimes," she said, "we have to joke so that people around us can deal with it."

At-Home Rehabilitation

The amputee's return home can be a particularly taxing period because of loss of the familiar surroundings of the hospital, and attenuation of the guidance and support provided by the rehabilitation team. Thus the attitude of the family becomes a major determinant of the amputee's adaptation. Family members should be involved in all phases of the rehabilitative process.[11,40]

During this phase, the full impact of the loss becomes evident. Some individuals experience a "second realization," with attendant sadness and grief.[52] Varying degrees of regressive behavior may be evident, such as a reluctance to give up the role of being a patient, a tendency to lean on others beyond what is justified by the disability, and a retreat to "baby talk."[53] Some resent any pressure put upon them to resume normal functioning. Others may go to the other extreme and vehemently reject any suggestion that they might be disabled or require help in any way. An excessive show of sympathy generally fosters the notion that one is to be pitied. In this phase, three areas of concern come to the fore: return to gainful employment, social acceptance, and sexual adjustment. Of immense value in all of these matters is the availability of a relative or a significant other who can provide support without damaging self-esteem.[31,32]

The mother of the young man who lost his arm as the result of an electrical injury spoke of the profound change that occurred in his behavior on his return home. He regressed to the point that she felt that she "had another baby in the house." The young mother who lost her hand in the paper shredder was concerned that people would look at her as though she were a "freak." She found her anxiety greatly relieved when both her children and their schoolmates took her amputation in stride and asked about it matter-of-factly. A middle-aged woman who underwent an amputation after a prolonged period of disability resulting from poliomyelitis found herself one day facing a sink full of dishes and a request from her husband that she wash them. She did so with tears running down her face and thoughts running through her mind of her husband as cruel and mean. Later, she recognized that it was "the best thing that he could have done for me" and was rather amused to learn that the scenario was contrived by her surgeon and her husband to encourage her independence. Equally helpful to her was her children's startled response on learning that their mother was receiving disability benefits. To them, she did not seem to be disabled at all and therefore did not need benefits. In fact, they were interested in the prosthesis and expressed the wish that perhaps they too could don and remove their limbs when they grew up.

The group members were unanimous in rejecting the "handicapped" label, and each thought that his or her affliction was lighter than those of the others. One of them said, "Most well-adjusted people prefer to accept what happened to them" and thus "would not trade with another amputee." All conceded that the adaptation would have been immensely more difficult without the active support of their families.

A subtle, but often overlooked, issue is the ease with which the disability can be concealed in social settings. One group member, for example, remarked that one advantage of a leg amputation over an upper limb loss was that it could escape detection in such settings.

Not surprisingly, amputees able to resume a full and productive life tend to fare best; this is much easier for those with marketable skills who sustain the amputation while still in vigorous health. For elderly amputees who have limited skills, particularly if they have other medical disorders, the probability of a full return to an active life is considerably diminished. Acceptance of a new, more leisurely way of living with reduced responsibility and pressure to be productive can partially or fully balance the loss of function in older amputees.[31]

Special Areas of Concern
Phantom Limb Sensations

The feeling that the amputated limb is present and moving is so common as to be regarded as a universal occurrence after surgery.[13,17,30,54] Phantom limb sensations tend to abate rapidly, however, so only a few individuals continue to perceive their limbs as still present and active 1 year after surgery. Many amputees, however, continue to have occasional experiences of itching or movement, sometimes after residual limb stimulation. Though rare, phantom limb sensation has been reported in both children and adults with congenital limb deficiencies and in those who sustain the limb loss at a very early age.[55-57] In general, phantom limb sensations present no particular problem. All members of the self-help group had experienced them at one time or another. Even 10 or 15 years after amputation, some of them still experienced an intermittent itch that, curiously, was relieved by scratching the prosthesis.

Phantom Limb Pain

Pain experienced in the missing limb is a much more serious issue than phantom limb sensations. At the University of Arizona, persistent phantom limb pain has been reported by fewer than 2% of amputees.[5]

Early work on phantom pain led to the assumption that antecedent and concurrent medical states as well as psychological factors combined to explain its existence. In the series of 2,284 amputees studied by Ewalt and associates[25] at the end of World War II, phantom limb pain was extremely rare and was noted in individuals who also showed psychopathology. These investigators wrote that pain "tended to come and to go with psychopathological symptoms, irrespective of what type of external treatment was carried on."

Parkes[17] found that phantom limb pain could be predicted by certain immediate postoperative phenomena such as the presence of residual limb pain, prior illness of more than 1 year duration, the development of residual limb complications, and, interestingly, other factors not related to surgery, such as continued unemployment and a rigid personality. Some amputees experience phantom limb pain in association with micturition, climatic changes, and emotionally disturbing events.[13]

Sherman and associates[58,59] argue that most amputees experience phantom limb pain to varying degrees and that it is probably a complex form of referred pain with a physiologic rather than a psychological etiology. Pinzur[54] regards phantom limb pain as a variant of sympathetic dystrophy. Preamputation pain has been shown to increase the incidence of phantom limb pain and residual limb pain.[60] There is general agreement that phantom limb pain and life stresses are related. In a study of 24 male amputees, Arena and associates[53] observed an isomorphic pain-stress relationship, namely, a roughly contemporaneous increase in phantom limb pain with increased stress and vice versa. The typical psychological profile of the amputee suffering phantom limb pain does not differ from that of the general population of chronic pain sufferers.[14] Thus, phantom limb pain, which can be serious and disabling, remains incompletely understood, but approaches the model of a chronic pain syndrome with evidence of physiologic and psychological components.

In the self-help group, only one member reported persistent phantom limb pain accompanied by residual limb pain. He underwent long and complicated procedures after the initial amputation, all designed to relieve his phantom pain. These included nerve stimulation, acupuncture, residual limb revision, and even spinal block. At the time of the interview, his only relief came from the use of oxycodone on a regular basis. So distressed was he by his pain that he had repeatedly entertained the fantasy of taking a gun and shooting his "leg" off to rid himself of it. Other members experienced fleeting episodes of pain described as a sensation like an electric shock or, as one put it, "like putting your finger in a 220 [volt] outlet." A few described cramping sensations and feelings of constriction that diminished over time. Two mentioned aching when the weather changed and rain was approaching. Several members of the group spontaneously volunteered the view that the support of the family members was of great help in reducing phantom pain when it occurred.

Body Image

Amputation requires a revision of body image. Dreams and the draw-a-person test can indicate perceptions about body image. Amputees who adapt well draw a person with a foreshortened limb or without any limb at all; those who adapt poorly draw the missing limb larger than the opposite limb or with increased markings.[33] Similarly, dreams that incorporate the prosthesis or do not particularly dwell on the missing part are consistent with a more positive adaptation. In one prospective study of 67 patients who had suffered severe hand trauma, much of the dreaming included nightmares of further injury or incapacity.[61] However, the frequency of such nightmares decreased significantly about 1 month postoperatively. It has been suggested that the amputee, in a sense, must contend with three body images: intact, amputated, and with prosthesis. Individuals who are unable to accept the last two are likely to reject the prosthesis and to experience difficulty in functional and social adjustments. Related to the issue of revised body image is concern with social appearances and acceptance by others. Even when considerable success is achieved in functional restoration, there often remains some shyness about revealing the amputated body to others. Social discomfort related to the amputation has been associated with the development of depression.[62]

The members of the group confirmed these observations and saw a connection between accepting one's new bodily configuration and accepting a prosthesis. One viewed her body more positively after amputation because her prosthetic leg worked better than the leg that she had lost. Most had come to regard their prosthesis as part of themselves, at times revealed in dreams. Nonetheless, despite their successful adaptation and ac-

ceptance of the new body image, all of them continued to experience self-consciousness in social situations. For example, they tended to walk more clumsily when they felt observed by other people in public. Members of the group described a pool party hosted by them to which they had invited their friends and relatives. However, the only people who actually went into the pool were the non-amputees.

Sexuality

Sexuality is an area of some anxiety for most amputees, especially those who are young.[7,10,18,63] Concern arises from the following sources: (1) fear that the body will not be accepted by the partner, (2) self-consciousness, (3) the loss of a functioning body part such as the hand, and (4) the loss of an area of sensation.

A prosthesis can provide functional restoration and some return to normal appearance in most situations, but it is absolutely of no use in the terms of sexuality. A comparison with the sexual experience of paraplegics is instructive. Those who suffer paralysis often enjoy preserved sensation in the affected part and continue to see their body as intact. They may also entertain hope of a return of function in the affected part. The amputee enjoys none of these advantages.

A recent study of lower limb amputees showed that even though most patients experienced difficulties in the areas of sexual arousal, sexual behavior, and orgasm, more than 90% reported a high interest in sex.[64] The investigators could not attribute the disparity between sexual activity and sexual interest to anxiety or depression.

With the many concerns and challenges facing the amputee, the rehabilitation team must be careful not to overlook sexual issues. Successful resumption of sexual activity may require the learning and practice of new sexual behaviors.[65] The members of the self-help group agreed that sexuality was an important issue that had

to be faced by each of them. Most reported success in facing it, mainly because of the supportive response of the partner. Yet, despite verbal and behavioral reassurance of the partner, several patients spoke of lingering difficulty in seeing themselves as adequate sexual partners rather than as repulsive sexual "freaks." As one group member put it, "There is still a small part that doesn't accept." The passage of time appears to aid in this adjustment. One member stated that 15 years after the event, her missing limb was "a nonissue" in the sexual sense. This was not the case for the 13-year-old girl who had expressed the concern that no boy would ever look at her. She lived for 2 years after the surgery but did not have occasion to go out on a date. She maintained the hope that one day she would do so and was greatly comforted by her brother-in-law, who told her that her amputation would "weed out the creeps."

Management of the Amputee

Based on research and the personal experiences of amputees reported here, several conclusions can be drawn regarding effective approaches to the management of the amputee. The self-help group referred to in this chapter agreed unanimously with the following management approaches. The strategies fall roughly into six areas: preparation, surgical technique, early prosthetic fitting and mobilization, the team approach, vocational and activity rehabilitation, and special approaches such as group support and psychotherapy.

Preparation

Although it is hard to prove statistically that preparation has a bearing on ultimate outcome,[30,31] common sense, clinical observation, and the reports of amputees all suggest that proper preparation is highly desirable.[4,18,32,39,40] Ferrari and associates[28] have found it beneficial to broach the subject of amputation with children no more than 2 to 3 days before the surgery because they feel that discussing the procedure too far in advance "can cause anguish and be intolerable to people so young." Preparation must include a clear explanation of the reasons for the amputation, the viable alternatives, if any, the exact surgical procedure, and the postoperative rehabilitative processes. Anticipating and dealing with the various issues that patients will face, even if these are not raised by the patients themselves, is of great help. Such issues include disposal of the limb, relationship with friends and family, degree of loss and return of function, work capability, costs of surgery and rehabilitation, sexual adjustment, and social impact. Among patients in whom disease is the reason for the amputation, many fear a relapse or a worsening of the course of the disease. This feeling of ever-present dread is called the sword of Damocles syndrome because the missing limb is a constant reminder of the disease.[28]

The amputation should be presented as a desirable lifesaving or life-improving option, rather than as a last resort or an indication of failure. Indeed, the patient's quality of life is sometimes better after an amputation than with limb-sparing treatments.[37,66] The term reconstructive surgery is preferable to amputation and these terms can both be used to describe the procedure.

Much of the preoperative preparation should be conducted by the operating surgeon. Although the information is widely available and may be imparted by any member of the team, no other person can communicate with the degree of authority and confidence needed by patients as they contemplate the imminent loss.

Surgical Technique

Obviously, good surgical technique is of the essence. Perhaps less obvious is the need for the senior surgeon to perform the surgery or to be involved intimately in its performance. It is an error to relegate this procedure to inexperienced hands. As Bradway and associates[30] indicate, "In our program, the senior surgical attending physician is directly involved in the performance of all amputations and supervises the entire process of amputation rehabilitation."

Early Prosthetic Fitting and Mobilization

There is little doubt that the earlier the prosthesis is applied, the better the results are in terms of functional capacity and psychological adaptation.[5,31] As Bradway and associates[30] describe, "Early prosthetic fitting and rehabilitation enable the patient to incorporate all of his physical and emotional efforts into recovery from the earliest possible moment, rather than allowing the patient to focus only on disabilities and pain." Introducing the patient to a successfully rehabilitated amputee may be of great assistance in this effort.[52] Of paramount importance to patients, and perhaps a predictor of prosthetic use, is the comfort and usefulness of the device.[67] The level of the amputation also seems to be a significant determinant in the ultimate use of appliances. Sturup and associates[68] observed a greater rate of prosthetic use among transradial amputees than among transhumeral amputees and a clear tendency toward nonuse of a prosthesis among younger amputees and those with an amputation of the nondominant arm. Durance and O'Shea[67] reported that amputees are least likely to use prostheses during leisure activities.

The Team Approach

A team approach is optimal for the rehabilitation of amputees and should include the surgeon, surgical nurses, prosthetist, physical therapist, occupational therapist, social worker, vocational counselor, and, if indicated, a psychiatrist or psychologist.[3,18,19,30,37,38,40,45] With a team with a variety of skills, each member can address one particular aspect of the patient's needs. As these needs evolve, flexibility and adaptation to new realities are required not only of amputees, but of those who help them. To the extent possible, the involvement of members of the family at all of these stages can be of tremendous help.[40] Perhaps the most valuable contribution of the team approach is the facilitation of a more rapid return to familiar surroundings and to independence. The prospective study by Ham and associates[36] of 223 amputees found that team management reduced hospital stays significantly and increased the long-term effectiveness of rehabilitation. No less important, as Dise-Lewis[10] indicated, is the role of the team in validating the amputee's right to be in control of his or her own rehabilitation and in providing a safe haven for emotional expression.

Vocational and Activity Rehabilitation

No approach to amputation can be considered successful without some resolution of the issue presented by the loss of skills, job, and livelihood. Even in the absence of pressing financial need, the loss of earning capacity may entail a profound loss of self-esteem, which brings with it a variety of adverse psychological phenomena. It is not essential that the person resume work, but it is essential that the person accept whatever new role and capacity can now be enjoyed.[18] This issue should be approached with an open mind. Some amputees prefer returning to employment, with all the security, stimulation, and structure that it presents. Others, thanks to personal wealth or to disability and retirement benefits, may choose not to be employed. As Kohl[18] wrote, "It is important that there be not a judgmental response from the staff toward those patients who do not seek paid employment."

Several investigators have attempted to find predictors of success in the rehabilitation of amputees. Pinzur and associates[45] suggested that psychological testing using standard personality inventories and measures of cognitive abilities may be helpful in deriving a scale of rehabilitation potential for amputees. Kullmann[69] observed that the Barthel index of activities of daily living had a direct correlation with the general condition of the amputee and the fitness of the prosthesis. Based on these results, the Barthel index may have prognostic value for outcome of the rehabilitation of amputees. But as Mendelson and associates[40] reported, any psychological testing should be deferred until the patient is physically and emotionally prepared to withstand the stress of its administration.

Regardless of vocational rehabilitation, resumption and maintenance of normal activities, including household chores, self-care, and social visits, will avert the vicious cycle of depression and disability. In their study of social and psychological factors involved in adjustment to amputation, Williamson and associates[41] observed a direct contribution of restriction of activity to depression.

Special Approaches

Increasingly, group support is part of the help provided to amputees.[3,43,52] One such modality is Schwartz's situation-transition group, which is different from many self-help groups for alcoholics, smokers, and overeaters in that "members are not required to espouse a particular moral or behavioral value system."[3] Whether a trained person leads the group or it is conducted entirely by its own members, the group experience is likely to be of great value to both the participants and their families. Amputee self-help groups shy away from self-pity or self-designation in terms of disability and emphasize strength and participation in a full and healthy life.[69]

Psychotherapy may be indicated for individuals who have difficulty moving through any of the stages described and who are unable to resume a normal existence to the extent possible for them. It is important to understand that the various stages of grief described by Parkes[11,29] and others may not be accomplished in the predictable sequence or within the expected period of time. Some individuals will continue to mourn the loss of a limb for a long time. Others may not deal with the issue immediately, instead returning to it at a much later date and exhibiting a delayed grief reaction. Vivid flashbacks have been reported as a common early reaction to amputation.[4,61] Reclusiveness, hypervigilance, and delusions are other manifestations of disturbances of body image.[4] With the possible exception of the use of low-dose, low-potency neuroleptic agents to extinguish flashbacks, the opportunity to ventilate feelings is probably the most effective therapeutic activity for the amputee and is a crucial phase that should not be aborted. Feelings of sorrow, anger, and anxiety must be expressed before further therapeutic work can be accomplished. Occasionally, family therapy may be indicated to assist in reaching the proper balance between the legitimate support amputees need and the independence they must regain. In addition, psychological problems that have been avoided or disregarded in the past may surface after the surgical procedure and be blamed on the procedure. This might occur in individuals who have had longstanding marital discord, chronic depression, anxiety disorder, drug dependence, alcohol abuse, and/or antisocial behavior.

These psychiatric challenges can be addressed therapeutically, without determining the extent to which they are related to the amputation. If such a determination becomes desirable, such as in complicated legal situations, the individual's history and former level of adjustment can be of great value in clarifying the issue. For most amputees, however, psychiatric consultation and therapy are not required.

With respect to phantom pain, biofeedback and relaxation appear to be useful adjuncts to medical care of the residual limb and measures to control pain. Neither psychotherapy nor psychoactive medicine appears to be effective in treating phantom pain.[59] A knowledge of the psychological aspects of amputation and sensitivity of members of the rehabilitation team, however, are indispensable.

Conclusion

The psychological adaptation to amputation involves many variables and stages. With the help of a skilled rehabilitation team and a support system, the amputee can adapt successfully to the challenge of amputation. Most members of the self-help group noted an improvement in the quality of their lives after surgery. As one member put it, "You become a more compassionate and less critical person towards others." Another, who had suffered greatly both before and after the amputation, said, "When you become an amputee, you become a better person because you have to work for everything."

Acknowledgments

This chapter was written with the assistance of Richard E. D'Alli, MD, and revised for this publication with the able help of Elizabeth Hilton and Pippa Newell, senior students at the University of Arizona College of Medicine.

Many individuals assisted in all aspects of preparing this chapter. I wish in particular to acknowledge my debt of gratitude to John Bradway, MD, who, as a third-year clinical clerk in psychiatry, piqued my interest in this area by preparing a paper on psychological adaptation to amputation, which in turn formed the basis of a report written by him, myself, and several others;[30] to James Malone, MD, for sharing his extensive knowledge and experience; to Joseph Leal, CP, who put me in touch with the amputee self-help group in Tucson; to Sharon Stites, leader and organizer of the self-help group; to Diane Atkins, occupational therapist and coordinator for the Houston Center for Amputee Services, who shared a wealth of experience with hundreds of amputees at that center; to Sybil Kohl, social worker at the Houston Center for Amputee Services, for her profound observations and reflections on the lives of amputees; to Jan Pankey and Sandy Levitt, third-year clinical clerks, who assisted me greatly in my meeting with the self-help group in Tucson; and to the eight members of the group who, although unnamed, were the source of information, guidance, and inspiration to all who study amputation and those who must adapt to it.

References

1. MacBride A, Rogers J, Whylie B, Freeman SJ: Psychosocial factors in the rehabilitation of elderly amputees. *Psychosomatics* 1980;21:258-265.

2. Randall GC, Ewalt JR, Blair H: Psychiatric reaction to amputation. *JAMA* 1945;128:645-652.

3. Whylie B: Social and psychological problems of the adult amputee, in Kostuik JP, Gillespie R (eds): *Amputation Surgery and Rehabilitation: The Toronto Experience.* New York, NY, Churchill Livingstone, 1981, pp 387-393.

4. Frierson RL, Lippmann SB: Psychiatric consultation for acute amputees: Report of a ten-year experience. *Psychosomatics* 1987;28:183-189.

5. Malone JM, Moore WS, Goldstone J, Malone SJ: Therapeutic and economic impact of a modern amputation program. *Ann Surg* 1979;189:798-802.

6. Boyle M, Tebbi CK, Mindell ER, Mettlin CJ: Adolescent adjustment to amputation. *Med Pediatr Oncol* 1982;10:301-312.

7. Tebbi CK, Maloon JC: Long-term psychosocial outcome among cancer amputees in adolescence and early adulthood. *J Psychosoc Oncol* 1987;5:69-82.

8. Lasoff EM: When a teenager faces amputation. *RN* 1985;48:44-45.

9. Frank RG, Kashani JH, Kashani SR, Wonderlich SA, Umlauf RL, Ashkanazi GS: Psychological response to amputation as a function of age and time since amputation. *Br J Psychiatry* 1984;144:493-497.

10. Dise-Lewis JE: Psychological adaptation to limb loss, in Atkins DJ, Meier RH III (eds): *Comprehensive Management of the Upper-Limb Amputee.* New York, NY, Springer-Verlag NY, 1989, pp 165-172.

11. Parkes CM: Determinants of disablement after loss of a limb, in Krueger DW (ed): *Emotional Rehabilitation of Physical Trauma and Disability.* New York, NY, SP Medical & Scientific Books, 1984, pp 105-111.

12. Williams GM: Restrictions of normal activities among older adult amputees: The role of public self-consciousness. *J Clin Geropsych* 1995;1:229-242.

13. Kolb LC, Brodie HKH: *Modern Clinical Psychiatry,* ed 10. Philadelphia, PA, WB Saunders, 1982, pp 574-576.

14. Sherman RA, Sherman CJ, Bruno GM: Psychological factors influencing chronic phantom limb pain: An analysis of the literature. *Pain* 1987;28:285-295.

15. Livneh H, Antonak RF, Gerhardt J: Psychosocial adaptation to amputation: The role of socio-demographic variables, disability-related factors and coping strategies. *Int J Rehabil Res* 1999;22:21-31.

16. Gallagher P, MacLachlan M: Positive meaning in amputation and thoughts about the amputated limb. *Prosthet Orthot Int* 2000;24:196-204.

17. Parkes CM: Factors determining the persistence of phantom pain in the amputee. *J Psychosom Res* 1973;17:97-108.

18. Kohl SJ: The process of psychological adaptation to traumatic limb loss, in Krueger DW (ed): *Emotional Rehabilitation of Physical Trauma and Disability.* New York, NY, SP Medical & Scientific Books, 1984, pp 113-148.

19. Parkes CM: The psychological reaction to loss of a limb: The first year after amputation, in Howells JG (ed): *Modern Perspectives in the Psychiatric Aspects of Surgery.* New York, NY, Brunner-Mazel, 1976, pp 515-532.

20. Tebbi CK, Petrelli AS, Richards ME: Adjustment to amputation among adolescent oncology patients. *Am J Pediatr Hematol Oncol* 1989;11:276-280.

21. Tebbi CK, Stern M, Boyle M, Mettlin CJ, Mindell ER: The role of social support systems in adolescent cancer amputees. *Cancer* 1985;56:965-971.

22. White S: Hidden posttraumatic stress disorder in the mother of a boy with traumatic limb amputation. *J Ped Psychol* 1991;16:103-115.

23. Osterman HM, Pinzur MS: Amputation: Last resort or new beginning? *Geriatr Nurs* 1987;8:246-248.

24. Shukla GD, Sahu SC, Tripathi RP, Gupta DK: A psychiatric study of amputees. *Br J Psychiatry* 1982;141:50-53.

25. Ewalt JR, Randall GC, Morris H: The phantom limb. *Psychosom Med* 1947;9:118-123.

26. Noble D, Price DB, Gilder R Jr: Psychiatric disturbances following amputation. *Am J Psychiatry* 1954;110:609-613.

27. Opalic P, Lesic A: Investigation of psychopathological state of patients depending on specific clinical characteristics of physical trauma. *Panminerva Med* 2002;44:11-17.

28. Ferrari A, Clerici CA, Spreafico F, et al: Psychological support in children and adolescents with cancer when amputation is required. *Med Pediatr Oncol* 2002;38:261-265.

29. Parkes CM: Psycho-social transitions: Comparison between reactions to loss of a limb and loss of a spouse. *Br J Psychiatry* 1975;127:204-210.

30. Bradway JK, Malone JM, Racy J, Leal JM, Poole J: Psychological adaptation to amputation: An overview. *Orthot Prosthet* 1984;38:46-50.

31. Friedmann LW: (ed): *The Psychological Rehabilitation of the Amputee.* Springfield, IL, Charles C Thomas Publishers, 1978, pp 17-23.

32. Kessler HH: Psychological preparation of the amputee. *Indust Med Surg* 1951;20:107-108.

33. Hansen ST Jr: Editorial: The type-IIIC tibial fracture: Salvage or amputation. *J Bone Joint Surg Am* 1987;69:799-800.

34. Weddington WW Jr, Segraves KB, Simon MA: Psychological outcome of extremity sarcoma survivors undergoing amputation or limb salvage. *J Clin Oncol* 1985;3:1393-1399.

35. Sioson ER: The elderly amputee with severe chronic obstructive pulmonary disease: Case reports. *J Am Geriatr Soc* 1990;38:51-52.

36. Ham R, Regan JM, Roberts VC: Evaluation of introducing the team ap-

proach to the care of the amputee: The Dulwich Study. *Prosthet Orthot Int* 1987;11:25-30.

37. Hamilton A: Rehabilitation of the leg amputee in the community. *Practitioner* 1981;225:1487-1497.

38. Marks L: Lower limb amputees: Advantages of the team approach. *Practitioner* 1987;231:1321-1324.

39. May CH, McPhee MC, Pritchard DJ: An amputee visitor program as an adjunct to rehabilitation of the lower limb amputee. *Mayo Clin Proc* 1979;54: 774-778.

40. Mendelson RL, Burech JG, Polack EP, Kappel DA: The psychological impact of traumatic amputations: A team approach: Physician, therapist, and psychologist. *Hand Clin* 1986;2: 577-583.

41. Williamson GM, Schultz R, et al: Social and psychological factors in adjustment to limb amputation. *J Soc Behav Personal* 1994;9:249-268.

42. Hughes J, White WL: Emotional reactions and adjustment of amputees to their injury. *US Naval Med Bull* 1946; 46(suppl):157-163.

43. Lipp MR, Malone ST: Group rehabilitation of vascular surgery patients. *Arch Phys Med Rehabil* 1976;57: 180-183.

44. Letter: Psychology of limb loss. *BMJ* 1989;299:1526-1527.

45. Pinzur MS, Graham G, Osterman H: Psychologic testing in amputation rehabilitation. *Clin Orthop* 1988;229: 236-240.

46. Caine D: Psychological considerations affecting rehabilitation after amputation. *Med J Aust* 1973;2:818-821.

47. Gingras G, Mongeau M, Susset V, Lemieux R, Chevrier JM, Voyer R: Psycho-social and rehabilitative aspects of upper extremity amputees. *Can Med Assoc J* 1956;75:819-823.

48. Hovgaard C, Dalsgaard S, Gebuhr P: The social and economic consequences of failure to replant amputated thumbs. *J Hand Surg [Br]* 1989; 14:307-308.

49. Letter: Psychology of limb loss. *BMJ* 1989;299:1526-1527.

50. Schubert DS, Burns R, Paras W, Sioson E: Decrease of depression during stroke and amputation rehabilitation. *Gen Hosp Psychiatry* 1992;14:135-141.

51. Bowker JH: Amputation rehabilitation: Critical factors in outcome. *J Ark Med Soc* 1981;78:181-183.

52. Kerstein MD: Group rehabilitation for the vascular-disease amputee. *J Am Geriatr Soc* 1980;28:40-41.

53. Arena JG, Sherman RA, Bruno GM, Smith JD: The relationship between situational stress and phantom limb pain: Cross-lagged correlational data from six-month pain logs. *J Psychosom Res* 1990;34:71-77.

54. Pinzur MS: Letter: Phantom pain: A lesson in the necessity for careful clinical research on chronic pain problems. *J Rehabil Res Dev* 1988;25:83.

55. Saadah ES, Melzack R: Phantom limb experiences in congenital limb-deficient adults. *Cortex* 1994;30: 479-485.

56. Vetter RJ, Weinstein S: The history of the phantom in congenitally absent limbs. *Neuropsychologia* 1967;5: 335-338.

57. Poeck K: Phantoms following amputation in early childhood and in congenital absence of limbs. *Cortex* 1964;1: 269-275.

58. Sherman RA, Ernst JL, Barja RH, Bruno GM: Phantom pain: A lesson in the necessity for careful clinical research on chronic pain problems. *J Rehabil Res Dev* 1988;25:vii-x.

59. Sherman RA: Stump and phantom limb pain. *Neurol Clin* 1989;7:249-264.

60. Nikolajsen L, Ilkjaer S, Kroner K, Christensen JH, Jensen TS: The influence of preamputation pain on post-amputation stump and phantom pain. *Pain* 1997;72:393-405.

61. Grunert BK, Smith CJ, Devine CA, et al: Early psychological aspects of severe hand injury. *J Hand Surg [Br]* 1988;13:177-180.

62. Rybarczyk BD, Nyenhuis DL, Nicholas JJ, Schulz R, Alioto RJ, Blair C: Social discomfort and depression in a sample of adults with leg amputations. *Arch Phys Med Rehabil* 1992;73:1169-1173.

63. Reinstein L, Ashley J, Miller KH: Sexual adjustment after lower extremity amputation. *Arch Phys Med Rehabil* 1978;59:501-504.

64. Bodenheimer C, Kerrigan AJ, Garber SL, Monga TN: Sexuality in persons with lower extremity amputations. *Disabil Rehabil* 2000;22:409-415.

65. Shell JA, Miller ME: The cancer amputee and sexuality. *Orthop Nurs* 1999;18: 53-64.

66. Sugarbaker PH, Barofsky I, Rosenberg SA, Gianola FJ: Quality of life assessment of patients in extremity sarcoma clinical trials. *Surgery* 1982;91:17-23.

67. Durance JP, O'Shea BJ: Upper limb amputees: A clinic profile. *Int Disabil Stud* 1988;10:68-72.

68. Sturup J, Thyregod HC, Jensen JS, et al: Traumatic amputation of the upper limb: The use of body-powered prostheses and employment consequences. *Prosthet Orthot Int* 1988;12:50-52.

69. Kullmann L: Evaluation of disability and of results of rehabilitation with use of the Barthel index and Russek's classification. *Int Disabil Stud* 1987;9:68-71.

Chapter 58

The Art of Prosthesis Prescription

John H. Bowker, MD

Introduction

The prescription of a prosthesis no longer involves simply matching a particular level of residual limb with a prosthesis designed for that level. There are so many choices, in fact, that prescription becomes as much an art as a science. This multiplicity of options is the result of a revolution in prosthetic design, manufacture, and fitting made possible by the introduction of new concepts in socket and joint design as well as a wider array of components and new materials, including heat-moldable plastics, lightweight metals, and carbon fiber–reinforced composites.

General Considerations
Contraindications

Before discussing the factors involved in prescribing a prosthesis, a review of the reasons for not prescribing one is useful. If the patient's overall health has deteriorated irrevocably to the point where the strength or coordination required to use a prosthesis is lacking, prescribing one is useless. The patient must have the mental ability to learn the use, limitations, and care of the prosthesis. At the highest levels of amputation in both the upper and lower limbs, the ability of a prosthesis to restore useful function decreases exponentially with progressive loss of limb length. Following

lower limb amputation, energy requirements for ambulation increase sharply with each more proximal anatomic level. These challenges to function are exacerbated by concomitant cardiopulmonary deficits.

Factors Affecting the Prescription

A large number of factors affect the prescription, some of which become apparent only when the parameters of the patient's life are examined. First and foremost, the prosthesis should meet the needs and desires of the patient vocationally, avocationally, and socially as much as possible. Because prostheses vary considerably in complexity and resistance to environmental hazards, the limb-fitting team should determine both the "gadget tolerance" and the ability of the amputee to provide the level of care required for different types of prostheses. If the amputee lives in a geographically remote location without ready access to a prosthetist for maintenance, repair, and replacement of a prosthesis, a simple design that the amputee can repair independently may be of prime importance. Climate can also play an important role. In areas of excessive humidity, steel parts tend to corrode and wood tends to rot. In areas of extreme aridity such as desert regions, fine sand particles will quickly wear out close-tolerance pros-

thetic joints. The cost of a prosthesis, both initial and ongoing, can also be a determining factor in the prescription. Some insurance companies, for example, will provide only one prosthesis for the life of the patient. Fiscal limitations at the local and state levels may mandate prescribing only a very simple prosthesis for indigent amputees, similar to those prescribed for amputees in developing countries. Local custom and knowledge can also affect both socket and component prescription.

Team Approach

The prescription of the most suitable prosthesis, taking into account the above factors, is most effectively accomplished by a team. The team should be both interdisciplinary and interactive, cooperating closely rather than working independently. Although the surgeon cannot be expected to perform the activities of other team members, he or she must be fairly knowledgeable in all areas of prosthetic rehabilitation to effectively coordinate the limb-fitting program. The primary function of the surgeon, aside from providing medical care, is to synthesize the findings and recommendations of the team, which ideally should consist of the patient and the patient's family, the surgeon, a physiatrist who specializes in amputee rehabilitation, the prosthetist who will make the limb, the therapist who will

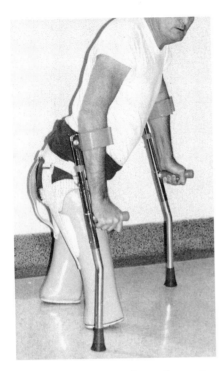

Figure 1 Bilateral transfemoral amputee walking with stubbies, which are nonarticulated sockets with rocker bottoms and pelvic suspension.

provide the training in prosthesis use, a psychologist and/or social worker who will help the patient through the adjustment period, and the insurance nurse, especially in worker's compensation cases. There is a widely held misconception that this sort of team is available only in large medical centers; on the contrary, an effective miniteam can be assembled in most small- to medium-sized cities. It takes only an interested surgeon, a local prosthetist, a therapist, a psychologist/social worker, and an insurance nurse to form a team. Once a surgeon expresses an interest in this type of work, other local surgeons are very likely to refer patients. By meeting once or twice a month at the surgeon's office or other designated location, team members can work more effectively than they can individually with no interchange of ideas. This approach also helps to improve prescription practices and tends to position the participants in leadership roles in this field.

Follow-up

It is obvious that an amputation affects the amputee for life; however, the need for regular preventive care is often forgotten. In addition to frequent follow-up visits immediately after the fitting is performed, amputees also need to be seen at 6- to 12-month intervals for the rest of their lives. Residual limbs change in volume with muscle atrophy and weight gain or loss, and prostheses require maintenance, repair, and periodic replacement. Failure to monitor these factors can result in damage to the residual limb. Prescription modifications may also be indicated as improved designs become available or when the patient's abilities or interests change.

Lower Limb Prosthetic Prescription
Indications

Reasons for fitting a lower limb prosthesis include eliminating the excess energy requirements of crutch walking and improving balance by restoring proprioceptive feedback through the residual limb–prosthesis interface. Equally important, the hands are freed for activities other than holding a walker or crutches. In short, the goal is to restore as much functional independence to the amputee as possible. This varies widely—from returning to all previous activities, including active sports, to the minimum acceptable rehabilitation goal of assisted transfer activities that help the caregiver as much as the amputee. Another considerable benefit is the restoration of the amputee's body image that a prosthesis may provide.

Contraindications

Cogent reasons also exist for *not* fitting lower limb prostheses, especially in dysvascular patients with bilateral transfemoral amputations. Fitting such debilitated amputees with articulated prostheses is rarely successful in the long term. By the time severe

vascular disease has necessitated bilateral transfemoral amputation, it has also affected the heart, brain, and other organs. Attempting to walk with two full-length articulated prostheses could prove hazardous to these patients because of the greatly increased cardiopulmonary stress associated with the loss of both natural knee joints. Younger bilateral traumatic transfemoral amputees are generally able to walk short distances in full-length prostheses with free knees, but they soon discover that using a lightweight wheelchair is not only less tiring but also much faster. Because walking is so physically demanding, for the sake of practicality most bilateral transfemoral amputees use wheelchairs for long distances. A nonambulatory patient may, however, request lightweight cosmetic prostheses, or a pair of pantyhose can be filled with sculpted foam and fitted with shoes to give a pleasing appearance while the patient is seated in a wheelchair.

Factors Affecting the Prescription

A bilateral transfemoral amputee who is interested in walking and can demonstrate sufficient cardiac reserve may be given a trial with "stubbies." These are simple, nonarticulated transfemoral sockets with rocker bottoms and pelvic suspension (Figure 1). Young traumatic bilateral transfemoral amputees will almost always demand a trial of ambulation; they should be encouraged to start with stubbies. After a variable training period during which the amputee can assess the energy required to walk while the team evaluates the amputee's motivation level, balance, and donning skills, the amputee may be able to use articulated limbs. In most cases, it is prudent to add feet and longer pylons to the stubbies before introducing prosthetic knees.

A unilateral dysvascular transfemoral amputee may not be able to muster the cardiopulmonary reserve to manage even household ambulation and will often request a wheelchair. Amputees with hip disarticulations or transpelvic amputations, typically younger trauma or tumor patients, often use a prosthesis for long-term community ambulation. Some patients, however, may find that the slower speed of prosthetic walking is the overriding factor in rejecting prosthesis use on most occasions. Major discomfort while sitting in the prosthesis may also become a factor in rejecting the prosthesis. If external aids are required for prosthesis use, the prosthesis provides little, if any, functional advantage over crutch walking without a prosthesis.

Patients should not be rejected for fitting of unilateral or even bilateral lower limb prostheses solely on the basis of age. Many elderly patients can be successfully fitted at the transtibial, Syme ankle disarticulation, or knee disarticulation level provided that they are physiologically sound and are mentally capable of comprehending the subtleties of sock adjustment necessitated by changes in residual limb volume (Figure 2). In borderline cases, transtibial amputees can be fitted with inexpensive preparatory prostheses to realistically assess their potential for ambulation and to facilitate transfers.

Many younger lower limb amputees, especially those with amputations at the transtibial level, will wish to resume previous sports activities. Should the amputee be interested in participating in any activities based on running, a variety of dynamic-response carbon fiber prostheses are available. Some amputees will benefit from prostheses designed for specific sports, including those made specifically for skiing, swimming, or sprinting. Because of these complexities, effective management is best achieved by a team as described above.

Blindness and hemiplegia are additional factors that may enter into the fitting of lower limb amputees, particularly diabetics. Once properly trained, blind amputees with unilateral or bilateral Syme ankle disarticulations or transtibial amputations

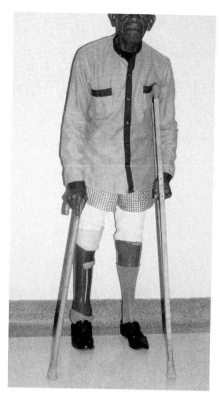

Figure 2 Ninety-year-old man with a right Syme ankle disarticulation and a left transtibial amputation. Like many elderly bilateral amputees with two intact knee joints, he became a successful limited community walker.

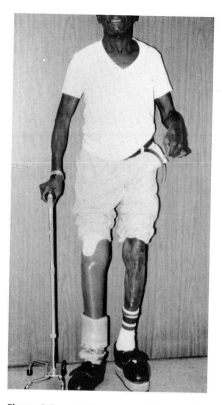

Figure 3 Seventy-three-year-old man with a long right transtibial amputation. As a result of a cerebrovascular accident, he has a left hemiparesis with moderate flexor patterning while walking. The left shoe lift and the right alignment device were removed upon completion of the prosthesis.

should be able to walk without assistance in familiar surroundings, though community ambulation may be safer with a companion. The fitting of blind unilateral transfemoral amputees should be approached with great caution. A free knee is usually contraindicated because of the loss of proprioceptive knee function. Patients with hemiparesis following a cerebrovascular accident can often walk with transtibial prostheses provided that they have adequate mentation and balance and no disruptive spasticity or severe extensor or flexor patterning (Figure 3).

The Amputee Mobility Predictor

Assessing the readiness, both physical and psychological, of an amputee for prosthetic fitting and training can be daunting. Patients, families, and even professional caregivers may have un-

realistic expectations of functional outcome. In addition, the societal and individual costs of inappropriate or unnecessary fittings can be enormous.

To provide some guidelines, Gailey and associates[1] have devised the Amputee Mobility Predictor (AMP) to measure an amputee's ambulatory potential with and without the use of a prosthesis. The evaluation consists of 21 simple task-oriented measurements that can be completed in less than 15 minutes. The resulting score can be reliably linked to the Medicare Functional Classification System for the purpose of prosthetic prescription. Neither the AMP instrument nor Medicare guidelines apply to bilateral amputees, however, whose unique situations require case-by-case review.

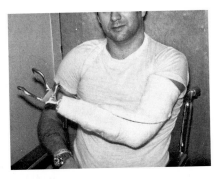

Figure 4 To prevent the development of complete one-handedness, an IPOP should be fitted whenever possible, as in this left transradial amputee.

Effect of Delayed Prescription

Delaying prosthetic fitting and training of the unilateral dysvascular amputee to prevent stress to a compromised remaining foot is not recommended, as this approach will result in months of avoidable deconditioning and tends to accustom the patient to wheelchair use. If the second foot is later amputated, simultaneous fitting as a debilitated bilateral amputee is much less likely to produce useful walking than if the patient had been fitted as soon as possible after the first amputation. The dysvascular amputee who loses one foot should therefore be made ambulatory with a prosthesis as rapidly as possible. If the second foot is lost, the patient will be an accomplished unilateral prosthesis user and will be more likely to learn to walk with two prostheses.

Upper Limb Prosthetic Prescription

The impact of hand loss is very different from the impact of foot loss. Awareness and use of the hands for grasping occur much earlier in infancy than the use of the lower limbs for walking. The hand has greater physical and psychological significance than does the foot. The function and cosmesis of the upper limb are much less completely replaced by a prosthesis than are foot function and cosmesis by a lower limb prosthesis.

Factors Affecting the Prescription

Successful fitting of the upper limb amputee depends largely on the patient's motivation, which is usually highest immediately after amputation. This is especially true in bilateral amputees, where the person is totally dependent on others for most activities of daily living, including dressing, eating, and toileting. It is useful, therefore, to fit bilateral upper limb amputees with immediate postoperative prostheses (IPOPs) whenever possible to provide prehensile tools that will restore significant independence.

The motivation of the unilateral amputee for prosthetic fitting is also highest immediately after amputation. The surgeon should use this window of opportunity to prevent the development of complete one-handedness by fitting an IPOP so that the amputee will awaken from surgery with a device in place to assist the intact hand (Figure 4). Two basic factors regarding these prosthetic fittings should be noted. First, successful fitting of the unilateral upper limb amputee is unlikely after the amputee has become fully functional with one hand, which usually occurs within the first 3 months. Second, prosthetic fitting is at the discretion of the unilateral amputee, although most upper limb amputees who are fitted early find that a prosthesis enhances their function. Early intervention, therefore, can best be provided by a specialized upper limb prosthetic team, which should include a behaviorist to assist the amputee in working through the grieving process.

The first step in prescription of a definitive upper limb prosthesis is determining the amputee's expectations. Because every amputee wants to receive a prosthesis with a hand that looks real, functions like the limb that was lost, is easily maintained, and is low in cost, it is important to provide a detailed explanation of what is realistically available. This discussion should include the basic differences between body-powered and myoelectric limbs, as well as the limits of prosthesis function versus function of an intact upper limb. The complexity of various prostheses must be explained, and the tolerance of the individual amputee for each should be ascertained. The amputee should understand that despite the obvious cosmetic advantages of myoelectric prostheses, they are very costly, they are heavier than most body-powered prostheses, and they require more maintenance. The patient should meet as often as necessary with team members, collectively or individually, to obtain information about the prosthesis and its use. The entire team should then meet again with the patient before actually ordering the prosthesis. With high bilateral amputation, consideration should be given to modifying the amputee's environment as much as possible for more effective function.

Blindness presents particularly difficult problems for the upper limb amputee because the dexterous control of any terminal device is highly dependent on visual feedback. Because of this, a blind bilateral transradial amputee will have great difficulty grasping objects independently with an active terminal device. In this situation, therefore, consideration should be given to a Krukenberg procedure on one or both sides. A blind unilateral upper limb amputee may find a passive prosthesis useful for holding a coat or carrying certain objects.

As with lower limb amputees, many upper limb amputees want to return to the sports and recreational activities in which they previously participated. These individuals have the option of using myoelectrically controlled hands or body-powered terminal devices featuring passive or active prehension. A variety of terminal devices designed for specific sports and recreational activities are available and should be carefully matched to the patient's needs and desires. Individuals who engage frequently in a variety of activities may require several different interchangeable terminal devices appropriate for those activities.

Payment Considerations

Because most upper limb amputations are traumatic and many are job related, third-party payment for prostheses plays an important role in prescription. Some insurers may require all upper limb amputees to be fitted with a lower cost body-powered prosthesis to demonstrate "adequate" motivation before being allowing a higher cost myoelectric limb. This approach does not take into account amputees whose amputation level makes the use of a body-powered prosthesis impractical. Nor does it suit the needs of those for whom cosmesis is an overriding concern, including individuals who meet the public in their daily work. Many of these amputees will refuse to consider any terminal device that does not reasonably resemble a hand. This attitude can be attributed to body image or, in many cultures, to societal acceptance. Therefore, the realistic preferences of the individual amputee with regard to function and cosmesis must be supported strongly by the rehabilitation team during negotiations with the third-party payer.

Another question often raised, especially by third-party payers, is the definition of what constitutes successful use of an upper limb prosthesis and what justifies its replacement over time. Is successful use defined by the number of hours of wear each day? Many amputees wear the prosthesis during working hours and remove it at home for comfort although it has been extremely useful at the workplace. Other amputees wear a myoelectric device at work and switch to a body-powered prosthesis for working in the garden after hours. Conversely, a manual laborer, such as a welder, may use a body-powered prosthesis or a myoelectric gripper at work and switch to a more cosmetic myoelectric hand prosthesis for social functions. Even part-time use of an upper limb prosthesis for specific vocational, avocational, or purely social purposes is a sign of acceptance of the prosthesis, making it worthy of initial provision and replacement as necessary. Some patients who have lost a limb from trauma or tumor at a high level may decide to forgo any prosthesis or to use a very light passive device if it is cosmetically acceptable.

Summary

The prescription of a prosthesis requires matching the needs and preferences of an amputee with the many prosthetic options available within the parameters of available funding. Contraindications to prosthetic fitting in terms of diminished physical or mental capacity must also be recognized. Many amputees may require two different prostheses to reach their full functional potential—for example, one designed for outdoor use and one for limited indoor use. Prosthetic prescription should be accomplished by a well-integrated interdisciplinary team, with the patient and family as active participants.

After the initial intensive effort involved in prescription, fitting, and training has been completed, follow-up should continue throughout the life of the amputee, with at least yearly evaluations by the appropriate lower or upper limb team. Prostheses wear out and sometimes break, and new designs, which might provide advantages to a given ampu-tee, become available. As significant advances in prosthetic research and development occur, a progressive team will keep their amputee clients appropriately informed of potentially useful changes in their prosthesis prescriptions. Recommending a change in a prescription, however, should be made only after thorough discussion of the amputee's individual needs and desires by the entire prosthetic team. As director of the team, the surgeon bears a particular responsibility, especially as prosthetic technology becomes increasingly complex and expensive. Change for its own sake often proves counterproductive, especially in older patients who are satisfied with their original prescription. For example, although a more complex transtibial prosthesis with an elastomeric liner and distal lock may provide improved suspension, many elderly amputees may find it harder to don than a simpler patellar tendon–bearing/supracondylar prosthesis. Patients should therefore be made aware of the possible impact of any change and should never be coerced to discard a previously successful prescription, no matter how outdated it may appear.

Acknowledgment

The author wishes to express thanks to Ms. Patsy Bain for her expert preparation of this manuscript.

Reference

1. Gailey RS, Roach KE, Applegate EB, et al: The Amputee Mobility Predictor: An instrument to assess determinants of the lower-limb amputee's ability to ambulate. *Arch Phys Med Rehabil* 2002;83:613-627.

Chapter 59

Rehabilitation Without Prostheses

Joan E. Edelstein, MA, PT

Introduction

Rehabilitation after amputation is not always synonymous with prosthetic fitting and use. Prosthetic technology does not serve all the needs of every person with limb absence, and even those who do use prostheses generally perform a few activities, such as bathing and donning undergarments, without an appliance. Some, particularly those with very proximal or very distal amputations, may choose to forgo prostheses altogether. Others, despite a trial experience with a prosthesis, may decide not to proceed with definitive fitting. And some people, particularly those with multiple disorders, cannot cope with the physical demands of prostheses. A few do not wear prostheses simply because they are unaware of current components and funding sources.[1]

Nonusers challenge designers to improve the prostheses so that future devices will allow greater function at less physiologic and financial cost. The clinician's responsibility is to guide every patient, regardless of whether or not the person wears a prosthesis, to the highest degree of personal, vocational, and recreational independence possible. This chapter outlines how patients can accomplish a wide range of activities without prostheses. Physicians and prosthetists should understand the function that can be achieved without prostheses in particular amputations. Even if patients do use prostheses, therapists

can incorporate the techniques in rehabilitation to help patients function better, both with and without a prosthesis.

Skills for Patients With Upper Limb Amputations

Many of the adapted clothing items, dressing aids, and utensils described here are available through catalogs such as those listed under Additional Resources at the end of this chapter.

Clothing Selection and Dressing
Unilateral Amputation

Each finger of the remaining hand has virtually independent grasping function.[2] Many garments and modifications suitable for adults with hemiplegia also serve the needs of people with unilateral amputations.[3-7] Adaptations should be as inconspicuous as possible, with accessories such as loops and Velcro tape the same color as the garment. Loosely fitting clothing is more convenient than snug apparel. When buttons are used, larger buttons are preferable because they are easier to manipulate with one hand than are small ones.[8] Alternatively, pressure-sensitive tape can be sewn under buttons to preserve the appearance of a buttoned front while facilitating dressing.[9] Snaps and mag-

netic closures are less cumbersome than buttons. Slippery fabric, rather than knitwear,[10] and front openings, rather than back or side openings, simplify dressing. Step-in skirts and dresses are easier to don than those that must be pulled on overhead, although overhead sweaters and shirts can be managed.[4]

Some people prefer simple dressing aids. A button hook and a zipper pull cord may be handy. To don and remove coats and shirts rapidly, the user can hold a dressing stick, which has a large hook at one end, in the antecubital fossa. The individual inserts the hook into a loop at the collar, retracts the shoulder girdle to create slack in the garment, and lifts the clothing off the torso. Initially, the person may use a mirror to guide the maneuver.

Socks can be donned by using the hand to spread the knitted top of the sock, introducing the foot into the sock, then pulling the sock into place with the teeth.[4] This method, of course, requires good hip joint mobility. Slip-on shoes are easier to manage than lace-ups, although models with Velcro straps are readily available. Some individuals replace regular laces with elastic ones. Many people, however, have no difficulty tying shoelaces with one hand;[11,12] lacing without crossing the ties aids tightening the laces because the end of the lace can be readily fashioned into a slip

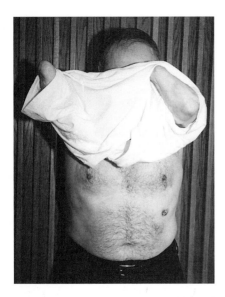

Figure 1 Man with traumatic bilateral transradial amputations dons cotton stockinette tee shirt by using his forearm to stretch the fabric near the hem to create a "pocket," which enables him to slide the shirt over his torso.

knot.[4,6,13] Putting on pants is easiest if they are placed on a bed near a wall. The patient sits on the bed, inserts one leg into a pants leg, and then leans against the wall to hold that side while putting the other leg into the garment.[7]

Managing a brassiere, especially one with a front closure, requires least effort if it is laid out on a bed. The woman lies supine over the garment, slips the amputated limb through one strap, then inserts the contralateral arm through the other strap. Velcro tape is easier to secure than are hooks and eyes.[4] Blouses and shirts are donned by first inserting the residual limb into one sleeve and then the opposite limb into the other. A buttoned cuff should be fastened before donning the shirt; securing the cuff button with elastic thread may be needed to allow room for the hand to slide easily through the cuff. A necktie can be knotted one-handed,[2] particularly if the narrow end of the tie is held to the shirt with a tie clasp. Pretied, clip-on neckties are another option. To don a glove, the individual can press it against the ipsilateral hip. Once the hand is partway into the glove, the amputee can use the back

of a chair to work the fingers into place.[6] A mitten is simpler to manage than a glove. A wristwatch with an expandable bracelet-type band goes on more easily than one with a buckled strap, although the latter can be managed.[14] To put on the bracelet watch, the patient lays the watch on a table and cups the fingers inside the band, then uses the table edge to slide the watch onto the wrist.[6] Adults will find that using a wallet with separate compartments for small and large denomination bills reduces the likelihood of making errors when shopping.[4]

Bilateral Amputation

Patients who have undergone bilateral amputations should be guided to make maximum use of the remaining portions of their limbs to perform daily activities, such as dressing. The antecubital fossae and, to a lesser extent, the axillae can be used to hold items. Objects may also be stabilized in the teeth and between the thighs. Some adults are limber enough to be able to grasp with the feet. A jeweler can resize wedding and other rings so they fit on the toes or can create a brooch from rings.[15]

The child with congenital bilateral limb deficiencies should be encouraged to manipulate with the feet.[16,17] The feet provide tactile sensation and considerable prehensile function, so manipulation with the feet can reduce reliance on adaptive equipment and help from others. The family and patient may require psychological support to overcome an aversion to seeing or using the feet to accomplish ordinary tasks.

Undergarments that can be put on and taken off by the person are especially important to fostering independence in both children and adults (Figure 1). Two tape loops can be sewn to the waistband of underpants. The amputee can then hang the underpants on two wall hooks installed at a height suitable for stepping into the pants. Once the underpants are on the torso, the individual can rise on the forefeet to release the loops.[3]

A single padded hook or wooden knob on the wall can aid dressing. One section of the trousers, skirt, or shirt is secured to the hook while the person maneuvers into the garment.[18] An alternative for donning both underpants and outer pants is to first place them on the floor; then, while seated, to insert the feet into the pants legs; and finally to raise the legs. Shaking the torso and legs causes the pants to slide down the raised legs, toward the waist. When the pants are at the buttocks, the individual uses friction between the floor and pants to work the garment into place. A fabric loop sewn to the waistband allows another means of independently donning trousers.[19] To accomplish this, the person with a transradial amputation slips the forearm through the loop to stabilize the waistband. Alternatively, the individual with a transradial or higher amputation can hold a rod with a hook at one end in the teeth or the antecubital fossa, then slip the hook through the loop.

A child with a phocomelic hand can manage underpants to which a tape has been sewn from the middle of the front waistband to the middle of the back waistband; the tape drapes over the front and continues to the back of the garment.[20] With a reacher, a stick with a hook at one end, the amputee can lower and raise the pants.[3]

Grooming and Hygiene
Unilateral Amputation

Although patients with unilateral amputation should have little difficulty with grooming activities, some prefer the convenience of scrub and denture brushes, nail files, and clippers stabilized with suction cups.[9,16] One could also stabilize a nail file or emery board between the thighs. Filling the cheeks with air to make the skin taut speeds shaving. By bathing at night, the person is ensured of having the skin dry before dressing. Either a wall-hung liquid soap dispenser or a soap bag made from a waffle-weave dishcloth[4] helps the cleaning process. Ridged caps on toiletries are easier to manage than are smooth-sided lids. Similarly, flip-top pill containers are far preferable to childproof bottle tops. Liquid antiseptic in squeeze bottle or spray form takes less effort to apply than coping with an individually wrapped adhesive bandage.

Bilateral Amputation

Individuals with bilateral transradial amputations can use a sponge mitt over one forearm for soaping and scrubbing. Alternatively, a terry cloth or waffle-weave cloth mitt can hold a bar of soap.[21] For cleansing while in the shower, the patient can loop one end of a strip of toweling over the showerhead by maneuvering with both residual limbs. The other end of the strip adheres to the tub floor by means of suction cups or the bather's foot. Most individuals can operate faucets with the feet, particularly if the faucet has a flange rather than a knob handle.[9,22] Similarly, flanged faucet handles at the washbasin are convenient. A terry cloth bathrobe simplifies drying oneself.[21]

Urination and defecation are made easier with the appropriate clothing that can be easily loosened or removed. For men and boys, the trouser zipper may be left partially open, covered by the hem of an overshirt. The individual can urinate independently, particularly if he does not wear undershorts. Defecation is aided if the client wears slacks with suspenders, rather than a belt. He can then pull the trousers down by grasping the pants leg with the toes. Some girls and women find that underpants modified with a split crotch facilitate toilet activity.[23] Undergarments designed for incontinence are another option to augment security.

Some patients regulate their diet so they can defecate at home in the morning or at night. Perineal cleansing can be accomplished by foot and trunk motion. Toilet paper is held in the toes or placed over the heel; the person then rocks over the foot.[9] Others drape paper over the rim of the toilet and straddle the bowl to wipe themselves.[24] A bidet or special toilet

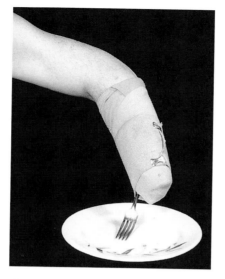

Figure 2 Fork secured to forearm with elastic bandage.

seat equipped with a water spigot and warm airflow is suitable for the home.

A vaginal tampon applicator for women with bilateral amputation[25] as well as other hygienic aids can be constructed easily.[26,27]

The patient with phocomelia can use a reacher stick with a padded hook or wire coil at one end to secure toilet paper.[28] Various grooming aids, such as a comb, hairbrush, and toothbrush, may be attached to a similar stick.

An electric floor model shoe buffer helps amputees take care of their shoes.

Dining
Unilateral Amputation

A commercial fork clip secures the utensil to the plate so that the contralateral hand can cut meat. A snap-on plate guard is useful for beginners because it serves as a stable area they can push food against. The rocker knife facilitates one-handed cutting; one model has prongs so that the user can spear food morsels.[24,29] Alternatively, patients can omit from their diet steak and other large pieces of meat they would have to cut. Techniques for buttering bread and opening a milk carton are easy to learn.[13] Chopsticks are another mode of one-handed dining.

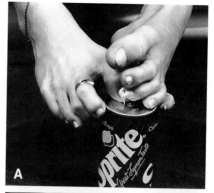

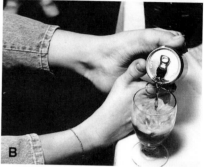

Figure 3 Persons with bilateral upper limb deficiencies or bilateral shoulder disarticulations use the feet for many activities, such as opening a can **(A)** and pouring from a can into a glass **(B)**.

Bilateral Amputation

A utensil holder designed for individuals with quadriplegia can be worn on the forearm of an amputee with at least one transradial-length residual limb. The holder accommodates a spoon, fork, and other objects. A fork or spoon can be strapped or bandaged to the forearm (Figure 2). If the residual limbs are long enough, the person does not need any device to hold eating utensils and can merely stabilize the fork or spoon between the ends of the residual limbs.[30]

Persons with bilateral upper limb deficiencies or bilateral shoulder disarticulations must use the feet for many activities such as opening a can and pouring from a can into a glass (Figure 3). Often, the toes become as dexterous as fingers, and independence in many eating activities can be achieved.

Striking a match (Figure 4) can also be accomplished by the toes. Toe dexterity such as this is achieved only

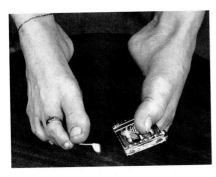

Figure 4 Striking a match can be accomplished by someone born without arms. Toe dexterity is possible only in a person with congenital absence of both arms or a person who has lost both arms at a high level at a very young age.

by those born without arms or those who have lost their arms at a high proximal level at a very young age.

Reading and Communication
Unilateral Amputation

The person with amputation of the right hand will find that writing with the left hand is easier on a table rather than on a right-armed writing desk. The individual should slant the paper in the opposite direction from that used by right-handers to avoid twisting the left arm into a cramped posture. Someone with unilateral amputation can use one-handed touch-typing methods devised for those with cerebral palsy.[31,32] Computer keyboards designed for unimanual use are readily available; they substitute a different letter configuration for the usual QWERTY key arrangement.[33] For telephone dialing, one can place the receiver on the desk. A commercial speaker phone or headband eliminates the need to stabilize the receiver against the shoulder with the head while writing a message. Many consumer phones include a speakerphone option that eliminates entirely the need to use the handset.

Bilateral Amputation

Many special equipment manufacturers offer book holders. The reader turns pages with the bare residual limb or a mouth stick; commercial

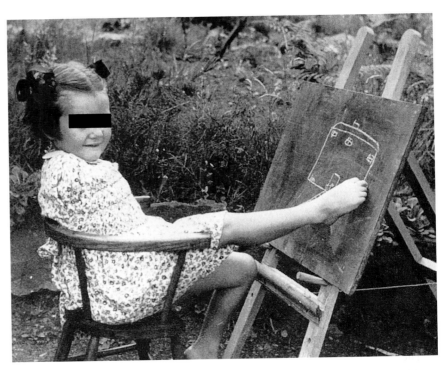

Figure 5 Child holding chalk in her toes to draw on a slate.

page turners are an expensive alternative. To write, the patient can secure the paper in a clipboard or use the transradial residual limb or the chin to nudge the paper into position. Some agile individuals can manage a commercial one-handed writing board that clamps the paper and has rubber feet to prevent the board from slipping on the table. The pen can be held in a forearm cuff, the teeth, or, if one is limber, the toes. The client with bilateral transradial or elbow disarticulation amputations can use both limbs to stabilize a pencil, pen, or crayon for writing and drawing or use the toes[30] (Figure 5). The beginner will find that a felt-tipped marking pen makes writing easier than a ballpoint pen. Touch-tone phones with oversized buttons are widely available and can be dialed easily using the tip of the residual limb or the olecranon.

Homemaking and Other Vocations
Unilateral Amputation

A full range of cooking is possible for the single-handed chef.[4] An apron with a semirigid plastic clip rather than fabric ties can be slipped onto the waist with one hand. A board with stainless steel holding pins secures potatoes and other firm vegetables so that one can peel with the sound hand. One-handed jar openers, beaters, mashers, and choppers, plus electric can openers are sold in most housewares stores.[13] Lightweight bowls and pans are easy to lift single-handed. A mixing bowl can be stabilized by placing it on a rubber mat[13] or setting it into a bowl holder or into a drawer that is closed snugly against the bowl. Eggs can be broken one-handed,[6] and separators can be used to separate whites from yolks.

Some chores such as folding laundry are aided by using the teeth as a holder. Child care tasks can be managed efficiently by using one hand while securing the infant against one's torso with the amputated limb or relying on the crib or other flat surface for stability.[34]

Sewing begins with threading the needle, which can be secured by slipping it into one's shirtsleeve, skirt, or trouser leg, or one can use an automatic needle threader. Left-handed scissors are sold in most needlecraft shops.[35] Embroidery and extensive sewing are less arduous if one uses an embroidery hoop on a floor stand, which frees the hand to wield the needle. A knitting holder clamped to a table facilitates one-handed knitting.

The residual limb makes an effective stabilizer in many carpentry and office tasks.[21] Nails can be set with one hand by holding the nail against the hammerhead and swiftly slamming it against the wood to be nailed.[24] Farm equipment and work-site modifications enable the amputee with unilateral amputation to accomplish most tasks efficiently.[36] Because farming and many other vocational and avocational pursuits involve operating a vehicle, using a spinner knob on the steering wheel should prove helpful.[24]

The adult with an amputation of the right hand can greet a visitor by extending the intact left hand with the forearm fully pronated.[37]

Bilateral Amputation

A reacher stick can help the amputee engage in light household tasks. Those with bilateral transradial amputations may make considerable use of the antecubital fossae for holding packages, which can then be opened with the teeth. The elbow or shoulder can flick a light switch on and off. With practice, even such fine motor tasks as threading a needle can be accomplished with just the residual limbs if they have sufficient length to oppose one another. The dexterity required to accomplish such tasks with the toes, however, develops only in persons with bilateral limb loss that was present at birth or that occurred at a very young age because they can achieve sufficient hip range of motion to bring the feet together at chest and face level and higher (Figure 6).

Sports and Recreation
Unilateral Amputation

One-handed card shuffling requires some dexterity.[38] Otherwise, the amputee can use a bowl or hat to hold the cards; commercial playing-card shufflers are inexpensive alternatives.

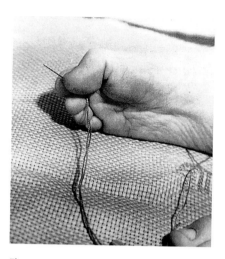

Figure 6 Sewing is accomplished by a bilateral upper limb amputee with toe dexterity. The needle is threaded by inserting the needle into a pincushion or into the fabric to stabilize the needle or by using a metal needle threader.

Simple devices aid the golfer, gardener, carpenter, and fishing enthusiast.[39] For example, a one-handed fishing vest holds the rod so that the user can cast and retrieve. An alternative is a broad waist belt fitted with a pocket to hold the pole. The camera tripod can be modified to support a bow for the archer who has unilateral amputation. Cameras designed for one-handed operation feature a pistol grip, a trigger to snap the shutter, and an automatic focus mechanism. The billiards player can use a mobile bridge to support the cue stick; mounted on two wheels, the bridge has a hole for the stick. Wrist disarticulation did not preclude a career as a major league baseball pitcher for Jim Abbott, who played for the Angels, Yankees, White Sox, and Brewers from 1989 to 1999.[40] Bicycle riding is easier for a cyclist with a transradial amputation if one end of a webbing strap is looped around the residual limb and the other end over the handlebar.[41] Children with transradial amputations can jump rope by securing the rope to the forearm of the residual limb with an animal harness made of webbing.[42] Golf can be played if simple modifications are made to the clubs.[43,44]

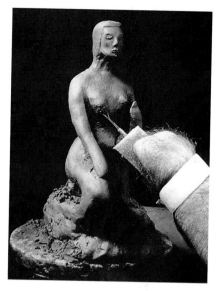

Figure 7 Sculpting tool secured to the forearm with an elastic webbing band.

Bilateral Amputation

Swimming, soccer, and kickball are obvious recreational choices for the child or adult with bilateral arm amputations at any level. A leather mitt riveted to the side of each aluminum ski pole accommodates the skier with transradial amputations. Bilateral longitudinal deficiencies do not preclude playing tennis.[45] One can shoot clay pigeons with a modified shotgun secured to the upper arm by an aluminum ring.[46] For those who enjoy creating sculptures, sculpting tools can be strapped to the forearm (Figure 7).

Music

Sometimes simple modifications or variations from customary performance practice can allow patients to play musical instruments.[47] Singing is a form of musical expression that needs no special equipment or technique.

Unilateral Amputation

The musician with transradial amputation can support a trumpet on the amputation limb, with an adapted neck strap, or on a custom-made stand. Although valves are designed for the right hand, they can be depressed with the left.

The French horn is particularly suitable for those with amputation. Conventional performance assumes valve control with the left hand; thus the player with right transradial amputation places the bare amputation limb in the bell. A cupped cardboard or plastic fixture mounted in the bell facilitates pitch regulation. A person with left amputation can play in reverse, although balancing the horn will be somewhat cumbersome. If the player develops a serious interest, an instrument with tubing coiled in reverse can be manufactured. Instrumentalists with left amputation can manage the larger brass instruments such as the tuba by supporting the instrument on the lap or on a commercial chair-stand and working the valves with the right hand.

Numerous ways of striking drums, xylophones, and other percussion instruments make them accessible to virtually all persons with amputation. The musician with transradial amputation holds the mallet or stick in the intact hand and has the other mallet secured to a snugly fitting leather cuff on the forearm. A double-headed drumstick enables the bass drummer to play while marching. Tambourines and bells are ideal for the person who can hold the instrument in the sound hand.

The player with transradial amputation can strum a guitar with a pick secured in a forearm cuff. Some musicians with transcarpal amputation who retain wrist motion hold the pick in the wrist. Those with left amputation reverse the strings and bridge and, for the steel-stringed guitar, the pick guard also. Commercial left-handed guitars are another option. The conventional guitar strap helps support the instrument, as does the footrest ordinarily used on the right side. The banjo and ukulele can be played in a similar manner.

One-handed performance on the piano and other keyboard instruments can feature music chosen from a large literature ranging from elementary to virtuoso pieces. Electronic keyboard instruments are another option for unimanual playing.

Bilateral Amputation

The musician with bilateral transradial amputation can sit and support the bell of a trumpet on the leg; either or both amputation limbs push the valves, depending on the desired note. The bugle can be held by a neck strap or floor stand; because it has no valves, pitch is determined solely by the musician's mouth. Assembling the instrument is accomplished by asking a friend to assist, or the player can use the broad, resilient surfaces of the transradially amputated limbs to stabilize the brass segments.

Borrowing from the one-man-band tradition, people with bilateral amputation can wear a rigid neck support for the harmonica to facilitate playing by moving the mouth along the instrument rather than the usual method of moving the instrument along the mouth. One or a pair of leather cuffs worn by a percussionist with bilateral transradial amputations enables playing the triangle, chimes, and gong suspended from a stand. Shaken instruments such as maracas can be secured with the cuffs, particularly if the handle is covered with friction tape to increase stability in the cuff. A snugly fitting sandal modified to hold a plastic pick enables one to play stringed instruments with the foot. Some guitarists are able to simply strum with the pick held in the toes.[48]

The piano and other keyboard instruments are accessible to children with phocomelia who play by sitting on a low stool so that they can extend their small limbs to reach the keys with bare fingers.

Skills for Patients With Lower Limb Amputations

The functional problems that attend lower limb amputation differ from those associated with loss of an upper limb. The person with a unilateral upper limb amputation who does not wear a prosthesis can accomplish daily and vocational activities rather easily, often without using assistive devices. Basic skills are, however, much more daunting for the person with bilateral upper limb amputations. In contrast, the person with unilateral or bilateral amputation of the lower limbs who does not wear prostheses is likely to have much more difficulty with certain tasks, especially ambulation, than those who use prostheses.

Clothing Selection and Dressing
Unilateral Amputation

The person who intends to ambulate with crutches should select a low-heeled shoe for the sound foot. Laces or a strap that fastens high on the dorsum of the foot will prevent the shoe from slipping off the foot when the leg swings forward.

Bathing
Unilateral and Bilateral Amputation

A bath chair with a plastic seat and rubber-tipped legs contributes to safety in the shower or bath. Some models have an extension that fits over the edge of the tub to aid transfer. Strategically placed wall-mounted bars increase safety during transfers. Waterproof shower prostheses are seldom ordered. Narang and associates[49] found that nearly all the adults they surveyed with lower limb amputations sat on the shower floor to bathe. The few who stood or used a stool, predominantly those with bilateral amputations, relied on grab bars to assist balance.

Ambulation
Unilateral Amputation

The person who does not wear a prosthesis may be able to manage with a pair of axillary or forearm crutches. Some individuals in good physical condition, with particular regard to the upper limbs, heart, and lungs, walk smoothly and efficiently for long distances with crutches. Young adults with hip disarticulation or transpelvic amputations sometimes opt for crutches because they can ambulate faster than with a prosthesis. For those who rely on a wheelchair, crutch walking may facilitate maneuvering in small or crowded rooms. Occasional use of crutches counteracts the negative consequences of prolonged sitting, such as the formation of contractures and pressure sores.

Crutches must be the proper length. The handpiece should be set at a point that permits the user's elbow to be slightly flexed. A resilient rubber or plastic foam handpiece cover reduces the risk of the hand slipping, especially if it is damp with perspiration. Alternatively, some individuals prefer to wear gloves to increase control of the crutches. The axillary piece, that is, the top bar of the axillary crutch, should be two finger widths from the axilla to avoid compression of the superficially located radial nerve. A resilient cover increases the friction of the axillary piece, which should be kept next to the chest. For both styles of crutch, the tip should be a large suction one to increase traction on the floor.

For good posture, the crutches must be kept parallel to the trunk to minimize pressure on the chest. The body should progress forward in a continuous manner. The walker moves the residual limb in the opposite direction from the contralateral leg, rather than maintaining the residual limb flexed, to create a rhythmic, swinging gait.[50]

Walking with crutches without a prosthesis is physiologically stressful and associated with markedly elevated heart rates for those with amputations, whether because of vascular disease or trauma. Heart rates are elevated to an average of 130 beats/minute among crutch users, comparable to the stress that jogging imposes on able-bodied persons.[51] Consequently, for most individuals, crutches should be considered only for traveling short distances.[52]

Forearm crutches are more compact than axillary crutches. Among subjects with transfemoral amputation, the use of forearm crutches resulted in a freely selected speed that was 15% to 40% slower than that chosen by able-bodied persons; energy cost per unit distance ranged from 48% to 70% greater than that for able-bodied persons. When the same subjects were tested with their prostheses, walking speed was 12% to 33% slower than able-bodied control subjects, at a metabolic cost 30% to 40% greater than normal.[52-54] A walker is a more stable alternative to a pair of forearm crutches.

Those whose balance is poor or whose arms are not strong require the added support of axillary crutches, rather than forearm crutches. Subjects with transfemoral amputations consumed approximately the same amount of energy whether walking with axillary crutches or with a prosthesis, although the pulse rate averaged 39% higher with the crutches.[52,55] Using a single axillary crutch often promotes a significant shift of body weight toward the crutch and exposes the walker to the risk of impinging axillary vessels and nerves.

Ascending stairs with one leg and a pair of crutches is somewhat less intimidating than descending, particularly if the aids are forearm crutches. One can increase safety by keeping the crutch tips close to the edge of the step with the crutches inclined toward the top of the stairs. Young adults consumed 49% more energy ascending stairs with axillary crutches than did able-bodied control subjects.[52] Those with transtibial amputations performed less efficiently with crutches than they did with prostheses. Crutch use was associated with greater energy cost and slower speed; subjects had to lead with the intact leg and then raise the crutches. With the prosthesis, they could climb step over step.[56] Young adults with transtibial amputation were 48% less efficient with crutches but only 29% less efficient with prostheses than were able-bodied adults.[57]

Hopping is another means that unilateral amputees who are in good physical condition use to move over relatively short distances. Even those who use a prosthesis may hop to get to the swimming pool from the locker room. The individual should endeavor to land lightly with a springy step on each hop to prevent spraining or fracturing the foot. The trunk should incline slightly forward, and the foot should be lifted from the ground as short a distance as possible.

To traverse very brief distances, the person may prefer to pivot on the foot, alternating between the heel and forefoot. The maneuver is less stressful than hopping.[50]

To operate an automobile, the driver with a right amputation should have a car equipped with a hand parking brake on the console between the driver's and passenger's seats. The motorist depresses the accelerator and brake pedal with the intact left foot. Another option is to have the car modified so that the accelerator is located to the left of the brake pedal.

Bilateral Amputation

Most people with bilateral lower limb amputation require a wheelchair for long-distance mobility, often as the primary mode of transport. The chair should have its rear wheels set back to compensate for the posterior shift of the user's center of gravity. While swing-out footrests are appropriate for those who wear cosmetic or functional prostheses, people who do not wear any prostheses can transfer to and from the chair more easily if there are no footrests (Figure 8). A reclining wheelchair relieves the discomfort of prolonged sitting.[58] An overhead trapeze bar facilitates moving from the bed to the wheelchair, particularly when elbow extensors are not strong enough to lift the body weight with the usual push-up maneuver. For other transfers, a wooden or plastic sliding board may be used. It bridges the gap between the wheelchair and the transfer goal, such as the bed. With the board in place, the individual can shift weight from one

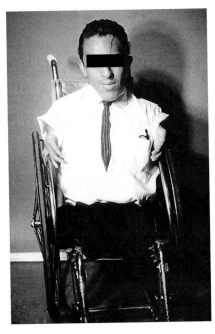

Figure 8 This adolescent with quadrimembral congenital limb deficiencies propels his wheelchair using the push rims repositioned medial to the tires. Note also the absence of footrests.

buttock to the other in a diagonal manner to maneuver from one surface to the next. Another option is a series of sturdy boxes of graduated height leading from the floor to the wheelchair seat. The person shifts from one box to the next with support by the buttocks and hands.[59,60]

Some who can tolerate weight bearing through the ends of the amputation limbs, such as a person with bilateral Syme or knee disarticulations, can walk either unassisted or with the support of short canes or crutches. Others may find a cart[26] or low platform on casters suitable for scooting about the home, with the hands used for propulsion.[59] Such a vehicle can be used in areas too narrow for a wheelchair to pass.

In an emergency, the person can negotiate stairs by sitting on the top stair, then lowering the trunk. Descent is controlled with the hands, which are placed on the tread or banister. Climbing stairs in this fashion is more difficult but is fortunately less likely to be required in emergency situations.

The automobile should be equipped with hand controls for safe operation. The controls, however, should augment rather than replace conventional foot controls so that other family members or a mechanic can drive the car.

Sports and Recreation

Numerous adaptations in equipment and technique enable many individuals with unilateral and bilateral leg amputations to engage in a wide variety of sports and other pastimes.[43]

Unilateral Amputation

Many people with amputations choose to swim and scuba dive without a prosthesis, but all swimmers must have a means of moving from the dressing room to the water's edge, such as by hopping or using crutches. Swimming provides superb recreation as well as good exercise.[58] Agile patients can play several sports while balancing on crutches, for example, kickball and soccer. Other sports that do not require the use of a prosthesis include mountain climbing, skiing, and sky diving.[39,61,62] Hiking over hilly terrain can be accomplished with the aid of a pair of long poles, enabling the climber to swing through the poles. Three-track skiing involves using a single ski under the intact lower limb and a pair of ski poles fitted with rudders distally. Skydiving requires the use of a sturdy harness securing the torso.

Bilateral Amputation

Swimming is popular with some people having bilateral amputation who use their upper limbs as the power source. The water enthusiast can obtain a wet suit or swim fins to fit the residual limbs. A plastic wheelchair is ideal for beach use. Many activities popular with people with paralysis also suit individuals with leg amputation who use a wheelchair. The seated individual can enjoy tennis, badminton, basketball, bowling, hockey,[58] and dancing. Other athletes play while sitting on the floor. Additional recreational pursuits suited to those with

bilateral leg amputation include horseback riding, motorcycling, skateboard stunts, and weight lifting. For example, the saddle on a horse or the motorcycle seat can be fitted with a molded seat into which the rider can lodge securely. Weight lifting can be done from a seated position on the floor.[61,62]

Summary

Adults and children with amputations and limb deficiencies can accomplish many personal activities without prostheses. Reasons for not wearing prostheses include the inordinate exertion of walking with prostheses, a preference for being unencumbered by devices, or because the person is not aware of financially, mechanically, or cosmetically acceptable options.

Those with unilateral or bilateral upper limb amputations can be guided to select clothing that is easy to don without prostheses. The clinic team should encourage the child with bilateral upper limb deficiencies to capitalize on the tactile and prehensile capabilities of the feet to develop proficiency in dressing as well as writing, feeding, and other skills. At all ages, the teeth are useful for grasping. Many nonprosthetic techniques enable adults and children to complete grooming and hygienic care and eat a varied diet gracefully. Writing and using a keyboard, important for school and vocations, can be done with simple adaptation of basic implements and thoughtful selection of computers and other equipment. Virtually all homemaking duties can be managed without prostheses, sometimes borrowing techniques developed for people with hemiplegia. A wide range of games, sports, musical endeavors, and other recreational pursuits are within the compass of those who do not wear prostheses.

Similarly, children and adults who do not wear lower limb prostheses can learn suitable clothing and safe bathing procedures. Alternatives to prosthetic locomotion include crutches, hopping and pivoting, and the operation of a wheelchair and automobile. Recreational pursuits for amputees without prostheses are burgeoning, with or without special equipment.

The techniques discussed here can help individuals not only perform basic activities of daily living but also enjoy recreational activities and achieve professional goals. The organizations and publications in the list of Additional Resources at the end of this chapter can serve as a springboard for expanding personal, vocational, and recreational opportunities.

References

1. Melendez D, LeBlanc M: Survey of arm amputees not wearing prostheses: Implications for research and service. *J Assoc Child Prosthet Orthot Clin* 1988;23:62-69.

2. Mayer T-K (ed): *One-Handed in a Two-Handed World: Your Personal Guide to Managing Single-Handedly.* Boston, MA, Prince-Gallison Press, 1996.

3. Berger PE, Mensh S (eds): *How to Conquer the World With One Hand: And an Attitude.* Merrifield, VA, Positive Power Publishing, 1999.

4. Cohn S (ed): *Do It One-Handed: A Manual of Daily Living Skills for Stroke Rehabilitation.* South Orange, NJ, Lenox House, 1996.

5. Danzig AL (ed): *Handbook for One-Handers.* New York, NY, Federation of the Handicapped, 1952.

6. Garee B (ed): *Single-Handed: Devices and Aids for One Handers and Sources of These Devices.* Bloomington, IL, Accent Special Publications, 1988.

7. Washam V (ed): *The One-Hander's Book: A Basic Guide to Activities of Daily Living.* New York, NY, John Day, 1973.

8. Gardner WH (ed): *Left Handed Writing Instruction Manual: Prepared for Use in the School, Clinic or Home.* Danville, IL, Interstate, 1958.

9. Heinze A: Videotape: *Use of Upper Extremity Prostheses.* Thief River Falls, MN, 1988.

10. Friedmann L: Functional skills in multiple limb anomalies, in Atkins DJ, Meier RH III (eds): *Comprehensive Management of the Upper-Limb Ampu-*

tee. New York, NY, Springer-Verlag, 1989, pp 150-164.

11. Stemack J: *Shoe Tying With One Arm.* http://amp-info.net/jenny-2.htm

12. Stemack J: *Shoe Tying With One Arm.* http://amp-info.net/jenny-1.htm

13. Bender LF (ed): *Prostheses and Rehabilitation After Arm Amputation.* Springfield, IL, Charles C Thomas, 1974.

14. Jandren S: *Putting a Watch On With One Hand.* http://amp-info.net/watch.htm

15. Baughn J: *How to Wear Wedding Rings Without Fingers.* http://amp-info.net/rings.htm

16. Kessler HH: Three cases of severe congenital limb deficiencies: Twenty-year follow-up. *Inter-Clin Info Bull* 1971;10:1-9.

17. Patton JG: Developmental approach to pediatric prosthetic evaluation and training, in Atkins DJ, Meier RH III (eds): *Comprehensive Management of the Upper-Limb Amputee.* New York, NY, Springer-Verlag, 1989, pp 137-149.

18. Wright B: Independence in toileting for a patient having bilateral upper-limb hemimelia. *Inter-Clin Info Bull* 1976;15:21-24.

19. Easley S: *Dressing Without Arms.* http://amp-info.net/abbidress.htm

20. Macnaughtan AKM: *Clothing for the Limb Deficient Child.* Edinburgh, Scotland, Princess Margaret Rose Orthopaedic Hospital, 1968.

21. Heger H: Adaptive devices for amputees and training of upper extremity amputees: A. Training of upper extremity amputees, in Banerjee SN (ed): *Rehabilitation Management of Amputees.* Baltimore, MD, Williams & Wilkins, 1982, p 255-295.

22. Cope PC, Hile J: A bathing assist. *Inter-Clin Info Bull* 1970;10:6-8.

23. Friedmann L: Special equipment and aids for the young bilateral upper-extremity amputee. *Artif Limbs* 1965;9:26-33.

24. Wellerson TL (ed): *A Manual for Occupational Therapists on the Rehabilitation of Upper Extremity Amputees.* Dubuque, IA, Wm C Brown, 1958.

25. Kuhn GG: Vaginal tampon applicator. *Inter-Clin Info Bull* 1977;16:13-15.

26. Ring ND: Miscellaneous aids for physically handicapped children. *Inter-Clin Info Bull* 1972;12:1-12.

27. Youll WJ: Toilet aid for people with lower limb disabilities. *Tech Aid Disabled J* 1983:13-15.

28. Friedmann L: Toileting self-care methods for bilateral high level upper limb amputees. *Prosthet Orthot Int* 1980;4:29-36.

29. Baughn B: *One Hand Knives.* http://amp-info.net/knife.htm

30. Phippen W, Hunter JM, Barakat AR: The habilitation of a child with multiple congenital skeletal limb deficiencies. *Inter-Clin Info Bull* 1971;10:11-17.

31. Smith LA: A method of typing for the handicapped: One-hand touch typing. *Cereb Palsy Rev* 1960;21:11-12.

32. Typewriting Institute for the Handicapped, 3102 West Augusta Ave, Phoenix, AZ 85021.

33. Patrick C: Dvorak eases single-hand typing blues. *InMotion,* July-August 1998, p 29.

34. May EE, Waggoner NR, Hotte EB (eds): *Independent Living for the Handicapped and the Elderly.* Boston, MA, Houghton Mifflin, 1974.

35. Robinault IP (ed): *Functional Aids for the Multiply Handicapped.* Hagerstown, MD, Harper & Row, 1973.

36. *Breaking New Ground: Identifying, Selecting, and Implementing Assistive Technology in the Agricultural Workplace.* West Lafayette, IN, Department of Agricultural Engineering, Purdue University, 1992.

37. Jandren S: *Shaking Hands.* http://amp-info.net/handshake.htm

38. Beck P: *Shuffling Cards One Handed.* http://amp-info.net/cards.htm

39. Lazerow AK, Nesbitt JA (eds): *The International Directory of Recreation-Oriented Assistive Device Sources.* Marina Del Rey, CA, Lifeboat, 1986.

40. White EE (ed): *Jim Abbott: Against All Odds.* New York, NY, Scholastic, 1990.

41. Gallagher N: *Daniel Gallagher.* http://amp-info.net//gallagher.htm#bike

42. Sobetski J: *Jump Rope Modified With a Ferret Collar.* http://amp-info.net/jumprope.htm

43. Miller K: Sports implications for the individual with a lower-extremity prosthesis, in Seymour R (ed): *Prosthetics and Orthotics: Lower Limb and Spinal.* Philadelphia, PA, Lippincott Williams & Wilkins, 2002, pp 281-312.

44. Beck P: *Patti Beck's Golf Strap.* http://amp-info.net/golfstrap.htm

45. Crawford R, Bowker M (eds): *Playing From the Heart.* Rocklin, CA, Prima Publishing & Communications, 1989.

46. Julavits J: Her sights are always high. *Times Union.* Jacksonville, FL, Sunday, March 17, 1996. http://www.amp-info.net/joyce.htm

47. Edelstein JE: Musical options for upper-limb amputees, in Lee MHM (ed): *Rehabilitation, Music, and Human Well-Being.* St. Louis, MO, MMB Music, 1989.

48. Melendez T, White M (eds): *A Gift of Hope: The Tony Melendez Story.* San Francisco, CA, Harper & Row, 1989.

49. Narang IC, Mathur BP, Singh P, Jape VS: Functional capabilities of lower limb amputees. *Prosthet Orthot Int* 1984;8:43-51.

50. Kerr D, Brunnstrom S (eds): *Training of the Lower Extremity Amputee.* Springfield, IL, Charles C Thomas, 1956.

51. Waters RL, Perry J, Chambers R: Energy expenditure of amputee gait, in Moore WS, Malone JM (eds): *Lower Extremity Amputation.* Philadelphia, PA, WB Saunders, 1989, pp 250-260.

52. Gonzalez EG, Edelstein JE: Energy expenditure during ambulation, in *Downey and Darling's Physiological Basis of Rehabilitation Medicine,* ed 3. Boston, MA, Butterworth-Heinemann, 2001, pp 417-447.

53. Fisher SV, Gullickson G Jr: Energy cost of ambulation in health and disability: A literature review. *Arch Phys Med Rehabil* 1978;59:124-133.

54. Ganguli S, Bose KS, Datta SR, Chatterjee BB, Roy BN: Biomechanical approach to the functional assessment for use of crutches for ambulation. *Ergonomics* 1974;17:365-374.

55. Erdman WJ II, Hettinger T, Saez F: Comparative work stress for above-knee amputees using artificial legs or crutches. *Am J Phys Med* 1960;39:225-232.

56. Ganguli S: Analysis and evaluation of the functional status of lower extremity amputee-appliance systems: An integrated approach. *Biomed Eng* 1976;11:380-382.

57. Datta SR, Roy BN, Ganguli S, Chatterjee BB: Mechanical efficiencies of lower-limb amputees rehabilitated with crutches and prostheses. *Med Biol Eng* 1974;12:519-523.

58. Karacaloff LA, Hammersley CS, Schneider FJ (eds): *Lower Extremity Amputation: A Guide to Functional Outcomes in Physical Therapy Management,* ed 2. Gaithersburg, MD, Aspen, 1992.

59. Engstrom B, Van de Ven C (eds): *Therapy for Amputees,* ed 3. Edinburgh, Scotland, Churchill Livingstone, 1999.

60. Holliday PJ (ed): Nonprosthetic care, in Kostuik JP, Gillespie R (eds): *Amputation Surgery and Rehabilitation: The Toronto Experience.* New York, NY, Churchill Livingstone, 1981, pp 233-257.

61. Kegel B: Physical fitness: Sports and recreation for those with lower limb amputation or impairment. *J Rehabil Res Dev Clin* 1985 (suppl 1):1-125.

62. Kegel B (ed): *Sports for the Leg Amputee.* Redmond, WA, Medic, 1986.

Additional Resources

Ability magazine
1001 W. 17th Street
Costa Mesa, CA 92627
http://abilitymagazine.com

Adaptability catalog
P.O. Box 515
Colchester, CT 06415-0515

Alberta Amputee Sport and Recreation Association
http://www.aasra.ab.ca

American Academy of Physical Medicine and Rehabilitation
Directory of Sports Organizations for Athletes with Disabilities
http://www.aapmr.org/condtreat/athletes3.htm

American Amputee Soccer Association
http://www.ampsoccer.org

Amputee Coalition of America
900 East Hill Road, Suite 285
Knoxville, TN 37915
http://www.amputee-coalition.org

Amputee Golfer Magazine
http://nagagolf.org/magazine.htm

Applied Technology for Independent Living catalog
4732 Nevada Avenue North
Crystal, MN 55428

Canadian Amputee Sports Association
http://www.interlog.com~ampsport/can_amputee.html

Canadian Association for Disabled Skiing
P. O. Box 307
Kimberley, BC VIA 249
Canada
http://www.disabledskiing.ca/

Challenged Athletes Foundation
2148-B Jimmy Durante Boulevard
Del Mar, CA 92014
http://www.challengedathletes.org/caf/

CLEO Living Aids catalog
3957 Mayfield Road
Cleveland, OH 44121

Disabled Sports USA
451 Hungerford Drive, Suite 100
Rockville, MD 20850
http://www.dsusa.org

Eastern Amputee Golf Association
2015 Amherst Drive
Bethlehem, PA 18015
http://www.eaga.org

Everest & Jennings Avenue catalog
3233 East Mission Oaks Blvd
Camarillo, CA 93012

Fashion Able for Better Living catalog
5 Crescent Ave
Rocky Hill, NJ 08553

Maddak Inc catalog
Pequannock, NJ 07440

Mainstream magazine
P.O. Box 370598
San Diego, CA 92137
http://www.mainstream-mag.com

National Amputee Golf Association
11 Walnut Hill Rd.
Amherst, NH 03031
http://www.nagagolf.org

National Sports Center for the Disabled
P.O. Box 1290
Winter Park, CO 80482
http://www.nscd.org/

National Wheelchair Basketball Association
http://www.nwba.org

One-Hand Typing Tutor
http://home1.gte.net/bharrell

Online Sports Links
http://www.activeamp.org

Special Living magazine
Post Office Box 1000
Bloomington, IL 61702
http://specialliving.com

Sport for Disabled Ontario
1185 Eglinton Avenue E
Suite 102
Toronto, Ontario M3C 3C6
Canada
http://www.sportsfordisabled.ca

Sport 'n Spokes magazine
2111 East Highland Avenue, Suite 180
Phoenix, AZ 85016
http://www.pvamagazines.com/sns/

Wheelchair Sports, USA
http://www.wsusa.org

Chapter 60

Special Considerations: Consumer Movement

Mary P. Novotny, RN, MS

Introduction

The current situation of professionals caring for amputees is a relatively new phenomenon that developed in the last century. Substitutes for limbs were first made by amputees themselves or by their family members to help rebuild their fragmented body image and self-esteem. Later, prostheses were made by tradesmen such as harness makers, armorers, carpenters, or blacksmiths as an extension of their other work. Finally, prostheses were made by skilled craftsmen who ultimately earned degrees, certifications, and licenses for the development of prostheses. Currently, there are organizations for advancing the business of developing prostheses, providing continuing education, lobbying for reimbursements, and regulating the various aspects of prosthetics.

Extraordinary improvements in surgical techniques, prosthetic technology, and rehabilitation efforts have considerably changed many aspects of limb loss and rehabilitation. Indeed, prostheses have evolved from crude supportive tree branches to technologically complex devices made of lightweight flexible materials, often controlled by microprocessors and/or myoelectric controls. With the advent of adequate prostheses and rehabilitation programs, amputation no longer needed to be labeled as a failure to preserve a limb, but could be viewed as the beginning of comprehensive restorative efforts.

By shifting the focus from disability to abilities, amputees became valued consumers of goods and services, as well as inventors who sought solutions to improve their lives. Amputees seeking better outcomes began advocating for themselves out of personal and economic necessity. The amputee consumer movement exemplifies the need to grow beyond the loss of a limb. Frankl[1] explored this reality in *Man's Search for Meaning*, which describes self-transcendence as the inherent characteristic of humans to reach beyond themselves and find meaning for their lives through their search. Frankl believed that people transcend difficulties by giving and receiving care, appreciating the world around them, accepting things that cannot be changed, and through creative works such as deeds, occupations, and relationships. So it is with consumers seeking to adapt to change and perhaps better themselves in the process.

In technologically advanced North America and Europe, consumerism has developed in response to social and cultural changes, information and technological advances, and shifting health care economics. Consumerism coupled with the information explosion substantially changed the role of the amputee from victim to a participant in the decision-making process. The impact of self-advocacy is demonstrated by the increased availability of patient-oriented educational literature, which represents a shift from the previous focus on publications pertaining to device technology, case studies, and research.

While the amputee consumer movement was occurring, health care was changing from a paternalistic medical model to a profit-oriented business model. To improve profitability, insurance companies and managed care organizations are attempting to replace professional decision making with tight regulations, price controls, and low-bid contracts, which are often in conflict with minimal standards of care. Reductions in benefits have forced health care professionals into the dilemma of trying to provide quality care with fewer resources. Without adequate funding, many amputees do not have access to the more technologically advanced prostheses.

This chapter (1) summarizes the evolution of amputee care, (2) reviews how developments by amputee consumers have changed the prosthetic industry, (3) explains the needs of amputees for adaptation, including acceptance of an altered body image, (4) reviews support programs, (5) discusses organizational models, and (6) summarizes the roles of trained peers and health care professionals in supporting amputees.

Evolution of Amputee Care and Prosthetics

Historically, limb deficiencies and disabling conditions were fraught with shame, guilt, and fear. Babies with congenital limb deficiencies were often killed or ostracized because they were perceived as being liabilities or spiritually unclean. King Montezuma II, an Aztec ruler, established an area for degrading the disabled within the royal zoo and botanical gardens. Amputation has also been used as a judicial punishment in several cultures—a practice that continues today.

Throughout medical history, amputation was only performed as a last resort to save lives. Armorers fabricated artificial limbs at the request of knights and royalty to camouflage lost limbs. Queen Vishpla was fitted with an iron leg to enable her to walk and return to battle.[2] Goetz Von Berlichingen (1480-1562), a German mercenary knight, was provided with an amazing mechanical prosthetic hand as was Admiral Barbarossa, who fought with the Spaniards in Bougie, Algeria in 1512.[3]

War often triggered government intervention to address the needs of veterans whose amputations resulted from the improved destructive power of war and evolving medical techniques. The first large-scale attempt at prosthetic replacement of limbs supported by the United States government was the Great Civil War Benefaction, which provided prosthetic devices to veterans of the Union Army in the American Civil War.

Initially, European universities began developing both the art and science needed for the development of prostheses. This process, however, lacked a thorough understanding of the underlying psychological needs of the amputee. Indeed, many curricula pertaining to the development of prostheses still lack a consideration of the amputee's alterations in self-image as they struggle to regain personal integrity and balance while affected by changes that they cannot control.

Consumerism
Impetus to Social Change

By the early 1900s, there was marked improvement in the survival of amputees. Persons injured in war or industrial accidents had better immediate care and more rapid evacuation to hospitals and rehabilitation centers. Centers with critical care units and trauma services saved many lives and salvaged function of residual limbs for thousands of people. Improved health care, industrialization, and postwar developments increased the number of amputee consumers who lobbied for services. Many amputees benefited from federal and state rehabilitation programs such as the Veterans Health Administration, Medicare, and Medicaid. A program to support research and development in prosthetics was launched by the National Academy of Sciences under the auspices of the Veterans Administration. In addition, expansion of health insurance coverage allowed prostheses to be more available to amputees.

Unfortunately, by the end of the 1980s, efforts to control rising health care costs through managed care imposed serious funding restrictions. New policies limited consumer choices and access to appropriate health care despite progress in research, professional care, and technology. These changes further stimulated the amputee consumer advocacy movement.

Possibly the issue that had the greatest influence on amputee consumerism was the perception of many amputees that health care professionals were perceived as experts and the amputee was supposed to remain dutifully subservient. This traditional view of medical care seemed an anachronism in the era of consumer empowerment and activism.

Individual Consumers Who Advanced Technology

Amputees soon began seeking ways to improve their lives. Many wanted more than the rudimentary replacement devices that provided limited function. The willingness of these individuals to challenge the status quo, and their zeal for devices that would make them more able than disabled, truly revolutionized prosthetics.

Bob Radocy was determined to make his life as normal as possible after losing his arm in an automobile accident when he was 21 years old. Having studied biology, engineering, and drawing, Radocy began sketching the kind of prosthesis he wanted while still lying in his hospital bed. When he was told that the standard split-hook would replace his arm, Radocy knew that no single device could serve his multiple needs. He was handicapped by the available technology. He began thinking that the design criteria were insufficient, and he decided to try to improve the situation. This decision changed his life and the lives of thousands of upper limb amputees who benefit from the multiple components that he designed. What began as a personal search for a better product resulted in vastly improved upper limb terminal devices, and changed the way amputees perceive themselves and their abilities.

Bruce Kania lived most of his life with the frustration of meshing an energetic lifestyle with the limitations of a prosthesis that did not meet his needs. As an active outdoorsman, Kania decided to seek better solutions for his prosthetic problems rather than being limited by the available devices. Eventually he worked with researchers to design a fabric-covered gel socket liner that allowed him to triple the amount of time that he could walk comfortably. The success of this type of gel liner has benefited thousands of amputees. In addition, Kania donates some of the proceeds from royalties on the liner to improve the quality of life for amputees.

Carl Caspers lost his leg in an accident while he was in high school. Severe tissue damage made wearing a prosthesis both difficult and uncomfortable. In his search for a more comfortable and functional socket, Caspers became a certified prosthetist and orthotist. His fascination with socket environments coupled with his inventive mind led Caspers and his team to discover the resilient cushioning properties of urethane, which he used to create an interface and socket design that controls the socket environment for the amputee wearer.

Van Phillips was 21 years old when his leg was severed just above the ankle. Because he had been so active, he felt handicapped and frustrated by the available unresponsive prosthetic feet. He began a search for a better alternative with the assistance of an aerospace engineer who had experience with composite materials. They analyzed the requirements for a prosthetic foot and ankle unit. This led to the design of a composite carbon fiber-resin material, which they formed into an L-shaped foot and ankle. When Phillips tested the spring-like foot/ankle unit by applying weight, the force compressed the spring and some force was returned at toe-off, putting more spring into his step. This design became the forerunner of the currently available dynamic response feet.

Competitive participants with high expectations were involved in promoting the development of functional, high-impact prosthetic devices made of durable lightweight materials capable of withstanding the stresses of athletic competition. The demands of athletic amputees provided the incentive for new product development and the expansion of the market for prostheses.

The common thread with these inventors was a desire for improvement of the status quo. Each one demonstrated the potential for positive adaptation based on individual characteristics including personality, self-image, life experience, and available resources. Unlike individuals who focus on the negative aspects of limb loss, successful individuals concentrate on available strengths and resources, and engage in adaptive rather than maladaptive behaviors. In some ways these resourceful inventors are comparable to amputees of previous centuries who either made prosthetic devices themselves or commissioned a craftsman to build something to their specifications.

Development of Amputee Support/Advocacy Programs

The growing demand for resources, information, and advocacy for amputee consumers prompted the development of several consumer organizations. War Amputations of Canada was the first nationwide amputee consumer organization in North America. This organization became a model for other organizations based on its success with regard to education and empowerment in areas such as veterans care and advocacy for children affected by amputation.

Since their first networking meeting in 1986, the leaders of amputee support groups in the United States recognized the serious need for a unified voice for amputee consumers. Their goals were to strengthen scattered support group programs, and to centralize resources for more effective support and dissemination of information to amputee consumers. This need led to the formation of the Amputee Coalition of America (ACA), which was incorporated in 1989. The ACA organized formal programs to fulfill its mission of outreach, education, and empowerment by developing resources for amputee consumers, establishing a network of trained peer volunteers, and assisting local amputee support groups.

By 1993, the ACA faced a new challenge. Proposed cuts in Medicare funding would severely limit reimbursement for prostheses and care of amputees. The elimination of reimbursement for necessary services and prostheses would affect both amputees and providers. An aggressive collaborative response was the only feasible solution. The ACA coordinated a campaign to write to federal policy makers and began an aggressive educational program to promote the benefit of prostheses. The ACA and the National Office of Orthotics and Prosthetics organized a reception with members of Congress that allowed amputees to demonstrate the necessity of their prostheses in leading productive and independent lives. This unified response resulted in a defeat of the proposed cuts in funding. The final result was the development of functional levels that provided guidelines for prosthetic prescriptions based on rehabilitation potential of amputees, rather than general classifications based on age, disease, or previous limitations.

As consumer problems with access to and funding for appropriate care and devices increased, advocacy was officially added to the mission of the ACA in 1995. To address the expanded mission, the ACA began advocating for funding to establish a national information center to handle requests for information related to limb loss, train peer visitors, and collect data.

In 1997, the ACA opened the National Limb Loss Information Center (NLLIC) in Knoxville, Tennessee, under a collaborative agreement with the Centers for Disease Control and Prevention (CDC). Touted as a model for other agencies, the NLLIC was the first collaboration between a private, nonprofit organization and the CDC. In 1999, a research partnership between the ACA and Johns Hopkins University to evaluate data on limb loss was also funded by the CDC. Through implementation of these programs, the ACA overcame fears that numerous agencies and organizations would not be able to collaborate on a national level. Continued funding and success will depend on maintaining credibility, continued communication with multiple agencies and organizations, producing mission-oriented results, and maintaining leadership of visionaries who are willing to change the status quo.

Theories on Body Image and Adaptation

Traditionally, medical care has focused on the physical issues of ampu-

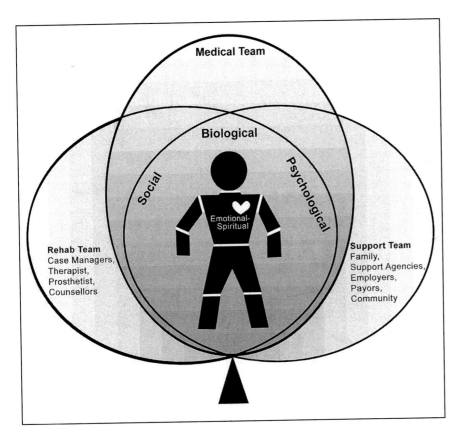

Figure 1 Interdisciplinary consumer care model.

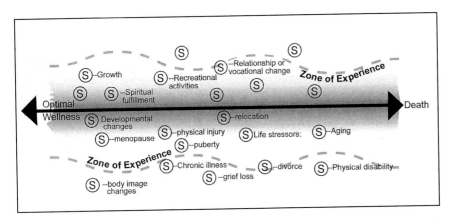

Figure 2 In this adaptation model, human beings are constantly responding to stimuli (circled S) along the health/illness continuum (↔).

approach unites amputees and professionals as partners in planning and achieving successful outcomes. Working together, the rehabilitation team, medical team, and support team can address biopsychosocial issues and promote positive adaptation.

Most literature pertaining to amputee rehabilitation focuses on physical aspects and issues pertaining to prostheses. Some theorists, however, including Sister Callista Roy, who proposed the Adaptation Model, suggest an integrated model of practice that highlights the relationship of biologic, psychological, and social aspects of health as they relate to individual adaptation to life changes.[4] The Roy Adaptation Model views humans as biopsychosocial beings, stressing the interrelationships between an individual's physical, psychological, and social well-being. An individual's response to stimuli in the environment is based on four modes: physiologic needs, self-concept, role function, and interdependence. Individuals have the capability of adaptive/positive response only when the stimuli are within their zone of experience. Individual responses are maladaptive when stimuli are outside their zone of experience. The goal of health care is to prevent or modify maladaptation by adjusting the stimuli, environmental factors, and/or resources to be within the patient's zone of experience (Figure 2). In a similar manner, transcendence theorists focus on the balance between physical and emotional health as determinants of outcomes in coping with illness.[5] Linking several of these concepts results in a consumer-centered health care model that integrates the medical, rehabilitation, and social networks with the patient/family unit to address the complex physical, psychological, and social needs associated with limb loss.

Any alteration in body image directly affects an individual's perceptions of attractiveness, capability, and normality. The factors involved in response to limb loss are complex and unique to each individual. Adaptation

tation, and prosthetics focused on devices. Neither discipline adequately addresses the psychosocial aspects of amputation, which profoundly influence outcomes. A multidisciplinary team that includes consideration of biologic, psychological, and social influences can enhance outcomes by addressing the holistic needs of the am-

putee consumer. The importance of keeping the amputee consumer at the center of the health care team is supported by body image and adaptation theories. With these models, the focus is shifted to reconstruction and rehabilitation following amputation rather than disability and disruption of physical integrity (Figure 1). This

to limb loss depends on a variety of factors including the meaning of the loss, physical changes surrounding the loss, level of self-esteem, premorbid personality, and associated environmental, psychological, and social resources. These complex issues are indicators of whether an amputee will approach or avoid a challenge, be a passive or active participant in care, and have an optimistic or pessimistic attitude towards life changes. Knowledge of body image and adaptation theories provides a perspective that can aid professionals in understanding some of the issues related to promoting positive adaptation to limb loss.

According to Schilder,[6] body image is the mental picture of one's body that is formed as a tridimensional entity and involves interpersonal, environmental, and temporal factors. He describes the development of body image as a dynamic process that is constantly affected by physical, psychological, and social factors. Schilder suggests that people continually construct, dissolve, and reconstruct their body image as well as the images of others. He also suggests that body image extends into the space around the individual. According to this theory, a firm object, rigid in its connection to the body, can be incorporated into the body image. In that way, a prosthesis can be incorporated into a reconstructed body image.

This concept was confirmed in a study at the University of Illinois with children and adolescents who were amputees. In this study, the amputees portrayed themselves with prosthetic devices, crutches, and even in wheelchairs when requested to complete a self-portrait. Because adaptation to change is based on an individual's need to develop, and later discard, the series of different selves, limb loss can provide the opportunity to redefine the concept, to learn new behaviors, and to master new tasks.[7] Therefore, amputees who are presented with a reconstructive framework with emotional support, physical training, and education are better able to adapt to

their limb loss than amputees who do not have these types of support.

If an amputee lacks adequate information, support, or coping skills, their problems may be compounded. New amputees have no reference point for the experience and often perceive disability in an excessively negative manner when confronted with alterations of body image and functional losses. Exposure to foreign terminology, baffling technology, and unfamiliar caregivers can also be negative factors. Fear of the unknown is an issue because so many of the stimuli bombarding the new amputee are outside of his or her zone of experience. Furthermore, the amputee's need to regain control and participate in decision making is often perceived as unimportant by health care professionals. Lacking adequate resources and support, these individuals may suffer from low self-esteem and fail to integrate positive changes, reconstruct a new body image, and regain their previous functional status. Without intervention and support to change, maladaptive behaviors can lead to mental and physical handicaps even in patients who had a medically successful amputation.

For optimal adaptation, amputees should be assessed with particular attention to perception and meaning of limb loss, roles, self-concept, and interdependence. Family members and significant others should be included in the assessment. Needs for education and support must be addressed so that the amputee and family members can be provided with useful information, strategies for effective functioning, social support, and an opportunity to participate in decisions regarding future care and needs.

An important aspect of positive adaptation is to use disequilibrium, the initial reaction to stress, as a motivator to learn new, more helpful behaviors. During this period, it is important that professionals and family members express positive attitudes regarding possibilities, rather than limitations. Although amputees benefit from professional help, they need

role modeling and peer support to increase skill mastery and confidence in problem solving, adaptive functioning, and resumption of sports, recreation, and other pursuits.

Many amputees also need a program of physical conditioning to build self-esteem, gain independence, and promote positive outcomes. Strength training exercises should be included in the preoperative and postoperative plan of care. Regaining balance and strengthening areas of weakness ensure that amputees do not become predisposed to problems of immobility, which complicate rehabilitation. To maintain focus and commitment, goals should focus on individual strengths, lifestyle, and interests. When there is a rapid return to normal activities, the amputee is less likely to experience prolonged depression and dependence. By avoiding delays and planning immediate follow-up with knowledgeable staff to review progress, the amputee should have maximum opportunity for a successful outcome.

Adaptation and Social Support

Amputees often indicate that although health care professionals provide medical information, they were aided the most by trained amputees. These trained amputee peers not only understand the complexities of dealing with a limb loss but are role models during a time of stress. In addition to dealing with the initial shock of losing a limb, an amputee must relearn many fundamental tasks. He or she can be greatly aided by another person who has succeeded in accomplishing the same goals that the new amputee is attempting to address. Routine functioning is often taken for granted, but the new amputee must struggle to adapt to the disruption of functioning caused by loss of a limb.

The usefulness of mutual, self-help support groups has been widely recognized, but has not been rigorously evaluated by statistical methods in controlled clinical trials. A major reason for this lack of documentation is the difficulty in completing a scientifically rigorous study on such a complex, multifactorial issue as limb loss. Challenges in the design and completion of studies to assess support of amputees include adequately controlling variables, developing appropriate end points, and correct use of statistical methods to ensure valid conclusions. Despite the lack of statistically validated studies, most professionals understand and accept that support and education help patients make complex transitions.

The results of studies of the effectiveness of social support in other situations, such as cancer and heart disease, are available and would likely apply to the support of amputees. One study used the Roy Adaptation Model to test the assumption that support leads to better adaptation to change.[8] This study examined adaptation of women to breast cancer and their participation in support groups. Data from structured telephone interviews with 70 women who participated in group social support and education on breast cancer were analyzed. Most women reported helpful adaptive physiologic, self-concept, role function, and independence with participation in a support group following treatment of breast cancer.[8] Other studies demonstrate that social support and quality of life are positively correlated in breast cancer patients. A 6-month randomized, controlled study showed that patients being treated for breast cancer who received early psychosocial support had a high acceptance of support and improved quality of life compared with patients in the control group who did not receive the support.[9]

Psychological state appears to be one of the best indicators of adjustment by cancer patients. Other findings indicate that the social contacts and social support from one's partner, family, friends, relatives, and medical professionals are important for survival.[10] A study at Stanford University demonstrated that greater quality of social support was associated with lower serum cortisol concentrations in women with metastatic breast cancer—a result that suggests healthier neuroendocrine functioning. A sample of 101 breast cancer survivors younger than 50 years demonstrated a positive correlation between perceived social support and quality of life.[11] In addition to known somatic factors, the 10-year prognosis for patients who had a myocardial infarction was adversely influenced by depression and lack of social support.[12]

Other positive correlations have been noted between support and network size, and between network size and the quality of life.[11] The interaction between personal and collective resources was studied among 230 kibbutz members in Israel. The combination of personal and collective resources is useful in avoiding functional limitation and becomes valuable in helping with recent life events. When stress affects social functioning, personal resources facilitate the mobilization of whatever collective resources are available.[13]

Studies have shown a direct relationship between religious involvement and/or spirituality and positive health outcomes such as mortality, physical illness, mental illness, and quality of life. Informing patients of available resources for spiritual care can provide reassurance, limit isolation, and facilitate recovery. Pastoral care departments in many hospitals have access to community resources that can make a valuable contribution to the holistic care of patients.[14]

Thus, research of a variety of conditions involving major life changes demonstrates that multidimensional support is highly beneficial to many individuals. Benefits of communicating with others who have similar problems include obtaining advice on adapting, shifting focus away from their own illness by helping others, and gaining insight as to what to expect. In many instances, motivation for seeking social support appeared to be a dynamic process with progression from receiving support to giving support.

Support Programs

Assuming that support is beneficial for those undergoing major life changes, it is useful to examine models and programs of support. Support services vary depending on their mission, resources, and location. Thus, although many programs provide information, resources, and peer support, the methods of support and focus differ.

The University of Wisconsin, for example, developed a social support network for breast cancer patients who communicate using computers. Participants indicated that anonymity within the support group fostered thoughtful interaction and enabled communication in ways that would have been more difficult in a face-to-face context.[15] On a more global scale, computers connect millions of people through e-mail, chat rooms, and informational websites. The ACA is staffed with information specialists to respond to requests for resources. In addition, trained peers associated with the ACA are available by telephone when local peer volunteers are not available. Common interests in sports and recreation also have led to the development of numerous sports and recreational programs for amputees seeking instruction, information, and peer support. The presence of a peer, role model, and/or guide seems to benefit amputees by reducing depression, decreasing anxiety, and reinforcing positive adaptive behaviors.

Some support groups are independent, but others work with professionals to increase visibility and to complement, rather than appear to compete with, rehabilitation teams. For example, some parent organizations, special camps for children and adolescents, veterans' organizations, and social clubs are cosponsored by rehabilitation centers and clinics. (See sidebar "Amputee Support Groups" on page 769.)

This model is particularly effective in establishing visibility and maintaining positive relationships between amputee consumers and professionals. Although consumer groups can be supported and guided by professionals, these groups should not be run by nonamputee professionals. Professionals involved in programs should not have the expectation of referrals and endorsements. This situation can lead to justifiable fear and anxiety among other professionals that the support group is merely a feeder organization, which can lead to competitiveness and program failure.

Discussions with patients and families should not include endorsements of devices and services. This is advertising, not education and empowerment. The goal of advocacy and support is to teach amputees how to obtain valid information and how to make choices, rather than telling them where they should go for care or service and what types of specific products should be requested. Fear regarding competition can be minimized if both amputee consumers and professionals recognize that the choice is always in the hands of the amputee consumer. Competent professionals have nothing to fear when consumers have realistic information and expectations.

Developmental Stages and Adaptation to Limb Loss

The need for psychosocial support for all amputees, regardless of age or gender, is supported by overwhelming evidence. Support is needed to address the profound changes in body image, self-esteem, role functioning, and interdependence that are associated with the loss of a limb. A balance between medical rehabilitation and social support is essential to achieving a positive adaptation to limb loss. Physical rehabilitation complemented by psychosocial support is vital and cost effective. Support should be made available to the amputee and family members as soon as possible, regardless of whether the involvement is through one-on-one peer contact, group programs, or support related to sports, recreation, or hobbies.

Although all amputees need support, the specific needs for information may vary by age and gender of the amputee. When a trauma center and the Veterans Hospital in Puget Sound, Washington, questioned amputees, they identified their main interests as (1) fit of the socket with residual limb, (2) mechanical functioning of the prosthesis, (3) nonmechanical qualities, and (4) advice about adaptation to life with a prosthesis with support from others.[16] Similar comments have been documented by other surveys in which amputees who acknowledged the assistance of health care professionals reported being helped most by peers who shared the experience of limb loss.[17,18]

Early Childhood

Children with congenital limb deficiency inhabit the only body they have ever known and it seems normal for them. Their world is dominated by parents, family, and friends who generally attempt to treat them as normal or who shield them from any emphasis on the missing limb. These children have minimal perception of their limb differences until they are confronted by peers and the public.

Initially it is parents who experience shock, the loss of their dream of a perfect child, guilt about the limb difference, depression, and sometimes even rejection of the child. To help parents and other families to adapt, they need counseling, information, and peer support to address current questions as well as future concerns. Experienced peers help the family recognize the normalcy of their confused feelings and focus on the overall health of their child. A peer group can demonstrate that the missing limb in no way diminishes the worth of the child and that, although there may be some limitations, child amputees should be treated as normally as possible. Without support and information, families become maladapted to an extent that affects the child throughout his/her lifetime.[19]

Family support groups formed because parents of children with congenital limb deficiencies wanted opportunities to share their experiences. Many parents lacked information and support at the time of the child's birth. They lacked the ability to explain the deficiency to family and friends. They sought information on how to address the child's questions, teach the child to handle questions, introduce their child into a new school system, and to prevent teasing from other children. These families are concerned about available services and the benefit of interdisciplinary treatment centers. Knowledgeable parents recognize that a symbiotic relationship between the professionals and families is helpful in identifying developmental problems, setting appropriate goals, and implementing solutions.[20-22] Health care professionals also learn from the children and parents. Parent groups raise public awareness, provide education about limb loss, and serve as models for adapting to life with disabilities. Some groups have newsletters or share information over the Internet.

Responses to parent groups are generally very positive. Successful models of support include informal gatherings when families and their children meet in a clinic setting or a home. These social outings are sometimes coordinated by nurses, social workers, and/or therapists. Regardless of the support group, parents can establish long-term, beneficial relationships with other families.

Adolescence

Many adolescents and young adults adapt more readily to limb loss than adults, even in the presence of medical complications such as cancer. Some of the greatest challenges of teenagers revolve around the need to be accepted within a society that places a high value on physical attributes and beauty.

Although many teenagers shy away from formal involvement with support groups, they may interact with peers in sports, recreation, camps, and other activities that focus on equal participation and independence. These activities provide feedback, role model identification, and promote positive self-image and self-esteem by focusing on abilities rather than disabilities.

Although school personnel may attempt to be supportive, many are not well informed about positive outcomes and abilities of individuals with limb loss. This lack of information can lead to overprotectiveness, anxiety, and possibly even reinforcement of negative behaviors. In some situations, adolescents need professional counseling. A team approach might involve a counselor, nurse, or social worker conferring with the amputee, their families, and school personnel. This approach can reduce problems by allowing teenagers to share their feelings and helping school personnel assist the amputee in regaining control of his/her life.[23]

Adulthood

As Gray discussed in *Men Are From Mars, Women Are From Venus,* men and women differ in their desire for and response to emotional support.[24] Women are more likely to seek support outside of marriage than men; however, women vary considerably in the kind of group they prefer. Some women find church groups most helpful; others prefer general support groups. These preferences may relate to training, the ability to deal with emotions, knowledge regarding empathy, and communication styles of the interaction. One study reported a lower risk of depression in women who were socially involved.[25] In contrast, men who received social support outside their marriages had an increased risk of depression.[25]

Senior Years

When amputations occur in the elderly, the medical complications of comorbid conditions such as diabetes mellitus, vascular problems, and heart disease compound the patient's physical adaptation. Psychological and social aspects are also dramatically affected. Entire families need information regarding pre- and postoperative care, skills to assist with rehabilitation, and emotional support throughout the experience. In many elderly patients, rehabilitation is complicated by isolation, lack of social support, and limited financial and social resources. The needs of these patients must be addressed immediately. An appropriate postdischarge placement should be provided until the individual can resume more independent functioning.

Significant Others

The need for involvement of family members is irrefutable. Because families are integral to the life of the amputee, they have a major impact on adaptation. Families can either promote rehabilitative efforts or enhance isolation, depending on styles of communication, problem-solving skills, and social support systems.

Trials of one psychoeducational support group indicate the need for interventions targeted at the significant other. Involved spouses had fewer mood disturbances, and reported greater confidence, support, and satisfaction with their spouses than those who had not been through the training program.[26]

Significant others, however, can hinder rehabilitation if they reinforce negative behaviors. Criticism and inappropriate advice impair adaptive responses. Some family members find it particularly difficult to separate their own needs from those of the amputee, thereby giving advice or criticism that undermines efforts at rehabilitation. Early, effective training and appropriate support for family members can promote positive adaptation for the new amputee by dispelling negative stereotypes, improving listening skills, and promoting empowerment rather than dependency.

Factors Contributing to the Success of Support Groups

The results of support programs can vary depending on leadership, culture of the community, and the presence or absence of professional support. Although it seems that support groups would flourish as complementary partners to the health care profession, many fail within the first few years. Causes of failure include lack of leadership and inadequate structure to sustain the group, meager resources, and failure to market services. But the greatest obstacle to success is underutilization by professionals who either lack the knowledge of the importance of support or who perceive amputee consumer advocates as a threat to their business. Some professionals prefer to focus on providing devices and fail to acknowledge that the psychosocial needs of amputees are at least as important, if not more so, than limb replacement in positive adaptation. Unfortunately, patients lacking referral to a support group or information about such resources as the NLLIC may never adapt to the changes imposed by limb loss and therefore never make a complete adjustment to living life fully after amputation.

The success of an amputee peer support program depends on focusing on a mission, developing collaborative partnerships between volunteers and professionals, and continuous follow-up to assess and improve program outcomes. An organization focused on its mission and with specific goals is less likely to fail than one trying to be all things to all people. Networking and building alliances with organizations that address other needs (eg, sports and recreation organizations or funding agencies) is far more effective than attempting to meet all the needs of the amputee within one organization.

The ability to develop collaborative relationships ensures that credibility and knowledge about the group among health care professionals is positive. This cooperation creates an environment of trust and rapport. For amputee patients and community agencies, the inclusion of emotional support, information, and affirmation benefits amputees and volunteers, and it strengthens linkages between the amputee consumer, the community, and the professionals. Professionals and peer support are perceived as complementary rather than competitive.

Roles of Trained Volunteers

The ACA provides training for volunteer peers and instructors that covers fundamental information on the role of peers, communication, and empathetic discussion of sensitive issues requiring judgment and tact. (See sidebar "The Peer Visitor" on page 770.) The role of a volunteer is to share experiences, information, and emotional support, thus empowering the new amputee and his or her family to make their own informed decisions. Trained volunteers can enhance positive adaptation and complement medical rehabilitation programs for amputees. Well-adjusted amputees can be role models demonstrating both function and quality of life despite the loss of a limb.

Amputees focused on returning to work may receive support from amputees who are similarly employed. Vocational organizations or others who have a stake in the amputee's outcome might also play a role. Numerous studies demonstrate that returning to work is a positive part of rehabilitation. For many individuals, work is related to identity, self-esteem, respect, and standing within the community. In addition, work provides social support, companionship, role fulfillment, and economic gains.[27]

Training is not intended to turn peer counselors into psychotherapists or professional problem solvers but to help volunteers develop the skills needed to assist other amputees. Volunteers need proper training to learn how to avoid excessive self-disclosure and/or giving inappropriate advice. Peer volunteers learn how to discuss their experiences about adapting to daily challenges without giving professional advice. Through constructive listening and exploring feelings, peers provide emotional support for the amputee facing alterations in body image, functional capabilities, and social interactions. Unlike professionals who have limited time for patient interaction, volunteers can interact with amputees and their families in a variety of settings.

The training program covers issues that should be referred to a professional for follow-up, such as possible litigation, avoidance of endorsements, discussions regarding inappropriate sexual and romantic content, and other topics that may exceed the capacity of a volunteer. Training should review the effects of endorsements and recommendations that can disempower the amputee who may seek answers and solutions from peer visitors. What works best for one amputee is based on a variety of issues; therefore, decisions must be considered on a case-by-case basis as outcomes vary.

Roles of Professionals

Health care professionals are divided in their opinions of the value of amputee and other self-help groups for several reasons. Unfortunately, some support groups mainly exist to satisfy the ego of the founder. Other groups may have good intentions but use untrained personnel who lack the skills to provide true benefits to amputees. A considerable number of health care professionals, however, are enthusiastic supporters of well-managed amputee support groups with trained visitors that offer genuine benefits to their patients.

For proactive health care professionals, numerous opportunities exist to build alliances with amputee groups. Professionals can serve as educators, make referrals of new amputees, provide resources and information, and assist with group discussions. They can also help with administrative functions such as obtaining financial support, developing newsletters, providing office space and services, and dispensing materials.

Professionals who are not directly involved with support groups can display literature and resources for amputees and families who visit their offices and facilities. Many facilities are developing patient information packets to distribute to new patients. Packets can include information about community and national resources.

Whether the interaction between patients and professionals occurs in a hospital, rehabilitation center, or prosthetic facility, collaboration can be advantageous for both support groups and professionals. This collaboration is not competitive as it involves mutual planning, implementation, and evaluation. Support groups for amputees are not intended to rival professional care and services; however, they can play a vital complementary role in rehabilitation at no expense to patients or health care professionals.

Involving the amputee consumers as members of the rehabilitation team includes devising a system of open and ongoing communication to discuss progress or problems. Any lack of resources, information, or support should be addressed appropriately. The amputee and his or her family, as well as medical, rehabilitation, and social support systems, should all contribute as members of the team. Successful adaptation is achievable if all team members collaborate to establish realistic goals, implement required measures, and continuously evaluate outcomes.

Summary

Long before the existence of technologically advanced methods and specialized health care professionals, amputees acted as their own advocates and sought solutions to improve devices to allow adaptation to limb loss. Many innovative prosthetic components would not exist without determined, dissatisfied consumers who were unwilling to accept discomfort and functional limitations. In a similar manner, amputees who were sports enthusiasts helped develop lighter weight, resilient, flexible materials for prostheses that tolerate long-term use in sporting activities.

Amputees who are educated and advocate for themselves are beginning to achieve better outcomes than ever before. Advances in medical care and prosthetics continue to improve clinical outcomes. In addition to medical advances, the shift in focus from disability to abilities is beginning to have a major impact for amputees. Rather than viewing amputation as the tragic end to an unsuccessful treatment regimen, health care professionals can regard amputation as a key element of a restorative effort.

Respect and collegiality are changing the relationship between amputees and health care professionals to that of a partnership. Unquestioned decision making by health care professionals is decreasing as empowered amputees and other consumers actively participate as members of the rehabilitation team. Amputee consumers are the only team members who interact with every health care provider and attend every office visit, meeting, and appointment. The changing attitudes of health care professionals has the potential for keeping consumers in the center of the comprehensive interdisciplinary health care model. The amputee is the reason for assessment, evaluation, fitting, technology, and research (Figure 1).

Professionals in medicine, rehabilitation, and prosthetics can gain invaluable allies by collaborating with information centers, support groups, and sports associations that provide assistance to amputees. Enhanced awareness of these resources is expected to increase referrals from professionals and use of their services. As consumer forums and advisory boards are beginning to communicate consumer needs to agencies and organizations, this information must be shared between professionals to further integrate consumer needs into prosthetic care, research, and education.

The availability of information via the Internet empowers amputee consumers to be involved in decision making. Although the literature previously focused on technical devices and research, information written in language understandable by the average person is now available to amputees and their families.

Unfortunately, a business model focused on financial results rather than on patient outcomes is replacing the medical model. This shift forces health care providers into the dilemma of trying to provide high quality care with fewer resources. Thus, amputees may not have access to the most technologically advanced prosthetics without appropriate reimbursement. Outcomes research to validate the importance of prostheses and the role of patient support are needed to help justify the reimbursement of these products and services.

Conclusions and Future Directions

To continue to make progress, consumers cannot rely on past accomplishments. Enforcement of the Americans With Disabilities Act, continued access to information and technology, and improvement of health care systems around the world require a unification of advocacy efforts as well as improved education and information and increased outreach. Health care professionals, particularly prosthetists, are robbing themselves of their most effective allies and advocates when they avoid involvement with amputee consumers.

Additional work is needed to ascertain how local amputee peer support and education groups can thrive and fulfill the important mission of education, advocacy, and empowerment. National organizations such as the ACA and War Amputations, with central resource databases and funding, demonstrate the greatest potential for longevity. By developing programs, resources, and techniques to assist local groups, national organizations can produce high quality educational pieces, deliver support effectively, and educate communities across the country.

Consumers adapting to a major lifestyle change must have readily accessible, easily understandable information and support. Any standard of care should include provisions to provide educational support services for amputee consumers and their families dealing with life changes. A global plan to improve access and available services is needed to coordinate resources around the world. Facilitating communication among professionals, informational resources, and consumers could help improve outcomes by making resources available to those in need.

Worldwide connections to a virtual library and resources facilitate access of both consumers and health care professionals to current information regarding technical resources, biomedical studies, rehabilitation, self-help information, prosthetic publications, consumer organizations, and funding sources. Virtual resources have the capability of networking consumers across the nation or the world, thereby eliminating the isolation of consumers, including those encumbered by location or mobility problems. As mentioned in *Prosthetics/Orthotics Research for the Twenty-first Century*,[28] a virtual library should be linked to consumer and professional programs, worldwide research and care centers, and online support groups to address the needs of isolated individuals who need easy access to resources. Virtual information on clinical issues, research, technology, and adaptive resources could potentially improve care worldwide.

Cooperative advocacy efforts are a win-win situation. Health care and disability coalitions have promoted legislation for patient rights (Table 1), the Americans With Disabilities Act, Veterans Administration Programs, the Paralympic Games, the National

Center for Medical Rehabilitation and Research, and the NLLIC. As federally funded priorities, these programs are increasing awareness, changing societal perceptions, and expanding opportunities for disabled persons to be recognized as successful and contributing members of society. Continued success depends on increased networking and collaboration to provide resources where needed. Improvements in communication, such as virtual resources, could facilitate this collaboration.

Success in prosthetics and rehabilitation depends on the ability of professionals to communicate, collaborate, and keep the amputee consumer the focal point of care. Amputee consumers must be integral to the development and implementation of medical, prosthetic, and allied health science curricula. Multidisciplinary professions that involve engineering, art, and science must have a common language and focus. That focus is the patient/consumer. Practitioners who understand practice management and use a staff of reimbursement experts can fail to maintain focus on the amputee consumer. Without consideration for the holistic needs of the amputee, prosthetic devices can become expensive engineering feats that may or may not address the specific needs of the user. Curricula that address interdisciplinary team communication, relationships between form and function, and the psychosocial needs of the user are imperative to educating practitioners capable of rebuilding lives instead of merely replacing limbs.

Finally, research that forms the basis for treatment plans is needed on an ongoing basis. Research involving consumers will help to ensure valid measures for improving the quality of life for persons with disability. Limitations in the methodology used to date should be addressed. Future studies must assess psychosocial needs and standards of care to address holistic needs of consumers in medical and rehabilitative settings. Collaborative studies will aid in securing clinical data, disseminating findings, and incorporating results into standards for quality that are valid for rehabilitation in a variety of cultures.

TABLE 1 ACA Consumer Bill of Rights and Responsibilities

All people who have experienced a disability have the right to:

Receive comprehensive, clear information about the medical, surgical, and rehabilitative aspects of care

Participate fully in all decisions concerning their health and well-being and the development of a personalized rehabilitation plan

Establish goals for optimal functioning, physical and emotional well-being, and prevention of secondary conditions and complications

Have access to peer support, funding information, and vocational/recreational resources

Be informed about appropriate and available prosthetic and orthotic services and devices, including new technologies

Become knowledgeable consumers of safe, effective products and services

Select from certified practitioners, and

Voice concerns about quality of care, billing practices, and services or products, and seek redress if the highest quality standards are not met

(Reproduced with permission from the Amputee Coalition of America, 1998.)

Additional Resources

The ACA provides gift certificates for free publications and membership to new amputees. The ACA has a toll-free number (1-888-AMP-KNOW) that makes it easy to obtain answers from a wide variety of resources listed through the NLLIC databases.

References

1. Frankl VE (ed): *Man's Search for Meaning: An Introduction to Logotherapy.* New York, NY, Pocket Books, 1963.

2. Sanders GT, May BJ (eds): *Lower Limb Amputations: A Guide to Rehabilitation.* Philadelphia, PA, FA Davis, 1986.

3. American Academy of Orthopaedic Surgeons: Historical development of artificial limbs, in *Orthopaedic Appliance Atlas: Artificial Limbs.* Ann Arbor, MI, JW Edwards 1960, Vol. 2, pp 1-22.

4. Roy C (ed): *Introduction to Nursing: An Adaptation Model.* Englewood Cliffs, NJ, Prentice-Hall, 1976.

5. Coward DD: Facilitation of self-transcendence in a breast cancer support group. *Oncol Nurs Forum* 1998; 25:75-84.

6. Schilder P (ed): *The Image and Appearance of the Human Body: Studies in the Constructive Energies of the Psyche.* New York, NY, International Universities Press, 1950.

7. LaFleur JF, Novotny MP: Study of human figure drawings by amputee children and verbalization of their general adjustment, in Krampitz SD, Pavlovich N (eds): *Readings for Nursing Research.* St Louis, MO, CV Mosby, 1981, pp 259-266.

8. Samarel N, Fawcett J, Krippendorf K, et al: Women's perceptions of group support and adaptation to breast cancer. *J Adv Nurs* 1998;28:1259-1268.

9. Scholten C, Weinlander G, Krainer M, Frischenschlager O, Zielinski CC: Difference in patient's acceptance of early versus late initiation of psychosocial support in breast cancer. *Support Care Cancer* 2001;9:459-464.

10. Sammarco A: Perceived social support, uncertainty, and quality of life of younger breast cancer survivors. *Cancer Nurs* 2001;24:212-219.

11. Turner-Cobb JM, Sephton SE, Koopman C, Blake-Mortimer J, Spiegel D: Social support and salivary cortisol in women with metastatic breast cancer. *Psychosom Med* 2000;62:337-345.

12. Welin C, Lappas G, Wilhelmsen L: Independent importance of psychosocial factors for prognosis after myocardial infarction. *J Intern Med* 2000;247:629-639.

Useful Websites

Amputee Coalition of America:
www.amputee-coalition.org

Center for International Rehabilitation:
http://www.cirnetwork.org

Center for International Rehabilitation, Research, Information, and Exchange:
http://www.cirrie.buffalo.edu

Disabled Sports USA:
http://www.dsusa.org

Landmine Survivors Network:
http://www.landminesurvivors.org

Limbless Association UK:
http://www.limbless-association.org

National Center on Physical Activity and Disability:
http://www.ncpad.org

O&P Digital Technologies sponsored site for resources for orthotics and prosthetics information:
http://www.oandp.com

Rehabilitation International:
http://www.rehab-international.org

War Amputations of Canada:
http://www.waramps.ca

13. Anson O, Carmel S, Levenson A, Bonneh DY, Maoz B: Coping with recent life events: The interplay of personal and collective resources. *Behav Med* 1993;18:159-166.

14. Mueller PS, Plevak DJ, Rummans TA: Religious involvement, spirituality, and medicine: Implications for clinical practice. *Mayo Clin Proc* 2001;76: 1225-1235.

15. Shaw BR, McTavish F, Hawkins R, Gustafson DH, Pingree S: Experiences of women with breast cancer: Exchanging social support over the CHESS computer network. *J Health Commun* 2000;5:135-159.

16. Legro MW, Reiber G, del Aguila M, et al: Issues of importance reported by persons with lower limb amputations and prostheses. *J Rehabil Res Dev* 1999; 36:155-163.

17. Geiger AM, Mullen ES, Sloman PA, Edgerton BW, Petitti DB: Evaluation of a breast cancer patient information and support program. *Eff Clin Pract* 2000;3:157-165.

18. Fitzgerald DM: Peer visitation for the preoperative amputee patient. *J Vasc Nurs* 2000;18:41-44.

19. Chepolis L, Thorp N: Networking families on a prosthetic clinic for children. *JACPOC Online Library* 1984; 19:80.

20. Cammack S: Integration of pediatric amputees and their parents with an adult amputee support group. *JACPOC Online Library* 1989;24:6.

21. Varni JW, Setoguchi Y, Rappaport LR, Talbot D: Psychological adjustment and perceived social support in children with congenital/acquired limb deficiencies. *J Behav Med* 1992;15: 31-44.

22. Tebbi CK, Stern M, Boyle M, Mettlin CJ, Mindell ER: The role of social support systems in adolescent cancer amputees. *Cancer* 1985;56:965-971.

23. Chalmers KI, Kristjanson LJ, Woodgate R, et al: Perceptions of the role of the school in providing information and support to adolescent children of women with breast cancer. *J Adv Nurs* 2000;31:1430-1438.

24. Gray J: *Men Are From Mars, Women Are From Venus.* New York, NY, Harper Collins, 1992.

25. Amato JJ, Williams M, Greenberg C, Bar M, Lo S, Tepler I: Psychological support to an autologous bone marrow transplant unit in a community hospital: A pilot experience. *Psychooncology* 1998;7:121-125.

26. Bultz BD, Speca M, Brasher PM, Geggie PH, Page SA: A randomized controlled trial of a brief psycho educational support group for partners of early stage breast cancer patients. *Psychooncology* 2000;9:303-313.

27. Quick JC, Murphy LR, Hurrell JJ Jr, Orman D: The value of work, the risk of distress, and the power of prevention, in Quick JC, Murphy LR, Hurrell JJ Jr (eds): *Stress and Well-Being at Work: Assessments and Interventions for Occupational Mental Health.* Washington, DC, American Psychological Association, 1992, pp 3-13.

28. Michael JW, Bowker JH: Prosthetics/ Orthotics Research for the Twenty-First Century: Summary 1992 conference proceedings. *J Prosthet Orthot* 1994;6:100-107.

Amputee Support Groups
From the Amputee Coalition of America

Paddy Rossbach, RN
Patricia Isenberg, MS
Douglas G. Smith, MD

A support group can play an important role in the recovery process for both recent and experienced amputees. The following factors appear to be integral to successful psychosocial adjustment to limb loss: (1) a strong support network of family and/or friends; (2) social support from outside the family/friend network, such as from a peer visitor and support group members; and (3) successful use of stress management and coping strategies.

Support groups can be an invaluable resource for the new amputee, a place to observe others who are successfully coping with limb loss and learn new coping strategies. The group can provide the opportunity to discuss or practice coping techniques in a supportive atmosphere.

Anyone interested in starting and maintaining a support group should first answer the four "W" questions: Where? When? Who? and Why?

Where: Look for a free space in the community such as a church community center, hospital, or independent living center. To establish the integrity of the support group, it should not be affiliated with a prosthetic facility or rehabilitation center. This does not preclude receiving space or supplies from such a group, but the support group cannot be seen as endorsing one practitioner or facility over another.

When: Decide on a regular meeting time and date that accommodates most potential group members. Support groups typically meet monthly for 1 to 2 hours.

Who: Will your group focus on the needs of new amputees, or will it focus more on experienced amputees? Will you include family members or caregivers? Are all ages welcome? Recruiting members will be a challenge, so be creative. Develop flyers to post in prosthetists' offices, hospitals, and rehabilitation centers. Write an article for the local newspaper. Contact the Amputee Coalition of America (ACA) to have your support group information added to the ACA database.

Why: To determine the type of meetings that will best meet the needs of your group, ask potential members. Do they want an open discussion group with a facilitator, social gatherings, or formal programs followed by discussion?

The ACA has found that groups with the most longevity share the following characteristics:

- Meet on a regular basis in a central location
- Offer a peer visitor program
- Have programs that are appropriate for a wide range of ages or clearly focus on one age group
- Offer both structured programs and social events for members
- Formalize the group's structure so that responsibilities are divided among a group of people.

The Peer Visitor
From the Amputee Coalition of America

Paddy Rossbach, RN
Patricia Isenberg, MS
Douglas G. Smith, MD

One of the most significant interventions an individual facing an amputation can have is a meeting with a trained peer visitor. A peer visitor is someone who has experienced an amputation, is living a full and productive life, and has completed a training program preparing him or her to visit another individual and his or her family facing a similar experience.

Good peer visitors are sensitive listeners who are trained in communication skills. They can facilitate the new amputee's own recovery and self-exploration so that they can make good decisions for themselves. Just being present tells the new amputee, "I've been where you are and I know you can find ways to make your life complete again." Peer visits, if done well, are shining moments.

An untrained peer visitor, on the other hand, can do more harm than good. Inexperienced peer visitors can mistakenly believe they are there to tell the new amputee, "Here's what you need to do." They may leave the meeting with the feeling that everything went well. Unfortunately, what they don't see is that the new amputee may actually feel worse, having been overwhelmed with information. What the person actually wanted from a peer visit was a chance to talk about confusion, pain, and feelings. Instead, they got yet another lecture telling them what to do. Feelings of being overwhelmed and helpless were made worse, not better.

A peer visitor should not try to think or act for the new amputee, as this fosters dependence and is considered "solicitous" behavior. In psychology literature, solicitous behavior is defined as behavior that appears positive but really undermines adaptive functioning. There is some evidence that solicitous behavior correlates with depression after limb loss.

Peer visitors are everyday people who typically are not professional counselors or therapists, and their purpose is not to give advice or solve problems. Rather, they serve as role models, offer emotional support, and provide information about resources available locally and nationally.

The Amputee Coalition of America (ACA), the leading national nonprofit consumer organization for the more than 1.2 million individuals living in the United States with the loss or absence of a limb, trains and certifies peer visitors. The ACA runs full-day seminars providing prospective peer visitors with a great deal of information, including the process of surviving to thriving, how to deal with grief, an understanding of cultural differences, when an individual's needs are beyond the capability of the peer visitor and should be referred to a health care provider, how to conduct a visit in a variety of settings including by phone, and most importantly how to communicate. The course stresses the different types of listening and the importance of each, and it teaches skills to encourage dialogue. In addition, subjects or actions that should be avoided during a visit are covered in great detail.

Each course participant is evaluated for knowledge, through pre- and posttesting, and suitability, through role playing and interaction during the session, before being certified by the ACA. Names of certified peer visitors are added to the National Peer Network database. Requests for a peer visitor are matched as closely as possible by several factors, including age, sex, and type of amputation. Personal visits are preferred. When these are impossible, phone visits can be conducted. The ACA evaluates the efficacy of the program periodically by asking visited individuals to fill out an evaluation form.

Section V

Pediatrics

Chapter 61

The Limb-Deficient Child

John R. Fisk, MD
Douglas G. Smith, MD

Introduction

Much of the *Atlas* deals with prosthetics, but the limb-deficient child needs much more than replacement limbs. Even the surgeon must follow a different set of rules when working with children. The child missing all or part of one or more limbs is a growing, developing, and learning individual. Equally important, limb-deficient children have parents and siblings who are learning along with them. Thus, those who work with limb-deficient children must consider many different factors beyond those involved with treating adults.

The child is not just a small adult. In addition to the obvious differences brought about by growth, children react differently to disabilities than do adults. The two major categories of pediatric patients with limb deficiencies are those with congenital deficiencies and those with acquired deficiencies (ie, those who underwent amputations). The child with a congenital limb deficiency has no sense of loss and nothing new to adjust to. Any prosthesis is seen as an aid, not a replacement, so if it does not truly aid the child, the child will reject it. In contrast, those who lose a limb because of trauma or disease experience a profound sense of loss and undergo a period of readjustment unless the amputation is performed when they are very young. How well these children manage this change greatly affects their acceptance of prosthetic limbs.

Epidemiology of Congenital Deficiencies

Congenital limb defects occur at an approximate rate of 0.3 to 1.0 per 1,000 live births. Because the United States does not have a formal and complete registry of birth defects, the number and types of limb deficiencies are not precisely known. Using hospital discharge information obtained from national surveys designed to sample 20% of the community, nonfederal, and short-term hospitals in the United States, Dillingham and associates[1] have estimated that between 1988 and 1996, the incidence of congenital limb deficiencies has remained fairly constant at approximately 26 per 100,000 (0.26 per 1,000) live births. The authors acknowledge that this rate is about one half of that reported by Froster[2] for British Columbia and Kallen and associates[3] for Sweden. Dillingham and associates[1] detail neither the specific types of limb deficiencies nor possible etiologies, but they do report that 58.5% of all limb deficiencies in newborns involve the upper limb. Among those, longitudinal hand deficiencies are the most frequent, accounting for 46.4% of upper limb abnormalities. Longitudinal toe reductions were the most common lower limb deficiencies found in newborns. Overall, multiple congenital limb deficiencies were identified in 17.8% of newborns with limb deficiencies.

In a study based on findings of the Active Malformations Surveillance Program and Brigham and Women's Hospital in Boston, McGuirk and associates[4] estimated a prevalence of 0.69 per 1,000 live births for all types of limb deficiency. They reported that limb reduction defects are much more common in the arms alone (70%) than in the legs alone (18%) or in both arms and legs (12%).

Finally, the National Birth Defects Prevention Study initial report by Yoon and associates[5] discusses the largest and broadest collaborative effort to identify infants with major birth defects in the United States and to evaluate genetic and environmental factors associated with the occurrence of birth defects. As of December 2000, 7,470 affected subjects and 3,821 control subjects had been enrolled. The data indicate that limb deficiency accounts for only 6% (452 of 7,470) of all the various types of birth defects when all anatomic systems are included.

Etiology of Congenital Deficiencies

After the initial shock, when sadness sets in, the ever-present question of "Why did this happen?" is on the minds of every relative of an infant with limb deficiency. Although a better understanding of the etiology of certain limb deficiencies has been gained in recent decades, in most cases the precise cause of the defect remains unknown.

In general, the causative events are categorized as genetic, vascular, amniotic, teratologic, and unknown, with the unknown category being the largest. Unfortunately, being told the cause of their child's difference is unknown is often just as frustrating for parents and families as if a known cause had been found. Brent[6] estimated in 1985 that 60% to 70% of all congenital limb deficiencies were of unknown etiology. He found that environmental causes were identified in 10% of malformations, maternal infections in 3%, maternal disease in 4%, uterine constraint in 2%, and exposure of the fetus to recognized drugs, chemicals, irradiation, or hyperthermia in 1%. Brent also surmised that 5% of malformations have a cytogenetic origin and that about 15% are due to a single gene mutation.

In 2001, McGuirk and associates[4] estimated that 32% of congenital limb deficiencies have no known cause and that 30% are of genetic origin. They broke down the latter into known hereditary disorders (15%), chromosomal disorders (6%), specific malformation syndromes (5%), and familial patterns (4%). They believed that 4% of congenital limb deficiencies were related to a teratogenic agent and 34% were of vascular origin. Although the possibility of identifying genetic abnormalities has increased, identification does not always reveal the reason for the genetic abnormality in a particular child.

Rasmussen (unpublished data, 2000) reported that the causes of more than 70% of birth defects are still unknown. Yoon and associates[5] wrote that "the specific genetic and environmental factors involved in the etiology of birth defects have, for the most part, eluded identification."

Genetic etiology is typically considered from the hereditary point of view, and therefore any genetic abnormality is assumed to be passed down from one or both parents. In limb deficiencies, however, the genetic defect often happens spontaneously, called a point mutation. With a point mutation, neither parent has, and therefore does not pass along, the genetic abnormality. This can be true even when the defect is known to have a future hereditary pattern, such as an autosomal dominant or autosomal recessive pattern.

In these situations, many families wonder if a specific factor, such as exposure to certain chemicals, was responsible for the event. Limb development begins in the 4th week of gestation and is nearly complete by the 8th week. If an outside agent is involved in transforming a specific gene, therefore, the exposure would have to occur within 8 weeks after conception, a time when most women do not know that they are pregnant. In most cases it is likely that no outside agent is to blame and that the genetic mutation simply happened for no reason we can identify with our current state of knowledge.

Agents responsible for birth defects may either have a direct impact on the tissue of the developing limb or induce a genetic abnormality that leads to the defect. Several toxins, medications, and even vitamins are known to affect limb development at early or later stages, the most notable being the medication known as thalidomide. This medication was prescribed between 1959 and 1962 to help relieve the nausea that is often associated with early pregnancy, but its inhibitory effect on angiogenesis resulted in many cases of phocomelia, a severe failure of development of the limbs. In very high doses, retinoic acid, or vitamin A, may also affect normal limb development. Therefore, the use of anti-acne treatments containing high doses of retinoic acid are not recommended in the childbearing period. Finally, Wang and associates[7] have reported that the periconceptual use of a multivitamin supplement might reduce the risk of transverse limb deficiencies.

Response to Limb Deficiency

Response to limb deficiency in children differs depending on whether the loss is congenital or acquired. Children with congenital deficiencies will try to do whatever other children do, and we find that the only limitations these children experience are those placed on them by adults. Left to their own devices, they are very adaptable. Amputees, on the other hand, want to be the same as they were before the amputation. They mourn the loss of the limb and are angry and resentful. Their motivation to use the deficient limb will be greatly influenced by their ability to resolve this inner turmoil.

Whether of congenital or acquired etiology, the child's limb deficiency is a great source of guilt for parents and other relatives. They will proceed through the stages of the universal grief process that Kübler-Ross[8] outlined. Initially they will experience shock, then denial and anger. Parents may approach their grief with bargaining, hoping to improve circumstances. They will also experience disappointment because their disabled child does not match their dreams. In time, with resolution and acceptance, they will develop more realistic expectations so that the child will receive needed support and nurturing. Health care professionals involved with families working through these stages must learn to recognize the changes as they occur and be prepared to alter their approach accordingly.

The Reverend Harold Wilke, born without arms and well-known for his work with disabled persons, once said that the most important action that his parents took while he was growing up was to decide to have another child. (Rev. Wilke, Annual Meeting of the Association of Children's Prosthetic/Orthotic Clinics, 1989).

That gesture showed him that they loved him sufficiently for who he was to risk having another child. Many of our patients' families, however, do not reach this point of adjustment; they never completely resolve their grief. The pediatric limb deficiency clinic team therefore must be concerned with not only the patient but also the parents and other relatives.

As children with limb deficiencies grow, they proceed through the same stages of development as do all children. In infancy, the accomplishment of normal motor milestones should be facilitated. A passive arm may offer balance or be a prop for sitting and crawling. A prosthetic leg becomes necessary when it is time to pull to stand. Developmentally oriented physical and occupational therapists are an invaluable part of the clinic team.

Adjustment to a Prosthesis

Little sound evidence exists to explain why some children adapt readily to a prosthesis and others reject anything that is placed on them. The difference between children's acceptance of upper and lower prosthetic limbs is well documented. Legs are required for mobility, and once the child realizes this, the prosthesis rarely comes off. Upper limb prostheses, on the other hand, are not always accepted with the same enthusiasm.

The upper limb prosthesis does not replace a missing arm to the same degree as a lower limb prosthesis replaces a leg. At best it is a tool, and if it does not enhance function, it will be rejected. Several authors[2,3] have studied the rejection of upper limb prostheses by children, but few conclusions have been reached. Clearly, cosmesis and function are two major concerns. A third factor, acceptance by the parents of the child's disability, may be even more important. A parent's acceptance of a cosmetic hand may have a far greater impact on whether it is worn than what the child

thinks of it. Children may also use prosthetic wearing practices to influence their relationship with their parents. For example, the prosthesis may become the object of rejection when a child is challenging parental authority, as in adolescence.

When limb-deficient children reach adolescence, they undergo the same intellectual and emotional changes as do other adolescents, but the limb deficiency makes this adjustment much more difficult. Frequently, adolescents reject their prosthesis when they are confronted with a new group of peers. They don't want to be "different." Once they are accepted into a group, they resume use of the prosthesis for greater function. This pattern can be seen sometimes with lower limb prostheses, but it occurs much more often with upper limb prostheses.

Children may continue to wear lower limb prostheses because they are needed for ambulation, but they may go to extremes to hide them. They may avoid swimming and wear clothes that mask the limb loss. These actions indicate that the child has not yet accepted his or her body image. Upper limb prostheses tend to be rejected outright when children experience frustration with themselves.

The Team Approach

There is no question that the child is not just a small adult and that a team approach is necessary to bring together professionals with expertise in addressing these concerns. In 1954, the need for an organized approach to the management of juvenile amputees across the United States was discussed at a meeting in Grand Rapids, Michigan. Subsequently, Gerald F.S. Strong, Chairman of the Prosthetics Research Board, appointed an interim committee of 10 members to pursue the issue. Charles H. Frantz, MD, chaired the first meeting at the University of California at Los Angeles in 1956. In 1959, the group officially became the Subcommittee on Child Prosthetic Programs within the National Acad-

emy of Sciences Prosthetics Research and Development Committee. The goal of the subcommittee was to raise the standards of prosthetic care for children in the United States. Before this time, prosthetic components were often not available in pediatric sizes. Prescriptions were withheld until the child started school and was then deemed to need a prosthesis.

To begin the dissemination of information and the establishment of clinical criteria, four major symposia were sponsored by the subcommittee to reflect the state of clinical expertise during the 1960s. By 1970, the subcommittee was charged to enlarge its sphere of activity to include children's orthoses and mobility aids. Under the guidance of Hector Kay, Assistant Executive Director of the Committee for Prosthetic Research and Development, the annual conferences were expanded to include cooperating clinic chiefs and their team members. The Association of Children's Prosthetic/Orthotic Clinics has held an annual interdisciplinary conference since 1972, and it is now the primary forum in North America for the exchange of information on the limb-deficient child. Members include not only individuals but also clinic teams, which stresses the importance of the team approach. As stated earlier, the limb-deficient child has multiple needs that can only be addressed by a team approach.

Surgical Considerations

Children and adults heal differently, and the skin of children, which is much more elastic than that of adults, better tolerates the stretching necessary to cover the end of the residual limb. Skin grafts often mature sufficiently to tolerate direct weight bearing as well as the shear forces experienced with socket wearing. The skin can also develop a callus and benefit from end bearing.

The skeletally immature child needs residual limb growth for good biomechanical function later. Growth potential differs in the child with a congenital deficiency and the child with an amputation. As a rule, the relative length discrepancy experienced in a congenital limb deficiency is maintained. One must not, however, leave this to chance. When planning the proper time for surgical intervention for a partial longitudinal deficiency of the femur (proximal femoral focal deficiency), the proper use of serial scanograms is necessary. With the newer techniques of limb lengthening and deformity corrections, proper documentation of growth potential is increasingly important.

Residual limb length is of vital concern for the child amputee, and the use of disarticulation rather than transosseous ablation should be considered to preserve as much length as possible. For example, because 70% of the growth of the femur comes from the distal femoral physis, a long transfemoral amputation in a 2-year-old results in a very short residual limb by the time the child becomes an adult. A knee disarticulation will avoid this problem. If a knee disarticulation is performed too close to the time of physeal closure, on the other hand, the relative retardation of physeal growth on that side may not be sufficient to avoid an overly long thigh. The solution to this dilemma is a distal femoral epiphysiodesis. This provides end-bearing ambulation with shorter length, allows transfemoral knee components, and provides good sitting and standing cosmesis.

Another reason to perform joint disarticulations rather than diaphyseal transections in children whenever possible is bony overgrowth, which frequently follows metaphyseal- or diaphyseal-level amputations. This is the major complication of amputation surgery in children, with an incidence variously reported in the range of 10% to 30%. Histologically, this is appositional bone growth of the remaining diaphysis and not growth from the remaining proximal physis. Various techniques of handling the bone and periosteum during amputation have failed to decrease the incidence of this complication. Silastic

caps or plugs have been tried, but the results are disappointing.[9,10] Marquardt[11] in Germany suggests transplanting a cartilaginous apophysis from the ilium or preserving an epiphysis from the amputated portion of the limb. Usually there is a bursal formation over the end of the bone, and it can become exquisitely tender. Occasionally, skin breakdown occurs and the bone may protrude. Socket modification can delay revision, but once the residual limb becomes sharply tapered, revision is necessary. This is often required repeatedly until skeletal growth ceases. The residual limb length is not shortened overall because the appositional growth has effectively added length to the bone.

One area where the option of preserving length at all costs must be carefully exercised is the posttraumatic partial foot amputation. For example, forefoot amputation caused by lawnmower injury frequently results in an infected residuum with plantar scarring. It is advantageous to be able to walk barefoot without a prosthesis, but making a functional partial foot prosthesis, especially for a less-than-optimal partial-foot amputation, is technically challenging. Concerns related to cosmesis, comfort, and function are very difficult to satisfy. Frequently, a Syme ankle disarticulation fitted with a prosthesis is the best option. This procedure leads to a cosmetically pleasing result in a child, in whom malleolar size is not a problem. Nevertheless, after investing much time and emotional effort to preserve length at all costs, the family is often unwilling to consider revision surgery as an alternative to a very clumsy partial foot prosthesis. This problem should therefore be carefully considered in the *initial* treatment of each partial foot amputation.

Prosthetic Considerations

Children have many unique prosthetic needs. As their minds and bodies grow, so do their residual limbs,

and frequent socket revisions or replacements are necessary to accommodate this growth. Lambert[12] reported on children followed up at the University of Illinois. He found they required a new lower limb prosthesis annually up to the age of 5 years, biannually from 5 to 12 years of age, and then once every 3 or 4 years until 21 years of age. The need for frequent and regular checkups by the clinic team is obvious.

The young and healthy tissue of a child's residual limb is different from that of the dysvascular tissue seen in many adult amputees. Consequently, alterations in fit are much better tolerated in children. Nevertheless, the frequent necessary changes present an economic concern. To lengthen the useful life of a prosthesis, materials should be used that are easily lengthened and modified, keeping in mind that the durability of children's prostheses is more important than their cosmesis. In that regard, soft covers, although cosmetically desirable, are easily damaged and therefore are not appropriate for the active child. Above all, prostheses must facilitate function, and those that the child must be careful of should be avoided.

In the past, prosthetic prescription was postponed to the purported ideal age at which a child could use an upper or lower limb prosthesis,[13] but now prostheses are prescribed at ages appropriate for specific terminal devices and feet. An effort has also been made to develop criteria for the prescription of costly myoelectric limbs for very young children. Some clinics are claiming that functional capabilities occur earlier than has been observed in sound limbs. Controlled studies are needed to evaluate the functional appropriateness of prescription ages. A recent collaborative study by a member of Shriners Hospital Clinics has demonstrated that very young children accept body-powered or electric-powered hands equally well.[14]

Lower limb components are being proposed for children on the basis of successes with adults. It remains controversial whether dynamic-response feet should be prescribed for children. Given the small body mass of the child and the frequent need for new limbs because of growth, the efficacy of these components needs to be demonstrated.

The epidemiology of traumatic amputations must be studied to learn how to provide a safer environment for children. Lawnmowers, farm implements, and recreational vehicles are all hazardous, especially to the inexperienced user.

The International Organization for Standardization (ISO) has adopted a definitive classification system for congenital limb deficiencies, as described in chapter 62. No longer is it necessary to learn a series of ancient language roots to describe patients; this new system, which uses only four basic terms—longitudinal, transverse, partial, and total—has been accepted by the International Society for Prosthetics and Orthotics and the Association of Children's Prosthetic/Orthotic Clinics. It will allow for a more concise database and the communication of statistics on an international basis.

Summary

The needs of limb-deficient children are indeed special. This section of the *Atlas* brings together state-of-the art information to help all the members of the clinic team provide better care for these children.

References

1. Dillingham TR, Pezzin LE, MacKensie EJ: Limb amputation and limb deficiency: Epidemiology and recent trends in the United States. *South Med J* 2002;95:875-883.
2. Froster UG, Baird PA: Congenital defects of lower limbs and associated malformations: A population based study. *Am J Med Genet* 1993;45:60-64.
3. Kallen B, Rahmani TM, Winberg J: Infants with congenital limb reduction registered in the Swedish Register of Congenital Malformations. *Teratol* 1984;29:73-85.
4. McGuirk CK, Westgate MN, Holmes LB: Limb deficiencies in newborn infants. *Pediatrics* 2001;108:E64.
5. Yoon PW, Rasmussen SA, Lynberg MC, et al: The National Birth Defects Prevention Study. *Public Health Rep* 2001;116(suppl 1):32-40.
6. Brent RL: Prevention of physical and mental congenital defects: Part A. The scope of the problem, in Marois M (ed): *Progress in Clinical and Biological Research*. New York, NY, Alan R Liss, 1985, vol 163A, pp 55-68.
7. Wang GW, Gaugher WH, Stamp WG: Epiphyseal transplants in amputations. *Clin Orthop* 1978;350:285-288.
8. Kübler-Ross E: *On Death and Dying*. New York, NY, Macmillan Publishing, 1969.
9. Swanson AB: Bony overgrowth in the juvenile amputee and its control by the use of silicone rubber implants. *Inter-Clin Info Bull* 1969;8:9-18.
10. Meyer LC, Sauer BW: The use of porous, high-density polyethylene caps in the prevention of appositional bone growth in the juvenile amputee: A preliminary report. *Inter-Clin Info Bull* 1975;14:9-10.
11. Marquardt TE: Plastische Operatione bei drohender Knochenburchspiesung am kindlichen Oberarmstumpf: Eine vorlaufige Mitteilung. *Z Orthop* 1976;114:711-714.
12. Lambert C: Amputation surgery in the child. *Orthop Clin North Am* 1972;3:473-482.
13. MacDonnell JA: Age of fitting upper extremity prostheses in children. *J Bone Joint Surg Am* 1958;40:655-662.
14. Patterson DB: Acceptance rate of myoelectric prostheses. *J Assoc Child Prosthet Orthot Clin* 1990;25:73-76.

Chapter 62

Terminology in Pediatric Limb Deficiency

John R. Fisk, MD

Introduction

As the world continues to shrink and as international communication becomes commonplace, an internationally accepted system of terminology that translates easily into different languages is of paramount importance. This was the goal of those who set out to devise a system of nomenclature for pediatric limb deficiencies.

Terminology for traumatic and surgical amputations in children follows the traditional practices used to name adult amputations. The problem arises with naming obvious failures of formation. To call such deficiencies congenital amputations, as had been done for many years, was recognized as inappropriate. In addition, some terms were based on Latin and Greek stems that did not translate consistently in languages with different origins. To remedy such problems, two different systems of nomenclature for congenital limb deficiencies were developed and came to be widely used, one in the United States and one in Germany.

In 1961, Frantz and O'Rahilly[1] published a system that, with slight modifications by others,[2,3] persists in the vocabulary of many practitioners in the United States. This system introduced such terms as amelia, hemimelia, and phocomelia. These terms also proved to have some drawbacks, however. For example, the term hemimelia means simply "half a limb." The question then arises as to whether the term should be applied to a missing longitudinal or transverse segment. These types of issues kept practitioners in Europe from accepting the Frantz and O'Rahilly system. In Germany, a different system of nomenclature developed. By the early 1960s, terms such as peromelia, ectomelia, and dysmelia, which never have been used in the United States, were recommended.[3,4]

In 1970, a working group of the International Society for Prosthetics and Orthotics met in Dundee, Scotland, with the goal of deriving a system of terminology that would gain wider acceptance. This method was published in 1974[5] and with only minor modification was ultimately accepted by the International Organization for Standardization (ISO) in 1989.

ISO Standard for Describing Limb Deficiencies Present at Birth*

International Standard 8548-1:1989,[6] which addresses limb deficiencies present at birth, is summarized here. The standard has three constraints:

1. The classification is restricted to skeletal deficiencies, where the majority of such cases are due to a failure of formation of parts.
2. The deficiencies are described on the basis of anatomic and radiologic characteristics only. No attempt is made to classify in terms of embryology, etiology, or epidemiology.
3. Classically derived terms such as hemimelia and peromelia are avoided because of their lack of precision and the difficulty of translation into languages that are not related to Greek.

Deficiencies are described as transverse or longitudinal. The former resemble an amputation residual limb in that the limb has developed normally to a particular level beyond which no skeletal elements are present. All other cases, in which there is a reduction or absence of an element or elements within the long axis of the limb, are classified as longitudinal.

Method of Description
Transverse Deficiencies

With transverse deficiencies, the limb has developed normally to a particular level beyond which no skeletal ele-

---

*Copies of standard 8548-1:1989 are available from the ISO Central Secretariat, 1, rue de Darembé, Case Postale 56, CH-1211 Geneva 20, Switzerland, http://www.iso.org, or from any ISO member body.

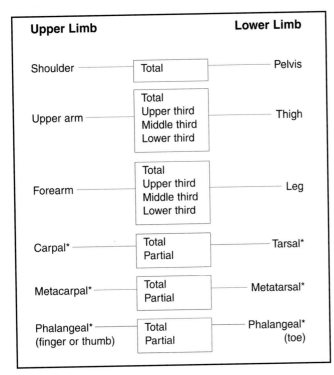

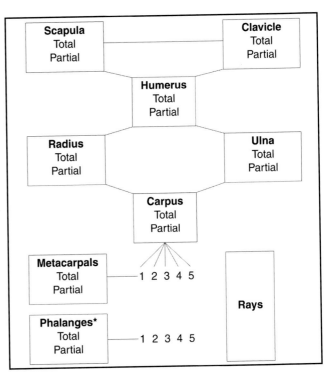

Figure 1 ISO designation of levels of transverse deficiencies of upper and lower limbs. Note that the skeletal elements marked with an asterisk are used as adjectives in describing transverse deficiencies; for example, transverse carpal total deficiency. A total absence of the shoulder or hemipelvis (and all distal elements) is a transverse deficiency. If only a portion of the shoulder or hemipelvis is absent, the deficiency is of the longitudinal type.

Figure 2 Description of longitudinal deficiencies of the upper limb using the ISO system. The asterisk indicates that the digits of the hand are sometimes referred to by name: 1 = thumb; 2 = index; 3 = middle; 4 = ring; 5 = little (or small). For the purpose of this classification, such naming is deprecated because it is not equally applicable to the foot.

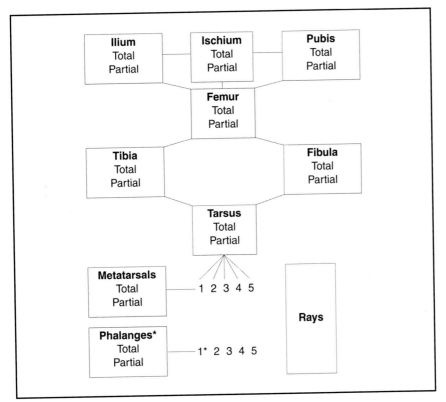

Figure 3 Description of longitudinal deficiencies of the lower limb using the ISO system. The asterisk indicates the great toe, or hallux.

ments exist, although there may be digital buds. Such deficiencies are described by naming the segment at which the limb terminates and then describing the level within the segment beyond which no skeletal elements exist; for example, "transverse deficiency, forearm, upper one third" (Figure 1). To describe deficiencies at the phalangeal level, another descriptor can be added to indicate the precise level of loss.

Longitudinal Deficiencies

With longitudinal deficiencies, there is a reduction or absence of an element or elements within the long axis of the limb. There may be normal skeletal elements distal to the affected bone or bones. The following procedure should be followed to describe such a deficiency (Figures 2 and 3):

1. Name the bones affected, from proximal to distal, using the name as a noun. Any bone not named is present and of normal form.

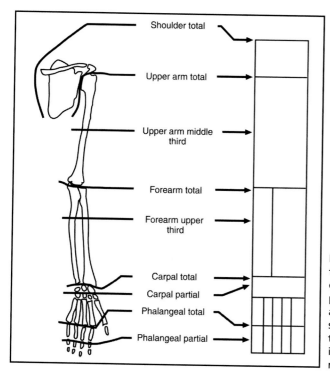

Figure 4 The Day system of recording deficiencies. Transverse upper limb deficiencies at various levels are shown on the skeleton and in Day's stylized version on the right.

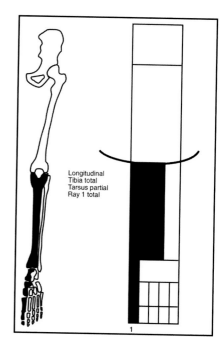

Longitudinal
Tibia total
Tarsus partial
Ray 1 total

Figure 5 An example of a longitudinal deficiency is shown on the skeleton and in Day's stylized representation on the right, which shows not only the original deficiency but also the treatment by knee disarticulation.

2. State whether each affected bone is totally or partially absent.

3. In the case of partial deficiencies, the approximate fraction and the position of the absent part may be stated.

4. For metacarpals, metatarsals, and phalanges, the number of the digit should be stated, with the number starting from the preaxial, radial, or tibial side.

5. The term ray may be used to refer to a metacarpal or metatarsal and its corresponding phalanges.

For example, for a fibular hemimelia and partial foot, the new terminology would be "partial longitudinal deficiency of the distal two thirds of the fibula, complete deficiency of the fourth and fifth rays of the foot."

The Day System

Day, a member of the original Kay committee of the International Society for Prosthetics and Orthotics that developed the system described above, devised a convenient method of recording deficiencies, which is shown in Figures 4 and 5. It is presented here for the consideration of the reader but should not be considered a part of the ISO nomenclature scheme.

References

1. Frantz CH, O'Rahilly R: Congenital skeletal limb deficiencies. *J Bone Joint Surg Am* 1961;43:1202-1224.

2. Nomenclature for congenital skeletal limb deficiencies: A revision of the Frantz and O'Rahilly classification. *Artif Limbs* 1966;10:24-35.

3. Henkel L, Willert HG: Dysmelia: A classification and a pattern of malformation in a group of congenital defect of the limbs. *J Bone Joint Surg Br* 1969;51:399-414.

4. Willert HG, Henkel HL: (eds): *Klinik und Pathologie der Dysmelie: Die Fehlbidungen an den oberen Extremitäten bei der Thalidomid-Embryopathie.* Springer-Verlag, Berling, NY, 1969.

5. Kay HW: A proposed international terminology for the classification of congenital limb deficiencies. *Inter-Clin Info Bull* 1974;13:1-16.

6. International Organization for Standardization: ISO 8548-1: Prosthetics and orthotics—Limb deficiencies, Part 1: Method of describing limb deficiencies present at birth. Geneva, Switzerland, International Organization for Standardization, 1989:1-6.

Chapter 63

Developmental Kinesiology

Joan E. Edelstein, MA, PT

Introduction

Understanding how infants without limb deficiencies grow, develop, and move can help families and clinicians determine approaches that are age appropriate for children with limb deficiencies. This chapter integrates norms established for normal children with the needs of children with congenital deficiencies or acquired amputations. A child is a growing, developing person, and clinical intervention, both in terms of prostheses and activities, should keep pace with and foster the emergence of the young person's abilities. Although growth and development begin at conception, this chapter addresses postnatal events.

Behavior is goal directed: the infant's curiosity leads to exploration of space visually, orally, aurally, and by means of hand movements, rolling, crawling, creeping, and walking. Cognitive and psychosocial factors interact with the infant's changing motor control, morphology, and physiology. For those with limb deficiency, intellectual functioning appears to be unrelated to the severity of the limb deficiency.[1] As casual observation in any playground or clinic confirms, children display considerable intersubject and intrasubject variability. Motor maturity appears to be influenced by trial and error, autonomous central pattern generators, and genetically predetermined central nervous system connections as the child solves the innumerable problems of dominating his or her universe.[2]

Contemporary evaluations of motor development, such as the Alberta Infant Motor Scale,[3] Bayley Scales of Infant Development,[4] Bruininks-Oseretsky Test of Motor Proficiency,[5] Denver II,[6] and the Pediatric Evaluation of Disability Inventory,[7] and screening tools developed by Bly[8] and Illingworth[9] present a relatively similar time frame for attainment of motor milestones. The Functional Status Inventory for Toddlers identifies developmental achievements by those with upper or lower limb deficiency.[10] Developmental targets can help guide prosthetic prescriptions[11,12] and treatment goals[13,14] (Figure 1).

Body Alignment

Because of the position that had been assumed within the uterus and the immaturity of the nervous system, the newborn displays a flexed posture.[15] When the newborn is placed prone, the arms and legs tuck under the torso, forcing weight onto the upper thorax. The head is turned to the side to facilitate breathing. From this position, an infant develops the ability to lift the head against gravity and to rotate it from side to side; these skills are accomplished, on average, within the first month after birth. The infant eventually lifts the head and upper trunk off the bed and comes to rest on the internally rotated forearms in the "on-elbows posture." Although infants now spend less time prone because of the current thinking that "back is best" when sleeping to avoid sudden infant death syndrome, normal infants learn to lift the head when given the opportunity to be prone. Six-month-old infants become proficient at pivoting on the abdomen to gaze at an interesting aspect of the environment. Stability in the prone position enables independent arm and leg movements to enhance exploration of space.[16]

In the supine position, the infant keeps the upper and lower limbs acutely flexed, with the ankles acutely dorsiflexed. Shoulders, elbows, and hands are also flexed. When the examiner extends the infant's limbs, they rebound back to flexion, indicating flexor tone, reflecting both the elasticity of soft tissues and central nervous system response. By the end of the first month, the newborn can keep the head in the midline position. At 3 months of age, the infant lies in extension, perhaps from increased control of the limb and trunk extensors as well as the effect of gravity.[15] By age 9 months, many infants discover side lying, either as a posture for playing or as a pause during the act of rolling from supine to prone.

With development, arm posture changes from flexion to abduction and extension when the head is in

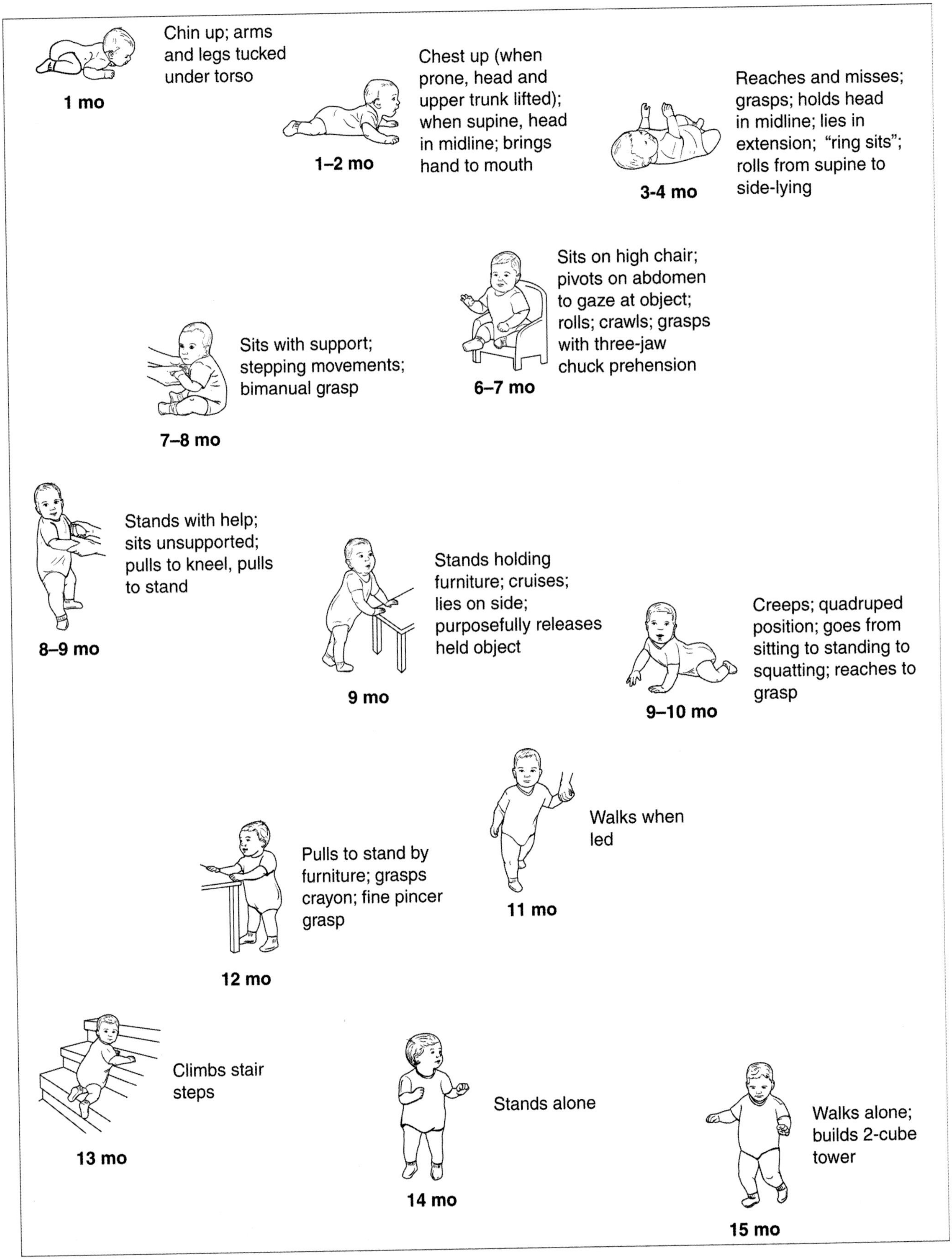

Figure 1   Normal developmental milestones in infants and young children.

midline. When the head is turned to the right, the infant exhibits an asymmetric tonic neck reflex posture. The right arm abducts and the right leg is extended. The left arm is externally rotated with the elbow flexed.

Culturally related practices may affect the development of skills. In the United States, for example, infants are often placed in the prone position during the day, whereas British infants are more likely to be supine, and skills in the preferred posture are likely to be more advanced.[16]

Sitting

Infants have enough muscle tone to support themselves when held in the seated or standing position; however, they are not able to sit or stand independently because their proprioception and balance coordination are immature. Initially, when the neonate is held in the sitting position, the head oscillates from extension to flexion. A 3-month-old infant should be able to hold the head steady in midline. At this age, infants are capable of "ring sitting," propping themselves forward on the hands with the head held in midline, the hips abducted and externally rotated, the knees flexed, and the soles touching. A few months later, the infant develops trunk control by briefly extending the trunk, abducting the shoulders, and flexing the elbows in a position called "high guard."[16]

By age 8 months, many infants can sit with support for 15 minutes or longer. At about the same time, the baby learns protective extension, bringing the hands to the supporting surface to prevent toppling forward. Unsupported sitting is common by age 8 or 9 months. The seated posture allows the infant to reach for, grasp, bang, and mouth objects. The infant gains skill at retrieving dropped toys by shifting weight laterally. Most clinics fit prostheses before the infant is 9 months old, but some recommend that the first upper limb prosthesis be fitted when the infant begins sitting,[17] and a few offer a prosthesis to those younger than 3 months.[18]

By age 9 months, the infant can move from sitting to the all-fours position, also known as the quadruped position, supporting weight on the hands and knees. This is a good position for rocking, which provides proprioceptive cues to the arms and legs and stimulates the vestibular system. A month or two later, the infant is proficient at sitting, capable of moving from prone to sitting, from sitting to the quadruped position, or from sitting to kneeling and then standing. The child can sit in a high chair, resting the feet on the footrest. "W" sitting, where the hips are internally rotated and the hips and knees are flexed, is often seen, although infants with dislocated hips should be discouraged from this posture. Some infants prefer side sitting.[16]

Standing

The first indication of standing is primary standing, in which the neonate maintains standing when supported. Usually, the feet are hyperadducted and may be plantar flexed. By age 4 months, primary standing abates and is replaced by "giving way," in which the infant, when supported, caves into hip and knee flexion. The standing posture (known as secondary standing) appears at about age 5 months. The hips are abducted, the knees extended, and the feet are plantigrade. When supported at the axillae, the infant will bounce up and down. Early stepping movements are likely at 7 months, if the infant is supported. These milestones are based on systematic observations of infants without limb deficiencies. Anecdotal evidence suggests that infants with lower limb deficiencies place the intact leg closer to the midline to achieve this milestone.

By age 8 months, infants become proficient at pulling to kneel and then pulling to stand, supporting themselves on the railings of the crib or other stable structures. Self-supported standing begins with flexed hips. Eventually the hip extensors contract to produce a more stable stance. Ini-

tially, arm strength enables the youngster to pull to stand and to travel laterally along the support structure. The infant will shift weight from side to side, stamping one foot and then the other. By age 10 months, the infant can switch from sitting to standing and back to squatting easily.[16]

Skeletal changes contribute to proficiency in standing. Femoral torsion progresses from retroversion of about 35° at birth to about 11° as an adult, contributing to stability of the femoral head in the acetabulum. The femoral-tibial axis changes from initial varus to valgus at age 2 to 3 years, then straightens. Development of normal cervical lordosis may be related to neck extensor activity. Limitation of hip extension reflects the usual tightness of the iliopsoas during the neonatal period. Neonates (those younger than 1 month) typically exhibit more external than internal rotation of the hip.[19]

Locomotion

Prenatal kicking, jumping, and responding to stimuli give way to postnatal stretching, kicking, and thrusting of the arms and legs and rotation of the head and trunk.[20] By the fourth month, infants can roll from supine to side-lying, turning the head and trunk in "log rolling" fashion. Rolling on a regular basis is uncommon until age 6 to 7 months.

When supine, the infant lifts the legs off the bed, bringing the feet toward the hands and mouth. The infant will tumble to the side, driven by the weight of the legs. Lifting the legs and extending and rotating the head prepare the youngster to roll independently, which ordinarily occurs by age 7 or 8 months. Another early maneuver is bridging, in which the infant places the feet on the supporting surface with the hips and knees flexed and extends the trunk and hip, raising the buttocks.

By age 4 months, the infant engages in push-up behavior when in the prone position, actively extending the neck, trunk, and elbows to support weight on the hands. At age 5 months, the push-up involves support by the hands and knees. From this posture, the infant can rock back and forth and side to side.[16]

Crawling, maneuvering across the floor with the hands while in the prone position, involves pushing and pulling with the arms and legs while the abdomen grazes the surface. This skill is typical of a 6-month-old infant.

Creeping, which is more sophisticated than crawling, is likely to appear by 10 months of age. It requires the infant to extend the trunk sufficiently to keep the abdomen off the floor while being supported by the hands and knees. The infant alternates movement of the right arm and left leg, and then pulls forward with the left arm and right leg. Some infants discover plantigrade creeping, supporting weight on the palms and soles. Infants with unilateral upper limb deficiency will perform a modified creeping maneuver, supporting themselves with the intact hand placed closed to the midline.

Another mode of locomotion is hitching, sometimes called scooting. The seated infant leans on one hand and externally rotates the ipsilateral hip while elevating the opposite leg. The youngster then plants the opposite foot and pushes with that leg to slide the buttocks across the support surface.

The 9-month-old infant will probably cruise, shifting weight from one foot to the other while supporting himself or herself with the hands on crib railings or other furniture. Weight is usually borne on the forefeet. Goal-directed ambulation begins at approximately age 10 months.[2] Another prewalking skill is clambering up stairs and low chairs, which demonstrates the ability to flex the hips independently and use the upper limbs for assistance.

By age 1 year, the child steps diagonally forward and sideward, which widens the walking base.[21] Independent walking is flat-footed with con-siderable trunk waddling.[22] Lateral trunk bending also serves to advance the leg. The beginning walker is somewhat top-heavy. The center of gravity is closer to the xiphoid process than to the sacrum,[15] necessitating holding the arms in "high guard" to aid stability; consequently, carrying a toy is difficult at this age.[23] Collapse into a fall is common, but the child is proficient at resuming upright balance.[4] The child takes short steps and keeps the trunk and limbs stiffly extended.[21]

At 18 to 20 months of age, the child relinquishes high guarding and parental hand support and becomes able to carry a toy while walking. Initial contact matures to heel loading. The base is more narrow, and the toddler can walk backward.[15] Stooping and rising are skillful.

During the second year of life, the child discovers jumping off a low box, running, ball kicking, and hopping.[24]

Children first rise from a chair by lifting the leg, flexing the trunk forward to enable sliding off the seat, and finally extending the hips and trunk. Skipping, which involves a step and a hop first on one foot and then the other, is not mastered until about age 6 years, although a younger child can balance on one foot for several seconds.[25] At about the same age, the youngster learns to kick, balancing on one foot while transferring force to the ball. The backswing appears first at the knee and later the hip. Follow-through and forward trunk lean are more sophisticated refinements.[16]

Rising from the floor is accomplished first by coming forward from supine, flexing and rotating the trunk. One hand reaches forward while the other pushes against the floor. The legs are placed wide apart in a squat and then to the upright stance. Rising matures by age 7 years,[16] as does gait.[26] Other ambulatory skills, such as cycling, skating, skiing, skateboarding, dancing, jumping rope, and stilt walking, become part of the child's motor repertoire.

Upper Limb Control

The newborn's grasp is reflexive without thumb activity.[15] Nevertheless, within a few days of birth, the neonate displays rudimentary eye-hand coordination when the trunk is supported and a moving target is presented.[27] When supine, the 1-month-old infant is apt to thrust the arms upward, although the hands are usually fisted. Between age 2 and 3 months, many infants attempt to bring a hand to the mouth.[4] This development is sometimes regarded as indicating readiness for fitting a passive prosthesis. The device satisfies parental needs for disguise of the limb deficiency, lengthens the deficient limb so that it can later interact with the intact limb, and assists the child's balance.[28] Eye-hand control becomes evident as the baby explores its body while supine. Infants can focus on an object held close to their face and will turn the head to track the item. Arm motion consists primarily of ballistic swipes and swats.[24] By age 3 to 4 months, the infant can turn the head beyond midline to follow an interesting target[20] and will grab an object within reach.[27] At 4 months, the infant can grasp a rattle voluntarily and enjoys noisy toys,[15] rotating and shaking them easily.[24]

The 5-month-old infant will have relaxed the fisted posture and will rotate the wrist to grab at a rattle or other small toy.[4] The infant swipes at brightly colored dangling objects, supporting himself or herself on the hands and knees and shifting weight to one hand while brushing or grabbing the toy with the other hand. When supported, the infant brings the hands together. Transferring an object from one hand to the other is done haphazardly. The infant gains skill at visually pursuing an object without necessarily relying on tactile feedback; this may indicate the desirability of prosthetic fitting before tactile dependence develops.[20]

At age 6 months, the infant still uses the whole hand to grasp a rod[4] but is increasingly able to grasp a cube with three-jaw chuck prehension.[25] Unlike a younger infant, the 6-month-old can differentiate among reach, grasp, manipulation, and release.[24] Functional reaching involves the perceptual ability to interpret the environment and then to orient the hand toward the object.[27] The infant has learned that the hands are extensions of oneself that facilitate bringing objects to the midline. This is the rationale for fitting the 6-month-old infant with a prosthesis.[29] At this age, many babies can sit securely and transfer an object from one hand to the other,[6,15,24] as well as hold an object in one hand while the other bangs it or picks at it.[24] Rudimentary elements of handedness appear,[25] although hand dominance is not fully established until age 2 years.[15]

Holding an object such as a spoon in each hand and bringing them to the midline is typical by age 8 months, but the infant cannot yet release one object to pick up another. Grip and load forces are coordinated sequentially. Upon initial contact with the object, the infant lingers before initiating adequate grip force and tends to press on the object before reversing the direction of force to lift it.[27] The infant is not yet able to anticipate the object's weight so as to select an appropriate target force. Grasping a crayon is likely by 1 year of age.[4] The 9-month-old infant starts to show true release, dropping one object to pick up another. The youngster can trap a moving object.[27] Within the month, the child uses the index finger for pointing and can release objects without simply dropping them.[15] The youngster can now use both hands for goal-oriented functions, such as opening a box with one hand and taking out its contents with the other.[24]

Integration of sitting and arm use is particularly evident at age 10 months, when the infant can reach as far forward as 10 inches without toppling. At 11 months, the infant can remove a cube from a cup, indicating improved eye-hand coordination as well as a sense of depth and dimen-

sion. Fine pincer grasp is expected at age 1 year.[15]

At 15 months, most children can build a two-cube tower, displaying excellent grasp, placement, and release as well as shoulder, elbow, and hand control.[25] A few months later, the child can turn pages in a book. By the second birthday, a child can usually turn single pages, fold paper, copy a vertical line,[15] and eat from a spoon.[24]

The 3-year-old child can build a 10-cube tower, may be able to build a bridge with blocks, and can copy a circle and a cross, which involves lifting the pencil from the paper at appropriate intervals.[25] A child of this age can also assist with hand washing and drying and can unbutton and unzip clothing.[15]

At age 4 years, the child can cut paper with scissors, button and lace clothing, and pour from a pitcher. Hair combing and tooth brushing are expected of the 5-year-old.[15]

A cookie crusher myoelectric prosthesis powered by a miniature electric circuit has been fitted to infants as young as 7 months.[30] A survey of 28 clinics revealed that more than one third of the patients were fitted before age 9 months, when sitting is well established, although a few infants received prostheses before age 3 months.[18] In another series, the average age of first myoelectric prosthesis fitting was 9 months, although half of the children received prostheses before they were 6 months old.[31]

The ability to throw a ball develops during the first year of life,[4] although catching is unlikely before age 3 years. Initially, the child will hold the arms in front of the trunk. Later, the child learns to follow the trajectory of the ball and to flex the arms to absorb the force of impact. Subsequent skills include refinement in grasp pattern, force, and accuracy in catching and throwing.[16]

The 2-year-old child usually can use the hand to hold paper in place while drawing. The 3-year-old child should be able to string beads and buttons.[4]

Prosthetic Considerations

Infants younger than age 2 years have been fitted with myoelectrically controlled prostheses.[32,33] For children with cable-controlled prostheses, terminal device activation before age 2 years is appropriate because the child is ready for bilateral grasp at this age. Prosthetic use discourages the child from developing compensatory unimanual motor control.[34]

Children with upper limb deficiencies have less strength, both on the deficient and on the opposite side, than do normal children.[35] Therefore, these factors should be considered in the design of prostheses and in the development of functional standards.

Myoelectric fitting and training at 3 years of age can proceed according to Hermansson's 14-step skill index, from wearing the prosthesis and using it as support to controlled grip while throwing overhead.[36]

Children with severe limb deficiencies may develop alternate skills, such as prehensile grasping with the head and shoulder or using the toes.[1] The hand function of young children with prostheses differs from that of children without deficiencies, and this should be considered when choosing developmentally appropriate prosthetic designs.[37]

Conclusions

Growth and development of motor skills proceed in an orderly sequence, although the age at which infants and children attain motor milestones varies. Fitting infants and children with equipment that exceeds their level of maturity can negatively affect their welfare, the parents' expectations and resources, and the efforts of the rehabilitation team. To support the child's progress, age-appropriate prostheses should be provided, and the child should be engaged in suitable activities.

References

1. French RW: Motor development and intellectual functioning: An exploratory study. *Inter-Clin Info Bull* 1973; 12:13-15.

2. Leonard CT: The neurophysiology of human locomotion, in Craik RL, Oatis CA: *Gait Analysis: Theory and Application.* St Louis, MO, Mosby, 1995, pp 46-64.

3. Piper MC, Pinnell LE, Darrah J, et al: Construction and validation of the Alberta Infant Motor Scale (AIMS). *Can J Public Health* 1992;83(suppl): 46-50.

4. Aylward GP: *Bayley Infant Neurodevelopmental Screen Manual.* San Antonio, TX, The Psychological Corporation, 1996.

5. Bruininks RH: *Bruininks-Oseretsky Test of Motor Proficiency. Examiner's Manual.* Circle Pines, MN, American Guidance Services, 1978.

6. Frankenburg WK, Dodds JB, Archer P, et al: The Denver II: A major revision and restandardization of the DDST. *Pediatrics* 1992;89:91-97.

7. Feldman AB, Haley SM, Coryell J: Concurrent and construct validity of the Pediatric Evaluation of Disability Inventory. *Phys Ther* 1990;70:602-610.

8. Bly L: *Motor Skill Acquisition in the First Year.* Tucson, AZ, Therapy Skill Builders, 1994.

9. Illingworth RS: *Basic Developmental Screening 0-4 Years.* Boston, MA, Blackwell Scientific Publications, 1990.

10. Pruitt SD, Seid M, Varni JW, Setoguchi Y: Toddlers with limb deficiency: Conceptual basis and initial application of a functional status outcome measure. *Arch Phys Med Rehabil* 1999;80: 819-824.

11. Cummings DR: Pediatric prosthetics: Current trends and future possibilities. *Phys Med Rehabil Clin N Am* 2000; 11:653-679.

12. Jain S: Rehabilitation in limb deficiency: 2. The pediatric amputee. *Arch Phys Med Rehabil* 1996;77:S9-13.

13. Clarke SD, Patton JG: Occupational therapy for the limb-deficient child: A developmental approach to treatment planning and selection of prostheses for infants and young children with unilateral upper extremity limb deficiencies. *Clin Orthop* 1980;148:47-54.

14. Patton JG: Developmental approach to pediatric prosthetic evaluation and training, in Meier RH, Atkins DJ (eds): *Functional Restoration of Adults and Children With Upper Extremity Amputation.* New York, NY, Demos, 2003.

15. Sobus KML, Karkos JB: Growth and development, in Gonzalez EG, Myers SJ, Edelstein JE, et al (eds): *Downey & Darling's Physiological Basis of Rehabilitation Medicine,* ed 3. Boston, MA, Butterworth-Heinemann, 2001, pp547-560.

16. Goldberg C, Van Sant A. Normal motor development, in Tecklin JS (ed): *Pediatric Physical Therapy,* ed 3. Philadelphia, PA, Lippincott Williams & Wilkins, 1999, pp 1-27.

17. Watts HG, Corideo J, Dow M: An upper-limb prosthesis for infants. *J Assoc Child Prosthet Orthot Clin* 1985; 20:55-56.

18. Sypniewski BL: Questionnaire survey concerning age at initial fitting. *Inter-Clin Information Bull* 1972;11:1-17.

19. Walker JM: Musculoskeletal development: A review. *Phys Ther* 1991;71: 878-889.

20. Fisher AG: Initial prosthetic fitting of the congenital below-elbow amputee: Are we fitting them early enough? *Inter-Clin Info Bull* 1976;15:7-10.

21. Stout JL: Gait: Development and analysis, in Campbell SK (ed): *Physical Therapy for Children.* Philadelphia, PA, WB Saunders, 1994, pp 79-104.

22. Gage JR: *Gait Analysis in Cerebral Palsy.* London, England, MacKeith, 1991.

23. Higgins JR, Higgins S: The acquisition of locomotor skill, in Craik RL, Oatis CA: *Gait Analysis: Theory and Application.* St. Louis, MO, Mosby, 1995, pp 65-78.

24. Campbell SK: The child's development of functional movement, in Campbell SK (ed): *Physical Therapy for Children.* Philadelphia, PA, WB Saunders, 1994, pp 3-38.

25. Prosthetic-Orthotic Education: *Management of the Juvenile Amputee.* Chicago, IL, Northwestern University, 1964.

26. Sutherland DH, Olshen R, Biden EN, Wyatt MP: *The Development of Mature Walking.* London, England, MacKeith, 1988.

27. Bradley NS: Motor control: Developmental aspects of motor control in skill acquisition, in Campbell SK (ed): *Physical Therapy for Children.* Philadelphia, PA, WB Saunders, 1994, pp 39-78.

28. Curran B, Hambrey R: The prosthetic treatment of upper limb deficiency. *Prosthet Orthot Int* 1991;15:82-87.

29. DiCowden MA, Ballard A, Robinette H, Ortiz O: Benefit of early fitting and behavior modification training with a voluntary closing terminal device. *J Assoc Child Prosthet Orthot Clin* 1987; 22:47-50.

30. Williams TW: One-muscle infant's myoelectric control. *J Assoc Child Prosthet Orthot Clin* 1989;24:53-56.

31. Menkveld SR, Novotny MP, Schwartz M: Age-appropriateness of myoelectric prosthetic fitting. *J Assoc Child Prosthet Orthot Clin* 1987;22:60-65.

32. Datta D, Ibbotson V: Powered prosthetic hands in very young children. *Prosthet Orthot Int* 1998;22:150-154.

33. Mifsud M, Al-Tennen I, Sauter W, et al: Variety Village electromechanical hand for amputees under two year of age. *J Assoc Child Prosthet Orthot Clin* 1987;22:41-46.

34. Trefler E: Terminal device activation for infant amputees. *Inter-Clin Info Bull.* 1970;9:11-14.

35. Shaperman J, Leblanc M, Setoguchi Y, McNeal DR: Is body powered operation of upper limb prostheses feasible for young limb deficient children? *Prosthet Orthot Int* 1995;19:165-175.

36. Hermansson LM: Structured training of children fitted with myoelectric prostheses. *Prosthet Orthot Int* 1991;15: 88-92.

37. Shaperman J, Landsberger S, Setoguchi Y: How toddlers hold objects: Designing a new hand and measuring grip function. *Orthop Trans* 1999;22:460.

Chapter 64

General Prosthetic Considerations

Donald R. Cummings, CP, LP

Introduction

The child with a congenital deficiency or acquired amputation presents a paradox to most practitioners. With or without a prosthesis, children continually accomplish things never expected or even considered possible. Their balance and dexterity are amazing, as is their preference for activities that seem totally inconsistent with limb absence, such as the double leg amputee who wants to be a running back or the transhumeral amputee who becomes a guitarist. Even veteran pediatric clinicians remain fascinated when a girl who is missing both arms uses her feet to put in her pierced earrings or sculpts or paints with her toes. Children have a miraculous capacity to adapt.

The development of a child into an adult is full of surprising twists and turns and unexpected outcomes. The same growth and change also characterize the practice of pediatric prosthetics. For those who provide prosthetic care for children with limb deficiencies, a few general observations and philosophies can be set forth, combined with a short but frequently debated list of standardized practices.

Pediatric Prosthetic Considerations

In most pediatric prosthetic clinics, about 70% of children younger than 15 years of age present with a congenital deficiency that can either be fitted with a prosthesis or for which amputation is the recommended treatment.[1] These presentations include deficiencies of the tibia or fibula; longitudinal deficiency of the femur, partial (LDFP, formerly called proximal focal femoral deficiency, or PFFD); amputations resulting from amniotic band constriction (Streeter's dysplasia); and various transverse or longitudinal absences of the upper and lower limbs.[2] (Many transverse absences are functional homologs of an amputation. Because no surgical or in utero ablation ever occurred, such conditions are not true amputations. However, perhaps for lack of a better replacement, the term has stuck.) Many children with congenital limb deficiencies will also demonstrate the biomechanical challenges that Aitken and Pellicore[3] described as being associated with their conditions—inadequate proximal musculature, unstable joints, malrotation, and limb-length differences. Multiple limb involvement occurs in perhaps 40% of cases.[4] Trauma (eg, motor vehicle accidents, burns, power tool or lawn-mower injuries) and cancer and other diseases account for the remaining 30% of amputations in children.

In addition to designing "typical" artificial limbs, prosthetists who work with children are often called upon to construct highly customized non-standard devices. One example is the equinus, or step-in, prosthesis that is fitted around an existing foot. McCollough and associates[5] described four situations for using such nonstandard prostheses: (1) surgical conversion has been refused; (2) surgical conversion has been delayed; (3) longitudinal deficiencies are being observed; and (4) amputation is not an option because the child's upper limbs are involved, requiring the child to use the feet to substitute for hand function.

Increasingly, children who might previously have required amputation for cancer may now present with an endoprosthesis combined with an amputation, or they may have undergone a rotationplasty.[6] A modified rotationplasty, which rotates the foot 180°, is sometimes performed for children with LDFP to enable their ankle to function as a knee.

Regardless of the etiology of their limb deficiency, most children are very active and participate in diverse activities ranging from soccer, baseball, dance, and swimming to playing instruments or video games, marching in a band, cheerleading, golfing, or rock climbing. Although many of these activities can be performed with conventional prostheses, children and adolescents often benefit from prostheses that are customized for specific activities. Thus the pediatric prosthetist is faced not only with a challenging array of conditions and levels, but also with meeting diverse needs that are complicated by the dynamic, ever-changing nature of pediatric clients.

The fact that children continually grow and change provides the prosthetist and clinic team with some unique opportunities. On average, a child may require a new prosthesis every year or two, creating the advantage of an accelerated learning curve. Opportunities to observe and improve upon what was done previously occur much more frequently than with adult prosthetic care. Thus the clinic team, patient, and family can work together to tailor each consecutive device to new and emerging needs and interests, as well as benefit from the experience of what succeeded in the past.

Conversely, the ongoing changes in children often require that the clinic team be patient enough to wait until the child is physically, intellectually, or emotionally ready for certain devices, interventions, or surgeries. For example, adequate space to accommodate a prosthetic knee or foot can be achieved through an epiphysiodesis; however, this must be done at the appropriate age in order to avoid an extremity that is disadvantageously short. During the interim, shoe-lifts or alternative components or designs will have to suffice. Similarly, certain prosthetic designs or components may be too heavy, complicated, fragile, or bulky for young children. Often the ideal prosthetic prescription has to be delayed until the child has matured enough for the application to be practical.

Initial Fitting Age

The child who needs a lower limb prosthesis is generally considered ready for fitting and early training when he or she begins pulling to stand. This developmental milestone, which even children with high or bilateral deficiencies will demonstrate, usually occurs between age 9 and 16 months.[7,8] Pulling to stand seems to be the ideal time for prosthetic fitting and early gait training to begin. If the

amputation is acquired at a later age, after the child has already been walking, the child should be fitted as soon as he or she is physically able.

The prosthetic prescription should reflect the child's developmental readiness. When fitting a toddler's first transfemoral or knee disarticulation prosthesis, for example, many clinics commonly incorporate a locked knee for its simplicity or exclude the knee joint altogether until the child has learned to walk safely.

Children who require an arm prosthesis are usually considered ready for their first prosthesis when they start to sit independently.[9] Traditionally, the first device has been a passive one, with the goal of enabling the child to sit, crawl, and perform some bimanual activities such as holding a bottle or toy. Around 2 years of age, most children are talking and also understand cause and effect. This seems to be the best time for them to be fitted with and trained to use a terminal device that can grasp.[10] Options at this stage include myoelectric hands or body-powered hooks. Elbows and elbow controls are generally considered only after the child has mastered use of the terminal device.

Strategies for Managing Growth

Although children will inevitably outgrow their devices, prosthetists, clinic teams, and therapists use numerous strategies to prolong the fit and function of pediatric prostheses. Most practitioners combine several strategies. Because children do not grow uniformly in length and girth, no single strategy will work every time. Descriptions of some of the most common strategies follow.[11]

Adjusting Prosthetic Socks

As children grow, they can wear fewer prosthetic socks or replace them with thinner socks. Because many gel liners are produced in several thicknesses, the same principle can often be applied to locking liners or gel liners.

Flexible Sockets

Modern flexible thermoplastic sockets, generally contained within an outer open frame, enhance comfort and suspension and often provide improved growth adjustability. The flexible material can be heated and stretched, sanded down, or replaced by a thinner socket. Pads may be added between the outer frame and socket and then removed later. In some cases, the material can also be made to "shrink." This not only enables growth expansion but also helps retain fit after edema reduction or limb atrophy.

Gel Liners

Liners constructed of thermoplastic gels, urethane, or silicone often provide a comfortable, protective interface for adolescents and many children. Currently most liners are not commercially available in size ranges that accommodate very small children. When used to suspend a prosthesis by means of a locking pin or lanyard, such liners may also avoid pressure over bony anatomy like the femoral condyles and can thus be considered "growth friendly." The locking versions have the disadvantage of being more difficult to modify for distal bone overgrowth or to fit over sharp, tapered residual limbs.

Slip Sockets

Prosthetists sometimes include one or two inner layers inside the prosthetic socket, which can be peeled out later to accommodate growth.[12]

Appropriate Materials and Components

Children with amputations are generally as active as their able-bodied peers. Consequently, their prostheses must be as durable as possible, while not restricting activity with excess weight, bulk, or impractical components or materials. Designs, components, and materials that can be switched out easily, that simplify lengthening, or that enable interchange to a larger or stronger component are preferred. Anything that is toxic, easily lost or swallowed, or difficult for a parent or child to apply and use should be avoided.

Staging

Some components are too large, require too much strength or range of motion, or are inappropriately complicated for young children. A good prescription plan should take into account the child's physical and intellectual readiness, the level and cause of amputation, age of onset, and the child's family and social dynamics.[13] In this context, the team often elects to stage, or gradually increase, the complexity of the device. This is partly based on development and partly based on what components, materials, or techniques can be practically applied. For these reasons, children younger than 2 years of age with transfemoral amputations are often fitted with a prosthesis that does not include a bending joint. Although this practice may be growing less common with the introduction of improved pediatric knees and therapy options, the long-standing concept has been to enable the child to learn to walk without the frustration of a knee joint that may buckle at unwanted times. The locked knee also reduces bulk and weight. Once the child has mastered basic walking, the knee can be added to consecutive prostheses. Upper limb prostheses are also often staged in their complexity. For example, a child with a transhumeral deficiency may be fitted first with a passive hand, or perhaps a friction elbow. The terminal device may not be activated until 2 years of age, followed a year or so later by the addition of a functional elbow, then finally, the elbow-lock control. As concepts and skills are gradually introduced and mastered, this incremental complexity should reduce the child's (and parents') frustration. Another parallel concept is to avoid "over-gadgeting" the child with excessive, often unnecessary options. Components and challenges should be added only when the child is ready to handle and benefit from them.

Education

Both the care providers and the child should learn to apply, remove, and care for the prosthesis. By watching how the child walks, examining the condition of the residual limb, and paying attention to any changes, the care providers should learn to recognize when relief over bony prominences, sock reduction, lengthening of the prosthesis, or other adjustments are likely to be needed, and they should then contact the prosthetist.

Follow-up

No design feature can replace appropriate follow-up. In general, follow-up with the physician and therapist should occur every 6 to 12 months. Devices generally will require growth adjustments by a prosthetist three or four times per year. Most pediatric limbs require replacement every 12 to 18 months during peak growing years, and perhaps every 1 to 3 years during adolescence.[14]

Most of these strategies are used in combination. For example, a prosthetist might fit a transtibial amputee with a silicone locking liner along with an overlying 5-ply prosthetic sock and modular components. Initially, as the child grows, sock thickness is reduced.[15] Later, the gel liner might be replaced with a thinner version. Concurrently, relief to the socket to accommodate growing bony prominences might become necessary, along with angular alignment adjustments beneath the socket adaptor, replacement of the pylon for a longer one, or interchange to a larger prosthetic foot.

Emotional Readiness

Children with congenital or acquired limb deficiencies are considered at risk for problems with psychological and social adjustment.[16] However, reports vary widely on how successfully they cope. Success seems to be related to the degree and quality of social support these children receive from parents, siblings, peers, and teach-

ers.[17] As with adults, children's emotions and self-acceptance can play a major role in how they perceive their limb loss, the role of their prosthesis, and their willingness to try new activities that may influence the prosthetic prescription.

In addition to their emotional maturity, children's life experiences, abilities, and interests are also constantly and often dramatically evolving. This can present the clinician with additional challenges. For example, a boy who has just received a new running prosthesis to achieve his goal of becoming a competitive sprinter may suddenly change his mind and decide to try out for the golf team instead. Children frequently subject their prostheses to activities and stresses for which they were never intended. Pediatric prosthetists often spend a lot of follow-up time cleaning sand, gravel, or water out of a child's prosthesis. Children with amputations will want to swim, run, climb, play sports, and ride bicycles—just like their peers. They will challenge the clinic team to find creative ways to enable them to meet their full potential throughout a dynamic array of interests.

Bone Overgrowth

Among children with acquired transdiaphyseal amputations, periosteal overgrowth is the most common surgical complication. Surgical methods to reduce this tendency have met with mixed results. Bone overgrowth results in a sharp, spiked protuberance. Through some advance planning, the prosthetist may be able to postpone the surgery.[3,18,19] However, overgrowth will require surgical revision once it becomes painful or erodes through the skin.

For any pediatric amputation other than a disarticulation, the prosthetist should either include a distal pad that can be replaced or modified when overgrowth occurs or have some other related contingency plan. In most cases, a new pad, socket modifications, or a new prosthesis will provide only short-term relief until a surgical revision becomes necessary.

Outgrowing a Prosthesis

Most growing children need a new prosthesis every 12 to 24 months. Follow-up and growth adjustments should occur every 3 to 4 months. Often the need for a new prosthesis is obvious—the child cannot fit into it at all or has lost it, or the prosthesis is beyond repair. These are good signs that the limb has been well used. At other times, the choice between ongoing repairs and adjustments or outright replacement is less obvious. Funding constraints may also complicate the process. To assist the team in making such decisions, a generalized list of indications for a new pediatric prosthesis follows.

When the prosthesis reaches a point at which no further length or growth adjustments can be made without risk of injury to the patient, a new prosthesis is indicated. Repairs or modifications may become so involved that they are cost or time-prohibitive. Often this is a judgment call based on the frequency of adjustments, the patient's frustration level, or limitations of components or materials.

The socket may no longer correspond to the child's anatomy. For example, if the fibular head and tibial tubercle have moved significantly out of the reliefs originally built for them in the socket, this is a sign that the child is outgrowing the prosthesis. If adjusting prosthetic socks or liner thickness along with extensive modifications cannot restore adequate fit, the prosthesis should be replaced.

Modern prosthetic components include weight and activity limits, torque settings, and time-based warranties. When the child's weight or activity level exceeds the manufacturer's specifications, the components or the entire prosthesis should be replaced.

The child's gait, posture, or joint alignment may change to the extent that a new prosthesis is required. This generally occurs more among young children following their first prosthesis or with children who have multiple limb involvement. Once the child exhibits significant gait or postural deviations that were not present when the device was delivered, the prosthetist can make only limited alignment alterations. At some point, the device may have to be disassembled and realigned, or replaced completely.

When angular changes can no longer be addressed through adjustments, the device should be replaced. For example, a child with a Syme ankle disarticulation for longitudinal deficiency of the fibula may exhibit increasing genu valgum. This could resolve on its own, or it may eventually require a surgical medial growth plate arrest (hemiepiphysiodesis). Regardless, the changing alignment is likely to require a new prosthesis.

Fitting and Fabrication Differences

The pediatric prosthetist must often evaluate alignment and fit primarily through trial and error, by observation, or by questioning the parents. Children, especially the very young, may lack the verbal skill or the abstract thought processes necessary to communicate their likes or dislikes about the prosthesis to the practitioner. Older children and adolescents have grown more experienced with their devices, have greater language skills, possess abstract thought processes, and can provide articulate feedback to the prosthetist or therapist. This makes the alignment and fitting process grow somewhat easier as the child matures.

So the child can gain confidence while alignment and fit are refined prior to the final fabrication of the device, pediatric prosthetists may allow the child to begin gait training on an unfinished prototype prosthesis. This also lets parents observe how the child functions with the device outside the hospital setting and often improves the feedback they can provide to the prosthetist. A prosthesis for an adult is intended to last many years; with pediatric patients, however, this goal is more short term in nature. Although the device should be reasonably durable, functional, adequately cosmetic, and safe, the child will outgrow it within a year or two. Attention to cosmetic finishing will vary according to individual preferences, but intricate, fragile, or highly cosmetic covers are likely to fail with this very active population. More often, pediatric prosthetists are asked to manufacture tough, durable covers that will tolerate the child's high activity level or to forgo the cover completely and provide devices that are brightly colored, uncovered, and look "sporty" or otherwise make a statement.

The Lower Limbs
Partial Foot

Children with congenital partial foot absences usually function quite well without surgical intervention. Most do not develop contractures and have few if any functional limitations. Their biggest challenge seems to be finding a shoe that fits, looks right, and is comfortable. For this group, soft slipper-style prostheses with padded toe fillers are generally fitted. If additional support is required, a thermoplastic arch support with a toe filler, or even something more rigid such as an ankle-foot orthosis (AFO) with a toe filler, may be provided.

For children with acquired partial foot amputations, my clinic prefers to start out with a thermoplastic AFO-style prosthesis that includes a padded cosmetic toe. This is recommended to enhance ankle stability, protect the wound site, and avoid any tendency for a contracture to develop. Arguably, it may lengthen stride by providing a longer, stiffer toe section. If no tendency toward contracture is evident, then less restrictive, more flexible slipper-style systems are recommended a year or so later.

Fibular Deficiencies

When corrective procedures are unlikely to succeed, a Syme procedure is often indicated for a complete or partially absent fibula. The prosthetist will encounter a few fitting challenges that are classically associated with this level. Although an ankle disarticulation has been performed, the fibula is wholly or partially absent, so the limb will not have the bulbous distal appearance associated with the Syme level. The child's heel pad and tibial malleolus may still be bulky and firm enough to suspend the prosthesis, but often some other form of suspension such as a cuff, sleeve, or locking liner will be needed. Most of these limbs can tolerate some loading of the distal soft tissues, but the heel pads have been known to migrate away, leaving only a thin layer of skin to cover the tapered malleolus. To reduce long-term stress on these tissues, a firm distal pad and patellar tendon–bearing (PTB) or total surface–bearing design should be emphasized. A sharp, prominent tibial crest along with anterior bowing of the tibia is often present. To protect these areas from injury, a protective socket interface, special padding, or other appropriate relief may be necessary. Fibular deficiency is often associated with a length discrepancy. This can actually be helpful because it allows more room for prosthetic ankles and feet, as well as distal pads and shuttle locks if indicated. Genu valgum is another common problem. Medial placement of the prosthetic foot may accommodate this for a while, but if the valgum becomes a cosmetic or functional concern, a hemiepiphysiodesis or tibial osteotomy may be required.[4]

Tibial Deficiencies

Although it has now fallen out of vogue, a Brown procedure (fibular centralization along with a Syme ankle disarticulation) was often performed in the past for complete absence of the tibia. The intent was to enable the fibula to remodel and take on the role of the tibia so that the child could be fitted with a transtibial prosthesis. To provide mediolateral knee stability, metal joints and a thigh corset were essential. Unfortunately, a high incidence of knee instability, recurrent deformity, and repeated surgical revisions was reported.[20] Thus, for complete absence of the tibia, knee disarticulation is now the procedure of choice.

The child with a knee disarticulation, even if it is bilateral, can usually be fitted prosthetically as soon as he or she is developmentally ready. By age 3 years, the child should be able to function well with an articulated knee. Barring any other health problems, a high activity level should be expected.[21] Many children with bilateral knee disarticulations find that they can learn to jog or run.

If the proximal tibia is present and a functional quadriceps mechanism exists, a slightly different scenario takes place. In this case, the surgeon may be able to centralize the fibula and then perform an ankle disarticulation. Afterward, the child can be fitted with a Syme prosthesis. The knee may need to be protected from injury by using metal joints and a thigh corset until the fusion and knee joint are stable.

Transtibial prostheses for children should generally include distal pads that can be adjusted for longitudinal growth or terminal bone overgrowth.[11] As with adults, limb length, skin condition, strength, and joint stability should dictate socket design, component selection, and alignment. Supracondylar socket designs, which grip over bony anatomy, should be used if indicated by limb length or stability. However, such systems are likely to need more frequent growth modifications than do other less restrictive designs. Gel, urethane, or silicone suspension sleeves and their variants are arguably more adjustable for growth over time because they do not grip over bony anatomy. Although sleeves and suspension liners are certainly appropriate for toddlers just learning to walk, prosthetists may find that they get torn or wear out so quickly during crawling that a waist belt or some other suspension is preferable.

Knee Disarticulation

Knee disarticulation, rather than any "through-the-bone" amputation, is the preferred transfemoral level for children. This procedure minimizes trauma, retains excellent hip muscle balance and insertions, preserves both femoral epiphyses, avoids osseous overgrowth, and usually enables distal load bearing. If tolerance of full distal weight bearing is maintained, knee disarticulation is generally considered to be functionally superior to a transfemoral amputation.[22]

Knee disarticulation in children has most of the same disadvantages associated with this level among adults, except that more options to correct the problems are available. The bulbous distal end, for example, is not usually as notable in children who have had the amputation early. The problem with matching knee centers and having fewer knee choices can be circumvented by performing a distal femoral epiphysiodesis at the appropriate age, thus eventually providing sufficient room for almost any commercially available prosthetic knee. Even with these problems, several prosthetic socket designs have been developed to enable suspension over the femoral condyles and to take advantage of the long lever arm and distal load tolerance of this level.

A knee disarticulation usually results in femoral length nearly equal to the opposite side. Standard single-axis knees can add at least 5 cm to the length of the prosthetic thigh. To avoid this problem, a polycentric knee that is designed for the knee disarticulation level should be used. Even the best of these, however, may lengthen the thigh by 25 to 30 mm. This discrepancy seems to be acceptable to most adults.[23] If an epiphysiodesis is planned to make more room for a prosthetic knee, a minimum of 3 cm of clearance should result, with somewhere between 7 and 11 cm achieved by adulthood, so that virtually any commercially available knee could be used.

Transfemoral

Growth and development complicate the prosthetic management of a child's transfemoral amputation. Traditional suction, the preferred method of suspension for most adults at this level, is usually not recommended for children younger than 7 years of age. Certainly there are successful exceptions; however, in general, the child should have the strength, cognitive understanding, patience, and maturity to apply a suction socket correctly—every time. If the parents or other care providers are still helping the child get dressed, they are likely to find that applying a suction socket correctly is too frustrating and time-consuming. Such sockets usually require stable limb volume. Any air space distally can result in negative pressures that may cause circulatory congestion and edema.[24] Growth of the child's limb and weight gain may result in frequent modifications or replacements of the suction socket in order to maintain a comfortable fit.

Although it is technically possible to fit younger children with suction sockets, it may create more problems than it solves until the child is at least 7 years old.[25] Thereafter, traditional suction sockets should still be prescribed judiciously until the child reaches adolescence. From the teen years on, suction sockets are generally tolerated and often preferred. As with adults, suction is not recommended in the presence of deep, fissured scars, frequent changes in volume (as with children undergoing dialysis or chemotherapy), extremely short residual limbs, or in the presence of upper limb deficiencies that would make donning of the socket burdensome.

Newer silicone, urethane, or other gel-like thermoplastic liners used in conjunction with shuttle locks, lanyards, or even flexible sockets and valves may be somewhat easier to don. The liner is rolled over the residual limb and then the child "steps" into the socket. Distally, a retaining pin or lanyard protrudes from the material and mates with a locking mechanism built into the socket, thus locking the limb onto the soft socket. To remove the prosthesis, the child either pushes a release button or pulls the cord out of the retaining lock. Growth adjustments may be facilitated by the use of socks over the liner. Although such systems are more common at the transtibial level, they hold great promise for earlier, more successful suction fittings in children with transfemoral amputations.[26]

For young children, the most traditional way to suspend a transfemoral prosthesis is with a Silesian belt. This fastens to the socket laterally above the greater trochanter, wraps around the child's pelvis and opposite iliac crest, and then attaches with Velcro or a buckle on the proximal anterior socket. The Total Elastic Suspension (TES) belt and other variations made of neoprene, spandex, or nylon work in a similar fashion. The neoprene is comfortable and growth-adjustable. Such belts can be used to assist suction or some other form of suspension, or they may be the sole means of suspension. For extremely short amputations, in the presence of rotational problems, weak hip abductors, obesity, or hip pathology, a traditional metal hip joint and pelvic band and belt may be indicated; however, this should be a last resort.

Although far more prosthetic knees are available for adults, a number of knee components engineered specifically for children have been introduced recently. Michael[27] has classified knee components into six categories, according to their function: manual locking, constant-friction (single-axis), stance control (weight-activated friction), polycentric (four-bar), fluid-controlled, and microprocessor-controlled knees. The knees may differ greatly in appearance, material, size, weight, or structural design, but their functional characteristics are very similar within each classification. Pediatric and adolescent knees are now available in most of these classes.

Manual Locking Knees

Although many classes of knees can be locked, this refers to a single-axis knee with a lock. Among adults, these are recommended only for patients who need maximum stability. For children just learning to walk, however, manual locking knees are often appropriate, particularly for children with bilateral amputations or deficiencies. The therapist, parents, or child can unlock such a knee for training purposes or to enable sitting or crawling. By 3 to 4 years of age, most children with a single amputation can learn to use an articulated knee without a lock. Those with high, weak, or bilateral absences may require locking knees for many years, if not indefinitely.

Constant-Friction (Single-Axis) Knees

Constant-friction knees have a single axis of rotation and some mechanism to apply friction at a constant rate. The friction controls the knee during swing phase and enables a smooth, controlled gait at a single, predetermined speed. Older children and adolescents who are active and constantly change their walking speed will generally prefer a hydraulic knee; however, only one or two choices are available for children or smaller adolescents.

Stance-Control (Weight-Activated Friction) Knees

Most stance-control knees are single-axis constant friction knees, but they also include a brake that is activated if the wearer's weight is applied during the first 20° of knee flexion. A few polycentric knees also provide a stance-control feature. In addition to the stability available through prosthetic alignment and the patient's hip extensors, this weight-activated brake provides an "anti-stumble" mechanism of sorts. Single-axis stance-control knees are generally recommended for new amputees, elderly, or debilitated amputees, or patients with short or weak residual limbs. The pediatric Total Knee (Ossur, Aliso Viejo, CA) is an example of a polycentric knee (see below) with stance control.[28] The enhanced stability of such knees is useful for fitting younger children with any level of amputation through or above the knee.

Polycentric (Four-Bar) Knees

Mechanisms in this class mimic the rocking, gliding motion of the anatomic knee joint, either through curved bearing surfaces or through a series of linkages. Polycentric knees have a moving center of rotation. This generally enhances control against buckling and so these knees are more stable than single-axis knees. Several variations have been designed specifically for knee disarticulation levels or long amputations. These allow the prosthetist to more closely match the patient's knee centers. Because the linkage "folds under" the amputee's thigh during flexion, some clinicians consider polycentric knees more cosmetically pleasing during sitting. Only a few polycentric knees are made for children younger than 10 years of age. Available features such as weight-activated stance control, spring-loaded extension assists, rubberized kneecaps to facilitate kneeling, and adjustable friction controls have made these popular choices in many pediatric clinics. Four-bar knees are recommended for children and adolescents with knee disarticulations or for any child with a transfemoral or even a hip disarticulation who needs extra knee stability. There are few if any contraindications to their use in children.

Fluid-Controlled Knees

Fluid-controlled knees may be either hydraulic or pneumatic and are available in both single-axis and polycentric configurations. The fluid, which may be liquid (oil), in the case of hydraulic units, or gaseous (air), in the case of pneumatic units, responds to changes in walking speed. Whether the amputee walks slowly or speeds up and runs, a smooth, controlled gait is the intended result. Some units

also provide resistance during stance, including features such as "lock" or "free-swing." Hydraulic knees are recommended for healthy, active adolescents. They would be ideal for young children, but only one or two downsized units exist.

Microprocessor-Controlled Knees

Microprocessor-controlled knees have been designed primarily for adults or older adolescents; no system specifically designed for younger children is presently available commercially. All use a microprocessor and some kind of feedback loop to control either a hydraulic or pneumatic knee. They have the benefit of far greater and more instantaneous responsiveness to situations the amputee may encounter during walking and a much wider range of adjustability. However, these knees share the disadvantages of greater expense, more stringent maintenance schedules, a power source that must be recharged, and higher susceptibility to damage from water.

Hip Disarticulation

The socket for a hip disarticulation prosthesis must generally wrap around the child's pelvis. The hip joint is positioned anteriorly and the knee posterior to the body's midline so that the prosthetic joints are stable during midstance or when the patient is standing. Although soft cosmetic covers are less durable for children in general, endoskeletal components are generally recommended at this level. Such systems keep the prosthesis light and also allow for long-term alignment changes. Toddlers or young children with a hip disarticulation may be fitted with an articulated hip only, along with a locked or nonarticulated knee. This facilitates early walking and sitting. Perhaps by 4 or 5 years of age, most children can learn to use an articulated knee effectively.[11] Because of their extra knee stability, polycentric knees—particularly those with stance control—are often advantageous for this level.

Longitudinal Deficiency of the Femur, Partial

Prosthetists are likely to see four orthopaedic methods of managing LDFP. Each will require a different prosthetic approach.

No Surgery

Sometimes no surgery is the best management option. This is particularly true for children with bilateral LDFP or with bilateral upper limb deficiencies occurring with LDFP. In most instances, children with bilateral LDFP should not have amputations. Most can walk independently; accordingly, ablating their feet makes them very dependent on prostheses. Still, they may benefit from a pair of extension prostheses for use at school or work.[29] Most children born with unilateral LDFP can bear weight comfortably on the affected side when they are not wearing their prosthesis, but they have to kneel or squat severely on the sound side in order to do this. These children are frequently fitted with equinus prostheses to compensate for leg-length discrepancies. The prosthesis raises them to the correct height and includes a prosthetic foot below the plantar flexed anatomic foot. The child's anatomic knee is usually included in the socket, and for cosmetic reasons, the foot is positioned in comfortable equinus. A waist belt or strap over the child's heel can suspend the prosthesis. Many can "self-suspend" simply by dorsiflexing the foot actively against the socket wall.

Although equinus prostheses are generally well accepted, the child's weak, unstable hip and extremely high knee and foot create cosmetic and functional challenges for the prosthetist. The limb may appear to lengthen during swing phase and shorten during stance phase. To counteract this piston action of the unstable hip, the prosthetic socket often extends to include the ischial tuberosity and gluteal musculature. As children wearing equinus prostheses mature, they may find it difficult to sit in a car or at a desk while wearing a prosthesis. In such instances, the prosthetist may choose to articulate the prosthesis by positioning a prosthetic knee joint below the child's foot, or by placing external metal knee joints on either side of the child's ankle.

Syme Ankle Disarticulation

The surgeon and family may decide on a Syme procedure alone. This might be recommended as an alternative to lengthening, when the femur is predicted to be 50% or greater than the sound side and the knee will function normally. A drawback to this approach is that the thigh on the amputated side will be visibly shorter. When the child sits, the relatively long prosthesis and short thigh are most visible. Despite this cosmetic disadvantage, the child will be able to control the prosthesis with his or her anatomic knee joint. Children who have had this procedure generally walk well as well as run and tolerate prosthetic fitting easily. As with LDFP in general, the abnormal hip and shorter, weaker hip abductors may produce a visible Trendelenburg lurch.

Syme Ankle Disarticulation With Knee Fusion

This combined approach is the most common surgical and prosthetic management option recommended for more severe cases of LDFP. A Syme procedure is performed and the child's knee is fused to form a single, straight limb. The knee fusion generally decreases the child's hip flexion contracture.[30,31] The limb is then fitted as a transfemoral amputation with some distal weight-bearing capability. Ischial or gluteal weight bearing is provided to lessen pistoning of the unstable hip. In some cases, as with other Syme prostheses, the malleoli and heel pad may be used to suspend the device. Pads, expandable sockets, and removable windows have all been used successfully, as have Silesian belts and various elastic or neoprene waist belts.[32]

Rotationplasty

Ideally, a rotationplasty turns the child's foot around 180°, thus enabling the ankle to function as a knee with a prosthesis. Rotationplasty has been used to treat LDFP as well as for limb salvage following tumor resection. For optimum function, the child's ankle joint should be normal and capable of an arc of motion of at least 60°.[25] By maturity, the child's ankle should be at the same level as the opposite knee.[33,34]

Bochmann[7] has described the ideal prosthetic design following rotationplasty. The child bears weight through the now anteriorly located sole of the foot, which is enclosed within a socket. The socket is positioned in equinus and provides extra space distally for growth of the toes. A soft socket liner is recommended. To stabilize the ankle and protect against injury, single-axis joints extend from the socket and attach to a corset or plastic thigh cuff. If necessary, ischial or gluteal support may be provided through an extended socket brim. The prosthesis is usually suspended by a heel strap or a waist belt. As with LDFP in general, the abnormal and weak hip may produce a Trendelenburg lurch when the child walks. Strength and remaining range of motion of an appropriately rotated ankle will determine the degree of functional knee control. Most children and adolescents who have this procedure will be very active; therefore, dynamic-response feet and sports-oriented components are recommended.

Bilateral Lower Limb Deficiencies and Amputations

When they are developmentally ready, even children with bilateral leg amputations will attempt to pull to stand. This is a good indicator that they are ready for their first prostheses. Fitting for bilateral transtibial absences is not much different than for unilateral absence. Keeping the child's overall height on the first pair

of prostheses several inches shorter than the child's estimated normal height may help the child learn to balance, but this is often not necessary. Children with bilateral knee disarticulations or higher amputations, however, usually will benefit from gradual progression in the height and complexity of the prostheses.

The young child with bilateral transfemoral amputations is usually first fitted with relatively short prostheses without functional knee joints. Alignment generally reflects the somewhat crouched appearance children exhibit when first walking: The hips are flexed and abducted, the knees are flexed, and the ankles are dorsiflexed. These prostheses generally include prosthetic feet, but if the amputations are extremely short or if fitting is complicated by developmental delays, the prosthetist may forgo feet in the interest of balance. Instead, some sort of crepe-lined stable soles may be used as a base of support. (These have been traditionally referred to as "stubbies.") In either case, relative shortening of the prostheses lowers the child's center of gravity. This provides for early successful standing balance and helps the clinic team evaluate prosthetic socket fit with the child in a safe, comfortable, weight-bearing position. This stage is usually quite temporary, ranging from a few days to a few months. The short nonarticulated prostheses may be lengthened over time as the child begins gait training.[35]

Deciding whether to fit shorter, nonarticulated prostheses or to add knees right away requires experienced judgment. Children with longer amputation levels (particularly knee disarticulations) and good upper limb strength usually progress quickly. They may be able to tolerate taller prostheses with knees almost immediately upon attempting to walk. In contrast, children with shorter amputation levels, or those who also have upper limb involvement, may require years of experience before they are able to use longer prostheses with articulated knees successfully. The transition to bending knees can be facilitated with options like manual locking knees, weight-activated friction knees, polycentric knees that provide greater stability, knee extension assists, walkers, crutches, canes, and, of course, prolonged physical therapy.

The Upper Limbs

Managing a child with a congenital upper limb deficiency differs significantly from managing an adult or adolescent whose limb deficiency is acquired through amputation. Children with congenital upper limb deficiencies generally possess a remarkable capacity for adapting to their situation. The dexterity and sensitivity they exhibit with the residual limb is often quite amazing. Children with high bilateral deficiencies may prefer not to wear prostheses at all. Children with bilateral upper limb deficiencies, for example, prefer to use their feet for functional activities. They may learn to operate prostheses impressively well, but they will usually revert to foot use when allowed to do so. Children born with a partial arm or hand will also function well by adapting their remaining limbs to their needs. Sensory discrimination with the residual limb is excellent. A prosthesis, adapted tool, or simple change to their environment (such as door handles instead of knobs) may help them functionally or cosmetically. The prescription of a prosthesis should take into consideration the unique efficiencies these children have already developed. If their current adaptations are not recognized, they may perceive a prosthesis as more of an imposition than a functional aid.

When appropriately designed and used, an upper limb prosthesis can be a helpful tool that a child may wear only intermittently for specific activities. This is in contrast to lower limb prostheses, which children usually quickly incorporate into their body images and tend to depend on daily for long periods of time. Often the cosmetic appearance of an upper limb prosthesis, which helps the child appear "like everyone else," may be the true underlying motivation for seeking a prosthesis.

The clinic team will generally want to plan upper limb prosthetic intervention around normal developmental milestones. Most centers fit upper limb prostheses when the child starts to gain sitting balance. This is usually between 3 and 7 months of age, when children develop two-handed skills.[36] The first prosthesis is usually passive. Between 1 and 2 years of age, when the child starts to speak, a functional terminal device is fitted. Choices include body-powered hooks and hands and myoelectric hands.

Transradial Deficiencies and Amputations

Regardless of the etiology, most young children with transradial amputations will learn to use the elbow effectively for prehensile activities. Although they can operate a prosthesis quite well, they will often have little functional need for one. If they use a prosthesis at all, it is generally for very specific activities. The challenge for the clinic team is often sifting through the array of choices to settle on something the child will actually use and benefit from.

Myoelectric hands are popular because of their good cosmetic appearance and the fact that the device usually requires no harness. Grasping and hooking functions are easily mastered. In the last 15 years, children younger than 3 years of age often have been provided with a myoelectric arm that is controlled through a single electrode positioned over just one muscle site. This system has been referred to as a "cookie crusher." All the child has to do is contract the muscle group below the electrode (preferably an extensor in the forearm), and the hand opens. As soon as the child relaxes, the hand will close. This enables even very young children to operate a myoelectric hand easily. The system should be converted within 1 or 2 years, so that the child learns to use two muscle groups, as with most adult myoelectric hands. A two-site system gives the child independent control of both opening and closing of the hand. Children as young as 3 years of age can learn to operate a hand with a two-site electrode system.[37]

A variety of body-powered terminal devices are also available for young children. A passive hand is usually fitted when the child begins to sit, followed by an activated hook at around 2 years of age. Devices such as tumbling mitts, ski pole attachments, baseball glove attachments, and numerous other sports or tool adaptations are available or can be customized to thread into a prosthetic wrist. Such devices meet the child's needs for very specific activities such as horseback riding, biking, or gymnastics. At other times, children and adolescents may prefer a cosmetic prosthesis. Peak desire for such a device seems to be when the child first starts school, when the child switches to a new school, or during early adolescence. There are few, if any, reliable predictors for which style of arm prosthesis a child will prefer or ultimately use as an adult. Clinics vary in their approach. A common protocol is to fit children with passive prostheses as they gain sitting balance, followed by prehensile training at 2 years of age. After that, prosthetic design and use are based on the child's needs and interests.

Higher Levels

A similar pattern exists for children with transhumeral deficiencies. The first prosthesis may include a passive elbow and passive hand. At around 2 years of age, either a myoelectric or cable-operated hand or hook is added. Once the child has mastered use of the terminal device, a functioning elbow (either electric or body-powered) is added. The final skill to be learned is usually locking and unlocking of an elbow. Most children should have the cognitive and physical ability to control all aspects of a transhumeral prosthesis by 4 or 5 years of age. However, they may lack sufficient strength, range of motion, and excursion to take full advantage of a body-powered system. Because of this, children and adolescents are often fitted with combination systems, or hybrids, consisting of body-powered and electronic components. Hybrid systems maximize all available control options and are especially helpful when fitting higher amputation levels or children with bilateral involvement.

Shoulder disarticulation and forequarter (interscapulothoracic) prostheses are even more challenging for children to wear and use effectively. The prosthetic shoulder joint is usually moved passively. The elbow may be passive, cable-operated, switch-controlled, or myoelectric. Children with this high level of absence generally lack the excursion necessary to operate an elbow. If an elbow is fitted, the prosthesis should generally be viewed as a "helper"; it will provide some protection for the amputation site and will fill out clothing, and it may provide some prehensile functions. The more function that is desired, the more likely that a hybrid system will be required.

The greatest challenge in prescribing prostheses for children with high or bilateral upper limb deficiencies is that success is difficult to quantify or predict. Children with transhumeral and higher amputations often reject prostheses, even though they can demonstrate excellent control of them. Whether or not a child will be a long-term user of an upper limb prosthesis, particularly if the amputation level is high, is highly individualized. However, several characteristics seem to play a role in a child's continuing prosthesis use. These factors include appropriate limb length, a clinical team with a high degree of experience and expertise in fitting pediatric upper limbs, good occupational training, an enthusiastic family commitment, and a pattern of consistent prosthetic wear by the patient.[36]

Summary

The growing, ever-changing nature of children presents a dynamic challenge to prosthetists and clinics treating children with limb deficiencies. Over the years, clinics have developed strategies for prescribing and fitting pediatric prostheses. The keys to success are listening carefully and frequently to the evolving needs of families and children and then remaining as flexible and open to change as possible.

References

1. Challenor YB: Limb deficiencies and amputation surgery in children, in Molnary GE (ed): *Pediatric Rehabilitation*. Baltimore, MD, Williams & Wilkins, 1985.

2. Day HJB: The ISO/ISPO classification of congenital limb deficiency, in Bowker JH, Michael JW (eds): *Atlas of Limb Prosthetics: Surgical, Prosthetic, and Rehabilitation Principles*, ed 2. Rosemont, IL, American Academy of Orthopaedic Surgeons, 2002, pp 599-622. (Originally published by Mosby-Year Book, 1992.)

3. Aitken GT, Pellicore RJ: Introduction to the child amputee, in *Atlas of Limb Prosthetics: Surgical and Prosthetic Principles*. St Louis, MO, CV Mosby, 1981, pp 493-500.

4. Gibson D: Child and juvenile amputee, in Banjerjee S, Khan N (eds): *Rehabilitation Management of Amputees*. Baltimore, MD, Williams & Wilkins, 1982, pp 394-414.

5. McCollough NC, Trout A, Caldwell J: Non standard/prosthetic applications for juvenile amputees. *Inter Clin Info Bull* 1963;2:7-14.

6. DiCaprio M, Friedlaender G: Malignant bone tumors: Limb sparing versus amputation. *J Am Acad Orthop Surg* 2003;11:25-37.

7. Bochmann D: Prosthetic devices for the management of proximal femoral focal deficiency. *Orthot Prosthet* 1980;12:4-19.

8. Kruger LM: Congenital limb deficiencies: Part II. Lower limb deficiencies, in *Atlas of Limb Prosthetics: Surgical and Prosthetic Principles*. St Louis, MO, CV Mosby, 1981, pp 522-552.

9. Patton J: Developmental approach to pediatric prosthetic evaluation and training, in Atkins D, Meier R (eds): *Comprehensive Management of the Upper-Limb Amputee*. New York, NY, Springer-Verlag, 1989, pp 137-149.

10. Shaperman J, Landsperger S, Setoguchi Y: Early upper limb prosthesis fitting: When and what do we fit? *J Prosthet Orthot* 2003;15:11-17.

11. Cummings D, Kapp S: Lower-limb pediatric prosthetics: General considerations and philosophy. *J Prosthet Orthot* 1992;4:203.

12. Gazely W, Ey M, Sampson W: Use of triple wall sockets for juvenile amputees. *Inter-Clin Info Bull* 1964;4:1.

13. Novotny M, Swagman A: Caring for children with orthotic/prosthetic needs. *J Prosthet Orthot* 1992;4:714-718.

14. Fisk J: Introduction to the child amputee, in Bowker JH, Michael JW (eds): *Atlas of Limb Prosthetics: Surgical, Prosthetic, and Rehabilitation Principles*, ed 2. Rosemont, IL, American Academy of Orthopaedic Surgeons, 2002, pp 731-734. (Originally published by Mosby-Year Book, 1992.)

15. Fillauer C, Pritham C, Fillauer K: Evolution and development of the silicone suction socket (3S) for below-knee prostheses. *J Pediatr Orthop* 1989;1:92.

16. Wallander J, Varni J, Babani L, Banis H, Wilcox K: Children with chronic physical disorders: Maternal reports of their psychological adjustment. *J Pediatr Psychol* 1988;13:197-212.

17. Varni J, Setoguchi Y, Rappaport L, Talbot D: Effects of stress, social support, and self-esteem on depression in children with limb deficiencies. *Arch Phys Med Rehabil* 1991;72:1053-1058.

18. Lovett R: Osseous overgrowth in congenital limb-deficient children. *J Assoc Child Orthot Prosthet Clinics* 1987;22:2-6.

19. Speer D: The pathogenesis of amputation stump overgrowth. *Clin Orthop* 1981;159:34.

20. Kruger L: Lower-limb deficiencies, in Bowker JH, Michael JW (eds): *Atlas of Limb Prosthetics: Surgical, Prosthetic, and Rehabilitation Principles*, ed 2. Rosemont, IL, American Academy of Orthopaedic Surgeons, 2002, pp 795-838. (Originally published by Mosby-Year Book, 1992.)

21. Loder R, Herring JA: Disarticulation

of the knee in children: A functional assessment. *J Bone Joint Surg Am* 1987; 69:1155-1160.

22. Hughes J: Biomechanics of the through-knee prosthesis. *Prosthet Orthot Int* 1983;7:96-99.

23. Oberg K: Knee mechanisms for through-knee prostheses. *Prosthet Orthot Int* 1983;7:107-112.

24. Bowker J, Keagy R, Poonekar P: Musculoskeletal complications in amputees: Their prevention and management, in Bowker JH, Michael JW (eds): *Atlas of Limb Prosthetics: Surgical, Prosthetic, and Rehabilitation Principles*, ed 2. Rosemont, IL, American Academy of Orthopaedic Surgeons, 2002, pp 665-688. (Originally published by Mosby-Year Book, 1992.)

25. Thompson G, Leimkuller J: Prosthetic management, in Kalamchi A (ed): *Congenital Lower Limb Deficiencies*. New York, NY, Springer-Verlag, 1989, pp 210-236.

26. Schuch M: Transfemoral amputation: Prosthetic management, in Bowker JH, Michael JW (eds): *Atlas of Limb Prosthetics: Surgical, Prosthetic, and Rehabilitation Principles*, ed 2. Rosemont, IL, American Academy of Orthopaedic Surgeons, 2002, pp 509-533. (Originally published by Mosby-Year Book, 1992.)

27. Michael J: Prosthetic knee mechanisms. *Clin Orthop* 1999;361:39-47.

28. *Total Knee™ Geometric Knee System*. Brochure by Century XXII Innovations, Inc, 1993, Ossur-North America, Aliso Viejo, CA.

29. Krajbich I: Proximal femoral focal deficiency, in Kalamchi A (ed): *Congenital Lower Limb Deficiencies*. New York, NY, Springer-Verlag, 1989, pp 108-127.

30. King R, Marks T: Follow-up findings on the skeletal lever in the surgical management of proximal femoral focal deficiency. *Inter Clin Info Bull* 1971; 11:1.

31. King R: Providing a single skeletal lever in proximal femoral focal deficiency. *Inter Clin Info Bull* 1966;2:23.

32. Tablada C: A technique for fitting converted proximal femoral focal deficiencies. *Artif Limbs* 1971;15:27-45.

33. Krajbich I, Bochmann D: Van Nes Rotation-plasty in tumor surgery, in Bowker JH, Michael JW (eds): *Atlas of Limb Prosthetics: Surgical, Prosthetic, and Rehabilitation Principles*, ed 2. Rosemont, IL, American Academy of Orthopaedic Surgeons, 2002, pp 885-889. (Originally published by Mosby-Year Book, 1992.)

34. Van Nes C: Rotation-plasty for congenital defects of the femur: Making use of the ankle of the shortened limb to control the knee joint of a prosthesis. *J Bone Joint Surg Br* 1950;32:12-16.

35. Hamilton E: Gait training: Part two. Children, in Kostuik J (ed): *Amputation Surgery and Rehabilitation: The Toronto Experience*. New York, NY, Churchill Livingstone, 1981.

36. Hubbard S, Kurtz I, Heim W, Montgomery G: Powered prosthetic intervention in upper extremity deficiency, in Herring J, Birch J (eds): *The Child With a Limb Deficiency*. Rosemont, IL, American Academy of Orthopaedic Surgeons, 1997, pp 417-431.

37. Baron E, Clarke S, Solomon C: The two stage myoelectric hand for children and young adults. *Orthot Prosthet* 1983;37:11-12, 22-23.

Psychological Issues in Pediatric Limb Deficiency

Alice L. Kahle, PhD

Introduction

Approximately 1 million children and adolescents in the United States have a chronic illness or disability that necessitates ongoing, comprehensive medical care.[1] Compared with other children in this group and with peers without physical disabilities, children with limb deficiencies and amputations generally show good adjustment and coping. In fact, child and adolescent amputees have been described as remarkably resistant to maladjustment.[2,3] Nevertheless, childhood limb deficiency, whether congenital or acquired, is emotionally significant. Even under optimal circumstances, coping with limb deficiency is undoubtedly challenging for the affected child and family.

This chapter focuses on the psychological adjustment of children with limb deficiencies. In the first part of the chapter, the effects of experiences and environment on the psychological adjustment of the child with a limb deficiency are discussed. In the second part of the chapter, practical techniques for supporting the adjustment in children with amputations and their families are presented.

Prenatal Diagnosis

What is the psychological impact of having advance knowledge that a child will be born with a congenital anomaly such as a limb deficiency? Some have speculated that prenatal diagnosis creates more stress for parents because it triggers fear and uncertainty. Others have argued that prenatal diagnosis allows parents to prepare themselves and others for the arrival of a child who will need specialized care. One study examined this question specifically in parents of children born with a range of congenital anomalies. Researchers found that 1 year after the child's birth, mothers who had prenatal information about their child's condition reported significantly higher parental burden and grief than parents who lacked advance knowledge of their child's anomaly.[4] Generalizations from these data need to be made cautiously because the sample of mothers who had prenatal information was very small (n = 8). Also, no prospective studies have directly compared the reactions of parents who had prenatal information about their child's limb deficiency with those of parents who learned of limb deficiency at the time of their child's birth. Even so, given the proliferation of prenatal diagnostic techniques, the findings point to the need to better understand how prenatal information affects parental coping.

Degree and Type of Limb Deficiency

The nature and extent of a child's limb deficiency certainly play a role in the child's psychological adjustment. Few studies, however, have compared adjustment outcomes based on the origin of the limb deficiency or the limb or limbs involved because researchers often pool data from children with different types of limb loss to achieve adequate sample sizes. Nevertheless, researchers typically do include some objective rating of degree of limb deficiency in their analyses. As is often seen in children with other chronic conditions,[5] the relationship between characteristics of the deficiency, such as the nature and severity of limb loss, and psychological outcome is more complex and less obvious than one might assume.

Condition Severity

Often, it is assumed that more severe deficiencies will have a greater impact on psychosocial outcome. Yet, most clinicians have worked with children with significant impairments who show exceptional emotional resilience as well as with children with more minor impairments who adjust poorly. These anecdotal observations mirror research findings in limb-deficient children and other children with chronic conditions or disabilities.

Studies examining the relationship between condition severity and psychosocial functioning of these youngsters and their families have produced mixed results. Some researchers have found a direct relationship between condition severity and adjustment outcomes. For example, parents of infants with multiple congenital anomalies reported significantly more personal strain than parents whose child had an isolated anomaly.[4] In addition, conditions with coexisting cognitive or intellectual impairments are associated with higher psychological morbidity than conditions that do not have these characteristics.[5]

When researchers examine patient groups within which there are fewer differences in condition severity, such as children with limb deficiencies, direct associations between degree of impairment and psychological adjustment tend to be weak, inconsistent, or insignificant. In a qualitative, retrospective study that included only parents of children with congenital limb deficiency, Kerr and McIntosh[6] found that the severity of limb loss was not related in a consistent way to the intensity of parents' emotional response at the time of their child's birth. In studies of self-esteem in children with limb deficiencies, the degree of limb deficiency was significantly correlated with self-esteem in adolescents,[7] but not in younger children.[8] Inconsistent findings have led researchers to hypothesize that the relationship between condition severity and adjustment may be mediated or moderated by the direct or indirect influence of a third variable, such as functional status.[9,10]

Etiology of the Amputation

In the pediatric population, limb deficiencies presenting at birth outnumber acquired amputations by more than 2 to 1.[11] Approximately 75% of acquired amputations are caused by trauma and 25% by disease processes. Some developing countries show exceptions to this pattern, especially countries with a history of conflicts in which land mines were used extensively. Land mine contamination can result in very high rates of childhood traumatic amputations.[12]

Although it seems intuitively obvious that emotional adjustment would depend on the etiology of the deficiency, studies show otherwise. In one of the few empirical studies to compare children with different limb loss etiologies, adolescents with acquired amputations were no different from those with congenital limb deficiencies in terms of their depressive symptoms, anxiety, or self-esteem.[7]

Children with a congenital limb deficiency may have longer to prepare for their limitations, which may facilitate patient and family adjustment.[13] For patients with acquired amputations, loss of function is usually abrupt. Patients may experience difficulties when they return to school, attempt to resume work or leisure activities, or begin to revise their self-image to incorporate their amputation.[3]

When amputations are necessitated by malignancy, the ultimate goal is patient survival. After amputation, patients may experience conflicted emotions. They may feel gratitude and relief at having survived but may also have a profound sense of loss. In addition, having experienced a life-threatening illness may produce post-traumatic stress symptoms in some patients,[14] and the fear that cancer will recur may further increase the patient's distress.[11]

Traumatic amputations are seen about twice as often in boys than in girls. Data from recent reviews indicate that, in North America, power lawnmowers are the most frequent cause of traumatic childhood amputations. Motor vehicle accidents, farm and commercial machinery injuries, and gunshot wounds also contribute.[12] Epidemiologic findings suggest that many traumatic amputations in children could have been prevented. For example, children often sustain their injury while playing near the hazard.[12] In a study of 74 children who sustained traumatic amputations, more than half were unsupervised at the time of their accident.[15] Thus, the circumstance of a traumatic amputation may leave the child or other family members with a sense of culpability. Feelings of guilt, regret,

and anger may disrupt adjustment as patients and family members deal with the realization that the amputation could have been avoided.

Amputation entails not just a physical loss but a multitude of potential emotional losses as well. Amputation may force children to alter aspirations, rethink vocational plans, or give up previously enjoyed hobbies or recreational activities. Because children with congenital limb deficiency never experience life without a disability, some authors have suggested that they may be less vulnerable to the feelings of grief and loss observed in patients with acquired amputations.[11] Nevertheless, clinical descriptions indicate that children with congenital deficiencies also grieve as they become aware of the implications of their impairment and consider what might have been were it not for their congenital anomaly.[16]

Maturation and Disability

People with disabilities are often encouraged to view the adjustments they must make as a matter of "management" rather than "mastery."[16] Adjusting to a disability should be seen as an ongoing, dynamic process rather than a task to be accomplished and then left behind. This view of psychosocial adjustment seems particularly relevant for children with disabilities. Like other children, children with limb deficiencies are very much "works in progress," responding to ever-changing coping demands created by normal transitions and disruptions in daily life. Concurrent with their efforts to adapt to their limb deficiency, they are also dealing with the same changes in physical, cognitive, and social development that other children experience. The positive adjustment outcomes seen in children with limb deficiencies are particularly striking because many of the developmental tasks of late childhood and adolescence depend on physical abilities.[3] Unfortunately, researchers have not documented how developmental maturation in the child with a disability affects adjustment and coping.

Early Development and Awareness of Disability

For children with congenital limb deficiency, awareness of their disability is a gradual learning process that depends on cognitive and social maturation. Based on her work with disfigured people, Bradbury[16] developed a useful model of how self-awareness of a physical deficit emerges. The model takes into account the influence of normal developmental changes and can be applied readily to limb-deficient children. The process begins as children develop the ability to recognize themselves and appreciate that their limbs are a part of their bodies. This first awareness of disability emerges early. For example, parents of infants with congenital hand differences report that their babies focus more on the deficient hand than on the typically formed hand.[16] Another consideration is that the parents' tendency to focus more on the deficient hand may contribute to the child's awareness of it. A child's awareness of a limb loss, however, does not necessarily mean that he or she is distressed by it. Typically, children first exhibit distress about their limb loss when they become aware that others notice it and respond negatively. Children may experience a grief reaction between the ages of 7 and 9 years, as they come to appreciate the permanence of their limb loss more fully and are able to consider its long-term implications.

Adolescence

Adolescence is the period that has received the most attention in the literature for its potential influence on the adjustment of youngsters with limb deficiencies. Adolescence is characterized by marked susceptibility to peer influence, a drive for independence from authority figures, and extensive psychological work devoted to development of a self-identity.[17] Because the most common malignant bone tumors of childhood are most likely to occur in children age 10 to 20 years,[18] pediatric patients who require amputation for malignancy are likely to be in their preteen or teenage years. Although these patients are generally less emotionally devastated than once thought, the experience of losing one's limb at a time when body image concerns are so prevalent undoubtedly has enormous psychosocial implications.[17]

For all adolescents with limb deficiencies, emotional difficulties may be instigated or exacerbated when struggles inherent in the passage to adulthood interact with the coping demands created by a physical impairment. Teens may experience more distress about their limb loss as their desire for acceptance from peers increases and they become more focused on perceived differences between themselves and others. Increased self-consciousness may lead some teens to attempt to conceal their amputation by avoiding activities that they think risk exposure. In doing so, adolescents may inadvertently increase their feelings of awkwardness and social ineptness as they curtail their opportunities to develop friendships and refine social skills. Eventually, this pattern may contribute to a self-fulfilling prophecy in which social development becomes delayed and expectations of rejection by peers are confirmed.

Adolescence is characterized by increased introspection. Teenagers with limb deficiencies may focus on the implications of the impairment. Some may become preoccupied with fears that they will always be rejected as a dating or marriage partner. Those with congenital limb deficiencies may feel conflicted about hopes of one day having a family because of fears that they may burden their offspring with a congenital defect. Open communication between the adolescent and the health care team is critical so that worries can be shared, questions can be addressed, and speculation can be replaced with factual information.

Accurate information about the long-term psychosocial outcomes in people who experience an amputation during childhood enhances the ability of health care providers to counsel youngsters and families who understandably are concerned about the future. Such information is most readily available for childhood cancer survivors who undergo amputation for treatment of the disease. A recent study examined the education, employment, insurance, and marital status of 694 survivors of pediatric lower limb bone tumors.[19] Participants consisted of 471 survivors who underwent amputation and 223 in whom the limb was salvaged. Full biologic siblings closest in age to the survivor served as a comparison group for the study. Overall, no difference between amputees and nonamputees were found. When compared with siblings, however, amputees had significant deficits in education and employment status. Of particular concern was the finding that both groups (amputees and nonamputees) were significantly more likely to experience difficulty obtaining health insurance compared with siblings. Unfortunately, similar large-sample studies of the long-term psychosocial functioning of youngsters with congenital limb deficiencies or other types of acquired amputations have not been presented.

Individual Characteristics

Many authors have identified the need to document sources of individual variation in the psychological adjustment of children with disabilities. Generally, studies of adjustment in children with physical health impairments have found that, compared with peers, children with chronic illness or disability are at increased risk of emotional disorders and social adjustment difficulties.[3] As a group, children and adolescents with limb deficiencies seem to be an exception, typically showing a low incidence of psychological problems. Given these findings, children with limb deficiencies are an ideal group to study for the factors that contribute to emotional resilience in children. Few researchers, however, have investigated how personal characteristics of the limb-deficient child contribute to positive or negative psychosocial outcomes. For example, among patients with acquired amputations, clinical experience suggests that premorbid psychological functioning is an important predictor of adjustment to amputation, but this relationship has not been investigated empirically.

One exception is a study by Varni and associates[20] that examined the relationship between temperament and psychological and social adaptations in children with limb deficiencies. The authors defined temperament as a set of inherited personal traits that appear early in life and provide a foundation for later personality development. They found that children with increased emotional lability exhibited lower social competence and greater internalizing and externalizing of behavior problems. In addition, they observed a significant interaction between child emotionality and family cohesion. When family cohesion was low, child emotionality accounted for significant additional variance in behavioral adjustment. Based on this finding, the authors stress that temperament should be considered within the context of family environment when assessing adjustment in pediatric limb deficiencies.

Family and Social Environment

Limb-deficient children both affect and are affected by the people they encounter day to day. The reactions of others to the child's limb deficiency and the manner in which the child incorporates these social responses play a significant role in the adaptive process.[3] First and foremost, children live within the context of a family, which has its own rules, organizing principles, and beliefs about health, development, and illness.[21] Several reviews have considered the impact of the child's limb deficiency on the family adjustment and coping.[22] Others examined the influence of parent and family functioning on the psychological outcomes in children with physical impairments.[23,24]

Initial Parental Response

Few events are as devastating to parents as the birth of a child with a limb deficiency.[25] Similarly, an acquired amputation presents a crisis for most families. Regardless of timing and origin, limb loss in a child usually evokes strong emotions in the family. The early days and weeks following the event are a formative period, with significant potential to influence the family's expectations, adjustment, and coping. A qualitative study of the recollections of parents of children born with congenital limb deficiencies provides insights about parents' initial emotional reactions and experiences with disclosure of their child's disability.[26] Participants included 34 fathers and 63 mothers. Parents recalled initial reactions of shock, devastation, disbelief, a sense of loss and isolation, and worry about the future implications of the child's limb loss. Researchers found that many parents remembered feeling dissatisfied with the manner in which disclosure was handled. Early complaints centered on parents' beliefs that they did not receive sufficient information about congenital limb deficiency at the time of their child's birth. Later, parents' primary concerns shifted to worries about how others would receive their baby.

When dealing with parents at the time of the birth of a limb-deficient child, good communication strategies should be followed. Parents should be provided with information about their child's diagnosis and treatment options without delay and preferably with all the child's primary caregivers present. Open questions should be used to encourage sharing of information and feelings; for example, "What concerns you about what we've discussed so far?" Families should be encouraged to share their emotional responses, and those responses should be acknowledged rather than dismissed. Specific information about resources should be provided, and at the end of the session, arrangements should be made for follow-up conversations.

Early in the treatment process, parents may be called on to make a decision about amputation versus limb-sparing procedures. Although the enormous emotional burden associated with such a decision is understandable, outcome studies have tended to focus on the medical rather than psychological sequelae. Limited data are available to guide parents in terms of psychological outcomes associated with these treatment options, and studies have not examined the parents' decision-making process or long-term satisfaction with their choice.

Gender differences in parental response to a child's disability have also been investigated. A study of parents of infants (age 2 to 12 months) born with congenital anomalies found similar overall rates of parental burden and grief for mothers and fathers. The pattern of strain, however, tended to vary by gender, with mothers reporting more personal strain.[4] In another study, mothers were more likely than fathers to experience feelings of guilt after the birth of a child with a congenital limb deficiency.[26] Although the limited number of studies precludes definitive conclusions, the findings suggest that both mothers and fathers are significantly affected but may experience strain differently.

Parental Adjustment and Behavior

There is support for the hypothesis that parental emotional adjustment, parental coping, and family functioning affect psychological adjustment in children with health impairments.[23] Three alternative pathways have been proposed by which parents may influence their child's adaptation to a stressful event: coaching and direct instructions in specific techniques or courses of action; modeling of coping styles and strategies; and general contextual influences, such as quality of family relationships and communication.[27]

Among physically healthy children, parental psychological distress and marital discord have been associated with vulnerability to psychological maladjustment. Recent studies have confirmed the importance of the marital relationship in predicting stress and adjustment in parents of children with disabilities, particularly for mothers.[28] To determine the impact of parental adjustment on children with limb deficiency, Varni and Setoguchi[29] examined depression, anxiety, and marital discord in parents of 54 children with acquired or congenital limb deficiencies. Parental distress and marital discord were found to be significant predictors of the children's emotions. Higher marital discord (whether reported by mothers or fathers) was associated with increased symptoms of anxiety and depression and lower general self-esteem in the child.

The presence of a child with a limb deficiency may create lasting changes in the family system or the marital relationship. Although some couples may draw together in the adversity, others may experience strain in their relationship, especially if partners have very different beliefs about their child's limb deficiency.[16] A study of marital satisfaction among parents of children with a variety of health problems found that 25% to 37% of parents reported significant marital distress compared with 17% of a control group consisting of parents of children without health impairments.[30] On the other hand, divorce rates among parents of children with disabilities are not significantly different from that in the population at large.[22]

Social Environment

One of the more robust findings in the literature on children's adjustment to disability is the significant influence of peer attitudes and behav-

ior. A study that examined the role of peers in shaping the adjustment of children with limb deficiencies focused on perceived social support,[10] meaning the child's own appraisal of the availability and adequacy of social support. The study included 49 children with limb deficiencies (42 congenital, 7 acquired) age 8 to 13 years. Adjustment was assessed using measures of depressive symptoms, anxiety, and general self-esteem. Perceived parent, teacher, and peer support were variously related to the adjustment measures. The study highlights the potentially powerful effects of the school environment. Perceived classmate social support was the only correlate that proved to be a significant predictor of outcome in all three adjustment domains. In describing limitations, the authors emphasize that because of the correlational nature of the study, neither directionality nor causation can be assumed; that is, the direction of the relationship between perceived social support and adjustment cannot be assumed. An alternative hypothesis would be that youngsters with better adjustment elicit more social support from their classmates. Also, the presence of an as-yet-unidentified mediator or moderator variable may help explain the relationship between perceived classmate support and adjustment. Despite limitations, this study provides preliminary evidence for the benefits of enhancing social support as a way to better help a child cope. For example, educating classmates about the disability may help reduce stigma.

Cultural Influences

According to a model presented by Wallander and Varni,[31] cultural factors may influence adjustment to disability via direct and indirect pathways. For example, cultural factors may shape the child's or family's appraisal of the limb deficiency and influence their understanding of the socially acceptable role of a disabled person. Other influences of culture may include variations in tangible resources, such as access to health care,

and experiences of marginalization and racism. To examine the role of cultural influences in the management of pediatric limb deficiency, researchers conducted a series of studies that compared satisfaction ratings of Mexican-American and Anglo-American parents who had a child who was fitted for a prosthesis.[32] They found that Mexican-American parents rated themselves as more satisfied with their child's prosthesis and with the prosthesis service than Anglo-American parents did. The authors hypothesized that the differences might be culturally based. For example, Mexican-American parents may have been more satisfied because of the high respect for health care professionals in this ethnic group.

Critique of the Literature

The literature on psychological adjustment in children with limb deficiency is sparse, and most studies are correlational. Thus, when significant associations are observed, researchers cannot make definitive conclusions about causation or the direction of influence. In addition, most studies assess child and family functioning at a single time in the child's life. Longitudinal studies that examine changes in child and family functioning over time and allow researchers to consider the influence of developmental maturation are greatly needed. Greater efforts to collect descriptive information about the educational level, social adjustment, occupational outcome, and marital status of adults who grew up with a limb deficiency would allow for comparisons to the general population and enhance the clinician's ability to accurately counsel (and perhaps reassure) concerned patients and families. Qualitative studies provide rich and interesting clinical information, but are limited by the absence of a scientifically rigorous design. Finally, as seen in the psychological literature in general,[33] many studies are dominated by a negative bias, focusing exclusively on maladjustment and its sources but failing to investigate factors that may contribute positively to resilience or growth.

Supporting Adjustment in Pediatric Patients and Their Families

Although pediatric health care providers may think they focus primarily on improving physical outcomes, their contact with a parent, child, or adolescent can also influence psychosocial functioning. This section focuses on how health care providers can engage with the families to support positive adjustment. At times, the extent or intensity of adjustment difficulties may warrant including a mental health professional as part of the health care team. How health care professionals can collaborate effectively with mental health consultants is discussed.

Understanding the Adjustment Process

Health care providers may assume that a family's psychological distress is proportional to the severity of the child's limb deficiency. Most studies, however, have not found a clear association between severity of limb deficiency and adjustment, so that assumption is likely to be inaccurate. In addition, if families sense that they are viewed as "overreacting," it may jeopardize their relationship with the health care team. Bearing in mind that patient/family adjustment is influenced by many interacting factors, health care providers may find it most beneficial to avoid preconceived notions about the psychosocial challenges of a patient's situation and, instead, resolve to meet families where they are.

Just as physical growth and development complicate surgical and prosthetic management of pediatric patients, cognitive and social maturation trigger ever-changing psychosocial demands for children with limb deficiencies. In addition, children with limb deficiencies influence and are influenced by the social environment in which they live. Nevertheless, it can be quite unsettling for the health care team when pediatric patients who had previously shown positive adjustment begin to exhibit distress related to their limb deficiency. Because the psychosocial demands of limb deficiency change with maturation and normal childhood transitions, some fluctuation in child and family adjustment is to be expected, even among those who have shown a remarkable ability to adapt. Recognizing the ongoing, dynamic nature of the adjustment process and anticipating fluctuations in adjustment may improve the ability of all parties to work together to overcome challenges.

Keeping the Lines of Communication Open

Establishing and maintaining an effective therapeutic relationship is essential to all work with patients and their families.[34] Open dialogue is often the first step. The medical culture is one of action and initiative, however,[35] because of time pressures and competing demands,[34] so health care professionals may not take the time to carefully listen to, acknowledge, and address the concerns of patients and families. Learning active listening, described as the foundation upon which all effective communication is built, is one way to overcome this tendency.

Using Active Listening Techniques

Active listening involves searching to understand the meaning underlying the words patients use.[36] Developing effective active listening skills requires practice, self-awareness, and awareness of how the patient is responding. When the techniques are used correctly, they pay dividends in terms of building a working alliance with patients and families. Health care providers can encourage patients to share concerns by maintaining eye contact, refraining from interrupting, and using verbal and nonverbal prompts. To ensure the patient that he or she has been heard and understood correctly, the health care provider can respond by summarizing, clarifying, or acknowledging feelings.[37] For example, patients and families are likely to feel more understood and supported when health care providers acknowledge the feelings of sadness and distress that limb deficiency can generate.

Gathering Information

Accurate and timely information can improve patient care. For example, children may limit wearing their prosthesis because of dissatisfaction with its comfort, performance, or appearance that they may be afraid to express. That can result in less independence and more disability than the child would otherwise have.[38] Health care providers can promote information exchange in face-to-face discussions with simple, open-ended questions.[36] For example, asking, "Would you describe a typical day with your new prosthesis?" is likely to elicit more information than asking, "Is the fit on your new prosthesis all right?" Following up with closed questions—those that can be answered with a few words or a simple "yes" or "no"—may be useful for obtaining specific information, but closed questions do not encourage the person to expand on what is said.[16] Practitioners might also consider using pencil-and-paper measures to gather information about patient satisfaction. The Child Amputee Prosthetics Project-Prosthesis Satisfaction Inventory (CAPP-PSI) is a brief parent report measure designed to assess parents' satisfaction with their child's prosthetic device in regard to fit, function, appearance, and service.[38] The CAPP-PSI has significant internal consistency and preliminary construct validity and does not appear to be contaminated by sociodemographic variables or the severity of a child's limb deficiency. Because some parents may feel more comfortable expressing concerns in writing, the CAPP-PSI may help identify dissatisfaction early.

Providing Information

Families consistently say that the support they appreciate and benefit from most is the information they receive from health care providers. Parents want the best for their child and value the knowledge that experienced health care providers can impart because it helps parents make informed decisions. Also, parents report that, as they gain knowledge about their child's condition and expected treatment, they feel more in control and less at the mercy of their child's disability. Kerr and McIntosh[26] provide specific recommendations for the initial discussion with parents about their child's limb deficiency. Although based on a qualitative study of parents of infants with congenital limb deficiency, most of their guidelines apply well to discussions with parents of children with acquired amputations. Kerr and McIntosh recommend that information be given as early as possible with both parents present, whenever feasible. They advise health care providers to be honest and empathetic, encourage parents to discuss their concerns, and advise parents of resources for additional information. Finally, these authors suggest that health care providers give opportunities for follow-up conversations frequently and without delay.

When providing information to children and adolescents, it is important to consider the patient's developmental status and readiness. A basic principle of pediatric prosthetics is to provide components only when the child is developmentally ready to use them.[11,39] A similar philosophy should apply to giving children information about their limb deficiency. Information about the child's condition, prognosis, or treatment should be tailored to the child's developmental level. Although all children will require at least some information to be adequately prepared, health care providers need to balance thoroughness with a step-by-step approach of giving information as it is needed to prevent patients from becoming overwhelmed by anticipatory worries.[17]

Empowering Families

Family-centered care involves more than "being nice" to patients and families.[36] It requires that health care providers adopt attitudes and behaviors that promote greater participation on the part of the family.[40] Health care providers empower patients and families by defining roles clearly, making patients active in their treatment, and partnering with families when making decisions and setting goals.[36] Empowerment assumes that most people are competent or have the capacity to become competent and will be enabled by experiences that create opportunities for competence to be displayed.[40] Health care providers can create a sense of empowerment in those they work with by providing information, apprising families of resources, and working with families to identify and implement a course of action. As patients develop experience in successfully overcoming difficulties, they gain confidence in their ability to cope with future adversities.

For those who work with pediatric limb deficiency, a relevant example might be parents who express concern that their school-age child is being excluded and teased by peers. As described above, perceived peer support has been associated with positive psychosocial outcomes in children with limb deficiency. An initial step toward empowerment might be to discuss these research findings with the parent and acknowledge the importance of helping the child develop supportive peer relationships. Next, the health care provider could inform the family of available resources. For example, several excellent books, such as those by Frankel[41] and Ross,[42] provide practical information on helping children deal with social difficulties

and develop friendship skills. Finally, with the support of the health care provider, the family could identify a course of action and determine what role, if any, the health care provider should play in implementing the plan. In the short-term, an empowerment approach may take more time and effort than a more "professionally directed" intervention.[16] However, the former approach is much more likely to enhance the family's sense of their own competence for handling future difficulties.

Fostering Independence

For children with physical disabilities, achieving autonomy may be a particularly important developmental issue.[43] Even the challenges parents normally face of ensuring the child's health and safety while facilitating the child's self-sufficiency are difficult to negotiate. Parents often report that they feel more conflicted or confused about the best child-rearing practices when it comes to parenting their child with a disability. For example, well-intended efforts to compensate for the child's vulnerability, shelter the child from the scrutiny of others, or protect the child from failure may contribute to the development of unnecessary dependence or interfere with the parent's ability to set appropriate limits.

Among other pediatric populations with health impairments, parental overprotection has emerged as a predictor of child maladjustment. Overprotectiveness has been described as an intrusive parenting style driven by the parent's anxiety. It is characterized by excessive physical or social contact, infantilization of the child, and excessive concern for the child's well-being.[43] Because more parental involvement than normal may truly be called for to manage a child's disability, it is easy to see how parents of children with disabilities may be at high risk for becoming overprotective.

Ultimately, children with disabilities must determine for themselves what their true limitations are. Although inappropriate dependence may emerge from the best intentions of caring parents, in the long run, it undermines self-esteem and sets families up for conflict. Because of their experience with many children who have similar physical limitations, health care providers may be in an especially good position to gently make families aware of the harmful effects of unnecessary dependence and guide parents toward practices that promote appropriate autonomy.

Recognizing the Need for Meaning and Control

People have an overwhelming need to find some kind of explanation for events that seem to have no obvious cause.[16] Because most pediatric limb deficiencies are congenital anomalies of unknown origin, many patients and families will never have a satisfactory answer to the "Why?" of their child's limb deficiency. In time, many parents reconcile themselves to this distressing reality, but some may remain so preoccupied by their search for an answer that it interferes with their adjustment process. As children with limb deficiencies mature, they may also wrestle with questions such as, "Why did God do this to me?" or "Why was I the only child in the family born with a missing limb?" Children with acquired amputations are vulnerable to the unsettling effects of the unanswered "Why?" as well. Questions like "Why weren't we more careful?" or "Why did I have to get cancer?" can haunt patients and families. The absence of definitive answers also can be distressing for health care providers who are accustomed to working with facts and certainties.

One of the most consistent findings in the vast literature on stress and coping is that stressors over which we feel we have no control are the most destructive. Health care providers can help families avoid the detrimental effects of perseverating on issues that cannot be changed by recognizing the need for meaning and control and encouraging families to

focus on what their child *can* do. Certainly, this is not meant to imply that parents' distress over their child's limitations should be dismissed or ignored. On the contrary, acknowledging feeling is essential to developing trust with families and often increases their receptiveness to any suggestions the health care provider might offer. If families remain focused on the unchangeable aspects of their child's situation, however, they are left without any choices. Once feelings are acknowledged and families begin to focus on their child's abilities, they can start to make choices, and their sense of control is increased.

Even simple choices like selecting the color for Velcro straps or incorporating the logo of a favorite sports team on a prosthesis can boost a child's sense of control. Making a decision to participate in a sport or other recreational activity can enhance self-confidence and help children develop physical, psychological, and social skills that will be enduring assets.[44]

As they mature, some youngsters may be drawn to organizations such as the US Paralympics or Wheelchair Sports USA because they enhance the youngster's sense of identity as a person with a disability. Others may derive meaning from being involved in relevant civic groups. Two examples are the Land Mine Survivors Network, an international organization that works to eradicate land mines and support land mine victims, and KaBOOM!, a nonprofit agency that partners with local communities to build safe, accessible playgrounds. As they discover their ability to help others, children may find their sense of vulnerability and helplessness to be diminished.

Other youngsters may choose to pursue activities that have no particular association with their limb loss because they prefer to deemphasize their disability or do not think of themselves as disabled at all. For example, some children favor an attitude toward their limitations that has been referred to as "healthy denial."

These youngsters take pride in their ability to "put their disability in its place" by minimizing its importance to their overall identity as a person.

When encouraging children with disabilities to pursue activities, health care providers and parents should take care to consider individual likes and dislikes and respect the child's personal choice. Although participating in sports can be extremely beneficial, some children with limb deficiencies will have little enthusiasm for athletics because of personal preferences that have nothing to do with their disability. Because sports programs for children with physical impairments tend to be better established than other types of recreational programs, health care teams may need to investigate local resources to identify alternative activities for children with other interests. The child's general orientation toward activities that accentuate or minimize their identity as a person with a disability should be considered. Personal preference should be accepted so long as the approach is meaningful to the youngster and contributes to his or her growth.

Providing Support for Mental Health

Although most children do not show prolonged maladjustment to their limb deficiency, they will have periods of increased distress related to it. In addition, health impairments can create a setting in which some children and families perform at their worst.[45] At times, the difficulties the child and family face may be beyond the scope of the existing health care team. When a counseling referral or consultation with a mental health professional seems warranted, there is much the referring team can do to foster a positive experience for all concerned.

Encouraging Additional Support

Resistance to psychological intervention, on the part of both families and health care teams, is not uncommon.[34] Health care providers can begin to destigmatize the process by first examining their own beliefs and expectations about mental health interventions. Hastily indicating that the patient should "consider counseling" or requesting a "psych consult" without first discussing the rationale with the patient and family will likely generate a negative reaction or erode the therapeutic relationship. Patients may assume that the health care provider believes that they are "weak" or "crazy" and feel hurt, insulted, or embarrassed.

In reality, significant adjustment difficulties are usually a normal reaction to an extraordinary situation rather than a sign of psychopathology. A competence-based approach, which views symptoms as well-intentioned attempts at adaptive functioning that have gone awry,[16,34] is usually appropriate. Health care providers can normalize the experience by telling the patient and family that they are going through an ordeal that would be a significant challenge for most people. Framing referrals in a way that shows shared responsibility for finding a solution to the presenting problem can strengthen the family's alliance with the health care team.[34] For example, a pediatric prosthetist could tell the family that he or she is an expert in designing and fitting a prosthetic device but would like assistance in helping the patient overcome self-consciousness about his or her appearance so that it does not interfere with treatment.

Groups

Support organizations or other therapeutic groups can expose patients and families to positive models, experience with problem solving and helping others, and opportunities to relate to peers.[46] The impact of parent-to-parent support was investigated in 63 families of children born with an upper limb deficiency.[6] Data were derived from in-depth interviews with parents. The researchers concluded that parent-to-parent contact fulfilled a support need that was not being met by other sources, reduced parents' sense of isolation and fears about the future, and helped parents resolve practical problems. Although the study is limited by its retrospective, qualitative design, it represents an important first step in discerning how parents of newborns with congenital limb deficiencies may benefit from contact with other families in similar circumstances.

When making a referral to a group, health care providers should anticipate that some patients and families may be reluctant to join because they feel there is a stigma attached to being part of an organization for people with disabilities. Attending these organizations' annual activities, such as a family picnic or a weekend family camp, can be an excellent way to expose families to positive models without requiring them to make a long-term commitment. For families who are interested in becoming involved with organizations that offer ongoing activities, multiple options are often available at the local as well as the national level. Before making referrals, health care providers should verify that organizations have adequate resources to support families and a facilitator who ensures that meetings are constructive and solution focused.

Summary and Conclusions

Although experiences of prolonged maladjustment are rare among children with limb deficiencies, most children and families will have periods of increased distress and challenge as they adjust. Health care providers can support positive psychosocial outcomes by acknowledging concerns and providing information and guidance that empowers the family and enhances their sense of competence and control. Ultimately, the best way for health care providers to help children with disabilities adjust positively is to develop accurate knowledge of the nature and causes of adjustment difficulties and then to develop and implement empirically sound interventions.[35] Clearly, additional research is needed to better understand factors that contribute to psychological risk and resilience in children with limb deficiencies and to guide preventive and interventional techniques to overcome adjustment difficulties.

References

1. Quittner AL, DiGirolamo AM: Family adaptation to childhood disability and illness, in Ammerman RT, Campo JV (eds): *Handbook of Pediatric Psychology and Psychiatry: Disease, Injury and Illness*. Needham Heights, MA, Allyn & Bacon, 1998, vol 2, pp 70-102.

2. Wallander JL, Thompson RJ Jr: Psychosocial adjustment of children with chronic physical conditions, in Roberts MC (ed): *Handbook of Pediatric Psychology*, ed 2. New York, NY, Guilford Press, 1995, pp 124-141.

3. Tyc VL: Psychosocial adaptation of children and adolescents with limb deficiencies: A review. *Clin Psychol Rev* 1992;12:275-291.

4. Hunfeld JA, Tempels A, Passchier J, Hazebroek JW, Tibboel D: Brief report: Parental burden and grief one year after the birth of a child with a congenital anomaly. *J Pediatr Psychol* 1999;24:515-520.

5. Hommeyer JS, Holmbeck GN, Wills KE, Coers S: Condition severity and psychosocial functioning in pre-adolescents with spina bifida: Disentangling proximal functional status and distal adjustment outcomes. *J Pediatr Psychol* 1999;24:499-509.

6. Kerr SM, McIntosh JB: Coping when a child has a disability: Exploring the impact of parent-to-parent support. *Child Care Health Dev* 2000;26:309-322.

7. Varni JW, Setoguchi Y: Perceived physical appearance and adjustment of adolescents with congenital/acquired limb deficiencies: A path-analytic model. *J Clin Child Psychol* 1996;25:201-208.

8. Varni JW, Rubenfeld LA, Talbot D, Setoguchi Y: Determinants of self-esteem in children with congenital/acquired limb deficiencies. *J Dev Behav Pediatr* 1989;10:13-16.

9. Wallander JL, Varni JW: Appraisal, coping, and adjustment in adolescents with a physical disability, in Wallander JL, Siegel LJ (eds): *Adolescent Health Problems: Behavioral Perspectives*. New York, NY, Guilford Press, 1995, pp 209-231.

10. Varni JW, Setoguchi Y, Rappaport LR, Talbot D: Psychological adjustment and perceived social support in children with congenital/acquired limb deficiencies. *J Behav Med* 1992;15:31-44.

11. Bryant PR, Pandian G: Acquired limb deficiencies: 1. Acquired limb deficiencies in children and young adults. *Arch Phys Med Rehabil* 2001;82(3 suppl 1):S3-S8.

12. Letts M, Davidson D: Epidemiology and prevention of traumatic amputations in children, in Herring JA, Birch JG (eds): *The Child With a Limb Deficiency*. Rosemont, IL, American Academy of Orthopaedic Surgeons, 1998, pp 235-251.

13. Atala KD, Carter BD: Pediatric limb amputation: Aspects of coping and psychotherapeutic intervention. *Child Psychiatry Hum Dev* 1992;23:117-130.

14. Kazak AE, Barakat LP, Meeske K, et al: Posttraumatic stress, family functioning, and social support in survivors of childhood leukemia and their mothers and fathers. *J Consult Clin Psychol* 1997;65:120-129.

15. Trautwein LC, Smith DG, Rivara FP: Pediatric amputation injuries: Etiology, cost, and outcome. *J Trauma* 1996;41:831-838.

16. Bradbury E: *Counselling People With Disfigurement*. Leicester, England, The British Psychological Society, 1996.

17. Fung AS, Lee PW: Sacrificing a limb for life: Psychological interventions in osteosarcoma. *Behav Cogn Psychother* 1996;24:283-286.

18. Himelstein BP, Dormans JP: Malignant bone tumors of childhood. *Pediatr Clin North Am* 1996;43:967-984.

19. Rajaram N, Neglie JP, Clohisy DR, et al: Education, employment, insurance, and marital status among 694 survivors of pediatric lower extremity bone tumors. *Cancer* 2003;97:2554-2564.

20. Varni JW, Rubenfeld LA, Talbot D, Setoguchi Y: Family functioning, temperament, and psychologic adaptation in children with congenital or ac-quired limb deficiencies. *Pediatrics* 1989;84:323-330.

21. Kazak AE, Segal-Andrews AM, Johnson K: Pediatric psychology research and practice: A family/systems approach, in Roberts MC (ed): *Handbook of Pediatric Psychology*, ed 2. New York, NY, Guilford Press, 1995, pp 84-104.

22. Benson BA, Gross AM: The effects of a congenitally handicapped child on the marital dyad: A review of the literature. *Clin Psychol Rev* 1989;9:747-758.

23. Drotar D: Relating parent and family functioning to the psychological adjustment of children with chronic health conditions: What have we learned? What do we need to know? *J Pediatr Psychol* 1997;22:149-165.

24. Lavigne JV, Faier-Routman J: Correlates of psychological adjustment to pediatric physical disorders: A meta-analytic review and comparison with existing models. *J Dev Behav Pediatr* 1993;14:117-123.

25. Ezaki M: Upper extremity deficiencies, in Herring JA, Birch JG (eds): *The Child With a Limb Deficiency*. Rosemont, IL, American Academy of Orthopaedic Surgeons, 1998, pp 381-385.

26. Kerr SM, McIntosh JB: Disclosure of disability: Exploring the perspective of parents. *Midwifery* 1998;14:225-232.

27. Kliewer W, Sandler I, Wolchik S: Family socialization of threat-appraisal and coping: Coaching, modeling, and family context, in Nestmann F, Hurrelmann K (eds): *Social Networks and Social Support in Childhood and Adolescence*. Berlin, Germany, Walter de DeGruyter, 1994, pp 211-291.

28. Trute B, Hiebert-Murphy D: Family adjustment to childhood developmental disability: A measure of parent appraisal of family impacts. *J Pediatr Psychol* 2002;27:271-280.

29. Varni JW, Setoguchi Y: Effects of parental adjustment on the adaptation of children with congenital or acquired limb deficiencies. *J Dev Behav Pediatr* 1993;14:13-20.

30. Quittner AL, DiGirolamo AM, Michel M, Eigen H: Parental response to cystic fibrosis: A contextual analysis of the diagnosis phase. *J Pediatr Psychol* 1992;17:683-704.

31. Wallander JL, Varni JW: Adjustment in children with chronic physical disorders: Programmatic research on a disability-stress-coping model, in La Greca AM, Siegel LJ, Wallander JL, Walker CE (eds): *Stress and Coping in Child Health*. New York, NY, Guilford Press, 1992, pp 279-298.

32. Varni JW, Pruitt SD, Seid M: Health-related quality of life in pediatric limb deficiency, in Herring JA, Birch JG (eds): *The Child With a Limb Deficiency*. Rosemont, IL, American Academy of Orthopaedic Surgeons, 1998, pp 457-473.

33. Seligman ME, Csikszentmihalyi M: Positive psychology: An introduction. *Am Psychol* 2000;55:5-14.

34. Kazak AE, Simms S, Rourke MT: Family systems practice in pediatric psychology. *J Pediatr Psychol* 2002;27:133-143.

35. Drotar D: Pioneers in pediatric psychology: Between two professional worlds. Personal reflections on a career in a pediatric setting. *J Pediatr Psychol* 2001;26:185-192.

36. Rollnick S, Mason P, Butler C: (eds): *Health Behavior Change: A Guide for Practitioners*. Edinburgh, Scotland, Churchill Livingstone, 1999.

37. Miller WR, Rollnick S: (eds): *Motivational Interviewing: Preparing People for Change*, ed 2. New York, NY, Guilford Press, 2002.

38. Pruitt SD, Varni JW, Seid M, Setoguchi Y: Prosthesis satisfaction outcome measurement in pediatric limb deficiency. *Arch Phys Med Rehabil* 1997;78:750-754.

39. Pruitt SD, Seid M, Varni JW, Setoguchi Y: Toddlers with limb deficiency: Conceptual basis and initial application of a functional status outcome measure. *Arch Phys Med Rehabil* 1999;80:819-824.

40. Dunst CJ, Trivette CM, Davis M, Cornwell J: Enabling and empowering families of children with health impairments. *Child Health Care* 1988;17:71-81.

41. Frankel FH: (ed): *Good Friends Are Hard to Find: Help Your Child Find, Make, and Keep Friends*. Los Angeles, CA, Perspective Publishing, 1996.

42. Ross DM: (ed): *Childhood Bullying and Teasing: What School Personnel, Other Professionals, and Parents Can Do*. Alexandria, VA, American Counseling Association, 1996.

43. Holmbeck GN, Johnson SZ, Wills KE, et al: Observed and perceived parental overprotection in relation to psychosocial adjustment in preadolescents with a physical disability: The mediational role of behavioral autonomy. *J Consult Clin Psychol* 2002;70:96-110.

44. Anderson TF: Aspects of sports and recreation for the child with a limb deficiency, in Herring JA, Birch JG (eds): *The Child With a Limb Deficiency*. Rosemont, IL, American Academy of Orthopaedic Surgeons, 1998, pp 345-352.

45. Simms S, Warner NJ: A framework for understanding and responding to the psychosocial needs of children with Langerhans cell histiocytosis and their families. *Hematol Oncol Clin North Am* 1998;12:359-367.

46. Plante WA, Lobato D, Engel R: Review of group interventions for pediatric chronic conditions. *J Pediatr Psychol* 2001;26:435-453.

Chapter 66

Occupational Therapy

Joanna G. Patton, OTR/L

Introduction

A sound clinical approach for the treatment of children with limb deficiencies and amputations incorporates principles of child development and the expertise of a multidisciplinary team. This chapter discusses the principles of child development as they relate to early prosthetic fitting, the role of a knowledgeable team in providing comprehensive care, and the occupational therapist's role in the patient/prosthetic evaluation and training process.

Children with unilateral upper limb loss can perform most, if not all, of their daily living activities without a prosthesis. This accomplishment is necessary and desirable for independence and flexibility in performing life skills. Use of a prosthesis is a choice made by the family and/or child. Gaining skill with the prosthesis takes time, patience, and practice.

Portions of this chapter are adapted with permission from Patton J: Developmental approach to treatment: Training the child with a unilateral upper extremity prosthesis, in Meier R, Atkins D (eds): *Functional Restoration of Adults and Children With Upper Extremity Amputation.* New York, NY, Demos Medical Publishing, 2004, pp 297-315.

Whether or not a prosthesis is part of the equation, the team and family need to work together toward a positive outcome for the child.

Unilateral Transradial Deficiency
Principles of Child Development

Sypniewski[1] reviewed the literature in 1972 and reported on the various rationales for early upper limb prosthetic fitting for children. Early fitting is clearly an important concept; however, considerable controversy exists as to which developmental milestones are most appropriate as a basis for treatment.

Shaperman and associates[2] administered a survey in 2002 titled "Developmental Indicators for Children's Unilateral Upper Limb Prosthetic Fitting: Congenital Transradial Deficiency." Of the 45 clinics that provided usable data, most relied on developmental milestones to determine when to fit the first infant passive prosthesis. Thirty-eight clinics cited the achievement of independent sitting balance as the most important readiness criterion. Clinicians feel that other indicators, such as the baby's ability to explore with the sound hand and the ability to hold an object in the elbow or against the body, are also very important. Early fitting is

preferred; two thirds of the clinics provided an infant prosthesis between 5 and 7 months of age.

In 1965, Brooks and Shaperman[3] conducted a study with a small sample of patients at the University of California, Los Angeles Child Amputee Prosthetics Project (CAPP). This research revealed that children who received their prosthesis before the age of 2 years developed better wearing and skill patterns than did children who received the prosthesis between 2 and 5 years of age.

In 1983, Scotland and Galway[4] reported on a long-term study of 131 children fitted with upper limb prostheses at the facility then known as the Ontario Crippled Children's Centre. Eighty-five patients with congenital limb deficiencies received their prostheses before 2 years of age. Only 19 patients (22%) had stopped wearing their prostheses at the time of the study. By comparison, more than 50% of the 31 patients who were fit after 2 years of age no longer wore a prosthesis.

Jain[5] contends that a child with a congenital limb deficiency who is not fit with a first prosthesis between 2 and 5 years of age develops compensatory techniques independent of a prosthesis and is therefore more likely to reject the prosthesis. Hubbard and associates[6] are emphatic about fitting before a child develops compensatory methods. They feel that fitting the first infant passive prosthesis between 3 and 6 months of age conditions the baby to wear the prosthesis and assists with gross motor development.

Clinical experience and practice at CAPP also demonstrate that habit patterns develop at an early age. Accordingly, if a family is interested in prosthetic fitting, providing the infant with a passive prosthesis when independent sitting balance is established seems to be a common-sense approach. Because the baby has progressed beyond the rolling stage, the prosthesis is less likely to hamper movement. Once the baby develops a wearing pattern, he or she learns to include it in age-appropriate gross motor activities. If the residual forearm is short, the prosthesis provides length and support to help the baby clasp large toys, creep on all fours, and pull to stand. By the time the child receives an active terminal device, he or she will have had an opportunity to become accustomed to wearing a prosthesis.[7]

Most clinicians agree that providing the first prosthesis when the child is entering the "terrible twos" can be a very negative experience and should be avoided if possible. A motivated child who is fitted at a later time has the potential to develop a good wear and use pattern. The child should not be denied the opportunity to receive a prosthesis simply because substitute patterns of function are already in place and habits are difficult to change. Outcome studies are needed to provide objective data that may resolve some of the issues related to when and what type of prosthesis to fit. Until then, opinions and approaches to prosthetic treatment will continue to differ.

The Team Approach

Early intervention and support are important for families. Whenever possible, family members should meet with an experienced multidisciplinary team soon after the baby's birth. Whether they are totally overwhelmed by the birth of a child with a limb deficiency or seem able to cope with the crisis, all parents benefit from the opportunity to discuss feelings, concerns, and expectations. With access to the World Wide Web, some parents obtain a great deal of information about their baby's deficiency and the potential treatment options before they come to the limb deficiency clinic. Family and friends are also a resource for the new parents, providing information that may or may not be appropriate. Team members will need to clarify misconceptions or misinformation about surgical and prosthetic interventions. After the first team visit, parents are asked to bring siblings and extended family members to the center so that everyone may receive accurate information about the treatment process.

The occupational therapist evaluates development and reassures the family that the baby with a transradial deficiency has the potential to develop normally unless there are other medical or neurologic problems unrelated to the limb deficiency. The child will be able to perform most activities of daily living—self-help, play, school, and recreational and vocational tasks—with and without the prosthesis. The family is encouraged not to overprotect the limb-deficient child but rather treat the child the same as other siblings or children in terms of performing daily tasks, receiving discipline, and going to regular school.[7]

The prosthetist and therapist also explain how children perform activities with and without a prosthesis. Some parents want a prosthesis for their infant; others question whether one is necessary. A child does not have to wear and use a prosthesis. Clinical experience reveals that children who have unilateral limb loss below the elbow are independent and functional without a prosthesis. Using a prosthesis does not change the central nervous system, nor does it alter the acquisition of developmental milestones. The child develops life skills through practice within the framework of his or her personality, natural abilities, and interests. Certainly the prosthesis can be beneficial by allowing the child to perform two-handed tasks away from the chest area at the midline of the body. Without the prosthesis, the child uses natural substitute grasp patterns such as clasping an object under the arm or against the body and using the residual limb as a stabilizer. The uncovered residual limb also retains full tactile sensation, which is a definite functional advantage.

The therapist and prosthetist will also provide information about state-of-the-art prostheses and clarify which type of components and control systems are available at the center where the child is receiving care. If the family has no insurance or access to other funding, prosthetic options may be limited.

Families need time to assimilate the information provided by the team because they are the ones who must make informed decisions concerning the prosthesis for the child. Even though the team provides information, support, and training, the parents are the ones who follow through on a daily basis. They help the child develop a consistent prosthetic wearing pattern and encourage use of the prosthesis to perform daily activities.[7]

Infant Prosthesis (No Active Control)

The prosthesis prescribed initially for infants is a lightweight transradial prosthesis with a nonactivated terminal device. An infant chest harness is used instead of the traditional figure-of-8 type (Figure 1). In some centers, use of a self-suspending supracondylar socket eliminates the need for a harness. The chief merit of a simple chest harness is that it provides enough suspension to prevent the socket from coming off when the baby crawls. The underside of the socket can be covered with a material that provides friction, to prevent the baby from sliding when the prosthesis is used for support on a hard, slick surface.[7]

Whenever possible, the parents should have the opportunity to select the type of prosthesis or at least the terminal device for their baby. Early options include a CAPP terminal device (TD) No. 1 (Hosmer Dorrance Corporation, Campbell, CA), a L'il E-Z Infant Hand (manufactured under a cooperative agreement between Los Amigos Research Education Institute and Therapeutic Recreation Systems [TRS], Inc, Boulder, CO; originally developed through a National Institutes for Disability & Rehabilitation Research grant), or the RSL-Steeper Infant Foam Filled Hand (Liberating Technologies, Inc, Holliston, MA). Other options may include the Alpha Infant Hand (TRS, Inc), the Infant 2 Hand (TRS, Inc), or an infant mitt.

The CAPP TD No. 1 has a large grasping surface, a 3-in-wide opening, and a good friction cover to provide a secure hold on an object. The manufacturer issues the terminal device with a regular spring. The prosthetist will need to change to a soft spring so that the toddler can open the CAPP TD with the sound hand.[8]

The thumb of the L'il E-Z Infant Hand opens easily to allow a toy or other item to be placed in the hand. Objects may also be inserted into the well or opening created by the index finger–thumb closure. No glove is required, and it is easily cleaned.

The Alpha Infant Hand has a passive holding capability and no glove. The hand is easy to clean. The Infant 2 Hand is a passive hand with a cup-shaped volar surface but has no capacity to grasp or hold an object.

The RSLSteeper Infant Foam Filled Hand is a lightweight hand that comes in several sizes and has a pleasing appearance. It does not provide grasp function.

Prosthesis Evaluation and Training

The prosthesis is evaluated by the prosthetist and therapist before delivery to the patient to ensure that it conforms to the prescription and standards of the clinic. The occupational therapist observes fit, comfort,

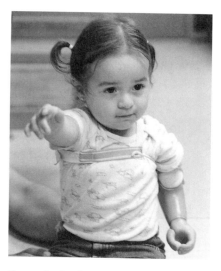

Figure 1 Passive transradial prosthesis with an infant harness.

and function of the prosthesis during normal use. Watching the baby move and play provides the opportunity to evaluate the stability of the socket and harness. Any signs of restriction or discomfort are reported to the prosthetist so that the necessary changes and adjustments can be made.

If possible, the therapist should see the baby and family two or three times during the first month to provide both information and support. Parents must be taught to correctly apply and remove the prosthesis; maintain the prosthesis in good condition by washing the harness, cleaning the inside of the socket, and using clean residual limb socks each day; encourage the baby to use the prosthesis in normal play activities; and identify when the socket and harness are tight, taking the child to the prosthetist for necessary adjustments.

Grandparents, siblings, babysitters, and other extended family members are encouraged to attend at least one session. Their cooperation with parents is vital in order to establish a consistent wearing pattern for the baby. Wearing the prosthesis the entire time the baby is awake is both reasonable and desirable. The prosthesis is removed at bed, bath, and nap times. Wearing patterns may vary with climate changes and individual parental needs.[7]

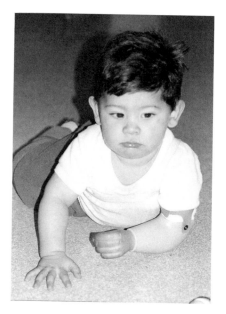

Figure 2 The baby includes the prosthesis to support his body weight.

When the baby receives the first prosthesis, body and arm movements may be awkward for the first few weeks. The family need not be overprotective but should provide assistance if the prosthesis becomes pinned under the baby's body or caught in furniture. The baby should be encouraged to include the prosthesis to stabilize body weight when creeping on all fours or when pulling to stand (Figure 2). Large balls or stuffed animals are presented so that the child learns to clasp objects between the sound arm and the prosthesis. If the terminal device has grasp function, the parents are asked to place a toy or cookie in the device. The 8- to 12-month-old child may try to remove the item or could totally ignore it. As the parents continue to place objects in the terminal device, the toddler becomes aware of the holding function and will mimic this behavior.[7] Gesell and associates[9] describe a similar developmental activity in which babies learn to place cubes in and out of a cup. This adaptive behavior becomes more meaningful and engrossing as the baby gets closer to 18 to 20 months of age. Use of a terminal device that has grasp capability provides the opportunity to learn about the holding function

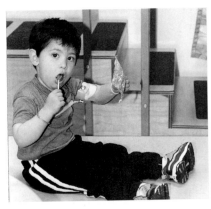

Figure 3 The child learns about the holding function of the terminal device (E-Z Infant Hand).

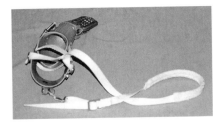

Figure 4 The first active prosthesis, with a CAPP TD No. 1 and a figure-of-8 harness.

even before the device is activated (Figure 3).

Readiness to Activate the Terminal Device

The control line or cable is added to the transradial prosthesis when the child demonstrates certain developmental behaviors that indicate the ability to learn how to use an active terminal device. Four criteria are used to determine readiness: (1) the child is able to follow simple directions that have no more than two steps; (2) the child demonstrates an attention span of at least 10 minutes; (3) the child demonstrates awareness that the terminal device can hold an object and attempts to open it with the sound hand and shows an interest in activities that require the use of two hands; and (4) the child shows some willingness to be handled, allowing the parent or therapist to move the arm (with prosthesis) through the control motion.[7]

Some of these behaviors become apparent near the child's second birthday and are based on principles of development. Pulaski[10] says "the child at two makes a transition from sensory motor experience to mental activity." The mental activity is demonstrated by the child's ability to follow simple directions and to understand cause and effect. In Shaperman and associates' survey,[2] these developmental criteria are also cited as im-

portant indicators that determine when to introduce an active control system. According to Gesell and associates,[9,11] the 2- to 2.5-year-old child starts expressing interest in constructive activity such as building with blocks and fitting simple toys together. Children may also demonstrate an elementary interest in imaginative play at this age. Introducing the active control line or cable at this time allows the therapist to capitalize on developmental skills and facilitate prosthetic training. However, these changes do take place during the "terrible twos," when behavior may be volatile and unpredictable. After the control line is added and everyone gears up for the training, the child may become uncooperative. The therapist and family members must remain flexible and patient. The formal training can be postponed, or alternative nonstructured training methods can be pursued. When the child reaches forward or leans over during play, tension on the control line will cause the terminal device to open. Calling attention to the inadvertent operation reinforces the learning process.[7]

Evaluation of the Prosthesis With the Active Terminal Device

If the child has outgrown the prosthesis, a new one is fabricated or the control line and figure-of-8 harness are added to the current prosthesis. The terminal device of choice is a voluntary-opening CAPP TD No. 1 (Figure 4). Some centers use the small Dorrance Hook or the voluntary-

closing TRS Adept Device or TRS Lite Touch Hand (TRS, Inc). Small size voluntary opening mechanical hands are also available but not recommended for the young child's first active terminal device. The hands are either too difficult to open or provide minimal pinch force, frustrating the child's attempt to learn terminal device operation.

Because the size and contour of the child's anatomy—as well as the range of motion and strength of the shoulder girdle—are certainly not the same as the adult's, the following components and adjustments should be standard in a child's prosthesis to maximize efficiency and ease of operation: (1) the cross point of the harness is stitched in the center of the back a little lower than C7 rather than toward the sound side; (2) the control attachment strap and lower axilla loop strap pass over the lower third of the scapulae; (3) the CAPP TD needs a soft spring, the 10X hook needs one quarter to one half of a rubber band, and both should open and close smoothly; (4) the cable housing is lined with Teflon to increase the efficiency of the cable system; and (5) the axilla loop is padded with Dacron felt and nylon tricot instead of plastic tubing for softness with skin contact.

Whenever a new prosthesis is issued, information about care and maintenance is reviewed. With their busy lives, parents sometimes forget to care properly for the prosthesis. Part of the ongoing treatment process is to impress upon families the importance of maintaining good personal hygiene and practicing the following procedures: (1) clean the inside of the socket nightly, and wash the harness at least weekly; (2) remove dirt or sand from the pulley system of the CAPP TD, using an air hose if necessary, and clean the ball bearing of the hook by immersing it in alcohol; (3) change the CAPP TD covers when they wear out, and remove all rubber bands from the hook when the elastic deteriorates, replacing them with new ones; (4) retread the neoprene lining of the hook when it wears out to maintain complete closure of the hook fingers; (5) clean the glove of a mechanical hand with alcohol or the manufacturer's glove cleaner; (6) adjust the wrist friction to prevent the terminal device from inadvertent movement during use; and (7) keep all appointments for repairs and harness adjustments.[7]

Control Motion Training

The occupational therapist teaches the child how to use the cable to open the terminal device. The child sits at a table and holds a toy in the sound hand. The therapist sits behind or beside the child, placing one hand on the child's shoulder (prosthetic side) and the other hand under the forearm of the prosthesis to move the shoulder into humeral flexion. As the terminal device opens, the child is encouraged to place the toy inside (Figure 5). During this procedure, the axilla loop causes pressure under the sound arm. Most children try to avoid the pull of the harness by moving the sound shoulder into extension. The result is slack in the control line, which prevents the terminal device from opening. To counteract the problem and minimize frustration, the therapist stabilizes the shoulder on the sound side and encourages the child to reach forward to place a toy in the terminal device. The therapist assists with the secure and correct placement of the toy and also moves the child's shoulder to the neutral position to relax tension on the control line in order to close the terminal device.[7]

Initially the arm and body movements are awkward when the child attempts to perform the control motion. The child may include the sound hand to manually open the terminal device or move the prosthesis forward to pull on the cable. The therapist definitely provides hands-on assistance during this period to help the child master and refine the components of controls training: (1) refine the control motion to open the terminal device (humeral flexion, not abduction); (2) insert an object or toy

securely into the open terminal device, holding on to the item until the device closes completely; (3) relax tension on the control line by extending the shoulder; (4) use the sound hand to remove the object from the terminal device and learn to actively release the item with the same control motion; (5) use the prosthesis to clasp or stabilize large items; and (6) learn the second control motion (biscapular abduction) to open the terminal device at the midline of the body.[7,12] Some children learn quickly and independently, but others need assistance.

Cooperative children can learn the control motion in two or three short training sessions a week for several weeks or months. Some children learn more quickly than others, and therapy goals are adjusted accordingly. Parents are always included in the therapy sessions and are given instructions to assist the child at home. Often they provide the only available ongoing training.

Although the focus is on learning the control motion, children often do not respond well to drills. Developmentally appropriate bimanual toys and games are preferable so that the child can relate the control motion to purposeful play. The therapist or parents should not ask the child to use the prosthesis to perform dominant hand skills such as stacking blocks or coloring with a crayon. The prosthesis is used to assist the sound hand. Appropriate activities that provide repetitive opening and closing of the terminal device may be used for this beginning phase of training, such as (1) stringing large wooden or plastic beads on a strong cord or leather lace, holding the bead in the terminal device and the cord with the sound hand; (2) holding a small container with a threaded cap in the terminal device, using the sound hand to unscrew the cap and remove a treat or toy; (3) holding a large felt-tip marker in the terminal device, loosening the cap to facilitate removal with the sound hand; (4) holding a Do-A-Dot Art paint bottle in the terminal de-

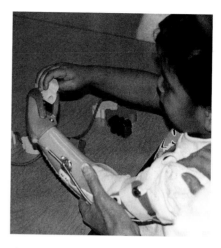

Figure 5 The therapist teaches the control motion for opening the terminal device.

vice, unscrewing the cap with the sound hand; or (5) holding matching picture cards in the terminal device, removing one at a time with the sound hand.[12]

Development of Prosthetic Skills

In the next phase of training, the child will focus on prosthetic skills that facilitate prehensile use of the terminal device. The child's ability to master the use of the prosthesis follows a developmental time line and coincides with the acquisition of other cognitive and motor skills. Because the child does not assimilate all facets of training at once, the therapist introduces the following skills as the child is ready to learn them: (1) placing an object securely and accurately in the terminal device, repositioning the object as needed; (2) refining the size of the terminal device opening, especially for small or thin items; (3) prepositioning or changing the position of the terminal device as required for different activities; (4) actively releasing an object from the terminal device using the control motion, learning to drop the object on the table or floor, actively tossing the object from the terminal device into space; and (5) actively grasping an object from a surface using the terminal device.

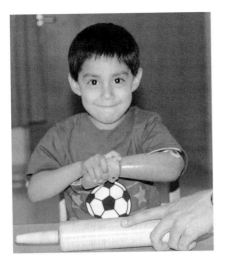

Figure 6 The child is reminded to preposition the terminal device.

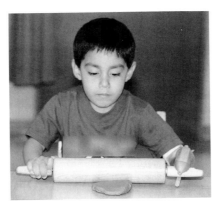

Figure 7 The CAPP TD No. 1 mimics the position of the sound hand.

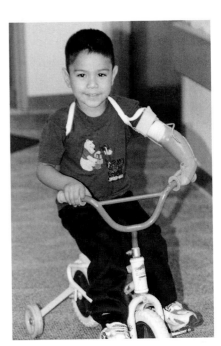

Figure 8 Riding a tricycle encourages the child to reach out with the sound hand and terminal device to grasp the handlebars.

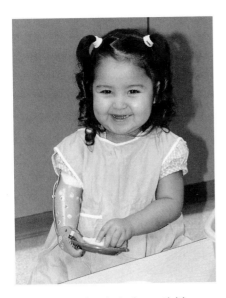

Figure 9 Two-handed play activities are used to integrate prosthetic skills into the functional use pattern.

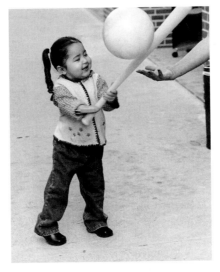

Figure 10 Outdoor play varies the play environment and encourages use of the prosthesis.

To assist the child in learning specific skills, the therapist demonstrates how to use the prosthesis to perform the activity and provides verbal instruction. The child practices the skill and integrates it into new activities. If the child has difficulty, the therapist asks how the task might be done another way.[12] This facilitates a trial-and-error approach before the therapist intervenes. If the child appears awkward when doing the task, the therapist corrects the method of performance. For example, many children avoid prepositioning the termi-

nal device. They attempt to substitute shoulder motion to place the terminal device in what they think is a good position of function. They must often be reminded to change the position of the terminal device in order to perform the task more efficiently (Figure 6). A helpful hint about the CAPP TD No. 1 is to position it so that it mimics the sound hand[13] (Figure 7).

The sound hand can always be used to place an object in the terminal device to complete a two-handed task. When the sound hand is occupied, knowing how to actively grasp an object from a surface with the terminal device is equally important. Likewise, to achieve fluid movement patterns with both arms, the child

learns to reach forward with both the terminal device and sound hand to grasp a stationary object in space. The child can practice this two-handed approach with toys such as a tricycle (Figure 8), rocking horse, seesaw, swing, shopping cart, doll carriage, wheelbarrow, and rolling pin.

Because the child's work is play, toys and games are always used to integrate prosthetic skills into the child's use pattern. The preschool youngster does well with activities that encompass imaginary play, such as a tea party, washing dishes (Figure 9), washing doll clothes and hanging them on a line, planting flowers or seeds in a pot, grocery shopping, and dress-up play with costumes and makeup. Other highly recommended activities include playing baseball with a plastic bat and large ball (Figure 10), as well as having fun outdoors on playground equipment.[7]

The goal of prosthetic use training is to help the child develop spontaneous and natural use. To achieve this level of performance, the child learns and refines the control motion to operate the component, acquires pros-

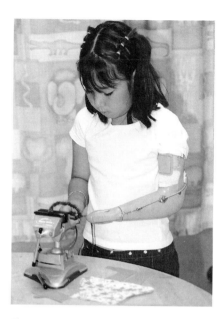

Figure 11 The child includes the prosthesis to perform complex fine motor tasks.

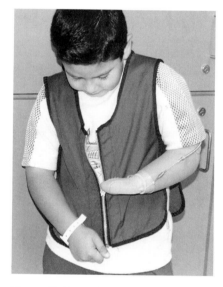

Figure 13 Use of the terminal device makes it easy to zip a jacket.

thetic skills that facilitate operation of the prosthesis, and includes the prosthesis and integrates the skills to perform complex motor tasks (Figure 11).

Although there is no magic in the training process, repetition and practice do help to build good habit patterns. The therapist can enhance training procedures by varying the work/play environment and providing creative activities. Activities of daily living are introduced as the

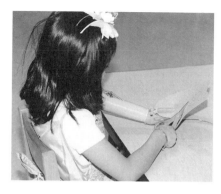

Figure 12 Learning to cut with scissors is an important kindergarten skill.

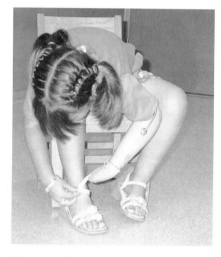

Figure 14 The child includes the terminal device to buckle her shoe.

child is ready to learn them. Before the child enters kindergarten, the therapist reviews specific prosthetic skills and self-help tasks. Practice with the following types of activities may help the child to function more independently in the classroom: holding paper to cut with scissors (Figure 12); opening and closing glue bottles and jars; opening milk cartons and packages of cookies; removing a coat or jacket; stabilizing clothing to zip a jacket or button a shirt (Figure 13); putting on and removing the prosthesis independently; tying shoelaces and buckling a shoe (Figure 14); and managing clothing when going to the bathroom.[7] Successful performance will vary depending on the child's abilities and motivation. Learning to tie shoelaces and going to the bathroom independently are difficult ac-

tivities for some children and require extensive practice.

The school-aged child learns additional skills that are a refinement of prosthetic use. To hold a soft or fragile object in the terminal device, the child controls the pressure grip by maintaining a slight amount of tension on the control line. This skill is important in order to hold a sandwich or to crack an egg without a mishap. The child with a voluntary-opening terminal device also learns to keep it closed when bending over or leaning forward to tie shoelaces. This skill is accomplished by moving the harness higher on the back to relieve tension on the control line. The child who has a voluntary-closing device will have greater control and find it easier to maintain the terminal device in a closed position when leaning forward.

The older child who receives a prosthesis for the first time must also learn to use it effectively. The training period is condensed if the patient has the cognitive and motor skills to understand instructions and assimilate information more rapidly. Assistance should be available at any developmental time period to help the child or teenager solve problems with daily living, recreational, athletic, or vocational activities. Prosthetic training may be conducted at the center where the prosthesis is prescribed or provided through some other therapy resource.[7,12]

No matter how much professional help is available, the role of parents or caregivers is essential. They can provide assistance that gives the child the potential for a successful prosthetic experience by attending therapy sessions to help the child with the prosthesis; reinforcing the prosthetic wearing pattern; encouraging the child to use the prosthesis at home, at school, and in the community; familiarizing the teacher and classmates with the prosthesis when the child enters school; supporting the child when teasing occurs; and encouraging the child to maintain a positive atti-

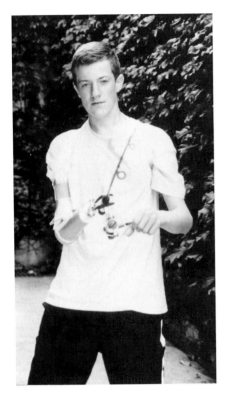

Figure 15 The configuration of the Dorrance hook and the rubber band loading provide a secure hold on an object.

tude about himself/herself and the prosthesis.

Functional Needs and Prosthetic Options

As children grow and develop, their interests and skill levels change. They also become more concerned about appearance. The therapist is usually aware of these needs and may be in a position to introduce different prosthetic components or recommend a change to an existing device. Early in the training period, the therapist or child will identify a need for more grip force. The child may become increasingly frustrated when he or she is unable to hold an object securely in the terminal device as resistance is applied by the sound hand. If the device is a CAPP TD No. 1, the Hosmer soft spring will be replaced with the regular spring. This exchange is made as soon as the child can generate enough operating force to pull against the increased resistance. A third and much

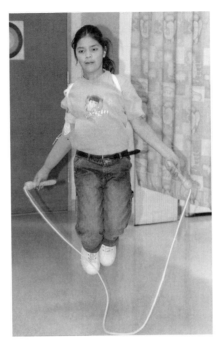

Figure 16 The child is able to securely hold the jump rope handles with the mechanical hand.

harder spring is available for the older school-aged child.[13]

The Dorrance voluntary-opening hook uses rubber bands to increase grip strength. For the young child, one fourth to one half of a band may be added at a given time depending on the youngster's available excursion and operating force. Some preteen and teenage boys may actually switch to a hook from some other device because they like the configuration, the fine tip grip, and the option of adding rubber bands to increase grip strength (Figure 15). The hook is especially versatile for grasping the handlebars of a bike, using tools, and performing heavy-duty work.

Voluntary-closing Adept terminal devices from TRS, Inc also provide a variety of benefits. Crandall and Hansen[14] reported that 16 transradial amputees of a group of 20 in their study who originally used voluntary-opening hooks switched to the Adept devices. The children cite several specific advantages of the voluntary-closing device. It provides increased grip force as well as greater control over the amount of force exerted to

do an activity. The voluntary-closing device also makes it easier to lift heavy objects and to grasp cylindrical shapes such as a bicycle handlebar or a baseball bat.

Electric hands with myoelectric control provide excellent grip force. When an older child at CAPP receives a first prosthesis or a preteen outgrows the CAPP TD No. 1, a mechanical hand as well as a hook are usually prescribed. The Otto Bock (Otto Bock, Minneapolis, MN) and Hosmer voluntary-opening mechanical hands and gloves are certainly cosmetically acceptable. Unfortunately, mechanical hands do not have the same power pinch as electric hands nor do they provide the same potential for function as the other body-powered devices already described. After the mechanical hand is issued, some patients prefer to use the prosthesis only as a stabilizer. They cite both limited grip force and opening as the reasons for not using the prehensile function. Other individuals may find the mechanical hand acceptable for grasp activities (Figure 16).

Sometimes a parent of a very young child will not accept any other device except one that looks like a hand. The Steeper 2-in mechanical hand is one available option. However, for the 2-year-old child who is just learning active operation of the cable-controlled device and for the therapist doing the training, this hand may provide more frustration than function. Excessive operating force is often needed to achieve minimal opening. The glove and configuration of the fingers also prevent the hand from closing completely. Whenever possible, it is prudent to wait until a child gains some control of the cable system before introducing a mechanical hand.[15]

Older children who are involved in school- or community-based athletic programs are sometimes required to remove the prosthesis for body-contact sports. If the terminal device is perceived to be a problem, the TRS Super Sport Hand (TRS, Inc) is a viable alternative; made of soft, flexible polymer, it is shaped like a cupped hand.[15] Using this device for sports in place of an electric or mechanical hand will often minimize costly repairs.

The types of prostheses and components that are offered in a particular amputee center may depend on the center's history and experience with certain components and control systems, research components developed in a particular center, and available financial resources and subsidized funding for prostheses and components. Nonetheless, patients and their families have an ongoing need for up-to-date information about new and available components and should have some input to the prescription process when possible.

Realistic Wear and Use Patterns With a Transradial Prosthesis

Wear and use patterns change during different life stages. Children who receive their first prosthesis as a baby have the potential to develop consistent prosthetic wear and use patterns. These children usually demonstrate good skills in kindergarten and beginning elementary grades. Play behaviors and the two-handed activities they engage in during this period reinforce use of the terminal device.

The preteen and teenage years are a time of transition; wear and use patterns begin to diminish. The teenager may choose not to wear the prosthesis at all, or only for selected activities. A passive cosmetic prosthesis or one with a sport device may be used for short periods to meet a specific need. Rather than include the prosthesis, the teenager often relies on the sound arm and hand—which now have increased strength and dexterity—for daily activities. If the terminal device or prosthetic control system does not provide the fine prehension or the needed grip force, this pattern is reinforced.

Children who receive their first prosthesis later in life may have difficulty adjusting to it because they may have developed and established alternative ways of performing activities. Too much thought and effort may be required to change existing habit patterns. However, some children will develop a natural, spontaneous use pattern and find the prosthesis to be extremely valuable. Experience demonstrates that certain factors influence this outcome. The best candidates to develop excellent long-term wear and use of prostheses are those who have a tolerance for wearing the prosthesis, have an aptitude for mechanical devices, demonstrate good motor planning and problem-solving abilities, and receive good support from family and peers.[15] These observations are based on clinical experience. Outcome studies now in progress may provide a more objective and realistic view of how children wear and use their prostheses.

Myoelectric Prostheses

Although a myoelectric prosthesis is suitable and appropriate for many children who have transradial and transhumeral limb deficiencies, the clinical practice of fitting this type of prosthesis is still a subject of controversy. Some centers prescribe myoelectric components exclusively; others provide a body-powered prosthesis first. The availability of funds for the more expensive myoelectric components often impacts prescriptions.

The technology for myoelectric components for children was applied in practice in the 1970s. In 1975, Dr. Rolf Sorbye collaborated with the Systemteknik AB Company in Sweden to produce the first child-sized electric hand.[6,15] Although this hand is no longer produced, other durable electric hands for children are manufactured by RSLSteeper, Variety Ability Systems (VASI, Toronto, Ontario, Canada), and Otto Bock.

Most parents view the myoelectric prosthesis as more desirable because of the advanced technology and natural appearance. Advantages of this type of prosthesis include the strong pinch force, elimination of the harness system, and the cosmetic appearance.

Once the child has mastered the control motion, the electric hand can be opened completely with very little effort while the arm assumes any position.[15,16] Operation of the prosthesis with a cable system and mechanical hand requires more strength and range of motion. It does not open fully or achieve the same grip force strength as the electric-powered hand.

Potential disadvantages of the myoelectric prosthesis are the heat and perspiration generated in the socket and the greater weight of the electric components. At first, all children complain about the hot, sticky feeling. The child with the short residual limb is more likely to feel muscle fatigue when lifting the electric prosthesis against gravity. These issues become less problematic with wear and use.[15]

Early Fit

Hubbard and associates[6] present a strong case for early fitting. At Bloorview-MacMillan Centre (Toronto, Ontario, Canada), which has an extensive electric-powered prosthesis program, babies receive an infant passive prosthesis between 3 and 6 months of age. The electric-powered prosthesis may be fit as early as 10 to 15 months of age. Their experience indicates that a child who is fit early and wears the prosthesis on a consistent basis usually demonstrates a more spontaneous and natural use pattern with the electric-powered hand. The child who is fitted at a later time tends to use the prosthesis primarily to stabilize objects. A similar outcome occurs in children who are fit with the infant prosthesis at 8 to 10 months and receive the cable system at 2 years of age.

CAPP Approach

Current practice at the Los Angeles Shriners Hospital CAPP program is to provide myoelectric prostheses for selected children with unilateral transradial limb deficiencies who demonstrate a full-time wear and use pattern with a body-powered prosthesis. The patient is at least 3 years of age before receiving the first myoelectric pros-

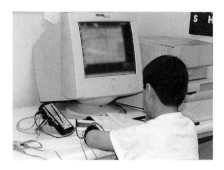

Figure 17 The MyoBoy (Otto Bock), a computerized tool to select muscle sites and train the child to separate the EMG signals.

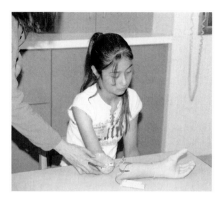

Figure 18 Myoelectric controls training using a temporary socket with electrodes attached to an electric hand.

thesis and must have the cognitive skills to learn to control muscle contractions separately. Parents and patients must show compliance with the treatment program and be able to keep required appointments at the hospital.[16] Once the candidate is chosen, the clinician determines if the child has suitable muscle sites. Components that include correct hand size and an appropriate control system are selected. Although we use digital controls at CAPP, proportional control systems are also available.

My experience indicates that most children 3 years of age and older are able to use the two-state, two-site control system. They learn to independently contract and relax two opposing muscle groups in order to control an electric hand. If for any reason the child cannot overcome cocontraction of the forearm muscles, the strongest muscle is selected to operate a one-muscle, two-function system. The child learns to vary the force of the muscle contraction so that the strong contraction signals the electric hand to open and a less forceful contraction signals the hand to close. This one-muscle system should not be confused with the single-site voluntary-opening system that is used with children younger than 2 years of age.[6,15,17]

Muscle Site Testers and Trainers

Several methods can be used to test for the best electromyographic (EMG)

signal from the residual forearm muscles. A large electric hand with electrodes may be used as a tester.[16] Although this method is a trial-and-error approach, it does produce results. Computerized evaluation training tools provide a precise and accurate way to select the optimum muscle sites and train the child to separate muscle contractions in order to operate an electric component.[6]

The MyoBoy from Otto Bock has a hardware interface that connects the electrodes to a personal computer and uses a Windows-based software platform. It allows the prosthetist or therapist to test the patient's ability to control a myoelectric system and locates the best electrode positions. The training mode enables the practitioner to adjust the electrodes so that the patient uses the EMG signals effectively to operate the electric component[18] (Figure 17).

MyoWizard and MyoAssistant are Windows-based software products produced by Bloorview-MacMillan Centre and distributed by Liberating Technologies-MyoWizard software uses microcomputer technology, allowing the prosthetist to select the appropriate control strategies for the patient on components that have programmable microprocessor-based systems. The MyoAssistant software gives the clinician the ability to evaluate the patient, adjust the control system and optimize it for the individual user, and train the patient to separate

the controls. As a cost-effective way to provide components that meet the changing needs of the developing child, manufacturers have begun to produce components that can be converted to more sophisticated control schemes as the child matures. For example, a single-site hand can be converted to operate with two electrodes with a simple exchange of a plug-in chip.

EMG Testing

To find the appropriate sites, the young child must learn how to contract the forearm muscles. One method is to use the sound limb for practice. An electrode, which provides the signal to open the hand, is placed over the forearm extensor muscles. The child extends the wrist and a signal is emitted. The other electrode is placed on the forearm flexor muscles. The child flexes the wrist and produces a signal.[16]

To select sites on the residual limb, the electrode is placed over the forearm flexors. The child is asked to wiggle or move the residual limb in a downward motion toward the flexor muscles to produce a signal. The process is repeated by moving the residual limb in the opposite direction to elicit a signal from the extensor muscles. Both electrodes are strapped on the residual limb and the child practices separating the EMG signals by operating an electric hand or generating a response on the computerized trainer. Electrodes may be repositioned to find the strongest signal. Sometimes the young child confuses the movement of the residual limb with flexion of the elbow. The therapist stabilizes the child's arm to prevent unwanted arm motions.[16]

Controls training is easier to accomplish when a temporary socket is made for the child. Electrodes are placed in the socket and then attached to an electric hand (Figure 18). The child practices three key activities—contracting and relaxing the muscles independently and on command, increasing the strength and repetition of the muscle signals, and refining the

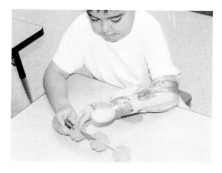

Figure 19 Temporary myoelectric prosthesis allows for evaluation of the fit and comfort of the socket during activity.

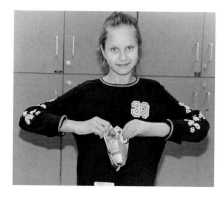

Figure 20 The myoelectric hand provides a secure hold when performing a task that gives resistance.

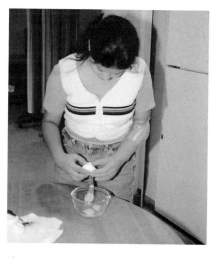

Figure 21 Two-handed activities used for functional use training with the myoelectric prosthesis.

control of opening and closing the hand in large and small amounts.[6,16]

To overcome the monotony of controls training, the child places toys in the electric hand or plays a simple game. The focus on purposeful activity improves attention and skill. If the child complains of excessive fatigue or demonstrates inadvertent operation of the hand, then the electrode gains (sensitivity to the signal) are adjusted. The child must be allowed to rest during the training process.

Once the child's control has improved, the socket is attached to a temporary forearm that is set up with the appropriate size electric hand. This temporary prosthesis (Figure 19) provides the opportunity to evaluate the fit, comfort, and suspension of the socket while the child performs activities under dynamic loading.[6,16] Several training sessions may be conducted with this unit before the definitive prosthesis is fabricated. If problems occur that do not seem related to training or the patient's performance, the clinician will need to evaluate the hand and control system.

When the final prosthesis is issued, the child must practice putting it on. The child either pushes the residual limb into the socket using a gel lubricant or pulls the tissue in with a nylon stocking threaded through a pull tube.[16] The child then performs activities to determine final comfort and function of the prosthesis. Finally, parents are taught how to care for the prosthesis; this includes cleaning the glove and socket as well as charging

the battery. Preferably, a lithium battery and charger will be provided. The lithium-ion battery can be charged every day no matter how much or how little it is used because it has no memory.[16,17] Nickel-cadmium batteries are still in wide use but are generally being replaced with lithium-ion batteries.

Prosthetic Skills and Functional Use

By the time the definitive prosthesis is issued, the child has usually learned to separate the signals and is able to open and close the hand; however, this is only part of the training process. The child must master specific skills in order to use the prosthesis effectively. The digital electric-powered hand opens and closes at a constant rate of speed; the child who has previously used a cable-operated system will notice the slower response time. To maintain a secure hold on an item, timing the placement of the object with the closure of the hand is important. The child also practices rotating the terminal device to place it in the best position for completing the task. If the cosmetic glove binds on the laminated forearm, the child will not be able to preposition the hand. The prosthetist can either shorten the glove or cut it and overlap the sections to provide freedom of movement.

The grip strength of the electric-powered hand allows a secure hold on an object when pushing or pulling it apart (Figure 20). However, excessive

force may cause contraction of forearm muscles that in turn causes inadvertent operation of the hand. To minimize this problem, the child practices activities that require firm grip and learns to limit the amount of arm motion when performing an activity that requires resistance. The prosthetist can also lower the electrode gains to make them less sensitive to the muscle signal as long as the adjustment does not interfere with the child's ability to control the hand.[16]

Age-appropriate bimanual activities as described in the training section above are used to reinforce prosthetic skills and to help develop a spontaneous functional use pattern (Figure 21). The number of training sessions is always adjusted to the needs of the child. The child who has worn a cable-operated prosthesis usually adapts quickly to the myoelectric prosthesis. The child with a short residual limb may need extra time to become accustomed to the additional weight.[16]

The myoelectric fitting and training procedures described in this section reflect the CAPP approach. Myoelectric programs vary according to the philosophy of the center. Those facilities that use cable-operated prostheses exclusively and fit the baby between 12 and 15 months of age may

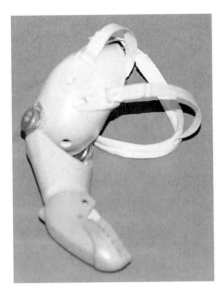

Figure 22 An infant transhumeral prosthesis with friction hinges.

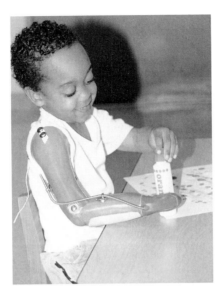

Figure 23 A transhumeral prosthesis with a single-control cable to activate only the terminal device.

have different treatment protocols.[6] When establishing a myoelectric program for the young child, different approaches should be evaluated and the expertise of practitioners with extensive experience with cable-operated prostheses should be employed. Centers that are excellent information resources include Bloorview-MacMillan Centre in Toronto, Ontario, Canada and the Institute of Biomedical Engineering at the University of New Brunswick (UNB) in Fredericton, New Brunswick, Canada. The myoelectric symposium held every 2 or 3 years at UNB focuses on research in cable-operated prostheses, technological advances, clinical application, and prosthetic training. Information is available from the Institute of Biomedical Engineering, UNB, PO Box 4400, Fredericton, NB, Canada E3B 5A3.

Transhumeral Deficiency
Early Fitting and the First Infant Passive Prosthesis

The prosthetic intervention described in this section reflects practice at the Los Angeles Shriners Hospital CAPP. For proponents of early fitting, the achievement of independent sitting balance is an appropriate developmental time frame for providing the infant with a passive prosthesis. The length, shape, strength, and range of motion of the residual limb will determine if fitting is either reasonable or beneficial. An infant with a short, weak limb may neither tolerate the weight of the prosthesis nor lift it to the midline of the body. If there is any potential for the prosthesis to interfere with gross motor skills, fitting should be postponed until the toddler stands and walks.

The length of the residual limb determines the type of prosthesis that should be provided. If the entire humerus is present, a laminated exoskeletal prosthesis is prescribed. Friction hinges or an outside elbow lock with manual pull-tab are generally used (Figure 22). For the shorter limb, an endoskeletal prosthesis is appropriate. This device will include some type of passive positional elbow unit with a piece of tubing for the forearm segment. Foam and a suitable covering are used for the cosmetic finish. Available terminal devices may include an infant passive hand, a mitt, a nonactive CAPP TD No. 1, or 10X hook. Weight should always be considered when selecting components for an infant.[7]

As long as the prosthesis does not interfere with mobility, the baby may wear it during the time he or she is awake. Parents need to develop a realistic but consistent wearing pattern and stimulate use of the prosthesis by assisting the baby to reach forward to clasp a large toy. They also need to place toys or food in the terminal device (which has a grasp function) so that as the baby matures, he or she will learn that the device can hold an object. Periodically the elbow should be unlocked and the forearm repositioned so that the baby becomes accustomed to having it moved. The baby with a short residual limb should not be expected to include the prosthesis for support to creep on all fours. To move from place to place, the baby will scoot on his or her bottom. If the residual limb has enough strength and length, the baby may use the prosthesis for balance.

Activation of the Terminal Device

Readiness criteria that determine when to activate the terminal device have already been described. Now that the child is ready to learn a new function, a single-control cable is added to the prosthesis to activate only the terminal device (Figure 23). The young child does not have sufficient range of motion or strength to operate a dual control system. With the single control cable, the same amount of cable excursion opens the terminal device whether the elbow is flexed or extended.[7]

Training Period

The training procedures have been discussed in detail earlier in this chapter. Two-handed play activities are used during training to refine the control motion, increase skill, and encourage spontaneous use of the terminal device (Figure 24). Prosthetic components must be prepositioned in order to make optimum use of the prosthesis and to place the terminal device in the best position for function. Initially the therapist and parents will need to preposition the terminal device and forearm. As children mature, they will learn to position the components by themselves. The training process always includes instruction for parents in all aspects of prosthetic interventions and care and maintenance of the prosthesis, as well as activities of daily living.

Most 3-year-old children learn to manually operate the elbow lock cable by pulling the billet with the sound hand. The ability to lock and unlock the prosthetic elbow precedes the awareness of when to change the position of the forearm. The therapist explains that the elbow is a positioning component and calls attention to the need to reposition the forearm when the play environment is altered. The child may either sit or stand to perform bimanual activities. The child manually unlocks the elbow, repositions the forearm, and supports it on the knee or table surface. This method maintains the desired position of the forearm and prevents it from dropping before the elbow is locked.[19]

When to Add the Dual-Control Cable and Activate the Elbow Lock

In a 1979 study, Shaperman[19] observed that children from 3.5 to 4.5 years of age were able to learn the elbow lift and lock sequence. Recent experience at CAPP indicates that it is easier for a child 4.5 to 5.5 years of age to meet all of the following readiness criteria necessary to learn the lift and lock sequence: (1) use the terminal device effectively and include it spontaneously to perform bimanual tasks, (2) operate the elbow lock billet manually to lock and unlock the elbow, (3) demonstrate the strength and range of motion to open the terminal device with the dual control system when the elbow is locked in 90° of flexion, (4) tolerate one to two rubber bands on the hook or use a medium spring on a CAPP TD No. 1, (5) understand the need to change the position of the forearm, and (6) dem-

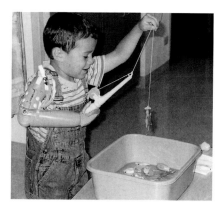

Figure 24 Prosthetic training to reinforce practical use of the prosthesis.

onstrate the cognitive ability necessary to understand instructions and the attention span needed to practice the lift and lock sequence.

Understanding the Dual-Control and Elbow Lock Cable System

The function of the dual-control and elbow lock cable systems is often misunderstood. The dual-control system has two functions; it lifts the forearm when the elbow is unlocked and opens the terminal device when the elbow is locked. The elbow lock cable system is separate and controls the locking mechanism.

The control motions needed to operate the dual-control cable are humeral flexion and scapular abduction. When the elbow is unlocked, the control motions lift the forearm. To maintain the forearm in flexion, tension is placed on the cable system by abducting the shoulder. The abduction position prevents the forearm from dropping as the humerus is extended. The extension motion triggers the separate elbow lock cable. Once the elbow is locked, humeral flexion moves the dual-control cable to open the terminal device.

Changes to the Prosthesis

The single control cable is replaced by the dual-control system. The elbow unit is either a positive-locking internal elbow or an outside elbow lock. The pull-tab on the elbow lock cable

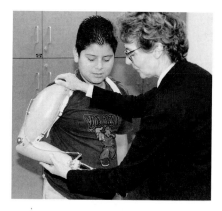

Figure 25 The therapist helps the child activate the elbow lock/unlock cable using the control motions of humeral extensions and scapular depression.

is attached to the elastic suspensor on the harness. A strap is placed on the underside of the elbow to limit flexion. It acts as a safeguard to prevent the forearm from striking the face because the child cannot control the force of forearm lift.[19]

Teaching the Forearm Lift and Elbow Lock Sequence

An older school-aged child or teenager will learn the combined operation of lift and lock with a few demonstrations. The young child learns these complex motions in stages, with assistance from the therapist. The elbow is unlocked and the child learns to control humeral flexion. Once the patient regulates the degree of forearm lift, the elbow stop is removed.[19]

Operation of the elbow lock is taught next. The elbow is unlocked and the forearm is supported in flexion. The humeral section is moved into extension, coupled with a downward motion to depress the scapula. The child listens for two clicks. The first click occurs when the elbow lock cable is triggered to lock the elbow. The second click is heard when the shoulder returns to a neutral position and the cable retracts. If the cable does not cycle properly, the mechanism will not operate to unlock the elbow. The therapist helps the child practice the lock and unlock motions with the forearm flexed and extended (Figure 25). Once this sequence is

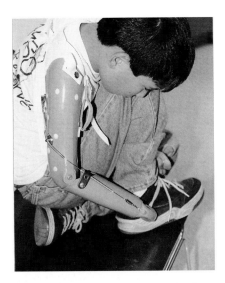

Figure 26 The child repositions the forearm of the prosthesis in order to reach his foot to tie shoelaces.

mastered, the shoulder abduction motion is introduced to maintain the forearm in flexion. Drill and repetition are used to practice the entire sequence of forearm lift and elbow lock and unlock. Because the elbow is a positioning component, its function has no relevance unless it is incorporated into age-appropriate two-handed tasks. Therefore, the child only begins to refine the lift and lock sequence when it is applied to purposeful activity. Changing the level of the work surface and varying the training activities provide the opportunity to reposition the forearm and use the grasp function of the terminal device (Figure 26). Most children avoid prepositioning prosthetic components unless it is absolutely necessary. With practice and verbal reminders, they learn to change the position of the forearm and terminal device but often prefer to compensate with body movements.[19]

Factors That Influence Realistic Wear and Use Patterns

The usefulness of the body-powered prosthesis is affected by its fit as well as the child's anatomy. The harness, cable systems, and socket design may prevent the child from reaching out

with the prosthesis. The work area for the terminal device is often restricted to the midline of the body at the waist level. The child's ability to lift the prosthesis against gravity and place the terminal device where it is needed depends on the length, range of motion, and strength of the residual limb. The child with a short, weak limb stabilizes the prosthesis against the body to open the terminal device. Often, the child cannot maintain the unlocked forearm in flexion and will use the sound hand to support the prosthesis and to trigger the elbow lock; the wear and use pattern in this situation will be limited. The child with a long residual limb, good shoulder motion, and secure purchase in the prosthetic socket can use the terminal device at face level and can also bend over to tie shoelaces. This child has the potential to operate the elbow and the terminal device more efficiently, usually wearing the prosthesis for longer periods and demonstrating good bimanual function.

Unilateral Upper Limb Shoulder-Level Deficiency
Early Prosthetic Intervention

The child who is missing an entire arm has a strong need for restoration of function. The shoulder disarticulation prosthesis does not realistically meet this need nor is it appropriate for every child. Parents are often disappointed to discover that the prosthesis is cumbersome and has limited use. Before recommending prosthetic fitting, several specific factors must be carefully considered. The shape and contour of the baby's trunk and shoulder girdle must provide enough surface area to suspend the socket, and the prosthesis must not interfere with the baby's mobility. The parents must decide if they want a prosthesis for their baby and are willing to follow through with the team's recommendations.

If fitting is appropriate, the baby may receive the first infant passive prosthesis when he or she sits or walks independently. The prosthesis of choice is a lightweight, endoskeletal type with a frame socket and non-active terminal device. A child with a limb deficiency—especially one missing an entire arm—has less skin surface from which to lose body heat. The shoulder disarticulation prosthesis compounds the problem because so much of the chest wall is covered, creating heat and perspiration. Large cutout areas in the socket will allow for some heat dissipation. The wearing pattern should be consistent in order for the baby to become accustomed to the prosthesis, but it does not need to be worn all day. The child needs time to cool off, move freely, and develop gross motor skills. When the baby does wear the prosthesis, the parents can place toys in the terminal device (if it can be opened) and periodically reposition the shoulder and elbow components.[12,15]

The Prosthesis With the First Active Terminal Device

Readiness criteria are used to determine when to activate the terminal device. The child must have the attention span and cognitive ability to learn and practice the complex control motions. Because limited strength and range of motion prevent reliance on chest expansion or scapular motion to move a cable system, a single-control cable attached to a thigh cuff or strap is used to open the terminal device—usually a CAPP TD No. 1. The thigh cuff is placed around the leg opposite the prosthesis, and the cable system runs diagonally across the child's back (Figure 27).

Training in Terminal Device Operation

The child stands between the therapist's knees. The pelvis is stabilized and the child flexes the trunk to open the terminal device. The therapist helps the child place and hold a toy in the terminal device until tension on the control line is relaxed.[7,12] This procedure allows the child early success in terminal device operation but does not provide the best position for performing activities. A more efficient method is to elevate and rotate the shoulder on the prosthetic side. Once children learn these motions, they can use the terminal device to perform activities at tabletop level.[7,12] Training procedures focus on refining the control motion and integrating terminal device operation into functional activities.

The therapist uses age-appropriate bimanual activities to refine the control motion, teach prosthetic skills, and develop functional use of the terminal device. The therapist also adjusts the thigh control strap as needed when the child changes from a standing to a sitting position during the initial training period and further adjusts all prosthetic components for optimum function. (All friction components must be tight enough to maintain their position when the child uses the terminal device.) The occupational therapist repositions all components to place the terminal device in the best position of function and provides instructions to parents in the care of the prosthesis, the adjustment and positioning of all components, and carrying out training recommendations.[7]

Options for Positioning the Forearm and Locking the Elbow

At CAPP, a nudge control is commonly used for locking and unlocking. To trigger the lock, the child uses the chin to depress the nudge lever. The device is placed on the socket within reach of the chin without poking the face or neck.[7] Most 3-year-old children learn to manually position the forearm with the sound hand and then lock the elbow with the nudge control.

The dual-control cable is added when the child has the strength and range of motion to use it effectively, usually between 4.5 and 5.5 years of

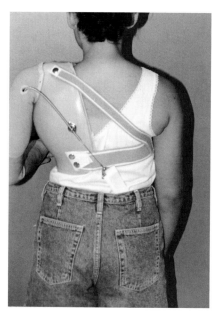

Figure 27 A shoulder disarticulation prosthesis with a thigh strap control. The thigh strap attaches to the leg opposite the prosthesis.

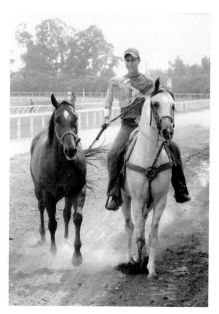

Figure 28 The patient uses a shoulder disarticulation prosthesis with a chest harness and dual-control cable in his daily activities.

age. The main concern is whether there is enough power and excursion for the cable to open the terminal device when the elbow is flexed at 90° or more. When the dual-purpose cable is provided, a flexion stop is placed under the elbow unit until the child is able to control the speed of forearm lift. Once the child is able to lift the forearm and maintain the position, the elbow can be locked by depressing the nudge control. If for any reason the child struggles to open the terminal device, return to the single-control cable is recommended. Older children may need to use the single-control cable to open the terminal device if they want a chest harness instead of a thigh strap. However, the teenager usually has sufficient strength and range of motion to move the dual-control system (Figure 28).

Use of External Power

Externally powered terminal devices are a viable option for children with shoulder disarticulation prostheses. Touch pads or switches are commonly used to control electric components. Myoelectric control is usually not effective because gross body motions

interfere with electrode placement on the chest wall. When the child receives the first active terminal device, the child-sized electric hook or small electric hand may be used.

The Hosmer electric hook has a small motor with a modified 10X hook. The motor tolerates about one full rubber band, which limits the pinch force. A single-function touch pad or push button is placed in the top part of the socket. The child hits the pad with the shoulder and the hook opens. When the child relaxes away from the pad, the rubber band action closes the hook. The pinch force provided by the hook is adequate for a 2-year-old but is insufficient for the needs of the school-aged child.[15] A child-sized VASI or RSLSteeper electric hand operated by a touch pad or switch is another option. The appearance of the hand is more pleasing and the grip is stronger than the hook. The pinch force of the smallest VASI 0-3 hand, for example, is 3.5 to 4.5 lb; the VASI 5-9 hand has a pinch force of 6 to 9.5 lb. By comparison, one rubber band on a hook is equivalent to 1 lb of pinch or grip force.

The Benefits and Disadvantages of Electric Components

The electric hand and hook open and close with the prosthesis in the same position. The potential area of function is greater because the electric terminal device can open directly in front of the waist or chest, away from the body, or out to the side. The electric hook and hand are easier to open and require less effort to operate than a terminal device with a thigh strap and cable system.[15]

Although electric components provide ease of operation, they are expensive and may require more maintenance. Depending on the component, additional weight is a factor. At CAPP, the child missing one arm rarely needs or uses an electric elbow. Positioning the elbow with the sound hand is often easier than dealing with the weight of an electric elbow.

Training Issues

The child must learn to refine the control motion by not hitting the touch pad or button during play. The prosthetist helps by adjusting the position of the control to prevent inadvertent operation. Because the electric hook and small electric hand open and close slowly, the child learns to place the object and wait until the terminal device closes completely before performing the activity. Parents are instructed to keep the prosthesis in good working condition by charging the battery correctly and preventing water and dirt from corroding the electric components.

Realistic Patterns of Use

The child with unilateral limb loss wears the electric- or body-powered shoulder disarticulation prosthesis a limited number of hours in a day. The prosthesis appears to be most useful during the preschool, kindergarten, and early elementary grades. It is usually worn during school hours and removed for outdoor play because children find that the prosthesis "gets in the way."

When the youngster enters middle school, he or she may choose not to wear a prosthesis. Weight, heat, and bulk are most commonly cited as reasons. The functional value of the prosthesis may also diminish in the teenage years. The youngster matures, motor skills increase, and the sound arm becomes stronger and more coordinated. This process allows the patient to perform tasks with one hand and to adapt more effectively. These changes are a growth experience for the teenager and not necessarily a failure of the prosthetic intervention. When appearance becomes important, the teenager may opt for a passive prosthesis with a cosmetic hand.

Conclusion

The child with a limb deficiency or amputation receives the best treatment from an experienced team that understands and addresses the medical, surgical, prosthetic, psychosocial, and life issues relevant to the patient and family. The prosthesis is only part of the treatment equation and not every child wants or needs one. When the first prosthesis is provided, the team should expect a reasonable amount of commitment from the patient and family. The parents need to establish a consistent prosthetic wearing pattern for the child for at least a year and follow the team's recommendations. There is no other way to build good habit patterns or determine whether the prosthesis has potential benefit.

As the child grows and develops, prosthetic wear and use patterns do change. The youngster who wears and uses the prosthesis daily may become a teenager who no longer needs one. Although many variables influence a successful prosthetic outcome, the patient is the one who ultimately makes the decision about wear and use.

References

1. Sypniewski BL: The child with terminal transverse partial hemimelia: A review of the literature on prosthetic management. *Artif Limbs* 1972;16: 20-50.

2. Shaperman J, Landsberger SE, Setoguchi Y: Early upper limb prosthesis fitting: When and what do we fit. *J Prosthet Orthot* 2003;15:11-17.

3. Brooks MB, Shaperman J: Infant prosthetic fitting: A study of the results. *Am J Occup Ther* 1965;19:329-334.

4. Scotland TR, Galway HR: A long-term review of children with congenital and acquired upper limb deficiency. *J Bone Joint Surg Br* 1983;65:346-349.

5. Jain S: Rehabilitation in limb deficiency: 2. The pediatric amputee. *Arch Phys Med Rehabil* 1996;77(suppl 3): S9-S13.

6. Hubbard SA, Kurtz I, Heim W, Montgomery G: Powered prosthetic intervention in upper limb deficiency, in Herring JA, Birch JG (eds): *The Child With a Limb Deficiency*. Rosemont, IL, American Academy of Orthopaedic Surgeons, 1998, pp 417-431.

7. Setoguchi Y, Rosenfelder R (eds): *The Limb Deficient Child*. Springfield, IL, Charles C Thomas, 1982.

8. Shaperman J, Sumida CT: Recent advances in research in prosthetics for children's prosthetics. *Clin Orthop* 1980;148:26-33.

9. Gesell A, Ilg FL, Ames LB, Bullis GE (eds): *The Child From Five To Ten*. New York, NY, Harper and Brothers, 1946, pp 35-366.

10. Pulaski MAS (ed): *Your Baby's Mind and How It Grows: Piaget's Theory for Parents*. New York, NY, Harper and Row, 1978, pp 87-186.

11. Gesell A, Haverson HM, Amatruda CS: *The First Five Years of Life: A Guide to the Study of the Preschool Child, From the Yale Clinic of Child Development*. New York, NY, Harper and Brothers, 1940, pp 108-110.

12. Clarke SD, Patton JG: Occupational therapy for the limb-deficient child: A developmental approach to treatment planning and selection of prostheses for infants and young children with unilateral upper extremity limb deficiencies. *Clin Orthop* 1980;148:47-54.

13. Shaperman J: The CAPP terminal device: A preliminary evaluation. *Inter Clin Info Bull* 1975;14:9-10.

14. Crandall RC, Hansen D: Clinical evaluation of a voluntary closing terminal device for below-elbow amputees.

J Assoc Child Prosthet Orthot Clin 1989; 4:71-73.

15. Patton J, Tokeshi J, Setoguchi Y: Prosthetic components for children, in Molnar G (ed): *Physical Medicine and Rehabilitation*. Philadelphia, PA, Hanley & Belfus, 1991, pp 245-259.

16. Baron E, Clarke SD, Soloman C: The two stage myoelectric hand for children and young adults. *Orthot Prosthet* 1983;37:11-24.

17. Schuch CM: Prosthetic principles in fitting myoelectric prostheses in children, in Herring JA, Birch JG (eds): *The Child With a Limb Deficiency*. Rosemont, IL, American Academy of Orthopaedic Surgeons, 1998, pp 405-416.

18. MYOBOY, Section VI, in MYOBOCK Course Manual. Minneapolis, MN, Otto Bock HealthCare, 2003.

19. Shaperman J: Learning patterns of young children with above-elbow prostheses. *Am J Occup Ther* 1979;33:299-305.

Chapter 67

Physical Therapy

Colleen Coulter-O'Berry, PT, MS, PCS

Introduction

Advances in pediatric prosthetic technology since the early 1990s have greatly enhanced the function and affected the physical therapy management of infants, children, and adolescents with congenital deficiencies and acquired amputations. Smaller and stronger articulating knees are available for infants (birth to 12 months of age) and toddlers (12 to 36 months of age),[1-3] and articulating ankles have been developed for toddlers.[4] Silicone liners and suspension sleeves are replacing the belts of the past. Biomedical engineers are developing ways to monitor and measure prewalking and walking activities of infants and toddlers.[1-3]

Advances in surgical reconstruction and in limb-sparing and salvage techniques have impacted the type of diagnoses requiring amputation and thus the physical therapy management of these children.[5] Families of children diagnosed with bone tumors and longitudinal deficiencies of the femur, tibia, or fibula are electing limb-sparing surgery instead of amputation. The physical therapist and prosthetist must be aware of these advances to assist each family in making educated decisions for their child.

The physical therapist's role is well defined in the management of children with traumatic or acquired limb loss. The primary goal is to restore function to its level before trauma or surgery through wound care; edema control; and range-of-motion, strengthening, and functional exercises.

Physical therapy management and goals are different for children with congenital limb loss. These children develop age-appropriate activities by incorporating the deficiency into all movements.[6] The deficient limb automatically takes part in the motor, sensory, and cognitive development of the child. Learning to move with the deficient limb is "normal" for the child. Regardless of the deficiency, the size, shape, flexibility, and strength of the deficient limb provide sensory and motor input that guides the child's motor development. Neurologically intact infants and toddlers with moderate to severe lower limb deformities will even attempt to pull to stand and cruise. The physical therapist needs to be knowledgeable in all areas of gross motor, fine motor, and cognitive development and have the ability to anticipate the limitations caused by the limb deficiency.[7] The physical therapist also must be aware of current pediatric prosthetic technology and surgical options available for the different classifications of limb deficiencies.

In the child with an acute trauma or recent surgery, the physical therapist is a primary provider of care. In children with congenital limb deficiencies, the physical therapist is an advocate, teacher, and mentor to the child and his or her family, anticipating immediate and future functional challenges. In most centers, the physical therapist sees the child, frequently acting as a liaison between the family, physician, prosthetist, nurse, and other team members. By acting as a teacher, the physical therapist empowers the parents to be the primary providers of therapy.

Home programs are necessary for optimal surgical and/or prosthetic outcomes. Many factors determine the frequency of physical therapy visits. These include the degree of limb deficiency; the child's age, flexibility, strength, associated medical and/or neurologic impairments, and developmental achievements; the distance the family lives from the center; and the family's ability to follow through with a home program. Videotaping therapy sessions is an excellent teaching tool for the parents and community-based physical therapists. Digital photography makes it easier to personalize therapy sessions, communicate with the community-based therapist, and document progress. Commercially available exercise manuals adapted for infants and children with limb deficiencies can provide excellent resources for home therapy programs.[8,9]

One of the main responsibilities of a physical therapist treating a child with a congenital limb deficiency is to support the surgical, prosthetic, and

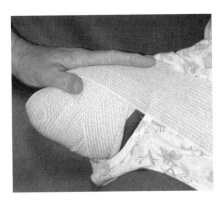

Figure 1 Elastic wrapping the residual limb of an 8-year-old child with a short transfemoral amputation level following revision for femoral overgrowth. The elastic bandage is wrapped around the waist for stabilization and high on the adductor area to control edema proximally.

therapeutic decisions made by the family and the limb-deficiency team. Preparing the child and family for the physical challenges ahead and anticipating the needs of the child helps the family make these important decisions. Maximizing a child's function within the degree of limb impairment is another important role of physical therapy. Physical therapy practices also include wound and skin care; edema control; and range of motion, strengthening, gait training, and age-appropriate functional activities.[7]

Postoperative swelling is common in children with congenital or acquired amputated or reconstructed limbs. A limb involved in multiple traumas typically has greater swelling and soft-tissue damage than a limb undergoing elective amputation and/or revision. Edema control begins with postoperative dressings and continues with elastic bandage wraps and shrinkers once the wound is healed. Properly applied dressings can control postoperative edema and facilitate prosthetic fitting.[10] The type of dressing is determined by the surgical procedure, the age and activity level of the child, parent preference, and distance of the child's residence from the center.

Soft dressings can work well with young children, but many centers pre-fer to provide the greater degree of protection offered by the rigid dressing for infants and toddlers undergoing amputations. The goals for the rigid dressing are to (1) protect the residual limb from additional trauma because infants and toddlers resume activity very quickly after surgery, (2) maintain bony alignment following revision, (3) reduce edema, (4) shape the residual limb, and (5) keep the dressing intact during the postoperative period as the swelling decreases.[10] The cast usually is changed within 2 weeks and may be followed by another cast or soft dressing and elastic bandage wrapping. Body spica casts and long leg casts are frequently used during reconstructive osteotomies requiring pins and plates. Soft dressings may be used in older children but need to be reinforced and reapplied frequently as the child's activity level increases. Elastic wrapping over the soft dressing can assist in early edema management.

Once the wound is healed, edema control is imperative. The principles for elastic wrapping in infants and children are about the same as those for an adult amputee. Differences include the size of the elastic bandages, use of tape strips to secure the shape of the elastic bandage as it is being wrapped, and extending the wrap around proximal structures to provide the greater stabilization needed for security because of the child's increased activity during the postoperative period (Figure 1). A soft elastic tubular sock is beneficial when put over the wrap as an additional barrier to keep the child from unwrapping the bandages and scratching at the incision and to secure the wrap in its place. Infants placed in soft dressings following surgery tolerate leggings and spandex bicycle-style shorts that are modified to be worn over the residual limb. These can provide additional control of the wrap and protection of the residual limb. Detailed written instructions need to be provided to the parents and caregivers. The techniques for elastic wrapping are described in chapter 48.

Children undergoing rotationplasty as treatment for trauma, tumors, or congenital anomalies require a unique wrapping technique to control edema and to shape the limb proximally. Typically there is significant swelling in the foot, ankle, and calf and there are extensive suture lines proximally. Delayed wound healing is of concern in children with cancer who are undergoing chemotherapy.[5,10] Figure 2 illustrates an effective technique for controlling edema following rotationplasty. The foot is wrapped incorporating the toes and ankle separately[11] as in an acute ankle sprain. The wrapping continues up the limb in a figure-of-8 configuration extending beyond the surgical site proximally. Shaping the proximal limb segment is imperative for optimal prosthetic fitting. Securing the wrap around the waist may be necessary to contain proximal tissues. The amount of compression increases with the child's tolerance to pressure and with wound healing.

Physical Therapy Treatments

Range-of-motion, strengthening, gait training, and functional activities depend on the child's age, medical and neurologic condition, and interests, as well as the family's ability to assist in the child's care. The following considerations should be made when developing therapy goals and home programs: (1) every child is unique and develops at his or her own rate; (2) the child with multiple limb loss has special needs, and treatment interventions must be prioritized; (3) the environment needs to be adapted to the child for maximal function; (4) the child with a limb deficiency may have associated medical, neurologic, or orthopaedic impairments that will influence function and intervention; and (5) surgical amputations and revisions may take place at different developmental ages; therefore, treatment should center around age-appropriate function.[6,7,12]

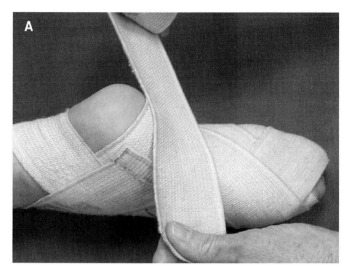
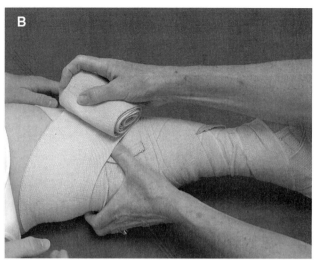

Figure 2 Elastic bandage wrapping techniques in a 12-year-old boy following rotationplasty. **A,** The foot and ankle are wrapped including the toes. **B,** The elastic bandage extends up the limb in a figure-of-8 pattern including the proximal thigh. An additional elastic bandage is necessary to continue around the waist for stabilization of the wrap and control of the edema proximally.

Infants (Birth to 12 Months)

When a child is born with a limb deficiency, a referral is made to the Limb Deficiency Center.[12-15] The family meets with the physician and team members to identify the infant's strengths and briefly outline possible future surgical, prosthetic, and therapeutic strategies that address the infant's physical impairments. The bond between the physical therapist and family begins at this point. Intervention should focus on assisting the infant to achieve motor and cognitive milestones in the context of his or her physical limitations.[7]

The infant with a congenital limb deficiency will benefit greatly from early intervention. Studies on the effectiveness of early physical therapy treatment have focused on the neurologically involved and/or developmentally delayed infant and toddler and not specifically on the child with a limb deficiency. Assumptions can be made that will support early physical therapy intervention for a child born with limb deficiencies. According to the American Physical Therapy Association and documented in the Competencies for Physical Therapy in Early Intervention,[16] early intervention is based on six important principles:

(1) the rapid growth and development in the first years of life provide the foundation for later development; (2) infants can actively interact, form attachments, and are capable of learning; (3) parents are the main providers of care and early learning experiences; (4) parents of children with special needs may require assistance or instruction in caring for their children; (5) the interaction between the biologic insult and environmental factors influences the developmental outcome; and (6) structured programming can improve the abilities of infants and young children.

Early intervention is recommended to provide optimal outcome and to prevent the development of secondary disability. Family-centered services provide for maximal intervention.[16] Exercise programs should be created with the parents' input when possible. Goals need to be age-appropriate, functionally based, and within the limits of the degree of limb deficiency. Well-informed and involved parents have a greater acceptance and understanding of their child's immediate and future surgical, prosthetic, and therapy needs. With positive parental input, the child is likely to become a successful prosthesis wearer.[6,13]

Intervention should begin with the evaluation of gross and fine motor development to establish baseline records of the infant's range of motion, strength, neurologic function, and movement patterns. Introducing the family to other families with children who have similar impairments is one of the most powerful interventions.[6,7,13] The impact of family networking is lasting and can help ease some of the parent's fears and concerns for the child's future. The therapist needs to monitor the amount of information given to parents. Not every parent is ready for all of the available information at the first visit. Too much information can increase the parent's anxiety and fears for the child's future by focusing on the disability rather than ability.

Families come to their first clinic visit with a multitude of questions and fears from information gathered from many sources about their child's deficiency. It is common to find that parents and extended family have engaged in conversations over the Internet with other families, each having opinions about the infant's care. Dolls with differing levels of amputations, samples of prostheses (similar to the child's first one), videos, and photographs of children wearing prostheses are useful teaching tools for parents

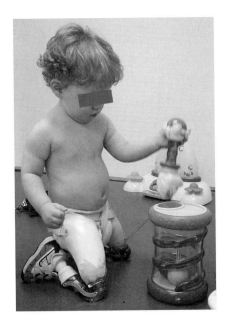

Figure 3 Sixteen-month-old child with congenital bilateral longitudinal deficiencies playing in kneeling position. Knee disarticulations were performed at age 9 months with prosthetic fitting at age 11 months. This child crawls, pulls to stand, cruises, and pushes a walker. The prostheses are not finished cosmetically because of the need for frequent alignment changes as he develops.

to help them understand the nature of their child's limb deficiency.

The development of the infant must be monitored to evaluate range of motion, functional strength, weight bearing, symmetry of posture, and movement as the infant learns to roll, sit, and pull to stand.[12,17] Asymmetry of movement is common. Exercises for positioning, handling, and play can be taught to parents and caregivers so they can foster equal movements as the infant develops.

Range-of-motion exercises are designed to minimize the development of contractures and to prepare the limb for future prosthetic fit and function. With certain levels of limb deficiency, characteristic contractures and deformities are present. Longitudinal deficiencies of the tibia and fibula are commonly associated with anomalies of the foot and ankle. These deficiencies can affect prosthetic and orthotic management as well as hinder gross motor develop-

ment. For example, foot contractures may rule out the future option of a rotationplasty in the infant with longitudinal deficiency of the femur, partial (LDFP, formerly called proximal femoral focal deficiency, or PFFD), or they can affect the results of future limb lengthening in the infant with longitudinal deficiency of the fibula. The parents should be instructed in range-of-motion and positioning exercises.[6,7,12,17] Hip and knee flexion contractures are common in children born with short residual limb segments of the femur and tibia, respectively, as a result of constrictive amniotic bands and in children who have had traumatic amputations as an infant.[6,7,12,17] Prosthetic fittings as early as age 6 months have been used to manage knee flexion tightness in an infant born with a very short unilateral transtibial amputation.[6,7]

The benefits of early fittings are threefold. First, flexion contractures are minimized. Second, symmetric bipedal weight bearing can be achieved for early age-appropriate standing activities. Third, the infant receives early sensory and proprioceptive feedback that truly prepares him or her for prosthetic fitting. An added benefit is that parents are involved early in the management of their child's care.[6,7] To maximize the benefits of the more anatomic prosthesis, it is recommended that the infant who would benefit from early prosthetic fitting have regular physical therapy to work on the transitions and activities that are preparatory for standing and walking.

Hip flexion, abduction, and external rotation contractures are anticipated in infants with LDFP and short transfemoral limb loss.[6,12,13] Knee instability is common in infants born with longitudinal femoral and tibial deficiencies. Again, instruction is given for positioning and range-of-motion exercises. Early prosthetic fittings can be considered if the loss is unilateral. Parents and caregivers can be taught how to maintain mobility at the hips, knees, and ankles during simple caregiving activities such as di-

apering, picking up the infant, dressing, feeding, and play.[6,7,13,18]

Parents are encouraged to move their infants to both sides and not to be afraid of further deformity or injury to the involved limb. They are taught to help the infant to come up and down from sitting, kneeling, and standing on both sides. Symmetry and balance of movements during early motor activities are precursors to weight shifting in standing, cruising, and walking.[6,7,12,17] Prosthetic fitting is recommended once the infant begins to pull to stand, typically around 8 to 12 months of age.[6,7,12,17-19] During this period, infants with longitudinal tibial and fibular deficiencies have undergone any necessary ablations and are ready for initiation of prosthetic fittings. Postoperative wound care, edema control, and range-of-motion exercises are imperative. Diligent elastic bandage wrapping is important to control swelling and to protect the limb because these infants are extremely active. Infants with knee disarticulation and transfemoral amputation levels have demonstrated the ability to control a prosthetic knee and incorporate knee functions in early developmental activities such as creeping and crawling, pulling to stand, and half kneeling and tall kneeling play[1-3] (Figure 3).

Matching an infant's function with available prosthetic components allows the infant to parallel normal development. Even infants with LDFP have demonstrated the ability to control prosthetic knee function in an unconventional prosthetic fitting with a short prosthetic tibia section using a hinged knee or internal knee, depending on the length of the limb segments[1,2] (Figure 4). Prosthetic alignment should take into account the developmental activities of the child and may need to be modified frequently as the infant develops and motor skills mature. The physical therapist and prosthetist should work closely together to address the alignment issues of the infant.

Infants born with multiple limb deficiencies with or without neurologic and medical involvement will require frequent therapy intervention and may take longer to acquire motor skills. Intervention should begin as soon as possible, focusing on all developmental parameters. Monthly monitoring is recommended to update home programs and to record changes in development, range of motion, and strength.[6,7,13,16]

Toddlers (12 to 36 months)

By the first year, the child should be pulling to stand and wearing a definitive prosthesis. The therapist and prosthetist should work closely together on prosthetic fit and function. Surgical intervention may be necessary at this age to correct deformities or perform a primary amputation. Postoperative management again is imperative for optimal prosthetic fit and function. When the toddler is ready for prosthetic fitting, instructions are given for donning and doffing, skin care, and wearing of the prosthesis. It is not unusual for infants and young children with knee disarticulations and transtibial amputations to reject their prostheses. Initially, the prosthesis interferes with mobility and hinders overall movements. Toddlers are more mobile in crawling and creeping activities without the prosthesis. It is not until the toddler spends more time in standing and cruising activity that the prosthesis is readily accepted. The use of articulating knees in infants and toddlers has diminished some of these frustrations because they allow them to engage in more normal gross motor functions, providing freedom and symmetry in patterns of movement. Gait studies in which toddlers are observed in developmental play situations are documenting prosthetic knee function during climbing up and sliding down a small slide, squatting in play, transitioning up to stand, and playing on the floor[1,2] (Figure 5).

A therapy program at this stage should stress symmetry of posture and movement and control of weight shifting over the prosthesis.[12,17] Developmental screening and assess-

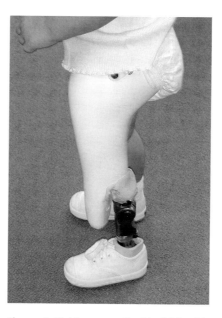

Figure 4 Eighteen-month-old child with LDFP fitted in a traditional high proximal socket for containment of the hip because of the LDFP. A knee unit is placed distally. Although there is a short tibial segment, the knee is used appropriately in gait and all functional developmental activities.

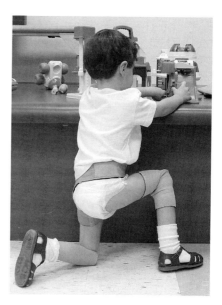

Figure 5 Two-year-old child with congenital bilateral tibial deficiencies playing in half kneeling position. Note the knee disarticulation level on the left side and Syme ankle disarticulation level on the right side. This child was fitted with an articulating knee unit at 11 months of age. He was walking independently by 15 months of age.

ment tools make excellent treatment guidelines and can assist in forming home programs.[7-9,20-23] Exercises should be fun and incorporated into the toddler's everyday play. Push toys and walkers are adjuncts to treatment. Most toddlers with single limb deficiencies do not require special assistive devices, but adaptations may be necessary to assist those with multiple limb loss in ambulation.

Toddler and Preschool Years (12 months to 6 years)

As the child begins walking with the prosthesis, treatment again focuses on age-appropriate activities. Activities such as marching to music, climbing on small gym equipment, and riding a tricycle are excellent gross motor activities. Home exercise programs still include range of motion to prevent the progression of contractures.

The frequency of therapy visits depends on the child's mastery of walking and the family's ability to follow through with the exercise program.

The physical therapist should monitor the child's development during clinic or prosthetic visits approximately every 4 to 6 months and make recommendations for changes of prosthetic components to parallel the child's motor development.[7,18] The prosthesis should be closely monitored for fit as the child grows. Technologic advances[4] have provided articulating ankles if the child's foot is longer than 17 cm. Feet with dynamic-response keels as well as feet that enable considerable adaptability to uneven terrain in all planes continue to become available in smaller and smaller sizes.

Physical therapy can take place at the child's preschool or home and is an effective means of educating the child's teachers, classmates, and other family members. The preschool staff will be less apprehensive about having a child with special needs if they are well informed and taught strategies on managing the prosthesis and adapting the environment as needed. Toilet training is a major obstacle at this age for children with transfemoral or knee disarticulation level prostheses. Typically, belts are required for suspension, making it difficult to pull pants up and down. Therapy can address this issue as well as dressing at home and in school. Surgical interventions may be introduced at this age. Van Ness rotationplasty may be performed for the child with LDFP. Following each surgical intervention, wound healing, edema control, pressure wrapping, and range-of-motion and functional strengthening exercises are implemented. The child may require additional physical therapy postoperatively until independent function is restored.

Elementary Years (6 to 12 years)

As children grow, they may receive technologically advanced prosthetic components that may require additional gait training and balance exercises.[1,2,7] At this age, amputations secondary to trauma or bone tumors occur.[5,6,18,19,24] Children with congenital limb deficiencies may undergo surgical revisions for overgrowth or to correct deformities. Rotationplasty may be a surgical option for children with distal femoral or proximal tibial tumors or those with LDFP. With each intervention comes a period of adjustment and retraining. Edema is controlled with elastic wrapping and/or shrinkers. Preprosthetic range-of-motion and strengthening exercises may be necessary. Postsurgical exercises begin to resemble those for adults, which are described in chapter 48. Gait training begins in parallel bars with multidirectional weight shifts and stepping patterns progressing to level surfaces with or without assistive devices. By the age of 7 years, the child's gait parallels that of an adult.[10,12,17] The child is able to participate actively in an exercise program and is less dependent on his or her parents. Outpatient physical therapy for this age group is best in a sports orthopaedic setting, using a developmental approach that moti-

vates and challenges them appropriately rather than a setting that is equipped for infants and younger children. School visits by the therapist are a helpful way of acquainting a child's teacher and classmates with his or her new prosthesis. Again, exercises should focus on age-appropriate activities, sports, and recreation.

Rehabilitation of the child with a rotationplasty is both challenging and rewarding. Children requiring rotationplasty from trauma or bone tumors without hip pathology have gait patterns similar to those with transtibial function. Children receiving rotationplasty for treatment of LDFP have issues relating to hip and knee instability that are addressed either surgically or with prosthetic fitting. Derotation may also occur in LDFP, requiring additional revision. These issues influence the gait pattern of the child. In both situations, range-of-motion and strengthening exercises of the hip, ankle, foot, and toes are imperative. Immediate postoperative management requires a 6- to 8-week period of immobility either in a cast or semirigid dressing. Healing may be delayed in children on chemotherapy for treatment of bone cancer.

Once the bone has advanced into the healing stage, elastic wrapping; range-of-motion exercises of the hip, foot, ankle, and toes; and isometric strengthening of the hip and ankle are initiated. Open- and closed-chain hip-strengthening and weight-bearing exercises can be initiated when the osteotomy site is healed. Healing time is different for every child and must be coordinated with the orthopaedic surgeon. Ankle, foot, and toe flexibility and strength are imperative for optimal prosthetic knee function. Flexibility and range of motion should precede strengthening. Ankle range of motion that is inadequate for the prosthetic knee function will interfere with proper gait, and in some children will cause pressure marks, skin breakdown, pain, and foot and midfoot breakdown. In extreme situations, rupture of the Achilles tendon has occurred. Tightness of the plantar

fascia will influence toe and foot function. Toes are excellent initiators of prosthetic knee motion and act to stabilize the foot inside the socket, but if the knee centers of the anatomic and prosthetic foot are not equal, tightness is created inside the foot because of the inability to flex the prosthetic knee.

Ankle dorsiflexion of 0° to 30° is adequate to operate prosthetic knee function. Optimal plantar flexion beyond 50° to 60° is desired.[6,7,12,17] The greater the plantar flexion, the more streamlined is the relationship of the foot with the proximal segment, creating a larger excursion of the prosthetic knee. Strength of the hip, ankle, foot, and toes leads to optimal prosthetic knee power following achievement of adequate range of motion. Exercises are necessary at speeds, excursions, and strengths common to knee function using the foot's anatomy in an opposite orientation (Figure 6).

Surgical management of limb-length discrepancies of the femur, tibia, and fibula is typically initiated at this age if the deficient limb is appropriate for lengthening. Limb equalization procedures can include lengthening the short limb, shortening the sound limb through epiphyseodesis or resection, or a combination of these methods. The goal is to have appropriate limb lengths at skeletal maturity. The challenge is to time the lengthening or growth arrest procedures appropriately to obtain minimal limb-length discrepancy. Scanograms, pelvic leveling with blocks, and the use of Mosely logarithmic growth charts are indispensable for predicting future discrepancies and timing appropriate interventions. The greater the projected discrepancy at maturity, the sooner the physician should act to obtain equalization. Limb lengthening procedures may be staged over several years, requiring extensive physical therapy and guidance for the child and family. Rehabilitation is extensive; goals for therapy include maintaining range of motion in the joints above and below the external fixator, strengthening of the limb, weight bearing, increasing endurance and overall conditioning, and restoring function and activity level during the application of the external fixator.[6,25,26] Good pin care can minimize major setbacks. These children should be kept as active as possible, going to school and participating in recreational activities as permitted. The lengthening process should be interrupted or stopped if there is hip or knee subluxation.[26] Hip stiffness and knee flexion range of motion less than 45° are relative indications to slow or stop the lengthening.

Table 1 gives examples of functional abilities of children with varying degrees of lower limb deficiencies. Although not comprehensive, this table provides therapists, prosthetists, and families with functional expectations for the children within the limits of the limb deficiency.

Adolescence (13 to 17 years)

Malignant bone tumors are most common in the first and second decades of life. Children and their families are faced with surgical options for limb salvage, amputation, or rotationplasty depending on the size, location, and characteristics of the tumor as well as the activity and functional levels, taking into account cultural, psychological, and family issues.[7] The physical therapist plays a vital role in educating the child and family about the functional outcomes of each surgical procedure.

The child who undergoes a limb salvage procedure faces numerous physical challenges. Physical therapy goals include regaining mobility and strength, progressive weight bearing, improving cardiovascular endurance, pain management, scar mobility, and independence in transfers. Age-appropriate activities, which include activities of daily living, are incorporated in the exercise program. The therapist must always remember, however, that the primary goal for a child with a bone tumor is to survive

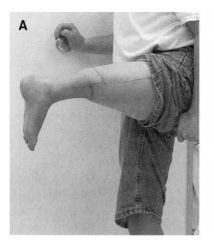
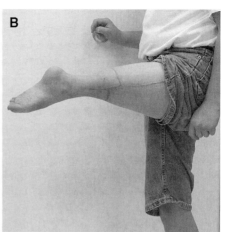
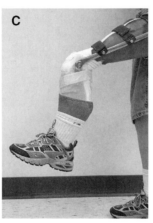
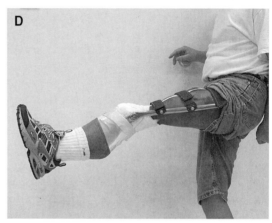

Figure 6 Use of the foot and ankle to power the prosthetic knee 12 weeks after surgery by a 15-year-old boy who underwent a rotationplasty because of osteosarcoma. **A,** The foot in plantar flexion. **B,** The foot in dorsiflexion. **C** and **D,** the same foot and ankle positions with the boy wearing the prosthesis. The prosthesis is not cosmetically finished because of the need for frequent alignment changes to accommodate gains in plantar flexion range of motion.

the malignancy. The aggressive nature of these tumors and the morbidity associated with their treatment may limit significantly the goals of physical therapy. Each limb salvage procedure is unique, and therapy must be under the close direction of the orthopaedic surgeon. Usually these children receive chemotherapy, which could delay the overall responses to healing and rehabilitation. Immediate postoperative fitting may be used when appropriate. Prosthetic technology has assisted these children to function with greater stability and balance. Physical therapy treatment includes edema control; wound healing; and range-of-motion, strengthening, and balance exercises necessary for prosthetic function.

Preadolescents and adolescents with congenital limb deficiency may undergo surgical reconstructions and revisions to correct deformities and overgrowth in limbs that are less than functional. Usually it is their choice, and improvement of function and cosmesis guided their decision. Limb lengthening, as described earlier, is continued for ongoing management of longitudinal deficiencies of the femur, tibia, and fibula when appropriate.

Phantom limb sensation is common in adolescents with acquired limb loss resulting from trauma and tumors[7,10,12,17] but is less frequent in those with congenital limb deficiencies following reconstructions or ablations. It typically does not interfere with function. Treatment guidelines

TABLE 1 Lower Limb Functional Outcomes Special Considerations in Children With Lower Limb Deficiencies

Unilateral Syme Disarticulation

No limitations in daily activities

Able to participate in age-appropriate activities and sports such as bicycling, skiing, dancing, gymnastics

No assistive devices

Unilateral Transtibial Level

No limitations in age-appropriate daily activities

Able to participate in sports and activities such as bicycling, skiing, dancing, gymnastics

No assistive devices

Bilateral Transtibial Level

Slight limitation on uneven surfaces, curbs, stairs

Participates in age-appropriate sports with limitations

May require adapted physical education, wheelchair sports

Rides bicycle with adaptations

No assistive devices for ambulation

Wheelchair as back-up

Unilateral Knee Disarticulation or Transfemoral Amputation Level

No limitations in age-appropriate daily activities

Requires adaptation to bicycle; may ride without prosthesis

Able to participate in sports; adaptations may be required

No assistive devices; crutches as a back-up

Bilateral Knee Disarticulation or Transfemoral Level

Some limitations on uneven surfaces, curbs, kneeling, stairs

Difficulty riding bicycle; needs adaptations

Adapted physical education

Wheelchair for sports and as a back-up

Limited in sports and age-appropriate activities

May use cane or Lofstrand crutches, although most do not

Unilateral Hip Disarticulation

Limitations on uneven surfaces, curbs, steps (Children with congenital deficiencies are quite functional; children with acquired loss have more difficulties.)

Bicycling is difficult with prosthesis; may ride without prosthesis

Limited in running and sports; requires adaptations in sports

Wheelchair for sports and as a back-up

May use cane in community, school, mall

May use crutches and no prosthesis

Bilateral Hip Disarticulation

Wheelchair used for primary mobility; power mobility may be necessary if associated upper limb involvement

Prosthetic use for standing and exercise

Requires assistive devices

Wheelchair sports

(Adapted from Coulter O'Berry C: Physical therapy management in children with lower extremity limb deficiencies, in Herring JA, Birch JG (eds): The Child With a Limb Deficiency. Rosemont, IL, American Academy of Orthopaedic Surgeons, 1997, pp 319-330.)

for phantom sensations are similar to those for adults. The most successful

treatment is appropriate prosthetic fitting and weight bearing.[10]

Learning to drive a car is a very age-appropriate activity for adolescents. The physical therapist should know of local resources to assess the adolescent's abilities and the need for adaptations and modifications to the car. Accessibility issues are more apparent as the adolescent prepares for college and independent living away from his or her family. Universities and colleges typically have a department dedicated to students with special needs and accessibility issues.[27,28]

Sports and Recreation

Children and adolescents of all ages with amputations or limb deficiencies should be encouraged to participate in sports and recreational activities with their peers. The psychological impact of sports cannot be underestimated.[6] Improving self-esteem and confidence, gaining independence, learning to win and lose, developing decision-making and problem-solving skills, and cooperating as a team member are a few of the benefits that a participant carries throughout life. Improvement in physical fitness; development of balance, strength, coordination, and motor skills; increased endurance; and weight control are also benefits of physical activity.[6] Over the past 10 years, sports and recreational programs have developed throughout the United States for individuals with all classifications of impairments. Laws have been passed that require children and adolescents to be educated in the least restrictive environments. Public law 94-142, the Individuals with Disabilities Education Act, provides free and appropriate education for children with disabilities.[6,12,17] Physical therapy and adapted physical education are included in this legislation. Special adaptations and sports prostheses are available, depending on the degree and level of impairment. Advances in prosthetic technology are assisting amputees to compete in major sporting events on national and international levels.[29-32] The United States Disabled Athletes Fund[33] is an excellent resource for geographically located programs. The Orthotic and Prosthetic Assistance Fund is another organization that provides financial and technologic assistance to individuals with physical disabilities who require orthotic and prosthetic services.[34] Exposing children and adolescents to these opportunities and referring them to local sports and recreational programs is one of the most important roles a therapist can have (Figure 7).

Multiple Limb Loss With and Without Neurologic Impairments

Infants, children, and adolescents with congenital or acquired multiple limb loss have special needs. They require more intensive and regular therapy interventions.[7,12,17] Typically there are delays in development; the severity of these delays depends on the degree of limb loss and other associated medical or neurologic impairments. Special mobility aids, wheelchairs, and adaptations to the environment may be necessary. Prioritization of surgical, prosthetic, and therapeutic interventions is required to meet the child's and family's goals. It is important not to overburden the child with all new prostheses at the same time.[6,7]

In an infant, child, or adolescent with both neurologic involvement and amputation, the neurologic impairment has a greater influence on function than the amputation in both acquired and congenital amputations. Examples of acquired limb loss with neurologic pathology include traumatic head injury with traumatic amputation; prematurity with intravenous infiltrate causing amputation; meningococcemia causing brain and musculoskeletal insults; and myelomeningocele (spina bifida) with amputation. Treatment should focus on neurologic function and balance of movements with the prosthesis to assist in stability and balance. Typically

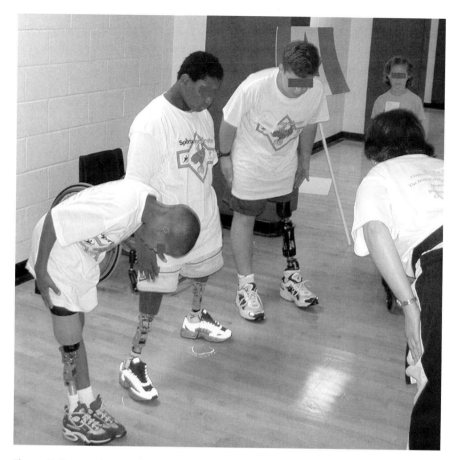

Figure 7 Karate class at a local sporting event for children with limb differences.

the prosthetic limb is the more sound and stable limb. Strong communication is necessary between the family, school, community, and limb-deficiency team for optimal outcomes.

Summary

Each infant, child, and adolescent is different and has expectations and goals unique to his or her needs. Many factors influence the goals when treating these patients. Age-appropriate functional activities that meet patient and family goals should guide physical therapy interventions. Treatments should be fun and meaningful. The therapist is a teacher, facilitator, and advocate for the infant, child, or adolescent in all settings.

References

1. Giavedoni BJ, Coulter-O'Berry C, Geil M: Movement masters. *Adv Dire Rehabil* 2002;11:43-44.

Additional Resources

Amputee Coalition of America
   1-888-267-5669
   (1-888-AMP-KNOW)
   www.amputee-coalition.org
Association of Children's Prosthetic-Orthotic Clinics
   (1-847-384-4226)
   www.acpoc.org

2. Giavedoni BJ: The use of prosthetic knees in infants and toddlers, in *Alignment*. Canadian Association of Prosthetists and Orthotists, 2000, pp 25-26.

3. Wilk B, Karol L, Halliday S, et al: Transition to an articulating knee prosthesis in pediatric amputees. *J Prosth Orthot* 1999;11:69-74.

4. College Park Industries Inc: TruPer Foot. Available at: http://www.college-park.com/CPStore/News.asp. Accessed May 26, 2004.

5. Dormans JP: Limb-salvage surgery versus amputation for children with extremity sarcomas, in Herring JA,

Birch JG (eds): *The Child With a Limb Deficiency.* Rosemont, IL, American Academy of Orthopaedic Surgeons, 1998, pp 289-302.

6. Morrissy RT, Giavedoni BJ, Coulter-O'Berry C: The limb-deficient child, in Morrissy RT, Weinstein SL (eds): *Lovell and Winter's Pediatric Orthopaedics,* ed 5. Philadelphia, PA, Lippincott Williams & Wilkins, 2001, vol 2, pp 1217-1272.

7. Coulter-O'Berry C: Physical therapy management in children with lower extremity limb deficiencies, in Herring JA, Birch JS (eds): *The Child With a Limb Deficiency.* Rosemont, IL, American Academy of Orthopaedic Surgeons, 1998, pp 319-330.

8. Jaeger L, Ascher G, Atlee J (eds): *Home Program Instruction Sheets for Infants and Young Children,* ed 3. Tucson, AZ, Therapy Skill Builders, 1987.

9. Diamant RB (ed): *Positioning for Play: Home Activities for Parents of Young Children.* Tucson, AZ, Therapy Skill Builders, 1992.

10. Seymour R (ed): Clinical use of dressings and bandages, in *Prosthetics and Orthotics: Lower Limb and Spinal.* Philadelphia, PA, Lippincott Williams & Wilkins, 2002, pp 123-142.

11. Taping, bandaging, orthotics, in Hunter-Griffin LY (ed) *Athletic Training and Sports Medicine,* ed 2. Rosemont, IL, American Academy of Orthopaedic Surgeons, 1991, pp 647-704.

12. Stanger M: Limb deficiencies and amputations, in Campbell SK, Palisano RJ, Vander Linden DW (eds): *Physical Therapy for Children.* Philadelphia, PA, WB Saunders, 1994, pp 325-351.

13. Gillespie R: Principles of amputation surgery in children with longitudinal deficiencies of the femur. *Clin Orthop* 1990;256:29-38.

14. American Academy of Orthopaedic Surgeons: *Atlas of Limb Prosthetics: Surgical and Prosthetic Principles.* St. Louis, MO, CV Mosby, 1981.

15. Krebs DE, Fishman S: Characteristics of the child amputee population. *J Pediatr Orthop* 1984;4:89-95.

16. Effgen SK, Bjornson K, Chiarello L, Sinzer L, Phillips W: Competencies for physical therapists in early intervention. *Pediatr Phys Ther* 1991;9:1-23.

17. Stanger M: Orthopedic management, in Tecklin JS (ed): *Pediatric Physical Therapy,* ed 3. Philadelphia, PA, Lippincott Williams & Wilkins, 1999, pp 378-428.

18. Tooms RE: The amputee, in Lovell WW, Winter RB (eds): *Pediatric Physical Therapy,* ed 3. Philadelphia, PA, Lippincott Williams & Wilkins, 1999, pp 378-428.

19. Krebs DE, Edelstein JE, Thornby MA: Prosthetic management of children with limb deficiencies. *Phys Ther* 1991; 71:920-934.

20. Bayley N (ed): *Bayley Scales of Infant Development.* New York, NY, Psychological Corporation, 1969.

21. Folio MR, Fewell RR (eds): *Peabody Developmental Motor Scales.* Nashville, TN, George Peabody College for Teachers, 1974.

22. Frankenburg WK, Dodds JB, Fandal AW (eds): *Denver Developmental Screening Test: Manual.* Denver, CO, University of Colorado Medical Center, 1970, revised.

23. Furuno S, O'Reilly K, Hoska C, et al: *Hawaii Early Learning Profile (HELP): Activity Guide.* Palo Alto, CA, VORT Corporation, 1979.

24. Kalamchi A (ed): *Congenital Lower Limb Deficiencies.* New York, NY, Springer-Verlag, 1989.

25. Catagni MA, Guerreschi F: Management of fibular hemimelia using the Illizarov method, in Herring JA, Birch JG (eds): *The Child With a Limb Deficiency.* Rosemont, IL, American Academy of Orthopaedic Surgeons, 1998, pp 179-193.

26. Paley D: Lengthening reconstruction surgery for congenital femoral defi-

ciency, in Herring JA, Birch JG (eds): *The Child With a Limb Deficiency.* Rosemont, IL, American Academy of Orthopaedic Surgeons, 1998, pp 113-132.

27. Ketchum AM: Best US colleges and universities for wheelchair accessibility. Available at http://www.geocities.com/ketchum/4/bestcollegesanduniversitiespg2.htm. Accessed May 26, 2004.

28. Haly J: College. Children's Hemiplegia and Stroke Association Web site. Available at: http://www.hemikids.org/college.htm. Accessed July 2004.

29. Radocy B: Upper-limb prosthetic adaptations for sports and recreation, in Bowker JH, Michael JW (eds): *Atlas of Prosthetics: Surgical, Prosthetic, and Rehabilitation Principles.* St Louis, MO, Mosby-Year Book, 1992, pp 325-344.

30. Michael JW, Gailey RS, Bowker JH: New developments in recreational prostheses and adaptive devices for the amputee. *Clin Orthop* 1990;256:64-75.

31. Anderson TF: Aspects of sports and recreation for the child with a limb deficiency, in Herring JA, Birch JG (eds): *The Child With a Limb Deficiency.* Rosemont, IL, American Academy of Orthopaedic Surgeons, 1998, pp 345-352.

32. Miller K: Sports implications for the individual with a lower extremity prosthesis, in Seymour R (ed): *Prosthetics and Orthotics: Lower Limb and Spinal.* Philadelphia, PA, Lippincott Williams & Wilkins, 2002, pp 281-310.

33. U.S. Disabled Athletes Fund, Inc: Available at: http://www.blazesports.com. Accessed June 4, 2004.

34. Orthotic & Prosthetic Assistance Fund, Inc: Available at: http://www.opfund.org. Accessed June 4, 2004.

Chapter 68

Acquired Amputations in Children

John P. Dormans, MD

Bülent Erol, MD

Christopher B. Nelson, CPO

Introduction

In children, about twice as many amputations are caused by trauma as by disease[1,2] (Table 1). The most common cause of traumatic injuries resulting in amputation is power machinery (such as lawnmowers), followed by vehicular accidents, gunshot wounds, explosions, railroad injuries, household accidents, and thermal and electrical injuries.[3-6] Of the disease processes resulting in amputation in children, malignant tumors are responsible for more than half, with the highest incidence occurring in the 12- to 21-year-old group. Vascular occlusion caused by meningococcemia or vascular catheterization, vascular malformations, neurogenic disorders, and a wide variety of other disorders are responsible for the remainder of amputations caused by disease.[7,8] In more than 90% of acquired amputations, a single limb is involved, and in 60% of those cases, it is a lower limb. Boys are affected more frequently than are girls, at a ratio of 3:2, probably because boys tend to engage in more hazardous activities.

Principles of Surgical Treatment

The evaluation and management of an acquired amputation must be approached differently in a child than in an adult for several reasons: (1) the child's bones (ie, the physes) continue to grow, (2) children heal better than adults do, (3) children risk residual limb bone overgrowth, and (4) children face different emotional and psychological problems in rehabilitation than adults do.[9]

Because children grow, discrepancies in limb length may become greater with time. The cardinal rule is to conserve as much limb length as possible and appropriate, consistent with the proper treatment.[3]

Because children heal better, surgical techniques that help conserve limb length but are not always successful in the adult may be successful in the child. For example, split-thickness skin grafts may help conserve limb length without compromising wound healing or subsequent prosthetic use and may be necessary to preserve length in some cases of trauma, burns, and meningococcemia[10,11] (Figure 1). Local rotation flaps or free vascularized flaps can provide excellent coverage. Open wounds may be closed successfully under slightly more tension in children than in adults; however, even in children, tissue tolerance has limits, so good surgical judgment must be used.

It is usually better to perform a disarticulation than a transmetaphyseal or transdiaphyseal amputation in a growing child to preserve the epiphyseal growth plate and ensure continued longitudinal growth of the remaining bone.[5,10,12] This is especially true for the femur, where 70% of growth occurs from the distal physis. Disarticulation also avoids terminal bony overgrowth and provides a sturdy, end-bearing residual limb, which enhances prosthesis use. Removing the cartilage from the bone end is not necessary in younger children (younger than 10 years) because the bony prominences of the epiphysis and metaphysis will usually not develop to adult proportions and will not interfere with fitting a prosthesis.[7]

Finally, children's psychological and emotional needs strongly influ-

TABLE 1 Causes of Acquired Amputations in Children in Order of Occurrence

Accidental and nonaccidental trauma

Power tools and machinery (lawnmowers)

Vehicular accidents

Gunshot wounds

Explosions/land mines

Railroad injuries

Household accidents

Thermal and electrical accidents

Disease

Malignant tumors (also, occasionally, aggressive benign tumors)

Vascular occlusions (meningococcemia, vascular catheterization)

Vascular malformations

Neurogenic disorders

Miscellaneous disorders

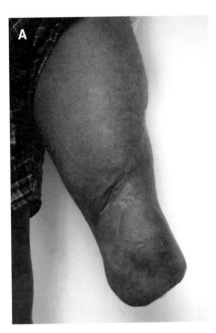

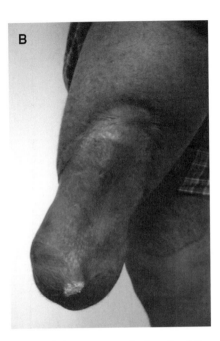

Figure 1 Split-thickness skin grafts are sometimes needed to preserve the length of the residual limb in children with traumatic amputations. Skin grafts can often help the surgeon achieve satisfactory coverage as seen in this patient who had a traumatic knee disarticulation from a train injury.

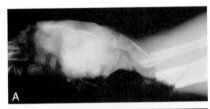

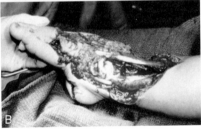

Figure 2 A 6-year-old boy with a mangled right lower limb. **A,** Radiograph obtained in the emergency department reveals a large intercalary shredding-type injury in the distal tibia and a comminuted, displaced fracture in the distal fibula. **B,** Photograph documents the extensive soft-tissue damage and open fractures.

ence the outcome of treatment. Young children depend on others for basic needs, so the quality of care parents or guardians provide is an important factor. Like all children with disabilities, children with acquired amputations are vulnerable to social isolation. Up to age 6 years, a child's understanding of a disability is general and incomplete, but around the age of 8 or 9 years, a child will come to understand the disability more completely.[13] As children develop, their appearance becomes important to their self-image, and physical differences can be an obstacle to healthy interaction with parents, teachers, friends, classmates, and others. Caregivers should keep in mind, however, that development of self-esteem is usually independent of the limb deficiency and can be encouraged through the social support of parents, teachers, friends, and classmates.

Traumatic Amputations

Children requiring amputation for trauma require special attention in their evaluation, stabilization, surgical treatment, postoperative management, and rehabilitation. When the injuries are extensive, it is important to know the patient's general condition and the details of the injury, especially how it occurred, as well as what the initial treatment was, how long the warm ischemic time was, how the amputated parts were handled, and what the child's tetanus status is. The patient's overall medical condition (assessed by the trauma ABCs) is the most important factor in initial evaluation, and in some cases, it will determine treatment.[14] Blood loss is often considerable with severe limb injuries, so early, aggressive volume resuscitation is required. For most replantation cases, blood transfusion is necessary, so blood typing and cross-matching should be done soon after the child arrives at the hospital.[15] Prophylactic antibiotics are recommended for traumatic amputations to reduce bacterial contamination of the wound, which is believed to be an important source of postoperative infections.[16] Radiographs are obtained in the emergency department or in the operating room, whichever is more appropriate (Figure 2, A).

In the operating room, the extent of injury is evaluated, including the orientation of the limb, the extent of devascularization, the amount and nature of contamination, and the damage to soft tissues. Consultation with other surgical specialists (eg, plastic, hand, vascular, and general surgeons) may be helpful at this point. Photographs are often very useful in documenting the extent of injury (Figure 2, B), for both medical and legal reasons. In treating a child with a mangled limb, the first decision that must be made is whether to reconstruct or to amputate. Many factors should be taken into consideration, such as the presence of neurovascular injury, warm ischemic time, wound contamination, and the extent of damage to the skin, bone, growth plates, articular cartilage, and muscle.[17,18] At present, no method can predict the success of limb salvage, so the decision depends on the surgeon's clinical judgment and experience. For certain severe injuries, early amputation may be the best option. The belief that amputation of a

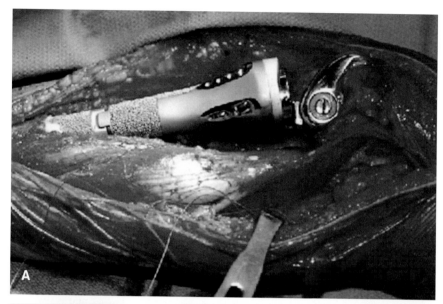

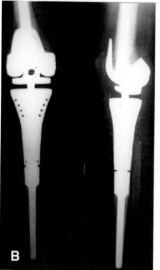
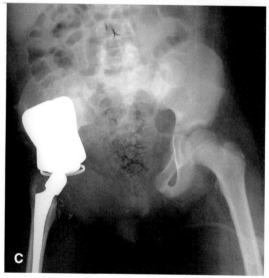

Figure 3 Local control of bone sarcomas of the limbs is usually achieved by resecting the tumor with wide surgical margins and limb salvage reconstruction with one of several different techniques. A 14-year-old patient with Ewing's sarcoma of the proximal tibia had wide resection and limb salvage reconstruction with an endoprosthesis as shown in an intraoperative photograph **(A)** and postoperative radiograph **(B)**. **C,** A 12-year-old boy with Ewing's sarcoma of the pelvis underwent limb salvage reconstruction with a saddle prosthesis, an endoprosthesis that was designed to reconstruct the pelvis after excision of malignant periacetabular tumors.

new classification of injuries was proposed, including shredding injuries (16 of 18 limbs), either intercalary or distal, and the less common paucilaceration injuries (2 of 18 limbs). Among the 4 salvaged limbs, shredding injuries were associated with poor results (infection, stiff joints, limb-length discrepancies), whereas paucilaceration injuries were associated with better results. Finally, the authors concluded that limb salvage may be appropriate in a small percentage of carefully selected patients, but that inappropriate attempts at limb salvage may contribute to long hospitalizations, a higher incidence of surgical complications, and increased pain and expense.

The level of lower limb amputation (ie, transfemoral or transtibial) significantly affects function. The energy expenditure for walking, functional outcome, and prosthetic function are poorer after a transfemoral amputation. These differences also apply to limb salvage surgery. Outcome after nerve repair above the knee is often poorer. On the other hand, reconstruction of vascular injuries is frequently easier above the knee. Reconstruction of both bone and soft tissue is easier above the knee because of the thick, well-vascularized soft-tissue envelope. As a result, limb salvage should be given more consideration for an above-the-knee injury than for one below the knee, unless the sciatic nerve is completely disrupted.

Function after salvage of an upper limb is better than for a lower limb, and the prognosis for function after amputation of an upper limb is usually poor. Criteria for salvage of the upper limb are, therefore, different from those for the lower limb.

Treatment of Sarcoma Affecting the Limbs

Most current sarcoma treatment protocols require complete removal of malignant tissue with wide surgical

mangled limb represents a treatment failure can result in costly, demoralizing, complicated, and sometimes lethal attempts at reconstruction of functionless limbs.[19]

In a study conducted at The Children's Hospital of Philadelphia of children with lawnmower injuries, 16 patients (18 limbs) were treated with an average follow-up of about 4 years.[5] All the injuries included extensive soft-tissue damage with open fractures and fracture-dislocations. All patients underwent aggressive attempts to salvage the limbs. The patients underwent an average of 4.9 operations each, and each had at least three débridements. The mean hospital stay was 24 days, at an average cost of $61,492. Most of the injured limbs (78%) required eventual amputation at different levels. From this study, a

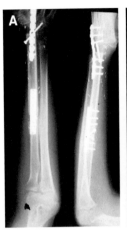
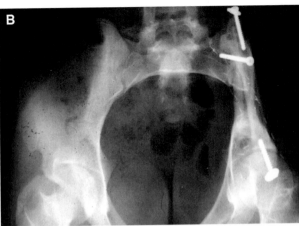

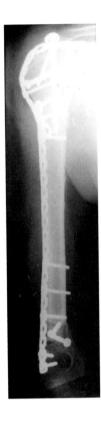

Figure 4 Radiograph shows allograft reconstruction in a 16-year-old girl who underwent resection with wide surgical margins of Ewing's sarcoma of the humeral diaphysis.

Figure 5 A, Postoperative AP and lateral radiographs of the forearm of a 16-year-old patient show limb salvage reconstruction with an autograft (free vascularized fibular autograft) following resection with wide surgical margins of a distal radial osteosarcoma. **B,** Another example of free vascularized fibular autograft reconstruction in a modified internal hemipelvectomy for Ewing's sarcoma of the pelvis.

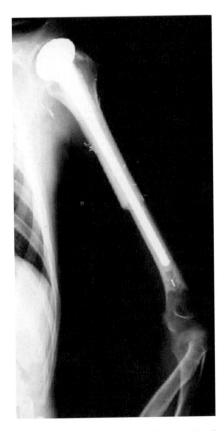

Figure 6 Limb salvage with combined (allograft-prosthesis composite) reconstruction following wide resection of a sarcoma of the humerus.

margins. This can be achieved by amputation or by resection and reconstruction. The success of chemotherapy, better imaging (especially MRI), and improvements in surgical technique have made limb salvage surgery increasingly common. After resection, reconstruction may be achieved with custom endoprosthetic devices (expandable or nonexpandable endoprostheses) (Figure 3), allograft reconstruction (Figure 4), autograft reconstruction (Figure 5), combinations of endoprostheses and bone grafts (allograft-prosthetic composites) (Figure 6), or bone transport reconstruction. Rotationplasty reconstruction is another option for patients with sarcoma of the lower limb (Figure 7). This technique allows better function than transfemoral amputation and better durability than endoprosthetic reconstruction.[20] Contraindications to limb salvage surgery include inability to obtain adequate wide surgical margins, poor response of the tumor to preoperative neoadjuvant chemotherapy, anticipated major limb-length discrepancy, inadequate soft-tissue coverage that cannot be satisfactorily addressed with modern plastic surgery reconstruction options, or widely displaced pathologic fracture.[20]

Although limb-sparing surgery is possible and indicated for most children with sarcomas of a limb, amputation is still occasionally needed. The standard principles of amputation surgery for children apply to amputation for sarcoma,[21] but there are some differences in management after amputation. After amputation for malignancy, prosthetic fitting and rehabilitation must be prompt to improve the child's chances of using a prosthesis successfully and having good function. Fitting these patients with prostheses immediately after surgery is controversial. Because body weight and residual limb size and volume fluctuate during chemotherapy, adjustable temporary sockets must often be used for a longer time. Psychological and physical rehabilitation after surgery for musculoskeletal tumors is often a lifelong process.

Vascular Problems Causing Acquired Amputations

Meningococcemia, perinatal limb ischemia, and vascular anomalies may require amputation in children. Patients with meningococcemia are at great risk for purpura fulminans, especially in regions where the disease is

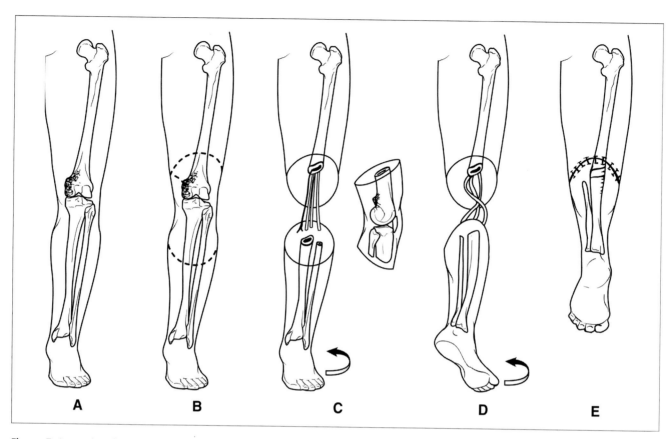

Figure 7 A rotationplasty reconstruction for malignant bone tumors of the distal femur. Following this procedure, with an appropriate prosthesis, the ankle joint serves the function of the removed knee joint. **A,** Preoperative status (distal femoral sarcoma). **B,** Skin incisions. **C,** Resected specimen with remaining limb and intact neuromuscular structures. **D,** Rotation component of procedure. **E,** Resultant limb after osteosynthesis and repair of soft tissues.

endemic.[22,23] Meningococcal-induced purpura fulminans is a thromboembolic condition that is an uncommon but potentially life-threatening sequela of sepsis induced by meningococcal infections that can cause gangrene leading to limb amputation. How the microvascular disease develops in this condition is not completely understood. Clinically, the condition is usually associated with rapid progression from nonspecific initial symptoms of fever, headache, lethargy, and vomiting to hemodynamic collapse and death in less than 12 hours. In a recent report of 113 patients with meningococcal C disease, purpura fulminans occurred in 25% of patients, and the mortality rate was substantially higher (50%) than in the nonpurpuric patients (1%).[24] In another large series of patients with meningococcemia (139 patients) who were treated over a 10-year period,

meningococcal-induced purpura fulminans developed in 16 (11%).[25] Four of these patients (25%) died within the first 36 hours after hospitalization.

Meningococcal disease may affect multiple limbs.[26] Despite the overall improvement in outcome for patients with meningococcal disease, the prognosis with meningococcal-induced purpura fulminans remains poor. About 50% of patients with this condition require amputation of two or more limbs.[25] Treatment must be individualized for each patient within general guidelines. The first is to help the patient achieve maximum function with the residual limbs, especially with the upper limbs, where sensation is so important to function.

Perinatal limb ischemia leading to vascular occlusion may also result in acquired amputations in newborns. Vascular occlusion may be related to

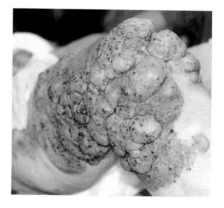

Figure 8 Patient with Klippel-Trenaunay syndrome had extensive involvement of the lower limb with vascular malformations. The patient eventually underwent hip disarticulation.

prematurity, polycythemia, sepsis, dehydration, umbilical artery catheterization, or other invasive procedures required to treat life-threatening illnesses.[7] Blank and associates[8] reported on 15 patients (16 ischemic

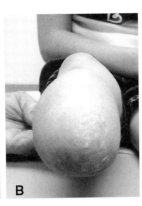 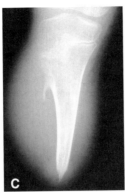 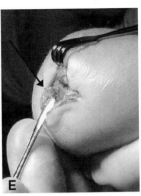 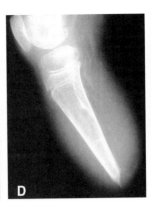

Figure 9 **A** and **B**, Clinical photographs of the residual limb of a 7-year-old girl who sustained a traumatic transtibial amputation on the right side when she was 5 years old. The distal tip of the limb was erythematous, warm, and tender to the touch. A small bursa and a spike of bone were palpable. AP **(C)** and lateral **(D)** radiographs show that the end of the tibia tapered distally to a narrow, sharp tip that was painful and threatening to pierce through the soft-tissue envelope. **E**, The patient underwent resection revision (*arrow*).

limbs), with an average gestational age of 30.8 weeks. The patients had limb ischemia caused by arterial thrombosis as a complication of arterial catheterization (8 patients), thromboembolism resulting from a hypercoagulable state (5 patients), intravenous infiltrate (1 patient), and in utero arterial thrombosis (1 patient). Ischemic events occurred at an average age of 5.4 weeks, and all patients required amputation, at a mean age of 8.5 weeks. Lower limbs were involved more often than the upper limbs (10 patients versus 5 patients). Eleven of the 15 patients (12 limbs) were followed for an average of 4.5 years and had good functional results. The remaining four died or were lost to follow-up.

Vascular malformations are associated with abnormalities in soft-tissue and skeletal growth. Klippel-Trenaunay syndrome is characterized by vascular malformation, musculoskeletal anomalies (finger or toe anomalies, scoliosis), and abnormalities of the cardiovascular, gastrointestinal, genitourinary, and central nervous systems. This syndrome is usually associated with overgrowth (hypertrophy) of soft tissue and bone in the involved limbs (mostly the lower limbs), causing size discrepancies[27] (Figure 8). For severely disfigured and dysfunctional limbs, reconstruction may not be an option, and amputation may provide a more

functional limb. The level of amputation is often dictated by the extent and severity of the vascular malformation.[28] Risks of surgery include infection, particularly in children with abnormal lymphatic drainage; delayed wound healing, which is common after transverse amputations; and increased blood loss for those with severe vascular anomalies.[29]

Proteus syndrome is another vascular, skeletal, and soft-tissue disorder characterized by vascular malformations and other anomalies. This condition also may cause hemihypertrophy resulting in significant limb-length discrepancy, and amputation may be required.

Complications of Amputation Surgery
Terminal Bony Overgrowth

Terminal bony overgrowth is the most common complication of surgical treatment of acquired amputation in skeletally immature children. It occurs in 4% to 35% of patients, depending on the age of the patient at the time of amputation and the bone involved.[30-32] This complication may follow transdiaphyseal and transmetaphyseal amputations and affects, in decreasing order of frequency, the tibia/fibula, humerus, and occasionally, the femur.[33,34] Contraction of the soft-tissue envelope as bones grow was initially thought to be the most

common cause of terminal bony overgrowth. Aitken[30] argued against this theory, however, and showed that overgrowth was primarily the consequence of local appositional bone growth (occurring at the end of the bone). Speer[35] demonstrated that occlusion of the medullary canal can lessen the likelihood that bony overgrowth will develop.

Children with terminal bony overgrowth usually present with pain on weight bearing or use of the prosthesis. The end of the residual limb may be tender, and inflammation, bursal formation, or protrusion of the bone end through the skin may be present (Figure 9). Commonly, the bony spike can be palpated within a small, tender bursa. Prosthetic modification and other conservative measures can be used if symptoms are mild and there is only a small amount of overgrowth. Prostheses should be designed to accommodate terminal bony overgrowth, especially if the child is young and the tibia or fibula is involved. This can be accomplished by incorporating a pad within the distal end of the socket that can be modified or replaced. Terminal bony overgrowth can also be managed by using a socket design and/or a donning procedure that maximizes distal soft-tissue coverage and minimizes axial tension between the transected distal end and the distal soft tissue and skin (Figure 10). Socket replacement is another

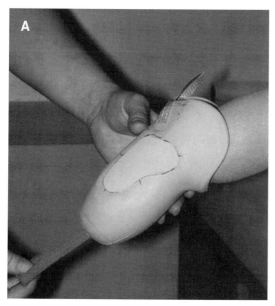

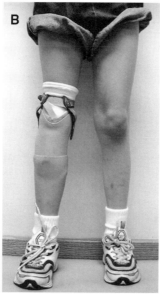

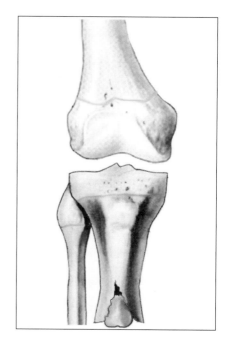

Figure 10 Prosthetic management of terminal bony overgrowth in an 8-year old girl with a transtibial amputation. **A,** A nylon sock is applied over the residual limb, leaving an equal length of sock distal to the limb. The end of the nylon sock is threaded through a hole in the distal end of the liner. Pulling on the end of the sock gradually draws the residual limb into the liner. **B,** After the patient reflects the nylon over the liner, she puts on the socket. This technique maximizes distal soft-tissue coverage and minimizes tension.

Figure 11 Diagram of the modified Marquardt technique for application of a biologic cap (usually an autologous tricortical iliac crest bone graft) to the distal tibia. *(Reproduced with permission from Davids JR, Meyer LC, Blackhurst DW: Operative treatment of bone overgrowth in children who have an acquired or congenital amputation. J Bone Joint Surg Am 1995;77:1490-1497.)*

option if other conservative measures are not successful.

A variety of surgical management strategies have been used to prevent terminal bony overgrowth. The standard treatment has been resection revision, which involves excising bursal and scar tissue and resecting the bony spike through more normal diaphysis or metaphysis (Figure 9, *E*). Although technically simple, this procedure sacrifices residual limb length and is often followed by recurrence of the bony prominence and bursa. Plugging the distal medullary canal with a synthetic and/or biologic device has not been particularly successful and has been associated with short- and long-term complications. Recognizing that overgrowth does not occur in children after disarticulation, Marquardt[36] and Marquardt and Correll[37] proposed placement of a biologic cap to treat overgrowth. For the child at risk for overgrowth, they developed a technique to transfer an autologous cartilage-bone graft, consisting of the distal tibial physis complex (metaph-ysis-physis-epiphysis–articular cartilage) or calcaneal apophysis, at the time of primary amputation. To manage established overgrowth, they recommended using the proximal fibular physis complex or iliac apophysis as a biologic cap. Recently, Davids and associates[34] modified this procedure by substituting a tricortical iliac crest graft as the biologic cap (Figure 11). Direct comparison of these three procedures (resection revision, synthetic capping, and biologic capping) showed that subsequent surgery for recurrent overgrowth was needed in 84% of resection revisions, 78% of synthetic caps, and only 31% of biologic caps.[34]

In a child with terminal bony overgrowth, it is best to wait as long as possible between surgical revisions or, if appropriate, to delay surgery until skeletal maturity. This helps preserve residual limb length and reduces the number of surgical revisions, thus minimizing the amount of "down time" for a child.

Residual Limb Scarring

Because children have greater healing potential and tissue resiliency, children with acquired amputations usually tolerate residual limb scarring from trauma, previous surgery, or skin grafting better than do adult amputees. Scarring alone seldom necessitates surgical revision of the residual limb, but it may require special prosthetic design to disperse weight bearing and diminish shear stress at the stump-socket interface. Congenital residual "nubbins" often negate suction and are sometimes recommended for removal. Deep, fissured scars may complicate or negate fitting with suction sockets. Minor modifications in the prosthetic socket will usually relieve symptomatic pressure that is concentrated over small areas of scarring in relatively non–weight-bearing areas of the residual limb. More extensive prosthetic modifications may be necessary if the scarred area is large or involves weight-bearing areas of the residual limb.

The Phantom Limb Phenomenon

The phantom limb phenomenon occurs frequently in children with acquired amputations. Phantom sensations are often described as the feeling that the absent part is present, can be moved, itches or tingles, and even that its position can be sensed. These are considered normal postamputation phenomena. Unpleasant or painful sensations, however, are often less common in children than in adults. These sensations may be similar to the pain the child had before the amputation and may occur in association with other unpleasant stimuli, such as headaches or bone or joint pain.

Some studies have reported that phantom sensations and pain are frequent, and others report they are rare. They may be triggered by a wide variety of stimuli, such as apprehension, happiness, being cold or ill, or not wearing a prosthesis.[7] The incidence and severity of symptoms depend somewhat on age. These sensations seem to be less frequent and less intense in children who undergo amputation before age 10 years.

Because the occurrence of phantom pain may be influenced by proper prosthetic fit, physical therapy-related activity, and family support, a team approach to evaluation and treatment is important. There is no one successful method to deal with phantom limb pain, just as there is probably no single cause, although the use of epidural catheters perioperatively has been shown to reduce the frequency and intensity of phantom pain.[38] Family and patient education is an important component and should start before the amputation whenever possible.[39]

Although less frequent in children than adults, phantom sensations and particularly phantom pain can be severe enough in children to affect the outcome of treatment and rehabilitation. These phenomena must be taken seriously and addressed early in the child's therapy.

Prosthetic Considerations
The Role of the Prosthetist

The unique needs of a child with an acquired amputation present a challenge to the prosthetist, who must formulate a prescription and treatment approach that will accommodate ongoing and rapid development. First, the prosthetist should know the complete history of the illness or have an account of the accident that led to the amputation. If the amputation is a result of a malignancy, the prosthetist should know whether postoperative treatments such as radiation or chemotherapy will be done and when they are scheduled. This information helps the prosthetist determine when to see the child and take the residual effects of therapy into account. If an amputation is the result of trauma, the mechanism and/or cause of the amputation can be important from a psychological standpoint. All clinic team members should be aware that strong feelings of guilt and anger from both the patient and family may be present and need to be carefully addressed. For example, one family member might blame another for "allowing" the accident to happen, or for not recognizing the illness soon enough. Children may experience guilt, and anger, or depression, yet not have the emotional maturity to express their feelings verbally. They may act out in other ways. Even while prosthetic fitting and rehabilitation are occurring, family dysfunction or deep emotional scars may be developing.

Because of the personalized, interactive nature of their service, prosthetists spend a great deal of time with the patient and family and often have a unique opportunity to listen to their feelings and concerns, observe nonverbal cues, and provide appropriate information and emotional support. The prosthetist may be the first to recognize when factors related to limb loss have stressed a family relationship, or that a patient is struggling with denial, anger, grief, fear, or depression. By being sensitive to such dynamics, the prosthetist can adjust the treatment approach accordingly. Referring the patient and family back to the clinic team for additional emotional support, counseling, or psychological intervention is also important. Amputee peer support groups, if locally available, are often great resources for additional information and the empathy that only another amputee can provide.

Obtaining a thorough social history on the child can help the prosthetist judge how the child will adapt to the challenges the injury poses. The child's support network is important to the success of rehabilitation. Family support and the child's emotional and cognitive status should be considered in developing the child's prosthetic prescription. Because the prosthetist must establish a working relationship with the family to encourage their involvement in the child's rehabilitation, he or she should get to know the family early in the treatment process and establish a sense of trust and reassurance with them and the patient. A family that knows what to expect will be better able to provide the support necessary for successful treatment.

Postoperative radiographs and surgical notes can provide valuable information to the prosthetist, such as the orientation and presence of bony anatomy and the type of procedure performed. An amputation in the case of a malignant musculoskeletal tumor, such as a hemipelvectomy in which the lower pelvic anatomy has been removed and the ipsilateral ilium retained, may require the prosthetist to resourcefully make use of the remaining bony and soft-tissue anatomy. In addition to providing a point of purchase for suspension of the prosthesis, the infrailial region of the remaining pelvis can be used as a load-bearing surface when the ischium is no longer present.

The prosthetist should perform a complete physical examination, including assessing sensation, strength, and range of motion in all joints of the extremities. He or she should also assess the condition of the residual limb, looking for presence of edema, the degree of soft-tissue coverage and firmness, damaged or sensitive skin, size, and length of limb, which are critical to developing the best prosthetic fit. Judging the stability of the major joints is important as well, because a contralateral ankle or knee that is weak or unstable can slow the treatment process. Contractures may be present in cases of severe trauma and should be addressed in a timely fashion with mobilization and physical therapy if possible. For example, an ipsilateral compound femoral fracture in a transtibial amputation can delay weight bearing for a significant amount of time and may lead to a knee flexion contracture.

Education and training are fundamental components of the prosthetic treatment process. At every visit, the prosthetist should teach the child and family how to manage the residual limb, including volume management of the residual limb and stretching. What to expect in recovery, including phantom limb phenomenon and the capabilities of the prosthesis, should be discussed to eliminate false expectations, decrease anxiety, and prevent hostility.

Socket Design and Suspension Systems

Prosthetic socket design takes into account differences in tissue compressibility, pressure tolerance, and the underlying bony structures of the residual limb. Depending on the amputation level, the socket design will use one or more weight-bearing methods (patellar tendon bearing, total surface bearing, ischial/gluteal) to support the residual limb. If the typical load-bearing areas are compromised, the prosthetist must consider alternative or adjunctive solutions.

Improving the skin-socket interface with one of the many available gel liners can help damaged areas tolerate pressure and shear forces. Typically, these liners are made of silicone or urethane and are considered "growth friendly" because they do not provide a rigid grip over the bony prominence. These liners require a certain degree of care, so the child's age, maturity, and family support need to be assessed before the prosthetist decides to use a liner. An accurately fitting socket with a silicone sandwiched sock or a nylon sock is often effective in reducing shear stress and pressure on a badly scarred residual limb.

The prosthetist can use other available tolerant load-bearing areas, such as the thigh, to minimize the adverse effects of the reaction forces placed upon the limb during ambulation. For example, for a child who has undergone a very short transtibial amputation with associated skin damage and loss of soft tissue, adding side joints and a corset to the transtibial socket will help unload the residual limb and protect the knee joint.

Some form of suspension is required to keep the prosthesis in contact with the residual limb, whether it is an integral part of the actual socket, as with supracondylar and suprapatellar supracondylar sockets, or a separate component of the prosthesis. Maximizing the suspension of the prosthesis will help diminish the effects of shear stress at the skin-socket interface. The prosthetist must consider the location and extent of the damaged skin and select a type of suspension that is both available for the particular amputation level and will not compromise the area of damaged skin.

Prosthetic Considerations for Different Levels of Amputation

Transfemoral Amputation

Depending on the child's age, loss of the distal femoral epiphysis can result in a significantly shorter residual limb, even with what may initially appear to be a long transfemoral amputation, by the time the child reaches skeletal maturity. Terminal bony overgrowth is also a possibility because of the natural tendencies of transected immature bones. The same modern transfemoral fitting and alignment practices used for adult sockets apply to pediatric designs.[40] Both quadrilateral and ischial containment socket designs are used in pediatrics, although for very young children, body fat and whether the child wears diapers often dictate the socket shape.

The most commonly used form of suspension for a child with an acquired transfemoral amputation is the Silesian belt or neoprene Silesian-type suspension belt.[40] These belts can be adjusted easily and work well when damaged skin is an issue. Suction suspension, however, is problematic in children younger than age 7 years because of their rapid growth.[41] Children quickly outgrow the intimate fit required for suction suspension, so it is not usually appropriate until later adolescence. As an alternative to suction suspension, silicone suction with a locking mechanism provides an intimate, but growth-adjustable form of suspension.[42] However, this system requires a degree of maturity and compliance on the part of the child, so it is usually not appropriate for children younger than age 10 years.[42] Silicone liners generally provide an excellent environment for compromised skin but may pose problems with scar tissue at the level of the proximal socket brim. In this case, a flexible socket, sock, or gel sock interface or a Silesian belt is a good alternative. Flexible inner sockets also maintain higher trim lines to account for longitudinal growth. They can be modified easily to allow for growth.

Knee Disarticulation

A knee disarticulation is a very functional amputation level in children. It offers the child some prosthetic advantages because it preserves the distal femoral epiphysis; avoids bone overgrowth; provides a load-tolerant distal end and a long, powerful femoral lever arm; allows excellent prosthetic suspension and rotational control; and lowers the metabolic cost of walking.[43] Although knee disarticulation is generally functionally superior to higher-level amputations, it may be somewhat less cosmetic, and the child may have fewer prosthetic knee options. The increasing number of pediatric polycentric knees available, however, has helped to minimize these disadvantages.

A knee disarticulation allows continued growth of that limb, and a longer residual limb is conducive to good prosthetic biomechanics. The length poses problems in selecting a knee mechanism, however. In these cases, a properly timed distal femoral epiphysiodesis will shorten the residual limb enough to allow any available knee mechanism to be chosen. Although this means an additional surgery, when it is planned for at the time of the initial amputation as a stage in therapy, the patient and family generally accept it well. This procedure has proved very beneficial in prosthetic design.

Knee disarticulation socket design for pediatric knee disarticulations is similar to that for adults. The ability and degree of end bearing will dictate the socket design. Tenderness over the distal end of the femur may preclude early end-bearing ambulation, but it should not delay rehabilitation or eliminate the possibility of future end bearing. Socket design can be modified to address this problem by leaving more proximal trim lines that allow ischial and gluteal weight bearing and by using end pads of various durometers or thicknesses. By varying the durometer or thickness of the distal end pad, the child's weight-bearing capabilities can be manipulated proximally and distally. However, the prosthetist must consider the new biomechanical stresses created by changing the weight-bearing location. The axis of rotation of the socket will change near the ischial tuberosity for

ischial bearing and at the end of the socket for end bearing. Therefore, the proper force couples must reflect these changes.[42]

Silesian or neoprene equivalent suspension is generally used for the very young child (< 10 years of age) or as an auxiliary means of suspension and/or rotational control for children with fragile skin or higher activity levels. As the child gets older, however, supracondylar suspension is preferred. The child's physical development and bony definition will dictate when the condyles can be used as a means of suspension and rotational control. The condyles usually become available at about age 3 years, but they can develop at different times and should be assessed on an individual basis.

Transtibial Amputation

Surgeons generally avoid transtibial amputations in children in favor of ankle disarticulations. Terminal bony overgrowth is a common complication of transtibial amputations. In some children, recurrent patellar subluxation dislocation or patella alta may develop, and this may be related to a valgus deformity of the residual limb.[44] However, the situation (eg, level of traumatic injury) sometimes necessitates a transtibial amputation to preserve the obvious benefits of a functional knee.

Although the principles of adult transtibial cast modifications generally apply to the pediatric patient, the smaller size of the child's limb must be considered. Cast modifications recommended in many prosthetic texts are expressed in inches or millimeters rather than as a percentage of overall circumference. Smaller limbs require less aggressive buildups or reliefs, in proportion to the child's smaller anatomy. Cuff suspension is a common means of suspension for the pediatric transtibial prosthesis because it is simple and easy to adjust. Cuff suspension is not a good option, however, for a child who has a very short residual limb, knee instability, or excessive scarring in the area of contact with the

cuff. In these conditions, side joints and a thigh corset with a waist belt may be a safe option because they avoid damaged skin around the knee and assist in load bearing if the load-bearing surfaces are compromised. Self-suspending (supracondylar and suprapatellar supracondylar) options can provide good suspension, but they require frequent adjustments for growth and are successful only when follow-up is regular.[42] Silicone suction with locking-pin or lanyard systems are growth friendly and can provide a good environment for the skin of the residual limb, but they require a certain maturity level on the part of the child.

Syme Ankle Disarticulation

A Syme ankle disarticulation generally offers excellent prosthetic suspension over the malleoli and satisfactory rotational control. It provides distal load bearing (in varying degrees) and a long lever arm and avoids terminal bony overgrowth. The greatest challenges are length, a bulbous distal end, and any angular deformities. Principles of this socket design for pediatric patients are similar to those for adults. Suspension for a Syme disarticulation can be achieved by using the malleoli. The three main socket design options are an inner removable liner, a medial window, and a bladder. A socket design that provides minimal friction during donning, such as a medial window, will reduce the risks of skin breakdown in this area. If skin damage is present over or around the malleoli, gel socks or sock/nylon combinations can minimize the shear forces created during ambulation and donning the prosthesis. Cuff suspension is used when the malleoli are underdeveloped or are intolerant and require additional suspension.

Physical or Occupational Therapy Management

Physical or occupational therapy is an integral component of the rehabilitation of a child with an acquired amputation. The therapist, physician, and prosthetist should be in agreement regarding the patient's treatment.

The primary role of the therapist is to be an educator. The education should involve the entire family and should be incorporated into virtually all aspects of the rehabilitation process. Parents have a great influence on a child's rehabilitation.

The therapist can help the parents prepare for the time when the child begins to interact with peers. Therapists can also educate teachers and classmates about the child's prosthetic function and limb deficiency to lessen the curiosity and inquisitiveness that can be uncomfortable for the patient. Preparing patients ahead of time can also help keep them from viewing going to school as a threatening event. This can be extremely important for the child's acceptance and socialization.

Returning to home and school are important aspects of the child's psychological and psychosocial development. Ideally, treatment programs should be home and community based rather than hospital or office based.[7] The child's condition will be permanent, so adaptation to the environment is important. The child should learn how to perform daily activities (toileting, eating, dressing, playing sports) in his or her normal environment. The child should not regard himself or herself as a medical problem, but rather as someone with a difference to which he or she can successfully adapt. Unnecessary hospital, clinic, or office visits are counterproductive to facilitate this goal of independence.

Edema control, wound healing, scar mobility, desensitization, range of motion, and strengthening as tolerated help prepare the child and the residual limb for prosthetic wear. When the incision has healed, grafts have matured, and residual limb volume has stabilized, the child is generally ready to be fitted with a prosthesis.

Physical therapy for a child with an acquired amputation should center on age-appropriate activities and include goals that are within the limits of the child's condition.[45] As the child grows, the therapist can help to design and modify age-appropriate play activities. With the approach of school age, emphasis switches to independence in activities of daily living, and later, fine motor skills that may be needed for classroom activities. Adaptations for sports are important, as is the advocacy role to allow the children to participate in all possible activities.

References

1. Aitken GT: The child with an acquired amputation. *Inter Clin Info Bull* 1968;7:1-15.

2. Lambert CN: Etiology, in Aitken GT (ed): *The Child With an Acquired Amputation.* Washington, DC, National Academy of Sciences, 1972.

3. Tooms RE: The amputee, in Morrissy RT (ed): *Lovell and Winter's Pediatric Orthopaedics,* ed 3. Philadelphia, PA, JB Lippincott, 1990, pp 1023-1070.

4. Tooms RE: Acquired amputations in children, in Bowker JH, Michael JW (eds): *Atlas of Limb Prosthetics: Surgical, Prosthetic, and Rehabilitation Principles,* ed 2. Rosemont, IL, American Academy of Orthopaedic Surgeons, 2002, pp 735-741. (Originally published by Mosby-Year Book, 1992.)

5. Dormans JP, Azzoni M, Davidson RS, Drummond DS: Major lower extremity lawn mower injuries in children. *J Pediatr Orthop* 1995;15:78-82.

6. Blazar PE, Dormans JP, Born CT: Train injuries in children. *J Orthop Trauma* 1997;11:126-129.

7. Morrissy RT, Giavedoni BJ, Coulter-O'Berry C: The limb-deficient child, in Morrissy RT, Weinstein SL (eds): *Lovell and Winter's Pediatric Orthopaedics,* ed 5. Philadelphia, PA, Lippincott Williams & Wilkins, 2001, pp 1217-1272.

8. Blank JE, Dormans JP, Davidson RS: Perinatal limb ischemia: Orthopaedic implications. *J Pediatr Orthop* 1996;16:90-96.

9. Dormans JP: Management of pediatric mutilating extremity injuries and traumatic amputations, in Herring JA, Birch JG (eds): *The Child With a Limb Deficiency.* Rosemont, IL, American Academy of Orthopaedic Surgeons, 1998, pp 253-265.

10. Aitken GT: Surgical amputation in children. *J Bone Joint Surg North Am* 1963;45:1735-1741

11. Cary JM: Traumatic amputations in childhood-primary management. *Inter Clin Info Bull* 1975;14:1-10

12. Aitken GT: The child amputee: An overview. *Orthop Clin North Am* 1972;3:447-472.

13. Dunn NL, McCartan KW, Fuqua RW: Young children with orthopaedic handicaps: Self-knowledge about their disability. *Except Child* 1988;55:249-252.

14. Alexander RH, Proctor HJ (eds): *Advanced Trauma Life Support Program for Physicians: ATLS,* ed 5. Chicago, IL, American College of Surgeons, 1993, pp 261-281.

15. Gupta A, Wolff TW: Management of the mangled hand and forearm. *J Am Acad Orthop Surg* 1995;3:226-236.

16. Breidenbach WC III: Emergency free tissue transfer for reconstruction of acute upper extremity wounds. *Clin Plast Surg* 1989;16:505-514.

17. Pozo JL, Powell B, Andrews BG, Hutton PA, Clarke J: The timing of amputation for lower limb trauma. *J Bone Joint Surg Br* 1990;72:288-292

18. Poole GV, Agnew SG, Griswold JA, Rhodes RS: The mangled lower extremity: Can salvage be predicted? *Am Surg* 1994;60:50-55.

19. Hansen ST Jr: Editorial: The type-IIIC tibial fracture: Salvage or amputation? *J Bone Joint Surg Am* 1987;69:799-800

20. Dormans JP: Limb-salvage surgery versus amputation for children with extremity sarcomas, in Herring JA, Birch JG (eds): *The Child With a Limb Deficiency.* Rosemont, IL, American Academy of Orthopaedic Surgeons, 1998, pp 289-303.

21. Rodriguez RP: Amputation surgery and prostheses. *Orthop Clin North Am* 1996;27:525-539.

22. Gedde-Dahl TW, Bjark P, Hoiby EA, Host JH, Bruun JN: Severity of meningococcal disease: Assessment by factors and scores and implications for patient management. *Rev Infect Dis* 1990;12:973-992.

23. Kirsch EA, Barton RP, Kitchen L, Giroir BP:: Pathophysiology, treatment and outcome of meningococcemia: A review and recent experience. *Pediatr Infect Dis J* 1996;15:967-978.

24. Powars D, Larsen R, Johnson J, et al: Epidemic meningococcemia and purpura fulminans with induced protein C deficiency. *Clin Infect Dis* 1993;17:254-261.

25. Herrera R, Hobar PC, Ginsburg CM: Surgical intervention for the complications of meningococcal-induced purpura fulminans. *Pediatr Infect Dis J* 1994;13:734-737.

26. Adams WP Jr, Hobar PC: Surgical treatment of meningococcal-induced purpura fulminans, in Herring JA, Birch JG (eds): *The Child With a Limb Deficiency.* Rosemont, IL, American Academy of Orthopaedic Surgeons, 1998, pp 447-454.

27. McCarron JA, Johnston DR, Hanna BG, et al: Evaluation and treatment of musculoskeletal vascular anomalies in children: An update and summary for orthopaedic surgeons. *Univ Pennsyl Ortho J* 2001;14:15.

28. Mackenzie WG, Gabos PG: Localized disorders of bone and soft tissue, in Morrissy RT, Weinstein SL (eds): *Lovell and Winter's Pediatric Orthopaedics,* ed 5. Philadelphia, PA, Lippincott Williams & Wilkins, 2001, pp 339-377.

29. Gates PE, Drvaric DM, Kruger L: Wound healing in orthopaedic procedures for Klippel-Trenaunay syndrome. *J Pediatr Orthop* 1996;16:723-726.

30. Aitken GT: Overgrowth of the amputation stump. *Inter Clin Info Bull* 1962;1:1-8.

31. Jorring K: Amputation in children: A follow-up of 74 children whose lower extremities were amputated. *Acta Orthop Scand* 1971;42:178-186.

32. Pellicore RJ, Lambert CN, Hamilton RC: Incidence of bone overgrowth in the juvenile amputee population. *Inter-Clin Info Bull* 1974;8:1-8.

33. O'Neal ML, Bahner R, Ganey TM, Ogden JA: Osseous overgrowth after amputation in adolescents and children. *J Pediatr Orthop* 1996;16:78-84.

34. Davids JR, Meyer LC, Blackhurst DW: Operative treatment of bone overgrowth in children who have an acquired or congenital amputation. *J Bone Joint Surg Am* 1995;77:1490-1497.

35. Speer DP: The pathogenesis of amputation stump overgrowth. *Clin Orthop* 1981;159:294-307.

36. Marquardt E: The multiple-limb-deficient child, in Bowker JH, Michael JW (eds): *Atlas of Limb Prosthetics: Surgical, Prosthetic, and Rehabilitation Principles,* ed 2. Rosemont, IL, American Academy of Orthopaedic Surgeons, 2002, pp 839-884. (Originally published by Mosby-Year Book, 1992.)

37. Marquardt E, Correll J: Amputations and prostheses for the lower limbs. *Int Orthop* 1984;8:139-146.

38. Danshaw CB: An anesthetic approach to amputation and pain syndromes. *Phys Med Rehabil Clin N Am* 2000;11:553-557.

39. Finnoff J: Differentiation and treatment of phantom sensation, phantom pain, and residual-limb pain. *J Am Podiatr-Med-Assoc* 2001;91:23-33.

40. Schuch CM: Modern above-knee fitting practice: A report on the ISPO Workshop on Above-Knee Fitting and Alignment Techniques May 15-19, 1987, Miami, FL. *Prosthet Orthot Int* 1988;12:77-90.

41. Thompson GH, Leimkuehler JP: Prosthetic management, in Kalamchi A (ed): *Congenital Lower Limb Deficiencies.* New York, NY, Springer-Verlag, 1989, pp 211-235.

42. Cummings DR: Prosthetic considerations for the child with a limb deficiency (lower extremity), in Herring JA, Birch JG (eds): *The Child With a Limb Deficiency.* Rosemont, IL, American Academy of Orthopaedic Surgeons, 1998, pp 307-317.

43. Pinzur MS: Knee disarticulation: Surgical procedures, in Bowker JH, Michael JW (eds): *Atlas of Limb Prosthetics: Surgical, Prosthetic, and Rehabilitation Principles,* ed 2. Rosemont, IL, American Academy of Orthopaedic Surgeons, 2002, pp 479-486. (Originally published by Mosby-Year Book, 1992.)

44. Mowery CA, Herring JA, Jackson D: Dislocated patella associated with below-knee amputation in adolescent patients. *J Pediatr Orthop* 1986;6:299-301.

45. Coulter-O'Berry C: Physical therapy management in children with lower extremity limb deficiencies, in Herring JA, Birch JG (eds): *The Child With a Limb Deficiency.* Rosemont, IL, American Academy of Orthopaedic Surgeons, 1998, pp 319-330.

Chapter 69

Hand Deficiencies

Terry R. Light, MD

Introduction

The birth of a child with an upper limb deficiency elicits a myriad of confusing parental emotions. Medical professionals should address parental concerns and expectations in an optimistic, compassionate, honest, and forthright manner. Parents may grieve that their infant is not the perfect child that they had anticipated through the course of the pregnancy. Some will voice anger that prenatal evaluations did not detect their child's abnormality. Many parents feel an intense need to "do something," either surgical or prosthetic, to make their child "normal" and whole. Conflicting advice from well-meaning friends and relatives may contribute to parental stress. When the child's condition is potentially hereditary, conflicts between the father's and mother's families may be heightened.

Some parents initially seek a cosmetic prosthesis to conceal their child's abnormality without regard to the functional impact of the prosthesis. The lack of success when a purely aesthetic prosthesis covers the sensate skin of an anomalous hand should be openly discussed. Although an aesthetic upper limb prosthesis may facilitate rehabilitation in the traumatic amputee, it is usually a hindrance to the congenital amputee possessing a mobile hand and wrist, even when fingers are absent. Aesthetic prostheses may become a source of conflict between parent and child if the child

regards the prosthesis as a hindrance to function. The child may feel that the prosthesis is to be worn merely to please parents who are embarrassed by his or her appearance.

If an active prosthesis is to be successfully integrated into the child's life, it must help the child either accomplish otherwise impossible activities or perform meaningful activities with greater facility.

Upper Limb Kinesiology

The hand allows children to explore their environment and to manipulate objects within that environment. The hand should be able to maneuver in space under volitional control and should be able to reach the body and the area in front of the body. Using both visual and tactile clues, a child must be able to aim the hand so that it can precisely approach an object. The object is then grasped by the closing fingers and adducting the thumb. The hand must also be capable of releasing the object from its grasp.

The two major types of grasp are precision prehension and power prehension.[1] Precision prehension is used to hold relatively small objects with modest force, whereas power prehension is used to hold larger objects, often with greater force. In pre-

cision prehension, the object is secured between the distal phalanx of the thumb and the index finger or within the thumb, index, and middle fingers. The fingers are usually extended at the interphalangeal (IP) joints, and the metacarpophalangeal (MCP) joints are partially flexed. The object itself usually does not contact the palm.

The three most common forms of precision grasp or pinch are palmar pinch, lateral pinch, and tip pinch. With palmar pinch, the flat palmar pads of the thumb and fingers secure opposite sides of the object being grasped. With lateral pinch, the palmar surface of the thumb's distal phalanx is brought against the radial border of the index finger. Because this posture is often used to grasp and twist a key, this pattern is also known as key pinch. Tip pinch provides contact with the distal end of the distal phalanx of the thumb with the distal phalanx of the index or of the index and middle fingers. Tip pinch is used to pick up small objects such as a pin or a dime from a tabletop.

Power prehension involves the ulnar digits (most often the ring and little fingers), whereas the radial digits (the index and middle fingers) are used primarily in precision prehension. Power grasp usually results in contact of the object against three surfaces: (1) the palmar aspects of the flexing fingers, (2) the palm of the hand, and (3) the thumb metacarpal or proximal phalanx. Although the distal phalanx of the thumb may wrap around the object, most thumb power is contributed by the stabilizing effect of the adductor pollicis, which buttresses the pressure transmitted from the fingers through the object.

The hand also plays an important role in nonprehensile activities. These activities usually involve the transmission of force through the terminal portion of the limb to another object. Nonprehensile activities include keyboarding or button pushing, pushing open a swinging door, throwing a punch, or striking a karate blow.

The hand may also be used to cradle or hold objects against the chest or to support objects such as a tray. Congenitally anomalous hands without prehensile capability are often used with great dexterity to perform these nonprehensile functions.

Other Considerations

As infants begin to explore their environment, they learn to use their unique physical capabilities to the best advantage. The young child's goal is to reach the cookie, grasp it, and bring it to his or her mouth. If this is most easily accomplished by one hand, the closest or most efficient hand will be used. If the object is large or if single-hand prehension is impossible, then both hands will be used together or the child will secure the object against the chest. When upper limb prehension is severely compromised, a child may become facile using foot prehension.

The child's growing awareness of his or her abnormality is usually the result of comments from playmates, siblings, or well-meaning adults. The child usually does not become self-conscious until about the age of 6 or 7 years. Peer pressure may cause the child with a unilateral abnormality to conceal the hand in a pocket or to reject an otherwise successful prosthesis.

Other points of psychological stress occur during adolescence when concerns arise over attractiveness. Feelings may be further complicated by impending marriage and the prospect of offspring with similar abnormalities. Access to knowledgeable genetic counseling is essential, particularly at that time.

Aesthetic considerations are important when weighing therapeutic alternatives in the management of congenital hand abnormalities. The hand and face are the unclothed areas of skin most often exposed to scrutiny. When anomalous parts have an abnormal appearance and do not contribute to function, they may be removed. In the perception of many, conversion of a malformed part to an amputation may result in an aesthetic improvement.

On occasion, the removal of a functionless part may facilitate prosthetic fitting. Approximately half of lower limb congenital amputees require surgical revision before prosthetic fitting, whereas only about 10% of congenital anomalous upper limbs fit for prostheses require surgical revision.[2] Consultation between the surgeon and prosthetist helps the surgeon to understand which anomalies will obstruct prosthetic donning and wear. Portions of the affected limb that are useful for prehension without a prosthesis should never be amputated. A prosthesis can be fit around a short phocomelic limb to allow the child to maintain functional capabilities without the prosthesis.

Clinical Presentation

Although congenital upper limb abnormalities are increasingly diagnosed by prenatal ultrasound, they typically are first diagnosed at birth. Parents often have a deep need to understand the nature of their child's abnormality and the potential treatments available. Early consultation with experienced physicians and therapists is helpful for most families.

Morphology

Conditions in which body parts are absent are referred to as failures of formation of parts. In most cases, the anatomic border between normal tissue and absent elements is indistinct and gradual; a blend of dysplastic and hypoplastic tissue typically forms a transition zone that may extend the entire length of the limb. The one condition in which there may be an abrupt transition, a result of highly localized intrauterine trauma to the growing limb, is early amniotic rupture sequence, which was previously termed congenital constriction band syndrome or amniotic bands (Figure 1). In these limbs, the anatomy proximal to the area of abnormality is usually perfectly normal.

Anomalies that extend the entire length of the limb are termed longitudinal deficiencies. When the preaxial border of the limb is involved, the condition is termed radial deficiency, and when the postaxial border of the limb is involved the condition is referred to as ulnar deficiency. These conditions are discussed in detail in chapters 70 and 71. Absence or hypoplasia of the thumb is often a component of radial deficiency. In some cases, thumb absence may be a component of ulnar deficiency.

Conditions in which the absence is most intense in the distal portion of the limb are usually referred to as terminal deficiencies (Figure 2). The entire limb, including the chest, must be evaluated to fully understand these abnormalities. Distal anomalies involving the hand, such as syndactyly, may be associated with chest abnormalities in children with Poland sequence.

Symbrachydactyly

The most common forms of terminal limb deficiency are related to the symbrachydactyly sequence of abnormalities.[3-5] The term symbrachydactyly literally refers to a hand with syndactylization of short fingers. The use of the expression symbrachydactyly sequence is confusing initially because many of the children grouped into this malformation sequence have neither syndactyly nor fingers. Symbrachydactyly represents the prototypic form for this group of terminal failure of formation abnormalities.

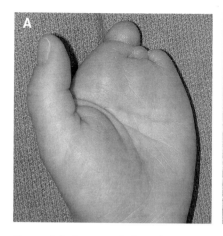

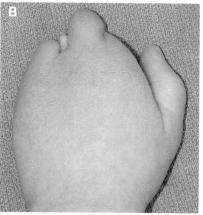

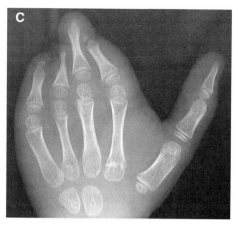

Figure 1 Early congenital amniotic rupture sequence with amputation and syndactylization of the index, middle, ring, and little fingers. **A,** Palmar view demonstrates interdigital sinuses. **B,** Dorsal view. **C,** AP radiograph shows tapering of the distal end of the proximal phalanx of the ring finger.

Many symbrachydactylous limbs have primitive digits, often termed nubbins. These bud-like, incompletely formed digits often include small finger nails. In many instances, digital flexor and extensor tendons insert into the nubbin, enabling children to pucker or withdraw the tip of the digit proximally into the residual limb. Manifestations may be as mild as slightly shortened middle phalanges or as severe as a very short forearm segment with digital nubbins protruding from its distal end (Figure 3). Children with intermediate forms may have only a thumb or only a thumb and little finger with small nubbins representing the undeveloped fingers. Mild hypoplasia of the ipsilateral humerus is common, as is dysplasia or hypoplasia of the forearm. When multiple digits are involved, the central three digits are usually the most profoundly affected. The symbrachydactyly sequence abnormalities are usually unilateral and nonhereditary. The left upper limb is involved more often than the right upper limb. Boys are more frequently affected than girls.

Imaging Studies

Radiographs of the entire upper limb should be obtained. Comparison views of the opposite hand may be useful in predicting the ultimate size of the affected part because its size in proportion to the unaffected side will

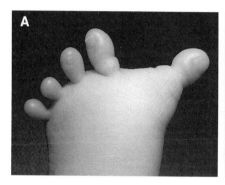

Figure 2 Terminal transverse deficiency characterized by persistent digital nubbins without bony phalangeal elements. **A,** Dorsal view. **B,** Palmar view.

likely not change even as the child grows. Radiographs of young children may underestimate the extent of bone formation, particularly in thin syndactylized fingers. Portions of the anomalous fingers and carpus often include unossified cartilage.

Classification

Digital absence may be simply described as thumb absence, index finger absence, middle finger absence, ring finger absence, or little finger absence. In many cases of terminal limb deficiency, the deficiency involves only part of the digit. The phalangeal elements may be absent, but the corresponding metacarpal is present. The extent of dysplasia in each ray should be assessed. A brief description of the more common forms of this condition is presented in Table 1.

Associated Findings

Poland sequence is the ipsilateral finding of symbrachydactyly and chest abnormality.[3-11] Interestingly, the proximal chest abnormality is more common with the milder, more distal forms of symbrachydactyly than with more profound limb abnormalities. The most frequently associated chest abnormality is absence of the sternocostal head of the pectoralis major muscle. More profound chest abnormalities include total absence of the pectoralis major muscle and rib abnormalities. Asymmetric nipple location may occasionally be seen. As girls mature, ipsilateral breast hypoplasia may be evident.

Functional Deficits

The functional deficits in children with symbrachydactyly are a direct

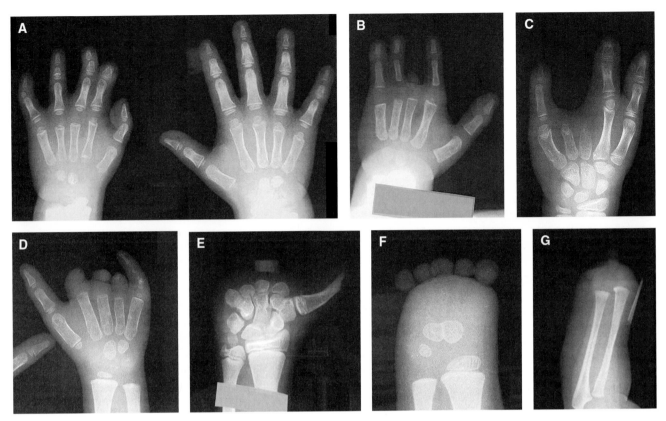

Figure 3 Unilateral symbrachydactyly may demonstrate variable morphology. **A,** Five-digit–type hand with biphalangeal thumb and biphalangeal fingers (left) is smaller than the opposite, normal hand. **B,** Four-digit–type hand with four biphalangeal digits and one digital nubbin. **C,** Three-digit–type hand includes a narrowed syndactylized web between the biphalangeal thumb and biphalangeal ring finger. **D,** Two-digit–type hand shows limited ossification of distal phalanx within the nubbin index, middle, and ring fingers. **E,** Monodigital-type hand consists of a widely abducted thumb metacarpal. **F,** Carpal-type hand with five soft-tissue nubbins. **G,** Wrist disarticulation-type hand with a single digital nubbin.

consequence of the degree of involvement as detailed in Table 1. In the more distal forms, prehension with digital independence is possible. Individual digital function may be compromised by syndactyly, IP joint instability, or angulation.

The absence of central digits may compromise hand dexterity and limit the child's ability to play certain musical instruments. Stable grasp and manipulative ability are diminished in a hand that has only two or three fingers. A two-digit hand is capable of prehension if the two digits can actively touch one another. Prehension requires that at least one of the digits is mobile and actively controlled. Hands with only a single digit are capable of nonprehensile activity such as pushing buttons or striking a letter on a keyboard.

Adactylous hands with wrist motion are used to cradle objects against the trunk and to hold objects in place for manipulation by the unaffected hand. The adactylous hand can hold a piece of paper in place while the other hand holds the pen or pencil to draw or write on the paper.

Differential Diagnosis

A hand that possesses only the thumb and little finger has, in the past, been referred to as an atypical cleft hand.[12,13] It is important to recognize, however, that these two-digit hands are unrelated to cleft hand, an autosomal dominant condition often with bilateral hand and foot involvement.

Surgical Treatment

Because symbrachydactyly is almost always unilateral, most affected children are remarkably facile at per-

forming activities of daily living. The extent of involvement determines the extent of function in the affected limb. Involved digits may be short and unstable. In some cases, an empty digital skin sleeve or nubbin is evident. Release of syndactyly between fingers with local skin flaps and full-thickness skin grafts increases digital independence.

Nonprehensile activities, such as typing, may be improved by the stabilization of unstable IP joints by capsulodesis, chondrodesis, or arthrodesis (Figure 4). Angulation of digits, usually the result of a trapezoidal middle phalanx, may be treated by simple closing wedge osteotomy.

When a soft-tissue digital sleeve is redundant and devoid of skeletal elements, puckering of the tip will demonstrate the insertion of extrinsic flexor and extensor tendons. In such digits, it is often possible to reconstruct a short, mobile digit by a simple nonvascularized proximal phalanx transfer from the foot to the hand (Figure 5).

The monodactylous hand consisting of only a mobile, actively motored thumb is capable of nonprehensile activities such as stabilizing a shoelace but incapable of either power or precision grasp. Construction of an ulnar-sided buttressing digit by distraction lengthening, toe-phalanx transfer, or free toe transfer may allow the hand to achieve meaningful prehension. A prosthesis that provides a passive ulnar-sided buttress may also make prehension possible.

When a mobile carpus is devoid of fingers, the microvascular transfer of both second toes has been suggested.[14] Even though this procedure is technically possible, the results are often disappointing because of the limited mobility of the transferred digits, making meaningful prehension unpredictable after a technically demanding intervention. Alternatively, Vilkki[15] and Foucher[16] suggested placing a single microvascular toe transfer on the distal radius in a position in which the mobile carpal segment can flex and extend in relation to the transferred toe. This unconventional digital position creates a more predictable prehension.

Syndactyly
Clinical Presentation and Classification

Syndactyly is the physical joining or tethering of fingers or toes. When syndactylization extends the entire length of a digit, the condition is termed complete syndactyly. When the web involves only part of the length of the digit, it is termed an incomplete syndactyly. When skeletal and nail elements of the syndactylized digits are separate, the syndactyly is said to be simple. When digital skeletal and/or nail elements are fused, the syndactyly is termed complex (Figure 6). Acrosyndactyly refers to syndactyly in which the ends of the fingers are joined, often as a result of early amniotic rupture sequence (formerly termed congenital constriction band syndrome). Syndactyly of the digits containing angulated phalanges is termed complicated syndactyly.[17]

Surgical Treatment

Surgical release of syndactylized digits will enhance digital independence, an important element of keyboarding. Even short digits consisting of only a proximal phalanx may benefit from separation. Index finger radial abduction may be increased and pinch improved when a short index finger is released from the middle finger. Syndactyly release must provide skin coverage of the adjacent lateral surfaces of the released digits and also create a proper web space floor. Because the surface area of two syndactylized digits is far less than the skin surface area of two separated digits, a full-thickness skin graft is necessary to supplement local flaps.

Many skin flap techniques have been advocated for the separation of syndactylized digits.[18-24] Successful surgical procedures cover the surface of both digits with durable skin, create an appropriate web space floor, and accommodate growth of the digit without secondary contracture (Figure 7). Effective techniques use skin flap tissue to create a sloping web space floor of true anatomic proportions, both in width and depth. This flap tissue may be derived either from

TABLE 1 Classification of Common Types of Digital Absence

Type of Hand	Characteristics
Symbrachydactyly	
Five digits with biphalangeal thumb	All fingers triphalangeal Incomplete simple syndactyly of the index, middle, and ring fingers
Five digits with biphalangeal thumb	Biphalangeal index, middle, and ring fingers Triphalangeal little finger Incomplete simple syndactyly of the index, middle, and ring fingers
Five digits with biphalangeal thumb	Monophalangeal index, middle, and ring fingers Biphalangeal little finger
Three digits with biphalangeal thumb	Nubbin index and middle fingers Monophalangeal ring finger Biphalangeal little finger
Two digits with monophalangeal thumb	Nubbin index, middle, and ring fingers Monophalangeal little finger
Monodigital with monophalangeal thumb	Nubbin index, middle, ring, and little fingers
Aphalangeal	
Adactylous with five metacarpals	Five nubbins
Adactylous with two metacarpals	Thumb metacarpal Little finger metacarpal Digital nubbins
Carpal	Digital nubbins No metacarpals or phalanges Mobile carpus
Wrist disarticulation level	Digital nubbins No wrist motion No carpal, metacarpal, or phalangeal elements
Short below-elbow level	Extremely short forearm Digital nubbins

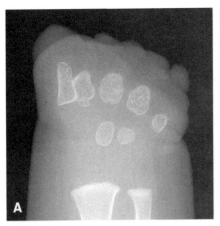
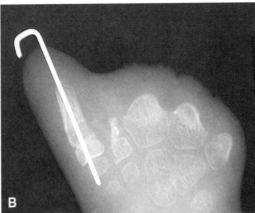
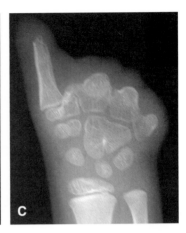

Figure 4 A, Adactylous hand with five small metacarpal elements has limited thumb metacarpal motion. **B,** Transverse osteotomy of the thumb metaphysis allowed insertion of intercalated bone graft from the adjacent index metacarpal. **C,** Additional length allowed improved monodigital function.

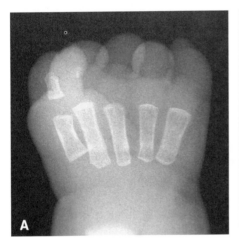
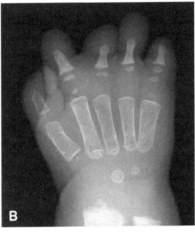

Figure 5 A, Monodactylous hand with monophalangeal thumb has empty finger skin sleeves. **B,** Nonvascularized toe phalangeal grafts from the third and fourth toe proximal phalanges enhance digital stability, length, and dexterity.

the dorsum of the hand, from the palmar aspect of the hand, or from a combination of both palmar and dorsal tissue. Dorsal flaps provide the best skin color match when the web space is viewed from the dorsum but may result in a hypertrophic scar across the interdigital commissure. A palmar flap provides a better commissure contour but results in the shifting of pink palmar skin into the web space. Because the web space is usually viewed from the dorsum, the difference in color is particularly noticeable in dark-skinned individuals.

The web space floor normally begins just distal to the MCP joint and slopes to the edge of the palmar com-

missure approximately one third the length of the proximal phalangeal segment. The web palmar commissure is supple enough to allow interdigital abduction of up to 45°.

Skin incisions on the palmar and dorsal surfaces of the syndactylized digits should be planned to avoid longitudinal scars crossing digital flexion creases because these scars tend to contract with growth. Zigzag incisions may be planned to interdigitate skin flaps to either achieve full closure of one digit or partial closure of two adjacent digits. Skin grafts are sutured in place. Interdigital dressings are maintained until all wounds have healed.

When multiple digits are syndactylized, surgeries should be staged to avoid releasing both sides of a digit during a single operation.

Early Amniotic Rupture Sequence
Clinical Presentation

Early amniotic rupture sequence, formerly referred to as congenital constriction band syndrome, amniotic bands, or annular bands, is a condition often characterized by upper and lower limb involvement and in some cases facial involvement.[25-27] Manifestations may include areas of ring-like narrowing of a digit or limb, amputation of the part distal to an encircling area of band formation, acrosyndactyly, and enlargement of the segment distal to the area of constriction. Because this condition represents an intrauterine injury that disrupts normal limb formation, the level of amputation is often through the diaphysis of a phalanx.

Surgical Treatment

Areas of band indentation may be effectively treated by excision of indented skin and constricting underlying fascia. A layered closure combined with local rotation flaps will improve contour of the limb or digit. When deep bands compress underlying nerves, compromising distal neurovascular function, decompression and nerve grafting may be helpful. Acrosyndactyly may be addressed using traditional syndactyly release techniques. If an interdigital sinus is present, it should be excised at the time of syndactyly release.

Complications

Because the level of amputation through the forearm or phalangeal bones often passes through the bone's diaphysis, bony overgrowth frequently occurs. Diaphyseal bony overgrowth results in tapered ends of fingers. The most distal bone grows faster than the soft-tissue coverage, resulting in tender, poorly padded finger tips or recurrent problems with prosthesis fit. Revision of the ends of these digits or limb ends should be generous to minimize the likelihood of recurrent overgrowth.

Polydactyly
Clinical Presentation

Polydactyly takes many forms. In black children, postaxial (ulnar) polydactyly is the most common form, whereas in white children, preaxial (radial) polydactyly is more frequent. Central polydactyly is less common than either preaxial or postaxial polydactyly.[28] Polydactylous digits are rarely supernumerary, that is, they rarely represent parts additional to a normal hand.[22] Most often, polydactylous digits are structurally abnormal.[29] The challenge of surgery is not

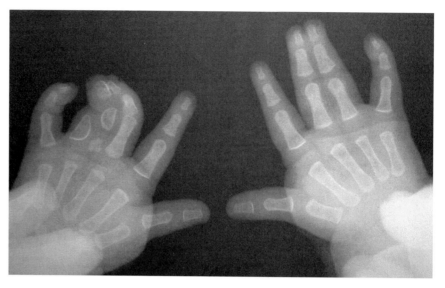

Figure 6 Syndactyly of both hands. On the left, a complete, complex central synpolydactyly is found, whereas the right hand demonstrates a complete simple syndactyly.

simply to remove sufficient tissue but rather to retain tissue sufficient to optimally reconstruct the retained digits.[30-33]

Surgical Treatment

Simply amputating one of the duplicate digits may result in an inadequate residual digit that is smaller than its counterpart on the opposite side. This effect can be decreased by soft-tissue coaptation (Figure 8). Incisions are planned to facilitate the coapting of soft tissues from both digits to provide optimal soft-tissue bulk. Angular deformity in either phalanx or metacarpal should be corrected by osteotomy. Surgical reconstruction aims to achieve a digit in

which the carpometacarpal, MCP, and IP joints are parallel. The longitudinal axis of the metacarpals and phalanges should be perpendicular to the three joints. Correction of angulation is usually achieved by a closing wedge osteotomy and secured by Kirschner wires. An opening wedge osteotomy using a segment of excised bone as intercalated graft is occasionally indicated.

Classification

Preaxial polydactyly takes many forms. Wassel[34] classified these abnormalities into seven categories, six of which involve biphalangeal thumbs (Figure 9). Type I deformities may present as simply a wide distal pha-

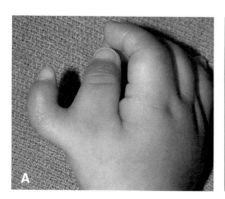
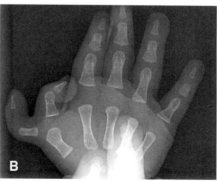
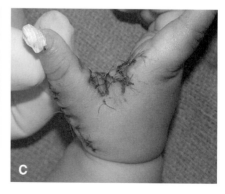

Figure 7 Thumb polydactyly consists of two biphalangeal digits and a narrow first web space. **A,** Clinical photograph. **B,** Radiograph. **C,** Reconstruction includes removal of skeletal elements of radial digit, reconstruction of the collateral ligament of the MCP joint and first web space release and Z-plasty.

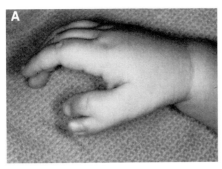

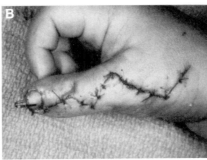

Figure 8 A, Wassel type IV thumb duplication preoperatively demonstrated angulation of the larger ulnar thumb MCP and IP joint levels. **B,** Surgical reconstruction of the thumb included a soft-tissue coaptation flap from the excised radial digit, a closing wedge osteotomy of the thumb metacarpal, and an opening wedge osteotomy of the proximal phalanx to achieve appropriate longitudinal alignment of the digit. The radial collateral ligament of the MCP joint was reconstructed and the abductor pollicis brevis muscle reinserted in the retained digit.

lanx and nail, in which case no treatment is indicated. If two nails are present, two treatment alternatives may be considered: (1) excision of one nail with the underlying bone or (2) central resection of adjacent nail borders and underlying bone, combined with longitudinal phalangeal osteotomies, to narrow the distal phalanx. The latter technique, known as the Bilhout-Cloquet procedure, requires care in nail matrix repair, articular surface alignment, and physeal alignment to avoid creating a stiff IP joint with a longitudinal nail ridge. Osteotomies should be performed distal to the physis to avoid growth disturbance.

Type II duplications consist of two undersized (compared to normal) distal phalanges seated atop a somewhat widened proximal phalangeal

distal articular surface. The more radial digital element has a collateral ligament along its radial border, whereas the ulnar digit has a collateral ligament along its ulnar border. The two digits abut with adjacent articular facets and are bound by pericapsular tissue. In most instances, it is preferable to excise the more radial digit because it is usually less well developed. The broad distal articular surface of the proximal phalanx may need to be tapered to a size appropriate to the distal phalanx. The collateral ligament that initially secured the radial aspect of the deleted radial digit must be retained to securely stabilize the radial aspect of the new IP joint. Retained flexor and extensor tendons must be examined to ensure that the course and insertion of residual tendons are centered.

Type III abnormalities are usually treated by deleting the radial digit. Type IV abnormalities usually require deletion of the radial digit, narrowing of the metacarpal head, and reconstruction of the collateral ligament. The intrinsic muscles that originally inserted into the more radial thumb are reinserted into the hood of the residual ulnar thumb component. Type V abnormalities usually require deletion of the more radial digit and reinsertion of the intrinsic muscle insertion into the residual ulnar digit. Type VI abnormalities may require shifting of the more distal portion of the radial digit onto the more proximal portion of the ulnar digit.

Central polydactyly often presents in combination with syndactyly.[28] Frequently an anomalous central digit lacks normal metacarpal development and is bound to the middle or ring finger. In these patients, the skeletal elements of the unsupported digit are excised, and skin flaps are designed to preserve or reconstruct normal web space contour and digital bulk. When formal ray resection is required, web space-preserving incisions should be used.

Postaxial polydactyly of the digit joined only by soft tissue may be treated by simple excision. When the most ulnar digit articulates with the metacarpal head in a fashion similar to that in the Wassel type IV thumb duplication, simple digital excision will result in an inadequate residual digit. It may be necessary to narrow the metacarpal head, but it should be

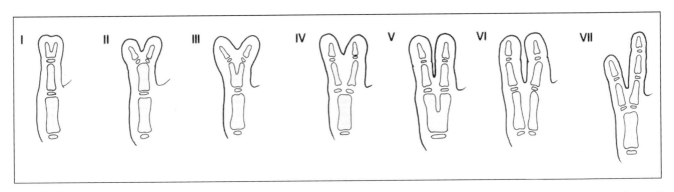

Figure 9 Wassel's original classification scheme for thumb polydactyly has been modified to demonstrate the most common form of thumb polydactyly (type IV), in which two proximal phalanges each possess separate secondary ossification centers.

recognized that the metacarpal head of the little finger, unlike that of the thumb, contains a physis and that care must be taken to preserve physeal growth. If the hypothenar musculature inserts into the more ulnar little finger, its insertion must be detached from the skeletal elements being resected and reinserted into the retained radial little finger. Similarly, the ulnar collateral ligament of the deleted digit must be retained and reconstructed to stabilize the ulnar aspect of the residual little finger MCP joint.

Ulnar dimelia (mirror hand) is an unusual abnormality characterized by duplication of the postaxial border of the hand with seven or eight fingers.[35] Neither the thumb nor the radius is present. Surgery on the preaxial proximal ulna is useful in expanding the arc of elbow flexion and extension but does not provide forearm rotation. Because there is an overabundance of flexor musculature and relative paucity of extensor musculature, release of the wrist flexion contracture may be necessary. Deletion of two or three digits with pollicization of one of the digits along the preaxial border will improve the aesthetic appearance of the hand and modestly improve function.[36]

Wrist Disarticulation

The Krukenberg procedure has been suggested as a reconstructive alternative for children with congenital absence of the hand, particularly in those with profound contralateral abnormalities, associated blindness, or a lack of access to prosthetic care.[37,38] The distal radius and ulna are surgically separated by division of the interosseous membrane and resurfacing the radial aspect of the ulna and the ulnar aspect of the radius. This creates a prehensile limb that will also allow prosthetic fitting. Because the cosmetic disadvantage of this procedure is substantial, it is rarely appropriate in patients with unilateral absence. This procedure is discussed in detail in chapter 17.

Short Transradial Amputation

This common level of terminal deficiency is effectively treated with prosthetic management. Surgical reconstruction is rarely necessary, even though Seitz[39] reported distraction lengthening of a very short ulna to facilitate suspension of a conventional myoelectric prosthesis. Initial prosthetic management begins with a passive hand. The sophistication of the prosthesis can be increased as the child matures.

Timing of Management

Surgical reconstruction of an anomalous hand can usually begin when an infant is between 6 and 12 months of age. In infants younger than 18 months, it is possible to operate on both hands during the same surgical anesthetic to minimize the number of anesthesia exposures. Children older than 18 months often are usually frustrated by the temporary postoperative immobilization of both hands.

Some procedures such as nonvascularized toe-phalanx transfer must be performed early for optimal revascularization and subsequent growth.[4,40] Children undergoing digit-shifting procedures such as pollicization or cleft hand reconstruction may benefit from early integration of the shifted digit into evolving patterns of grasp.

Systemic consideration may cause surgery to be delayed until children are older. For example, children with thrombocytopenia with absent radius (TAR) syndrome have low platelet counts at birth, but these usually gradually increase with age. Surgical reconstruction usually should be delayed until the child's platelet count is at least 60,000/mm^3. Centralization of the wrist, which is typically done within the first year of life, may sometimes be delayed in these children until 3 or 4 years of age.

Decisions regarding the reconstruction or deletion of digits or digital nubbins are best made when children are young. It is inappropriate to place the burden for deciding whether a digit is to be deleted on an adolescent. Parents should not be encouraged to allow children to "decide for themselves when they are older" because this serious decision places inappropriate pressure on adolescents.

References

1. Light TR: Kinesiology of the upper limb, in *Atlas of Orthotics*. St. Louis, MO, Mosby-Year Book, 1985.

2. Aitken GT, Pellicore RJ: Introduction to the child amputee, in *Atlas of Limb Prosthetics*. St. Louis, MO, Mosby-Year Book, 1981.

3. Blauth W, Gekeler J: Symbrachydaktylien: Beitrag zur Morphologie, Klassifikation und Therapie. *Handchirurgie* 1973;5:121-174.

4. Buck-Gramcko D: The role of nonvascularized toe phalanx transplantation. *Hand Clin* 1990;6:643-659.

5. de Smet L, Fabry G: Characteristics of patients with symbrachydactyly. *J Pediatr Orthop B* 1998;7:158-161.

6. Beals RK, Crawford S: Congenital absence of the pectoral muscles: A review of twenty-five patients. *Clin Orthop* 1976;119:166-171.

7. Goldberg MJ, et al: Poland's syndrome: A concept of pathogenesis based on limb bud embryology. *Birth Defects* 1977;13:103-115.

8. Ireland DC, Takayama N, Flatt AE: Poland's syndrome. *J Bone Joint Surg Am* 1976;58:52-58.

9. Ireland DCR, Takayama N, Flatt AE: Poland's syndrome. A review of forty-three cases. *J Bone Joint Surg Am* 1976; 58:52-58.

10. Poland A: Deficiency of pectoralis muscle. *Guys Hosp Rep* 1841;6: 191-193.

11. Wilson MR, Louis DS, Stevenson TR: Poland's syndrome: Variable expression and associated anomalies. *J Hand Surg [Am]* 1988;13:880-882.

12. Barsky AJ: Cleft hand: Classification, incidence and treatment. *J Bone Joint Surg Am* 1970;23:269.

13. Miura T, Suzuki M: Clinical differences between typical and atypical cleft hand. *J Hand Surg [Br]* 1984;9: 311-315.

14. Kay SP, Wiberg M: Toe to hand transfer in children. Part 1: Technical aspects. *J Hand Surg [Br]* 1996;21: 723-734.

15. Vilkki SK: Advances in microsurgical reconstruction of the congenitally adactylous hand. *Clin Orthop* 1995; 314:45-58.

16. Foucher G: The "stub" operation: Modification of the Furnas and Vilkki technique in traumatic and congenital carpal hand reconstruction. *Ann Acad Med Singapore* 1995;24:73-76.

17. Dobyns JH, Wood VE, Bayne LG: Congenital hand deformities, in Green DP (ed): *Operative Hand Surgery*. New York, NY, Churchill Livingston,1988.

18. Bauer TB, Tondra JM, Trusler HM: Technical modifications in repair of syndactylism. *Plast Reconstr Surg* 1956; 17:385-392.

19. Eaton CJ, Lister GD: Syndactyly. *Hand Clin* 1990;6:555-575.

20. Ashmead D, Smith PJ: Tissue expansion for Apert's syndactyly. *J Hand Surg [Br]* 1995;20:327-330.

21. Flatt AE: Treatment of syndactylism. *Plast Reconstr Surg* 1962;29:336-341.

22. Light TR: Congenital anomalies: Syndactyly, polydactyly and cleft hand, in Peimer CA (ed): *Surgery of the Hand and Upper Extremity*. New York, NY, McGraw-Hill, 1996.

23. Toledo LC, Ger E: Evaluation of the operative treatment of syndactyly. *J Hand Surg* 1979;4:556-564.

24. Upton J: Congenital anomalies of the hand and forearm, in McCarthy J, May JW, Jr, Littler JW (eds): *Plastic Surgery*. Philadelphia, PA, WB Saunders, 1990, vol 8.

25. Foukes GD, Reinker K: Congenital constriction band syndrome: A seventy year experience. *J Pediatr Orthop* 1994;19:973-976.

26. Jones KL: *Smith's Recognizable Patterns of Human Malformation*. Philadelphia, PA, WB Saunders, 1988.

27. Ogino T, Saitou Y: Congenital constriction band syndrome and transverse deficiency. *J Hand Surg [Br]* 1987;12:343-348.

28. Tada K, Kurisaki E, Yonenobu K, et al: Central polydactyly: A review of 12 cases and their surgical treatment. *J Hand Surg [Am]* 1982;7:460-465.

29. Marks TW, Bayne LG: Polydactyly of the thumb: Abnormal anatomy and treatment. *J Hand Surg* 1978;3: 107-116.

30. Cheng JCY, Chan KM, Ma GFY, et al: Polydactyly of the thumb: A surgical plan based on ninety five cases. *J Hand Surg [Am]* 1984;9:155-164.

31. Ezaki M: Radial polydactyly. *Hand Clin* 1990;6:577-588.

32. Miura T: Duplicated thumb. *Plast Reconstr Surg* 1982;69:470-479.

33. Tada K, Yonenobu K, Tsuyuguchi Y, et al: Duplication of the thumb: A retrospective review of two hundred and thirty-seven cases. *J Bone Joint Surg Am* 1983;65:584-598.

34. Wassel HD: The results of surgery for polydactyly of the thumb. *Clin Orthop* 1969;64:175-193.

35. Barton NJ, Buck-Gramcko D, Evans DM: Soft-tissue anatomy of mirror hand. *J Hand Surg [Br]* 1986;11: 307-319.

36. Barton NJ, Buck-Gramcko D, Evans DM, et al: Mirror hand treated by true pollicization. *J Hand Surg [Br]* 1986; 11:320-336.

37. Bora FW, Nicholson JT, Cheema HM: Radial meromelia: The deformity and its treatment. *J Bone Joint Surg Am* 1970;52:966-979.

38. Swanson AB: The Krukenberg procedure in the juvenile amputee. *J Bone Joint Surg Am* 1964;46:1540-1548.

39. Seitz WH: Distraction osteogenesis of a congenital amputation at the elbow. *J Hand Surg* 1989;14:945-948.

40. Goldberg NH, Watson HK: Composite toe (phalanx and epiphysis) transfers in the reconstruction of the aphalangic hand. *J Hand Surg* 1982;7:454-459.

Chapter 70

Radial Deficiencies

Terry R. Light, MD

Introduction

Congenital differences associated with preaxial abnormalities of the upper limb have been variously termed longitudinal radial deficiency, radial hemimelia, radial dysplasia, radial aplasia or hypoplasia, preaxial deficiency, congenital absence of the radius, or radial clubhand. The chief morphologic finding in this condition, as the name implies, is partial or total absence of the radius.

Morphology

Shoulder, elbow, wrist, and hand abnormalities are common. In some children, radial dysplasia is evident as an element of phocomelia, which is characterized by a severely shortened or absent humeral component, resulting in a hand that is close to the shoulder. Characteristic anomalies of the forearm in children with radial dysplasia include shortening, bowing of the ulna, and profound radial deviation of the hand on the ulna. The ulna in children with radial dysplasia is usually approximately two thirds of the length of the normal ulna (Figure 1). At skeletal maturity, the normal ulna is approximately 28 cm long, whereas the untreated ulna in an adult with radial dysplasia is approximately 18 cm.[1] The ulna in the radial-deficient limb may be curved or bowed. Bowing is primarily believed to be a postnatal phenomenon caused by musculotendinous forces across the radial aspect of the ulna.

The ipsilateral humerus is often short. The elbow may demonstrate a flexion contracture or may be stiff. Careful physical and radiographic examination will distinguish a true elbow joint flexion contracture from curvature of the ulnar shaft. The hand may be missing some digits or demonstrate dysplasia in the digits along the preaxial portion of the hand. The thumb may be hypoplastic or absent, and the index finger is often stiff and may be syndactylized to the middle finger.

Imaging Studies

Because the shoulder, elbow, forearm, and hand may demonstrate abnormalities, initial evaluation should include radiographs of the entire upper limb, including AP and lateral views of the forearm. The extent of radial ossification is used as the basis for classifying the extent of radial deficiency. Radiographs of the hand help

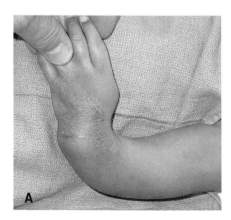
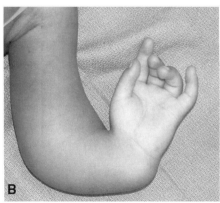
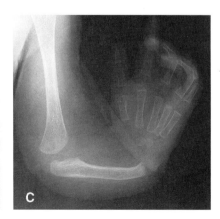

Figure 1 Uncorrected Bayne type IV radial-deficient forearm. **A,** Dorsal view. **B,** Palmar view. **C,** AP radiograph.

TABLE 1 Bayne Classification of Radial Deficiencies	
Type	Characteristics
0	Hypoplasia of the radial carpus (scaphoid); radius of normal length
I	Radius slightly shorter than normal; physis evident both proximally and distally
II	"Radius in miniature": normally shaped but small radius with a proximal and distal physis
III	Partial aplasia of the radius; absence of the distal part of radius, including the distal epiphysis
IV	Total absence of radius

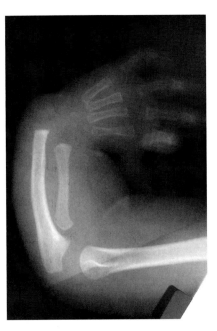

Figure 2 Bayne type II radial-deficient limb has a short, small radius and both a proximal and distal physis.

evaluate associated thumb deficiencies.

Some authors measure the angle between the long axis of the ulna and the hand to define the extent of soft-tissue tightness along the preaxial surface of the forearm.[2] These measurements are valid only if the hand is positioned in a standardized fashion. Because the primitive articulation of the carpus against the radial border of the ulna does not constrain rotation of the hand on the ulna, positioning of the hand in a standardized fashion relative to the forearm is surprisingly difficult. Rotation of the ulna must be uniformly controlled by positioning the flexed elbow in a lateral position on the x-ray plate to ensure a reproducible measurement of the hand and forearm.

Classification

The classification of radial deficiency initially proposed by Bayne (Table 1) includes radially deviated wrists with normal radii[3] (Figure 2). Because the carpus is unossified at birth, type 0 limbs should be suspected in patients in whom the wrist is deviated radially despite a radiographically normal radius. Even though the diaphysis of the normal radius is ossified at birth, the dysplastic radius may not be. Limbs without radiographic evidence of a radius early can demonstrate ossifica-

tion of the radial anlagen on subsequent postnatal radiographs or may, at surgical exploration, reveal an unossified tethering anlage. In such cases, a limb initially classified as type IV may be reclassified as type III.

Associated thumb deficiency is classified by Manske's modification of Blauth's[4] system. The thumb hypoplasia and aplasia classification system suggested by Blauth has been reinterpreted by other authors.[5-8] Thumb aplasia and hypoplasia has been divided into five different grades.

Grade I thumbs are slightly smaller or narrower than normal but possess all normal anatomic structures. The thumb metacarpal is often narrow. Function is nearly normal and diagnosis is often not established until adolescence or adulthood.

Grade II thumbs are smaller than normal. The thenar intrinsic muscles are hypoplastic, the metacarpophalangeal (MCP) joint is unstable, and the first web space is narrow. Thumb flexion may be limited because of cross connections between the extensor pollicis longus and the flexor pollicis longus along the radial aspect of the thumb.

Grade III thumbs are small, short, unstable, and have deficient thenar musculature. In addition, the extrinsic muscles are absent or rudimentary, and the metacarpal is small and narrow. Manske distinguished grade IIIA thumbs with a stable carpometacarpal joint from grade IIIB thumbs in which there is absence of the proximal thumb metacarpal and consequent instability of the basilar thumb joint.

Grade IV thumbs consist of a digit with one or two hypoplastic phalanges without tendon or muscle connected to the hand by a narrow skin bridge attaching the thumb to the hand in the region of the metacarpal neck of the index finger. Because of the narrow connection to the hand, the term "floating thumb," or "pouce flotant," is often used. Grade V is characterized by total thumb aplasia or absence.

Although the extent of thumb dysplasia often is greater in more severe cases of radial dysplasia, this is not always the case. For example, children with thrombocytopenia with absent radius (TAR) syndrome have type IV radial dysplasia with either normal or type I thumbs.

Typical Deficits

Radial dysplasia may be unilateral or bilateral. When bilateral, the extent of radial dysplasia is not necessarily symmetric. Even though finger motion may be deemed satisfactory, functional problems abound. The uncorrected hand curls back along the forearm, unable to effectively reach out away from the body. This abnormal hand position requires the patient to move very close to the object that he or she wishes to manipulate with his or her hand. Given the lack of radial carpal support, the wrist is unstable, and the grip is weak. The extent of thumb dysplasia will determine the extent to which pinch or grasp activities are compromised. In addition, the upper limb is short compared with the normal unaffected limb.

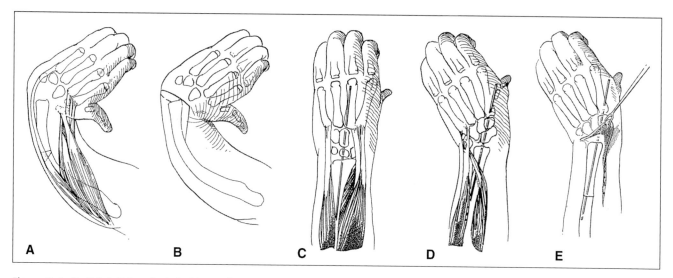

Figure 3 **A,** Radial-deficient limb, lacking radial carpal support, is held in radial deviation by short dysplastic extrinsic flexor and extensor muscles. **B,** L-shaped skin excision provides exposure of dorsal soft tissues and ulnocarpal articulation. **C** and **D,** Centralization places the hand in line with the forearm; radialization shifts the carpus toward the ulna and obtains fixation in the index metacarpal. **E,** Skin flap is recontoured after ulnocarpal stabilization. *(Reproduced with permission from Light TR: Centralization for radial dysplasia, in Blair WF, Steyers CM (eds): Techniques in Hand Surgery. Baltimore, MD, Williams & Wilkins, 1996, pp 1144-1151.)*

Etiology

The incidence of radial dysplasia ranges from 1 in 30,000 to 1 in 100,000 live births.[9,10] Many times, radial dysplasia is an element of a syndrome or an association. Often, however, the forearm and hand abnormalities are isolated findings, and the etiology remains unknown. Thalidomide is the only teratogenic agent conclusively linked to radial dysplasia;[11] a total of 60% of children whose mothers took thalidomide had evidence of radial dysplasia. The role of other environmental factors remains unproved.

A number of conditions include radial dysplasia as part of the clinical presentation, including the VATER/VACTERL association, Holt-Oram syndrome, Fanconi pancytopenia syndrome, and TAR syndrome. Children with VATER (sometimes referred to as VACTERL) association may have a number of the following characteristics: **v**ertebral abnormalities, imperforate **a**nus, **t**racheo**e**sophageal fistula, **r**adial deficiency, **r**enal abnormalities, defects in **c**ardiac development, and other **l**imb abnormalities.[12,13] Holt-Oram syndrome is an autosomal dominant condition in which a cardiac septal defect occurs in addition to radial dysplasia.[14,15] Fanconi anemia is an autosomal recessive condition in which radial dysplasia is associated with pancytopenia that becomes more severe as the child matures.[14,16] The radial dysplasia may be as modest as thumb hypoplasia or as severe as absence of the radius. Bone marrow transplant has substantially improved the prognosis for affected children. Children with TAR syndrome, another autosomal recessive disorder, commonly have thrombocytopenia, in addition to total bilateral absence of the radius and slightly hypoplastic well-developed thumbs.[17] The relatively severe thrombocytopenia at birth improves as the child matures. Some of these children also demonstrate humeral, elbow, tibial, and knee abnormalities.[18]

Management
Surgical Centralization

The aim of treatment is to enhance function while improving cosmesis. The uncorrected radial-deficient limb is short, unstable, and awkwardly positioned in space. Surgical centralization repositions the hand at the distal end of the ulna, corrects bowing of the ulna, and stabilizes the articulation between the forearm and the hand (Figure 3). This repositioning allows the hand to more effectively reach out and interact with the environment. The force of the finger flexors of the stabilized hand is concentrated on finger flexion rather than on twisting the hand into a flexed, radially deviated position with less powerful finger flexion.

Following successful centralization, the amount of motion at the wrist and the carpometacarpal joints is limited.[19] Thus, centralization is contraindicated in a limb with a stiff elbow because stabilizing the hand at the distal end of the forearm will make it impossible for a child to bring his or her hand to the mouth. Limbs with profound shortening of the humerus (phocomelia) are also unlikely to benefit from centralization.

Effective surgical stabilization of the hand at the distal ulna requires rebalancing of tendon forces across the wrist. Before centralization is performed, the soft tissues along the radial side of the ulna should be as supple as possible. In most children, this may be achieved by a combination of parental stretching, forearm splinting, and serial casting.

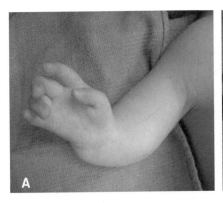
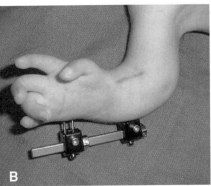

Figure 4 A, Soft tissues of the uncorrected hand were deemed too tight to allow single-stage repositioning of the hand and carpus on the distal ulna. **B,** Soft-tissue relaxation is achieved through volar soft-tissue release and gradual distraction lengthening.

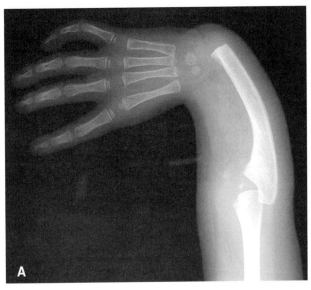
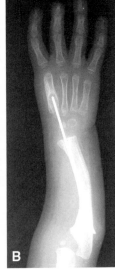

Figure 5 A, Uncorrected, radially deviated hand articulates against the radial side of the distal ulna. **B,** The hand and carpus are repositioned on the articular surface of the distal ulna.

flexor side fascia. The distractor is gradually elongated until the carpus has been pulled distally beyond the distal ulnar epiphysis. The device is retained for an additional 4 to 5 weeks while soft tissues readjust and relax from the effects of distraction. The device is then removed, and conventional wrist stabilization can be performed.

Centralization of the hand on the distal ulna requires exposure of the distal ulnar articular surface and the articular surface of the proximal carpal row (Figure 3). Carpal bones are resected as necessary to seat the carpus on the end of the ulna. The articular surface of the distal ulna may be minimally recontoured. Tight soft tissues, which may include a fibrous anlage, must be released.[25] The classic centralization procedure aligns the middle finger metacarpal with the axis of the ulna.

Modifications to Centralization

Because centralization has been associated with an extremely high incidence of recurrent radial deviation deformity, a number of modifications have been proposed. Radialization, the modification of centralization suggested by Buck-Gramcko,[26] places the hand in a position of ulnar deviation, with internal pin fixation through the metacarpal shaft of the index finger, across the radial carpus, and into the ulna. The alignment of the wrist in ulnar deviation, as suggested by Buck-Gramcko, diminishes the tendency for recurrent radial deviation (Figure 5).

Some surgeons try to maintain pin fixation indefinitely in an attempt to achieve a forearm of maximal length with a stiff wrist at skeletal maturity.[2,27] Others attempt to create a mobile wrist by removing pin fixation within the first 6 months after wrist stabilization.[19,25] If a mobile wrist is achieved by early pin removal, the risk for postoperative deformity is markedly increased in the presence of unresolved motor imbalance. Long-

Parents are instructed to apply gentle pressure to bring the hand toward the axis of the ulna for 5 to 10 minutes four to five times a day. Forearm splinting should begin in the newborn period. Splints may be applied along either the radial or ulnar border of the forearm. Those applied along the radial forearm push the hand radially, whereas those fitted along the ulnar border of the forearm pull the hand toward the axis of the ulna.[20,21] Splints may be removed throughout the day to allow the child opportunities for unconstrained use and exploration. Splints should not cover the fingers or prevent tactile awareness of the hand. In children who do not tolerate splinting, serial casting may be effective in loosening or elongating the soft tissues along the radial aspect of the forearm.

When stretching, splinting, and casting prove ineffective in sufficiently loosening the radial soft tissues to allow centralization, distraction may be achieved with a distraction fixator[22-24] (Figure 4). At the time of fixator application, a limited soft-tissue release is helpful. A longitudinal incision over the volar radial aspect of the wrist allows release of the flexor carpi radialis tendon, as well as release of the tight

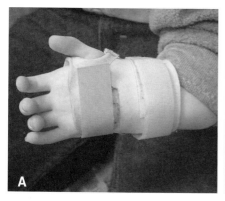
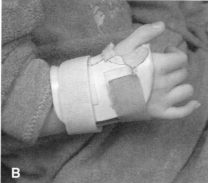

Figure 6 Palmar **(A)** and dorsal **(B)** clinical photographs showing the postoperative splint worn after removal of pin fixation of the wrist.

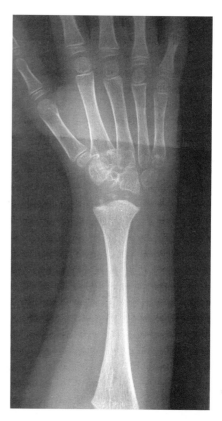

Figure 7 With time, the mechanical force of the repositioned hand leads to broadening of the distal ulna.

term bracing may be particularly helpful in these situations to allow ulnocarpal articular remodeling and ultimately minimize long-term postoperative deformity (Figures 6 and 7).

In most patients, satisfactory alignment is preserved through childhood.[28] If the deformity recurs and the hand resumes a flexed, severely radially deviated position, surgical arthrodesis of the ulna to the distal carpal row can be performed at adolescence or adulthood.[29]

Thumb Reconstruction

When thumb dysplasia is associated with radial deficiency, hand function may be enhanced by thumb reconstruction. In patients with types 1, 2, and 3A thumb dysplasia, reconstruction improves the function of the native thumb by addressing deficits, including narrowing of the first web space, instability of the MCP joint, and inadequate intrinsic-extrinsic function. Web space narrowing may be addressed by soft-tissue release and a dorsal rotation flap. MCP joint instability requires soft-tissue plication, chondrodesis, or arthrodesis. Inadequate extrinsic thumb extensor tendons are effectively treated by extensor indicis proprius tendon transfers, whereas inadequate opposition is treated by opponensplasty. Extrinsic flexor tendon deficiency is often associated with cross connections between the radially placed flexor pollicis longus tendon and the extensor mechanism. Tenolysis and repositioning of

the flexor pollicis longus may modestly improve thumb interphalangeal joint flexion.[30]

Types 3B and 4 thumbs are so dysplastic that reconstruction is not attempted; the thumb is amputated, and the index finger is pollicized. In type 5 hands (ie, with no thumb), the index finger is pollicized.[31] Pollicization of the index finger shortens and rotates the metacarpal and repositions the distal portion of the finger in the posture of a normal thumb, articulating along the radial aspect of the carpus.[32,33] In most instances of radial deficiency, the index finger is relatively stiff with limited MCP joint flexion.

Because of the underlying dysplasia in the index finger, the results of pollicization in radial dysplasia are not as good as the results in children with a normal forearm.[34-36] Nonetheless, the procedure is worthwhile in children with radial dysplasia because the pollicized finger is particularly helpful in buttressing large objects and facilitating cylindrical grip. After pollicization, many children with radial dysplasia will continue to use ring to little finger pinch for small precision activities.

Summary

Longitudinal radial deficiency is a relatively common congenital difference of the upper limb. It is often associated with systemic abnormalities and occasionally associated with other

musculoskeletal abnormalities. Function and appearance are enhanced by ulnocarpal stabilization and thumb reconstruction. When the thumb is severely dysplastic, pollicization of the index finger will enhance function.

References

1. Vilkki SK: Distraction and microvascular epiphysis transfer for radial club hand. *J Hand Surg* 1998;23:445-452.

2. Manske PR, McCarroll HR Jr, Swanson K: Centralization of the radial club hand: An ulnar surgical approach. *J Hand Surg* 1981;6:423-433.

3. James MA, McCarroll HR Jr, Manske PR: The spectrum of radial longitudinal deficiency: A modified classification. *J Hand Surg* 1999;24:1145-1155.

4. Blauth W: Der hypoplastiche Daumen. *Arch Orthop Unfallchir* 1967;62: 225-246.

5. Buck-Gramcko D: Congenital absence and hypoplasia of the thumb, in Strickland JW (ed): *The Thumb.* Edin-

burgh, Scotland, Churchill Livingston, 1994, pp 45-65.

6. Kleinman WB: Management of thumb hypoplasia. *Hand Clin* 1990;6:617-641.

7. Manske PR, McCarroll HR Jr, James M: Type III-A hypoplastic thumb. *J Hand Surg* 1995;20:246-253.

8. James MA, McCarroll HR Jr, Manske PR: Characteristics of patients with hypoplastic thumbs. *J Hand Surg* 1996; 21:104-113.

9. Geek MJ, Dorey F, Lawrence JF, Johnson MJ: Congenital radius deficiency: Radiographic outcome and survivorship analysis. *J Hand Surg [Am]* 1999;24:1132-1144.

10. Urban MA, Osterman AL: Management of radial dysplasia. *Hand Clin* 1990;6:589-605.

11. Lamb DW: Radial club hand: A continuing study of sixty-eight patients with one hundred and seventeen club hands. *J Bone Joint Surg Am* 1977;59: 1-13.

12. Beals RK: VATER association: A unifying concept of multiple anomalies. *J Bone Joint Surg Am* 1989;71:948-950.

13. Quan L, Smith DW: The VATER association: Vertebral defects, anal atresia, T-E fistula with esophageal atresia, radiala and renal dysplasia: A spectrum of associated defects. *J Pediatr* 1973;82:104.

14. Goldberg MJ: *The Dysmorphic Child: An Orthopaedic Perspective.* New York, NY, Raven Press, 1987.

15. Holt M, Oram S: Familial heart disease with skeletal malformations. *Br Heart J* 1960;22:236-242.

16. Fanconi G: Familial constitutional panmyelocytopathy, Fanconi's anemia (F.A.): I. Clinical aspects. *Semin Hematol* 1967;4:233-240.

17. Dell PC, Sheppard JE: Thrombocytopenia, absent radius syndrome: Report of two siblings and a review of the hematologic and genetic features. *Clin Orthop* 1982;162:129.

18. Schoenecker PL, Cohn AK, Sedgwick WG, Manske PR, Salafsky I, Millar EA: Dysplasia of the knee associated with the syndrome of thrombocytopenia and absent radius. *J Bone Joint Surg Am* 1984;66:421-427.

19. Bayne LG, Klug MS: Long-term review of the surgical treatment of radial deficiencies. *J Hand Surg* 1987;12: 169-179.

20. Butts DE, Goldberg MJ: Congenital absence of the radius: The occupational therapist and a new orthosis. *Am J OT* 1977;31:95-100.

21. Kennedy SM: Neoprene wrist brace for correction of radial club hand in children. *J Hand Ther* 1996;9:387-390.

22. Kessler I: Centralization of the radial club hand by gradual distraction. *J Hand Surg* 1989;14:37-42.

23. Nanchahal J, Tonkin MA: Pre-operative distraction lengthening for radial longitudinal deficiency. *J Hand Surg* 1996;21:103-107.

24. Smith AA, Greene TL: Preliminary soft tissue distraction in congenital forearm deficiency. *J Hand Surg [Am]* 1995;20:420-424.

25. Watson HK, Beebe RD, Cruz NI: A centralization procedure for radial clubhand. *J Hand Surg* 1984;9:541-547.

26. Buck-Gramcko D: Radialization as a new treatment for radial club hand. *J Hand Surg* 1985;10:964-968.

27. Lamb DW, Scott H, Lam WL, Gillespie WJ, Hooper G: Operative correction of radial club hand. *J Hand Surg* 1997; 22:533-536.

28. Bora FW, Osterman AL, Kaneda RR, Esterhai J: Radial club-hand deformity: Long term follow-up. *J Bone Joint Surg Am* 1981;63:741-745.

29. Rayan GM: Ulnocarpal arthrodesis for recurrent radial club hand deformity in adolescents. *J Hand Surg* 1992;17: 24-27.

30. Graham TJ, Louis DS: A comprehensive approach to surgical management of the type IIIA hypoplastic thumb. *J Hand Surg [Am]* 1998;23:3-13.

31. Kozin SH, Weiss AA, Webber JB, Betz RR, Clancy M, Steel HH: Index finger pollicization for congenital aplasia or hypoplasia of the thumb. *J Hand Surg [Am]* 1992;17:880-884.

32. Buck-Gramcko D: Pollicization of the index finger: Method and results in aplasia and hypoplasia of the thumb. *J Bone Joint Surg Am* 1971;53: 1605-1617.

33. Light TR, Forseth M: Pollicization of the index finger. *Atlas Hand Clin* 2000; 5:47-64.

34. Harrison SH: Pollicisation in cases of radial club hand. *Br J Plast Surg* 1970; 23:192-200.

35. Manske PR, Rotman MB, Dailey LA: Long-term functional results after pollicization for the congenitally deficient thumb. *J Hand Surg* 1992;17: 1064-1072.

36. Sykes PJ, Chandraprakasam T, Percival NJ: Pollicization of the index finger in congenital anomalies: A retrospective analysis. *J Hand Surg* 1991;16:144-147.

Chapter 71

Longitudinal Ulnar Deficiency

Julian E. Kuz, MD
James Engels, MD

Introduction

Congenital postaxial deficiencies of the upper limb have been variously termed ulnar hemimelia, ulnar aplasia/hypoplasia, postaxial deficiency, congenital absence of the ulna, or ulnar clubhand. The current standard term is longitudinal ulnar deficiency, partial or complete. The chief morphologic finding, as the name implies, is partial or total absence of the ulna.

Clinical Morphology

In longitudinal ulnar deficiency, associated shoulder, elbow, wrist, and hand differences are common. Characteristics of the forearm include shortening and increased bowing of the radius. The shoulder may be internally rotated. The elbow may present with either flexion or extension contractures or with a synostosis. The radial head may be dislocated, and the elbow complex may be unstable. Associated hand differences can include absence, syndactyly, thumb hypoplasia or absence, malrotation of digits, web-space contracture, and ectrodactyly.[1] In longitudinal ulnar deficiency, unlike radial longitudinal deficiency, the hand is usually reasonably aligned at the wrist level.

Imaging Studies

Standard plain radiography of the shoulder, arm, elbow, forearm, wrist, and hand may be necessary for assessing this condition. An AP view of the forearm will delineate the ulnar deficiency and allow the condition to be defined according to a published classification system. AP and lateral radiographs of the elbow can demonstrate radial head dislocation and instability, and AP and lateral views of the hand will help determine thumb deficiencies and syndactyly components. In skeletally immature children, allowances need to be made for bones that are not yet ossified.

Classification Systems

Numerous classification systems have been proposed for longitudinal ulnar deficiency (Table 1), but because of the variable involvement of the shoulder, elbow, wrist, and hand, no system is entirely satisfactory. Those of Kummel,[2] Ogden and associates,[3] and Bayne[4] have been used to describe the ulnar deficiency and/or elbow difference involved. Kummel's classification is based on elbow morphology, Ogden's system focuses on the ulnar deficiency, and Bayne's system (Figure 1) combines elements of both. Swanson and associates[5] and Broudy and Smith[6] noted numerous radial-sided hand differences in these patients. Ogino and Kato[7] proposed a classification system of hand differences based on the number of missing ulnar rays in the hand, ignoring differences on the radial aspect of the hand. Cole and Manske[1] based their classification system of ulnar deficiency on changes of the thumb and first web. A combination of systems, though cumbersome, may prove to be most useful because it yields the most detailed description. An example of how classification systems can be combined is illustrated in Figure 2. We prefer to classify ulnar deficiencies using Bayne's system, with the hand subclassified according to Cole and Manske.

Typical Deficits

Because most patients will have a unilateral deficiency, function is usually good. Patients with severe flexion contractures at the elbow, however, especially bilateral, will have difficulty with activities of daily living such as perineal hygiene, toileting, and some dressing activities. Patients with concomitant hypoplastic or absent thumbs will have weak pinch and grasp and will have difficulty handling large objects. Differences involving a combination of severe internal rotation of the shoulder and forearm pronation will cause difficulties with hand-to-mouth and hand-to-head motions, perineal care, and bimanual activities.

TABLE 1 Classification Systems for Longitudinal Ulnar Deficiencies

Kummel

Type	Characteristics
A	Normal radiohumeral joint
B	Radiohumeral synostosis
C	Dislocation of the radiohumeral joint

Ogden

Type	Characteristics
I	Hypoplasia of otherwise normal ulna with a distal epiphysis
II	Partial aplasia (absence of distal part of ulna, including the distal epiphysis)
III	Total aplasia

Bayne

Type	Characteristics
I	Hypoplasia; distal epiphysis present
II	Partial aplasia; distal epiphysis absent
III	Total aplasia
IV	Radiohumeral synostosis with total aplasia of the ulna

Cole and Manske

Type	Characteristics
A	Normal thumb and first web space
B	Mild first web and thumb deficiency
C	Moderate to severe first web and thumb deficiency (loss of opposition, malrotation, thumb index syndactyly, absent extrinsic tendon function
D	Thumb absent

Blair and associates[8] assessed the functional status of patients with ulnar hemimelia. The investigators measured total active joint motion (elbow + forearm + wrist) to be 46% of normal, power grip averaged 27% of the contralateral limb, and prehension was "generally well performed." Using the affected limb, patients finished timed tests an average of 11.6 seconds slower than they did using the contralateral limb. Patients with the most impaired function were those with radiohumeral synostosis and those with absence, deformity, or contracture of digits. Johnson and Omer[9] compared patients' function with standards for the general population. Total active motion for elbow, forearm, and wrist was 54% of normal. Power grip averaged 18% of normal (for those patients who could perform this function), and key pinch, 41%. Most difficulties with prehension were with grasping spheres and large cylinders.

Incidence and Etiology

The incidence of longitudinal ulnar deficiency is often reported as 1 in 100,000 live births.[10] In a series of 2,758 patients, Flatt[11] reported that 28 patients presented with this diagnosis, making it one of the least common forms of longitudinal limb deficiencies. Among the 28 patients, 25% had bilateral deficiency, and the ratio of longitudinal ulnar deficiency to radial longitudinal deficiency was 1:4.5. The male-to-female ratio was 3:2. Two other series place the ratio of ulnar deficiency to radial deficiency at 1:3.[9,12] Left-sided occurrence is more common.[9]

The etiology of isolated ulnar deficiency remains unknown. Ulnar defi-

ciencies may also be interpreted as a disturbance arising from the C8 sclerotome, according to the neurocrest cell theory postulated by McCredie.[13] A teratogenic process or defective gene causes a defect or deficiency in the mesenchymal cells of the limb bud before the limb bud forms. Ogino and Kato[7] induced ulnar deficiencies in Gunn-Wistar rats by giving busulfan to gravid rats on the ninth gestational day. Some of the ulnar-deficient rats had other associated musculoskeletal abnormalities. They were similar in proportion and extent to those seen in humans. Ogden and associates[14] had similar results when they treated gravid Gunn-Wistar rats with acetazolamide. Genetic studies suggest the existence of a limb deficiency gene for ulnar deficiencies, and the 6q21 locus has been linked to some cases of ulnar ray deficiencies.[15,16] Several syndromes have been described that suggest a genetic component, but few studies demonstrate a familial pattern.[17] Despite our current knowledge, the exact roles of the possible environmental and genetic factors remain unclear.

At least 11 syndromes include hypoplasia of the ulna, including Miller, Pallister-Hall, Pillay, and Schinzel-Giedion syndromes; Weyers' oligodactyly; Reinhardt-Pfeiffer and Langer mesomelic dwarfism; and the best known, Cornelia de Lange syndrome, which includes radial ray defects, brachymetacarpia, clinodactyly, absence of digits, Kirner deformity, growth failure, hirsutism, mental retardation, and microbrachycephaly.[18,19] Also described have been femoral-fibular-ulnar deficiency syndrome, ulnar-fibular dysostosis syndrome, and ulnar-mammary syndrome.[17,20,21] Longitudinal ulnar deficiency is associated with other musculoskeletal differences, including radial deficiencies, fibular hypoplasia, partial longitudinal deficiency of the femur, congenital coxa vara, phocomelia, cleft palate, polydactyly, and transverse absence of the upper extremity at the wrist level.[5] Congenital dysplasia of the hip, absent patella, tibial ray deficiency,

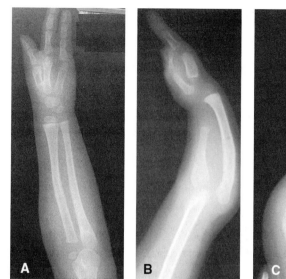
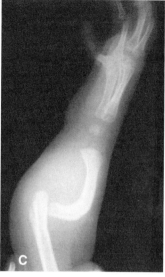
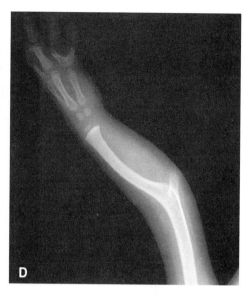

Figure 1 Bayne's classification of longitudinal ulnar deficiency. **A,** Bayne type I. No significant shortening of the ulna is present, and the distal epiphysis is present. The ulnar metacarpals are absent. There is contracture of the thumb web space consistent with a type B difference in Cole and Manske's classification system. **B,** Bayne type II: There is significant bowing of the radius, a dislocated radial head, and a shortened ulna. The ulnar anlage is acting as a tethering force. **C,** Bayne type III: The ulna is absent, and the radial head is dislocated. This type is considered to be the rarest. **D,** Bayne type IV: Radiohumeral synostosis is present. The thumb is a type C difference in Cole and Manske's classification system and shows significant hypoplasia and web space contracture.

and scoliosis have also been reported.[20] In 29% to 40% of cases, associated contralateral limb anomalies occur, including phocomelia, complete longitudinal deficiencies, ectrodactyly, and radial ray deficiencies.[20]

Treatment and Functional Considerations

Treatment is aimed at improving function. Cosmetic benefit should be pursued only if a simultaneous improvement in function may be achieved. In most reported series, the investigators advocate conservative treatment of most anomalies occurring around the humerus, elbow, forearm, and wrist. Splinting helps maintain wrist position, but clinical studies showing efficacy in preventing deformity are lacking. The greatest benefits seem to accrue from well-recognized procedures performed on the hand to enhance function.

Patients with severe internal rotation of the shoulder with a pronation difference of the forearm may benefit from an external rotation osteotomy

of the humerus. In some cases of bilateral rotational differences of the forearm, a rotational osteotomy of the forearm can be considered. When a painful, unstable elbow exists with poor forearm rotation, a one-bone forearm procedure can be performed.[22-24] Radial head resection can be considered for patients with a painful prominence and a stable ulnohumeral joint. Patients with radiohumeral synostosis[25] and pterygium cubitale (Figure 3) rarely benefit from surgery because it produces no useful increase in range of motion. On rare occasions, a radiohumeral synostosis can be osteotomized to achieve a different static position if the patient requires it for functional activities.[11] Elbow disarticulation with prosthetic fitting is usually not appealing to patients but can be considered in patients with severe flexion differences.[22,26]

Resection of the ulnar anlage remains controversial. There is no clear documentation in the literature of decreasing deformity at the wrist or elbow with resection.[1,22] Nevertheless, some clinicians believe it is worthwhile to perform another procedure in the region to provide at

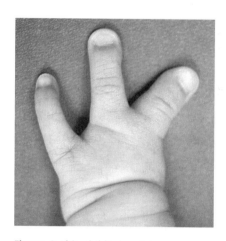

Figure 2 This child's hand has a severe thumb web space deficiency. Radiographs of the forearm demonstrated mild hypoplasia of the ulna with an epiphysis present. Therefore, the hand can be classified as a Bayne type I ulna with a Cole and Manske type C hand.

least short-term correction of the ulnar-deviated wrist.[6,11,27] Routine resection is not recommended.[6] Johnson and Omer[9] believe the natural history indicates that the risk of progression of deformity is slight, so there is little need for anlage resection. The literature does not support isolated radial head resection for functional improvement.[11,22]

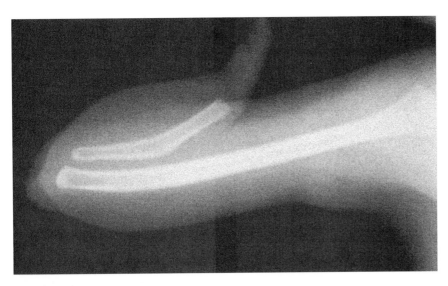

Figure 3 A Bayne type III forearm with severe pterygium cubitale.

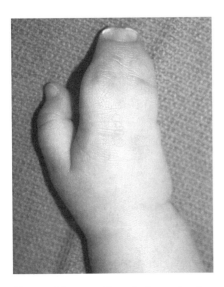

Figure 4 Preoperative photograph of a child with longitudinal ulnar deficiency. The hand has a complete complex syndactyly with a conjoined distal phalanx and synonychia. The ulna is mildly hypoplastic, and the thumb web space is of normal depth. This would be classified as a Bayne type I ulna with a Cole and Manske type A hand.

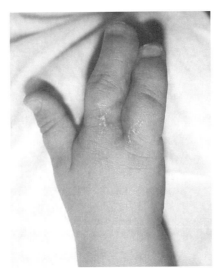

Figure 5 Early postoperative photograph of the same child in Figure 4. A syndactyly reconstruction was performed using full-thickness skin flaps and grafts. Nail fold reconstruction and synonychia/distal phalanx separation were performed using flaps designed from the adjacent finger pulp.

As stated previously, the largest number of surgeries in these patients are of the hand. Syndactyly release (Figures 4 and 5), rotational osteotomies, pollicization, opponensplasty, contracture release, and web-space deepening have all been reported.[1,6] These procedures have obvious merit in a patient if grasp, pinch, release, and accommodation of the hand can be improved.[8] Ilizarov's techniques of distraction lengthening for the forearm and humerus for ulnar deficiency have been used in unilateral cases. Distraction gains length for cosmesis and function. These techniques can also be used to create a single-bone forearm in instances of elbow or forearm instability, particularly with significant radial shortening.[25,28-30] These procedures are complex, and the surgeon may encounter many problems. The complications can be significant, despite reported good results.[28,29] No long-term clinical studies demonstrate functional outcomes using lengthening techniques in patients with longitudinal ulnar deficiencies.

Nonsurgical treatment methods involve prostheses or splinting. As mentioned above, elbow disarticulation with prosthetic fitting can help improve function in a patient with severe bilateral elbow contractures, but neither pediatric patients nor their parents accept this well. In a patient with a monodactylous hand and a mobile, actively controlled wrist, a forearm-based opponens post may provide functional grasp. Splinting should be considered in any difference that is thought to be progressive. Some advocate serial casting of Bayne types I and III deficiencies to correct wrist differences. This is usually a long arm cast that can position both the wrist and elbow.[9,11] No controlled studies have determined whether this is effective, however. Splinting pterygium cubitale is difficult and usually does not successfully modify the contracture.

Summary

Longitudinal ulnar deficiency is a relatively rare congenital deficiency of the upper limb. It is associated with other musculoskeletal abnormalities, but not usually with systemic abnormalities, as have been noted with radial deficiencies. The ulnar deficiencies range from absence of an ulnar digit with a normal ulna to complete ulnar aplasia. Elbow, wrist, and hand differences are common. Many classification systems exist, but the ideal system will likely combine the several systems that individually describe the elbow, ulna, and hand differences.

Most patients have acceptable function, despite elbow and forearm deficiencies. For this reason, surgery should be performed only if the patient presents with pain or significant functional loss because of gross and/or fixed malpositioning of the hand. The standard tenets of surgery for the hand manifestations associated with this condition should be followed carefully. Progression of the difference does not seem to be a great concern. Resection of the ulnar anlage or radial head is not routinely recommended.

References

1. Cole RJ, Manske PR: Classification of ulnar deficiency according to the thumb and first web. *J Hand Surg [Am]* 1997;22:479-488.

2. Kummel W: Die Missbildungen der Extremitaeten durch Defekt, Verwachsung und Ueberzahl. *Bibliotheca Medica* 1895;3:1-83.

3. Ogden JA, Watson HK, Bohne W: Ulnar dysmelia. *J Bone Joint Surg Am* 1976;58:467-475.

4. Bayne LG: Ulnar club hand (ulnar deficiencies), in Green DP (ed): *Operative Hand Surgery.* New York, NY, Churchill Livingstone, 1982, vol 11, pp 245-257.

5. Swanson AB, Tada K, Yonenobu K: Ulnar ray deficiency: Its various manifestations. *J Hand Surg [Am]* 1984;9: 658-664.

6. Broudy AS, Smith RJ: Deformities of the hand and wrist with ulnar deficiency. *J Hand Surg [Am]* 1979;4: 304-315.

7. Ogino T, Kato H: Clinical and experimental studies on ulnar ray deficiency. *Handchir Mikrochir Plast Chir* 1988;20: 330-337.

8. Blair WF, Shurr DG, Buckwalter JA: Functional status in ulnar deficiency. *J Pediatr Orthop* 1983;3:37-40.

9. Johnson J, Omer GE: Congenital ulnar deficiency: Natural history and therapeutic implications. *Hand Clin* 1985;1: 499-510.

10. Birch-Jensen A: (ed): *Congenital Deformities of the Upper Extremities.* Odense, Denmark, Andelsbogtrykkeriet, 1949, pp 46-47.

11. Flatt AE: (ed): *The Care of Congenital Hand Anomalies,* ed 2. St Louis, MO, Quality Medical Publishing, 1994, pp 411-424.

12. Manske PR: Longitudinal failure of upper-limb formation. *J Bone Joint Surg Am* 1996;78:1600-1623.

13. McCredie J: Neural crest defects: A neuroanatomic basis for classification of multiple malformations related to phocomelia. *J Neurol Sci* 1976;28: 373-387.

14. Ogden JA, Vickers TH, Tauber JE, Light TR: A model for ulnar dysmelia. *Yale J Biol Med* 1978;51:193-206.

15. Gurrieri F, Cammarata M, Avarello RM, et al: Ulnar ray defect in an infant with a 6q21;7q31.2 translocation: Further evidence for the existence of a limb defect gene in 6q21. *Am J Med Genet* 1995;55:315-318.

16. Reynolds JF, Wyandt HE, Kelly TE: Denovo: 21q interstitial deletion in a retarded boy with ulno-fibular dysostosis. *Am J Med Genet* 1985;20: 173-180.

17. Temtamy SA, McKusick VA, Bergsma D, Mudge JR, Paul NW, Greene SC: (eds): *The Genetics of Hand Malformations.* New York, NY, Liss, 1978, pp 48-50.

18. Goldberg MJ: (ed): *The Dysmorphic Child: An Orthopaedic Perspective.* New York, NY, Raven Press, 1987.

19. Jones KL: (ed): *Smith's Recognizable Patterns of Human Malformation,* ed 4. Philadelphia, PA, WB Saunders, 1988.

20. Schmidt CC, Neufeld SK: Ulnar ray deficiency. *Hand Clin* 1998;14:65-76.

21. Czeizel AE, Vitez M, Kodaj I, Lenz W: Causal study of isolated ulnar-fibular deficiency in Hungary, 1975-1984. *Am J Med Genet* 1993;46:427-433.

22. Mulligan PJ: The elbow, in Gupta A, Kay SPJ, Scheker LR (eds): *The Growing Hand: Diagnosis and Management of the Upper Extremity in Children.* London, England, Mosby, 2000, pp 197-202.

23. Straub LR: Congenital absence of the ulna. *Am J Surg* 1965;109:300-305.

24. Kitano K, Tada K: One-bone forearm procedure for partial defect of the ulna. *J Pediatr Orthop* 1985;5:290-293.

25. Jacobsen ST, Crawford AH: Humeroradial synostosis. *J Pediatr Orthop* 1983;3:96-98.

26. Lovett RJ: The treatment of longitudinal ulnar deficiency. *Prosthet Orthot Int* 1991;15:104-105.

27. Marcus NA, Omer GE Jr: Carpal deviation in congenital ulnar deficiency. *J Bone Joint Surg Am* 1984;66: 1003-1007.

28. Villa A, Paley D, Catagni MA, Bell D, Cattaneo R: Lengthening of the forearm by the Ilizarov technique. *Clin Orthop* 1990;250:125-137.

29. Tetsworth K, Krome J, Paley D: Lengthening and deformity correction of the upper extremity by the Ilizarov technique. *Orthop Clin North Am* 1991; 22:689-713.

30. Smith A, Greene T: Preliminary soft tissue distraction in congenital forearm deficiency. *J Hand Surg [Am]* 1995;20:420-424.

Chapter 72

Humeral Deficiencies

Mary Williams Clark, MD
Chris Lake, CPO

Introduction

Habilitation of the individual with upper limb deficiency can be a challenge for the entire therapeutic team. The evolution of prosthetic components as well as changes in treatment styles and protocols have led to significant differences in patient care throughout North America as well as internationally. In addition, many rehabilitation professionals seldom treat children and are much more familiar with the unique characteristics of limb deficiencies in adults. Rehabilitation care of children can differ widely from that of adults. Adults with upper limb deficiencies have prosthetic, functional, and personal rehabilitation goals that may remain quite consistent over their lifetimes. In contrast, the focus of pediatric prosthetic management changes throughout the patient's childhood and up to when he or she enters adulthood. This focus may initially revolve around play activities and mobility and later transition into ˉtivities of daily living and communication. As the child matures, social acceptance and independence increase in importance. Ultimately, the patient's chief concerns become vocational, educational, and family pursuits.

Medical Considerations

Both congenital and acquired humeral deficiencies occur less frequently than do forearm or lower limb deficiencies, and the prosthetic challenges are greater.

Congenital Deficiencies

Congenital deficiencies at and above the elbow are classified according to International Organization for Standardization (ISO) terminology (see chapter 62) as transverse or longitudinal. The through-elbow equivalent is termed a "transverse deficiency, forearm, total." The transhumeral level is "transverse deficiency, arm," with the level of loss noted as lower, middle, or upper third (eg, "transverse deficiency, arm, upper third"). All other congenital arm differences are classified as longitudinal, with the absent part(s) listed as total or partial (absence) from proximal to distal.[1]

Congenital absences are usually sporadic in nature, but some—particularly those including radial absence—may be inheritable.[2] Upper limb differences, especially bilateral, also may be part of an identified syndrome, warranting a thorough physical examination and family history as well as efforts to rule out other congenital problems. For example, bilateral phocomelic upper limbs with all digits present (Figure 1) are now well recognized as occurring in patients with thrombocytopenia absent radius (TAR) syndrome. Early recognition of this diagnosis in neonates is extremely important so that the physician can monitor and treat platelet levels, preventing bleeding problems, strokes, etc.

The clinician should always search for other silent problems associated with limb differences. In the case of TAR syndrome, for example, the frequent knee dysplasia may ultimately become much more troublesome than the arms. Because limbs and kidneys share the same developmental stage, from the fourth to seventh weeks of

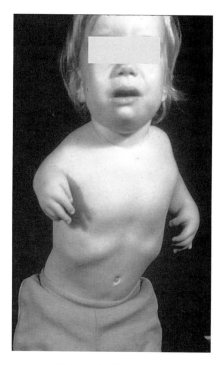

Figure 1 Child with TAR syndrome. There are five digits on each hand, but thumbs usually are not opposable.

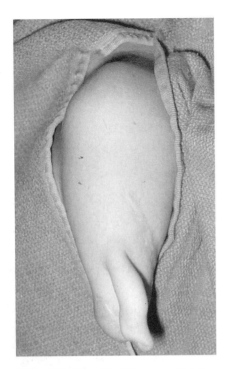

Figure 2 Child with left congenital humeral deficiency and phocomelic digit. (ISO classification: longitudinal humeral deficiency, partial; radius/ulna, total; carpal, total; rays 1–4, total; bifid distal phalanges.)

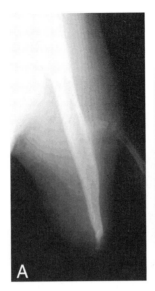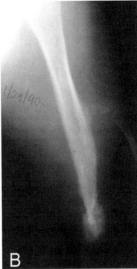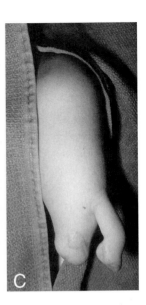

Figure 3 A, Radiograph of a 10-year-old boy with congenital humeral deficiency (ISO classification: longitudinal humeral deficiency, partial; radius/ulna, total; carpal, total; rays 1–4, total; ray 5, partial with bifid distal phalanges). Note the bony humeral overgrowth. The radiograph was taken after multiple overgrowth resections and before capping. **B,** Two months after capping from iliac crest. Note that the end is no longer pointy and a "bulb" of new bone has formed. **C,** One year after capping (before removal of stitch granuloma).

gestation, and both are of mesodermal origin, ultrasound images should be obtained to identify kidney problems in all children with significant limb differences.

Longitudinal congenital limb differences above the elbow often include hands or digits in phocomelic patterns, with distal elements attached to a more proximal arm segment or to the shoulder or chest wall (Figures 2 and 3). The residual or vestigial digits may well have active motor function; however, the potential strength of these digits, or even the presence of active muscle, may not be apparent at birth. Any degree of digit function may prove extremely useful to the older child or adult once it is developed. The child's future function should not be compromised by premature amputation of any digits. Small, seemingly useless digits—even the small nubbins of incomplete fingers—may be invaluable later, allowing the child to manipulate small items, use prosthetic switches, or perform other functions.[3]

Acquired Deficiencies

Children who acquire a transhumeral limb loss past infancy may be more likely to use a prosthesis than those with congenital absence because they have not yet developed compensatory one-handed skills or foot-use skills. This also may be true of patients with bilateral acquired amputations at the elbow or above; however, at this level and with bilateral amputations, prostheses are primarily a tool for specific functions. Foot function, if available, should always be encouraged in children missing both upper limbs.

Traumatic losses may involve more proximal injury than the level of the amputation, eg, brachial plexus injury associated with amputations in lawnmower or other high-speed rotary injuries. This can complicate retraining for function, with or without prosthetic fitting.

Surgical Considerations

Children who lose one or both arms to disseminated intravascular coagulopathy (DIC), also known as purpura fulminans, may have areas of skin loss and scarring as well. This may influence fitting decisions, suspension options, and other factors. Surgeons should wait as long as possible before performing amputation in these children because the necrosis is rarely septic, and recovering tissue beneath dry eschar may allow preservation of considerably more length than initially apparent. Also, the frequent growth plate injuries from DIC, which can result in physeal bars, must be recognized and treated before they cause deformity and/or limb shortening.[4]

Malignant or locally aggressive tumors may require upper limb amputations. For these patients, the postoperative course and decision making may be altered by concomitant chemotherapy and/or radiation therapy. They will have an extended treatment team, including oncologic surgeons and oncologists. Rehabilitation team treatment goals, decisions, and schedules will need to be closely coordinated through clear communication.

Although distal bony overgrowth, or terminal appositional bone, can occur in limbs with congenital deficiencies, this happens less frequently than in acquired limb loss. It occurs more commonly in the humerus than in the other long bones. Distal bony overgrowth becomes symptomatic when the spike of distal bone produces a tender bursa or progresses to protrude through the skin. The standard surgical treatment has been resection of the distal bone, using a medial or lateral incision to avoid thin, tender scar directly distal. These procedures often become "birthday operations," occurring every year or so as the patient grows. More recently, surgeons have been performing capping, as described initially by Marquardt and Correll[5] and modified by Davids,[6] to decrease the number of revision operations needed (Figure 3).

Marquardt also pointed out that an anterior angulation osteotomy of the distal humerus in a distal-third or lower transhumeral amputee can facilitate rotational control of a body-powered prosthesis.[7]

Treatment

The challenges of treatment are to restore function and to remember not only that "cosmesis is a function" (AB Swanson, personal communication, 1988) but also that function can be cosmetic. In other words, a limb—no matter how different it appears from the usual form—is less noticeable when it is functioning (Figure 4).

Tactile sensation, or sensibility, is key to upper limb function. Presently, there is no effective way to provide sensibility prosthetically, despite promising ongoing research over the past 25 to 30 years. However, with the increasing use of microprocessors, pursuit of sensory feedback is likely to yield some commercially available products within the decade. Although prosthetic advances continue to decrease the weight of the prosthesis, lessen noise, and improve comfort, because of the complexity of upper limb function, upper limb devices cannot provide or restore function to the extent that lower limb prostheses do at their level. As Dr. Robert

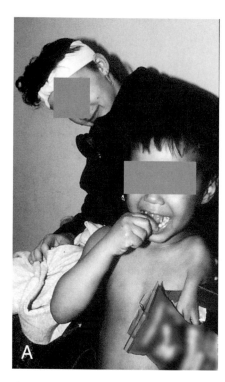 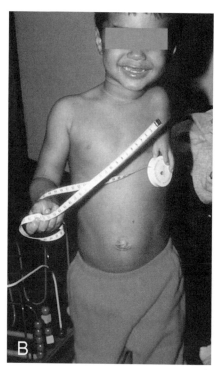

Figure 4 Child with phocomelic left arm. **A,** Holding a bag of chips with smaller arm. **B,** Using a tape measure.

Gillespie pointed out in 1981, "In the case of the upper extremity…the combination of strength and incredibly fine dexterity which characterize the human hand are painfully lacking in any currently available prosthesis. Furthermore, the quality of sensation is so vital to dexterity that a feeble pair of digits in the end of a very short arm are likely to be of more use to the patient than would an elaborate prosthesis."[8] This situation will likely continue for some time to come.

The functional challenges to children with upper limb loss vary with age and increase with more proximal level of loss. Children with a congenital or early acquired unilateral upper limb loss, even at the transhumeral level or higher, quickly become independent in skills of daily living without a prosthesis. However, if fitted with a prosthesis early, they will learn for themselves which tasks are easier to accomplish with a prosthesis and will determine their own unique wearing preferences.[9]

Children with bilateral upper limb loss have more significant challenges

and will benefit from developing foot function, if they have usable (prehensile) feet. They may also benefit from prosthetic fitting of one or both arms, but their families should understand from the beginning that the child's feet can become his or her hands.[10] The foot can become so dexterous that many people who watch the child will forget that the child is using a foot, not a hand (Figures 5 and 6).

This means that the feet need to be free to be used from the beginning and the child should be encouraged to use them. As Herring said, these children "should wear socks as often as the rest of us wear gloves—that is, only when outside in the cold."[11] Shoes that are easy to slip in and out of facilitate this function. For children with quadrimembral limb differences, it is equally important to maintain the feet, ie, refrain from amputating—even if amputation would make fitting lower limb prostheses easier—until it is clear that the feet will not be necessary for prehension.

Many families of children who lose arms or are born without one or both arms are immediately interested in re-

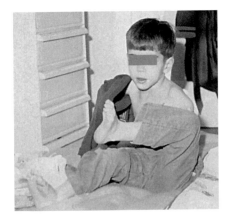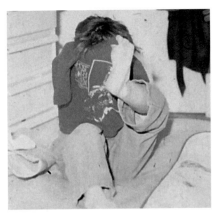

Figure 5 Boy with bilateral congenital humeral deficiencies, partial, donning shirt with feet.

storing how the children looked or were expected to look. This is an emotional response that the treatment team must thoroughly understand; the treatment team must gently but promptly help the patients and families realize that full cosmetic or functional restoration of an upper limb is simply not possible. Even the best cosmetic and functional prosthetic hands available do not approach the appearance of a normal hand in function. Acceptable cosmesis varies widely from person to person. Simply having something to fill the sleeve may be enough to meet the emotional needs of an individual or family at a particular time. At another time, that same person or family may find that an active prosthesis will provide an ease of function not otherwise attainable.

Prosthetic Considerations

Clinical studies reveal varying levels of results and patient acceptance of upper limb prostheses, complicating the decision as to which type of rehabilitation protocol might be appropriate for a particular individual. In addition to multiple component, design, and control options, there are varied approaches across the country, from early-fit programs guided by age of the patient to programs that fit specific prostheses only when requested by the family. These approaches are very different, illustrating that there appears to be no one most appropriate method of treating a child with an upper limb deficiency, particularly at the humeral level.

To facilitate a successful prosthetic outcome, occupational therapy must be incorporated throughout all phases of pediatric upper limb prosthetic treatment. Visits to the therapist and prosthetist to monitor function and provide additional training related to the child's development should occur several times a year. The complete involvement of parents and family as an integral part of the rehabilitation team is absolutely critical to success, and the team needs to be aware of changes in the patient's needs as his or her development progresses.

General Prosthetic Options

Prosthetic options for the pediatric transhumeral level include passive, body-powered, electronic (including options such as myoelectric and various switching strategies), hybrids that combine electric and body power, and customized or activity-specific prostheses. Alternatively, the decision not to fit a prosthesis unless and until the child finds a reason to use one is of course realistic and defensible. Most of these approaches are described well in other chapters, whether devoted to pediatric or adult upper limb prosthetic designs. These options are ex-

actly the same general options that are available for the transradial level or any upper limb absence. At the transhumeral level, the key differences are socket design and the child's missing elbow.

Transhumeral Socket Designs for Children

At the heart of transhumeral prosthetic management is the socket. The socket lays the foundation for the prosthesis and should be viewed as the starting point for appropriate prosthetic management. In contrast to adults, in whom atrophy often occurs through prosthetic use, limbs of pediatric patients are growing both in circumference and length. Some initial atrophy may be seen in acquired limb loss, however. Another potential socket problem with the humeral level deficiency in children is that the humerus has a greater tendency for bony overgrowth than do other bones.

Many authors have offered suggestions for dealing with these growth issues, including the use of removable layers (the "onionized" socket approach) originally proposed by Sauter and associates[12] for radial level deficiency. These are also known as slip sockets and can be used in some cases at a transhumeral level (Figure 7). More recently, Schuch[13] mentioned use of the Utah Dynamic Socket for the pediatric patient. This socket design, described by Andrew,[14] provides a much more progressive socket approach. This advance is similar to the transition that has occurred from quadrilateral transfemoral socket designs to more anatomic ischial containment designs.

The Utah Dynamic Socket and its variations have several unique features (Figure 8). These socket designs do not extend up to or past the acromion as do traditional humeral designs. This lateral socket trimline is often between the axilla and the acromion, allowing more range of motion for humeral abduction. Its aggressive contours within the deltopectoral and

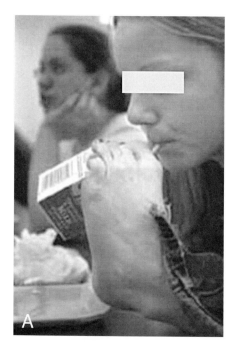

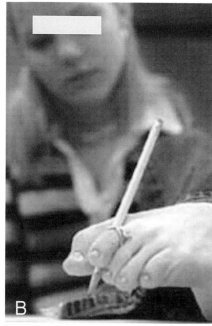

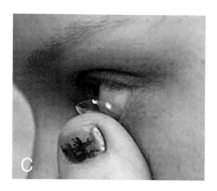

Figure 6 Young woman with total bilateral congenital transverse upper limb deficiencies. **A,** Drinking milk at school. **B,** Writing. **C,** Putting in contact lens. *(Reproduced with permission from* The Flint Journal/*Lisa DeJong, Flint, MI.)*

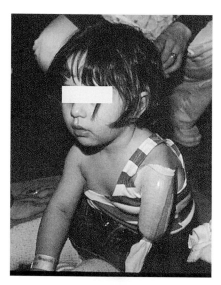

Figure 7 Two-year-old girl with traumatic high transhumeral amputation in initial socket fitting. Socket was made multilayered for growth (slip socket). Note similar trimline to Figure 8, *B.*

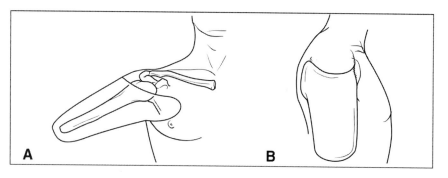

Figure 8 Range of motion and comfort are enhanced with the dynamic anatomic contoured socket. **A,** The dynamic anatomic contoured socket stabilizes the humerus and allows for less restrictive range of motion during abduction. **B,** The aggressive anterior-posterior contours help stabilize the socket against rotation, thus reducing harnessing requirements.

scapular anatomic regions enhance rotational stability, often resulting in less restrictive harnessing.

Anderson[15] noted that the use of thermoplastics with the pediatric population allows for ease of adjustments for growth. Combining this progressive socket design with the use of thermoplastics (inner flexible liners and outer rigid frames), residual limb changes resulting from growth

can often be accommodated. Retention of a bivalve duplication of the patient's socket can help with growth modifications (Figure 9). A positive model of this bivalve mold is then poured, and modifications can be made as growth dictates. By adding plaster in regions of bony growth, the inner flexible socket can then be heated and reformed about the newly rectified model. This flexible socket is then placed inside the prosthetic frame, allowing for growth of the residual limb. This method allows for specific adjustments as needed instead of global expansion of the prosthetic interface.

The use of gel locking liners has provided an effective means of suspension and growth management for the pediatric amputee (Figure 10, *A*). Often the prosthetic socket will be fabricated with a predetermined amount of socks that can be removed from the fitting as a child grows. Also, as the child grows, the silicone liner expands (Figure 10, *B*), maintaining suspension and comfort to the residual limb. Removable distal pads are another way of adapting the sock to growth or bone overgrowth. The primary goal of socket management is to provide a stable prosthetic interface that maintains suspension and

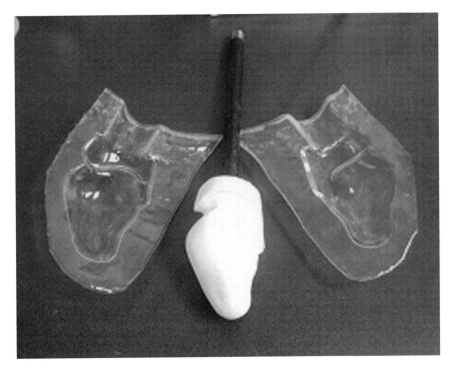

Figure 9 The bivalve model socket (the transradial model is shown here) is formed by vacuum-forming over the positive model, using two pieces of copolyester with the film intact. The film prevents the plastic from sticking together during the vacuuming and facilitates easy removal from the positive model.

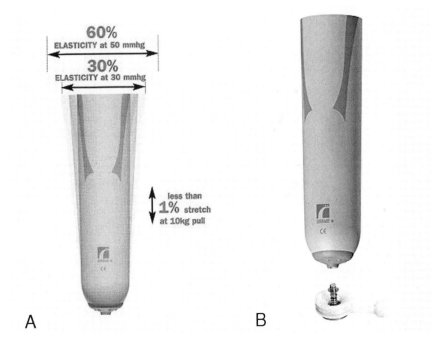

60%
ELASTICITY at 50 mmhg

30%
ELASTICITY at 30 mmhg

less than
1% stretch
at 10kg pull

A   B

Figure 10 The increased use of silicone suspension sleeves with upper limb patients has influenced manufacturers to fabricate liners specifically for the individual with upper limb deficiency. **A,** This liner specifically made for upper limb deficiency has enhanced elasticity that can accommodate circumferential growth. Reinforcement within the liner prevents excessive elongation under load. **B,** Upper limb liners use smaller, low-profile shuttle locks, which allow use with children in whom component clearance is important. (Courtesy of Ossur).

comfort as the child's residual limb develops.

Elbow Control Options

Regardless of the terminal device (passive, myoelectric, hook, etc), the child with a transhumeral level deficiency has the added challenge of lacking an anatomic elbow with which to move and place the terminal device in space. As with adults, the length of the child's residual limb makes a difference. For example, an elbow disarticulation provides greater rotational control than is possible at higher levels, as well as a longer lever arm for operating the prosthesis and the added benefit of epicondyles over which to suspend the socket. If the child intends to use a body-powered terminal device for prehension, then it follows that the shorter the level of amputation, the greater the challenge.

Few prosthetic elbows are truly designed for children. Most are just downsized versions of the adult components. Essentially the same choices are available—outside hinges for longer levels, passive or friction elbows, body- or electric-powered.

When fitting infants, many centers will choose not to provide a movable elbow at all. They will simply preflex the elbow at 90° or more so that the passive hand or other terminal device is ideally positioned for bimanual activities such as holding a bottle. Later, when there is sufficient space and the child has adapted to using the terminal device, an appropriate movable elbow can be added. Friction elbows allow the child, parent, or therapist to flex or rotate the elbow against adjustable friction settings in order to optimize the position of the terminal device for a certain activity. The child can learn to do this either by reaching over with the other hand or by other means such as nudging the prosthetic forearm against an object or another part of the body, such as the leg. The passive friction elbow is ideal for training a young child to use a terminal device before learning to use a cable-operated or electronic elbow. It is also a reasonable long-term alter-

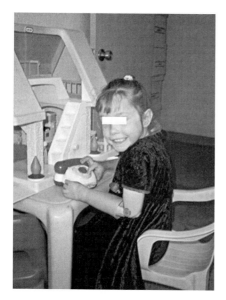

Figure 11 Child using a hybrid prosthesis, with a body-powered elbow and an electric-powered hand.

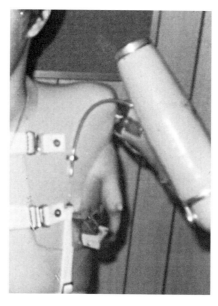

Figure 12 Boy with bilateral upper limb deficiencies and single left phocomelic digit, which can control prosthetic switches. (The prosthetic arm is abducted and its elbow is fully flexed to allow a better view of the digit.)

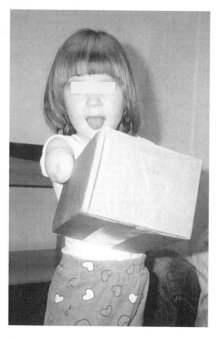

Figure 13 Girl with right congenital transverse humeral deficiency, distal third, holding box.

native, mostly for unilateral amputees who do not wish to bother with the added cables, harnesses, or extra weight of other elbows. Friction elbows are available in pediatric, adolescent, and adult sizes. Disadvantages are obvious; the elbow functions less naturally and can be moved only in the ways described. Also, the friction setting may give way against heavier objects held in the terminal device.

Elbow options, such as electric-powered, body-powered, or hybrid combinations of an electronic hand and body-powered elbow or vice versa, are described in other chapters in this book. Hybrid designs (Figure 11) offer particular advantages to children around age 5 or 6 years, who are capable of being trained to use a completely body-powered terminal device and elbow system yet may lack sufficient strength or excursion to move the arm through its complete range of elbow flexion and terminal device operation.[16-18]

Terminal device operation should generally be taught before elbow function. Criteria for determining when children are ready to learn to use a terminal device are described in chapter 66, which also describes the sequence of progression for a child

from a preflexed or locked elbow to one that is controlled by cable and harness. When to use an electronic elbow is less clear, but is likely to follow the same readiness criteria. Often an electronic elbow is added when the child needs and understands how to control an elbow, yet lacks the means to do so other than with a motorized system.[13,17]

Unique Considerations and Options

Although the recommendations in this chapter are general, there are some unique considerations for children, specifically those with phocomelic limbs and/or bilateral absences. A child with a phocomelic limb (Figure 12) may be able to use hand or digit function to operate the prosthesis by using switches or Force Sensing Resistor technology.[3] The phocomelic limb often retains prehension and sensation, even though some can be flail or very weak. Therefore, the team should carefully consider whether prosthetic use is appropriate versus the sole use of the phocomelic limb.

For the patient with bilateral humeral deficiency, debates about fitting one limb or both are common. Herring[11] discusses the use of active grasp with the residual limb (Figure 13). Children who can reach the midline with their limbs are more likely to be able to feed themselves independently, in contrast to those with shorter reach.

Children with multiple limb absence have decreased body surface area and therefore experience difficulty with heat dissipation. This may limit the amount of body surface that can be safely and practically covered with prostheses. It is also important to not overwhelm a child with technology. Pediatric specialists often hold to the motto of "keep it simple" for children. Just because varying levels of limb presentations can be fitted with electronics and different assistive devices does not necessarily mean that this should be done or that it is appropriate for every person. For the individual with bilateral upper limb loss and normal feet, the use of the feet in activities of daily living must be encouraged and taught (Figures 5 and 6).

Conclusion

Because the perceptions of children and their parents of the need to use a prosthesis will change as the child grows, it is important to monitor and evaluate the child's needs from infancy through adulthood. The use of different outcome measures and evaluation tools can aid in this task.[19,20]

As children develop, they may opt to discontinue prosthetic use for a time or permanently. The treatment team needs to understand the variability of the child's needs over time and appreciate the fact that most children with upper limb deficiencies will at some point want not to use a prosthesis, or to use it only for certain activities. The experienced comprehensive prosthetic team realizes that this may not necessarily indicate a failure of the prosthesis; rather, it is often just a developmental stage of the child. Failure can result when the prosthetic team does not continue to follow the patient, leading to missed developmental milestones and opportunities when a prosthesis, prosthetic modification, or therapy technique could enhance the maturing child's function.

Prompt adjustment for growth as well as accommodation for the patient's current circumstances are key. Other team members must be available for the patient and family when they want to discuss changes or a new or different need. They should work toward satisfying that need, whether the answer is prosthetic, an adaptation of the child's environment, specific tools, or training. The answer to a functional problem is not always purely prosthetic. Experienced team members may have new options to offer, but very often the patient can be instructive to the team.

There is currently a renewed focus on development of new upper limb prosthetic components for the pediatric population. The use of microprocessors in electronic components provides several new benefits. Research protocols require a more comprehensive analysis of the variables that affect upper limb prosthetic use in children. Rehabilitation team responsiveness, comfort of the prosthesis, age-appropriate attention, and psychological issues should all be thoughtfully considered. Experience and expertise are critical to the success of pediatric upper limb deficiency programs.

Acknowledgments

We are grateful to Don Cummings, CP; Sheila Hubbard, OTR; John Miguelez, CP; and Joanna Patton, OTR, for content review and professional input. We also thank Julie Lake for literary review and editing and Jerry King for help with pictures.

References

1. Schuch CM, Pritham CH: International Standards Organization Terminology: Application to prosthetics and orthotics. *J Prosthet Orthot* 1994;6: 29-33.

2. Goldberg MJ (ed): *The Dysmorphic Child: An Orthopedic Perspective.* New York, NY, Raven Press, 1987, pp 301, 324-357.

3. Sullivan RA, Celikyol F: The functional use of phocomelic and digital appendages. *Inter-Clin Info Bull* 1976; 15:1-8.

4. Adams WP Jr, Hobar PC: Surgical treatment of meningococcal-induced purpura fulminans, in Herring JA, Birch JG (eds): *The Child With a Limb Deficiency.* Rosemont, IL, American Academy of Orthopaedic Surgeons, 1998, pp 447-454.

5. Marquardt E, Correll J: Amputations and prostheses for the lower limb. *Int Orthop* 1984;8:139-146.

6. Davids JR: Terminal bony overgrowth of the residual limb: Current management strategies, in Herring JA, Birch JG (eds): *The Child With a Limb Deficiency.* Rosemont, IL, American Academy of Orthopaedic Surgeons, 1998, pp 269-280.

7. Marquardt E: The multiple limb-deficient child, in American Academy of Orthopaedic Surgeons (eds): *Atlas of Limb Prosthetics: Surgical and Prosthetic Principles.* St. Louis, MO, CV Mosby, 1981, pp 595-641.

8. Gillespie R: Congenital limb deformities and amputation surgery in children, in Kostuik JP, Gillespie R (eds): *Amputation Surgery and Rehabilitation: The Toronto Experience.* New York, NY, Churchill Livingstone, 1981, p 115.

9. Hubbard SA, Kurtz I, Heim W, Montgomery G: Powered prosthetic intervention in upper extremity deficiency, in Herring JA, Birch JG (eds): *The Child With a Limb Deficiency.* Rosemont, IL, American Academy of Orthopaedic Surgeons, 1998, pp 417-431.

10. Wilke HH (ed): *Using Everything You've Got.* Chicago, IL, National Easter Seal Society for Crippled Children and Adults, 1984.

11. Herring JA: Functional assessment and management of multilimb deficiency, in Herring JA, Birch JG (eds): *The Child With a Limb Deficiency.* Rosemont, IL, American Academy of Orthopaedic Surgeons, 1998, pp 437-445.

12. Sauter WF, Dakpa R, Galway R, Hubbard S, Hamilton E: Development of layered "onionized" silicone sockets for juvenile below elbow amputees. *J Assoc Child Prosthet Orthot Clin* 1987; 22:57-59.

13. Schuch CM: Prosthetic principles in fitting myoelectric prostheses in children, in Herring JA, Birch JG (eds): *The Child With a Limb Deficiency.* Rosemont, IL, American Academy of Orthopaedic Surgeons, 1998, pp 405-416.

14. Andrew JT: Elbow disarticulation and transhumeral amputation: Prosthetic principles, in Bowker JH, Michael JW (eds): *Atlas of Limb Prosthetics: Surgical, Prosthetic, and Rehabilitation Principles,* ed 2. Rosemont, IL, American Academy of Orthopaedic Surgeons, 2002, pp 255-264. (Originally published by Mosby-Year Book, 1992.)

15. Anderson T: Thermoplastic and lamination, in *Pediatric Orthotics and Prosthetic Pediatric Management Certificate course.* American Academy of Orthotics and Prosthetics, 2001.

16. Brenner CD: Electronic limbs for infants and pre-school children. *J Prosthet Orthot* 1992;4:24-30.

17. Lake C, Miguelez J: Comparative analysis of microprocessors in upper limb prosthetics. *J Prosthet Orthot* 2003;15: 48-63.

18. Wise M: Upper extremity prosthetic rehabilitation, in Lusardi MM, Nielsen CC (eds): *Orthotics and Prosthetics in Rehabilitation,* ed 2. Philadelphia, PA, Butterworth-Heinemann, in press.

19. Wright FV, Hubbard S, Jutai J, Naumann S: The prosthetic upper extremity functional index: Development and reliability testing of a new functional status questionnaire for children who use upper extremity prostheses. *J Hand Ther* 2001;14:91-104.

20. McCarthy ML, Silberstein CE, Atkins EA, Harryman SE, Sponseller PD, Hadley-Miller NA: Comparing reliability and validity of pediatric instruments for measuring health and well-being of children with spastic cerebral palsy. *Dev Med Child Neurol* 2002; 44:468-476.

Chapter 73

Foot Deficiencies

Mary Williams Clark, MD

Introduction

Partial foot deficiencies in children may be congenital or acquired. Congenital differences and deficiencies that are acquired in utero may be associated with other anomalies in syndromes and may or may not be heritable; therefore, thorough examination of the child is important. Syndromes known to involve foot deficiencies include ectrodactyly-ectodermal dysplasia-clefting, Adams-Oliver, and a group of syndromes (Moebius and six others) known together as oromandibular-limb hypogenesis spectrum.[1-3] Hand deficiencies are also common with these syndromes. Split-hand/split-foot syndrome, often inherited in an autosomal dominant pattern, may require special shoes, orthotic assistance, or occasionally prosthetic assistance (Figure 1).

Acquired losses of the foot in children and young adults are most frequently the result of accidental trauma; for example, lawnmower accidents affect more than 9,000 children per year in the United States. Loss of toes and larger parts of the feet also result from gunshot wounds, frostbite, and burns.[4,5]

Malignancies account for another large segment of lower limb loss in children. Only a small number of these children lose just part of a foot.

Vascular causes of partial foot loss include disseminated intravascular coagulopathy (DIC), also known as purpura fulminans, and other ischemic incidents. Intrauterine amputations occur because of amniotic constriction bands and often involve the feet. Other prenatal limb losses may be related to vascular anomalies, disruption by emboli, abnormalities in perfusion, hypotension, or hypertension.[6]

Incidence

In an 18-year survey of more than one million births in British Columbia, foot deficiencies were documented in 0.26 cases per 10,000 live births.[7] Among these patients, 26% also had anomalies outside of the musculoskeletal system. The reported incidence of all reduction deformities of limbs (ICD-9 classifications 755.2 through 755.4) was 0.25 in 1,000 total births in Hungary in a 6-year study that included stillbirths.[8]

Levels of Deficiencies

Congenital absences of toes, rays, and/or tarsal bones often occur with bony coalitions in the remaining part of the foot. The split-hand/split-foot syndrome produces variations of deficiency; some patients will need orthoses or prostheses and some will require surgical modification to facilitate shoe wear (Figure 2).

Congenital deficiencies at midtarsal (Chopart) and tarsometatarsal (Lisfranc) levels occur and may be developmental or the result of amniotic rupture sequence. Bands also may produce irregular longitudinal levels, missing toes, or missing parts of metatarsals and their rays. Lawnmower accidents and DIC also can destroy portions of the foot in irregular ways.

Surgical Techniques for Children

In children younger than 8 or 9 years of age, after trauma or DIC, it is often best to maintain all viable parts of the foot rather than convert the remaining foot to a standard partial-foot level. These children usually heal rapidly and are still growing; therefore, they may retain good function with the remaining part of the foot.[9-11] Tendons should be salvaged and rebalanced if necessary, taking care to preserve the anterior tibialis tendon. The anterior tibialis tendon should be attached to a remaining navicular or talar neck. In young children, this can be done with suture; in an older child, it can be placed in a drill hole. An Achilles tendon lengthening (percutaneous) should be considered to help prevent future equinus deformity. The foot should be casted in approximately 5° of dorsiflexion and be subtalar-neutral.

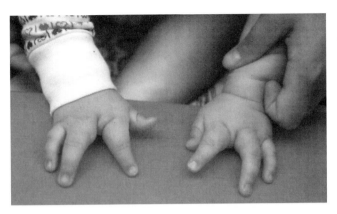
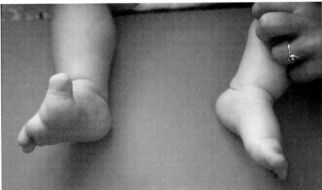

Figure 1 A 2-year-old boy with bilateral split hands and split feet. No special footwear is needed at this age.

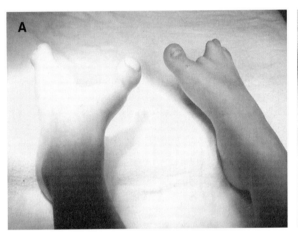
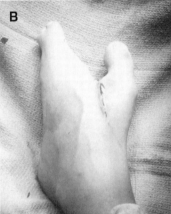
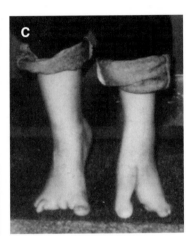

Figure 2 **A,** A 9-year-old boy with split-hand/split-foot syndrome is no longer able to wear his left shoe because of the fixed angle of rays from the midfoot, with a midtarsal coalition. **B,** Narrower foot after midtarsal resection. **C,** Several months after surgery, the patient is able to wear regular shoes and can toe-stand.

Marquardt[12] points out that transfer of the anterior tibialis alone to the talus may leave the calcaneus unbalanced by the pull of the remaining triceps surae, producing instability of the subtalar joint. He recommends placing the common extensor tendons into the anterior calcaneus.

If diaphyseal transection and loss of a metatarsal or phalanx has occurred, salvage of any available metatarsal head (or a phalanx with an intact joint surface) may allow capping of the diaphyseal end of the bone to prevent future distal overgrowth problems (Figure 3, *A*). Parts of the injured foot that cannot be covered by remaining skin can often granulate well in a vacuum-assisted closure system.[13-15] Thin split-thickness grafts that contract later can be used, pulling more mobile remaining skin to cover weight-bearing surfaces (Figure 3, *B* and *C*).

Heel pads often are amputated in lawnmower injuries, while some of the forefoot remains. The preserved dorsal, medial, or even lateral skin of the foot can be moved as a flap, and careful prosthetic fitting will allow weight bearing and hypertrophy. Early postoperative weight bearing can be facilitated by a temporary reinforced "orthoprosthesis" that is constructed with closed-cell moldable foam.

Prosthetic Treatment

The growth potential of children, the rapidity of their healing, and their relatively low body weight all facilitate prosthetic fitting of a partial foot. They may be managed with relatively simple prostheses or "prosthoses" (a combination of foot orthosis with a prosthetic section). As the child grows, the foot remnant becomes proportionally shorter compared with the normal intact foot, and the prosthesis may need to provide greater support. Body weight over the weight-bearing area of the foot increases, and modifications may become necessary for skin protection, better rollover during gait, and/or a more natural appearance. Commonly used prosthoses associated with selected levels of absence are summarized below.

Toe or Longitudinal Partial Ray

Young children may need only a soft insert (toe filler) in the shoe. Others may not even require that, showing

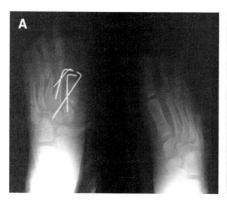
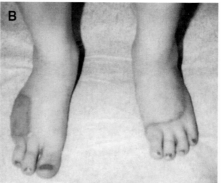
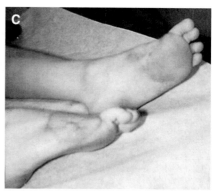

Figure 3 In a lawnmower accident, a 5-year-old girl sustained multiple open fractures and toe amputations, including loss of the distal four fifths of the first left metatarsal and the right lateral two toes with metatarsal heads. The amputated toes were brought from the scene of the accident in saline gauze. The left first metatarsal head with its cartilage intact was salvaged and used to cap the residual base of the first metatarsal to try to prevent distal bony overgrowth. The physis at the base of the first left metatarsal was grossly intact. **A,** Postoperative radiograph. Photographs taken 3 months after the injury show the healed left dorsalis pedis rotation flap covering the capped first metatarsal remnant and healed right lateral split-thickness skin graft **(B),** which is shrinking dorsally and pulling plantar skin over the weight-bearing surface **(C).**

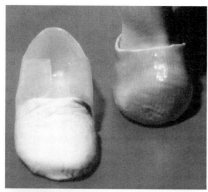

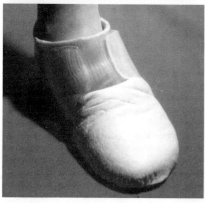

Figure 4 A 3-year-old girl sustained a Lisfranc-level amputation in a lawnmower accident. Distal plantar skin was used for closure. This low-profile partial foot prosthesis for Lisfranc level has a flexible silicone liner and copolymer slipper with distal filler attached.

no significant differences in gait, including running. As the child's height, weight, and disproportional foot shortening increase, a slipper-type University of California Biomechanics Laboratory (UCBL) shell or a molded plastic ankle-foot orthosis (AFO) with a custom filler may be needed.

Transmetatarsal

For transmetatarsal absences, children will need a UCBL orthosis with a toe-piece attached or an AFO. A stiffer yet still flexible distal footplate is necessary to allow good transition to late toe-off in gait.

Lisfranc (Tarsometatarsal) and Chopart (Midtarsal)

Several designs exist for these levels, including slipper-style low-trimline prostheses.[16,17] These often work well in young children (Figure 4), who often need to transition to a higher, sturdier prosthesis as they grow, such as an AFO with forefoot filler or a split rigid laminate with a prosthetic foot.

Summary

Acquired and congenital foot deficiencies in children may need prosthetic management to achieve optimal function. A prosthesis may work well in younger children (younger than 8 or 9 years), but the design may need to be modified to a different type as the child's weight and height increase. Surgical modification may also become necessary. Children injured at older ages may be best served by amputation at standard adult levels, that is, the midtarsal, tarsometatarsal, or Syme level.

References

1. Goldberg M: *The Dysmorphic Child: An Orthopedic Perspective.* New York, NY, Raven Press, 1987, pp 33-36, 333-335, 348-350.

2. McKusick VA (ed): *Mendelian Inheritance in Man: A Catalog of Human Genes and Genetic Disorders,* ed 12. Baltimore, MD, Johns Hopkins University Press, 1998.

3. Smith GA: American Academy of Pediatrics, Committee on Injury and Poison Prevention: Technical report. Lawn mower-related injuries to children. *Pediatr* 2001;107:E106. http://pediatrics.aapublications.org/cgi/content/full/107/6/e106. Accessed June 23, 2004.

4. Setoguchi Y, Rosenfelder R: *The Limb Deficient Child.* Springfield, IL, Charles C. Thomas, 1982, pp 46-47.

5. Letts M, Davidson D: Epidemiology and prevention of traumatic amputations in children, in Herring JA, Birch JG (eds): *The Child With a Limb Deficiency.* Rosemont, IL, American Academy of Orthopaedic Surgeons, 1998, pp 235-251.

6. Weaver DD: Vascular etiology of limb defects: The subclavian artery supply disruption sequence, in Herring JA, Birch JG (eds): *The Child With a Limb Deficiency*. Rosemont, IL, American Academy of Orthopaedic Surgeons, 1998, pp 25-27.

7. Wilson GN: Heritable limb deficiencies, in Herring JA, Birch JG (eds): *The Child With a Limb Deficiency*. Rosemont, IL, American Academy of Orthopaedic Surgeons, 1998, pp 39-43.

8. Czeizel A, Tusnády G: *Aetiological Studies of Isolated Common Congenital Abnormalities in Hungary*. Budapest, Hungary, Akademiai Kiadó, 1984, p 12.

9. Cummings DR, Kapp SL: Lower-limb pediatric prosthetics. *J Prosthet Orthot* 1992;4:198-206.

10. Graves SC, Brodie JT: Amputations below the knee, in Mizel MS, Miller RA, Scioli MW (eds): *Orthopaedic Knowledge Update: Foot & Ankle 2*. Rosemont, IL, American Academy of Orthopaedic Surgeons, 1998, pp 305-314.

11. Greene WB, Cary JM: Partial foot amputations in children: A comparison of the several types with the Syme amputation. *J Bone Joint Surg Am* 1982;64:438-443.

12. Marquardt E: Die Chopart-Exartikulation mit Tenomyoplastik. *Z Orthop* 1973;111:584-586.

13. Argenta LC, Morykwas MJ: Vacuum-assisted closure: A new method for wound control and treatment. Clinical experience. *Ann Plast Surg* 1997;38:563-576.

14. Mooney JF III, Argenta LC, Marks MW, Morykwas MJ, DeFranzo AJ: Treatment of soft tissue defects in pediatric patients using the V.A.C. system. *Clin Orthop* 2000;376:26-31.

15. Webb LX: New techniques in wound management: Vacuum-assisted wound closure. *J Am Acad Orthop Surg* 2002;10:303-311.

16. Clark MW, Rosenberger R: Abstract: Low-profile partial foot prosthesis. *J Assoc Child Prosthet-Orthot Clin* 1986;21:27.

17. Pullen JJ: A low profile paediatric partial foot. *Prosthet Orthot Int* 1987;11:137-138.

Chapter 74

Fibular Deficiencies

Gerard L. Glancy, MD

Introduction

Fibular deficiency is a congenital abnormality of unknown etiology characterized by shortening of the leg and deformity of the foot, both of which are usually apparent at birth. The condition is neither inherited nor transmissible and is regarded as an isolated, sporadic occurrence. Fibular deficiency may also have a very mild "forme fruste" presentation in which the feet are normal. This condition may not be noticed until later in life, when limb-length discrepancy is observed (Figure 1).

Initial Evaluation

Initial evaluation begins with a complete orthopaedic examination. Particular attention should be paid to the status of the ankle and foot, limb-length discrepancy, and any associated conditions. The foot should be evaluated with respect to the number of rays, the alignment and motion of the hindfoot, and the stability of the ankle. A stiff hindfoot implies the presence of a tarsal coalition. Because fibular deficiencies are accompanied by a delay in the ossification of the bones of the foot, the tarsal coalition may not be visible on radiographs until later in life. Fewer rays and greater ankle valgus are associated with more severe fibular deficiency.[1] In one reported series of patients, all feet with three toes or less had tarsal coalitions.[2] A ball-and-socket ankle

results as an adaptive change to tarsal coalition. The tibia may have a bow with a dimple over the apex. The apex of the bow is usually anteromedial (procurvatum).

AP and lateral radiographs of both of the entire lower limbs, including the hips, knees, and ankles, are usually sufficient to classify and formulate a treatment plan. The determination of the initial length discrepancy, which is calculated as a percentage difference from the opposite side, is of particular importance (Figure 2). In general, fibular deficiencies follow a Shapiro type I pattern, in which the percentage of limb-length difference remains constant throughout the child's growing years.[3] The percentage of tibial shortening does not correlate with the degree of fibular absence.[1,2] On occasion, MRI may be helpful to determine the status of unossified foot bones or the presence of a cartilaginous anlage of an unossified fibula.

Associated Problems

The affected limb may also demonstrate hypoplasia of the lateral femoral condyle and laxity of the knee. The anterior cruciate ligament (ACL) is frequently deficient,[4] and the patella may be small and high riding. The condition most commonly associated with fibular deficiency is partial longitudinal deficiency of the

femur (LDFP, previously called proximal focal femoral deficiency, or PFFD). The presence of LDFP compounds the problem of overall extremity length. Clubfoot, a variety of hand anomalies, and congenital kyphosis or scoliosis also may occur. Other organ systems are usually not affected.

Classification

The classification of Achterman and Kalamchi[1] (Table 1) divides fibular deficiency into two types. In type 1 the fibula is present, and in type 2 it is absent. Letts's classification (Table 2) accounts for the projected discrepancy in length at maturity and considers the conditions of the foot and ankle[5] (Figure 3). The severity of the length discrepancy does not necessar-

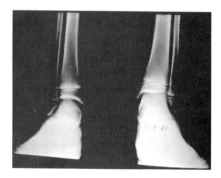

Figure 1 AP radiograph of a 12-year-old patient with "forme fruste" fibular deficiency shows mild limb-length discrepancy and a ball-and-socket ankle.

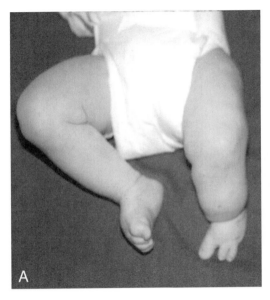
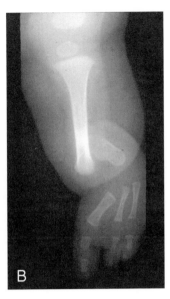

Figure 2 Child with fibular deficiency. **A,** Clinical photograph showing the three-toed valgus foot and the prominent anterior/medial bow of the tibia with a dimple. **B,** Radiograph of the affected leg.

TABLE 1 Achterman and Kalamchi Classification of Fibular Deficiencies

Type	Characteristics
1	Fibula present
1a	Physis of proximal fibula distal to proximal tibial physis Distal fibular physis proximal to dome of talus
1b	Only partial fibula present
2	Fibula absent

TABLE 2 Letts Classification of Fibular Deficiencies

Type	Characteristics
A	Affected side < 10% shorter than opposite side Discrepancy projected to be < 6 cm at maturity Foot nearly normal Minimal femoral shortening
B	Affected side 10% to 20% shorter than opposite side Discrepancy projected to be 6 to 10 cm at maturity Minimal foot deformities Minimal femoral shortening
C	Affected side ≥ 30% shorter than opposite side Discrepancy projected to be ≥ 10 cm at maturity Severe foot deformity Severe femoral shortening
D	Bilateral fibular deficiency or partial longitudinal deficiency of the femur

ily correspond with the presence or absence of a fibula, and some limbs with severe projected shortening can have a reasonably good ankle and foot (ie, minimal valgus, no instability,

and plantar grade) (Figure 4). The most important determinant for treatment is projected length discrepancy. Type A fibular deficiency would be treated with a shoe lift and type B

with leg equalization procedures. For type C, most experts recommend amputation of the foot, though this is controversial.

The Birch classification focuses on the quality of the foot (Table 3). If the foot is or can be surgically treated to meet the criteria above, then management of the limb-length discrepancy is determined by the projected discrepancy at maturity. Thus, a Birch type IA foot would have an epiphysiodesis, if anything at all. A type IB foot would have either an epiphysiodesis or a single episode of lengthening. A Birch type IC foot could have one or two episodes of lengthening or an amputation. A Birch type ID foot could be considered for more than two episodes of lengthening, but in these cases amputation is most commonly recommended.

Stanitski and Stanitski[3] have recently proposed a new classification system based not only on fibular appearance but also ankle morphology (horizontal, valgus, or spherical), number of rays, and the presence of a tarsal coalition. They believe that the presence or absence of a fibula should not be the sole determinant of treatment options;[6,7] if a stable ankle with a mobile foot that can withstand more than one lengthening procedure is present, good limb function will ultimately result.

As noted in Letts's classification, the problem most commonly associated with fibular deficiency is LDFP. If LDFP is combined with fibular deficiency, the length discrepancy issues are magnified, as is the likelihood of knee instability because of congenital absence of the ACL. LDFP usually follows a Shapiro type I pattern, but it also sometimes follows a Shapiro type II or III pattern.

Treatment Options

Available options include no treatment, the use of a shoe lift or a step-in nonstandard (equinus) prosthesis, epiphysiodesis, ankle reconstruction, limb lengthening, and foot amputation. Before a treatment plan

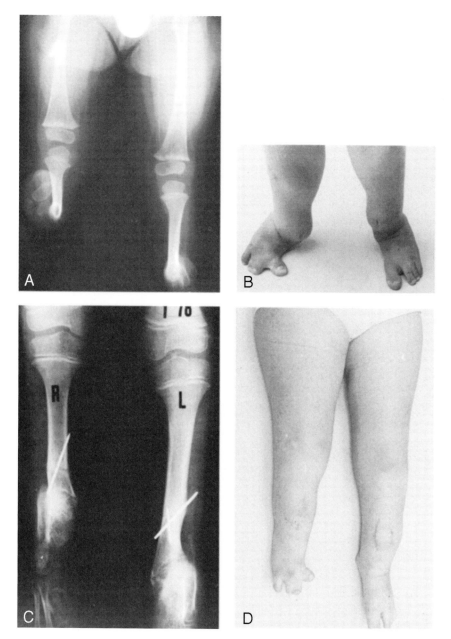

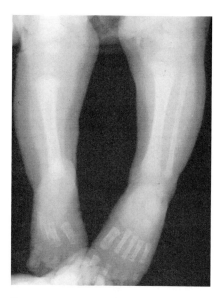

Figure 4 AP radiograph of a patient with type II Kalamchi, type B Letts, Birch type IC fibular deficiency. Note the absent fibula, 20% growth inhibition, and five-toed equinovarus foot.

Figure 3 A, AP radiograph of a patient with a Letts type D or Birch type II fibular deficiency shows a longitudinal deficiency of the fibula bilaterally with some shortening of the right femur and considerable shortening of the right tibia. B, Clinical photograph shows classic anteromedial bowing of the lower limbs with a dimple of the skin and absence of the fifth ray, severe equinus, and a valgus deformity at the ankle. C, AP radiograph obtained after bilateral tibial osteotomy for correction of the deformity. D, The realigned tibias are now much more amenable to prosthetic restoration. Note that differences in the knees persist because of shortening of the right femur.

found that all adult amputees were unable to obtain funding for prostheses.

No Treatment

Parents may refuse treatment for their child for a variety of reasons. One common situation is when the appearance of the foot is nearly normal. The limb-length inequality may not look severe, and the parents may fail to understand that it will become worse with further growth. There may be cultural norms that preclude acceptance of amputation.[6] Some parents want to wait "until the child is able to enter into the decision process." Unfortunately, by the time this occurs, both parent and child are reluctant to give up the foot, regardless of lack of function and severity of limb-length discrepancy. An equinus contracture is also well established by this time, making limb equalization more difficult. A child who is older than 15 years and has a limb with more than 20% shortening and severe ankle equinus should not have a lengthening procedure.[6]

If the parents decide that the child will not be treated, the child may be fit with a nonstandard step-in prosthesis

is determined, parents should be fully informed of the options. They should have an opportunity to meet other families who have a member with fibular deficiency of a similar severity that has been treated. They should also meet with a knowledgeable physical therapist who can provide additional information regarding expectations during the child's growing years. If amputation is selected, preoperative discussions with the intended prosthetist are valuable. Cost considerations may also have an impact on the final decisions regarding treatment, although Birch and associates[8]

TABLE 3 Birch Classification of Fibular Deficiencies

Type		Characteristics
I		Functional foot
	A	0% to 5% predicted limb-length inequality at maturity
	B	6% to 10% predicted limb-length inequality
	C	11% to 30% predicted limb-length inequality
	D	>30% limb-length inequality
II		Nonfunctional foot
	A	Functional upper extremity
	B	Nonfunctional upper extremity

Adapted from Birch JG, Lincoln TL, Mack PW: Functional classification of fibular deficiency, in Herring JA, Birch JG (eds): The Child With a Limb Deficiency. Rosemont, IL, American Academy of Orthopaedic Surgeons, 1998, p 166.

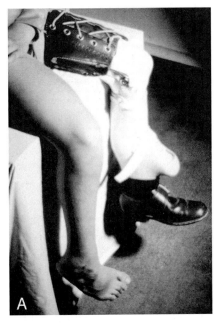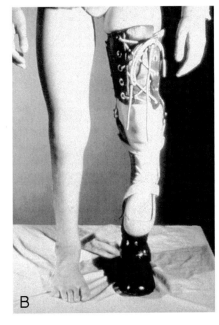

Figure 5 Lateral **(A)** and anterior **(B)** photographs show a nonstandard step-in prosthesis used in patients who elect to forgo surgical treatment. Despite its noncosmetic appearance, the prosthesis is both functional and durable.

If the parents decide that the child will not be treated, the child may be fit with a nonstandard step-in prosthesis (Figure 5). Although this approach may complicate fitting and limit component choices and is not as cosmetic as a Syme or Boyd procedure, the child will nonetheless be able to participate in most normal activities.

Epiphysiodesis

Epiphysiodesis on the longer limb is indicated when the fibular deficiency is mild (Letts type A). An appropriately timed epiphysiodesis will be sufficient in situations in which the discrepancy is predicted to be less than 5 cm. Epiphysiodesis is most often performed with very mild types of fibular deficiency, which are characterized by minor limb-length discrepancy with minimal dysplasia of the lateral aspect of foot and a ball-and-socket ankle, as shown in Figure 1.

Limb Lengthening

Limb lengthening is indicated when the discrepancy is expected to exceed 5 cm but be less than 10 cm at maturity. This applies to patients with Letts type B fibular deficiencies and some with type C deficiencies. The Birch type IB and IC and perhaps ID also apply. Before deciding on foot preservation and limb lengthening, a careful evaluation of the status of the foot and adjacent joints (ankle and knee) is needed. Compared with lengthening performed for conditions with other etiologies, limb lengthening for congenital shortening is associated with a greater incidence of difficulties both during and after the lengthening process.[9] Of particular concern is the response of the ankle and knee joints to the lengthening process because significant loss of motion can result. Procedures to lengthen a limb with a projected discrepancy of more than 30% are associated with a high rate of complications.[10] Congenital discrepancies greater than 15 cm are rarely amenable to lengthening. Although the technical details of limb lengthening are beyond the scope of this chapter, it should be noted that several surgical procedures will be required during childhood. The lengthening program of Catagni[6] may require up to five operations. The first procedure, a soft-tissue release of the ankle, is performed at 3 to 6 months of age. At 5 to 6 years of age, the first tibial lengthening with a foot frame is performed. At 8 to 10 years of age, a second lengthening, which may include femoral osteotomy for lateral condyle hypoplasia, is completed. Finally repeat lengthening is performed, if necessary, at 12 to 13 years of age and at maturity. An ankle arthrodesis may be required. A child with a stable ankle, no tarsal coalition, four or five rays, and a projected discrepancy of less than 20% may be a candidate for lengthening regardless of the presence or absence of a fibula (Figure 3).

Amputation of the Foot

For patients with Letts type C and D or Birch type ID or II fibular deficiencies, the value of early amputation of the foot has been well established.[8,11-15] A Syme[16] or Boyd[17] procedure will produce a tough, resilient residual limb

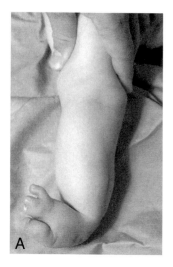
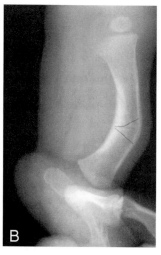
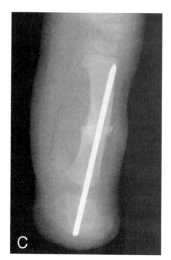
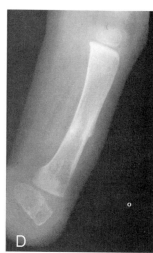

Figure 6 Child with severe fibular deficiency—Kalamchi type II, Letts type C, or Birch type ID. **A,** Clinical appearance. **B,** Radiographic appearance. Note the severe tibial bowing. **C,** Radiographic appearance of affected leg after simultaneous Boyd procedure and correction of tibial bowing. **D,** Radiograph obtained 3 months postoperatively. Amputation is timed to coincide with age of expected independent ambulation (approximately 1 year old patient is ready for the first prosthesis).

that can be fit with a standard prosthesis.[18] This is likely to be the only operation ever performed on the child's limb. The child will be able to participate in all normal activities of childhood and avoid the physical and emotional trauma associated with multiple surgical procedures.[8,10,11]

The decision to amputate should be made early and the procedure performed just prior to the age when the child starts walking (between 12 and 18 months of age). The retained heel pad allows the child to ambulate about the house without a prosthesis. Because the Syme and Boyd procedures are essentially disarticulations, they avoid the inherent problems with transtibial amputation in children, specifically residual limb overgrowth. Strict adherence to meticulous surgical technique[13] will increase the likelihood of success. If a Syme procedure is chosen, the flares of the malleoli do not need to be narrowed because they are already hypoplastic. The most common complication of the Syme procedure is instability or migration of the heel pad.[12,19] Heel pad migration can be reduced by suturing the extensor tendons into the heel pad[20] and stabilizing the heel pad with a Steinmann pin through the pad into the tibial shaft for 4 to 6 weeks post-

operatively. Because the amputation is performed for severe projected discrepancy, it is usually unnecessary to excise the distal tibial epiphysis. Late ossification of the calcaneus may require excision.[12]

The Boyd procedure has the advantage of stabilizing the distal weight-bearing heel pad. This procedure also results in a longer residual limb, although the end of the residual limb may be more bulbous. This can create difficulties with prosthetic fit, especially donning and doffing the prosthesis, but it provides a good means of prosthetic suspension. The calcaneus should be stabilized with a Steinmann pin for 4 to 6 weeks postoperatively to promote union to the distal tibia. Consideration should be given to excising the distal tibial physis to anticipate the need for additional space to accommodate a prosthetic foot.[19]

Additional Procedures at the Time of Amputation

If severe tibial bowing (more than 30°) is present, this should be corrected by osteotomy at the time of the amputation, especially if the bowing is likely to result in difficulties with prosthetic fitting (Figure 6). The fibular anlage should be excised if it is be-

lieved to contribute to tibial deformity. Excision does not seem to decrease the likelihood of later development of knee valgus.[19]

Prosthetic Considerations

The typical initial prescription for a child who has had a Syme or Boyd procedure will be a total contact socket, an expanded polyethylene foam liner, and a soft distal end pad with a window, if necessary, to facilitate donning and doffing the prosthesis and to improve suspension (Figure 7). Children younger than 4 years may require additional suspension devices such as a neoprene sleeve (Figure 8). It is also possible to extend the socket into a patellar tendon-bearing configuration with a suprapatellar strap or even a waist belt for additional suspension. As the child matures, the shin of the residual limb may thin out, and the distal portion may grow more bulbous, thus providing more "adult-like" suspension options. A windowed socket generally works well. Alternatives include an internal bladder, which the child "pushes past" to don and doff the prosthesis, or the use of suspension pads worn inside the socket. Because

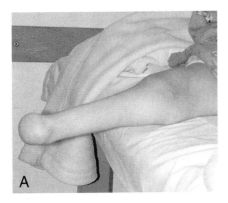
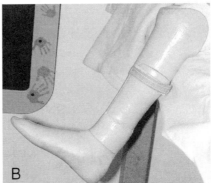
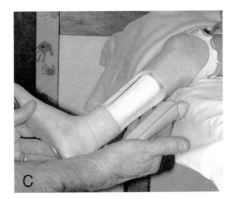

Figure 7 A, Appearance of the residual limb after a Syme ankle disarticulation. **B,** Typical prosthesis for a child with a Syme ankle disarticulation. **C,** Window for suspension.

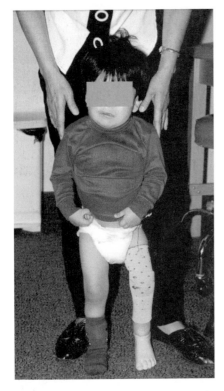

Figure 8 Young child with a Syme ankle disarticulation using a prosthesis with an added neoprene sleeve to improve suspension.

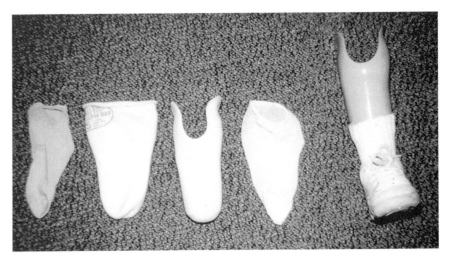

Figure 9 Oversized socket and various residual limb socks. An oversized socket may be prescribed to accommodate growth, with residual limb socks used to provide a snug fit.

children by nature will be rough on the prosthesis, it should be especially durable, simple, and repairable. Transition to roll-on locking liners is very dependent on the individual child's cognitive skills and developmental maturity and the shape of the residual limb.

Whether children younger than 10 years are likely to enjoy the benefits of a more modern dynamic-response foot is a question that war-

rants further study. Articulated ankle/foot combinations are subject to higher maintenance in children and therefore should be used judiciously. Furthermore, the need for frequent prosthetic changes to accommodate growth, the high demand placed on the prosthesis by the active child, and the cost may impact the prescription for prosthetic feet. It is encouraging that more manufacturers are addressing the needs of pediatric clients and that the number of choices of prosthetic feet is increasing.

The child's leg grows longitudinally more than circumferentially. Changes in the socket will be necessary every year until approximately 5 years of age and then every other year until 12 years of age. At 13 years of age, a new prosthesis will be re-

quired every 2 to 3 years until 21 years of age.[21] More mileage may be obtained from each prosthesis by starting with the socket a little long and using a shoe lift in the opposite side. A slightly oversized socket can be accommodated by extra residual limb socks or a growth liner (Figure 9). Components should be reused wherever possible.

Special Problems
Genu Valgum

The prosthetist can adjust the alignment to accommodate a mild valgus of less than 15° (Figure 10). If the valgus is greater, especially if accompanied by medial knee laxity, an osteotomy of the proximal tibia is indicated (Figure 11). If the valgus develops relatively slowly during the child's growth, then a medial proximal tibial epiphysiodesis may suffice.[22] Hypoplasia of the lateral femoral condyle can be a contributing factor and may be severe enough to require osteotomy. Weight-bearing radiographs, including the hips, knees, and ankles, with the child in the prosthesis, may be helpful to accurately assess the alignment.

Ligamentous Laxity

Knee instability may be sufficiently severe to require a thigh lacer and outside knee hinges. This problem is compounded when partial LDFP is present and the ACL is absent.

Length of Residual Limb at Maturity

Because Letts type B and C and Birch type IC and ID fibular deficiencies are expected to result in significant limb shortening at maturity, the residual limb is usually short enough to accommodate contemporary ankle/foot combinations. At maturity, 3.5 cm is required from the end of the residual limb to the prosthetic foot to maintain equal limb length. Occasionally, a residual limb associated with fibular deficiency will be too long. If this is detected prior to maturity of the child, an epiphysiodesis can be performed.[23]

Considerations for Rehabilitation

Rehabilitation is really a misnomer for children with fibular deficiency and their families. More appropriate terms are prehabilitation and habilitation.

Prehabilitation

Prehabilitation begins at birth and consists of education of the parents regarding treatment options and long-term expectations for both childhood and adulthood. Relieving the parents of any guilt feelings and helping them accept the condition are essential. Most children with fibular deficiencies enjoy a normal childhood and lead productive adult lives.[8,10,11] This outcome is facilitated by an emotionally mature parental response.

Habilitation

Habilitation is an ongoing process regardless of whether the treatment in-

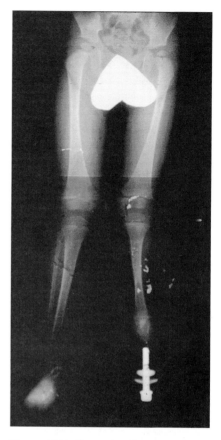

Figure 10 Radiograph of a patient with mild genu valgum that has been accommodated by prosthetic alignment.

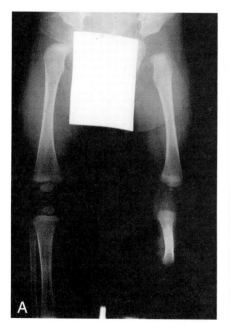

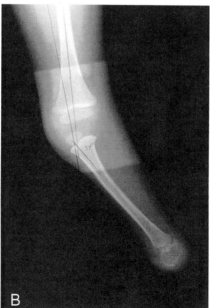

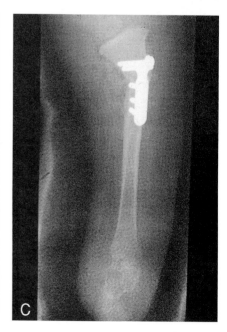

Figure 11 A, Radiograph of a child with Kalamchi type II or Letts type C fibular deficiency treated with a Boyd procedure at age 14 months. **B,** A valgus deformity developed by age 4 years, as shown in this radiograph. **C,** Radiograph after a corrective osteotomy was performed. The clinical postoperative appearance is shown in Figure 8.

volves limb lengthening or foot amputation. Surgery is but one of many events in optimizing the functional outcome. If the family chooses to forgo treatment, nonstandard prostheses will be required almost yearly. The child with a foot amputation will also require frequent prosthetic changes to accommodate growth. The physician needs to help ensure that the fit and alignment of the prosthesis fulfill the recommended prescription. The physical therapist needs to ensure that the function of the prosthesis is optimized. All of these determinations are the responsibility of the health care team. It is particularly helpful to consult a prosthetist who is familiar with children and fibular deficiency. Growth of the residual limb and incipient alignment issues need continuous monitoring. The child should be encouraged to participate in any normal childhood activities of interest, including athletic activities. Costs associated with the prostheses and procedures must be anticipated. Fearing increased out-of-pocket expenses, parents may delay steps required to optimize prosthetic fit during growth.

Conclusion

Fibular deficiency is a challenging condition that presents at birth and requires treatment throughout the child's growing years. Accurately classifying the condition is important so that appropriate treatment options can be chosen. Treatment can be optimized by educating parents in all aspects of care. This requires the input of the physician, the therapist, and the prosthetist. With optimal care, the outcome can be a childhood with pleasant memories and a productive adulthood.

References

1. Achterman C, Kalamchi A: Congenital deficiency of the fibula. *J Bone Joint Surg Br* 1979;61:133-137.

2. Stanitski DF, Shahcheraghi H, Nicker DA, Armstrong PF: Results of tibial lengthening with the Ilizarov technique. *J Pediatr Orthop* 1996;16:168-172.

3. Stanitski DF, Stanitski CL: Fibular hemimelia: A new classification system. *J Pediatr Orthop* 2003;23:30-34.

4. Miller LS, Bell DF: Management of congenital fibular deficiency by Ilizarov technique. *J Pediatr Orthop* 1992;12:651-657.

5. Drennan JC: *The Child's Foot and Ankle.* New York, NY, Raven Press, 1992.

6. Catagni MA: Management of fibular hemimelia using the Ilizarov method. *Instr Course Lect* 1992;44:431-434.

7. Birch JG, Lincoln TL, Mack PW: Functional classification of fibular deficiency, in Herring JA, Birch JG (eds): *The Child With a Limb Deficiency.* Rosemont, IL, American Academy of Orthopaedic Surgeons, 1998, pp 161-170.

8. Birch JG, Walsh SJ, Small JM, et al: Syme amputation for the treatment of fibular deficiency: An evaluation of long-term physical and psychological functional status. *J Bone Joint Surg Am* 1999;81:1511-1518.

9. Cheng JC, Cheung KW, Ng BK: Severe progressive deformities after limb lengthening in type II fibular hemimelia. *J Bone Joint Surg Br* 1998;80:772-776.

10. Herring JA, Barnhill B, Gaffney C: Syme amputation: An evaluation of the physical and psychological function in young patients. *J Bone Joint Surg Am* 1986;68:573-578.

11. McCarthy JJ, Glancy GL, Chang FM, Eilert RE: Fibular hemimelia: Comparison of outcome measurements after amputation and lengthening. *J Bone Joint Surg Am* 2000;82:1732-1735.

12. Anderson L, Westin GW, Oppenheim WL: Syme amputation in children: Indications, results, and long-term follow-up. *J Pediatr Orthop* 1984;4:550-554.

13. Wood WL, Zlotsky N, Westin GW: Congenital absence of the fibula: Treatment by Syme amputation: Indications and technique. *J Bone Joint Surg Am* 1965;47:1159-1169.

14. Krajbich JI: Lower-limb deficiencies and amputations in children. *J Am Acad Orthop Surg* 1998;6:358-367.

15. Choi IH, Kumar SJ, Bowen JR: Amputation or limb-lengthening for partial or total absence of the fibula. *J Bone Joint Surg Am* 1990;72:1391-1399.

16. Syme J: Amputation at the ankle joint. *Lond Edinb Mon J Med Sci* 1843;3:93-96.

17. Boyd HB: Amputation of the foot, with calcaneotibial arthrodesis. *J Bone Joint Surg* 1939;21:997-1000.

18. Eilert RE, Jayakumar SS: Boyd and Syme ankle amputations in children. *J Bone Joint Surg Am* 1976;58:1138-1141.

19. Fulp T, Davids JR, Meyer LC, Blackhurst DW: Longitudinal deficiency of the fibula: Operative treatment. *J Bone Joint Surg Am* 1996;78:674-682.

20. Davidson WH, Bohne WH: The Syme amputation in children. *J Bone Joint Surg Am* 1975;57:905-909.

21. Jain S: Rehabilitation in limb deficiency: II. The pediatric amputee. *Arch Phys Med Rehabil* 1996;77(suppl 3):S9-S13.

22. Boakes JL, Stevens PM, Moseley RF: Treatment of genu valgus deformity in congenital absence of the fibula. *J Pediatr Orthop* 1991;11:721-724.

23. Osebold WR, Lester EL, Christenson DM: Problems with excessive residual lower leg length in pediatric amputees. *Iowa Orthop J* 2001;21:58-67.

Chapter 75

Tibial Deficiencies

Michael L. Schmitz, MD
Brian J. Giavedoni, MBA, CP
Colleen Coulter-O'Berry, PT, MS, PCS

Introduction

Congenital longitudinal deficiency of the tibia is characterized by partial or complete absence of the tibia with a relatively intact fibula. It is an uncommon condition, occurring in approximately 1 per 1 million births,[1] and may have a genetic origin.[2] Skeletal anomalies of the affected limb include an abnormal knee joint, variably shortened leg, an equinovarus foot, and longitudinal deficiencies of the foot may also occur.[3-9] Although the clinician may have difficulty distinguishing tibial deficiencies from fibular deficiencies on initial radiographs, the clinical picture is always revealing. Tibial deficiencies are characterized by equinovarus positioning of the foot on the affected limb, whereas with fibular deficiencies, the foot will be positioned in equinovalgus (Figure 1).

Classification

A classification system should aid the clinician in choosing the most effective interventions for a given problem, provide information useful for counseling the patient and parents about prognosis, and serve as a basis for future studies of the patient population. Ideally, the classification system should further define the deficiency by variables that are known to affect outcome and that help to identify effective interventions. The identification of these determinant variables must be reproducible to allow researchers to appropriately define populations for study.

The variables that have the greatest effect on outcome in tibial deficiency include the presence or absence of extensor power across the knee joint, the length of the leg segment, the extent of foot and ankle involvement, and associated anomalies. Although the first classification system for lower limb congenital deficiencies was published in 1961,[10] and Jones and associates[4] described a system specific to tibial deficiencies in 1978, no single system includes all the variables listed above. The two classification systems specific for tibial deficiencies indirectly describe these variables, but they do not assess them directly.

The most widely used classification system is the one described by Jones and associates,[4] which is based on radiographic evaluations (Figure 2). In this classification, type 1 is characterized by absence of the tibia on radiographs. In type 1a, the distal femoral epiphysis is abnormal and there is no evidence of any tibial anlage. In type 1b, the distal femur is normal and the proximal tibial anlage is present but not yet ossified. This cartilaginous proximal tibia will not be apparent on radiographs but can be visualized directly with surgical inspection[11] or with arthrography, ultrasound,[12] or MRI. The distinction between types 1a and 1b is important because pres-

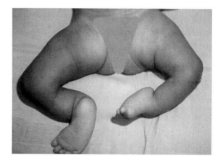

Figure 1 Clinical appearance of bilateral tibial deficiencies. Note the variably shortened legs, equinovarus feet, and longitudinal deformities of the feet. Note the flexion contracture seen bilaterally.

ervation of the knee joint may be possible in a patient who has type 1b deficiency. With type 2 deficiencies, the proximal portion of the tibia is visualized on radiographs, but the tibia is shortened, often significantly. Type 3 is a very rare condition in which the distal tibia is visible on radiographs but not the proximal tibia. Over time, the amorphous proximal segment will develop representative knee and ankle joints.[8] In type 4 deficiencies, the tibia is shortened and a distal tibiofibular diastasis is present (Figure 3).

The Jones classification is useful for describing patients retrospectively when only radiographic evidence is available. This classification neglects several determinant variables, however, including such clinically important features as motor power across the knee joint, the amount of limb

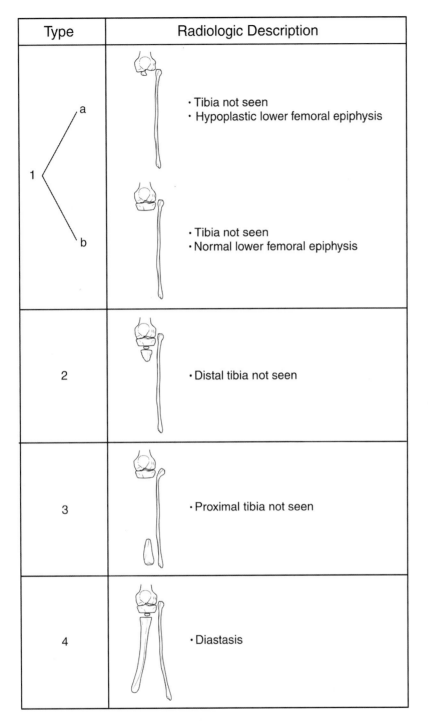

Type	Radiologic Description
1 a	• Tibia not seen • Hypoplastic lower femoral epiphysis
1 b	• Tibia not seen • Normal lower femoral epiphysis
2	• Distal tibia not seen
3	• Proximal tibia not seen
4	• Diastasis

Figure 2 The Jones classification of tibial deficiencies. *(Reproduced with permission from Jones D, Barnes J, Lloyd-Roberts GC: Congenital aplasia and dysplasia of the tibia with an intact fibula: Classification and management.* J Bone Joint Surg Br *1978;60: 31-39.)*

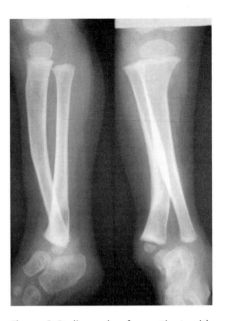

Figure 3 Radiograph of a patient with Jones type 4 or Kalamchi and Dawe type III deficiency. Note the diastasis at the ankle and the proximal subluxation of the talus.

shortening, and foot abnormalities. Although Jones and associates[4] propose that a tibial remnant is always present in a patient with type 1b deficiency, Williams and associates[9] noted no tibial remnant on surgical explora-tion of amputated limbs classified as type 1b dysplasia based on radio-graphic evidence.

Kalamchi and Dawe[5] described three categories of deformities based on both radiographic and clinical findings (Figure 4). This system improves upon the Jones classification by describing important clinical variables including knee extensor power, knee flexion contracture, and foot deformities. Foot deformities are not described independently, however, and there is no comment on length discrepancy. In this system, type I deficiencies are characterized by no tibia visible on radiographs, a hypoplastic distal femur, a significant knee flexion contracture, an equinovarus foot that occasionally lacks medial rays, and no active quadriceps action. Type II deficiencies are characterized by a proximal tibia with a relatively normal articulation and a normal distal femur. Knee flexion contractures are variable, ranging from 25° to 45°, and correlate with the degree of development of the proximal tibia. Active knee extension can usually be elicited. In type III dysplasias (Figure 3), the knee joint is normal and has intact active extension, but a diastasis of the distal tibiofibular syndesmosis is present. The amount of diastasis will vary, but the talus will always be proximally subluxated with the foot in a varus position.

The various classification schemes address deformities of the tibia and knee joint, but none directly addresses the associated foot abnormalities. Although radiographic evaluation has demonstrated the absence or duplication of medial rays (Figure 5), surgical dissection of amputated specimens has revealed several other abnormalities in the foot.[9,13] The most common abnormalities are coalitions, including a complete subtalar coalition.[10,13-17] The ankle articulation may be abnormal, with either a wide diastasis or a sagittally oriented joint.[13] Muscle, tendon, and vascular development is often quite abnormal.[13,15,16] Although these anomalies are not addressed by the classification schemes, they are important and have an impact on selection of treatment and prognosis.

Associated Abnormalities

Tibial deficiencies are associated with other types of skeletal abnormalities.[2,4,5,8,13,18,19] According to data from the four largest patient series,[4,8,19,20] which included 113 patients, the most common associated abnormalities were found in the hip and the hand. Among hip abnormalities, developmental dysplasia of the hip was most common, followed by proximal femoral focal dysplasia, coxa valga, and shortened femur. The most common deformity of the hand was lobster-claw deformity, followed by thumb abnormalities. Spinal abnormalities were observed in 21% of the patients in one series, with the most common being a hemivertebra or hypoplastic vertebra.[8] Kalamchi and Dawe[5] and Jones and associates[4] reported visceral abnormalities including hernias, imperforate anuses, abnormal kidneys, and cardiac abnormalities.

Etiology

The etiology of tibial deficiency remains unknown. Exposure to the ter-

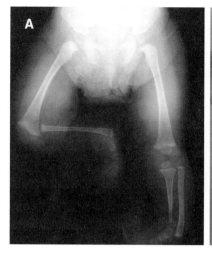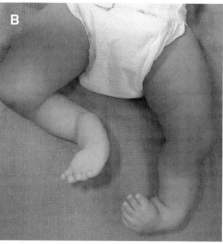

Figure 4 Radiograph (**A**) and photograph (**B**) of a patient with a Kalamchi and Dawe type I deficiency on the right (Jones type 1b), with no tibia visible on radiographs, a significant flexion contracture, and an equinovarus foot deformity. The left leg represents a Kalamchi and Dawe type II deficiency (Jones type 2), with a relatively normal knee joint and variably shortened tibia.

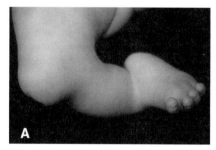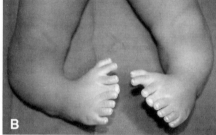

Figure 5 Tibial deficiencies may be accompanied by deficiency (**A**) or duplication (**B**) of the rays of the foot.

atogen thalidomide has been reported.[4] Dissections of amputated specimens have demonstrated a persistence of embryonic vascular patterns in both fibular and tibial deficiencies.[15,16] One investigator has postulated that some sort of iatrogenic insult during the fifth or sixth week of gestation is responsible for the cessation of normal arterial development and subsequent limb abnormality.[15]

An association between tibial deficiency and other congenital anomalies[2,4,5,8,13,18,19] as well as the observed incidence of deformities in family members[2,4,8,18,21] suggests that tibial deficiency may have a genetic transmission. Clark[2] documented an autosomal dominant inheritance pattern with variable penetrance in a report

of a kindred. Autosomal dominant inheritance patterns suggest a 50% risk of inheritance in children of affected parents, but this pattern is not always seen. A variable penetrance could explain how individuals may be affected genetically but have a normal phenotype.

Treatment

Treatment of tibial deficiency is directed toward functional optimization of the affected limb to allow the child's development to parallel that of an unaffected child as closely as possible. Close cooperation between the prosthetist and surgeon is required to address limb shortening and abnormalities in the knee, ankle, and foot. Working with a physical therapist is essential to maximize the functional gains facilitated by surgical interventions and changes in prostheses.

Before considering specific treatment measures, the surgeon should evaluate not only all aspects of the deficient limb but also the entire patient, including associated abnormalities, which in some situations will dictate treatment. Treatment of the affected leg of children who also have an associated partial longitudinal deficiency of the femur, for example, is often dictated by treatments that address the femoral deficiency.[8,21]

Even tibial deficiency without associated abnormalities can present a difficult problem for the orthopaedic surgeon. The functional determinants that must be addressed can include a variable limb-length discrepancy, abnormal knee function with potential laxity and/or stiffness, an abnormal ankle articulation, and an abnormal foot that may have compromised motor function. These determinants have a profound effect on surgical options, prosthetic designs and fittings, and rehabilitation. Treatment measures should not only address these problems but do so with a minimum of iatrogenic morbidity.

Complete Tibial Deficiency and Absent or Poor Knee Extensor Power

Surgical limb reconstruction is not possible in patients with complete tibial deficiency and absent or poor knee extensor power. Early knee disarticulation and prosthetic fitting, however, may allow good function for Jones type 1a or Kalamchi type I deficiencies. Aitken[19] was an early proponent of amputation for abnormalities of the lower limbs, and subsequent reports by other authors have confirmed the efficacy he initially reported.[4,5,8,20]

The disarticulation is usually performed shortly after the child begins to pull to stand. The timing of this procedure is designed to allow the child development that is parallel to that of children without a deficiency.

Patients are usually discharged the following day with a rigid dressing, a cast, or a soft compressive dressing. The surgical site is examined 5 to 7 days postoperatively, and sutures are removed approximately 2 weeks postoperatively. Wrapping with an elastic bandage to control edema is initiated at the time of suture removal. Ideally, the residual limb should be wrapped for shrinkage before the prosthetic fitting. Compression garments can usually be applied 2 to 3 weeks postoperatively, and prosthetic fitting can be started about 4 to 6 weeks postoperatively. An epiphysiodesis later in life can be used to shorten the femur on the affected side to allow greater latitude in selection of mechanical knee components.[8]

Complete Absence of the Tibia With Good Extensor Power

A fibular centralization procedure has been advocated for the patient with complete absence of the tibia and good extensor power at the knee.[1,3,22] The goal is a long residual limb, ending at the distal transtibial level, rather than a knee disarticulation. The technique of creating a femoral-fibular articulation without fusion was originally described by Myers[23] and was popularized by Brown.[1,11,22] The proposed advantages include preservation of knee function and leg length to aid in limb length equalization. The abnormal foot is usually addressed with an ablative procedure to facilitate prosthetic fitting either at the time of the original surgery or later, when the child begins to pull to stand.[1,3-5,7,8,11,20,22]

Some authors[3,11,21,22] have reported good results with the Brown procedure, but more often poor results and the need for significant revision surgery have been reported.[5-8,20,21] Brown later refined the patient selection for the procedure,[22] specifying that the patient must have good quadriceps power, full passive extension of the knee, and the potential for walking (with no significant as-

sociated abnormalities), and must be younger than 1 year of age at the time of the procedure. Specific contraindications include poor quadriceps function and fibular bowing. Even when these guidelines for patient selection are followed, a significant number of patients require additional procedures including knee disarticulation, flexion contracture release, and knee fusion.[5-8,20,21] A review of all cases reported in the English literature found uniformly poor results when patients were evaluated objectively.[24] The most common problem following the Brown procedure was a recurrent and progressive knee flexion contracture or varus-valgus instability.[6-8,20,21,24]

Proponents of the Brown procedure note that because the salvage procedure for an unsuccessful fibula transfer is a knee disarticulation,[25] little is lost in attempting the procedure if there are no contraindications. However, the need for revision compared with the uniformly excellent result seen with knee disarticulation has led several clinicians to abandon the Brown procedure and recommend primary ablation.[6,7,20,24]

Partial (Proximal) Tibia Present

Jones type 1b and Kalamchi type II tibial deficiencies are characterized by the presence of some proximal tibia. Although it may not be initially visible on radiographs, the extent of the proximal tibia can be assessed by MRI, ultrasound, or direct surgical exploration.[12] Patients with these deficiencies usually have good quadriceps function, and the deficiency is usually amenable to a synostosis of the fibula to the proximal tibial segment. The foot and ankle are typically deformed and ablated with a Syme procedure. This maximizes length and preserves a proprioceptive knee and motor power across the joint. Ablation of the foot allows for prosthetic fitting to equalize limb lengths. In some patients (Jones type 1b), the proximal tibial segment is not sufficiently developed to support synostosis when the child begins to pull to stand. In these instances, the foot should be ablated and the patient fitted with a prosthesis until a synostosis can be performed. In patients with proximal tibial segments clearly visible on radiographs (Jones type 2 or Kalamchi type II), the synostosis and foot ablation can be performed simultaneously. Regardless of when the synostosis is performed, it is important to create proper surgical alignment of the limb for future prosthetic fitting (Figure 6).

It is important to neutralize knee alignment at the time of synostosis because significant knee laxity often persists after the procedure. Patients with these deficiencies often have difficulty with prosthetic fitting because the fibular head is prominent after synostosis. Resection of this prominence at the time of the initial procedure will allow better prosthetic fitting.

Proximal Tibia Absent, Distal Tibia Present

Jones type 3 deficiencies are rare. The distal segment of the tibia is visible on radiographs, with a proximal segment that remains cartilaginous. The few reported cases had active quadriceps function and functioned well with preservation of the knee, ablation of the foot, and fitting with a transtibial prosthesis.[4,8]

Proximal Tibia Present, Distal Diastasis

Kalamchi type III and Jones type 4 deficiencies exemplify the importance of assessing the functional determinants in tibial deficiencies. This deficiency presents as a spectrum of involvement, with the severity of ankle deformity and shortening commensurate with the amount of tibial hypoplasia.[26] The knee is well formed with active quadriceps function. The foot may be relatively well formed, and the ankle may appear salvageable, but some deformities have such significant tibial hypoplasia that ankle reconstruction is not possible.[26] Even in the presence of a salvageable ankle

and foot, significant limb-length discrepancies persist.[4,8,26,27]

Although leg lengthening can be successful in patients with Kalamchi type III and Jones type 4 deformities, some initially successful ankle reconstructions can eventually require Syme procedures for significant limb-length discrepancies. Schoenecker and associates[8] reported that patients who retained ankle reconstructions did so either because deformities on the contralateral side required prosthetic fitting or because successful limb lengthening was accomplished. Wehbe and associates[28] reported a successful reconstruction in a patient who did not require limb equalization because of deformities on the contralateral side.

Prosthetic Management

Prosthetic intervention and design depend on the type of anomaly, the surgical revision performed, and the resultant anatomy and function of the residual limb. Although the complete absence of the tibia is the most anatomically abnormal clinical presentation, it is the easiest to fit prosthetically. Generally, surgical intervention results in a distal weight-bearing limb that can be fit with a knee disarticulation–type socket. The residual limb usually has a normal hip and either a small bulbous or a tapered end. In either case, the socket is non-ischial weight bearing, and suspension can be in the form of a segmented socket that incorporates an expandable inner material that is donned and then inserted onto a rigid socket. The bladder-style socket is a viable alternative to the segmented liner, but it is usually less adjustable and therefore better suited to adults. Rotational control of the limb within the socket is achieved through proper modification of the proximal socket area to ensure a well-formed gluteal impression and even contouring over the femoral condyles. A standard Silesian belt is still the suspension system of

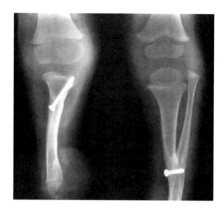

Figure 6 Radiograph of a patient with Jones type 1b (left) and type 2 (right) deficiencies (both Kalamchi and Dawe type II deficiencies) treated with synostosis of the fibula to the tibial remnant and foot ablation. Both limbs were fitted with transtibial prostheses. *(Reproduced with permission from Morrissy RT, BJ Giavedoni, Coulter-O'Berry C: The limb-deficient child, in Morrissy RT, Weinstein SL (eds): Lovell & Winter's Pediatric Orthopaedics, ed 5. Philadelphia, PA, Lippincott Williams & Wilkins, 2001, vol 2, pp 1217-1272.)*

choice for infants and toddlers. The total elastic suspension (TES) belt, however, is becoming a popular choice for suspension in this young population because it offers maximal stability around the hip, helps control rotation, and is accommodating to diapers and pull-ups. TES belts are extremely effective in infants and toddlers with associated femoral and hip anomalies who lack hip stability and control. Belt suspensions can be discontinued with growth and development of the bony distal femoral condyles and other anatomic prominences necessary for purchase and as the toddler gains strength and control of his or her movements. A silicone liner suspension using a distal shuttle attachment or a pull-through strap is becoming more popular for use with pediatric amputees and can be used as a combination liner/suspension system. The liner thickness can be increased or decreased to accommodate growth. Generally, liners are available in 3-mm, 6-mm, and 9-mm thicknesses. These, combined with prosthetic socks of various plies, allow the prosthetist to compensate for volu-

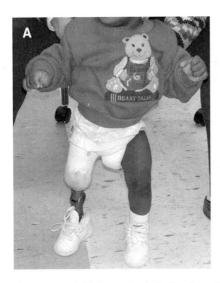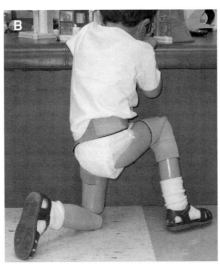

Figure 7 **A,** Initial prosthetic fitting for a 10-month-old child incorporating a single-axis constant-friction articulated knee. **B,** A 2-year-old transitioning to stand with a single-axis constant-friction articulated knee with an internal spring assist.

metric changes that occur with growth.

In recent years, manufacturers have produced a greater variety of prosthetic knees for pediatric patients. Traditionally, all children requiring a prosthetic knee were fitted at age 3 to 6 years,[29] suggesting that children must reach stages or achieve developmental milestones before they can be fitted for specific components, such as articulated knees. Wilk and associates,[30] however, advocate the use of articulating knees as early as age 17 months, and Giavedoni and associates[31] advocate the use of articulated knees in infants at about age 10 months or when the child begins pulling to stand. Through clinical observation, it was noticed that infants and toddlers could play in the half kneel and tall kneel positions, squat symmetrically to pick up toys, and stand from the floor or a small chair with excellent control of flexion and extension of the prosthetic knee.

In our experience, all children with transfemoral amputations and knee disarticulations are fitted with articulated knees with the first prosthesis (Figure 7). We have made four major clinical observations pertaining to the treatment of children in this age group: (1) The child achieves normal progression from crawling, pulling to stand, and early ambulation; (2) the articulated knee prevents the development of unfavorable compensatory gait patterns; (3) the articulated pediatric knee is usually small enough to be used in the prostheses of infants and toddlers; and (4) the use of external knee joints is an adequate alternative to internal knees when there are space limitations.

Benefits can be seen with the early use of articulated knees even if the child presents with inadequate hip movement to stabilize the knee, poor motor control of the limb, and lack of physical space. The use of external joints (space issues), TES belts for stabilization (weakness, paralysis, and motor control issues), and proper alignment of the prosthesis (weakness and motor control) can compensate for these impairments. It is also important that the child receive consistent physical therapy and have a supportive, involved family.

If the deficiency is bilateral, requiring bilateral knee disarticulations or one knee disarticulation and a Syme procedure on the opposite limb, early mobility aids must be considered. Traditionally, "stubbies" (above-knee sockets attached to rocker feet) have been prescribed for the child with bilateral knee disarticulations. By placing the child close to the ground, bal-

ance can be slowly mastered. The prostheses are gradually lengthened until they are proportionate with the body. Some clinics bypass traditional stubbies by incorporating pediatric knees and solid ankle–cushion heel (SACH) feet in the initial prosthesis. Overall, height is kept as low as possible to encourage early ambulation. As mentioned, the child quickly learns to balance, using hip extension to maintain balance and to prevent the knees from collapsing.

In the child with a different degree of bilateral tibial deficiency in each limb, the limb requiring a knee disarticulation with prosthetic knee fitting may be more stable than the knee-sparing side, offering more control and balance in gait. This is because ablative procedures that spare the knee do not address the cruciate and collateral ligament deficiencies. These deficiencies cause instability that may have a profound effect on prosthetic fit and function. The knee laxity is controlled by design of the trim lines of the proximal socket, use of external suspension sleeves, and increased strength through growth and development of the muscles. External joints and a thigh lacer are options for patients in whom more conservative treatment does not provide adequate stability.

Children with bilateral tibial deficiencies requiring bilateral Syme procedures with or without osteotomies will present ongoing challenges of progressive valgus deformities at the knee and bowing of the fibula and remaining tibia. These deformities tend to be asymmetric and are a challenge to every prosthetist and orthopaedic surgeon.

Alignment in the pediatric patient differs from that of the adult amputee in several ways. In general, the younger the infant, the greater the flexion of the socket and the greater the hip abduction angle. Prostheses are generally worn over diapers, and this must be taken into consideration when modifying the prosthesis. Diapers also tend to increase the abduction angle of the socket in relation to the knee and foot. Socket design for the pediatric knee disarticulation prosthesis is similar in most aspects to the design of prostheses for adults. Accommodation for hypoplastic femoral condyles is discussed later in the chapter.

External suspension sleeves greatly assist knee stability and control. The thickness of various materials, such as neoprene, relative to the child's size provides a fairly high degree of stability not generally attainable in adults. Several types of sleeves are available, offering varying degrees of flexibility. A more flexible silicone sleeve that allows for crawling, creeping, and tall-kneel and half-kneel play is appropriate for infants. A flexible sleeve also allows for easier transitions from sitting to standing. However, these sleeves tend to wear down quickly in infants and young toddlers who creep as their primary means of locomotion. Once the child is standing and cruising, a less flexible neoprene sleeve offers greater knee stability and control. This makes a thigh lacer and side joint unnecessary except in patients with very severe knee laxity.

In patients with deficiencies in which a tibial segment has been preserved or the fibula has been joined to the tibial remnant, a modified transtibial prosthesis is used. The medial and lateral walls are kept proximal and fitted snugly to the femoral condyles (supracondylar transtibial prosthesis) to aid in control and support of the knee compartment. In many instances, the proximal anterior brim of the prosthesis is designed to enclose the patella (supracondylar/suprapatellar prosthesis); this design aids in the control and stability of the knee and prevents a hyperextension moment.[32] As a measure of last resort, external side joints and a thigh lacer may be used when knee stability and control are beyond the design capabilities of the sockets described above. Use of a thigh lacer at such a young age, however, will inevitably lead to thigh muscle atrophy.

Patients with congenital tibial deficiencies pose unique fitting and suspension problems not often found in patients with traumatic amputations. Patients with tibial deficiency with knee disarticulation revision generally have hypoplastic femoral condyles, requiring fitting similar to that of the transfemoral amputee. Suspension cannot be achieved by locking proximal to the condyles through the use of a bladder or segmented liner configuration. In such cases, a silicone liner, Silesian belt, or TES belt is required. At the Syme level, knee instability because of ligamentous laxity can be controlled and protected by the use of higher medial and lateral socket brim walls. Generally, the walls rise to the level of the proximal border of the patella, ensuring enclosure of the knee and helping to reduce medial or lateral rotational moments.

Rehabilitation

Infants and children with tibial deficiencies, especially bilateral deficiencies, require close monitoring of their development and prompt referral to early intervention programs. The goal of the team treating the child with a limb deficiency is to have the patient's development parallel that of a child with normal limbs. Physical therapy is described in the physical therapy chapter of this text.

These infants not uncommonly have dislocated hips, hand deficiencies, or radial/ulnar deficiencies that will affect early gross and fine motor development. The therapist is instrumental in assisting the team in prioritizing both surgical and prosthetic interventions.

Children with bilateral deficiencies tend to walk later than do those with unilateral deficiencies. Infants with bilateral knee disarticulations who are fitted with prosthetic knees at the first prosthetic fitting can learn excellent control of prosthetic knees with exercises and activities that parallel those of normal development.[31] However, infants and toddlers who undergo bilateral knee disarticulations early in their development are very functional without prostheses because they walk on the ends of their residual limbs. They become easily frustrated with initial prosthetic fittings because the additional weight and bulk of prostheses slow them down.[33] These children must be encouraged to wear prostheses consistently, however, so that they can learn to pull to stand, come up and down from a seated position, and, eventually, walk. Therapy should focus on early gross motor activities that lead to standing and walking. The infant must learn to roll, sit, and creep in the prostheses. Parents, prosthetists, and therapists need to be aware of these frustrations and developmental challenges and consider them when establishing appropriate functional goals for the child.

Children with bilateral knee disarticulations usually do not require assistive devices to walk. These children can participate in sports and recreational activities within limits, but these limits should be based on the patient's level of functioning, not by the extent of limb loss. Children with bilateral limb loss should have a manual wheelchair to use as a backup when not wearing their prostheses or after surgical revisions. A wheelchair is also indicated for long-distance mobility, use on rugged terrain, or when competing in wheelchair sports.[33]

References

1. Brown FW: The Brown operation for total tibial hemimelia, in Aitken GT (ed): *Selected Lower-Limb Anomalies: Surgical and Prosthetics Management.* Washington, DC, National Academy of Sciences, 1971, p 20.

2. Clark MW: Autosomal dominant inheritance of tibial meromelia: Report of a kindred. *J Bone Joint Surg Am* 1975;57:262-264.

3. Christini DC, Levy EJ, Facanha FA, Kumar SJ: Fibular transfer for congenital absence of the tibia. *J Pediatr Orthop* 1993;13:378-381.

4. Jones D, Barnes J, Lloyd-Roberts GC: Congenital aplasia and dysplasia of the tibia with an intact fibula: Classification and management. *J Bone Joint Surg Br* 1978;60:31-39.

5. Kalamchi A, Dawe RV: Congenital deficiency of the tibia. *J Bone Joint Surg Br* 1985;67:581-584.

6. Epps CH Jr, Tooms RE, Edholm CD, Kruger LM, Bryant DD III: Failure of centralization of the fibula for congenital longitudinal deficiency of the tibia. *J Bone Joint Surg Am* 1991;73: 858-867.

7. Loder RT, Herring JA: Fibular transfer for congenital absence of the tibia: A reassessment. *J Pediatr Orthop* 1987;7: 8-13.

8. Schoenecker PL, Capelli AM, Millar EA, et al: Congenital longitudinal deficiency of the tibia. *J Bone Joint Surg Am* 1989;71:278-287.

9. Williams L, Weintroub S, Getty CJ, Pincott JR, Gordon I, Fixsen JA: Tibial dysplasia: A study of the anatomy. *J Bone Joint Surg Br* 1983;65:157-159.

10. Frantz CH, O'Rahilly R: Congenital skeletal limb deficiencies. *J Bone Joint Surg Am* 1961;43:1202-1224.

11. Brown FW: Construction of a knee joint in congenital total absence of the tibia (paraxial hemimelia tibia): A preliminary report. *J Bone Joint Surg Am* 1965;47:695-704.

12. Grissom LE, Harcke HT, Kumar SJ: Sonography in the management of tibial hemimelia. *Clin Orthop* 1990; 251:266-270.

13. Turker R, Mendelson S, Ackman J, Lubicky JP: Anatomic considerations of the foot and leg in tibial hemimelia. *J Pediatr Orthop* 1996;16:445-449.

14. Grogan DP, Holt GR, Ogden JA: Talocalcaneal coalition in patients who have fibular hemimelia or proximal femoral focal deficiency: A comparison of the radiographic and pathological findings. *J Bone Joint Surg Am* 1994;76:1363-1370.

15. Hootnick DR, Levinsohn EM, Randall PA, Packard DS Jr: Vascular dysgenesis associated with skeletal dysplasia of the lower limb. *J Bone Joint Surg Am* 1980;62:1123-1129.

16. Miller LS, Armstrong PF: The morbid anatomy of congenital deficiency of the tibia and its relevance to treatment. *Foot Ankle* 1992;13:396-399.

17. Wolfgang GL: Complex congenital anomalies of the lower extremities: Femoral bifurcation, tibial hemimelia, and diastasis of the ankle. Case report and review of the literature. *J Bone Joint Surg Am* 1984;66:453-458.

18. Pashayan H, Fraser FC, McIntyre JM, Dunbar JS: Bilateral aplasia of the tibia, polydactyly, and absent thumb in father and daughter. *J Bone Joint Surg Br* 1971;53:495-499.

19. Aitken GT: Amputation as a treatment for certain lower-extremity congenital abnormalities. *J Bone Joint Surg Am* 1959;41:1267-1285.

20. Epps CH Jr, Schneider PL: Treatment of hemimelias of the lower extremity: Long-term results. *J Bone Joint Surg Am* 1989;71:273-277.

21. Jayakumar SS, Eilert RE: Fibular transfer for congenital absence of the tibia. *Clin Orthop* 1979;139:97-101.

22. Brown FW, Pohnert WH: Abstract: Construction of a knee joint in meromelia tibia (congenital absence of the tibia): A fifteen-year follow-up study. *J Bone Joint Surg Am* 1972;54:1333.

23. Myers TH: Congenital absence of tibia: Transplantation of head of fibula: Arthrodesis at the ankle joint. *Am J Orthop Surg* 1905;3:72-85.

24. Loder RT: Fibular transfer for congenital absence of the tibia (Brown procedure), in Herring JA, Birch JG (eds): *The Child With a Limb Deficiency.* Rosemont, IL, American Academy of Orthopaedic Surgeons, 1998, pp 223-229.

25. Simmons ED Jr, Ginsburg GM, Hall JE: Brown's procedure for congenital absence of the tibia revisited. *J Pediatr Orthop* 1996;16:85-89.

26. Sedgwick WG, Schoenecker PL: Congenital diastasis of the ankle joint: Case report of a patient treated and followed to maturity. *J Bone Joint Surg Am* 1982;64:450-453.

27. Garbarino JL, Clancy M, Harcke HT, Steel HH, Cowell HR: Congenital diastasis of the inferior tibiofibular joint: A review of the literature and report of two cases. *J Pediatr Orthop* 1985;5: 225-228.

28. Wehbe MA, Weinstein SL, Ponseti IV: Tibial agenesis. *J Pediatr Orthop* 1981; 1:395-399.

29. Stanger M: Limb deficiencies and amputations, in Campbell SK, Palisano RJ, Vander Linden DW (eds): *Physical Therapy for Children.* Philadelphia, PA, WB Saunders, 1994, pp 325-351.

30. Wilk B, Karol L, Halliday S: Characterizing gain in young children with a prosthetic knee joint. *Phys Ther* 1999; 10:20.

31. Giavedoni BJ, Coulter-O'Berry C, Geil M: Movement masters. *Adv Direct Rehabil* 2002;11:43-44.

32. Morrissy RT, Giavedoni BJ, Coulter-O'Berry C: The limb-deficient child, in Morrissy RT, Weinstein SL (eds): *Lovell & Winter's Pediatric Orthopaedics,* ed 5. Philadelphia, PA, Lippincott, Williams & Wilkins, 2001, vol 2, pp 1217-1272.

33. Coulter-O'Berry C: Physical therapy management in children with lower extremity limb deficiencies, in Herring JA, Birch JG (eds): *The Child With a Limb Deficiency.* Rosemont, IL, American Academy of Orthopaedic Surgeons, 1998, pp 319-330.

Chapter 76

Femoral Deficiencies

Kenneth J. Guidera, MD

Cara D. Novick, MD

Janet G. Marshall, CPO

Introduction

Longitudinal deficiency of the femur, partial (LDFP) is the new term for what was previously called proximal focal femoral deficiency (PFFD). LDFP is a complex congenital absence of part or all of the femur that is associated with other lower limb soft-tissue and osseous abnormalities. It may be unilateral or bilateral, and involvement of the hip joint is variable, ranging from normal to a complete absence of both sides of the joint. The challenges facing the orthopaedic surgeon and the prosthetist are significant, with treatment options ranging from limb ablation and prosthetic fitting to limb salvage with limb lengthening.

Etiology

LDFP tends to arise spontaneously without a clear-cut genetic pattern of inheritance. Various embryologic and teratologic etiologies have been proposed. These include vascular epiphyseal disruption, infection, and medications such as thalidomide.[1,2] Most cases appear to arise sporadically, although Sen Gupta and Gupta[3] have reported a possible linked mode of inheritance in one family. Bailey and Beighton[4] have proposed an autosomal recessive pattern of inheritance. Sorge and associates[5] described five patients with mixed patterns of inheritance and/or spontaneous presentation. There are some reports of occur-

rence in twins, siblings, and third-degree relatives. The disorder of femoral hypoplasia and unusual facial features does appear to have an autosomal dominant inheritance. Although there is no clear increased risk in children of affected individuals, genetic counseling is recommended. Boden and associates[6] performed a histologic study of growth plates from a fetus with LDFP. They noted failure of migration and organization with abnormal architecture and disorganized vascular invasion.

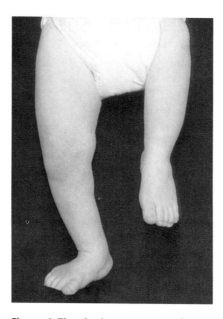

Figure 1 The classic appearance of LDFP. Note the shortened lower limb and ship's funnel–shaped thigh.

Clinical Presentation

The patient presents with a shortened lower limb. The thigh is thickened and funnel-shaped ("ship's funnel" appearance)[7,8] and fibular deficiency, foot deformity, or other lower limb anomalies may be present (Figure 1). Associated skeletal congenital anomalies have been reported in 61% to 92% of patients with LDFP, with fibular deficiency being the most com-

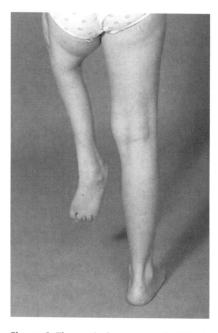

Figure 2 The typical posture of LDFP is flexion, abduction, and external rotation, with the affected foot at midtibial position. This patient has had a Van Nes derotational osteotomy.

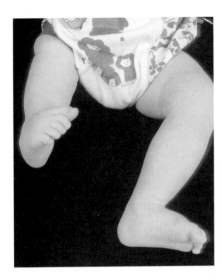

Figure 3 Foot and fibula abnormalities may be associated with LDFP as shown here, with talipes equinovarus but all foot rays present.

TYPE		FEMORAL HEAD	ACETABULUM	FEMORAL SEGMENT	RELATIONSHIP AMONG COMPONENTS OF FEMUR AND ACETABULUM AT SKELETAL MATURITY
A	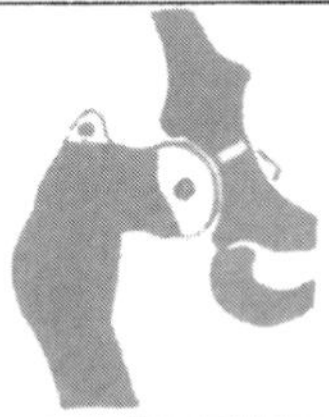	Present	Normal	Short	Bony connection between components of femur Femoral head in acetabulum Subtrochanteric varus angulation, often with pseudarthrosis
B	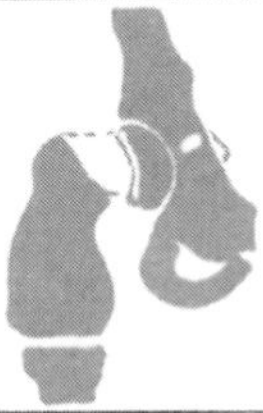	Present	Adequate or moderately dysplastic	Short, usually proximal bony tuft	No osseous connection between head and shaft Femoral head in acetabulum
C	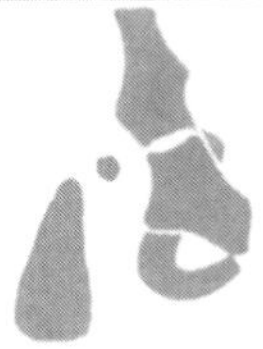	Absent or represented by ossicle	Severely dysplastic	Short, usually proximally tapered	May be osseous connection between shaft and proximal ossicle No articular relation between femur and acetabulum
D	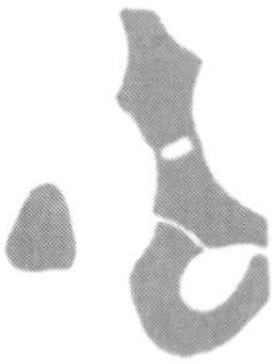	Absent	Absent Obturator foramen enlarged Pelvis squared in bilateral cases	Short, deformed	(none)

Figure 4 Aitken classification of LDFP. *(Reproduced with permission from Herring J, Johnson C, Rathjen K, et al: Tachdijian's Pediatric Orthopaedics. Philadelphia, PA, WB Saunders, 2002, vol 3, p 1758.)*

mon. The spine, heart, and upper limbs may also be involved.[9,10] The deficiency may be bilateral in up to 15% of patients. When both limbs are affected, limb acetabular dysplasia is likely to be more severe.

The affected lower limb is generally held in a flexed, abducted, and externally rotated position. This is caused by a combination of osseous deformity and soft-tissue contracture. The classic position of the thigh actually makes the limb appear smaller, as do the associated fibular deficiency and foot anomalies. Frequently, the foot on the involved side is at the midtibia position of the uninvolved side, making early ambulation difficult (Figure 2). Children, however, are adaptable, and they tend to use modified gaits, such as walking on the knee on the sound side, or flexing the sound side hip and knee.[11]

The knee is frequently involved and may be unstable, with a flexion contracture and severe femoral shortening. Genu valgum is common. The knee may be so proximal as to be buried in the thickened thigh tissue. Angulation of the distal femoral condyles at the knee may enhance the deformity and instability. The cruciate ligaments may be absent, and anteroposterior in-

stability as well as subluxation or dislocation are common.[12,13]

Frequently, the leg has an associated partial or complete fibular deficiency with a foot and ankle valgus deformity accentuating the femoral shortening (Figure 3). The foot may have absent lateral rays, as is typical with fibular deficiency. Grogan and associates[7,8] noted an association of both LDFP and fibular deficiency with talocalcaneal coalition. A nonfunctional foot may influence the decision for amputation versus limb salvage.

Classification

Numerous classification systems have been devised to categorize LDFP. The most commonly used system is the Aitken classification.[14] In this system,

LDFP is classified into four types by radiographic appearance of the proximal femur and acetabulum (Figure 4).

In type A, the femoral head and acetabulum are present but the femur is shortened. A lucency representing a pseudarthrosis in the proximal femur is seen on radiographs; this may unite by the time the child reaches skeletal maturity. Varus of the proximal femur may be present. In type B, the proximal femur is more deficient, but the acetabulum is present and usually well formed. The femoral head may ossify late, but the discontinuity between the head and shaft persists through skeletal maturity. In type C, there is little or no femoral head, and the acetabulum is severely dysplastic or absent. An ossified tuft is present on the proximal end of the femur. In type D, the femur is extremely short, with the head absent and the acetabulum severely dysplastic or absent, and there is no tuft on the proximal femur. This classification system is limited because, as ossification occurs, the classification type may change, making comparisons over time difficult.[11,15-17]

The Fixsen and Lloyd-Roberts classification[18] may be more useful prognostically and therapeutically. This system describes three types based on the appearance of the proximal ossified shaft, the site and nature of shaft sclerosis, and the nature of the acetabulum. The classification system of Gillespie and Torode[19] is clinically based and treatment oriented, dividing patients into two groups with different treatment recommendations. Many patients, however, fall somewhere between these two groups, so Gillespie has modified the system to comprise three groups. Paley[20] devised a classification system based on factors influencing lengthening, including femoral and acetabular structure and hip and knee mobility. No classification system is universally acceptable and applicable. Each of the systems has strengths and limitations and may be applicable for different purposes.[1,2,7,8,11-14]

Treatment Options

Treatment options for LDFP are even more numerous than classification systems. Several important orthopaedic issues should be considered when formulating a treatment plan. These include ultimate limb-length discrepancy, joint instability, inadequacy of musculature, and malrotation. Functional needs, cosmesis, and bilaterality must also be considered. A shoe lift is generally not an adequate long-term solution (Figure 5).

Nonsurgical Management

Patients may be managed nonsurgically with equinus prostheses. This is feasible in patients with close to 50% of femoral length. The prosthesis is designed to accommodate the foot in plantar flexion. For children with a

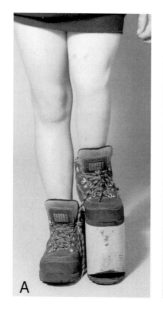
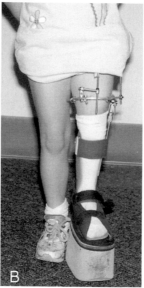

Figure 5 Most limb-length discrepancies with LDFP are too severe to be treated with a shoe lift. A, Patient with LDFP wearing shoe lift. B, Patient during limb lengthening. The shoe lift is progressively shortened.

short or absent femur managed this way, a knee joint may eventually be added, and the prosthesis must be modified over time for growth.[1,2,11,14]

Surgical Management
Early Osteotomy and Derotation

The possibility of early surgical intervention for improved function has been investigated. Tonnis and Stanitski[21] immobilized three patients in squatting casts for 3 months during infancy. Consolidation was achieved and the growth plates developed normally. The patients were subsequently treated with valgus osteotomy and derotation of the proximal femur. The earlier this was done, the earlier growth began. The authors felt that this ultimately resulted in a reduced limb-length discrepancy, making eventual limb lengthening easier.

Ankle Disarticulation

Another treatment option is ankle disarticulation with or without knee arthrodesis, creating a functional transfemoral amputation. The initial fitting takes place when the patient is approximately 1 year of age and is expressing interest in standing (Figure 6). A modified Syme disarticulation or Boyd amputation will create a residual limb suited for prosthetic fitting or weight

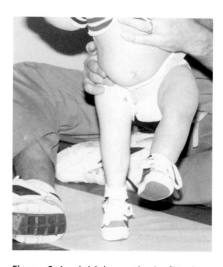

Figure 6 An initial prosthesis fitted at approximately age 1 year. A knee joint may be added later.

bearing (Figure 7). A Syme procedure is a through-ankle disarticulation that maintains the heel pad. A Boyd amputation retains the calcaneus, which is fused to the tibia. If the knee is not fused, flexion may occur during weight bearing and lead to further instability during gait. In addition, the knee in LDFP may have laxity or valgus deformity. A knee fusion can eliminate this in unstable knees, creating a functional transfemoral amputation. Knees that are stable and in good position can be controlled with the prosthesis without arthrodesis.[11,15,16]

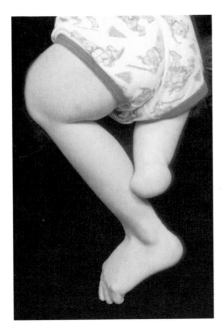

Figure 7 A patient with bilateral LDFP after a Syme procedure on the right. The heel pad is maintained for weight bearing and prosthetic fitting.

Rotationplasty

Rotationplasty is another alternative, enabling the use of a below-the-knee prosthesis[1,2,11,15,21,22] (Figure 2). Rotationplasty was first described in 1930 by Borggreve, who performed a rotation through the femur. Van Nes[22] described his technique in 1950, rotating the foot 180° through the tibia so that the toes point posteriorly and the ankle functions as a knee. The ankle must have at least a 60° arc of motion and should be at the same level as the opposite knee. The gastrocnemius-soleus complex acts as an extensor of the new knee and can help to limit heel rise of the prosthetic lower segment. The rotationplasty may gradually derotate with growth, making repeated surgeries necessary.

Several modifications have been described. Torode and Gillespie[23] rotate the tibia and arthrodese the knee, achieving 120° of rotation through the knee and the remainder through a tibial osteotomy. Kritter[15] described a one-stage tibial rotationplasty, using a section of fibula as graft to maintain stability and alignment. He found less derotation than reported with other techniques. Krajbich[24] further modified the procedure, achieving all of the rotation through the knee and performing a knee arthrodesis. Muscles crossing the knee are rerouted to pull in a straight line. A segment of femur is removed as well as the distal femoral growth plate.[24]

The decision whether to perform amputation or rotationplasty may depend on appearance and function. Rotationplasty is thought to be cosmetically unacceptable to many patients because of the reversed foot. Prosthetic fitting may also be difficult. However, many patients are pleased to have an ankle functioning effectively as a knee.[1,2,11,15,22,23,25]

Results

Studies have also been undertaken to evaluate differences in gait and energy consumption after various procedures. Fowler and associates[26,27] used motion analysis to compare 9 patients who had Syme procedures with 10 patients who had Van Nes rotationplasties and found improved gait, enhanced prosthetic knee function, and fewer compensatory mechanisms in patients who had Van Nes rotationplasties. Even those patients who used the subtalar joint rather than the ankle joint had fewer compensatory mechanisms than did patients who had Syme procedures. Patients with Van Nes rotationplasties demonstrated decreased energy consumption even if rotation occurred. In addition, patients with Syme procedures walked more slowly. Alman and associates[16] compared nine rotationplasties with seven Syme procedures in terms of perceived appearance, gross motor function, and metabolic energy expended. The authors found no difference in motor function or perceived appearance. Rotationplasty was associated with a more energy-efficient gait.

Other Techniques

Hip stability is another factor to be considered. If hip stability can be achieved, the resultant gait may be more satisfactory. Several techniques have been described to address hip instability. Steel and associates[28] described an iliofemoral fusion with femoral shortening and arrest of the epiphysis. The femur is flexed, and the knee acts as a hip joint. The main problem is limited hip flexion, abduction, and adduction, interfering with activities of daily living.

The pseudarthrosis must be considered as well. Goddard and associates[17] investigated the natural history of this instability in 78 femurs in 68 patients. Subtrochanteric instability was found to fuse spontaneously in 30% of patients, and it responded well to surgical intervention. Bony fusion was difficult to obtain with cervical instability.

Brown[29] described rotating the femur 180° and fusing it to the pelvis in neutral to slight adduction and neutral to slight external rotation. The medial hamstrings are attached to the anterior or lateral muscles. The gastrocnemius-soleus complex acts as a hip flexor and knee extensor, with the reversed knee functioning as a hinged hip.

Some authors have described subtrochanteric valgus osteotomy in patients with Aitken type A or B femurs to improve hip stability, femoral head ossification, and gait. This procedure involves resection of the pseudarthrosis and fixing the femoral head and neck in a valgus position of 155° to 170° on the femoral diaphysis. The results of this procedure are mixed. Koman and Meyer[30] reported improvement in patients with type A femurs, whereas Richardson and Rambach[31] reported less satisfactory results.

Many different treatment options are available for LDFP. Treatment must take the unique anatomy and goals of each patient into consideration, including psychological and cosmetic aspects. No matter which procedure is performed, there will be residual shortening, weakness, and Trendelenburg lurch. The treatment choice must therefore be individualized to minimize gait abnormalities.

Limb Reconstruction

Deciding between limb reconstruction and amputation is difficult. To be considered for limb reconstruction, the patient must have adequate musculature for ambulation, a stable knee, and a functional foot. The limb-length discrepancy should not be too severe (25 cm maximum at end of growth). The foot must be plantigrade (after surgical correction, if necessary) and have enough rays to be suitable for weight bearing (Figure 8). Significant deformity of the ankle or shortening of the tibia secondary to fibular hemimelia may hamper attempts at limb reconstruction and ambulation and may compound the shortening of the deficient femur. Gross hip instability may impair attempts at ambulation and require a prosthesis that extends above the hip to provide stability. Patients affected bilaterally may not need limb salvage or lengthening because of the symmetry of the deformity. Last, the patient and family must be psychologically equipped to handle the pressures of multiple surgical procedures and one or more protracted lengthenings.

Surgical Techniques

Various surgical approaches have been proposed for limb salvage in LDFP. Tonnis and Stanitski[21] proposed early spica cast immobilization to achieve consolidation and better alignment of the growth plate. This was followed by a valgus osteotomy with derotation and, later, a minimal femoral lengthening. Saleh and Goonatillake[32] recommended early axis correction and joint stabilization before femoral lengthening averaging 4 cm achieved by repeated short lengthenings. Conejero Casares and associates[33] recommend initial lengthening for LDFP and a congenitally short femur and were able to accomplish this in a single procedure in 75% of patients. They cautioned that the patient must be carefully evaluated preoperatively for other congenital anomalies, axial malalignments,

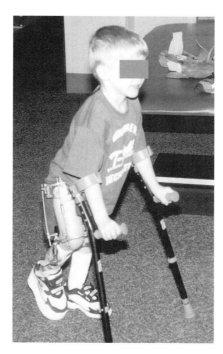

Figure 8 A patient undergoing femoral limb lengthening ambulating on crutches. Note knee flexion contracture and AFO attachment.

joint instability, and patient and family cooperation. Many of their patients have undergone two or three lengthenings over their growing years. The authors have not found this to be psychologically damaging to patients who regard the procedures as an "investment" (Figure 9). Paley[20] recommends a complete soft-tissue release ("super hip" procedure) with a proximal femoral valgus osteotomy, a pelvic osteotomy, and femoral lengthening.

In our experience, limb salvage and lengthening should be reserved for the patient and family who are highly motivated and cooperative because numerous procedures are required, extending over several years. The foot and ankle need to be stable, other anomalies such as partial longitudinal deficiency of the fibula corrected, and contractures released. During the lengthening, attention must be paid to range of motion, pin care, frame stability, and bone regeneration. Knee joint stiffness is common, and a vigorous physical therapy

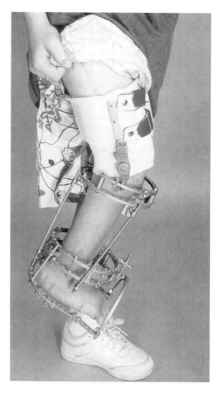

Figure 9 Patient with severe LDFP undergoing tibial lengthening after a previous femoral lengthening. This patient required a total of three lengthenings. An orthosis is attached to the Ilizarov frame to control knee motion and stability. The foot is incorporated to correct talipes equinovarus deformity.

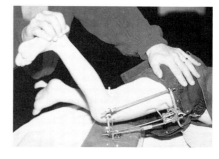

Figure 10 Patient undergoing physical therapy to prevent knee joint stiffness.

program is essential (Figure 10). Failure to adequately address any of these issues can result in a difficult or unsuccessful lengthening. For any patient who does not meet these criteria, or has a failed lengthening, an amputation and prosthetic fitting may be the best option.

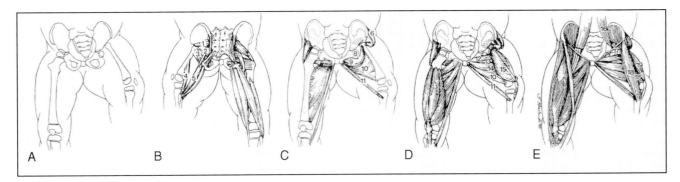

Figure 11 In LDFP, all muscle groups are present, but sizes and orientation are quite variable. **A,** Osseous tissues. **B,** Soft tissues, layer 1. **C,** Soft tissues, layer 2. **D,** Soft tissues, layer 3. **E,** Soft tissues, layer 4. 1 = piriformis, 2 = sciatic nerve, 3 = short external rotators, 4 = biceps femoris short head, 5 = biceps femoris long head, 6 = gluteus medius, 7 = gluteus minimus, 8 = dissociated femoral head, 9 = obturator externus, 10 = adductor magnus, 11 = gracilis, 12 = pectineus, 13 = adductor brevis, 14 = adductor longus, 15 = vastus medialis, 16 = psoas, 17 = femoral neurovascular bundle, 18 = sartorius, 19 = rectus femoris. *(Adapted with permission from Pirani S, Beauchamp RD, Sawatzky B: Soft tissue anatomy of proximal femoral focal deficiency. J Pediatr Orthop 1991;11:563-570.)*

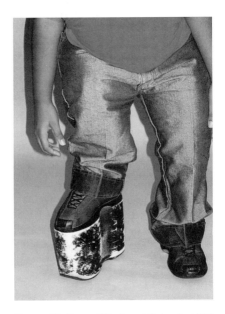

Figure 12 Shoe lift for bilateral LDFP with an asymmetric presentation.

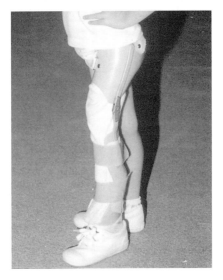

Figure 13 Prosthesis using a thigh cuff and outside hinges with foot in equinus incorporated in a weight-bearing socket and prosthetic foot beneath.

Prosthetic Treatment

LDFP presents unique anatomic challenges for prosthetic fitting. The Aitken categories of A, B, C, and D help to organize the required prosthetic treatment in accordance with the severity of levels of involvement. Because the soft-tissue anatomy surrounding the bony abnormalities of LDFP differs from normal and compensates for gait deviations, it presents challenges for socket design. A clear understanding of the clinical picture of LDFP is required before prescribing a prosthesis. The approaches differ, depending on whether the deficiency is unilateral or bilateral. If the deficiency is bilateral, the orthopaedic surgeon should determine if it is symmetric and check for concurrent anomalies such as fibular deficiency, upper limb involvement, or contractures because these factors may alter the indicated treatment. The timing of surgical intervention should be coordinated with prosthetic treatment for optimal success. All of these factors need to be dealt with separately and thoroughly in order to recommend the best prosthesis, both cosmetically and functionally.

The clinical presentation of LDFP reveals a short femoral section held in a flexed, abducted, and externally rotated position and a flexed knee. Pirani and associates[34] explored the musculature of the four categories of LDFP in six patients through MRI and confirmed the presence of all soft-tissue structures that are in a normal leg (Figure 11). The differences are in their sizes and orientation, as a result of the abnormal osseous formations of each category. The authors suggested that despite the lack of osseous formation, the hip is stable because the musculature transfers the weight across the hip, similar to the function of the rotator cuff in the shoulder. Hypertrophy of the sartorius helps explain the "tailor" positioning of the leg. The authors postulated that, by fusing the knee, the sartorius changes its primary function to a hip flexor, and the contracted hamstrings will then extend the hip, thus improving the gait. The abductors remain weak, leading to a Trendelenburg gait. A better understanding of the total anatomy present in LDFP helps identify gait deviations and the indications for prosthetic treatment.

Bilateral Deficiency

When LDFP is bilateral, as it is in approximately 15% of patients,[35] it is usually Aitken type D. Typically, the choice of treatment is to do nothing if the deformity is symmetric and the

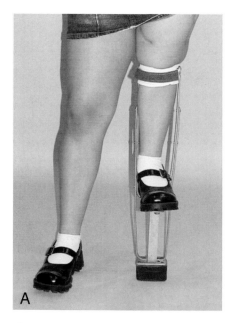
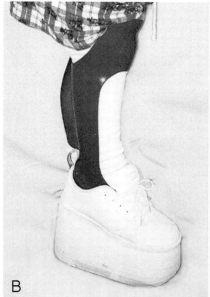
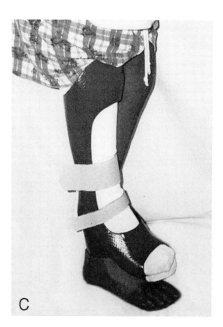

Figure 14 Various designs for orthoses and prostheses for leg-length discrepancies without amputations. **A**, Skate orthosis. **B**, Floor-reaction AFO in equinus with a shoe lift. **C**, Laminated floor-reaction AFO with attached prosthetic foot.

patient is functional. If the patient desires to be a more normal height, then a stilt-like prosthesis can be fabricated to incorporate the foot. A knee joint can be successfully incorporated with proper alignment and training. If a limb-length discrepancy is present, then a simple shoe lift is the easiest treatment (Figure 12).

Aitken Type A

Unilateral Aitken type A with a stable hip and shortened femur is the mildest form of LDFP. Treatment depends on the total length of the femur compared with the opposite side and must take into consideration any associated anomalies. Occasionally, a shoe lift can be the definitive treatment, giving symmetry to the legs and facilitating a normal gait.[36] Frequently, however, a more significant discrepancy is present that requires a "prosthosis" as a solution (Figure 13). One design[37] incorporates a plantigrade ankle-foot orthosis (AFO) that is attached to a pylon with adjustable pyramid components for alignment, connected to a solid ankle–cushion heel (SACH) or Seattle foot.

If a fibular deficiency that results in a valgus ankle deformity is present,

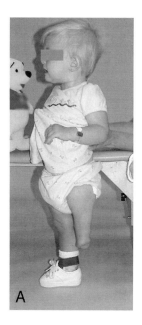
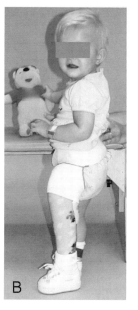

Figure 15 A, One-year-old patient without prosthesis standing with assistance. **B**, One-year-old patient with first prosthesis without a knee, for beginning ambulation.

then the orthosis will contribute stability. Another design places the anatomic foot in an equinus position to reduce the height difference and cosmetically conceal the foot. An anterior panel over the dorsum of the foot and proximal tibia help to unload the pressure of weight bearing. Either a lift or a pylon extension with a prosthetic foot at the base completes the "prosthosis" (Figure 14). Commonly, the

leg-length discrepancy is significant or anomalies are severe enough to require amputation. If a Syme ankle disarticulation can be performed and there is enough femoral length, then a Syme prosthesis is adequate. The only trade-off is that the knee on the amputated side will be considerably higher. This may require femoral lengthening or an epiphysiodesis of the opposite side to equalize knee heights.

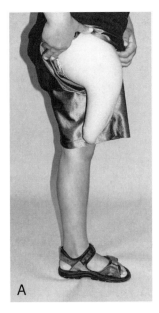
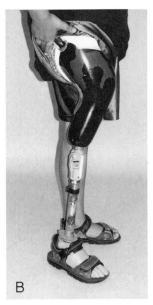
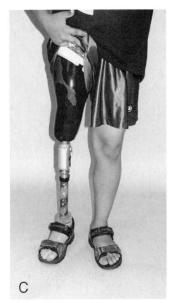
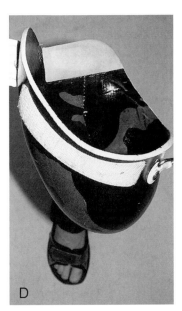

Figure 16 A, Patient with LDFP with limb length at knee on sound side. **B,** Lateral view of an unconventional endoskeletal construction LDFP above-knee socket using a dynamic foot and Silesian belt for suspension. **C,** Anterior view showing that knee heights are equivalent, allowing for a hydraulic knee. **D,** Top view to illustrate medial wall alignment orientation to toe out.

Aitken Types B, C, and D

Aitken types B, C, and D, although anatomically different, have common prosthetic solutions. Soon after birth, the surgical decision to amputate is made. Consultations are conducted that include the family, surgeon, prosthetist, therapists, and, ideally, another experienced family having a child with the same diagnosis. Typical treatment is a Syme procedure that leaves the affected side at approximately the same level as the knee on the opposite side. Surgery is recommended during the first year to enable the child to begin walking at an age-appropriate time. A knee joint may be introduced with the first prosthesis or later, at approximately 2 to 3 years of age, when there is more space to accommodate the component and the child can better follow gait training instructions (Figure 15).

The affected side presents clinically with the hip in a flexed, abducted, and externally rotated position with the knee flexed. The prosthetic socket for the residual limb resembles a ship's funnel to incorporate the resultant bundled musculature of the shortened femur and the intended position

of the tibia. The shape varies with the length of the femur and the category of LDFP. The Syme procedure offers a bulbous end for some weight bearing and possible suspension of the prosthesis. Fibular deficiency, however, is a commonly associated anomaly that reduces the bulbous shape of the leg and can also result in a genu valgum deformity that must be contained within the socket.

The design of the socket is unconventional because of the unique shape of a limb affected by LDFP. The most important goal is to maintain a total-contact fit for maximum transfer of load to supplement end bearing. Ischial containment or ischial weight-bearing is attractive, but this compromises the position of the anterior wall as a counterforce because of the unique anatomy of the thigh. Encompassing part of the gluteal fold may result in shared ischial/gluteal weight bearing, but it remains a challenge. The anterior wall encloses the bundle of muscles, the bulk of which is inversely proportionate to the length of femur and the attitude of flexion/extension at the knee (Figure 16). When the knee has been fused surgically, the anterior thigh bulk is re-

duced; the lateral wall can remain high for hip stability. In this situation, the medial wall needs to accommodate the rather rounded conical shape as well as the externally rotated position. When a good fit has been achieved, toddlers and adults can ambulate with comfort. The prosthetist should be aware that he or she is fitting a modified above-knee prosthesis around a thigh that may be weak, bulky, and unstable.

Suspension of a LDFP prosthesis may use means traditionally used to suspend other prostheses. The choice of suspension depends on the patient's anatomic architecture. The use of an expanded polyethylene foam liner or a window for the Syme conversion may be adequate if a bulbous end is present. An inner flexible bladder is another option. Usually a Silesian belt or total elastic suspension (TES) belt is the main or auxiliary form of suspension with a three-ply fit and hard socket construction. Suction sockets are generally not a realistic approach because of the unique shape of the residual limb. Because of length restrictions, liners with shuttle locks are rarely used. A hip joint with a pelvic band is also uncommon, but

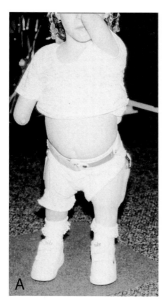
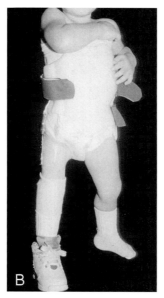
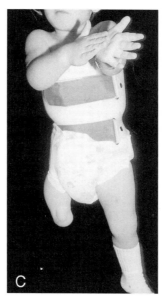
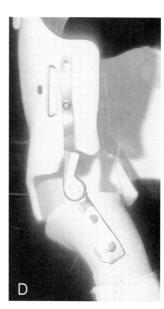

Figure 17 Some patients with very short residual limbs and unstable hips need hip joints for stability. **A,** A hip joint using a stabilizing extension on the contralateral side. **B,** Patient with LDFP and scoliosis treated with a thoracolumbosacral orthosis (TLSO). **C,** A TLSO incorporated for scoliosis and pelvic stability. **D,** Modified hip joint for flexion assist.

it may be indicated for a grossly unstable hip or extremely short residual limb (Figure 17).

The residual limb length poses ongoing challenges for the prosthetist. When implementing the first knee, outside hinges are usually the only way to match knee height to the opposite side. The knee centers may be so asymmetric that the distal thigh protrudes beyond the outside hinges when the child sits with the knee flexed. When space allows, a four-bar knee offers advantages in cosmesis, durability, and function, but placement is still often lower than the opposite side. In other cases, in order to compensate for length, a four-bar knee is helpful (Figure 18). Cosmetic consideration is a difficult challenge during growth. More severe categories of LDFP with less hip stability can benefit from a hydraulic knee, which offers better control in gait. The space allowed dictates the sophistication of the components. Because the leg affected with LDFP grows at a slower rate than the sound side, it may match the opposite knee height naturally. However, if an epiphysiodesis is necessary to achieve symmetric knee height by skeletal maturity, the surgeon must predict the growth of the leg. If the affected leg is

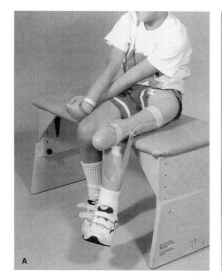
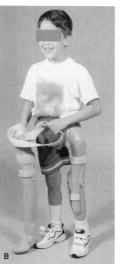
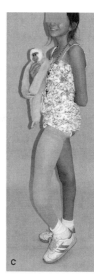

Figure 18 Patients with long residual limbs extending below the knee center on the unaffected side. **A** and **B,** Outside hinges for asymmetric knee heights functionally improve gait but have poor cosmesis. These are indicated for young patients, to allow growth time until revision or epiphysiodesis is considered. **C,** A four-bar knee in endoskeletal construction reduces the difference but does not resolve the cosmetic and stride-length problems.

significantly longer at skeletal maturity, a transtibial revision should be considered to equalize the knee height. The surgical plan should allow adequate space for componentry.

Revisions to a Syme ankle disarticulation after skeletal maturity occasionally help to equalize the knee height. Adequate room for compo-

nents should be considered to match the knee on the opposite side. A proximal tibial epiphysiodesis may be a better alternative. However, with any transtibial amputation, there is a risk of bony overgrowth that may necessitate another revision. This is why the transtibial amputation should be avoided unless necessary.

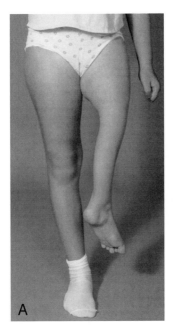
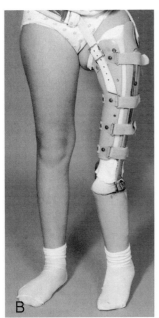
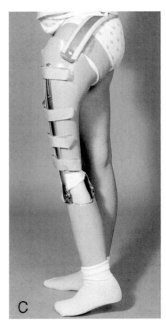
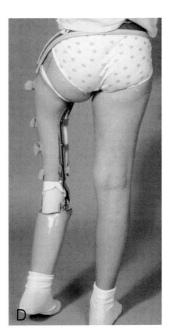

Figure 19 A, Patient with LDFP with Van Nes rotationplasty. **B,** Anterior view of unconventional socket with outside knee joint thigh lacer and Silesian belt suspension. **C,** Lateral view to illustrate alignment and cosmesis of foot in the socket. **D,** Posterior view of prosthesis.

Gait patterns for LDFP vary with the severity of the deformity. The more normal the hip joint and the longer the femur, the smoother the gait that will result. When the knee is fused in extension, a longer, more stable lever arm is created. Pirani and associates[34] suggested that, with a fusion, the function of the sartorius muscle is changed to a primary hip flexor, and the hip is extended more effectively by the hamstrings, resulting in an improved gait with increased knee stability. Because of the unique stabilizing musculature surrounding the hip, the telescoping of the femur is more limited than would be expected. There is a gluteus medius lurch caused by weak abductors on the affected side. Stride length is affected if knee heights are not the same. Vaulting to clear the toe is also a common gait deviation. Because the thigh is abducted, flexed, and externally rotated, the leg is advanced by the adductors and sartorius, coupled with a pelvic twist. In spite of these deviations, the resultant ambulation is quite effective and pain free.

The Van Nes rotationplasty poses another socket challenge for the prosthetist (Figure 19). The foot is encompassed in a below-the-knee socket in a weight-bearing equinus position, with joints and thigh lacer for support and suspension. The construction is usually exoskeletal, with an appropriate foot for the patient's activity level. Studies comparing patients with Van Nes rotationplasty with patients who have undergone Syme procedures showed that the former expend less energy during walking, have smoother gaits, and vault less at faster speeds.[26] However, there may be a tendency for the foot to derotate over time, necessitating a revision. The most obvious challenge is to make a prosthesis that is functional as well as cosmetically acceptable.

Summary

LDFP is a complex lower limb deficiency. The condition involves more than just a short femur, because the soft tissues, growth plates, and the other portions of the lower limb are frequently involved. Associated conditions, such as partial longitudinal deficiency of the fibula, complicate the condition and its treatment.

Treatment modalities range from amputation to limb salvage and limb lengthening. Prosthetic challenges include abnormal limb configuration, musculature, and joint alignment. The prosthetist must be able to fit limbs ranging from "ship's funnel" thighs to Van Nes derotations. Advancements in prosthetic orthopaedics have benefited this population with better components, improved materials, gait analysis, and surgical procedures.

The complexity of the condition necessitates a team approach to treatment with frequent reevaluations involving the surgeons, prosthetists, therapists, and, most important, the patient and family. The desires and abilities of the patient and family must be considered for any outcome to be successful and fruitful.

References

1. Bryant DD III, Epps CH Jr: Proximal femoral focal deficiency: Evaluation and management. *Orthopedics* 1991; 14:775-784.

2. Epps CH Jr: Proximal femoral focal deficiency. *J Bone Joint Surg Am* 1983; 65:867-870.

3. Sen Gupta DK, Gupta SK: Familial bilateral proximal femoral focal deficiency: Report of a kindred. *J Bone Joint Surg Am* 1984;66:1470-1472.

4. Bailey JA II, Beighton P: Bilateral femoral dysgenesis. *Clin Pediatr* 1970;9: 668-674.

5. Sorge G, Ardito S, Genuardi M, et al: Proximal femoral focal deficiency (PFFD) and fibular A/hypoplasia (FA/H): A model of a developmental field defect. *Am J Med Genet* 1995;55: 427-432.

6. Boden SD, Fallon MD, Davidson R, Mennuti MT, Kaplan FS: Proximal femoral focal deficiency: Evidence for a defect in proliferation and maturation of chondrocytes. *J Bone Joint Surg Am* 1989;71:1119-1129.

7. Grogan DP, Holt GR, Ogden JA: Talocalcaneal coalition in patients who have fibular hemimelia or proximal femoral focal deficiency: A comparison of the radiographic and pathological findings. *J Bone Joint Surg Am* 1994;76:1363-1370.

8. Grogan DP, Love SM, Ogden JA: Congenital malformations of the lower extremities. *Orthop Clin North Am* 1987;18:537-554.

9. Hillmann JS, Mesgarzadeh M, Revesz G, Bonakdarpour A, Clancy M, Betz RR: Proximal femoral focal deficiency: Radiologic analysis of 49 cases. *Radiology* 1987;165:769-773.

10. Schatz SL, Kopits SE: Proximal femoral focal deficiency. *AJR Am J Roentgenol* 1978;131:289-295.

11. Herring JA: Congenital lower limb deficiencies: Proximal focal femoral deficiency, in Herring JA (ed): *Tachdjian's Pediatric Orthopaedics*, ed 3. Philadelphia, PA, WB Saunders, 2002, pp 1756-1775.

12. Sanpera I Jr, Fixsen JA, Sparks LT, Hill RA: Knee in congenital short femur. *J Pediatr Orthop* 1995;4:159-163.

13. Sanpera I Jr, Sparks LT: Proximal femoral focal deficiency: Does a radiologic classification exist? *J Pediatr Orthop* 1994;14:34-38.

14. Aitken GT: Proximal femoral focal deficiency: Definition, classification, and management, in Aitken GT (ed): *Proximal Femoral Focal Deficiency: A Congenital Anomaly*. Washington, DC, National Academy of Sciences, 1968, pp 1-22.

15. Kritter AE: Tibial rotation-plasty for proximal femoral focal deficiency. *J Bone Joint Surg Am* 1977;59:927-934.

16. Alman BA, Krajbich JI, Hubbard S: Proximal femoral focal deficiency: Results of rotationplasty and Syme amputation. *J Bone Joint Surg Am* 1995;77:1876-1882.

17. Goddard NJ, Hashemi-Nejad A, Fixsen JA: Natural history and treatment of instability of the hip in proximal femoral focal deficiency. *J Pediatr Orthop* 1995;4:145-149.

18. Fixsen J, Lloyd-Roberts G: The natural history and early treatment of proximal femoral dysplasia. *J Bone Joint Surg Br* 1974;56:86-95.

19. Gillespie R, Torode IP: Classification and management of congenital abnormalities of the femur. *J Bone Joint Surg Br* 1983;65:557-568.

20. Paley D: The International Center for Limb Lengthening: Lengthening reconstruction surgery for congenital femoral deficiency. Available at www.lifebridgehealth.org/limblengthening. Accessed 7/1/03.

21. Tonnis D, Stanitski DF: Early conservative and operative treatment to gain early normal growth in proximal femoral focal deficiency. *J Pediatr Orthop* 1997;6:59-67.

22. Van Nes CP: Rotation-plasty for congenital defects of the femur: Making use of the ankle of the shortened limb to control the knee joint of a prosthesis. *J Bone Joint Surg Br* 1950;32:12-16.

23. Torode IP, Gillespie R: Rotationplasty of the lower limb for congenital defects of the femur. *J Bone Joint Surg Br* 1983;65:569-573.

24. Krajbich I: Proximal femoral focal deficiency, in Kalamachi A (ed): *Congenital Lower Limb Deficiencies*. New York, NY, Springer-Verlag, 1989, pp 108-127.

25. Friscia DA, Mosley CF, Oppenheim WL: Rotational osteotomy for proximal femoral focal deficiency. *J Bone Joint Surg Am* 1989;71:1386-1392.

26. Fowler E, Zernicke R, Setoguchi Y, Oppenheim W: Energy expenditure during walking by children who have proximal femoral focal deficiency. *J Bone Joint Surg Am* 1996;78: 1857-1862.

27. Fowler EG, Hester DM, Oppenheim WL, Setoguchi Y, Zernicke RF: Contrasts in gait mechanics of individuals with proximal femoral focal deficiency: Syme amputation versus Van Nes rotational osteotomy. *J Pediatr Orthop* 1999;19:720-731.

28. Steel H, Lin PS, Betz RR, Kalamchi A, Clancy M: Iliofemoral fusion for proximal femoral focal deficiency. *J Bone Joint Surg Am* 1987;69:837-843.

29. Brown KLB: Rotationplasty with hip stabilization in congenital femoral deficiency, in Jerring JA, Birch JG (eds): *The Child With a Limb Deficiency*. Rosemont, IL, American Academy of Orthopaedic Surgeons, 1998, pp 103-109.

30. Koman LA, Meyer LC: Proximal femoral focal deficiency: A 50-year experience. *Dev Med Child Neurol* 1982;24: 344-355.

31. Richardson EG, Rambach BE: Proximal femoral focal deficiency: A clinical appraisal. *South Med J* 1979;72: 166-173.

32. Saleh M, Goonatillake HD: Management of congenital leg length inequality: Value of early axis correction. *J Pediatr Orthop* 1995;4:150-158.

33. Conejero Casares JA, Florez Garcia MT, Salcedo Luengo J, Amaya Alarcon J, Boudet Garcia J, Gonzalez Herranz J: Alargamiento oseo en malformaciones congenitas de miembros inferiores. *An Esp Pediatr* 1991;34:293-298.

34. Pirani S, Beauchamp RD, Li D, Sawatzky B: Soft tissue anatomy of proximal femoral focal deficiency. *J Pediatr Orthop* 1991;11:563-570.

35. Stormer SV: Proximal femoral focal deficiency. *Orthop Nurs* 1997;16:25-31.

36. Sutherland DH (ed): *Gait Disorders in Childhood and Adolescence*. Baltimore, MD, Williams & Wilkins, 1984.

37. Devens MF: Treatment of proximal femoral focal deficiency by using a hybrid orthotic and prosthetic design. *J Prosthet Orthop* 1999;11:29-32.

Chapter 77

Absence of the Lumbar Spine and Sacrum

James T. Guille, MD
S. Jay Kumar, MD

Introduction

The term lumbosacral agenesis, or agenesis of the lumbar spine and sacrum, encompasses an uncommon condition characterized by the absence of one or more lumbar vertebrae along with a total or partial absence of the sacrum. The etiology of this condition is not fully understood, although it is believed to be caused by disruption in the development of the caudal portion of the bony spine and spinal cord, possibly by prenatal exposure to various substances such as solvents. The causes of this disruption in development are not fully understood, but a mutation in a homeobox gene may be responsible.[1] Although we have not observed any patients with a relative having the same condition, this has been reported by others.[2]

Although a history of maternal type 1 diabetes mellitus and maternal insulin use during pregnancy has been reported, a causal relationship between agenesis of the lumbar spine and sacrum and diabetes has not been identified. Inconsistencies exist in the reporting of specifics such as type of diabetes (type 1 or type 2) and the maternal consumption of insulin. Nevertheless, the reported prevalence of cases of sacral agenesis with some association with diabetes ranges from 14% to 50%.[3-8] Rusnak and Driscoll[9] reviewed 1,150 children born to mothers with diabetes and found that only three had sacral agenesis. No correlation has been reported between the severity of deformity and the presence of maternal diabetes mellitus.

Clinical Presentation

The term distal spinal agenesis has been proposed as a replacement for lumbosacral agenesis, but this has not received widespread acceptance.[5] We question the use of this terminology because up to one half of patients have involvement of the cervical spine. Thus, a wide variety of appearances can present in different individuals. The head may be large if hydrocephalus is present. Most patients will have a shortened trunk, depending on the amount of missing vertebral elements. Some authors believe that this shortened trunk predisposes the patient to respiratory distress and compression of the abdominal contents; however, this has never been proved by any objective study to our knowledge. Regardless, many of these patients develop a barrel-shaped chest with flaring of the ribs to accommodate the lungs and other organs. The classic buddha-like posture is usually seen in patients with near or total absence of the lumbar spine (Figure 1). Other conditions that may be observed include narrowed transverse diameter of the pelvis, atrophy and dimpling of the buttocks, a short intergluteal fold with horizontal anus, tapered atrophic lower limbs, and flexed, abducted, externally rotated hips.[10] The upper limbs are usually normal, but musculoskeletal abnormalities in the lower limbs, such as flexion contractures of the hip and knee and foot deformities, are common and depend on the level of paralysis. The tapered lower limbs have been described as resembling the appearance of a "siren" or "mermaid."

Imaging Studies

All patients with lumbosacral agenesis should have radiographs of the entire spine. For older children, AP and lateral views taken while the patient is

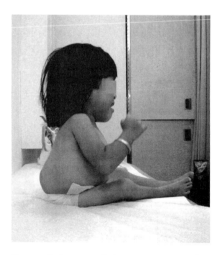

Figure 1 Characteristic appearance of a child with absence of the lumbar spine and sacrum.

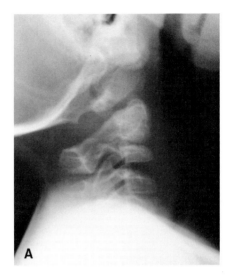
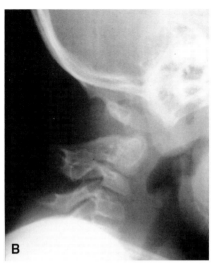

Figure 2 Extension (A) and flexion (B) lateral cervical spine radiographs showing occipitalization of the atlas with a hypoplastic dens.

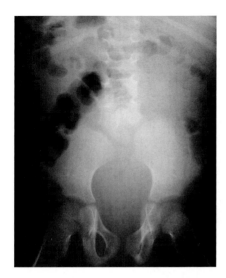

Figure 3 Radiograph showing the type A pattern, in which the vertebral column articulates in the midline with the pelvis. These patients have an excellent potential for ambulation.

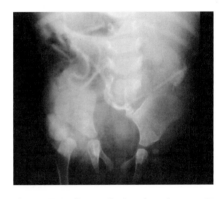

Figure 4 Radiograph showing the type B pattern, in which the vertebral column articulates with one of the ilia, shifted away from the midline.

TABLE 1 Renshaw Classification of Sacral Agenesis

Type	Characteristics
I	Partial or total unilateral sacral agenesis
II	Partial sacral agenesis with a partial but bilaterally symmetric defect and a stable articulation between the ilia; first sacral vertebra is normal or hypoplastic
III	Variable lumbar and total sacral agenesis; ilia articulate with the sides of the lowest vertebra present
IV	Variable lumbar and total sacral agenesis; caudal end plate of the most distal vertebra rests above either fused ilia or an iliac amphiarthrosis

sitting are recommended. Given the 50% prevalence of anomalies of the cervical spine, ranging from simple vertebral body fusion to atlantoaxial instability (Figure 2), routine screening is warranted.[4,11] Scoliosis is present in approximately one half of patients, and serial radiographs are used to document progression of a curve. The presence of hip dysplasia can be ruled out with an AP radiograph of the pelvis. MRI of the entire spine is necessary to look for occult intraspinal lesions and to determine the extent of the spinal dysraphism. Myelography is preferred in cases of severe spinal deformity or when

stainless steel spinal instrumentation precludes the use of MRI. In addition to studies of orthopaedic importance, shunt studies and imaging of the brain may be requested by the neurosurgeon, and renal ultrasound evaluations may be used by the urologist.

Classification

Two classifications of lumbosacral agenesis in the orthopaedic literature are popular today. The first is the four-part classification of Renshaw,[3] which was published in 1978 (Table 1).

More recently, Guille and associates[4] proposed a simple three-part classification in an effort to identify patients with ambulatory potential. These patients were then further subdivided into those with and those

without a myelomeningocele. By identifying these patients, the authors hoped that measures could be taken early to address anomalies of the lower limbs that would prohibit ambulation. All of the patients in the series had partial or total absence of the lumbar spine with total absence of the sacrum. In the type A patients, there was either a slight gap between the ilia or the ilia were fused in the midline, one or more lumbar vertebrae were absent, and the caudad aspect of the spine articulated with the pelvis in the midline (Figure 3). All patients with the type A pattern who did not have a myelomeningocele were able to ambulate, regardless of their motor level. In type B patients, the ilia were fused together, some of the lumbar vertebrae were absent, and the most

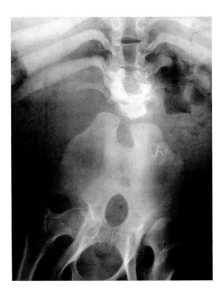

Figure 5 Radiograph showing the type C pattern, in which the vertebral column does not articulate with the pelvis.

caudad lumbar vertebra articulated with one of the ilia (Figure 4). None of these patients were functional ambulators. In type C patients, there was total agenesis of the lumbar spine, the ilia were fused together, and there was a gap between the most caudad intact thoracic vertebra and the pelvis (Figure 5). None of these patients were functional ambulators.

Typical Defects

As mentioned, a wide variety of spinal deformities occur in these patients. There can be partial to total absence of both the lumbar spine and sacrum. Approximately 25% of patients will have an associated myelomeningocele. Absence of a normal lumbosacral junction results in increased motion in this area. The cause and management of this motion is the subject of much debate.[12-14] Some investigators have termed this spinal-pelvic instability and believe that excessive motion occurs at the abnormal intersection, causing further shortening of the trunk and requiring use of the hands to support the upper body. Various techniques of spinal-pelvic fusion and fixation to stabilize

the area and increase the height of the trunk and volume of the abdomen have been described. Other investigators believe that the motion that occurs in this region provides for increased mobility and substitutes for restricted hip flexion.

Associated Findings and Abnormalities
Visceral Anomalies

Visceral anomalies, especially those involving the genitourinary and lower gastrointestinal systems, such as imperforate anus, are common.[8,15,16] Accordingly, most patients have a neurogenic bowel and bladder. Varying degrees of renal agenesis can be present, along with renal dysfunction. Inguinal hernias, cleft lip and palate, undescended testes, and cardiac anomalies are other visceral abnormalities that have been reported.

Anomalies of the Cervical Spine

The cervical spine is another area that is commonly affected in these children. Although abnormal findings on radiographs of the cervical spine have been noted in some reports, not until recently have investigators recommended routine radiographic screening of the cervical spine in all patients with lumbosacral agenesis. Guille and associates[4] observed that anomalies of the cervical spine, most commonly isolated congenital fusions, were present in 9 of 18 patients. A recent unpublished review of 60 patients from the same institution showed a similar prevalence (JT Guille, MD, Alfred I. duPont Hospital for Children, Wilmington, DE, 2003). The role of routine MRI scans of the cervical spine in these patients has yet to be defined.

Neuromuscular Findings

All patients with lumbosacral agenesis have neurologic compromise secondary to the spinal dysraphism. Corre-

sponding neural elements are also absent or anomalous, resulting in various motor and sensory deficits as well as bowel and bladder dysfunction. We believe it is difficult to predict motor and sensory levels based on the radiographic appearance of the spine. Some investigators believe that it is important to identify the last vertebra with an intact laminar arch (LILA) or bilaterally visible pedicles. This vertebra should be differentiated from the caudad vertebra that articulates with the pelvis or ilia. Part of the confusion arises from the fact that in the literature this landmark has been variously referred to as "nubbin," "last normal vertebra," "last intact vertebra," or "last recognizable vertebra," with no clear definition provided. The identification of this vertebra is important, as Phillips[15] noted that the level of involvement was best described by the most caudal normal vertebral body, which "usually corresponds well with the degree of motor impairment," but the term "normal" was not defined. The association between the most caudal normal vertebral body and the degree of motor impairment has been reported by some, but not all, investigators. This landmark has been said to be a more reliable predictor of motor power and sensory level in children with only a myelomeningocele.[17] Many patients with lumbosacral agenesis, on the other hand, will have multiple anomalous lumbar vertebrae that may have intact neural elements providing motor and/or sensory function.

Differential Diagnosis

The differential diagnosis includes the various forms of spinal dysraphism, caudal regression syndrome, and congenital vertebral anomalies. Many of these conditions can coexist in the same patient. For example, a patient may have absence of the sacrum and lumbar vertebrae, thoracic hemivertebrae Lund scoliosis, and a myelomeningocele.

Treatment Options

The orthopaedic management of children with lumbosacral agenesis has always been controversial. For the more severely affected lower limbs, amputation at the subtrochanteric level or knee disarticulation and subsequent prosthetic fitting has been advocated.[10,18,19] Other authors believe that these patients have satisfactory sensation and proprioception in their lower limbs and have stated that patients perceive preservation of the limbs to be essential for them to have a complete body image.[2,14] Frantz and Aitken[18] and Russell and Aitken[19] reported that amputation allowed the patient to sit better and to ambulate effectively with the hands. Renshaw[3] believed that amputation may be the treatment of choice in patients with severe contractures of the lower limbs. Winter[20] stated that the bone harvested from amputation could be used for bone graft during spinal reconstruction. Andrish and associates[14] and Banta and Nichols[2] advocated leaving the lower limbs alone in these patients because they provide stability for sitting, often maintain proprioception and protective sensation, and provide the patients with a better body image. We do not advocate routine amputation. We believe that soft-tissue releases that are performed early and selective corrective osteotomies can obviate the need for amputation in most patients.

In an effort to stabilize the spinal-pelvic junction, Perry and associates[12] advocated fusion of the lumbar spine to the pelvis. Others have reported that spinal-pelvic instability is not a problem in their patients.[14] In our experience, patients function well without a spinal-pelvic fusion. Some authors believe that spinal-pelvic fusion allows the hands to be free from supporting the body, protects the viscera from compression, and allows more effective stretching of contractures of the lower limbs. This reasoning has been used more recently by several authors who have described modified techniques with modern instrumentation.[20-22] Although we have no experience with spinal-pelvic fusion, we believe that patients who have hip flexion contractures will have difficulty with sitting and ambulation if the spine is fused to the pelvis. Andrish and associates[14] described nine patients with spinal-pelvic instability who had no visceral compression and whose ambulation was enhanced by the fact that they had a mobile spinal-pelvic junction. Banta and Nichols[2] suggested that lumbar-pelvic instability did not have to be treated surgically and that a brace could be used if support was needed.

It has been reported that hip dislocation, severe knee flexion contractures, and popliteal webbing are more common in patients with a high-level (first lumbar) lesion.[2,7] In our study, we could not correlate the presence of hip dysplasia with the level of spinal involvement or motor power.[4] We believe an attempt at hip reduction and later reconstruction should be made only in patients who have ambulatory potential. Hip and knee flexion contractures should be corrected early with stretching; soft-tissue releases or supracondylar extension osteotomies of the distal femur are done later, if necessary, in patients who have a potential to ambulate. Banta and Nichols[2] stated that complete correction of knee flexion contractures needs to be obtained and that deformity can recur even after complete correction. In children older than 8 years, anterior knee physeal stapling may be performed to prevent recurrence of the deformity. In our opinion, hip and knee deformities should be addressed at the same setting.

Most patients have bilateral rigid foot deformities; a clubfoot is most common. An initial attempt at stretching and casting should be tried in most patients. If the condition does not respond and if the patient has ambulatory potential or if shoe wear is difficult, soft-tissue releases may be performed. If inadequate correction is obtained from this procedure, osteotomies or fusions may be required.

In our study, we could not correlate the presence of scoliosis with the pattern of deformity or motor level, other than finding it more prevalent in children with an associated myelomeningocele.[4] Van Buskirk and Ritterbusch[5] found that scoliosis was present in 13 of 19 patients (68%) and was more common in patients with extensive spinal involvement. Forty-six percent of their patients had congenital scoliosis. Scoliosis in these patients needs to be observed carefully, as bracing is impractical because of the body habitus. Consideration should be given to arthrodesis for progressive curves or curves that interfere with ambulation or sitting. The use of rigid segmental instrumentation can obviate the need for postoperative immobilization in most patients. Fusion of the cervical spine is performed for patients who have instability.

Rehabilitation

Most patients with ambulatory potential initially will require hip-knee-ankle-foot orthoses (HKAFOs) with dial locks at the hips and knees. Children are best fitted with braces between the ages of 12 and 18 months. As the ambulatory potential improves and the lower limb deformities are corrected, most children with type I lumbosacral agenesis can walk with knee-ankle-foot orthoses (KAFOs) or ankle-foot orthoses (AFOs) with a standard walker. Braces may be tried in children who have the type II condition, but these children are never functional walkers.[23,24] It is futile to brace children with the type III condition with the intent of ambulation, especially if they have a myelomeningocele and fixed abduction-external rotation contractures of the hips.

A parapodium and braces may be used to achieve upright posture (Figure 6). A bucket-type prosthesis is needed for patients who have undergone bilateral subtrochanteric amputation. These children will generally ambulate with crutches and a swing-through gait. Because of issues of

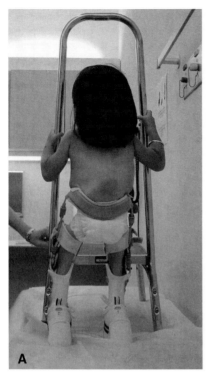
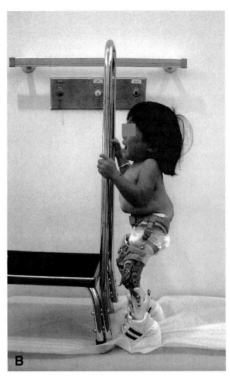

Figure 6 Posterior **(A)** and lateral **(B)** photographs of a child with type III lumbosacral agenesis. The child is able to stand in HKAFOs with support but is unable to ambulate functionally.

practicality and the high energy consumption required for prosthetic gait, prosthetic fitting for these children is controversial and challenging. A wheelchair with seating modifications (padding and cut-outs) provides the most optimal and efficient means of transportation for most patients with absence of the lumbar spine and sacrum.

Summary

Most patients with lumbosacral agenesis, especially those with large areas of the spine and sacrum absent, have marked disability. The etiology of this condition remains unknown. When the condition is recognized, it is of the utmost importance that the physician evaluate organ systems other than the musculoskeletal system for congenital anomalies and dysfunction. The cervical spine should be screened radiographically for vertebral anomalies and atlantoaxial instability. The upper limbs are usually normal, but the lower limbs are af-

fected by paralysis and contractures. Surgical treatment of the lower limbs is indicated in patients with ambulatory potential or to facilitate brace and shoe wear. The role of spinal-pelvic fusion and lower limb amputation remains controversial.

References

1. Ross AJ, Ruiz-Perez V, Wang Y, et al: A homeobox gene, HLXB9, is the major locus for dominantly inherited sacral agenesis. *Nat Genet* 1998;20:358-361.

2. Banta JV, Nichols O: Sacral agenesis. *J Bone Joint Surg Am* 1969;51:693-703.

3. Renshaw TS: Sacral agenesis: A classification and review of twenty-three cases. *J Bone Joint Surg Am* 1978;60:373-383.

4. Guille JT, Benevides R, DeAlba CC, Siriram V, Kumar SJ: Lumbosacral agenesis: A new classification correlating spinal deformity and ambulatory potential. *J Bone Joint Surg Am* 2002;84:32-38.

5. Van Buskirk CS, Ritterbusch JF: Natural history of distal spinal agenesis. *J Pediatr Orthop* 1997;6:146-152.

6. Passarge E, Lenz W: Syndrome of caudal regression in infants of diabetic mothers: Observations of further cases. *Pediatrics* 1966;37:672-675.

7. Phillips WA, Cooperman DR, Lindquist TC, Sullivan RC, Millar EA: Orthopaedic management of lumbosacral agenesis: Long-term follow-up. *J Bone Joint Surg Am* 1982;64:1282-1294.

8. Blumel J, Evans EB, Eggers GWN: Partial and complete agenesis or malformation of the sacrum with associated anomalies: Etiologic and clinical study with special reference to heredity. A preliminary report. *J Bone Joint Surg Am* 1959;41:497-518.

9. Rusnak SL, Driscoll SG: Congenital spinal anomalies in infants of diabetic mothers. *Pediatrics* 1965;35:989-995.

10. Frantz CH: Complete absence of the lumbar spine and sacrum, in Aitken GT (ed): *Selected Lower-Limb Anomalies: Surgical and Prosthetics Management.* Washington, DC, National Academy of Sciences, 1971, pp 29-48.

11. Guille JT, Sherk HH: Congenital osseous anomalies of the upper and lower cervical spine in children. *J Bone Joint Surg Am* 2002;84:277-288.

12. Perry J, Bonnett CA, Hoffer MM: Vertebral pelvic fusions in the rehabilitation of patients with sacral agenesis. *J Bone Joint Surg Am* 1970;52:288-294.

13. Dal Monte A, Andrisano A, Capanna R: The surgical treatment of lumbosacral coccygeal agenesis. *Ital J Orthop Traumatol* 1979;5:259-266.

14. Andrish J, Kalamchi A, MacEwen GD: Sacral agenesis: A clinical evaluation of its management, heredity, and associated anomalies. *Clin Orthop* 1979;139:52-57.

15. Phillips WA: Sacral agenesis, in Weinstein SL (ed): *The Pediatric Spine: Principles and Practice*, ed 2. Philadelphia, PA, Lippincott Williams and Wilkins, 2001, pp 193-201.

16. Wilmshurst JM, Kelly R, Borzyskowski M: Presentation and outcome of sacral agenesis: 20 years' experience. *Dev Med Child Neurol* 1999;41:806-812.

17. Trivedi J, Thomson JD, Slakey JB, Banta JV, Jones PW: Clinical and radiographic predictors of scoliosis in patients with myelomeningocele. *J Bone Joint Surg Am* 2002;84:1389-1394.

18. Frantz CH, Aitken GT: Complete absence of the lumbar spine and sacrum. *J Bone Joint Surg Am* 1967;49: 1531-1540.

19. Russell HE, Aitken GT: Congenital absence of the sacrum and lumbar vertebrae with prosthetic management: A survey of the literature and presentation of five cases. *J Bone Joint Surg Am* 1963;45:501-508.

20. Winter RB: Congenital absence of the lumbar spine and sacrum: One-stage reconstruction with subsequent two-stage spine lengthening. *J Pediatr Orthop* 1991;11:666-670.

21. Rieger MA, Hall JE, Dalury DF: Spinal fusion in a patient with lumbosacral agenesis. *Spine* 1990;15:1382-1384.

22. Dumont C-E, Damsin J-P, Forin V, Carlioz H: Lumbosacral agenesis: Three cases of reconstruction using Cotrel-Dubousset or L-rod instrumentation. *Spine* 1993;18:1229-1235.

23. Hoffer MM, Feiwell E, Perry R, Perry J, Bonnett C: Functional ambulation in patients with myelomeningocele. *J Bone Joint Surg Am* 1973;55:137-148.

24. Huff CW, Ramsey PL: Myelodysplasia: The influence of the quadriceps and hip abductor muscles on ambulatory function and stability of the hip. *J Bone Joint Surg Am* 1978;60:432-443.

Chapter 78

Multiple Limb Deficiencies

Hugh Watts, MD

Introduction

Children with limb deficiencies have special problems not shared by adult amputees, and the difficulties mount exponentially for children with multiple limb involvement (Figure 1). Therefore, the care of such children should take place in special treatment facilities.

The term multiple limb deficiencies covers many possibilities, ranging from the child missing two minor toes and a single finger on the nondominant hand to the child born with no arms or legs. Children may have multiple limb deficiencies either because they were born with the deficiencies or as a result of an accident or illness. Common sense is required to recognize and treat appropriately the varied needs of these children.

Congenital Multiple Limb Deficiencies

Limb deficiencies may refer not just to the absence of a limb but also to anomalies of the extremities that might require a prosthesis or modification of a prosthesis for one of the involved limbs. For example, a child with the most severe form of thrombocytopenia and absent radius (TAR) syndrome may have phocomelic upper limbs and fusion of both knees due to congenital synchondroses. These children cannot effectively use their feet to replace the limited hand

function because their knees do not bend sufficiently to allow the foot to reach the mouth. If bilateral knee disarticulations are performed, the child would be able to sit in a chair more easily but would be unable to get up from the floor after a fall because his or her arms are too short to help.

Of children with congenital limb deficiencies, 30% have multiple limb involvement (15% with two limbs, 5% with three limbs, and 10% with all four limbs).[1-3] By contrast, only 10% of children with acquired amputations have a loss of more than a single limb. Because approximately 60% of children seen in amputee clinics have congenital conditions,[2,4] children with multiple limb deficiencies represent a significant population that cannot be overlooked. Children who sustain traumatic amputations are probably underrepresented in these statistics because they are treated in the community and not in pediatric amputee centers, particularly if they have lower limb amputations, which are easier to manage in a less specialized facility.[5] This also relates to the widely held belief that limb deficiencies in children more often involve the upper limbs. Among children who have acquired amputations, only 40% will involve the upper limb; however, of children presenting to amputee clinics, in those with congenital conditions the upper limb is twice as likely to be involved.[2]

Associated Anomalies

The old medical school adage "If there is one congenital anomaly look for other anomalies" is relevant to this discussion. The limbs form at 4 to 7 weeks of gestation, as do organs such as the kidneys and heart. Therefore, a thorough examination for associated anomalies is mandatory. The clinician should start at the head and work downward, checking the cranial nerves, especially VII; the palates (soft and hard); and the eyes and ears for placement and formation. Then examine the chest, checking for the proper

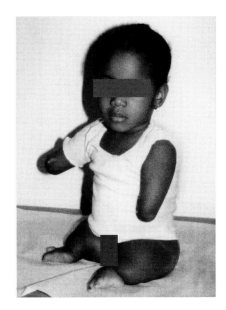

Figure 1 Child with multiple limb deficiencies.

number and placement of nipples, and examining the pectoral muscles. Check for a heart murmur and examine the anus for normal formation. Carefully check the other limbs: even minor abnormalities could change the diagnostic (and possibly prognostic) category from single-limb to multiple-limb. Look for petechiae or bruises that might suggest TAR syndrome. Ask the mother and the nurses in the newborn nursery about the infant's sucking and swallowing to assess for tracheoesophageal abnormalities. If the infant's urination is abnormal, renal anomalies might be suspected.

Renal ultrasound and chest radiographs to evaluate the heart should be ordered for all limb-deficient infants. Any child with a radial limb deficiency should also have a complete blood count and differential blood count, including a platelet count.

Anomalies in the central nervous system (CNS) or one of the receptive senses (vision or hearing) have a particular importance. Children are generally extremely adaptable, but if the CNS is involved, the child's adaptive capacity may be compromised.

Acquired Multiple Limb Deficiencies

Not all multiple limb involvement is congenital. One devastating condition is purpura fulminans, commonly caused by meningococcal disease, with resultant disseminated intravascular clotting. The condition can follow other bacteremias (eg, with pneumococci) or viremias (eg, chicken pox). The child is normal one moment, and, several hours later, without warning for the family, may become a multiple limb amputee. Train accidents can be another cause of multiple limb loss. A common scenario is that of a child trying to hop a train at the after-end ladder, losing his or her grip, and being spun around the back end of the railway car and thrown down on the tracks in front of the following car. This commonly results in the loss of two or more limbs.

The age at which the child sustains a traumatic amputation can greatly affect the outcome. Older children who lose limbs often do not adjust to the loss as well as do children who start life with congenital losses. Often, older children are disappointed with the function of bilateral upper limb prostheses because they have experienced normal-functioning limbs.

Special Needs of the Multiple Limb–Deficient Child

This *Atlas* can generally be seen as a resource, providing practical, how-to advice. Children with multiple limb loss, however, present special challenges to the professionals who work with them. As Fisk pointed out, the knowledge gained by treating one child with multiple limb deficiencies does not necessarily transfer to another because each is unique: "When you have seen one, then you have seen just one" (J Fisk, MD, personal communication, 2002).

Prosthetic Components

Children with multiple limb deficiencies have a greater need for specialized prosthetic components than do those with single limb deficiencies. Several characteristics of prosthetic components need to be considered in relation to the special needs of the child with multiple deficiencies.

Size and Weight

Prosthetic components for adults usually come in large, medium, and small sizes, with perhaps an extra small size that is usually appropriate for smaller women. Children, however, need an array of sizes, to fit a tiny 1-year-old up to a teenager of almost adult proportions. Although competition has encouraged many manufacturers to address this niche market, it is not economically feasible for manufacturers of prosthetic components to fabricate and store large stocks of multiple-sized items that have a low turnover. Hence, some

such components may need to be individually crafted. The weight of prosthetic components is an issue not only because of the smaller muscle mass available to move the prostheses but also because children with multiple limb deficiencies find that minor difficulties with one prosthesis may adversely affect the functioning of another.

Heat Retention

Wearing a limb prosthesis can be hot, especially in warm climates. Children who have to wear two, three, or even four prostheses may not have enough bare skin to disperse heat adequately. Also, prostheses for higher levels of limb deficiency demand greater energy expenditure by the child, compounding the heat problem. This is a particular problem if the child has a hip or shoulder disarticulation requiring a prosthesis that covers a considerable area of the trunk. Body temperature may become significantly elevated. Even reasonable normal activity may be prohibitive in any season, and especially so in the summer, and the child may understandably refuse to wear the prostheses.

Integration of Prosthetic Components

Children with multiple limb deficiencies frequently require custom-designed components. This typically requires custom fabrication. For example, an 8-year-old boy who was born with bilateral hip disarticulations and an absent left hand was able to walk on bilateral lower limb prostheses by using a regular forearm crutch with his normal right arm and by having a specially made crutch built as the terminal device of the left upper limb prosthesis. For use when the boy was not walking, the left arm prosthesis included a quick-disconnect wrist that let him easily exchange the crutch for a hook. Fabrication of such special items is labor intensive and costly. Yet such challenges provide the stimulus to creativity that those dealing with these children find very satisfying.

Donning and Doffing

Often, too little attention is paid to the child's ability to don and doff the prostheses independently. The child with multiple deficiencies may wear such an array of devices that it can be difficult for a parent, let alone the child, to apply them all. If the child is to become an independent adult, this aspect must be considered. Obviously, this need will depend on the child's age and psychosocial development and the relationships within the family. Many parents are reluctant to let go of their own need to assist the child and must be encouraged by the clinic staff to do so. Prostheses appropriately designed for ease of donning and doffing may help. Examples might be the use of Velcro pull tabs on belts and harnesses that can be easily grasped with a prosthetic hook for donning a suction socket, or a total elastic suspension (TES) belt for those wearing transfemoral prostheses.

Wheelchair Use

The various components need to be integrated with the child's possible need for a wheelchair. If a powered wheelchair is not necessary, a standard chair is preferable because the exercise it requires can help with the common problem of obesity. If a powered chair is necessary, its size and weight must be considered. It will usually be necessary for the parents to have a van modified with a lift or ramp to accept the chair because power chairs are so heavy. For adolescents of driving age, the van will need to be modified to allow the wheelchair user to operate the vehicle.

For the most severely involved children, such as those missing both arms and both legs, the wheelchair may need to be adjustable to almost floor level. This allows the child to crawl or roll onto the seat, and then raise the seat to a level more functional for table activities. Such wheelchairs are individually fabricated and are very costly.

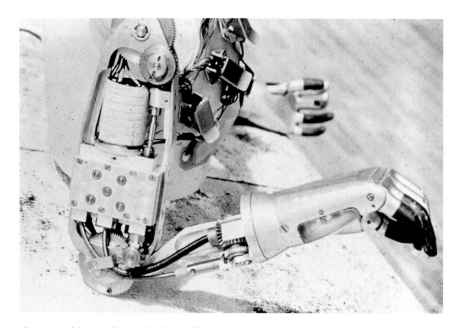

Figure 2 This prosthesis, developed for a bilateral high-level upper limb amputee, is unlikely to be worn by a child born with absence of both upper limbs because it will be hot, heavy, and provide little sensory feedback. It exceeds a child's gadget tolerance.

Gadget Tolerance

Members of the rehabilitation team or the family may devise a complicated mix of equipment, especially electronic, to allow the child to perform an array of activities. Often these devices outstrip the child's needs and desires. In spite of their adaptability, children will not tolerate having a large number of highly technical mechanical devices applied to them. This is commonly called "poor gadget tolerance" (Figure 2). Children often function much better without the equipment. An electronic replacement for an upper limb may cause amazement when seen on television but is infrequently accepted in the long term by a child with multiple limb deficiencies. Many reasons have been given for this, but factual information is lacking. Most children find it hard to articulate why they prefer not to wear upper limb prostheses. It has been speculated that the excessive heat buildup, high energy consumption, discomfort, and most importantly the lack of sensory feedback are important factors in prosthesis rejection. Others have speculated that children born with a limb deficiency may lack an appropriate representation in the brain for the absent limb. Regardless of the reasons, the lack of willingness among children to wear upper limb prostheses has been frustrating for those working to develop improved upper limb prosthetic components for this population.

Funding

Given the need for multiple prostheses, special wheelchairs, and vans for the child's transportation, the major limitation experienced by the family of a child with multiple limb deficiencies is likely to be the ability to pay for all the ancillary equipment. Some government agencies may help, as will a number of charitable organizations. Sadly, those with personal experience note that cute, verbal children are usually most likely to benefit from these sources.

Accessibility to the classroom and assistants to help these children (especially with toileting while they are at school) are more common since the passage of legislation ensuring educational opportunities for all.

Developmental Capabilities

As is true of able-bodied children, the developmental capabilities of children with limb deficiencies are constantly changing. Unlike able-bodied children, however, those with multiple limb deficiencies face greater challenges, and the adaptation required may be overwhelming. Although there have been reports of successful fittings of toddlers with a unilateral prosthesis incorporating an articulated knee, the child with multiple limb loss faces a greater challenge. Mastering two articulated lower limb prostheses is very difficult, and if upper limb deficiency is present, the child's ability to avoid injury in a fall is compromised. It is much simpler, therefore, for these children to learn to use nonarticulated limbs. The child's intellectual development as well as physical coordination and strength are important in planning the prosthetic program. A 5-year-old cannot be expected to manage myoelectrically controlled hands with the same dexterity as a 12-year-old. Prosthetic components for children need to be appropriate to the developmental age of a child and for the degree of multiple challenges they may face. Surprisingly, this principle is often forgotten.

Age of First Fitting

Some have advocated fitting children younger than 6 months of age so that the child can be trained to develop bimanual eye-hand coordination. Current practice, however, is to wait until a child is beginning to develop sitting balance, usually at about 5 to 6 months of age. The first fitting may occur later in a child with multiple limb loss, however, if developmental delay or other health needs intervene.

Age of Activation of Terminal Devices

The age at which the terminal devices in a child's prostheses should be activated will depend on the child's psychomotor development. Ordinarily, the terminal device is mounted at the time the prosthesis is first applied. At first, the therapists and parents open the device and place objects in it so that the child can understand the

principle of the device. If a myoelectric prosthesis is to be used, some clinics will fit the child very early (at 12 to 24 months) with a simpler single-electrode system, which alternately controls opening and closing. If a body-powered prosthesis is to be used, the activating cable is usually connected at about 18 to 24 months of age, when the child is more developmentally ready. Once again, the major factor in the timing of these decisions is the child's developmental readiness. In children with multiple limb deficiencies, the timetable may need to be extended.

Sports and Recreational Activities

Children learn by playing. A child with multiple limb deficiencies is no different. Such children may have an even greater psychological and physical need for active play both because they have few activities to help them burn calories and because food is often offered to these children in sympathy by parents and siblings. This is especially true for children with multiple high-level deficiencies, in whom the propensity for obesity should be counteracted with exercise and caloric limitation. Children with lower level deficiencies who wear prostheses and are very active may burn energy at a rate such that they need additional calories to maintain normal weight.

Although parents sometimes worry that swimming is not safe for children with multiple limb deficiencies, swimming is a good sport for amputees, and can be readily done by those with no legs. Even children with missing arms and legs can perform a porpoise-like trunk motion that will propel them through the water. Clearly, supervision is necessary, but many swim groups welcome the challenge of helping these children.

Skiing is another favorite sport among amputees because it gives them an opportunity to experience the exhilaration of speed. Clearly, the child will need help, and prostheses may need to be modified. An extra socket may be needed to protect the

residual limb and keep it warm when no prosthesis is worn. For ski poles, modified forearm crutches are fitted with small ski tips ("outriggers"). Of course instruction is important to help the child use these new pieces of equipment. If skiing "tri-track" or "three track," is unrealistic, a child with multiple limb deficiencies could learn to ski seated in a special frame mounted over a single ski, called a monoski, which is what paraplegics use.

Amputees can learn to participate in sports of all kinds at special centers. Parents often need to be encouraged to let their children participate because it is natural for them to be overprotective. This may require an active effort on the part of the clinic team to reassure parents. A referral to a recreational therapist may be beneficial.

Sexuality

Children with multiple limb deficiencies will undergo normal sexual maturation and have normal concerns about sex. These children face many of the same issues as their able-bodied peers, but their sexual development is often complicated by added concerns about their altered body image and how they will be accepted by a potential partner. Do the patients we care for suddenly change from children into adults overnight on their 21st birthdays? Who is going to talk to them about this? Adult amputees do discuss issues of sexuality among themselves. Clinic team members are often squeamish about discussing sexuality, but they should not shy away from facing this issue. They need to provide the developing child with appropriate information or counseling. Adult men without arms or legs have fathered children, limbless women have given birth to children, and both have successfully raised children.

Adolescents with congenital deficiencies commonly worry about passing their condition on to potential offspring. Such worries are generally unfounded, but a referral to a genetic counselor may provide valuable insight and, in most cases, will relieve the anxiety.

Psychological Needs of the Child and Family

One would expect that multiple limb deficiency would exact a heavy toll on a child's psyche. Surprisingly, studies have shown that these children do well psychologically.[6-10]

A long-term prosthetic treatment plan may be easier to accomplish in a child than in an adult who is employed and cannot afford to miss work. On the other hand, intervening during childhood means that more people are involved with the prosthetic management: the patient, the parents, and, frequently, two sets of grandparents as well. Issues such as the need for a "conversion amputation" or the child's refusal to wear upper limb prostheses may require more skillful diplomacy with the grandparents than with the parents. Both the parents and grandparents should know that it is their right, and it is in the best interests of the child, for them to be appropriately informed. There is usually no need to rush into elective conversion amputations until everyone is comfortable with the need to proceed.

The need for cultural sensitivity has come to assume more importance in recent decades. Some cultures are much more resistant to conversion amputation, though the clinic team may see the need as obvious. These cultural differences can be compounded because of misunderstandings caused by language translation. Putting the child's family in contact with other families who share the same cultural traditions can often be an enormous help.

Special Aspects of Upper Limb Absence
Scoliosis

Children with upper limb deficiencies have an increased chance of developing scoliosis, either congenital or idiopathic.[11-15] If the scoliosis should become progressive, the curves are notoriously resistant to bracing, if for no other reason than such braces are difficult to wear for a child with upper limb absence. If spinal fusion is being considered, the possible impact on the child's ability to reach the mouth with the feet should be considered carefully because most of these children choose to use their feet rather than prostheses. Decisions should be made based on advantages and disadvantages to the child's lifetime functioning rather than on the basis of radiographic findings alone.

Use of Upper Limb Prostheses

Children born without one or both upper limbs can be extraordinarily capable of functioning. They can readily be taught to feed themselves and perform many tasks using their feet and toes (Figure 3). Objects can be grasped between the chin and shoulder or between a very short humeral stump and the chest wall.[16] The sensory feedback provided by using feet or residual limbs is an advantage over any prosthesis. The increased energy consumption required to manipulate a prosthesis can be a problem in the multiple limb–deficient child. Also, the recent focus on high-technology components for adults has not found a significant place in prosthetics for children because of the high costs. These factors can lead to difficulty when trying to convince a child to wear an upper limb prosthesis because the child may be more facile, especially initially, without the prosthesis. In fact, most children who are born without arms will not wear prostheses throughout their lifetime.[17-19] The percentage of such children who use prostheses may depend on the enthusiasm of the clinic team for fitting such children and may also depend on the age at which such children are first fitted.[20]

Although there are some notable exceptions, in spite of all of the developments in the field of modern prosthetics, the lack of proprioception, the

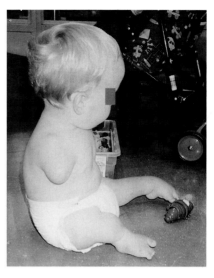

Figure 3 This child readily uses his feet to replace the function of the hands.

weight, and the discomfort of heat retention are such that children find that they function better without prosthetic help. By the time they reach adulthood, they are able to do almost everything for themselves, including driving an automobile, with their feet.

These comments relate to children born without arms. Children who lose their arms to trauma are much more likely to struggle to replace the limbs they were accustomed to.

With this in mind, common sense and a need to carefully husband limited financial resources might lead the team to not prescribe any upper limb prostheses. Other factors should be considered, however. For example, at some point in their lives, especially during adolescence, children born without arms may request simple cosmetic arms to be used for special occasions.

Initially, most parents are desperate to try to fit their child with prosthetic arms. As a consequence, a trial of prosthetic fitting may be a necessary stage that a family must go through so that they can personally experience the rejection of the prostheses by the child. Consequently, the prescription of a set of arm prostheses with expensive myoelectric components may not be a practical way to begin. There may be a temporary need, however, to provide lifelike passive hands for an infant so that a parent will not reject the child.

Because these children will probably not use prosthetic arms and will function by using the feet in place of the hands, it is important to know the status of the motion and muscle control of the hips, knees, ankles, and toes. Careful examination is essential because congenital anomalies are frequently associated with other anomalies.

The occupational therapist's skills in upper extremity prosthetic training may play a limited role in the child's care if, in the long run, the child will not wear prostheses. The therapist's important role will be to teach the child how best to substitute the feet for the missing arms and how to use adaptive equipment creatively. The ability to shrug the shoulders can be useful for grasping objects between the side of the neck and the upper scapula. The use of assistive devices (for example, a mouth stick for typing) can help the older child deal with the world. Toileting is a major problem for the child without arms, especially if the child wants to be able to use public restrooms, such as in a mall while shopping with friends.

Computers may change the lives of children with upper limb absence. Computers can be used as controllers to activate remote switches (eg, turning lights on and off or answering a telephone), although control of the computer keyboard is still a problem. Voice-control software has not yet proved to be as effective with children as with adults.

Summary: A Hypothetical Scenario

Consider a girl born with no arms, a little nub of a right lower limb, and a very short left lower limb with multiple congenital anomalies. She can move her left foot well with good control, but she cannot reach her mouth with her foot, and she does not have enough strength to hold a long-handled spoon to feed herself.

Options for this child's care might be to fit her with bilateral upper limb prostheses that are switch-controlled by the left foot or the chin. She could also be fitted with bilateral lower limb prostheses (a modified hip disarticulation prosthesis on the right, and a modified transfemoral prosthesis on the left). The transfemoral prosthesis would be modified to have a manual lock activated by her left foot to provide stability when walking yet the ability to bend the knee for sitting. She would initially be provided with short prostheses ("stubbies") to reduce the fear of falling while learning to use the prostheses.

Alternatively, the girl could be fitted with an electric-powered wheelchair. The powered wheelchair could become the platform on which extra heavy-duty batteries could be mounted to power a robotic arm that the girl could manipulate with her left foot. The wheelchair could also be fitted with a computer deck that the girl could control with a small penlight laser attached to a headband or by voice control. This would allow her to use her computer to answer her phone, control household light switches, and even do her homework by modem.

Which would be the best option for this child? The chance that the girl will use prostheses is slim. She has very little body surface area from which to lose heat, so she will find the prostheses not only cumbersome, but also unbearably hot. The energy expenditure required for her to get up and walk on the prostheses would be tremendous. Even if she could be fitted and taught how to walk, the prostheses would not be used to realistic functional advantage. In addition, with no arms, she would not be able to rise to her feet from a sitting position.

The second approach (using a computer and robot arm fitted to a wheelchair) is currently possible, but the technology is in its infancy. This approach would be most likely to succeed if each piece of equipment is added a step at a time.

An important point is that conventional prostheses attached to the body in a way that approximates the anatomic limb may not always be the best choice. The goal should be the replacement of function, not necessarily the missing anatomic parts. The choice of treatment will depend on the child, the family's understanding, the financial resources available to the child, and the medical facilities available. Both options may need to be tried before the family and child recognize the futility of the approach.

Unfortunately, there is no simple road map for treating the child with multiple limb deficiencies. A willingness to listen, coupled with creativity and sensitivity, should be the hallmark of the clinic team involved in the care of these children.

References

1. Tooms RE: Congenital amputee, in Morrissy RT (ed): *Lovelll and Winter's Pediatric Orthopedics,* ed 3. Philadelphia, PA, JB Lippincott, 1990, pp 1023-1070.

2. Krebs DE, Fishman S: Characteristics of the child amputee population. *J Pediatr Orthop* 1984;4:89-95.

3. Wilson JG, Brent RL: Are female sex hormones teratogens? *Am J Obstet Gynecol* 1981;141:567-580.

4. Kay HW, Fishman S (eds): *1018 Children With Skeletal Limb Deficiencies.* New York, NY, New York University Post-Graduate Medical School, Orthotics and Prosthetics, 1967.

5. Davies EF: BR, Clippinger FJ: Children with amputations. *Inter-Clin Info Bull* 1969;9:6-19.

6. Pruitt SD, Varni JW, Seid M, Setoguchi Y: Prosthesis satisfaction outcome measurement in pediatric limb deficiency. *Arch Phys Med Rehabil* 1997;78: 750-754.

7. Varni J, Setoguchi Y: Perceived physical appearance and adjustment of adolescents with congenital/acquired limb deficiencies: A path-analytic model. *J Clin Child Psychol* 1996;25:201-208.

8. Varni JW, Rubenfeld LA, Talbot D, Setoguchi Y: Determinants of self-

(reBULabs,)

esteem in children with congenital/acquired limb deficiencies. *J Dev Behav Pediatr* 1989;10:13-16.

9. Tyc V: Psychological adaptation of children and adolescents with limb deficiencies: A review. *Clin Psychol Rev* 1992;12:275-291.

10. Bryant PR, Pandian G: Acquired limb deficiencies: I. Acquired limb deficiencies in children and young adults. *Arch Phys Med Rehabil* 2001;82(suppl 1): S3-S8.

11. Makley JT, Heiple KG: Scoliosis associated with congenital deficiencies of the upper extremity. *J Bone Joint Surg Am* 1970;52:279-287.

12. Heyman JH, Ivankovich AD, Shulman M, Millar E, Choudhry YA: Intraoperative monitoring and anesthetic management for spinal fusion in an amelic patient. *J Pediatr Orthop* 1982;2: 299-301.

13. Herring JA, Goldberg MJ: Amelia and scoliosis. *J Pediatr Orthop* 1985;5: 605-609.

14. Lester DK, Painter GL, Berman AT, Skinner SR: Idiopathic' scoliosis associated with congenital upper-limb deficiency. *Clin Orthop* 1986;202: 205-210.

15. Samuelsson L, Hermansson LL, Noren L: Scoliosis and trunk asymmetry in upper limb transverse dysmelia. *J Pediatr Orthop* 1997;17:769-772.

16. Herring JA: Functional assessment and management of multilimb deficiency, in Herring JA, Birch JG (eds): *The Child With a Limb Deficiency*. Rosemont, IL, American Academy of Orthopaedic Surgeons, 1998, pp 437-445.

17. Crandall R, Tomhave W: Pediatric unilateral below-elbow amputees: A retrospective analysis of 34 patients given multiple prosthetic options. *J Pediatr Orthop* 2002;22:380-383.

18. Davidson J: A survey of the satisfaction of upper limb amputees with their prostheses, their lifestyles, and their abilities. *J Hand Ther* 2002;15: 62-70.

19. Kruger LM, Fishman S: Myoelectric and body-powered prostheses. *J Pediatr Orthop* 1993;13:68-75.

20. Scotland TR, Galway HR: A long-term review of children with congenital and acquired upper limb deficiency. *J Bone Joint Surg Br* 1983;65:346-349.

Chapter 79

Surgical Modification of Residual Limbs

Hugh Watts, MD

Introduction

Children with limb deficiencies frequently need surgical modification of their residual limbs. Sometimes the limb anomaly is so severe that fitting a prosthesis is either extremely challenging or completely impossible (Figure 1). At other times, the deficiency can result in a nonfunctional limb. Some attempts at surgical reconstruction (eg, medial transposition of the fibula with total absence of the tibia) have such poor results that the child will function much better if the limb is amputated. This surgery is usually called *conversion amputation.*

Modifying a residual limb to improve function may include fusing of several limb segments because this retains length and gives the child a single rigid lever to propel the prosthesis. This is characteristically done in surgery for longitudinal deficiency of the femur, partial (LDFP, formerly called proximal femoral focal deficiency, or PFFD), in which the very short femoral segment is fused to the tibia.[1,2]

Physicians commonly believe that conversion amputations should be done before the age of about 1 year, when a child is less likely to miss the part removed. However, one of the drawbacks of surgery at this age is that it is often very difficult for parents to accept the need to remove limbs. They frequently hope that the deformity can somehow be corrected, thereby avoiding amputation. This reluctance to proceed is not a major problem for the child, and a delay of several years is acceptable because children are sufficiently adaptable. It should be noted, however, that 2 years of age is a bad time to do an elective amputation, because that age—the "NO!" year—is a bad time to try almost anything.

Conversion Amputations at the Ankle

Conversion amputations at the ankle for children are best done by leaving the end of the residual limb covered with cartilage to avoid terminal bone overgrowth. This can be accomplished in several ways.

Syme Procedure

The Syme procedure is a simple ankle disarticulation; its advantage over a Boyd procedure is its simplicity. Disadvantages of the Syme procedure are more theoretical than actual. One disadvantage is that some surgeons tend to make the skin incision too curvilinear, putting the posterior flap at risk of vascular compromise. Many surgeons worry that the heel pad will migrate proximally, obviating end-weight bearing, but this heel pad migration can be minimized by dividing

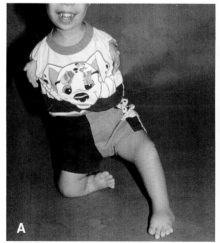
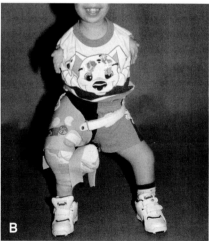

Figure 1 Boy with thrombocytopenia and absent radius (TAR) syndrome. **A,** The right lower limb is very deformed. **B,** The limb required a complex prosthesis that was used until the parents accepted the need for a conversion amputation.

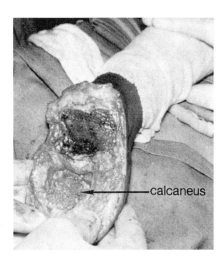

Figure 2 Intraoperative photograph of a McCollough amputation shows the thin section of the posterior calcaneus, which will be rotated 90° to be attached to the distal tibia. (*Courtesy of N.C. McCollough, III, MD.*)

the Achilles tendon above its insertion into the calcaneus and skin of the heel. Even if heel pad migration takes place, children's skin is so responsive to altered weight bearing that the skin will soon become thickened and callused. This phenomenon of skin thickening is frequently seen in children with untreated clubfeet who have been walking on the dorsum of their feet and who develop immense callosities there. Another potential disadvantage is that if the Syme procedure is performed during infancy, the distal tibia and fibula may become somewhat penciled, making them less optimal for end-weight bearing.

Boyd Amputation

The Boyd amputation removes the talus and the distal foot while retaining the calcaneus, which is then fused to the distal tibia or secondary center of ossification at the tibia. This has the potential to prevent any heel pad migration and the very real advantage of providing a bulbous end that can be used for self-suspension. This latter advantage can be a cosmetic disadvantage. The determining feature is the child's age. If the child has little growth left in the distal tibia on the

unaffected side, the bulbous tibial end on the affected side produces an unsightly bulge in the prosthetic shank. If, however, there is a great deal of growth left in the unaffected side, the bulbous end of the amputated side will end up at the level of the normal gastrocnemius-soleus muscles and can be readily masked in the prosthesis. The disadvantage of performing a Boyd amputation is the potential for nonunion or malunion of the tibia and the calcaneus. An additional nuisance is using pins to fix the fragments and subsequently having to remove them; using a screw instead of pins minimizes these problems.

McCollough Amputation

McCollough[3,4] described an operation in which a thin segment of the posterior calcaneus was rotated 90° to fuse it to the distal tibia (Figure 2) to prevent heel pad migration. This procedure leaves a less bulbous residual limb than a Boyd amputation. Although this may be a cosmetic advantage, the lack of a bulbous end does not allow for prosthetic self-suspension and shares with the Boyd procedure the potential disadvantage of nonunion or malunion. The procedure described by McCollough did not find favor among orthopaedic surgeons and has been largely abandoned.

Terminal Overgrowth

The overgrowth of amputation residual limbs in children is an ongoing problem, occurring in congenital limb deficiencies as well as posttraumatic amputations. The problem occurs most commonly in the humerus, the fibula, and the tibia. Pellicore and associates[5] and Abraham and associates[6] found that 15% of their pediatric patients who underwent amputations before age 12 years required revision, whereas no revisions were necessary if the amputations were performed at a later age. However, if a child has once had a residual limb revision, overgrowth can recur between ages 12 years and 20 years.

The problem manifests first by a protrusion, then a sore, at the end of the residual limb. If left untreated, the bone can penetrate the skin. Radiography performed at this time will demonstrate that the end of the bone has a sharply tapered point. Each surgical residual limb revision results in loss of school and recreation time during the process of healing of the limb and fabricating of a new socket.

The overgrowth is not a result of stimulation of the physis proximally but of the development of appositional new bone on the end of the residual limb. Proximal epiphysiodesis has been tried as a means of stopping the overgrowth without success.[6-8]

The easiest way to manage the problem is to avoid it by performing amputations through a joint where possible, so that the end of the bone is covered by its normal cartilage. If this is not possible, several other maneuvers (described later in this chapter) that have been used with varying success can be performed.

Overgrowth at the end of an amputation residual limb must be differentiated from soft-tissue retraction in children who have had amputations because of tumors and who have undergone postoperative chemotherapy. Healing of the fascia is adversely influenced by chemotherapy, causing the muscles to draw proximally, leaving the bone protruding subcutaneously.[9] Residual limb revisions performed while the child is undergoing chemotherapy will likely have to be repeated; several revisions may lead to an unfortunately short residual limb. It is better to wait until 3 to 6 months after the chemotherapy to perform a definitive procedure.

Simple Residual Limb Revisions

Simple residual limb revisions can succeed; however, recurrence is usual after about 18 months.[10] Surgical procedures that provide a smooth periosteal surface around the end of the bone appear to be somewhat more successful.

Silastic Caps

Silastic end pieces (either stemmed plugs that fit into the medullary cavity or caps that fit over the end of the diaphyseal bone) have been abandoned[11] because of frequent breakage and dislodgment. Metal and high-density polyethylene caps have also produced disappointing results (E. Marquardt, MD, personal communication).

Ertl Procedure

Ertl[12] described a procedure for revising transtibial residual limbs resulting from war injuries in which the distal fibula was fused to the distal tibia to create a potential end-weight bearing residual limb. This technique has subsequently been advocated to reduce the incidence of terminal overgrowth in children who have to undergo residual limb revision. Two reviews of this procedure have led to opposite results.

Drvaric and Kruger,[13] who reviewed their experience at the Shriners Hospital for Children in Springfield, MA, found that bony healing occurred in all of their revisions but spiking recurred anyway. This led them to abandon the procedure. Gates,[14] who learned the technique at the same institution as Drvaric, recently reported very favorable results and recommended Ertl as the procedure of choice. Gates stated, "I don't know why the results are so different. I cast my children longer, but that would more likely make a difference in healing than in recurrence. I am very meticulous about the periosteal closure, and that may be important in this process."

Biologic Capping

In 1984, Marquardt[15] introduced the concept of a "biological cap." A segment from the proximal fibula that included the epiphysis was inverted and fitted into the end of the distal tibia. The fibula was excised extraperiostially to prevent bone regrowth. Although the proximal fibular physis is not expected to grow, the cartilage enveloping the joint provides a smooth nonosseous surface to prevent osteoblastic reaction. Marquardt also described the use of iliac crest cartilage, an obvious choice if there is no proximal fibula.

Davids and associates[16] used apophyseal cartilage from the iliac crest and doubled the interval between residual limb revisions. My associates and I prefer to use the proximal fibula and invert its diaphysis into the tibial or humeral medullary canal. This has been very effective, with only four recurrences of overgrowth in 30 children in 5 years of follow-up.[17] Peroneal nerve injury has not occurred. Such an injury would be of no consequence in a child with below-knee deficiency, but it could have consequences if a fibular cap was used for the humerus. Laxity of the lateral collateral ligament does not occur because a segment of that ligament extends from the femur to the tibia.

Biologic capping should be considered when transosseous amputations are required. It may be possible to salvage an epiphyseal cap from part of the discarded specimen (eg, the first metatarsal head, the talar head, or the calcaneus) which could then be attached to the end of the cut bone.[18] The cartilage-capped piece of bone does not have to be living, but possible infection or tumor contamination must be kept in mind.

Longitudinal Deficiency of the Femur, Partial

Most children with LDFP live with the affected knee held in flexion. They will often sit on the thigh section of their prosthesis, which decreases their control and power over the prosthesis and aligns the vertical axis of the prosthesis lateral to the center of gravity, causing the child to lurch laterally when weight bearing. Function is greatly enhanced if the femur is fused to the tibia.[1,2] This can be done at the level of the bony secondary centers of ossification, which permits continued growth at one or both physes. This choice not only makes for a better single-segment residual limb but also brings the line of weight bearing closer to the body's center of gravity (Figure 3), resulting in much more functional prosthetic wearing. The fusion must be done with the knee in full extension. Initially, there may be enough of a hip flexion contracture that the residual limb cannot come to neutral, but this quickly stretches out. This procedure was slow to be accepted but is now considered routine.

Technique of Knee Fusion

Knee fusion should be delayed until the proximal tibial ossification can be visualized easily with plain radiography, usually between the ages of 18 months and 2 years. An anterior approach is easiest. The patellar ligament is sectioned, and the patella may be removed along with the menisci and cruciate ligaments. The cuts through the femur and tibia are determined by calculating expected residual limb length (see below). The femoral resection is usually just proximal to the distal physis; division of the gastrocnemius is at the level of the insertions to the posterior femoral condyles. The peroneal nerve and posterior neurovascular bundle are protected throughout the resection.

If the proximal physis is to be spared, a knife is used to shave off the articular cartilage of the proximal tibia to expose the ossific nucleus to its widest diameter. A Rush rod (Berivon, Meridian, MI) is introduced retrograde, exiting along the lateral aspect of the proximal femur. It is then withdrawn and replaced antegrade to fix the fusion in good alignment. The Rush rod should extend through the proximal tibial physis as centrally as possible. I have not observed growth arrest, but cross Kirschner wire fixation above the tibial physis is an alternative method of fixation. The resected distal femur and the patella can be harvested for supplemental bone grafting, if necessary, and the wound closed over suc-

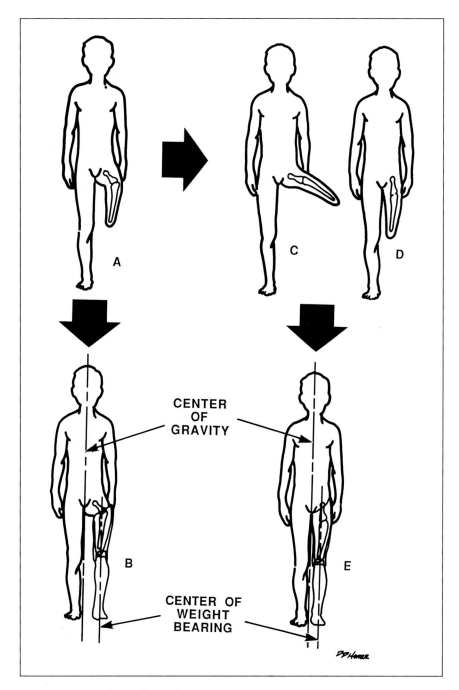

Figure 3 Fusion of the affected knee in a child with LDFP. **A,** The child before knee fusion. **B,** The child fitted with a transfemoral prosthesis. Note that the weight-supporting line of the affected leg is far lateral from the center line and leaves an unattractive lateral thigh bulge as well as a gap between the thighs. **C,** The same child has undergone a knee fusion in extension. **D,** The side with the fused knee is gradually brought to a neutral hip position. **E,** When this leg is fitted with a prosthesis, the position of the weight support line is now more medial, which requires less leaning to the left when the child stands and removes the cosmetically unattractive lateral thigh bulge and gap between the thighs.

Residual Limb Length
Conversion of LDFP to an Above-Knee Level

One distinct characteristic of children with LDFP who undergo conversion to an above-knee level is that the residual limb is *too long*. At the time of knee fusion, the distal femoral or proximal tibial physis (or both) should be considered for excision. This decision is often difficult for the orthopaedic surgeon, who may fear that the limb will be much too short.

Generally, the length of the tibia of the affected side is close to normal (80% of children with LDFP achieved > 92% of the length of the normal side tibia).[19] In adults, the tibia is approximately 10 cm shorter than the femur in men and 9 cm shorter than the femur in women. This means that the tibia on the affected side (if at normal length) is at the appropriate length for an ideal residual limb, if one allows a minimum of 7 cm difference in the knee heights plus 2 to 3 cm of flesh on the end of the bone for the placement of a standard internal mechanical knee joint in the prosthesis. Therefore, if *any* segment of the femur remains on the affected side, the residual limb will be too long. This extra length is often not recognized before a knee fusion is performed. Therefore, the overall surgical plan must include the excision of parts of the physes around the knee at the time of the knee fusion. The "thigh" segment, after a Syme disarticulation or Boyd amputation with a knee fusion, can be a little short rather than a little long and still provide ample leverage to propel a prosthesis adequately.

Length Measurements

Scanography and orthoradiography are difficult to perform for children with congenital anomalies of the lower limbs because the knees and ankles may be at markedly different levels on each side. Separate radiographs for each limb may be required. Furthermore, because flexion deformities at the knee are so common in

tion drainage. A Syme disarticulation or Boyd amputation can be performed at the same time, although many surgeons delay this stage for 6 weeks for fear that the proximal surgery might cause sufficient swelling to compromise the healing of the distal amputation. This is my preference.

children with congenital anomalies, it may be necessary to take lateral views of the limbs. If this is done, a separate radiograph of the femur and the tibia should be obtained so that each one is taken in line with the ruler. Alternatively, trigonometric calculations can be used to calculate the actual limb lengths.

Classically, all growth data are measured in relation to bone (or skeletal) age rather than to chronologic (or calendar) age. Data are characteristically measured using the standards in the atlas of selected radiographs of the left hand and wrist developed by Greulich and Pyle.[20] Children with limb deficiencies often have either no left hand or a left hand with a considerable deformity. What then? If the right hand is available, it can be used with a very small margin of error. Radiographs of the knees have been compared with standard radiographs of normal knees at different bone ages, but because these are not related to the data generated from the radiographs of the wrist, they are best not used. Furthermore, children with limb deficiencies often have anomalies in the knee, so this option is rarely useful. Bone age estimates have a considerable measurement error. Commonly, the estimate of bone age is just an educated guess, so chronologic age is used. The estimate should be made based on which result will be less of a problem for the child—overcorrection or undercorrection.

Predicting Future Growth

The problems of estimating limb-length discrepancies in children are well covered in standard pediatric orthopaedic texts; however, the materials describe children with both femurs and both tibias intact. For these children, most orthopaedic surgeons use estimates made from Moseley's[21] straight-line graph, which does not separate growth of the femur from that of the tibia. In children with limb deficiencies, however, the orthopaedic surgeon is faced with making an appropriate decision for children with problems not covered in the usual

texts. For children with congenital deficiencies, the Anderson-Messner-Green charts[22] are more helpful.

Even if all of the lower limb bones are present, it is important to be able to estimate what the limb-length discrepancy will be *at maturity* in children who have severe deficiencies so that appropriate long-range planning can be done. For example, in a child with a congenital short femur, the question needs to be resolved when the child is an infant whether later lengthening is appropriate or whether the parents should be counseled to have their child undergo a conversion amputation for prosthetic fitting. It was initially demonstrated by Amstutz[23] and now has become an accepted principle that the growth of a congenitally short limb will progress at the same proportional rate as the difference between the limbs at the time of birth. For example, if the short femur is 50% of the length of the unaffected side at birth, it can be expected to be 50% of the length of the unaffected side at skeletal maturity. This principle is especially useful in surgical planning for infants.

For estimating potential limb-length discrepancy for limb-deficient children, the Green-Anderson growth remaining charts[24] are usually the most useful. These charts have five lines for the femur and five for the tibia. The central line is the mean, above and below which are lines for +1 and −1, and +2 and −2 standard deviations. The standard deviation lines are developed from the Anderson-Messner-Green charts,[22] which most orthopaedic surgeons seldom use. These charts give the total length of the femur or tibia at any given bone age for each sex. The bone on the unaffected side is measured by scanogram and then compared (at the appropriate bone age) with the Anderson-Messner-Green charts to find out whether the rate of growth on the child's unaffected side is at the mean or at +1 or +2 or −1 or −2 standard deviations from the mean. This information is then used to select the appropriate line on the growth re-

maining charts for the unaffected side. To determine the amount of growth remaining for the short side, the amount of growth remaining for the unaffected side is multiplied by the proportional difference between the sides. For example, if the growth remaining for the unaffected side is 10 cm, and the short side is growing at 50% of the rate of the unaffected side, the growth remaining for the short side is 5 cm.

The Green-Anderson charts are based on measurements at specific landmarks not commonly used by orthopaedic surgeons. The femur is measured from the top of the femoral head to the bottom of the lateral femoral condyle ossification (not the medial condyle). The tibia is measured from the midpoint of a line drawn across the proximal condyles (not the tibial spines) to the midpoint of the distal articulating surface ossification.

Integration With Other Anticipated Surgery

Children with limb deficiencies frequently have other anomalies. A few centimeters in length can be gained through a proximal femoral osteotomy, changing the femoral neck from varus into valgus. A major potential problem in leg length is the requirement for fusing the knee in children with LDFP. The knee is usually in flexion, but it should be fused in extension. When the limb is brought into extension, there is considerable gain in length. Conversely, there may be loss of bone at subsequent surgery. At the time of rotation osteotomies (eg, Van Nes procedures for LDFP), a wafer of bone is often excised to facilitate the rotation. The amount of bone excised can be greater if one needs to reduce the length. If knee fusion is part of the plan, a segment of bone, together with the epiphysis of the distal femur, the proximal tibia, or both, can be resected at the time of surgery. All of these aspects need to be integrated into the initial surgical plan.

Intercalary Amputations: Turnaround Procedure for Tumor Resection

Significant differences exist between the turnaround and Van Nes procedures. In the turnaround procedure, the hip joint and surrounding muscles are normal, and the bones grow at a more predictable rate.

Ordinarily, the distal tibia on the affected side grows at approximately one half the rate of the distal femur on the unaffected side. In planning for resection surgery, scanography should be performed and the bone age estimated both preoperatively and from the Anderson-Messner-Green growth remaining chart to calculate how much further growth remains in the distal femur on the unaffected side at the time of surgery. The resection side should be left long. As an estimate, plan to position the tip of the lateral malleolus (which is a reasonable estimate of the location of the former ankle joint, which is now the "knee") of the resected side beyond the level of the knee joint on the unaffected side divided by half the distance that the normal femur has yet to grow. For example, if the unaffected distal femur has 8 cm to grow, the resection side should be left 4 cm longer so that the joints will align at skeletal maturity.

Van Nes Procedure

Growth in patients with LDFP is harder to predict because the tibia on the affected side may not grow at a normal rate. Serial scanograms are needed to establish the growth rate of the affected side. Surgeons also need to plan for the effects of excising one or more physes (that of the distal femur and possibly the proximal tibia) and the need for one or more rotation procedures. At the time of the final rotation, the distal tibia should be left long (and will usually need to be left longer than for a turnabout procedure for tumor patients, as described above). The added length should be the difference between the growth remaining in the unaffected distal fe-

mur and that remaining in the affected distal tibia. Growth remaining can be estimated based on the assumption that the unaffected distal tibia grows at half the rate of the unaffected distal femur, but this value must be multiplied by the ratio of the length of the deficient tibia to the unaffected tibia. The following example estimates length for a child with an unaffected femur estimated to have 9 cm of growth remaining, an affected tibia measuring 20 cm, and an unaffected tibia measuring 30 cm. If the tibias were normal, then the Van Nes side would be fixed longer by half of the femoral growth remaining, ie, 4.5 cm. However, in our example, where the affected tibia is not growing normally but instead at two thirds the rate of the unaffected tibia, the growth remaining on the affected distal tibia is half of 9.0 cm multiplied by two thirds, ie, 3 cm. Therefore, at the time of the Van Nes procedure, the deficient side should be left longer by 6 cm (ie, 9 cm − [{9 cm × ½} × 2/3]).

Surgery About the Hip

In the past there has been a great deal of focus on the radiographic appearance of the bone of the upper femur, and the cartilage and soft tissues have been overlooked. If absolutely no acetabulum has developed, the management decisions regarding length are the same as described in the earlier discussion. If, however, the acetabulum is satisfactorily formed and there is some element of a secondary center of ossification of the proximal femur in the acetabulum and some segment of the upper femur that are not joined, surgery may be considered. Surgery should be delayed until the two fragments are ossified enough to be fused. More complications occur from proceeding before there is adequate bone stock than by delaying surgery.

The distal femur can be fused to the pelvis to use the knee joint as a replacement for the hip joint.[25] Theo-

retically, this provides the advantage of a stable hip, but the knee joint has limited rotation as well as abduction and adduction, so the long-term outcome is questionable. Although several authors[25,26] have reported using this procedure, most surgeons believe it is not useful. Femoral fusion to the pelvis can be performed at the time of rotation if the Van Nes procedure (rather than excision of the knee) is the chosen treatment. When the distal femur is fused to the pelvis, the distal femur will grow anteriorly, but the hip joint will not be at a mechanically appropriate place. Therefore, a distal femoral epiphysiodesis should be performed at the same time.

Lengthening Residual Limbs

For a child with a very short residual limb, even small gains in length may provide a lever adequate for a less extensive prosthesis. The potential advantages include decreased energy consumption, improved prosthetic control, decreased heat retention, increased comfort, fewer components requiring repairs, and decreased cost.

Children with upper limb loss, especially congenital loss, commonly choose not to wear a prosthesis. Longer residual limbs may permit grasping of objects in the midline between the residual limbs for bimanual activity without a prosthesis. Furthermore, adding a longer distal segment can allow objects to be grasped between a lengthened humeral residual limb and the chest or between a lengthened forearm and upper arm, even if a prosthesis is never worn.

The goal of lengthening posttraumatic amputation residual limbs or short congenital residual limbs is not new.[27,28] The interest in Ilizarov's technique[29] of callus lengthening has brought new enthusiasm for the idea. Although Ilizarov is known to have lengthened several amputation limbs, the exact experience is not well documented.[28-32] Ilizarov commented that "the author's method can be used

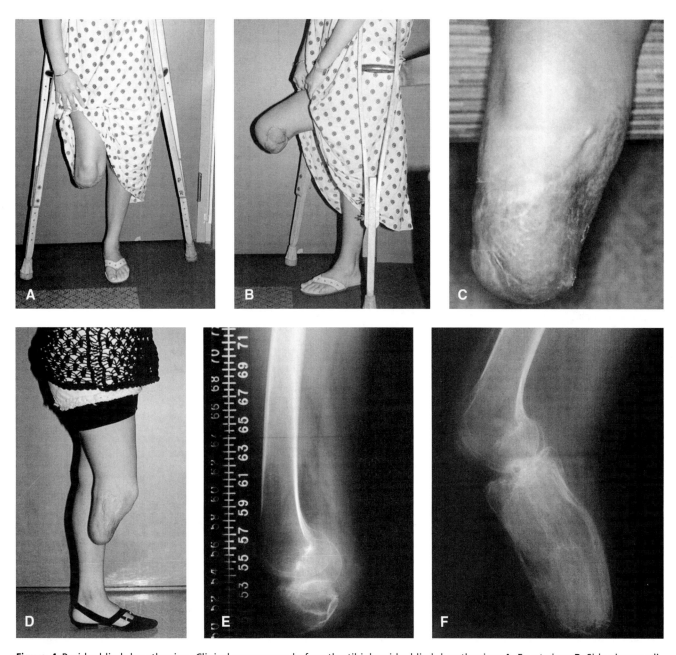

Figure 4 Residual limb lengthening. Clinical appearance before the tibial residual limb lengthening: **A,** Front view. **B,** Side view medially. Clinical appearance after the tibial residual limb lengthening. **C,** Front view. **D,** Side view laterally. **E,** AP radiograph before the tibial residual limb lengthening. **F,** Lateral radiograph after the tibial residual limb lengthening.

to lengthen amputation residual limbs for improved prosthetic fitting."[33]

Twelve adult cases have been reported in the English literature.[34-40] In children, Watts[41] reported lengthening of 32 short amputation residual limbs in 27 patients (12 femurs; 4 tibias; 12 humeri; 2 ulnas; 2 feet) (Figure 4). All were lengthened by gradual distraction using the biology described by Ilizarov[42] but using several

different distracting devices. The choice of device was determined by the anatomy of the very short segments. Lengths achieved averaged 8.7 cm, representing 110% of the preoperative length.

Children who underwent lengthening of their femurs or tibias achieved sufficient length to permit fitting with a prosthesis at one level more distal than before lengthening.

Two children with partial foot amputations no longer required partial foot prostheses.

It was more difficult to assess outcomes in children who underwent lengthening of their upper limbs. Three patients underwent lengthening with the anticipation that a prosthesis would not be used. All became able to grasp objects between the lengthened residual limb and trunk.

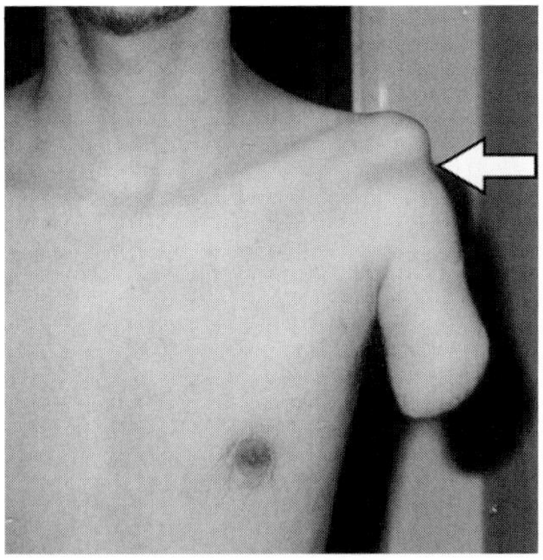

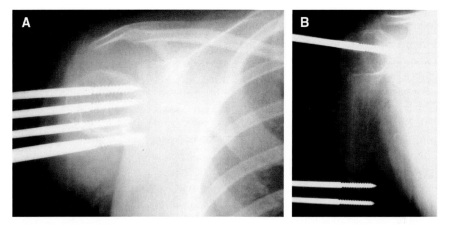

Figure 5 Subluxated humeral head. This 16-year-old boy sustained a left traumatic transhumeral amputation at age 7 years. Note the deltoid muscle atrophy and the marked subluxation of the humeral head.

Figure 6 A, Radiograph before residual limb lengthening of a boy age 14 years who sustained a bilateral transhumeral amputation at age 9 years. Note that the top of the humerus is not abutting the acromion. **B**, Radiograph after humeral residual limb lengthening. Note that the humeral head is now abutting the acromion. The amount of bone lengthening is greater than the lengthening of the residual limb available for prosthetic fitting.

These are functions that are useful in the presence of water or dirt, which may damage prostheses. Of the remaining patients, all but one are "wearers" of their prostheses but not constant "users."[43]

The lengthening procedures produced no deep wound infections, but pin tract infections and oozing were virtually universal. Pain was usually mild to moderate during lengthening, but one child required hospitalization on two occasions for 3 days each. One child undergoing lengthening of her femoral residual limb for a congenital lesion sustained a dislocation of the femoral head that was managed successfully by closed reduction and the application of a spica cast for 6 weeks. She retained full range of motion. One boy with a very short ulnar segment suffered loss of motion of the elbow when the osteotomy was made too proximally (just at the level of the coronoid process) so that, as the fragments separated, the proximal ulna was forced proximally, which partly enlarged the joint. One patient who underwent lengthening of bilateral short transtibial residual limbs required hamstring lengthening bilaterally as a result of knee flexion contractures that developed during the lengthening.

Criteria useful for assessing lengthening of intact limbs may not be appropriate for lengthening amputation residual limbs. For example, children who have sustained proximal amputations of the humerus usually have weak deltoid muscles, with a resulting inferior subluxation of the humeral head (Figures 5 and 6). At the beginning of lengthening, the bone can be elongated as much as 3 cm before the upper end of the humerus abuts against the acromion. It is only at this point that further lengthening starts to change the effective length of the residual limb distally. In some femoral residual limb lengthenings, the bone can be lengthened several centimeters with loss of the flabby soft tissues at the end of the residual limb. In such a case, the residual limb may not have lengthened as much as the bone, yet this residual limb may be more easily fitted to a prosthesis and provide the child with better prosthetic control. Using percentages to gauge increases in bone or residual limb length may be a misleading measure of technical results because the initial residual limb lengths are often so small (ie, a 3 cm tibial residual limb lengthened 100% may not be worthwhile).

Assessment of the functional results is more challenging, especially for children with short upper residual limbs. Lower limb function is more easily assessed. One question is whether energy consumption is decreased by residual limb lengthening. Waters and associates[44] estimated that, for lower limb amputees, each distal level of amputation increases the gait velocity by 20% and halves the oxygen consumption per meter. They studied a limited number of patients, however, and the lengths of the residual limbs were not reported. No data indicate whether an amputee with a femoral residual limb of 20 cm would function significantly better with a residual limb of 30 cm, for example.

A child with a short femoral residual limb usually has an abductor lurch. The lurch decreases with longer residual limbs. Gait laboratory analyses are needed to document the residual limb length at which the lurch significantly decreases. Comparing the gaits of children with various femoral residual limb lengths might not be valid because of the differences in age, size, and muscle strengths. It might be preferable to study each child before and after lengthening, but even this may result in misinterpretation because of the very long treatment time. Consequently, for such studies, it would be preferable to evaluate patients who have reached maturity.

Assessing functional results in children with upper limb deficiency is difficult. Children with congenital upper limb deficiencies frequently choose not to use prostheses. I believe it is worthwhile to lengthen upper residual limbs. Longer residual limbs may allow for grasping objects in the midline for "bimanual" activities without a prosthesis. Some functions, especially toileting, may be greatly enhanced by having longer residual limbs. One child who had both humeral residual limbs lengthened at my institution became able to manipulate the zipper on the fly of his trousers so that he could use public toileting facilities without help.

Many surgeons who have lengthened amputation residual limbs have had problems maintaining skin coverage, especially in those residual limbs resulting from burn injuries. Myocutaneous free flaps have been used. One potential problem with flaps is the limited sensation. If a residual limb has limited or no sensation, an upper limb prosthesis may not add function. In one girl who sustained a short transradial amputation because of a fire, I lengthened the bone under an abdominal flap. When length had been achieved, the flap was cut free. The child subsequently did not use her prosthesis because she said the lack of sensation made her prosthesis "feel weird." Two years later, as a teenager, she became a full-time wearer and user. She now has some sensation, but the change in prosthetic wearing might have been driven by her desire for cosmesis as she matured.

I have tried other strategies with indifferent success. In one patient I tried concomitant skin lengthening, using stockinette attached to the thigh with Super Glue, but found that the glue did not hold successfully. I have not yet tried attaching the stretcher to the skin by sutures or hooks.

I have not found tissue expanders to be useful. Tissue expanders need to be superficial to the fascia, so the skin coverage provided has not been able to withstand the abuses of prosthetic wear. The major problem with tissue expanders is the prolonged time between the start of lengthening and the fitting of the final prosthesis. Over a lifetime of prosthetic wear, the process seems to be a good investment of time. Nevertheless, this prolonged treatment time can be very frustrating for everyone. We have tried to obviate the problem of the long wait for a prosthesis by fabricating a temporary leg that can be worn around the pins of the external fixators. This has been successful in patients with femoral and tibial residual limb lengthenings.

Lengthening a residual limb over an intramedullary rod might allow for fitting as soon as sufficient length has been gained. Alternatively, after the length has been achieved, the external fixator could be replaced with an interlocked intramedullary rod. My associates and I have been reluctant to try these techniques, however, for fear of creating a severe bone infection during a treatment that we still consider investigational.

A very short humeral residual limb that is unused for several years after an amputation results in a very weak deltoid muscle and subluxation of the humeral head. This has been a problem, especially in children who have sustained traumatic amputations. It may be beneficial to strengthen the deltoid before lengthening.

The age at which to start lengthening has been an issue. In a child with an open physis proximal to the level of the amputation, subsequent growth itself might provide an adequate residual limb without lengthening. My associates and I have waited to lengthen such a residual limb until we were able to document an absence of useful growth proximally.

Bone fixation has not proved to be a major problem. Before lengthening, most of the bones of the residual limb have become porotic from disuse. On the other hand, the forces required to effect the lengthening of a short residual limb appear to be less than those needed for lengthening intact bones. It has been necessary to change pin locations in only one child who was

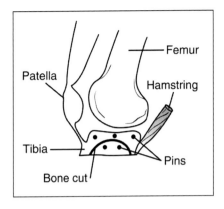

Figure 7 The cut in the proximal tibia is designed to leave the insertions of the quadriceps and hamstring muscles attached to the proximal fragment so that they will not be dragged distally during the residual limb lengthening.

undergoing lengthening of a congenital femoral deficiency.

I do not believe that one apparatus works best for all lengthenings. The apparatus I have used for a given bone has been predicated on my desire to select the smallest apparatus (for weight considerations) that will provide an adequate lengthening excursion. For femoral residual limbs, we have settled on using the small Wagner lengthener; for tibial lengthenings, a large Hoffmann; and for humeral residual limbs, the small Hoffmann. When performing lengthenings, it is essential that the cuts in the bone be designed to allow the bone fragments to elongate without dragging the adjacent tendons with them. Such bone cuts may need to be oblique, stepped, or a complex shape. For example, in a short tibial residual limb, the cut in the bone needs to leave the patellar tendon and the hamstring tendons attached to the proximal segment, not to the distal one. Thus the cut is half-barrel–shaped, made from medial to lateral (Figure 7).

As experience with residual limb lengthening improves, strategies for acute amputation surgery may change accordingly. In limb replantations, some surgeons have found it useful to shorten a limb sufficiently to allow soft-tissue approximation. The same principle could be used at the time of initial amputation. Good skin coverage could be achieved by shortening the bone in anticipation of lengthening after healing is complete. This would be especially useful if it preserves a knee joint rather than proceeding immediately to a knee disarticulation because the tibial residual limb might be too short to be useful.

Lengthening of short amputation residual limbs can be successful in children but requires different techniques from those used for standard limb lengthenings. The lengthening has potential to improve the function of amputees over a lifetime, but further research is needed to prove the value of the surgery. Many experiences with children should be applicable to adult amputees, except those with limbs lost to vascular disease, and might alter the strategy for amputation surgery during the acute phase.

Other Considerations
Limb Length in Knee Disarticulations

One of the disadvantages of a knee disarticulation is the lack of room below the residual limb to fit a standard prosthetic knee joint. For a person with a unilateral knee disarticulation, this results in markedly different knee heights, which can be cosmetically unappealing, especially when the patient is sitting. Some have speculated that this may also increase energy consumption. Special short knee joints to decrease the problem increase prosthetic expense.

It is believed that 7 cm is the ideal amount of space below the residual limb end to fit a standard knee joint. However, the soft tissue covering the bone end may well occupy another 1.5 to 2 cm, so it is preferable to set a goal of a 10-cm difference of the bone ends at maturity.

In children, however, this can readily be obviated by an appropriately timed distal femoral epiphysiodesis on the affected limb. The key is planning, both in thinking about the

issue and by getting adequate data to estimate the growth rate of the affected limb. Menelaus[45] showed that the growth of the distal femur could be roughly estimated to be 10 mm per year of growth. Femoral growth ends in boys at approximately 16 years of age, and in girls at approximately 14 years of age. This provides a rough guide to femoral growth in an otherwise normal child who sustains a posttraumatic amputation. Factors may be present, however, suggesting that the involved limb may not have reasonably normal growth. Many children with congenital deficiencies who undergo conversion amputations at the knee disarticulation level may experience decreased growth. This, in itself, may obviate the need for shortening altogether. But proper data, as discussed earlier in the section on predicting future growth, will be more useful.

Humeral Flexion Osteotomy for Rotation Control

Individuals who wear a transhumeral prosthesis may be unable to raise the arm above shoulder height, especially when the prosthetic elbow is flexed, because the prosthetic socket will spin on the humeral residual limb so that the terminal device moves in the direction of the floor. Marquardt[46] recommended a 90° flexion osteotomy in the midhumeral shaft to eliminate this problem. In children, such an osteotomy soon remodels to the point that there is insufficient bend to prevent the socket from slipping. As a consequence, the procedure has largely been abandoned in children.

Krukenberg Procedure

Several orthopaedic surgeons worldwide have promoted the Krukenberg procedure, in which the two long bones of the forearm are split apart, allowing each to function separately so that the amputee is able to grasp objects as if using a pincers (see chapter 17). Advocates of the procedure point out the advantages of improved

function, the lack of need for continuing prosthetic replacement and repair, and especially retention of sensation. These features make the operation attractive in rural or developing regions. Critics of the procedure believe that the resulting limb is unsightly and an added indignity to the injured person. The procedure has much wider acceptance in Europe than in the United States, where the operation has been restricted to those who have bilateral amputations and are also blind (as might happen if a child picked up an unexploded land mine, thinking it was a toy). In these children, retaining sensation is critical. This debate is characterized by the intense emotion generated on both sides.

Although health care professionals in the United States frequently object to the cosmetic outcome of a Krukenberg procedure, laypersons do not share that opinion. Schwartz and Watts[47] surveyed 226 laypeople aged 8 to 82 years after they viewed a video of a 5-year-old child performing various tasks with the Krukenberg residual limb and with an upper limb prosthesis fitted over the residual limb. Teenagers and older adults found the Krukenberg residual limb less appealing, although they thought that function was better. Children and young adults did not find the procedure a cosmetic disadvantage and agreed that function was better. Most respondents said that they would prefer to see a child in public at a restaurant using the Krukenberg residual limb rather than a prosthesis.

This might be explained by Swanson and Swanson's[48] concept of *active versus passive cosmesis*. *Passive cosmesis* refers to appearance at rest, whereas *active cosmesis* refers to appearance in motion. An example is a paralyzed hand: at rest, it appears quite normal; however, with attempts at use, it is obvious that it does not function normally and is not as acceptable. The Krukenberg is similar in that the extraordinary dexterity it allows makes it seem more natural because of its usefulness to the patient. In the

Schwartz and Watts survey, approximately half of those questioned would choose a Krukenberg procedure for themselves if they had an appropriate upper limb amputation. Schwartz and Watts stated that "Since the functional advantages of the operation are great, the Krukenberg should be considered as an option for any child with an upper limb amputation, or congenital deletion, at or distal to the level of the midforearm. It gives the patient an autonomous, functional upper limb with sensory feedback." Furthermore, it does not prohibit the use of a prosthesis that can be worn over the Krukenberg residual limb.

Genu Valgum in Fibular Deficiency

In children with complete fibular deficiency, hypoplasia of the lateral femoral condyle is very common. This results in a valgus knee and may require a very large and unsightly medial offset of the prosthetic foot to accommodate the deficiency. The amount of offset will vary with the length of the tibial residual limb. Eventually, the leg usually requires surgical straightening.

Straightening can be accomplished by either an osteotomy of the distal femur or by stapling of the distal medial femoral physis. The choice between these techniques has been debated. Medial physeal stapling is a simple, quick procedure and well accepted in the treatment of nonamputee children with angular anomalies.[49,50] For amputees, the experience is limited,[51] with complete straightening reported in four of five children needing angular correction. Straightening takes place over a considerable time, however, because the distal femur grows only approximately 1 cm per year. In addition, there is the fear that growth may not recur when the staples are removed, leading to further shortening in an already short femur, thus producing more knee-height difference. This latter concern can be obviated if the procedure is delayed until near the end of growth. For children with severe genu valgum, this may be too late because of increasing medial knee pain. A distal femoral osteotomy is a considerable procedure and keeps the child out of a prosthesis for 2 to 3 months until the fixating hardware is removed, the swelling resolved, and a new prosthesis fabricated. My associates and I prefer to proceed to a femoral osteotomy with overcorrection to allow for further angular change as growth continues.

Terminal Residual Limb Modification for Self-Suspension

One of the advantages of a knee disarticulation, Syme disarticulation, or Boyd amputation is the possibility of a distal residual limb that is larger in diameter than the shaft just proximally, so that a self-suspension system can be used. Reports of surgical attempts to provide such a residual limb in transcortical amputations are anecdotal. My associates and I have fixed the excised malleolae onto the lateral aspects of the end of a femoral residual limb that did provide this function in one child, but long-term follow-up is unknown.

Terminal Modification for Conversion to End-Weight Bearing

Surgical modifications that might permit self-suspension (ie, a broader distal end) could allow for some end-weight bearing in an otherwise transcortical amputation. Children with untreated clubfeet soon develop a very tough callus on the dorsum of their feet, which allows them to bear weight on skin not designed to do so. An otherwise intact limb that requires transcortical amputation cannot be expected to be end bearing immediately, however. Ertl[12] designed his procedure for war amputees with transtibial amputations to enhance end-weight bearing. The operation has had some popularity for adult amputees, but I am unaware of any study describing its use in children for that purpose. My associates and I have experience with one child for whom the plantar half of the calcaneus was fixed to the distal femoral residual limb. End-weight bearing was gradually increased to the point that 50% of body weight could be tolerated. The long-term follow-up is unknown, however.

Toe-to-Hand Transfers

Patients with lower limb deficiencies often have concurrent hand anomalies. Surgeons should keep in mind that a toe-to-hand transfer is now a well-established procedure. Before any lower limb parts are removed and discarded, possible uses in upper limb reconstruction should be considered.

Summary

For patients with amputations, prosthesis wear may be made more comfortable and function may be enhanced if the residual limb is surgically modified. Similarly, children with congenital limb deficiencies may also benefit from surgical modification of the limb. Yet little attention has been focused on this issue. Patients will be better served if this oversight is corrected.

References

1. King R: Providing a single skeletal lever in proximal femoral focal deficiency: A preliminary case report. *Inter Clin Info Bull* 1966;6:23-28.

2. King R: Follow-up findings on the skeletal lever in the surgical management of proximal femoral focal deficiency. *Inter Clin Info Bull* 1971;11:1-4.

3. McCollough NC: Early opinions concerning the importance of bony fixation to the heel pad in the juvenile amputee. *Inter Clin Info Bull* 1964;3:10.

4. McCollough NC III, Shea JD, Warren WD, Sarmiento A: The dysvascular amputee: Surgery and rehabilitation. *Curr Probl Surg* 1971;1-67

5. Pellicore R, et al: Incidence of bone overgrowth in juvenile amputee population. *Inter Clin Info Bull* 1974;13:1.

6. Abraham E, Pellicore RJ, Hamilton RC, Hallman BW, Ghosh L: Stump overgrowth in juvenile amputees. *J Pediatr Orthop* 1986;6:66-71.

7. Beekman F: Amputations during childhood. *Surg Clin North Am* 1938;18:425-431.

8. vom Saal F: Epiphyseodesis combined with amputation. *J Bone Joint Surg* 1939;21:442-443.

9. Watts HG: Special considerations in amputations for malignancies, in *Atlas of Limb Prosthetics: Surgical and Prosthetic Principles*. St. Louis, MO, Mosby-Year Book, 1981, pp 459-463.

10. Davids JR: Terminal bony overgrowth of the residual limb: Current management strategies, in Herring JA, Birch JG: *The Child With a Limb Deficiency*. Rosemont, IL, American Academy of Orthopaedic Surgeons, 1998, pp 269-280.

11. Swanson A: Silicone-rubber implants to control the overgrowth phenomenon in the juvenile amputee. *Inter Clin Info Bull* 1972;11:58.

12. Ertl J: About amputation stumps. *Chirurg* 1949;20:218-224.

13. Drvaric DM, Kruger LM: Modified Ertl osteomyoplasty for terminal overgrowth in childhood limb deficiencies. *J Pediatr Orthop* 2001;21:392-394.

14. Gates P: The Ertl procedure for prevention of terminal overgrowth in children, in *Association of Children's Prosthetic and Orthotic Clinics*. Toronto, Canada, 2002.

15. Marquardt E: Plastic surgery in imminent bone perforation at the infantile humerus stump: Preliminary report. *Z Orthop Ihre Grenzgeb* 1976;114:711-714.

16. Davids JR, Meyer LC, Blackhurst DW: Operative treatment of bone overgrowth in children who have an acquired or congenital amputation. *J Bone Joint Surg Am* 1995;77:1490-1497.

17. Bernstein R, Watts H: Modified Marquardt procedure for terminal overgrowth in children. *69th Annual Meeting Proceedings*. Rosemont, IL, American Academy of Orthopaedic Surgeons, 2002.

18. Benevenia J, Makley JT, Leeson MC, Benevenia K: Primary epiphyseal transplants and bone overgrowth in childhood amputations. *J Pediatr Orthop* 1992;12:746-750.

19. Watts H: Length of the PFFD stump after a Symes: How long is enough? *Shrine Surgeons Annual Meeting Proceedings*. Philadelphia, PA, 1994.

20. Greulich WW, Pyle SI (eds): *Radiographic Atlas of the Skeletal Development of the Hand and Wrist*, ed 2. Stanford, CA, Stanford University Press, 1959.

21. Moseley CF: A straight-line graph for leg-length discrepancies. *J Bone Joint Surg Am* 1977;59:174-179.

22. Anderson M, Messner MB, Green WT: Distribution of lengths of the normal femur and tibia in children from one to eighteen years of age. *J Bone Joint Surg Am* 1964;46:1197-1202.

23. Amstutz HC: The morphology, natural history, and treatment of proximal femoral focal deficiencies, in Aitken GT (ed): *Proximal Femoral Focal Deficiency: A Congenital Anomaly*. Washington, DC, National Academy of Sciences, 1969, pp 50-76.

24. Anderson M, Green WT, Messner MB: Growth and predictions of growth in the lower extremities. *J Bone Joint Surg Am* 1963;45:1-14.

25. Steel HH, Lins PS, Betz RR, Kalamchi A, Clancy M: Iliofemoral fusion for proximal femoral focal deficiency. *J Bone Joint Surg Am* 1987;69:837-843.

26. Browne KLB: Rotationplasty with hip stabilization in congenital femoral deficiency, in Herring JA, Birch JG (eds): *The Child With a Limb Deficiency*. Rosemont, IL, American Academy of Orthopaedic Surgeons, 1998, pp 103-109.

27. American Academy of Orthopaedic Surgeons (ed): *Atlas of Limb Prosthetics: Surgical and Prosthetic Principles*. St. Louis, MO, Mosby-Year Book, 1981.

28. Shatilov OE, Rozhkov AV: Lengthening of short stumps of the leg in children at the expense of rupture of the growth zone. *Ortop Travmatol Protez* 1972;33:58-60.

29. Ilizarov GA, Shevtsov VI, Kaliakina VI, Okulov GV: Methods of shaping and lengthening the foot. *Ortop Travmatol Protez* 1983;11:49-51.

30. Rozhkov AV, Startseva TE, Batenkova GI, Lukashevich TA, Kudriavtsev VA: Method of reconstructing a short stump of the foot by the distraction method. *Ortop Travmatol Protez* 1983;5:48-5031.

31. Rozhkov AV, Iankovskii VM: A method for lengthening a very short stump of the leg and its prosthesis. *Ortop Travmatol Protez* 1988;10:61-63.

32. Voinova LE: Characteristics of surgical preparation of invalids for prosthesis after amputation of the upper limbs. *Ortop Travmatol Protez* 1984;11:10-14.

33. Ilizarov GA: Clinical application of the tension-stress effect for limb lengthening. *Clin Orthop* 1990;250:8-26.

34. Eldridge JC, Armstrong PF, Krajbich JI: Amputation stump lengthening with the Ilizarov technique: A case report. *Clin Orthop* 1990;256:76-79.

35. Fealy MJ, Most D, Struck S, Simms GE, Hui K: Femur lengthening with a vascularized tibia bone flap. *Ann Plast Surg* 1996;37:140-146.

36. Kour AK, Seo JS, Pho RW: Combined free flap, Ilizarov lengthening and prosthetic fitting in the reconstruction of a proximal forearm amputation: A case report. *Ann Acad Med Singapore* 1995;24(suppl 4):135-137.

37. Latimer HA, Dahners LE, Bynum DK: Lengthening of below-the-knee amputation stumps using the Ilizarov technique. *J Orthop Trauma* 1990;4:411-414.

38. Moss AL, Waterhouse N, Townsend PL, Hannon MA: Lengthening of a short traumatic femoral stump. *Injury* 1985;16:350-353.

39. Persson BM, Broome A: Lengthening a short femoral amputation stump: A case of tissue expander and endoprosthesis. *Acta Orthop Scand* 1994;65:99-100.

40. Younge D, Dafniotis O: A composite bone flap to lengthen a below-knee amputation stump. *J Bone Joint Surg Br* 1993;75:330-331.

41. Watts HG: Lengthening of short residual limbs in children, in Herring JA, Birch JG (eds): *The Child With a Limb Deficiency*. Rosemont, IL, American Academy of Orthopaedic Surgeons, 1998, pp 281-288.

42. Ilizarov G, Trokhova V: Surgical lengthening of the femur. *Ortop Travmatol Protez* 1973;34:73.

43. Kruger LM, Fishman S: Myoelectric and body-powered prostheses. *J Pediatr Orthop* 1993;13:69-75.

44. Waters RL, Perry J, Antonelli D, Hislop H: Energy cost of walking of amputees: The influence of level of amputation. *J Bone Joint Surg Am* 1976;58: 42-46.

45. Menelaus MB: Correction of leg length discrepancy by epiphysial arrest. *J Bone Joint Surg Br* 1966;48: 336-339.

46. Marquardt EH: Angulation osteotomy of the humerus, in Bowker JH, Michael JW (eds): *Atlas of Limb Prosthetics: Surgical Prosthetic and Rehabilitation Principles*, ed 2. Rosemont, IL, American Academy of Orthopaedic Surgeons, 2002, pp 852-854. (Originally published by Mosby-Year Book, 1992.)

47. Schwartz A, Watts H: Non-medical opinion concerning the cosmetic appearance of the Krukenberg procedure. *Association of Children's Prosthetic and Orthotic Clinics Annual Meeting Proceedings.* Banff, Canada, 2000.

48. Swanson AB, Swanson GD: The Krukenberg procedure in the juvenile amputee. *Clin Orthop* 1980;148:55-61.

49. Bowen JR, Leahey JL, Zhang ZH, MacEwen GD: Partial epiphysiodesis at the knee to correct angular deformity. *Clin Orthop* 1985;198:184-190.

50. Zuege RC, Kempken TG, Blount WP: Epiphyseal stapling for angular deformity at the knee. *J Bone Joint Surg Am* 1979;61:320-329.

51. Crandall R: Surgery on the physis to correct stump deformity in the lower extremity pediatric amputee: A review of eleven patients (12 stumps). *Association of Children's Prosthetic and Orthotics Clinics Annual Meeting Proceedings.* St. Petersburg, FL, 2003.

Appendix

Terminology in Acquired Limb Loss

John H. Bowker, MD

Throughout this *Atlas*, the authors have endeavored to use the internationally accepted nomenclature for congenital limb deficiencies and acquired limb amputations developed by Technical Committee 168 of the International Organization for Standardization (ISO) based in Geneva, Switzerland. Since this new terminology was introduced in 1989 and 1993, it has rapidly gained worldwide acceptance because it facilitates communication among health care workers. The nomenclature for congenital limb deficiencies, published as ISO 8548-1, is well described in chapter 62. The subject of this appendix is terminology solely applicable to acquired limb loss.

ISO Standard Nomenclature for the Lower Limb

ISO 8548-2 describes the nomenclature for acquired loss of the lower limb, related to each successive level.[1] Division through a long bone is considered a true amputation, whereas severance through a joint is termed a disarticulation. The level is named according to the bone or joint divided; thus, an amputation through the tibia is termed *transtibial* rather than *below-knee* because the latter term has no precise meaning other than that accorded by common usage in English. Because such terms have no precise meaning in other widely used languages, such as Mandarin, which are not based on Latin, Greek, or Germanic roots, the use of ISO terminology is encouraged to facilitate international communication. The levels are as follows:

Ankle (Syme) disarticulation
Transtibial amputation
Knee disarticulation
Transfemoral amputation
Hip disarticulation
Transpelvic amputation

ISO Standard Nomenclature for the Upper Limb

Acquired loss of the upper limb is described by level in ISO 8548-3, using the same distinction between transosseous amputation and disarticulation as in the lower limb.[2] The levels are as follows:

Partial hand amputations (These may be further subclassified according to exact level within the hand.)
Wrist disarticulation
Transradial amputation
Elbow disarticulation
Transhumeral amputation
Shoulder disarticulation
Forequarter amputation

The standards from which the above nomenclature is abstracted also contain a great deal of information of use to caregivers pertaining to methods of evaluating the configuration and condition of individual residual limbs.

References

1. International Organization for Standardization: ISO 8548-2: Prosthetics and orthotics—Limb deficiencies, Part 2: Method of describing lower limb amputation stumps. Geneva, Switzerland, International Organization for Standardization, 1993.

2. International Organization for Standardization: ISO 8548-3: Prosthetics and orthotics—Limb deficiencies, Part 3: Method of describing upper limb amputation stumps. Geneva, Switzerland, International Organization for Standardization, 1993.

*Copies of standards 8548-2:1993 and 8548-3:1993 are available from the ISO Central Secretariat, 1, rue de Darembé, Case Postal 56, CH-1211, Geneva 20, Switzerland, http://www.iso.org, or from any ISO member body.

Index

Page numbers in *italics* indicate figures.

A

A.A. Marks rubber foot, 11
Absence of the lumbar spine and sacrum, *917,* 917-922
    associated findings, 919
    classification, 918-919
    differential diagnosis, 919
    neuromuscular findings, 919
    rehabilitation, 920-921
    treatment options, 920
    typical defects, 919
Achterman and Kalamchi classification, 889, *890*
Acrylic materials, 309
Actinomycetes, 50
Active prehensile devices, 117-119
Activities of daily living (ADLs)
    at-home rehabilitation, 731-732
    bilateral amputees, 746
    communication, 748
    dining, 747-748
    functional use training and, 281-283, *283*
    getting dressed, 745-746
    grooming, 746-747
    hand prostheses, *282*
    homemakng, 748-749
    hygiene, 746-747
    lower limb amputees, *665*
    partial hand devices and, *306*
    pediatric prostheses and, 817-820
    prosthetic/orthotic effectiveness and, 297
    reading, 748
    steps needed, 383
    transtibial amputations, 503-504
    use of feet in, *747, 748*
Activity-specific prostheses. *See* Task-specific prostheses
Acute vascular insufficiency, 37
Adactyly, *858*
Adamantinoma, *64*
Adaptation
    developmental stages and, 763-764
    model, *760*
    social support and, 761-762
    theories on, 759-761
Adaptive Knee, 667
Adductor magnus muscle, 360, 362, *534, 538*

Adductor roll, 551
Adept voluntary-closing devices, 120, 820
Adjustable heel foot, *510*
Adjustment
    by children, 777
    parental, 804-805
    process of, 806
    support for, 806-808
Adjustments, prosthetic, 348
Adolescents
    adaptation and, 763-764
    chronic pain, 718
    physical therapy, 837-838
    psychological aspects, 727, 803
Adults, adaptation and, 764
Advocacy programs, 759, 766
Aerobics, prosthesis use and, 329-330
Aesthetics, 303-310
Age/aging
    adaptation and, 763-764
    bimanual activities, 823
    initial fittings, 790
    prosthetic use and, 382-383
    psychological response and, 727
    recreational activities and, 642
    transtibial amputations and, 503
Agility drills, 654, *654*
Aitken classification, *906,* 911-914
Alberta Infant Motor Scale, 783
Alginate impression technique, *214*
Alignment
    biomechanics, 510–513
    developmental kinesiology, 783-785
    dynamic, 512-513
    knee prostheses, 530-531
    plantar flexed, *626*
    postoperative, 832
    residual limb fractures and, 697-698
    sports prostheses, 328
Allografts
    harvesting, 61
    reconstruction using, *844*
        femur, 63-64
        humerus, 61-62
        pelvis, *62,* 62-63
        postoperative management, 64-65

        radius, 62
        scapula, 61
        skeletal, 61-62
        tibia, 64
Alpha Infant Hand, 815
Aluminum, prosthetic use, 13
Ambulation. *See also* Gait; Walking
    with assistive devices, 597-598
    lower limb amputations, 750-752
    physical therapy and, 591
American Academy of Orthotists and Prosthetists (AAOP), 17
American Board for Certification in Prosthetics and Orthotics (ABC), 17
American Civil War, 12, 16, 77-79
    amputation levels, *79*
    amputations, 4-5, 69
    amputee care, 77-79
    chloroform use, 9
American Expeditionary Force, 80-81
"American" leg, 11, 16
American Orthotic and Prosthetic Association, 16, 17
American Pain Foundation, 723-724
American Red Cross, 79
Americans with Disabilities Act, 766
Amniotic bands, 858–859
Amp-U-Pod camera accessory, 336, *336*
Amputation surgery
    American Civil War, 77-79
    costs, 69-71
    creation of control sites, 185-188
    general principles, 21-30
    goals, 21
    history of, 3-19
    indications for, 3-5
    mortality related to, 7-8
    postoperative management, 26-29
    preprosthetic therapy, 275-276
    rigid dressings, 27-28
    soft dressings, 27
    staged procedures, 86
    stages of care, 246-248
    team approach, 21-22
    transtibial, 6, *6*
    World War I, 79-82
    World War II, *83,* 83-84

Amputations
  blood vessels, 25
  bone tissue management, 25-26
  in children, 841-852
  etiology of, 802
  indications, 90
  late, 90
  levels of
    decision-making process, 22
    selection, 37-41
  limb salvage versus, 22
    infections, 47-53
    trauma, 69-75
    tumors, 55-67
    in vascular disease, 31-45
  muscles
    myodesis, 24
    myofascial closure, 23
    myoplasty, 23-24
    tenodesis, 24
  nerves, 24-25
  open, 26
  open fractures and, 90-91
  predicting need for, 91
  psychological aspects, 32-33
  revisions, 26
  skin
    fasciocutaneous flaps, 23
    grafts, 23
    long-term concerns, 23
    scars, 22-23
  staged, 26
  transtibial, 8
  vascular repair failure and, 91
  Vietnam War, 88
  wound closure, 26
Amputee Activity Survey (AAS), 591
Amputee clinic teams, 17
Amputee Coalition of America, 759
  amputee support groups, 769
  Consumer Bill of Rights and Responsibilities, 767
  insurance coverage and, 327
  The Peer Visitor, 770
Amputee Golf Grip, 330, 330
Amputee Mobility Predictor, 593, 594-595, 741
Amputees
  ages of, 381
  bilateral, 403-404
  early ambulation program, 87
  evolution of care, 758
  first year care, 28-29
  gait, 367-384
  long-term follow-up, 87-88
  lower limbs, 92-93
  management of, 733-735
  mechanisms of injury, 90-90
  postoperative positioning, 596-597
  realistic goals, 33
  refugee care, 90
  soldiers, 91-92
  veterans, 381
  wartime care, 77-97, 81
Analgesia, history, 8-9
Anatomic suspension
  expandable inner walls, 412-413
  fenestrations, 412

  hidden panels, 412
  overview, 416, 417
  supracondylar wedges, 413
Anderson-Messner-Green charts, 935
Anesthesia, 5, 8-9, 220
Angiography, 38
Angle osteotomies, 185
Anglesey Leg, 11, 13, 79
Animated Prosthetics, 348
Anitiproliferative agents, 341
Ankle block anesthesia, 49
Ankle Brachial Pressure Index (ABPI), 38-39
Ankle disarticulation
  case studies, 478-479
  contraindications, 461-462
  early prosthesis, 474
  functional outcomes, 465-467
  indications, 461
  infection control, 464
  outcomes, 467
  preoperative considerations, 462-465
  surgical management, 459-471
  Syme, 15
  technique, 464-465
  variants, 467-469
Ankle-foot mechanisms, 650-653
  classification, 415
  component selection, 626
  motion, 375-376, 653-654, 668
  overview, 419
  prosthesis based on, 455
  single-axis ankle-foot, 415-416
Ankle joint function, 355-358
Ankle prostheses
  overview, 419
Ankle prosthesis design, 474-475
Ankles
  motion, 368
  reference data, 356
  single-limb support, 371-372
Annular bands, 858-859
Anterior closing wedge osteotomy, 241
Anterior cruciate ligament deficiency, 889
Anthropomorphic hands, 344
Antibiotics
  autograft reconstruction, 64-65
  history, 8
  prophylaxis, 73, 483
Anticoagulant therapy, 37
Antiseizure drugs, 722
Antisepsis, 8. See also Infection control
APRL voluntary-closing hands, 120, 121
APRL voluntary-closing hooks, 120
"Arbeitsprosthese" (work prostheses), 16
Arcuate field maximum, 101
Arms. See also Forearms
  complete electronic systems, 346-347
  myoelectric control, 178-179
  swings, 612
Army Medical Museum, 79
Army Prosthetics Research Laboratory, 14
Arterial duplex angiography, 38
Arteriovenous shunts, nonnutritional, 35
Association of Child Prosthetic and Orthotic Clinics (ACPOC), 17, 775
Association of Limb Manufacturers of America, 16

Atasoy-Kleinert volar V-Y technique, 199
Atheromatous disease, 482
Athletics. See Sports
Atmospheric pressure suspensions
  elastomeric knee sleeves, 411
  hypobaric socks, 411
  internal roll-on locking liners, 409-410
  overview, 416, 417
  suction sockets, 409-410
Attachment systems, 678
Autoamputations, 36-37, 430
Autografts, 59, 844
Autologous cartilage-bone graft, 847
Automatic Forearm Balance unit, 128, 128, 163
Autonomy, psychological response and, 727-728
Avocational prostheses, 327
Axilla loop, 132, 133

B

Back-lock features, 119
Back-up prosthesis units, 277
Bacterial folliculitis, residual limbs, 706
Balance, 590, 603, 605-606, 606, 751
Ball-and-socket shoulder joint, 129, 129
Ball roll exercise, 605
Ball sports, 329-330, 634
Bandages, wrapping, 832, 833. See also Dressings
Barthel Index, 592
Base of support (BOS), 590, 606, 607
Baseball Glove Attachment, 335, 335
Battle wounds. See American Civil War; Korean War; Vietnam War; World War I; World War II
Bayley Scales of Infant Development, 783
Bayne classification, 864, 864, 870, 871
Beaufort transtibial prostheses, 13
Bed mobility, 590
"Behelfsprosthese" (temporary prostheses), 16
Belgrade Hand, 183
Bent-knee peg leg, 15
Bent-knee prostheses, 688
Berlichingen, Goetz von, 11
Bicycle riding, 332, 568, 638
Bilateral friction-brake knees, 420-421
Bilateral prostheses
  elbow units, 317-318
  upper limbs, 311-325
    components, 315-316
    harnessing, 314-315
    patient evaluation, 311-312
    prototypes, 321, 321
    socket design, 313-314
    staging of care, 312-313
    terminal devices, 315-316
  wrist units, 316-317
Bilateral transradial harnesses, 134
Bilhout-Cloquet procedure, 860
Bill of Rights and Responsibilities, 767
Billiards adaptors, 336-337
Bimanual stabilization, 210
Biologic capping, 933
BIONs, development of, 182
Biopsies, intraosseous, 55
Birch classification, 892

Biscapular abduction, 141, *320*
Bivalve model socket, *880*
Black Iron Master, 334, *335*
Blind patients
    benefits of sensation, *323*
    Krukenberg procedure, *187*
    prosthesis prescription, 742
Blisters, residual limbs, *707*
Blood vessels
    amputation surgery, 25
    interosseous, 25
Bluetooth technology, 667
Bly legs, 79
Body alignment
    developmental kinesiology, 783-785
Body image, 733, 759-761
Body-powered components, 117-130
    body-control motions, 279, 280
    controls, 319-320
    definitive prostheses, 225-227
    donning and doffing, 278
    elbow units, 163-164, 226, *294*
    hand units, 210, *282*, 345
    harness designs, 226
    hook-type, 277, *295*, 316, 322
    locking elbow, 246
    partial hand prostheses, 214
    pediatric, 797
    practice, 281, *297*
    preparatory/training prostheses, 225, *225*
    shoulder prostheses, 266
    shoulder units, 163-164, *266*
    signal acquisition, 347
    socket designs, 226, *268*
    for sports activities, 328
    training, 278
    upper limbs, 131-143
    wear and use patterns, 826
    wrist components, 226
    wrist units, *322*
Body weight
    prostheses for children, *815*
    transpelvic amputations/hip disarticula-
        tions, 572
    volume-adaptible sockets, *520*
Bona-Jaeger procedure, 442
Bone grafts, 243. See also Allografts; Autografts
Bone spurs, 691-693, *692*, 717, 719
Bone tissue
    coverage, 6-7
    growth in children, 776
    knee disarticulations, 520-521
    length
        preservation of, 185
        prosthesis design and, 243-244
    necrosis, *234*
    overgrowth, 696, 791-792, 846-847, *847*,
        932-933
    problematic prominences, 691-693
Bone wax, 25
The Book of Wound Surgery (Brunschwig), 9
Boston Arm, 183
Boston Digital Arm Systems, 164, *164*, 165,
    166, 166-167
Boston Elbow III, 183
Bowden cable system, 13-14, 126, 225, *225*, 297
Bowling Ball Adaptor, 331, *331*

Boyd amputation, *469, 470*, 907, 932
Brachial plexus injuries
    clinical evaluation, 285
    complete, *291*, 291-293
    infraclavicular socket, 271-272
    level of injury, 290-293
    neurotization, 288-289
    orthosis design, *297*
    postganglionic, 293
    preganglionic, 290-291
    rehabilitation, 295-296
    reliable EMG sites, *294*
    severe, 258, *259*
    surgical management, 286-293
Braiding, 615, *616*
Brånemark prosthetic attachment system, *674*,
    674-680
Bruininks-Oseretsky Test of Motor Proficiency,
    783
Bulkhead units, 128
Bunions, *437*
Burgess technique, 482
Burns
    amputations associated with, 698-699
    high-voltage, 219
Bursitis, 690, *691*
Button hooks, 745

C

C-Sprint running foot, *652*, 652-653
Cable systems. *See also* Bowden cable system
    body-powered, 117
    cable length, *132*
    dual control cables, 825
    grippers, 315-316
    housing, 132, *132*
    housing modifications, 135, *135*
    prehension devices, 188
    Spectra cables, 324
    split housing, *136*
Calcaneotibial arthrodesis, 467-468, *468*
California, University of, Berkeley, 14-15, 85
Camera, adaptor accessory, 336-337
Canadian ankle disarticulation prostheses, 475
Canadian hip disarticulation prostheses, 565
Canadian-type plastic socket, 565
Candidal infections, 707
CAPP terminal devices, 119, *120*, 815, *816*, *818*
CAPP voluntary-opening hands, 121, *122*
Capping, 877
Carbon-reinforced fabrics, 328
Carpus
    amputation through, *219*, 219-222
    components, 110
    wrist motion and, 110-111
Casts
    hip dislocations, 567-568, *569*
    negative wrap, 550
    postoperative, 832
    pressurized systems, 665
    transpelvic amputations, 567-568
    transpelvic prostheses, *569*
    transtibial amputations and, 499
    vacuum system, 665
Cauterization, 4, 7, 25
Cellulitis, residual limbs, *706*

Center of gravity, 622-625
Center of mass (COM), 590, 606, *607*, 609
Centri Electric Hands, 152-153, *153*
Charcot deformity, 48
Charcot neuroarthropathy, 482
Charcot neuropathy, 47-48, *48*
Cheetah running foot, 651, *651*
Chemotherapy, choice of, 55-56
Child Amputee Clinic Chiefs, 17
Child Amputee Prosthetics Project, 119, 806-
    807, 813, 821-822
Child Prosthetic Studies, 17
Childbirth, in lower limb amputees, 571-572
Childcare tasks, 748
Children. *See also* Specific deficiencies
    acquired amputations in, 841-852
    adaptation and, 763
    adjustment to prostheses, 777
    bony outgrowth, 696, *696*
    causes of acquired amputations, *841*
    chronic pain, 718
    developmental kinesiology, 783-788
    developmental milestones, *784*
    durability of prostheses, 420
    elbow disarticulation, 244
    Electrohand 2000, 344
    fibular deficiencies, 461, 792-793
    fittings, 790, 792
    general prosthetic considerations, 789-799
    knee disarticulations, 518, 519-520, 793
    limb-deficient, 773-777, 779-781
    lower limb amputations, 403, 796-797
    managing growth, 790-791
    maturation and disability, 802-804
    multiple limb loss, 839
    occupational therapy, 813-829
    organizations for, 17
    outgrowing prostheses, 792
    partial hand amputations, 203
    passive transradial prostheses, *815*
    psychological adaptation, 727
    psychological issues, 801-811
    rehabilitation, 851
    rubber knee sleeves, *412*
    school sports, 328
    single-axis knees, *420*
    split liners, *528*
    staging components, 791
    tibial deficiencies, 793
    transfemoral amputations, 794
    transhumeral amputations, 239
    upper limb deficiencies, 797-798
Chimerism, hematopoietic, 341
Chondrosarcomas, 60, *62*
Chopart disarticulations, *430*, 443-445, *444*,
    445
Chronic pain, management of, 711-726
Chronic Pain Grade, 718, 720
Cineplasty
    control sources and, 186-187
    effects of, 85-86
    forearm muscle, *186*
    history, 6
    introduction, 85
    pectoral, 186
    Vanghetti-Sauerbruch-Lebsche muscle
        tunnel, 186

Claviculectomy, 256-257
Clear test sockets, 271
Clostridial myonecrosis (gas gangrene), 50, 52
Clothing selection, 745-746
Clubfoot, 889
Coaching, disabled athletes, 659
Cold intolerance, 200
Cole and Manske classification, 869, 870
Colostomy bags, 572
Committee on Artificial Limbs, National Research Council, 85
Committee on Prosthetic Research and Development (CPRD), 17
Competencies for Physical Therapy in Early Intervention, 833
Computer Aided Design—Computer Aided Manufacturing, 15
Computer-aided prosthetic laboratory (CAPL), 662
Congenital absences. See also Congenital deficiencies
    digital, 857
    humerus, 875
    lumbar spine and sacrum, 917, 917-922
    multiple limbs, 881
    shoulder, 271
    transmetatarsal, 887
Congenital arteriovenous fistulae, 460-461
Congenital constriction band syndrome, 858-859
Congenital deficiencies. See also Congenital absences; specific limbs
    aesthetic considerations, 308
    classification, 777
    degree and type, 801
    epidemiology of, 773
    etiology, 773-774
    humeral, 875-876, 876
    multiple limbs, 923-924
    prosthetic considerations, 776-777
    psychological aspects, 801-811
    quadrimembral, 312, 752
    response to, 774-775
    transverse upper limb, 879
    upper limb, bilateral, 312
Congenital kyphosis, 889
Constant-friction knees. See Single-axis knees
Constant-friction wrist units, 123-124
Consumer movement, 757-770
    advanced technology and, 758-759
    interdisciplinary model, 760
    social change and, 758
Contact dermatitis, 703, 703-704
Contact forces, signal acquisition, 347
Contoured Adducted Trochanteric-Controlled Alignment Method (CAT-CAM), 403
Contractures
    abduction, 689
    absence of the lumbar spine and sacrum, 920
    equinus, 442, 445
    flexion, 526, 622
    flexion-abduction, 689
    impact of, 687-690
    in infants, 834
    knee extension, 688
    knee flexion, 520, 520, 688, 688, 689

soft dressings and, 27
    transtibial amputations and, 687-688
    upper limbs, 690
Control motion training, 817
Control sources
    nerve-graft systems, 187
    neuromuscular reorganization, 187-188
    osteointegration, 188
    shoulder disarticulation prostheses, 190
Control systems
    activation, 825
    bilateral prostheses, 190-192
    biomechanics, 214-215, 247-248
    body inputs to, 176-183, 347
    body position-type, 319
    body-powered devices, 131-143
    contact forces in, 347
    elbow units, 189, 880-881
    extended physiological proprioception (EPP), 320
    externally powered hands, 343-344
    force sensing resistors, 321
    goals, 174-175
    implants, 181-183, 347-348
    integrated, 177
    liner transducers, 319, 320
    microprocessors, 665-668
    modulated, 177
    multifunctional, 183-185, 184
    myoelectric prostheses, 320
    myoelectric signals acquisition, 347
    neuroelectric, 181-183
    new developments, 348
    sensors, 347-348
    servo, 320-321
    sites/sources, 185-188
    switches, 320
    training, 279-283, 280
    transhumeral prostheses, 135, 135-137
    transradial prostheses, 188-189
    unilateral limb loss, 188-190
    upper limb prostheses, 318-319
Conversion amputations, 931-932
Coordination
    physical therapy and, 590
    residual limbs, 690
    training, 605-606
Coping strategies, 728
Cosmesis
    developments, 668
    longitudinal humeral deficiencies, 877
    sports prostheses, 328
Cosmetic gloves, 122, 122
Critical limb ischemia (CLI)
    acute vascular insufficiency and, 37
    angiography, 35
    incidence, 31
    nonsurgical management, 34
Crutches, 399-400, 613, 751
Cultural influences, 805
Cup walking drill, 649, 649
Curbs, climbing, 613
Current cut-off circuits, 152
Custom production gloves, 122, 122
Custom-sculpted gloves, 122, 122
Customary walking speeds, 397, 400, 400-401
Cutaneous horns, residual limbs, 707

Cutaneous papillomas, residual limbs, 707, 708
Cysts, 690-691, 704-706, 705, 717

D

Dacron grafts, 36
Dance, prosthesis use and, 329-330
Day System, 781
Débridement, salvaged limbs, 73-74
Decubitis ulcers, 559, 560
Deep peritoneal nerve ligation, 24
Deep vein thrombosis, 40
Degloving, foot and ankle, 432
Dental alginate, 213
Denver II, motor development evaluation, 783
Depressive disorders, 720-721
Depth-ischemia foot grading system, 47, 48
Dermatoses, chronic, residual limbs, 707
Desensitization, 276, 598
Desoutter Brothers design, 13
Development of skills, 817-820
Developmental Indicators for Children's Unilateral Upper Limb Prosthetic Fitting, 813
Developmental kinesiology, 783-788, 802-804
Developmental milestones, 784, 925-926
Diabetes mellitus
    amputation decisions, 22
    diabetic foot, 48-50, 49, 50
    dry gangrene, 434
    folliculitis, 706
    foot ablations and, 429
    infected MTP joint, 441
    infections, 47, 48-50
    limb care check list, 602
    lower limb amputations, 42
    maternal, 917
    neuropathy, 48
    osteomyelitis and, 438
    peripheral vascular disease and, 31
    postoperative management, 446, 483-484
    ray amputations, 439, 440
    skin disorders, 707
    Syme ankle disarticulations, 460
    toe disarticulations, 436
    transmetatarsal amputations, 442
    transtibial amputations and, 482
    wet gangrene and, 435
    wound healing and, 462
Diabetic dermopathy, 707
Diagnostic sockets, 269-270
Diaphyseal bone covering, 25
Diffuse tissue glycation, 462
Digital absence, types of, 857
Digital Twin Hand, 149-152
Digits, terminal transverse deficiency, 855. See also Fingers; Toes
Dining, adaptations, 747-748
Disseminated intravascular coagulopathy (DIC). See Purpura fulminans
Distal pads, 508-509, 528
Distal stump edema, 702
DMC Plus Hand, 149-152
Doppler ultrasound, 38, 40, 48
Double-axis shoulder units, 128
Double-ring harnesses, 315
Dressing, garments, 745-746, 750

Dressings
    changes, 446
    compressive, 27, 599
    figure-of-8 wrapping, *275*
    goals, 832
    postoperative, 596
    rewrapping, 687
    rigid, 27-28
    salvaged limbs, 74
    semirigid, *688*
    soft, 27
    stockinette over, *224*
    transtibial amputations, 505, *506*
Drive mechanisms, 345
Driving automobiles, *331*
Drum stick adaptor, 337, *337*
Dry gangrene
    ankle disarticulation and, 460
    diabetes and, *434*
    foot, 432-433
    lupus and, *433, 438*
    peripheral vascular disease and, 36, *37*
Dual control cables, 825
Duplex ultrasound angiography, 462
Durable Medical Equipment Regional Carrier
    K Codes, 593
Dynamic elastic response foot (DERF), 403
Dynamic Foot, 678
Dynamic Mode Control Plus Hand, 154
Dynamic Mode Control principle, 348
Dynamic-response feet, *418*, 418-419, *419*, 425,
    653
Dynamometers, hand, 197
Dysvascular disease, 381. *See also* Peripheral
    vascular disease

E

E-400 mechanical elbow, 317
E-Z Infant Hand, *816*
Early amniotic rupture sequence, 858-859
Early congenital amniotic rupture, *855*
Early postoperative prostheses, *225*
Economic considerations, 33, 69-71, 728
Eczema, residual limbs, *704*
Edema, 702-703
    control of, 836
    distal stump, *702*
    postoperative, 832
    residual limbs, *706*
Edinburgh Arm, 183, *346, 347*
Education. *See also* Patient education; Training
    amputation surgery, 9
    of families, 833-834
    information gathering, 806-807
    in prosthetics, 17-18
Elastic bandages, *246*, 687
Elastic liners, 475
Elastic sleeves, 228
Elastic suspension belt, *553*
Elastomeric knee sleeves, 411
Elastomeric liners, 29, 348
Elbow disarticulation
    osteotomy procedure, *244*
    surgical management, 240
    transhumeral amputation and
        bone length, 243-244

    patient evaluation, 243
    prosthetic management, 243-249
    surgical management, 239-241
    traumatic, *240*
Elbow flexion/terminal devices
    control cables, 135-136, *137*
    split cable housing, *135*
Elbow joints. *See also* Elbow disarticulation
    disarticulation, 6
    extension, 109, 279
    flexion, 108, *108*, 279
    motion, 108-109
Elbow lock control straps, 139, *142*
Elbow locks, 163, 825
Elbow units
    Automatic Forearm Balance unit, *128*
    bilateral prostheses, 317-318
    body-powered, 163-164, 189
    electric, 164-169, 189
    endoskeletal design, 130
    flail-arm hinge, 128, *128*
    flexible hinges, 125, *126*
    flexion assists, 128
    friction, 128
    harness, *131*
    inside-locking hinges, 127-128
    lock control cables, 136, *136*
    outside-locking hinges, 127
    passive friction, 128
    polycentric hinges, 125, *126*
    positioning, 279
    prototype, *346*
    residual limb-activated locking hinges,
        126-127
    rigid hinges, 125
    single-axis hinges, 125, *126*
    sockets, 246
    split cable housing, *136*
    stability, 297
    step-up hinges, 125-126, *126*
    transradial amputees, 125-127
Elderly patients
    adaptation and, 764
    peripheral vascular disease and, 32
    psychological adaptation, 727, 729
    split liners, *528*
Electric Elbow Lock, *163*, 164
Electric Greifer, 155-156, *156*, 162
Electric Hand, *149*, 149-152, 153-154, *154, 161*,
    162, *343*
Electric Hands, 154-155
Electric-powered components, 145-171
    body-powered elbows, 163-164
    cost and maintenance, 228–229
    definitive, 227-229
    prehension mechanisms, 145-160
    preparatory/training prostheses, 226-227,
        227
    prescription of, 277
    terminal components, 315-316
    wrist mechanisms, 160-163
Electric Terminal Devices, 149, 158, *158*, 162
Electric Wrist Rotator, *161*, 161-162
Electrical burns, high-voltage, 219
Electrohand 2000, 344
Electromechanical switches, 151
Electromyography (EMG), 178

    brachial plexus injuries, *294*
    functional testing, 341
    testing, 822-823
    upper limb motion, 103, 104
    use in training, 280-281
Emotional readiness, children, 791
Empowerment, of families, 807
Endoskeletal construction, 129-130
Endoskeletal transfemoral prostheses, *13*
Endurance, physical therapy and, 603
Energy expenditure
    bilateral amputees, 403-404, *404*, 622
    at customary walking speeds, 397
    ground-reaction forces and, 477-478
    level of amputation and, *401*
    prosthesis type and, 403
    unilateral amputees, *404*
    walking, 395-407, *398*
Energy sources, walking, 395-397
Envelope of action, 101
Epidermoid cysts, 690-691, 704-706, *705*
Epiphysiodesis, 892
Equinus contractures, 442, 445
Equinus prostheses, 795-796
ErgoArm Electronic Plus, 163-164
ErgoArm Hybrid Plus, *162*, 163
Erosion, residual limb, *702*
Ertl osseoperiosteal tibiofibular synostosis, *493*
Ertl procedure, 88, 93, 691, 933
ES Hand, 183, 185
Evacuation hospitals, WWII, 83
Exercises, categories, 641-642
Expanded polytetrafluoroethylene (PTFE)
    grafts, 36
Extended physiological proprioception (EPP),
    176, 320
Externally powered components. *See also*
    Electric-powered components
    electronic arm systems, 346-347
    hand prostheses, 210
    hook-type, 345
    microswitch controls, 293, *293*
    new developments, 343-345
    partial hand prostheses, 214
    shoulder disarticulation prostheses, 827
    shoulder prostheses, 267, *267*
    for sports activities, 328
    switch control harness, 143

F

Fair-lead cables, *318*
Falling, controlled, 615-616
Families
    children with multiple limb deficiencies,
        927-928
    clinic visits, 833-834
    empowerment of, 807
    participation in therapy, 831
    psychological issues, 33, 804-805
    support for adjustment, 806-808
Farmer's hooks, 119
Fasciocutaneous flaps, 23
Feedback loops
    artificial reflexes and, 173-174, *174*
    cable and harness systems, 266
    EMG signals and, 344

Feet. *See also under* Diabetes mellitus; Foot
    amputations; Foot deficiencies; Gait
    clubfoot, 889
    depth-ischemia foot grading system, 47, *48*
    diabetic foot, 48-50, *49, 50*
    dry gangrene, 432-433
    foot ablations and, 429
    infection, 434-436
    joint function, 358
    manipulation by, 746
    normal function, 449
    peripheral vascular disease, 429
    silicone reconstruction, *542*
    trauma to, 430
    use in place of hands for ADLs, *747, 748*
    wet (infective) gangrene, 433-434
Femoral deficiencies. *See also* Longitudinal
    deficiency of the femur, partial
    Aitken classification, 911-914
    bilateral, *908,* 910-911
    classification, *906,* 906-907
    clinical presentation, 905-906
    etiology, 905
    limb lengthening, *909*
    muscle groups, *910*
    pediatric, 905-915
    surgical management, 907-908
    treatment options, 907
Femurs. *See also* Longitudinal deficiency of the
    femur, partial; Transfemoral amputations
    allograft reconstruction, *63,* 63-64
    chondrosarcoma, *60*
    force distribution, *544*
    protruding, *693*
    residual, *378*
Fenestrations, 412
Fibular centralization procedure, 900
Fibular deficiencies
    associated problems, 889
    children, 792-793
    classification, 889-890, *890, 891, 892, 893,*
        895
    evaluation, 889
    infant with, *890*
    pediatric, 889-896
    prosthetic considerations, 893-894
    rehabilitation, 895-896
    treatment options, 890-892
Field Book of Wound Surgery (Gersdorff), 9
Field hospitals, WWII, 83
Fields of motion, definition, 101, *101*
Fifth ray resections, 202
Figure-of-8 harnesses, 116, 132-133, 137-140,
    246-247, *816*
Figure-of-9 harnesses, 116
Fine motor tasks, *819*
Finger prostheses, 305-306
Fingernails, silicone, *305, 309*
Fingers
    amputations, 202-203
    flexion, 112, 115
    range of motion, 111-114
    ray amputations, *204*
Fingertips
    amputation zones, *198*
    Atasoy-Kleinert volar V-Y technique, *199*
    injuries, 198

Kutler lateral V-Y technique, *200*
    replantation, 198
Fitting
    age of, 926
    for children, 790
    considerations, 321-323
    early, 821, 834
    hip dislocations, *569*
    hip prostheses, *568*
    knee prostheses, 530-531
    pediatric issues, 792
    poor, 695-696
    psychological adaptation and, 734
    scarring and, 409
    single-axis constant-friction knee, *902*
    sockets, 550-551
    timetable, *224*
    transpelvic prostheses, *568, 569*
    transtibial prosthesis, 510-511
Fixation, salvaged limbs, 74
FK-506 (tacrolimus), 341
Flail-arm hinge prostheses, 128, *128*
Flail arm orthoses, 294-295, *295, 296*
Flash fires, skin damage in, 699
Flex-Foot, 371
    floor contact pattern, *372*
    Modular III, 367
    opposite limb demand, 372-373
    power spike, 374
    running with, 645
    terminal stance, 373
    weight acceptance, 373
Flex-Sprint, 645, 651-652, *652*
Flexible hinges, 125, *126*
Flexible-keel feet, 418, *418, 419*
Flexible passive mitts, *118*
Flexible transfemoral sockets, 549
Flexible-walled sockets, 15
Flexion abduction joints, *129*
Flexion contractures, 622
Flexion-Friction Wrist, 162
Flexion wrists, 124, *124*
Floor-reaction AFO, *911*
Floor to standing movement, 616
Fluid-controlled knees, 422, *424,* 566, 795
Fluorometry, 40
Foam liners, *508*
Foam panels, *412*
Folliculitis, residual limbs, 707
Fontaine classification, *31, 32*
Foot amputations
    fibular deficiencies and, 892-893
    level selection, 430-431
    loss of function and, 450
    partial, 688-689
    postoperative care, 431-434, 444-446
    preoperative assessment, 431
    prostheses, 308
    prosthetic assessment, 450-456
    prosthetic management, 449-457
    surgical management, 429-448
Foot deficiencies
    incidence, 885
    levels of, 885
    pediatric, 885-888
    prosthetic treatment, 886-887
    surgical techniques, 885-886

Foot disarticulations, 429-448, 449-457
Foot fillet procedures, 493-494
Foot prostheses. *See also* Ankle-foot
    mechanisms
    aesthetic considerations, *309*
    alignment, 512-513
    ankle motion of, *368*
    biomechanics of, 509
    components, 476
    energy peaks, 375
    hamstring action, *370*
    hip disarticulation prostheses, 570
    knee kinetics with, *374*
    knee motion with, *369*
    microprocessor controlled, *668*
    overview, *419*
    selection of, 509-510
    stance phase, *374*
    transpelvic prostheses, 570
Force measurement sensors, 343-344
Force Sensing Resistor controls, 321, 344
Force Sensing Resistors, 214, 347
Forceps kinematics, 343
Forearms
    body control motions, 279
    flexion, *317*
    pronation, *110,* 279
    rotation, 109-110
    supination, *111,* 279
Forequarter amputation. *See* Scapulothoracic
    amputations
Fork strap, 413
Forks, adaptations of, *747*
Forme fruste fibular deficiency, *889*
Four-bar knees, *627,* 795, 913
Four-function forearms, *317*
Four-function wrists, 125
Fractures, residual limb, 697-698
Frames, 269, *269, 550*
Free Flex Hands, *330*
Free-functioning muscle transfer, 289-290, *290,*
    292, 292
Freestyle Swimming accessory, 335, *335*
"French" leg, 12
Friction elbows, 128, 880
Friction wrist units, *123*
Frostbite, *430*
Functional activities. *See also* Activities of daily
    living (ADLs); Occupational therapy;
        Physical therapy
    children, 820-821, 823-824
    chronic pain and, 717-718
    physical therapy and, 603
Functional Ambulation Profile, 593
Functional deficits, in children, 855-856
Functional Independence Measure, 593
Functional outcomes, 591, *838*
Functional Reach Test, 593
Functional use training, 281-283
Funding, multiple limb deficiencies, 925. *See*
    also Economic considerations; Insurance
    coverage
Fungal infections, residual limbs, *706,* 706-707

G

Gadget tolerance, 925

Gait
  advanced training, 612-616
  amputee, 367-384
  amputee stride characteristics, 382, *382*
  biomechanics, 476-479
  cycle, 353-354, *354*
  electromyographic activity, 535
  hip disarticulation and, 611-612
  hip function in, 360-362
  knee function, 358-360, 376-377
  normal, 353-365, *356*, 622
    basic studies, 14
    foot joint function, 358
    knee function, 358-360
    phases, *354*, 354-355
    sound limb stepping, *610*
    swing limb advancement, 357-358
  Syme ankle disarticulation and, 611-612
  tasks, *355*
  training skills, 606-611
  transfemoral amputations, 375-381, 541-545
Gait analysis
  amputee stride characteristics, *382*
  electromyographic activity, 535
  full body, *387*
  pain management and, 719-720
  visual, 385-394
Gait training, 606-611, *623*
Gangrene. *See* Dry gangrene; Gas gangrene; Wet gangrene
Gas gangrene (clostridial myonecrosis), 50, 52
Gas-operated hand, 181
Gastrocnemius muscles
  in ankle function, 357
  knee disarticulations and, 517
  in total limb function, 364
Gel liners, 508, *570*
  adjustments, 790
  bilateral amputees, *629*, 629-630
  lower limb amputees and, 637
  use for children, 794
Genu valgum, 894-895, *895*, 941
German Society for Technical Cooperation [Deutsche Gesellschaft fuer technische Zusammenarbeit (DTZ)], 17
Giant cell tumors, 59, *60*, 63
Gluteal ring, *568*, *569*
Golf, prosthetics for, 330-331, *568*, *637*, 656-657
Golf Pro, 330, *330*
Gracilis muscles
  free-functioning muscle transfer, 290, *290*
  in hip function, 362
  in knee function, 360
  in total limb function, 364
Graft-host junctions, 59
Graft-versus-host disease (GVHD), 341
Green-Anderson growth remaining charts, 935
Griefer prehensor, *191*, 324
Grip
  force control, 281
  power, 197
  prehension force and, 147
Grip prehensors, *331*, *332*
Grip voluntary-closing terminal device, 120, *120*

Grippers, cable-driven, 315-316
Grooming, personal, 746-747
Ground-reaction forces, 477-478
Growth
  management of, 790-791
  prediction of, 935
Guitar adaptor accessory, *337*
Gunshot wounds, 78-79, 286
Gunshot Wounds of the Extremities Requiring Amputation (Guthrie), 9

H

Hair, prosthesis development, *309*, 309-310
Half-and-half sockets, 314, *314*
Hall effect, 344
Hallux, wooden prosthesis, 10, *10*
Hamstring muscles
  artificial insertions, *939*
  in hip function, 360, 362
  in knee function, 358
  persons with transtibial amputations, *370*
Hand amputations
  complications, 204-205
  Krukenberg procedure, 231-237
  partial
    finger components, 185
    patient evaluation, 209-210
    prosthetic management, 209-217
    prosthetic options, 210-212
    staging of care, 212
    surgical management, 197-207
    transmetacarpal-level, *209*
    transverse, 216, *216*
Hand deficiencies, pediatric, 853-862
Hand dynamometers, 197
Hand-like devices, 149-155
Hand prostheses
  anthropomorphic, 344
  body-powered, 210, *282*
  full-hand, aesthetics, 307
  hook power grips, 116
  internal armatures, 306
  iron, 10, *11*
  manipulation using, 281
  molds for, *306*
  myoelectric, *180*, *282*
  new developments, 343-346
  opposition posts, *212*, *322*
  partial
    aesthetics, 306-307
    articulated design, *215*
    body-powered, 214
    components, 213-214
    fitting considerations, 321
    socket design, 213
    staging of care, 212
    suspension, 213
    wrist-driven, *215*
  passive, 210, *211*, *212*, 213-214
  power grips, 115
  for sports, *330*
Hands
  functional activities, 115-116, 197-198
  range of motion, 111-115, *112*
  reconstruction, 203-204
  spherical grip, 115-116

transplantation, 339-342
Hansen's disease, 50, 482
Hard sockets, 508
Harnesses
  axilla loop, *132*
  bilateral transradial, *134*, 323
  bilateral upper limb, 314-315
  body-powered devices, 132-143
  double-ring, *315*
  figure-of-8, 137-140, *816*
  modification, 246
  ring-type, 139
  shoulder disarticulations, 140-143, *141*, *316*
  shoulder saddle, *134*
  for sports activities, 328
  switch control, 143
  upper limb prostheses, *133*
Heel pads, 5, *474*
Heel strike, 353
  prosthetic foot selection, 509
  prosthetics and, 476
  torque, *543*
  transfemoral amputees, *391*
  transtibial amputees, *388*
Hematopoietic chimerism, 341
Hemiatrophy, *467*
Hemicorpectomy. *See* Translumbar amputations
Hemipelvectomy, 62
Heterotopic ossification, 698, 717, 719
Hidden amputations, *442*
High-profile design prostheses, *454*, *455*, 455-456, *456*
Hills, training on, 614
Hindfoot amputations, 25
Hinges
  elbow units, 125-128
  step-up, 317-318
  suspensions, 414-415, *416*, *417*
Hip disarticulation
  in children, 795
  gait training, 611-612
  indications, 557-559
  level of, 559-560
  patient evaluation, 566
  postoperative management, 563-564
  preoperative care, 559
  prosthetic management, 15, 565-573
    casting, 567-568
    follow-up care, 570-571
    lifestyle considerations, 571-572
    suspension, 568-569
  socket design, 566-567, *568*
  surgical management, 557-564
  suspension, 567-569
  technique, 560-562, *561*
Hip flexion bias system, *571*
Hip flexion contractures, 526
Hip joint and pelvic belts, 414-415, 552
Hip-knee-ankle-foot orthoses, 920
Hip prostheses, intelligent, *667*, *668*
Hip spica casts, 92
Hips
  abduction contracture, *689*
  endoskeletal joints, 566-567
  function, 360-362, 526
  mechanical joints, 569-570

motion patterns, *377*, 377-378
muscular control, *380*
reference data, *361*
stability, 908
surgery about, 936
Hirase classification, 198, *198*
Homunculus, 713, *713*
Hook-type terminal devices, 116, *118*, 277,
    345-346, *346*
    functionality, 265
    voluntary-closing, 119-121
    voluntary-opening, *118*, 119
Horner's syndrome, 285, *287*
Houghton Scale, 592
Humeral deficiencies
    acquired, 876
    congenital, *876*
    pediatric, 875-883
    prosthetic considerations, 878-881
    surgical considerations, 876-877
Humeral flexion osteotomy, 940
Humerus. *See also* Transhumeral amputations
    allograft reconstruction, 61-62
    appositional outgrowth, *696*
    external rotation, 102
    internal rotation, 108
    proximal, *60*, *270*
    subluxated head, *938*
Hybrid prostheses, *881*
    knees, 422-423, *423*
    shoulder, 266
Hydraulic actuators, 345, 376
Hydraulic knee control cylinder, *423*
Hydraulic knees, 422, 665-667
Hydrostatic sockets, 508
Hygiene, personal, 278, 702, 746-747, *747*, 750
Hyperbaric oxygen, *685*
Hyperemia, reactive, 702
Hyperglycemia, 462. *See also* Diabetes mellitus
Hypobaric socks, 411, *411*

I

Icelandic Roll-On Suction Socket (ICEROSS),
    410, *410*
Ilizarov technique, 243, 872, 936
Imler prostheses, *454*
Immediate postoperative prosthesis (IPOP),
    246, 498, *506*, 596, *742*
Immunosuppression, 340-341, 462
Imperial hand, 121
Implantable myoelectric sensors (IMESs), 182,
    347
Implants
    femoral, *675*, *676*
    myoelectric sensors, 182, *182*, 347
Independence, fostering of, 807-808
Index finger prostheses, *305*
Index ray amputation, *202*
Individuals with Disabilities Act, 838
Infant Foam Filled Hand, 815
Infants
    developmental milestones, *784*
    elbow units, 880
    hand deficiencies, 854
    physical therapy, 832-835
    prostheses, 814-815

transhumeral prostheses, *824*, 824-826
Infection control, 8, 464, 498
Infections
    diabetic foot, 48-50
    foot ablations and, 429
    MRSA, 37
    peripheral vascular disease and, 36-37
    residual limbs, *706*
    salvage versus amputation, 47-53
    staged amputations and, 26
    transfemoral amputations, 536
    types of, 50
    wet (infective) gangrene, 433-434
    wound healing and, 684-685
    WWI amputees, 81
Inferior checkrein effect, 102
Informed consent, 33-34
Infraclavicular socket, *264*, 265, 269, 271-272
Infrainguinal vein grafts, 34
Insensate skin, 695
Inserts, soft, 508. *See also* Liners
Inside-locking hinges, *127*, 127-128
Insoles, modified, *451*
Instantaneous center of rotation (ICOR), 421
Intelligent hip joint, 667-668, *668*
Intelligent Knee, 376
Intelligent Prosthetic Plus, 666
Intercalary amputations, 271, 936
Intercalary reconstruction, 59
InterClinic Information Bulletin (ICIB), 17
Interfaces
    design, 629
        pressures during locomotion, 662-664
        suspension and, 528-529
Interim prostheses, *213*
Intermittent claudication (IC), 31, 691
Internal armatures, 306
Internal roll-on locking liners, 409-410
International Association for the Study of
    Pain, 711
International Committee of the Red Cross, 17,
    90
International Committee on Prosthetics and
    Orthotics (ICPO), 17
International Organization for Standardization
    (ISO), 661, 777, 779-781, 875
International Society for Prosthetics and
    Orthotics, 779
Interscapulothoracic/transhumeral amputa-
    tions, *315*
Intertriginous dermatitis, residual limbs, 707
Iodine (I-125) clearance, 40
Iron hands, 10
Ischemia, 429, 432-433, 719. *See also* Peripheral
    vascular disease
Ischemic rest pain, 34
Ischial containment sockets, 15, 543-545, 547-
    548, *548*, *549*

J

Joints. *See also* specific joints
    contractures, 27, 687-690
    preservation of, 185
    range of motion, 244, 276
Joints and lacer suspension, 414
Jones classification, *801*, 897, 898

Journal of Prosthetics and Orthotics, 17
*Journal of Rehabilitation Research and
    Development*, 17
*Journal of the Association of Child Prosthetic and
    Orthotic Clinics*, 17

K

Kalamchi and Dawe classification, 898, *898*,
    899
Karlsruhe Hand, *344*, 344-345
Kinesiology, 101-116, 783-788, 853-854
Kinetic Concepts, Inc., 74
Klebs-Löfler bacillus, 81
Klippel-Trenaunay syndrome, *845*, 846
Knee disarticulations
    advantages, 517-518
    benefits, *521*
    bilateral, *522*
    children, 793
    indications, 518-520
    limb length and, 940
    nonambulatory patients, 520
    postoperative management, 523
    prosthetic considerations, 849-850
    prosthetic management, 525-532
    socket design, 527-529
    staging of care, 527
    stubbies and, 902
    surgical management, 517-523
    technique, 520-523
Knee extension contracture, *688*
Knee flexion contractures, 520, *520*, 688, *688*,
    689
Knee fusion, 933-934, *934*
Knee prostheses
    case studies, 531-532
    components, 529-530
    fitting, 530-531
    fluid-controlled, 422
    four-bar, *627*, *628*
    hybrid, *422*, 422-423
    manual lock, 421-422
    mechanisms, 420-423
    microprocessor controls, 173, 628, 665-667,
        795
    motion patterns, *376*
    options, 654
    overview, *424*
    pneumatic swing-control, 14, 376
    polycentric, 421
    selection, 626-627
    single-axis knees, 420
    stance-control, 420-421
    types, 529-530
Knee rotation adapters, 655
Knees
    instability, 541-543, *542*
    joint surface contact, *368*
    motion, *369*
    preservation of, 482
    reference data, *359*
    salvage, 621-622
    selection, 570
    single-limb support, 371-372
    transtibial amputations, 504-505
Kneewalker peg legs, 5, 10, *11*, 12, *13*, 16

Korean War, 69, 86
Kritter irrigation system, *50*, 445, *446*
Krukenberg procedure, 231-237, 742, 861,
    940-941
    blind patients, *187, 323*
    contraindications, 232
    description, 94
    dressings, *234*
    fasciocutaneous flaps, *232*
    indications, 231-232
    muscular envelope, *233*
    myodesis attachment, *232*
    postoperative care, 232, 234
    postoperative complications, 234
    ray coverage, *233*
    rehabilitation, 234-235, *235*
    split-thickness skin grafts, *233*
    technique, 232-233
Kummel classification, 869, *870*
Kutler lateral V-Y technique, *200*
Kyberd's Southampton Hand, 345

L

Land mines, 84, 86, 90
Landsmeer's concept of coordination, *114*
Lange silicone prosthesis, *454*
Lanyard systems, 529
Laser Doppler velocimetry, 40, 431
Lateral agility drill, 649, *649*
Lateral pinch, 853
Lateral speed weaves, 653, *653*-654
Lawnmowers, foot ablations, *430*
Leiomyosarcomas, *61*
Leprosy, amputations, 3
Letts classification, *890*
Level section, history, 5-6
Lever principle, *544*
Lichenified areas, 703, *703*
Light guide spectrophotometry, 40-41
Limb length
    discrepancies, 836-837
    fibular deficiencies, 891-892
    preservation of, 14
    prosthesis fitting and, 526
    residual limbs, 934-936
Limb lengthening, 892, *909*, 936-941, *937, 938*.
    See also Ilizarov technique
Limb salvage. *See also* Salvaged limbs
    allograft/prosthesis composite, *844*
    amputation versus, 22, 31-45
        infections, 47-53
        trauma, 69-75
        tumors, 55-67
    costs, 69-71
    femoral deficiencies, 909
    scoring indices, 71-72
    war wounds, 90
Limb Salvage Index, 72
Liners
    distal pads and, *528*
    elastomeric, 29
    flexible plastic, *636*
    gel, 508, *570*, 629
    hand prostheses, 213
    hip dislocation prostheses, 569

roll-on
    advantages, 245
    hand prostheses, *306*
    locking, *228*, 409-410
    skin contacts, 348
    split, *528*
    transpelvic prostheses, 569
Liposarcomas, *57*
Lisfranc disarticulation, *433*, 442-443, *443, 887*
Lite Touch Hand, 345
Load
    gait biomechanics, 476-479
    normal foot function, 449
    spreading of, *315*
    sustentaculum tali, *453*
    during walking, 399
Loading response, 388, *392*, 509
Lock control cables, 136, *136*
Lock-Grip hands, 121
Locking shoulder joint, 169, *169*, 324
Locking shoulder joints, *129*, 318
Locomotion
    development, *784*, *785*-786, 925-926
    interface pressures, 662-664, *663*
    prosthetic ambulation, 400-401
Longitudinal deficiencies
    congenital bilateral, *834*
    present at birth, *780*, 780-781
    prosthetic considerations, 789
    ulnar, *869*-873, *872*
        etiology, 870-871
        incidence, 870-871
        treatment, 871-872
Longitudinal deficiency of the femur, partial
    (LDFP), 795-796, 933-936. *See also* Femoral
    deficiencies
    bilateral, *908*, 910-911
    classification, *906*, 906-907
    limb lengthening, *909*
    muscle groups, *910*
    posture, *905*
    presentation, *905*
    treatment options, 907-908
Lordosis, lumbar, 625, *625*
Low back pain, 696-697, 716
Lower Extremity Assessment Project (LEAP),
    73, 91
Lower limb amputations. *See also* specific
    amputations
    activities of daily living, 665
    aesthetic considerations, 308-309
    bilateral, 629-630, 796-797
    biomechanics, *533*, 533-534
    children with, 403
    children with congenital deficiencies,
        792-797
    definitive amputee management, 92-93
    functional outcomes, *838*
    high-energy trauma, *71*
    levels, 381-382
    prosthetic prescriptions, 740-741
    regional considerations, *698*
    skills for, 750-752
    stride characteristics, *382*
    total limb function, 362-364, *364*
    unilateral, 399-400
    walking, 395-407

Lumbar lordosis, 625, *625*
Lumbar spine and sacrum, absence of, 917-922
Lumbar sympathectomy, 34-35
Lumbosacral agenesis, 917-922, *921*
Lupus erythematosus, *433, 438*

M

Madura foot, 50
Magnetic resonance angiography, 38
Mallet toes, 436
Mangled Extremity Severity Score (MESS), 72,
    73, 91
Mangled Extremity Syndrome Index (MESI),
    72, *72*
Manual lock knees, 421-422, *424*
Manual locking knees, 794
Manufacturers, contact information, *338, 660*
Marquardt angulation osteotomy, 240, *240*,
    241, 847, 877
Marquardt tenomyoplastic modification, *444*
McCollough amputation, 932, *932*
Medical Outcomes Survey, 592
Medical Outcomes Survey Health Status Pro-
    file, 481
Medicare Functional Classification Levels
    (MFCL) system, 593, 741
Meningococcemia, 844-845
Mental health, support for, 808-809
MICA shoulder joints, 192
Michigan Crippled Children's Commission, 17
Microprocessor-controlled swing phase con-
    trols, 15
Microprocessor controls
    future of, 667
    hydraulic knees, 376
    knees, 173, 423, 628, 795
    lower limb prostheses, 665-668
Microswitch controls, 293, *293*
Midstance
    biomechanics, 476
    body alignment and, 478
    prosthetic foot selection, 509
    visual analysis, 389, *392*
Midtarsal disarticulation, 443-445, *444*
Miller vein cuff technique, *36*
Mobility, prosthesis prescription, 741-742
Mobilization, adaptation and, 734
Model 55-SS lyre-shaped hook, 119, *120*
Modularity, prosthesis control, 177
Molds, hand prostheses, *306*
Monodactyly, *858*
Monofilament testing, 341
Moseley's straight-line graph, 935
Motor-Drive Lock/Unlock Actuator, 169, *169*
MRSA. *See* Methicillin-resistant *Staphylococcus*
    aureus (MRSA)
Muenster sockets, 228
Multiaxial ankle-feet, 417-418, *418, 419*
MultiControl Plus Electric Hand, 154-155, *155*
MultiControl Powered Gripper, 158-159, *159*
Multidirectional turns, 614-615
Multifunctional prostheses, *319*
Multiple check-socket prostheses, 29
Multiple limb absence, 881

Multiple limb deficiencies
　　acquired, 924
　　congenital, 923-924
　　doffing prostheses, 925
　　donning prostheses, 925
　　prostheses, 924-925
　　special needs, 924-927
Muscle transfers, 289-290, 295
Muscles
　　atrophy, 534-535
　　myodesis, 24
　　myofascial closure, 23
　　myoplasty, 23-24
　　stabilization, 23-24, 244
　　strengthening, 276
　　tenodesis, 24
Musculoskeletal complications, 683-700, 717
Musical instrument adaptor accessory, 336-337
MyoBoy, *822*
Myodesis
　　attachment, *232*
　　closure, *686*
　　control sources and, 185-186
　　history, 7
　　muscle stabilization, 24
Myoelectric prostheses
　　brachial plexus injuries and, 293-294
　　children, 821
　　controls, 320
　　cost, 742
　　custom silicone cover, *308*
　　donning and doffing, 278
　　hand, *282*, 797
　　pediatric, 828
　　practice with, 281
　　temporary, *823*
　　training, 278, 280-281, *822*
　　wrist, *322*
Myoelectric signals
　　acquisition, 347-348
　　control systems, 247
　　definitive electronic prostheses, *228*
　　feedback, 344
　　forearm muscles, 15
　　implantable sensors, *182*
　　muscle transfers and, 295
　　non-hand prehensile devices, 157
　　pattern recognition, 184
　　preprosthetic myoelectric training, 227
　　processing, *178*
　　prostheses control, 177-181
　　transradial prostheses, 188
　　Utah Arm controls, *190*
　　voltage, 179
Myoelectric testing, 276
Myoelectrodes, 151
Myofasciocutaneous flap technique, *492, 493*
　　knee disarticulations, *522*, 522-523
　　long posterior, *487*, 487-490, *488, 489, 490*
Myoplasty
　　control sources and, 185-186
　　muscle stabilization, 23-24
　　transtibial amputation, *686*
　　wrist disarticulation and, *221*
Myoprehension, *190*
Myotesting, 263-264

N

N-Abler terminal devices, *118, 334*
Nail deformities, 205. *See also* Fingernails,
　　silicone
National Academy of Sciences, 14, 17
National Birth Defects Prevention Study, 773
National Center for Medical Rehabilitation
　　and Research, 767
National Commission on Orthotic and Pros-
　　thetic Education, 17
National Federation of State High School As-
　　sociations, 328
National Limb Loss Information Center, 759
National Office of Orthotics and Prosthetics,
　　759
National Research Council, 85, 148
National Sporting Goods Association (NSGA),
　　642
Necrosis
　　AIDS and, *433*
　　burn injuries, 698
　　distal bone, *234*
　　marginal, 683-684, *684*
　　skin flaps, 234
　　transtibial amputation, 694
Necrotizing fasciitis, 50, *51,* 51-52
Negative wrap casts, 550
Nerve-graft systems, 187
Nerve grafts, 287, *294*
Nerve root avulsions, 285, *287*
Nerve roots as donors, 289, *289*
Nerves, sectioned, 24-25
Neuroarthropathic changes, 47-48
Neuroelectric control systems, 181-183
Neurogenic pain, 693-694
Neurologic impairments, 839
Neuromas
　　formation, 24, 693
　　painful, 204-205, 716-717, 719
　　symptomatic, 24
Neuromuscular reorganization, *187,* 187-188
Neurotization, 288-289
New Brunswick system, 188
Ninhydrin sweat test, 198
NISSSA score, 72, 91
Nitrile rubber finger linings, 119
NU-VA Synergetic Prehensor, 156-158
Nudge control units, *129, 143*
NY Electric Elbows, *164,* 165, *165,* 165-166
NY Prehension Actuator, *159,* 159-160

O

Oberlin transfer, 290
Observational gait analysis, 385-394
Occupational therapy
　　children with limb deficiencies, 813-829
　　multiple limb deficiencies, 928
　　postprosthetic, 270-271
　　rehabilitation for children, 851
Ogden classification, *870*
Ontario Crippled Children's Center, 813
Opposite limbs, 372-373, 380-381, 599-600
Opposition posts, *322*
Optical-acoustical sensors, 344
Orthopaedic and Prosthetic Appliance Journal, 17
Orthopaedic Hospital of Copenhagen Knee, 15

Orthotic and Prosthetic Assistance Fund, 839
Osseointegration, 188, 305, 664, 673-681
Osseointegration Prosthesis Rehabilitation for
　　Amputees, 679
Osseoperception, 679
Osteomyelitis
　　chronic, 49-50, 50, *51,* 484
　　diabetes mellitus and, *438*
　　transpelvic amputations and, *560*
Outside-locking hinges, 127, *127*
Oxygen cost, *395,* 396-397, *404*

P

Pain, 711-726
　　after hand amputations, 204-205
　　conceptual models, 712-713
　　definition, 711
　　low-back, 696-697
　　multidimensionality, 711-712
　　neurogenic, 693-694
　　phantom limb, 714-715, 732-733, 848
　　postoperative, 498
　　prosthesis-related, 717
　　psychological distress and, 720-721
　　residual limbs, 691
　　risk of, 718
　　sources of, 716-717
　　treatment, 721-722
Pain management
　　assessment of pain, 720
　　clinical assessment, 718-719
　　history of analgesia, 8-9
　　interventions, 722-723
　　medical assessment, 719
　　orthotic assessment, 719-720
　　prosthetic assessment, 719-720
　　revision amputations for, 26
Pain-stress relationships, 732
Papillomas, cutaneous, residual limbs, 707
Paralympic Games, 766, 808
Parmelee's endoskeletal transfemoral prosthe-
　　ses, *13*
Passive friction elbow, *128*
Passive hands, 117, *118*
Passive mitts, *118*
Passive terminal devices, 117, *118*
Patellar tendon-bearing (PTB) prosthesis, 11,
　　15
Patellar tendon-bearing (PTB) sockets, 507,
　　511, 512, 513, 514
Patellar tendon-bearing (PTB) strap, 413, 414
Patient assessments, 621. *See also* Occupational
　　therapy; Pain management; Physical ther-
　　apy
　　ankle disarticulation and, 473-474
　　arterial circulation, 431
　　bilateral upper limb loss, 311-312
　　dynamic alignment, 386
　　expectations and, 277-278
　　foot prostheses and, 450-456
　　functional outcomes, 591
　　hand transplantation, 339-340
　　knee disarticulations, 525-527
　　lifestyles, 382-383, 633
　　observational gait analysis, 385-386
　　performance-based, 592-596

physical capabilities, 327
pre-ankle disarticulation, 462-465
prosthesis use, 382
self-report, 591-592
static alignment, 385-386
transtibial amputations, 503-505
upper limb deficiencies, 209-210
Patient compliance, 304, 446
Patient education, 598, 600. *See also* Occupational therapy; Physical therapy
Patient expectations, 277-278
Patient Health Questionnaires, 721, *721*
Pectoral cineplasty, 186
Pediatric Evaluation of Disability Inventory, 783
Pediatric patients. *See* Adolescents; Children; Infants; Preschool children; School children; Toddlers
Peg legs
    kneewalker, 5, 10, *11*, 12, *13*, 16
    transtibial, *10*
    use of, 5
    waterproof prostheses, *639*
Pelvis. *See also* Transpelvic amputations
    allograft reconstruction, *62*, 62-63
    function, 362
    in gait, 543
    motion, 378, *378*, 607-608
    transverse rotation, *610*
Percutaneous transluminal angioplasty, 34
Perimalleolar designs, 454-455
Perimeter Frame, 269, *269*
Perinatal limb ischemia, 844, 845
Peripheral vascular disease
    classification, 32
    Fontaine classification, *31*
    foot ablations and, 429
    indications for amputation, *32*
    knee disarticulations, 519
    limb salvage versus amputation, 31-45
    pain, 719
    tests
        angiography, 38
        Ankle Brachial Pressure Index, 38-39
        Doppler ultrasound, 38
        fluorometry, 40
        laser Doppler velocimetry, 40
        light guide spectrophotometry, 40-41
        radioisotope clearance, 39-40
        scanning Doppler velocimetry, 40
        segmental pressures, 38-39
        thermography, 40
        transcutaneous oxygen partial pressures, 39
    transfemoral amputations, 536
Phalangization, 186-187
Phantom limbs
    adolescent patients, 837-838
    non-painful sensations, 713-714
    pain, 498, 713-716, 732-733
    sensations, 732, 848
Philadelphia Arm, 183
Phocomelic arms, *877*
Phocomelic digits, *881*
Physical therapy, 589-619
    ankle/foot performance, 653-654
    for children, 831-840, 851

gait skills, 606-611
home programs, 831
postoperative evaluation, 589-590
postoperative treatment, 596-598
preoperative aspects, 589
preparing for sports, 658-660
preprosthetic exercises, 601-605
    for sports and recreation, 641-660
transfers, 597
wheelchair propulsion, 597
Pirogoff procedure, 467-469, *469*
Plantar ulcers, *48*
Plastisol, 119
Pneumatic knees, 376, 422, 665-667
Pneumatic sensors, 347
Point localization, 197
Poland sequence, 855
Polycentric hinges, 125, *126*
Polycentric knees, 421, *421*, *422*, *518*, 530
    fitting, *526*
    overview, *424*
    pediatric users, 795
    selection, 627
Polydactyly, 859-861
Polyvalent gangrene antitoxin, 52
Popliteal-to-distal anterior tibia/dorsalis pedis bypass, *35*
Positional rotators, *423*, 425
Positive-locking components, 317
Posterior myofasciocutaneous flaps, 6, *6*, 10
Postoperative management. *See also* specific procedures
    amputations, 26-29
    autograft reconstruction, 64-65
    first year care, 28-29
    immediate/early prostheses, 246
    WWI amputees, 81-82
Postoperative prostheses. *See* Immediate postoperative prosthesis (IPOP)
Postural abnormalities, 258-260
Pott's Anglesey Leg, *13*
Power ball pumps, 668
Power grips, 115, 197, 853
Power options. *See* Body-powered components; Externally powered components
Power Swing Ring, 331, *331*
Precision, prehensile activities, 115
Precision grasp, 853
Precision prehension, 853
Predictive Salvage Index (PSI), 72
Pregait training, 605-606
Prehensile activities, 115, 197
Prehension devices
    cable-controlled, 188
    controls, *131*
    electric-powered, 145-160
        hand-like devices, *148*, *149*, 149-155
        manufacturers, *147*
        mechanical characteristics, 145-146
        non-hand-like devices, *148*, 155-160
        prehension force, 146
        speed of movement, 148-149
        width of opening, 147-148
    functionality, 265
Preparation, of amputee, 601-605, 729, 733-734. *See also* Physical therapy; Psychological adaptation

Preparatory prostheses, 225, *225*
Preparatory/training prostheses
    body-powered components, *225*
    electric-powered components, *227*
    electronic, *225*, 226-227
    myoelectric transradial, *228*
Preprosthetic therapy, 227, 275-276, 601-605
Prescriptions
    delayed, 742
    infant prostheses, 814-815
    payment considerations, 743
    for prostheses, 739-743
Pressure-sensitive tape, 745
Pressure sensitivity, 197
Preswing limb advancement, 372
Preswing (toe-off)
    prosthetic foot selection, 509
    transfemoral amputees, *393*
    transtibial amputees, *390*
Progressive hemiatrophy, 461
Prostacycline analogues, 34, 37
Prostheses. *See also* specific needs; specific types
    back-up units, 277
    body-powered components, 117-130
    care of, 278-279, 598
    choice to wear, 265
    cleaning of, 279
    component choices, 29, 276-278
    control of, 173-195, *177*
        design considerations, 175
        goals, 174-175
        muscle bulge, 181
        myoacoustic signals, 177
        myoelectric signals, 177-181
        tendon movement, 181
        transducers, 177
        variables, 175-176
    design history, 10-16
    doffing, 278, 599
    donning, 278, *278*, 599
    early intervention, 223-224
    electric-powered components, 145-171
    endoskeletal, 129-130
    energy expenditure, 399-400
    feedback in, *174*
    fitting, 222
    history of, 9
    ISO testing, 661
    management goals, 210
    metal, 60-61
    prescription of, 739-743
    prototypes, 321
    provisional, 92-93
    reflex action, 173
    WWI amputees, 82
    WWII progress in, 84-85
Prosthesis Evaluation Questionnaire, 592, 720
Prosthetic gait, 385-394
Prosthetic Gait Training Program, 608-611
Prosthetic Profile of the Amputee (PPA), 591
Prosthetic skills
    children and, *818*
    development of, 817-820
    pediatric patients, 823-824
Prosthetic socks, 790
Prosthetic training, 275-284

Prosthetics and Orthotics International, 17
Prothosis, *271*
Provisional prostheses (pylons), 92-93
Proximal focal femoral deficiency. *See* Longitudinal deficiency of the femur, partial
Psychological adaptation
    emotional readiness, 791
    stages of, 730-732
Psychological aspects
    aesthetic prosthetics, 303-310
    age and, 382-383
    amputation, 32-33
    bilateral upper limb amputees, 313
    bilateral upper limb loss, 311-312
    of chronic pain, 717-718
    coaching disabled athletes, *659*
    etiology of amputation, 802
    functional use training and, 281-283
    goal setting, 591
    maximizing independence, 276
    multiple limb deficiencies, 927
    of pain, 712-713
    pediatric limb deficiency, 801-811
    transtibial amputations, 499
Psychological counseling, 244
Psychological responses, determinants of, 727-729
Psychosocial support, 728
Pylons, shock-absorbing, 425

Q

Quadriga, 205
Quadrilateral sockets, 545-547, *546, 547,* 554
Quality of life, 69-71, 717-718. *See also* Activities of daily living (ADLs); Psychological adaptation
Quick-disconnect wrist units, 124, *124, 228,* 247
Quick-release couplers, *638*

R

Radial deficiencies, 863-868, *864, 865, 866. See also* Transradial amputations
Radial dysplasia, 863, *864, 865*-867
Radialization, 866-867
Radiohumerus interosseous distances, *109*
Radioisotope clearance, 39-40
Radius
    allograft reconstruction, 62
    deficiencies, *863,* 863-868
Ramps, training on, 614
Range of motion, 590, 603, 834
Rate of oxygen consumption
    bilateral amputees, 625
    customary walking speeds and, *400*
    definition, *395*
    loading and, 399
    walking speed and, 398, *399*
Ray amputations
    feet, *439, 439*-441, *440,* 452, *542*
    finger, 202, *202, 204*
Ray resections, *203*
Reamers, 675

Recreation
    child participation in, 838-839
    lower limb amputees, 642-643, 752
    multiple limb deficiencies, 926
    physical therapy for, 641-660
    popular activities, *643*
    prosthetic adaptations, 327-338, 633-640
    rehabilitation and, 749
Redundant tissue, *247*
Referrals, support groups, 809
Reflexes, artificial, 173, 184
Rehabilitation. *See also* Occupational therapy;
    Physical therapy; specific procedures
    absence of the lumbar spine and sacrum, 920-921
    aesthetic prosthetics, 304
    at-home, 731-732
    bilateral upper limb amputees, 313
    brachial plexus injuries, 295-296
    for children, 851
    Civil War amputees, 79
    communication devices, 748
    fibular deficiencies, 895-896
    in-hospital, 731
    Krukenberg procedure, 234-235
    longitudinal humeral deficiencies, 876
    Osseointegration Prosthesis Rehabilitation for Amputees, 679
    pain interventions, 723
    plan formulation, 268
    postprosthetic phase, 270-271
    prosthesis design and, 244
    psychological adaptation and, 729, 730
    PVD management, 33
    rotationplasty, 836
    shoulder-level amputations, 263
    tibial deficiencies, 903
    upper limbs, 224-229
    vocational activities, 734-735
    without prostheses, 745-755
Reintegration to Normal Living Index (RNL), 591
Renshaw classification, *918*
Replantation
    elbow disarticulation and, 239
    fingertips, 198-201
Residual digits, 305-306
Residual limb-activated locking hinges, 126-127, *127*
Residual limbs
    abducted, *534*
    alignment, *215*
    care check list, *602*
    care of, 278-279
    children, 776
    compressive dressings, 599
    desensitization, 276
    elastic bandage, *246*
    erosion, *702*
    femoral, 541
    first year care, 28-29
    foot forces, *452*
    fractures, 697-698
    humeral neck, *264*
    hygiene, 278
    interaction with sockets, 662-665
    joint range of motion, 276

    length, 402-403, *842,* 895, 934-936
    limb lengthening, 936-941, *937, 938*
    maturation, 27
    motor control, 690
    MRI reconstruction, *535*
    osseointegration, 673-681
    pain, 691, 715-716
    poor prosthetic fit, 695-696
    positioning, *597*
    postoperative care, 538-539
    preprosthetic therapy, 275-276
    pressure tolerance, 511
    protection of, 210
    reconstruction, 21
    scarring, 847-848
    self-inspections, 278
    shaping, *211,* 276, 685-687
    shrinkage, 276, *506*
    simple revisions, 933
    skin breakdown, *508,* 701-710
    strength exercises, *604*
    surgical modification of, 931-943
    tapered, *488*
    terminal modification, 941
    tolerance for shear, *636*
    transtibial amputations, 504, *504*
    ulceration, *702*
    wrapping, *600*
    xeroradiograph, *475*
Resisted elastic kicks, *605*
Resistive gait training, *612*
Respiratory exchange ratio (RER), *395,* 396, 397-398
Restorationists, cosmetic, 122
Revascularization, 33-34
Rhomboid paralysis, 285
Rigid hinges, 125
Ring ray resections, 202
Rocker feet, 12
Roll-on liners, 245, *306*
Rotasafe device, *678, 679*
Rotational wrist units, *125*
Rotational wrists, 124-125
Rotationplasty, 58, *58,* 796, 836, 908, *914*
Roy Adaptation Model, 760, 762
Rubber knee sleeves, *412*
Running. *See also* Sprinting
    biomechanics, 644-646
    lower limb amputees, *635, 637, 637,* 643-644
    with prostheses, 646-647, *647*
    skills, 646
Rutgers University multifunctional hand, 181

S

S-type Swing Only hydraulic knee, 654
Sabolich-style frames, *550*
Sacrum, lumbar spine and, absence of, 917-922
Sagittal flap technique, 521-522
Salvaged limbs, 73-74. *See also* Limb salvage
Sandia National Laboratories, 667
Saphenous vein femoroposterior tibial bypass grafting, 36
Sarcomas, *843,* 843-844

Scalding, foot and ankle, *432*
Scandinavian Flexible Socket, *550*
Scanning Doppler velocimetry, 40
Scapula
    abductors, *105*
    adductors, *106*
    allograft reconstruction, 61
    depressors, *106*
    downward rotation, *106*
    elevators, *106*
    protractors, *105*
    retractors, *106*
    upper limb elevation, 102
    upward rotation, *105*
Scapular abduction, 142-143, 279
Scapular winging, *287*
Scapuloectomy, 257
Scapulohumeral joints
    adductors, *105*
    elevators at, *104*
    extensors, *107*
    flexors, *107*
    rotation at, *108*
    rotators at, *104*
Scapulothoracic amputations
    anterior approach, 254-255, *255*
    appearance following, *254*
    description, 251
    myoelectric prostheses, 280
    posterior approach, 255-256, *256*
    procedure, 254
Scapulothoracic joints, 102
Scars
    adherent, *708*
    fitting and, 409
    postamputation, 22-23
    residual limbs, 847-848
    from vascular surgery, 687, *687*
Seattle Foot, 367, 373-374, 645
Seattle Lite foot, 380
Seattle Orthopaedic Group, 667
Segmental pressures, 38-39
Self-help groups, 730-731, 735, 761-762
Self-suspending prostheses, *328*, 941
Self-suspending sockets, 314, 323
Semmes-Weinstein monofilaments, 197
Sensation. *See also* Pain; Phantom limbs
    blind patients, *323*
    physical therapy and, 590
SensorHand, 149-152, *150*, 173
SensorHand Speed, 344
Sensors, 182, *182*, 343, 347-348
Sepsis, 26. *See also* Infections
Servo control systems, 247, 320-321
Sexuality, 733, 926-927
Shock absorbers
    hip disarticulation prostheses, 570
    sports prostheses, 654
    transpelvic prostheses, 570
    vertical, 628, *628*
Shock-absorbing pylons, 425, *571*, *636*
Shoulder complex
    amputation levels, 252-258
    body control motions, 279
    "high" shoulder, 259
    intercalary resection, 257-258
    internal resection, 257-258

    motion, *101*, 101-105, *102*, *103*
    rotary capability, 107-108
Shoulder disarticulations
    bilateral
        control systems, *191*
        fitting prostheses, 323
    chest harness, *827*
    in children, 798
    claviculectomy, 256-257
    en bloc resections, 256-258
    endoskeletal prosthesis design, 130
    harnesses, 140-143, *142*
    internal amputations, 256-258
    modified, *252*, 252-253
    myoelectric prostheses, 280
    postural scoliosis and, *259*
    prosthetic components, 264-265
    residual limbs, *264*
    scapuloectomy, 257
    thigh strap control, *827*
    transhumeral amputations and, 192
    true, *252*, 252-253
    unilateral prostheses, 190
Shoulder-level amputations
    bilateral, *272*, 272-273
    interim prosthetic phase, 268-270
    postprosthetic phase, 270-271
    postural abnormality following, 258-260
    preprosthetic phase, 263-264
    prosthetic management, 263-273
    rehabilitation, 263
    surgical management, 251-261
Shoulder-level deficiencies, 826-828
Shoulder-level prostheses, *272*, 272-273
Shoulder prostheses, 128-129
    ball-and-socket joint, 129, *129*
    body-powered, *266*
    design considerations, 267-268
    externally powered components, 267
    hybrid designs, *266*, 266-267
    locking joints, *191*, *317*
    passive, 265, *266*
    positioning, 279
Shoulder spica casts, 93
Shrinker socks, *498*, 687, *687*
Shuttle locks, 410
Sickness Impact Profile, 592, 718
Sidestepping, 614
Sierra voluntary-opening hand, 121
Sierra Wrist Flexion Units, 162
Silastic caps, *933*
Silesian belt, 413-414, *414*, 794, 849, 901
Silesian belt suspension, *552*
Silicone bladder ankle disarticulation prostheses, *475*
Silicone bladders, 475
Silicone prostheses, 455, *455*
Silicone reconstruction
    advantages, 307
    color, 310
    creation, 213
    finger prostheses, 305
    fingernails, *305*, 309
    foot, *542*
    myoelectric prostheses, *308*
    toenails, 309
    toes, *451*, 451-452

Silicone suspension sleeves, *228*, 880
Single-axis ankle-foot, 12, *415*, 415-416, 419
Single-axis constant-friction knee, *902*
Single-axis hinges, 125, *126*
Single-axis knees, 420, *420*, 424, 518, 794
Single-axis shoulder units, 128
Single-limb squatting, 615
Single-limb support
    amputees, 371-372
    ankle, 355, 357
    full-body gait analysis, *387*
    knee function, 358
    total limb function, *363*, 363-364
Sinus formation, 690
Sitting, developmental milestones, 785
6-minute walk test, 593, 596
Skeletal reconstruction, 58-61, *60*
Skew flap technique, *493*
Skin
    adherence, 186, 694-695
    in amputations, 22-23
    care, 598
    color changes, 310
    fasciocutaneous flaps, 23
    grafts, 23
    hygiene, 702
    insensate, 695
    problems, 701-710
    quality, 244
    scars, 22–23
    self-inspections, 278
    transtibial amputations, 504
Skin grafts
    decision-making, 23
    foot and ankle, *432*
    Krukenberg procedure, *233*
    split-thickness, 694-695, *842*
    tolerance for shear, *636*
Skin perfusion, 431
Slapping gait, 47
Slip socket adjustments, 790
Slipper-type elastomer prosthesis (STEP), *454*
"Smart" prostheses, 667
Smoking, 429, 691
Social environment, 805, 848. *See also* Psychological adaptation
Social support, 33, 761-762. *See also* Support groups; Support programs
Socioeconomic forces, 16-17, 69-71
Sock regulation, 598-601
Sockets
    adjustments, 790
    alignment biomechanics and, 510-513, *546*
    center of rotation, *531*
    cleaning, 279, 702
    clear test, *271*
    design
        bilateral upper limb prostheses, 313-314
        body-powered components, *268*
        electronic prostheses, 227-228
        humeral prostheses, 878-880
        knee disarticulations, 527, 850
        pediatric patients, 849
        principles of, 545
        shoulder-level amputations, 268-269
        suspension systems, 245

tibial prostheses, 507-509
    translumbar prostheses, 584-586, *586*
diagnostic, 269-270
elbow disarticulation prostheses, *246*
fit, *245*, 511, *528*, 550-551
flexible, *245, 248*, 549
half-and-half, *314*
hand prostheses, 213
hard, 508
hip disarticulation prostheses, 566-567
humeral prostheses, *879*
hydrostatic, 508
indications, 549-550
infraclavicular, *264*
inner, 509
ischial containment, 545, 547-548, *548, 549*
lamination, 15
leather, *526*
limb interaction with, 662-665
looseness, 695
new developments, 348
oversized, *894*
patellar tendon–bearing (PTB), 507
pediatric, *835*
PTB supracondylar-suprapatellar, *505*
quadrilateral, 545-547, *546, 547*
self-suspending, 314
sports prostheses, 648-649
stability exercises, 649-650
suction, 409-410
temporary, 29
tightness, 695
total surface-bearing (TSB), 507
transducer sites, 663
transfemoral designs, 545-551
transpelvic prostheses, 566-567
volume-adaptable, *520*
Soft belt liners, 552
Soft inserts, 508
Soft tissues
    conservation, 185-186, 244
    coverage, 504, 521, *693*
    excessive, 685, *685*
    force transmission and, 664-665
    reconstruction, 185-186
Soft voluntary-closing hands, *120*
Soft voluntary-opening hands, 121, *122*
Solid ankle–cushion heel (SACH), 15
    description, 416-417, 418
    design, *418*
    development, 367
    energy expenditures and, 403
    floor contact pattern, *371*
    opposite limb demand, 372-373
    overview, *419*
    Syme amputations and, 93
    terminal stance, 373-374
    weight acceptance, 373
Sound side stepping, *612*
Southampton Adaptive Manipulation Scheme (SAMS), 348
Southampton Hand, 345
Spectra control cables, 324
Spectrophotometry, light guide, 40-41
Spherical grip, 115-116
Spica casts, 92, 93, 832
Split-hand/split-foot syndrome, 885, *886*

Split hook devices, 119
Split-socket prostheses. *See* Step-up hinges
Sports
    child participation in, 838-839
    lower limb amputees, 752
    multiple limb deficiencies, 926
    physical therapy for, 641-660
    prosthetic adaptations, 327-338, 633-640, 647-649
    rehabilitation and, 749
    safety in, 327-328
    terminal devices, 329-330
    transtibial amputations, 503-504
Sports prostheses
    ankle/foot options, 650-653
    knee options, 654
    knee rotation adapters, 655
    lower limb
        alignment, 634
        choice, 634
        design, 634-637
        dynamics, 634-635
        impact reduction, 635-637
        physical preparation, 633-634
    shock absorbers, 654
    socket design, 647-648
    socket stability, 648-649
    suspension, 647-648
    torsion adapters, 655
Spring-lift assist devices, 128, *129*
Springlite foot, 380
Sprinting, foot options, 651. *See also* Running
Squamous cell carcinomas, 50, *708, 709*
Squatting, single-limb, 615
Stainless steel reinforcement, 328
Stance-control knees, *420*, 420-421, *424*, 794-795
Stance-phase knee flexion, 627-628
Standing, developmental milestones, 785
Staphylococcus, 81, 484, 705. *See also* Methicillin-resistant *Staphylococcus aureus* (MRSA)
Steeper-2 in mechanical hand, 820
Step Activity Monitor, 592-593
Step counters, 592-593
Step-up hinges, 125-126, *126*, 317-318
Stereognosis. *See* Tactile object recognition
Stockinette, over dressings, *224*
Stool stepping exercise, *608*
Stovepipe prostheses, 475
Strain gauges, 151, 343
Strap suspensions, 413-414, *416, 417*
Strength, 590, 603, *604. See also* Patient assessments; Physical therapy
Streptococcus sp., 81, 484, 705
Stubbies, 404
    bilateral amputees, *623*
    bilateral prostheses, *623*
    knee disarticulations and, 902
    transfemoral amputations, 623-625, *740*
    trial use, 740
Stumble controls, 665
Subcritical limb ischemia, 32
Subintimal angioplasty, 34
Suction sockets, 85, 245, 409-410, *410*
Suction suspension, 13, 551-552
Sudomotor function, 197, 198

Support groups, *769, 809*, 848. *See also* Social support
Support programs, *759*, 762-765. *See also* Psychological adaptation; Social support
Support straps, *132, 137-138*, 137-140
Supracondylar amputation, 517
Supracondylar cuffs, 413, *414*
Supracondylar wedges, 413
Suprapatellar cuff, *414*
Surfaces, uneven, 613
Surgical complications, 729
Suspension belts, elastic, *414*
Suspension liners, 15, 228, *228*
Suspension systems
    anatomic, 412-413
        expandable inner walls, 412-413
        fenestrations, 412
        hidden panels, 412
        overview, *416, 417*
        supracondylar wedges, 413
    atmospheric pressure, 409-411, *416*
        elastomeric knee sleeves, 411
        hypobaric socks, 411
        internal roll-on locking liners, 409-410
        suction sockets, 409-410
    design, 245, 629, 849
    finger prostheses, 305
    foam liners and, 528
    foam panels, *412*
    hinge, 414-415, *416*
    hip dislocation prostheses, 567-569, *568-569*
    interfaces and, 528-529
    liners, 552
    new developments, 348
    options, 409-420
    patient education, 598-601
    split cylindrical, 528
    sports prostheses, 647-648
    strap, 413-414, *416, 417*
    suction, 551-552
    transfemoral prostheses, *417*, 551-552, *552*
    transpelvic prostheses, 568-569
    transtibial prostheses, *416*
SUVA grasp stabilization system, 348
Sven Hand, 183
Swedish Total Knee, 677, *678*
Swelling, postoperative, 832. *See also* Edema
Swing limb advancement
    full-body gait analysis, *387*
    gait, 357-358
    hip function in, 362
    knee in, 360
    total limb function in, 364-365
    visual analysis, *390*
Swing'N'Stance, 654, *655*
Switches, 177, 320
Sword of Damocles syndrome, 734
Symbrachydactyly, 854-857, *856*
Syme ankle disarticulation
    advantages and disadvantages, *473*
    bone tissue management, 25
    in children, 792-793, 796
    for congenital arteriovenous fistulae, *461*
    conversion, 931-932
    description, 459, *459*
    Elmslie's modification, *465*

failure rate, 87
femoral deficiency and, 907-908
fibular deficiencies and, 893, *894*
gait mechanics, 368
gait training, 611-612
heel pad shift, *686,* 686-687
with knee fusion, 796
mature, *468*
outcomes, *468*
procedure, *463, 466*
prosthesis prescription, 741, *741*
running biomechanics, 646
running skills, 646
socket design, 850
staging of care, 473-474
traumatic injury, *431*
wartime amputees, 93
xeroradiograph, *475*
Syme prostheses, 15
aesthetic considerations, 308-309
medial-opening, 476
posterior-opening, *412*
Syndactyly, *855, 857-858, 859,* 872
Synergetic Prehensor, 149
System Electric Hands, 149-152

T

Tactile gnosis. *See* Tactile object recognition
Tactile object recognition, 197
Tactile sensitivity, 197
Tandem walking, 615
Tarsometatarsal amputations, *453,* 453-456
Tarsometatarsal disarticulations, 442-443
Task-specific prostheses
hand, 210, *213*
lower limb amputees, 637
modified tools, *214*
shoulder units, 267, *267*
Team approaches, 729-730, 739-740, 743, 775, 814
Tenodesis, 24, 214-215
Tenomyoplastic operations, 443-444
Terminal devices
activation, 824, 926
anthropomorphic, 329-330
Child Amputee Prosthetics Project, 815
grip prehensors, *331-333, 334*
positioning, 279, *280, 818*
readiness for activation, 816
Terminal overgrowth, 932-933
Terminal stance
prosthetic feet and, 373-374
prosthetic foot selection, 509
visual analysis, *389, 393*
Terminal swing, *394*
Terminal transverse deficiency, *855*
Tests. *See* Patient assessments
Tetanus prophylaxis, 52, 73
Thigh lacer with side joints, *414, 415*
Thoracolumbosacral orthosis, *913*
Thrombocytopenia with absent radius syndrome, 861, 875, *875, 931*
Thumb prostheses, 306
Thumb web space deficiency, *871*
Thumbs
amputations, 201-202

dysplasia, 864
field of motion, *114,* 114-115
opposition of, *115*
polydactyly, *859*
reconstruction, 865
Wassel's type IV thumb, *860*
Tibial arteriogram, *463*
Tibial deficiencies. *See also* Transtibial amputations
allograft reconstruction, 64, *64*
associated anomalies, 899, *899*
bilateral, *835,* 902
children, 793
classification, 897-899
etiology, 899
knee extensor power and, 900
pediatric, 897-904
prosthetic management, 901-903
treatment, 899-901
Tikhor-Linberg procedure, 257-258, 271
Tilt table, 623, *623*
Tilting table prostheses, *565*
Tinea corporis, residual limbs, 706
Tinea cruris, residual limbs, 706
Tinel's sign, 341, 693, 719
Tip pinch, 197, 853
Tissue engineering, 341-342
Titanium
bone tolerance to, 674
intraosseous, 673
reinforcement with, 328
use of, 15
Toddlers, physical therapy, 835
Toe amputations, 308, 451-452, *452*
Toe-box jumps, 653, *653*
Toe-to-hand transfers, 203, 941
Toenail reconstruction, 309
Toes, *451*
deficiencies, 886-887, *887*
disarticulations, 436-438, *437*
dry gangrene, *37*
pressure measurements, 39
pulsed-wave assessment, 39
spacers, *451*
wet gangrene, *50,* 446
Torque absorbers, 423, *423,* 425, 628-629
Torsion adapters, 655
Total-contact PTB transtibial socket, 15
Total Elastic Suspension (TES) belt, 794, 901
Total Knee, 794-795
Total surface-bearing (TSB) sockets, 507
Totally Modular Prosthetic Arm with High Workability (TOMPAW), 347
Training. *See also* Patient education; Physical therapy
activities of daily living, 281-283
amputation surgery, 9, 41
balance and, 605-606, *606*
cardiovascular endurance, 603
coaching disabled athletes, *659*
coordination and, 605-606
early, 278-279
elbow lock sequence, 825-826
energy expenditure and, 396-397
forearm lift, 825
functional use, 281-283
gait skills, 606-611

general conditioning, 601
infant transhumeral prostheses, 824-825
motion control, 817
with prostheses, 275-284, 815-816, 828
in prosthetics, 17-18
range of motion, 603
repetition and, 819
strengthening, 603
terminal device operation, 826-827
volunteers, 765
Transcarpal electronic hands, *213, 344*
Transcarpal Hands, 151-152, *152, 152*
Transcutaneous oxygen partial pressures (TcPO$_2$), 39
Transducers
dynamic, 661
liner, *319*
prostheses control, 177
socket sites, 663
Transfemoral amputations
abduction contractures, *689*
alignment devices, *545*
benefits, *521*
bilateral, 89, 693
center of mass, 609
children, 794
flexion-abduction contractures, 689
gait deviations, 375-381, *391-394*
healed, *539*
hip motion patterns, *377,* 377-378
history, 7, 11
indications, 536
interface pressures, 663, *663*
ischial containment sockets, 553, 554
knee options, 654
management, 92-93
muscular control of hip, *380*
osseointegration in, 673-681, *679,* 679-680
other limb demand, 380-381
postoperative care, 538-539
postoperative positioning, 596
prosthetic considerations, 849
prosthetic management, 541-555
quadrilateral sockets, 554
residual femur alignment, *539*
residual femur motion, *378*
residual limb biomechanics, 541-545
residual limb wrapping, *601*
selection, 39
stair climbing, 613
stubbies, 623-625
stubby use, *740*
support moment, *381*
surgical approaches, 535-536
surgical management, 533-540
technique, 536-538
transportation casts, 92
war amputees, 88-89
xerogram, *535*
Transfemoral amputees
gait, 376-377
pelvic motion, 378, *378*
trunk motion, 378, *379*
Transfemoral prostheses, *13,* 308-309
flexible socket-rigid socket design, *550*
history, *12*
Silesian belt suspension, *552*

suspensions, *417*, 551-552
Transfer prostheses, 597
Transfers, physical therapy and, 590-591
Transhumeral amputations
    axillary discomfort, 139
    bilateral
        harnesses, 139-140, *140*
        pediatric patient, *312*
    elbow disarticulation and
        level of amputation, 239
        prosthetic management, 243-249
        surgical management, 239-241
    endoskeletal prosthesis design, 130
    flexible wall socket, 248-249
    myoelectric prostheses, 280
    redundant tissue, 248
    shoulder disarticulations and, 192
    shoulder fusion and, 293-294
    surgical management, 240-241
Transhumeral deficiencies, 797-798
Transhumeral harnesses, 137-140, *140*
Transhumeral prostheses
    aesthetics, 307-308
    body-powered elbow, *245*
    control systems, *135*, 135-137, 189-191, *191*
    fitting considerations, 322-323
    hybrid, *189*
    infants, *824*, 824-826
    passive elbow, *308*
    unilateral, 189-190
Translumbar amputations
    complications, 578-579
    follow-up evaluations, 581-582
    outcomes, *576*, *580*, *581*
    patient appearance, *583*
    patient selection, 575-583, *579*
    postoperative management, 579-581
    prosthetic management, 583-588
    surgical management, 575-582
    surgical technique, 576-578, *578*
Translumbar prostheses, *586*
    ambulatory, *586*, 586-587, *587*
    independent transfer to, *584*
    sitting, 584, *584*, *585*
    socket design, 584-586
Transmetacarpal amputations, *209*, *215*, 215-216, 452-453
Transmetatarsal absences, 887
Transmetatarsal amputations, 441-442, *442*
Transmetatarsal prostheses, *453*
Transosseous division, 3
Transpelvic amputations
    indications, 557-559
    level of, 559-560
    patient evaluation, 566
    postoperative management, 563-564
    preoperative care, 559
    prosthetic management, 565-573
        follow-up care, 570-571
        lifestyle considerations, 571-572
    socket design, 566-567
    surgical management, 557-564
    technique, *562*, 562-563
Transpelvic prostheses, 567-568, *568*
Transplantation
    hands, 339-342, *340*
Transportation casts, 92

Transradial amputations
    bilateral, *221*, 323-324, *746*
    blind patients, *323*
    in children, 797
    limb length preservation, 185
    myoelectric prostheses, 280
    short, *861*
    surgical management, 221-222
    traumatic, *221*
    wrist disarticulation and, 219-230
Transradial amputees
    elbow units, 125-127
    endoskeletal prosthesis design, 130
    myoelectric forearm signals, 15
Transradial control systems, 131-132
Transradial deficiencies, 797, 813-814
Transradial harnesses
    bilateral, 134
    figure-of-8, *132*, 132-133
    heavy-duty, 134
    modifications, 134-135
Transradial prostheses, *12*
    aesthetics, 307
    bilateral, 190
    control systems, 188-189
    definitive electronic prostheses, *228*
    fitting considerations, 321-322
    myoelectric, *180*, *308*
    passive, *308*, *815*
    preparatory/training, *227*
    wear and use patterns, *821*
Transtarsal amputations, *453*, 453-456
Transtibial amputations, *8*
    amputee gait, 367-375
    anesthesia, 486-487
    bilateral prostheses, *616*, *623*
    bone treatment, 496-497
    closed amputations, 487-494
    contractures, 687-688
    contraindications, 483
    crutches, 613
    in diabetes mellitus, 497
    excessive soft tissue, *685*
    fascia treatment, 495
    fixation, *494*
    flaps, 490, 491, *491*, *492*, 493
    fractures after, 697
    gait deviations, 388-390
    inappropriate beveling, *683*
    indications, 482-483
    nterface pressures, 663, *663*
    knee flexion contractures, 688
    level selection, 484-485, *486*
    long fibula, *692*
    muscle treatment, 495
    myoplasty, *686*
    nerve treatment, 495-496
    open amputations, 494, 495, 496
    patellar dislocations and, 697
    postoperative care, 483-484, 497-499
    postoperative positioning, 596-597
    prosthesis prescription, *741*
    prosthetic feet, *370*
    prosthetic management, 503-515
    running and, *644*, *645*, *648*
    running biomechanics, 646
    short, *497*

sinus formation, 690, *690*
skin adherence, 694
skin treatment, 494-495
split-thickness skin graft, *694*
staging of care, 505-507
stair climbing, 613
surgical management, 481-501
suspensions, 850
sutures, *684*
transportation casts, 92
traumatic, *497*, *846*
types of, *487*
war amputees, 88
Transtibial amputees, bilateral, 622
Transtibial peg legs, *10*
Transtibial prostheses, *12*
    aesthetic considerations, 308-309, *309*
    Beaufort, *13*
    fitting, 510-511
    suspension, *416*
Transverse deficiencies, 779-780, *780*, *881*
Traumatic amputees
    acute vascular insufficiency, 37
    bilateral lower limb, 621
    energy expenditure, 401-402, *402*
    foot ablations, 430
    high-energy amputation rates, *71*
    limb salvage *versus* amputation, 69-75
    pediatric, 842-843
    wound healing and, *684*
Trinity Amputation and Prosthesis Experience
    Scale (TAPES), 720
Triple-axis shoulder units, 128
Trochanter knee-ankle relationships, 542-543
Trunk
    load on, 399
    motion, 378, *379*
    passive rotation, *612*
Tumbling, prosthesis use and, 329-330
Tumors. See also *Specific* tumor types
    adductor compartment, *558*
    adolescent patients, 837
    chemotherapy, 55-56
    limb salvage *versus* amputation, 55-67
    pelvic resections, 559
    resection, 57-58
    rotationplasty, *845*
    staging, 55, *55*
    surgical treatment, 56, 876
    transfemoral amputations, 536
"Two-load" hooks, 119, *120*
Two-point discrimination, 197

U

Ulceration, *708*
    chronic, 708
    depth, 47
    diabetes and, 707
    formation, 47
    plantar, 48
    residual limbs, *702*, *706*
Ulnar hemimelia, 870
Ultrasonic motors, 345
United States Children's Bureau, 17
United States Disabled Athletes Fund, 839
Universal shoulder joints, *129*

Upper limb amputations
   bilateral, 877, *878*
   prosthesis prescription, 742-743
   regional considerations, *699*
   rehabilitation, 745-750
Upper limb deficiencies. *See also* specific
      deficiencies
   bilateral, *881*
   in children, 797-798
   congenital postaxial, 869-873
Upper limb prostheses
   bilateral, 308, 311-325
   body-powered components, 117-130
   body-powered devices, 131-143
   considerations, 305-308
   control, 175-176, 785-786
   early intervention, 223-224
   elevation, *107*
   endoskeletal, 129-130
   function prerequisites, 296-298
   kinesiology, 853-854
   multiple limb deficiencies, 927-928
   new developments in, 343-349
   rehabilitation, 224-229
   shoulder complex, 101-105
   trends in, 223
Upper limbs. *See also* specific limbs
   contractures, 690
   motion, *101*, 105-107, *107, 108*
Utah Arm, 183, *190*
Utah Arm 2, 164, *164*, 167-168, *168*, 181
Utah Dynamic Sockets, 878

V

Vacuum casting, 665
Vaduz hand, 181
Valley Forge Army General Hospital, 87, *88*
Van Nes rotationplasty, *914, 936*
Vanghetti-Sauerbruch-Lebsche muscle tunnel
      cineplasty, 186
Varus deformity, 461
Vascular amputees, 401-402, *402*
Vascular anomalies, 844-846
Vascular compromise, 685
Vascular disease, 31-45, 37-41. *See also* Periph-
      eral vascular disease
Vascular malformations, 846
Vascular occlusion, 845
Vascular salvage procedures, 35-36, 91, 485
Verrucae, viral, 707
Verrucous hyperplasia, *708*, 708-710, *709*
Vertical ground-reaction force, *353*
Vertical shock units, 628

Veterans Administration
   courses, 17
   NU-VA Synergetic Prehensor and, 156
   Programs, 766
   Prosthetics Research Laboratory, 14
   Rehabilitation Research and Development
      Service, 185
   research funding by, 85
Vibration thresholds, 197
Vietnam War, 69, 86-89, 481
Vilkki procedure, *323*
Vocational activities. *See also* Occupational
      therapy; Physical therapy; Task-specific
      prostheses
   psychological adaptation, 728
   rehabilitation, 730, 734-735
   training, 283
Voluntary-closing devices
   hands, *120,* 121, 820
   hooks, 119-121, *120*
Voluntary-opening devices
   developmental modifications, 820
   function, 117-118
   hands, 121-122
   hook-type terminal devices, *118,* 119, 316
   sports prostheses, 3332
Voluntary-opening hand, 121

W

Waist belts, 142, *142*, 413, *552*
Walking, 751
   amputees, *404*
   average distances, 398-399
   customary speeds, 397-398
   energy expenditure, 395-407
   fast customary speeds, 398
   knee disarticulation and, 518
   phases, *666*
   pressure points, 512
   residual limb length and, 402-403
   speeds, 397
   toe disarticulation and, 437
War Amputations of Canada, 759
Warts, viral, residual limbs, 707
Warty keratoses, residual limbs, 707
Wasada hand, 183
Wassel's classification, *860*, 860-861
Waterproof prostheses, 638-639
Weight acceptance, 362-363, 368-371, *387*
Weight-activated friction brakes, 15
Weight-activated friction knees. *See* Stance-
      control knees
Weight-bearing capability, *387*, 503

Wet (infective) gangrene
   ankle disarticulation and, 460
   in diabetes, *461*
   diabetes mellitus and, *435*
   feet, 433-434
   great toe, *50*
   peripheral vascular disease and, 37
   toes, *446*
Wheelchair propulsion, 597, 925
Wooden sockets, 11
World War I, 6-7, 16-17, 69, 79-82, *80, 81*
World War II, 7, 17, 69, 82-85, *84*
Wound closure
   chronic osteomyelitis, 49-50
   postoperative, 26
Wound Data and Munitions Effectiveness
      Team (WDMET), 86-87
Wound dressings. *See* Dressings
Wound healing
   assessment, 40, 484
   chemical burns and, 699
   delayed, 683, *684*
   graft-host junctions, 59
   potential for, 462
   rates of, 442
   vascular compromise and, 37, 685
Wrinkle test, 198
Wrist disarticulation
   definitive electronic prostheses, *228*
   procedure, 861
   prosthesis fitting timetable, *224*
   residual limb, *220*
   surgical management, *220*
   transradial amputation and, 219-230
Wrist units
   articulated, *210*
   bilateral upper limb prostheses, 316-317
   electric-powered components, 160-163
   fitting, rehabilitation and, 222
   flexion, *125,* 162-163
   nonarticulated, *210*
   postoperative, *221*
   prosthesis positioning, 279-280
   prosthetic, 122-125
   quick disconnect, 155
   range of motion, *322*
   shoulder disarticulation prostheses, 265
Wrists
   extension, *113*
   motion, 110-111
   range of motion, *112*

X

Xenon (Xe-133) clearance, 39

Index of Manufacturers

Aesthetic Concern, 122

Alfred Mann Foundation, 182

Becker Mechanical Hand Corp, 120, 121

Bergomed AB, 347

Berivon, 933

Bioengineering Centre, Edinburgh, 346

Bloorview-MacMillan Center, 822, 824

Centri AB, 146, 147, 152–153

Charles A. Blatchford & Sons, LTD, 15, 376, 666, 667

Child Amputee Prosthetics Project, 119

College Park Industries, 371

Fillauer, Inc, 338, 550

Free Handerson Co, 333

Gröpel, 348

Hosmer Dorrance Corp, 118, 120-130, 146, 147, 155, 159–160, 162, 164, 165, 180, 318, 323, 324, 331, 335, 336, 338, 815-817, 820, 824, 827

Howmedica, 61

Instituto Nazionale Assicurazione contro gli Infortuni sul Lavoro (INAIL), 345

Integrum AB, 679

Kingsley Manufacturing Co, 367–368

Liberating Technologies, Inc, 129, 147, 162, 164-167, 169, 183, 190, 192, 318, 324, 815, 822

Liberty-Collier, 191

Los Amigos Research Education Institute, 815

Mauch Laboratories, 654, 655, 660

Motion Control, Inc, 146, 147, 153–154, 155, 158, 161, 162, 164, 181, 183, 190, 343, 345, 348

Ossur, 367, 368, 425, 635, 645, 651, 652, 655, 660, 677, 795

Otto Bock, 15, 16, 122, 128, 129, 146, 147, 149, 155, 156, 160–162, 173, 178, 180, 181, 189, 191, 213, 246, 324, 344, 346, 348, 367, 376, 380, 420, 422, 654, 655, 660, 678, 820, 821, 822

Oxford Orthopaedic Engineering Centre, 345, 348

Rimjet Corp, 318

Robin-Aids, 191, 330

RSLSteeper, 146, 147, 154–155, 158–159, 163, 164, 189, 821, 827

Seattle Systems, Inc, 367, 373, 374, 380, 645, 660, 667

Systemteknik AB, 821

T/Wright Archery, 338

Texas Assistive Devices, LLC, 118, 213, 214, 333, 334, 338

Therapeutic Recreation Systems (TRS), Inc, 118, 120, 330-338, 345, 815, 816, 820

VASI (Variety Ability Systems), 821, 827

Wright Bow Brace, LTD, 334